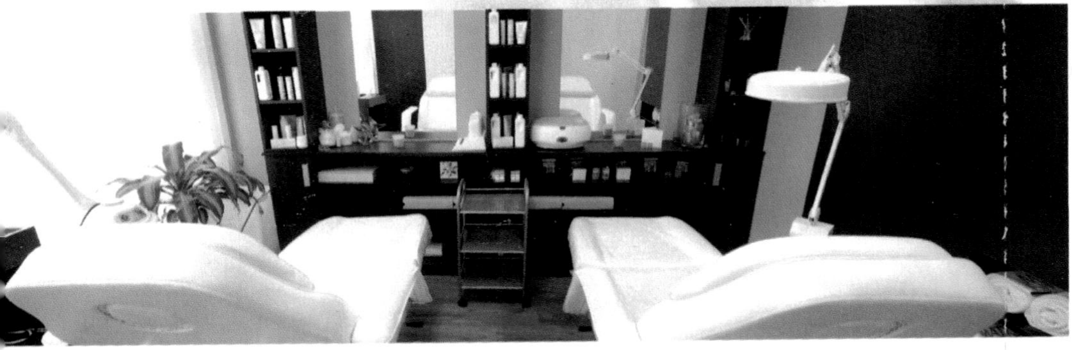

Milady's Standard Esthetics

ADVANCED

Milady's Standard Esthetics

ADVANCED

Editorial Contributor
Judith Culp

Contributing Authors

Efrain Arroyave, M.D.
Linda Bertaut
Helen Bickmore
Jon Canas
Roque Cozzette
Janet M. D'Angelo
Sallie Deitz
Michelle Eldridge
Ramona Moody French
Judy Garcia
Jimm Harrison
Patricia Heitz
Pamela Hill, R.N.
Jane Iredale
Mark Lees
Sheila McKenna
Anne Miller
Sandra Alexcae Moren
Patricia Owens
Peter T. Pugliese, M.D.
Melanie Sachs
Christian Sterling
Laura Todd
David Vidra

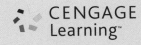

CENGAGE Learning™

Australia • Brazil • Japan • Korea • Mexico • Singapore • Spain • United Kingdom • United States

CENGAGE Learning™

Milady's Standard Esthetics: Advanced, First Edition

Judith Culp, Efrain Arroyave, M.D., Linda Bertaut, Helen Bickmore, Jon Canas, Roque Cozzette, Janet M. D'Angelo, Sallie Deitz, Michelle Eldridge, Ramona Moody French, Judy Garcia, Jimm Harrison, Patricia Heitz, Pamela Hill, R.N., Jane Iredale, Mark Lees, Sheila McKenna, Anne Miller, Sandra Alexcae Moren, Patricia Owens, Peter T. Pugliese, M.D., Melanie Sachs, Christian Sterling, Laura Todd, and David Vidra

President, Milady: Dawn Gerrain

Publisher: Erin O'Connor

Acquisitions Editor: Martine Edwards

Product Manager: Jessica Burns

Editorial Assistant: Elizabeth Edwards

Director of Beauty Industry Relations: Sandra Bruce

Senior Marketing Manager: Gerard McAvey

Marketing Specialist: Erica Conley

Production Director: Wendy Troeger

Content Project Manager: Angela Iula

Senior Art Director: Joy Kocsis

Library of Congress Control Number: 2009920985

ISBN-13: 978-1-4283-1975-2
ISBN-10: 1-4283-1975-1

Milady
5 Maxwell Drive
Clifton Park, NY 12065-2919
USA

Cengage Learning products are represented in Canada by Nelson Education, Ltd.

For your lifelong learning solutions, visit **milady.cengage.com.**

Visit our corporate website at **cengage.com.**

Notice to the Reader
Publisher does not warrant or guarantee any of the products described herein or perform any independent analysis in connection with any of the product information contained herein. Publisher does not assume, and expressly disclaims, any obligation to obtain and include information other than that provided to it by the manufacturer. The reader is expressly warned to consider and adopt all safety precautions that might be indicated by the activities described herein and to avoid all potential hazards. By following the instructions contained herein, the reader willingly assumes all risks in connection with such instructions. The publisher makes no representations or warranties of any kind, including but not limited to, the warranties of fitness for particular purpose or merchantability, nor are any such representations implied with respect to the material set forth herein, and the publisher takes no responsibility with respect to such material. The publisher shall not be liable for any special, consequential, or exemplary damages resulting, in whole or part, from the readers' use of, or reliance upon, this material.

Printed in the United States of America
2 3 4 5 DOW 13 12 11 10

Contents at a Glance

PART 1
ORIENTATION

1 CHANGES IN ESTHETICS 3

PART 2
GENERAL SCIENCES

2 INFECTION CONTROL .19

3 ADVANCED HISTOLOGY OF THE CELL AND THE SKIN BY PETER T. PUGLIESE, M.D. 53

4 HORMONES 87

5 ANATOMY AND PHYSIOLOGY: MUSCLES AND NERVES 103

6 ANATOMY AND PHYSIOLOGY: THE CARDIOVASCULAR AND LYMPHATIC SYSTEMS . . 121

7 CHEMISTRY AND BIOCHEMISTRY 137

8 LASER, LIGHT ENERGY, AND RADIOFREQUENCY THERAPY 155

PART 3
SKIN SCIENCES

9 NUTRITION AND STRESS MANAGEMENT. 187

10 ADVANCED SKIN DISORDERS: SKIN IN DISTRESS 200

11 SKIN TYPING AND AGING ANALYSIS 235

12 SKIN CARE PRODUCTS: INGREDIENTS AND CHEMISTRY 249

13 BOTANICALS AND AROMATHERAPY 281

14 INGREDIENTS AND PRODUCTS FOR SKIN ISSUES 305

15 PHARMACOLOGY FOR ESTHETICIANS 323

PART 4
ESTHETICS

16 ADVANCED FACIAL TECHNIQUES 349

17 ADVANCED SKIN CARE MASSAGE 390

18 ADVANCED FACIAL DEVICES 435

19 HAIR REMOVAL. 475

20 ADVANCED MAKEUP 518

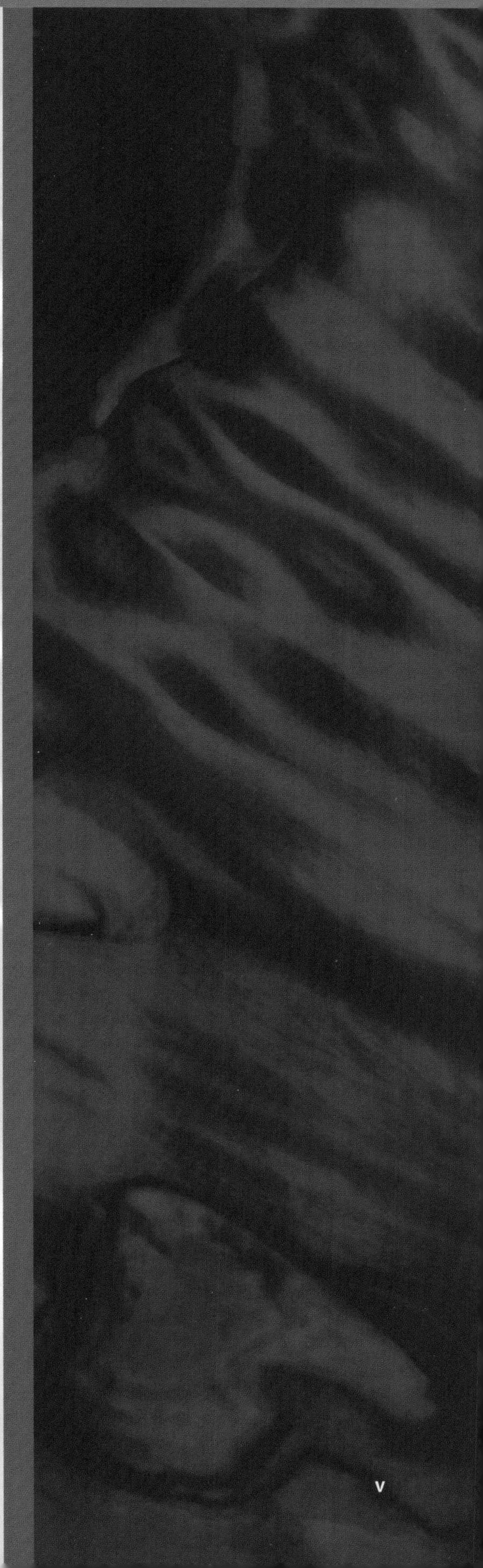

PART 5

SPA AND ALTERNATIVE THERAPIES

21 SPA TREATMENTS 563

22 ALTERNATIVE THERAPIES 600

23 AYURVEDA THEORY AND TREATMENTS 627

PART 6

MEDICAL

24 WORKING IN A MEDICAL SETTING 661

25 MEDICAL TERMINOLOGY. 672

26 MEDICAL INTERVENTION 688

27 PLASTIC SURGERY PROCEDURES 709

28 THE ESTHETICIAN'S ROLE IN PRE- AND POST-MEDICAL TREATMENTS 732

PART 7

BUSINESS SKILLS

29 FINANCIAL BUSINESS SKILLS 747

30 MARKETING 764

REFERENCES AND RESOURCES 781

GLOSSARY 787

INDEX 813

Contents

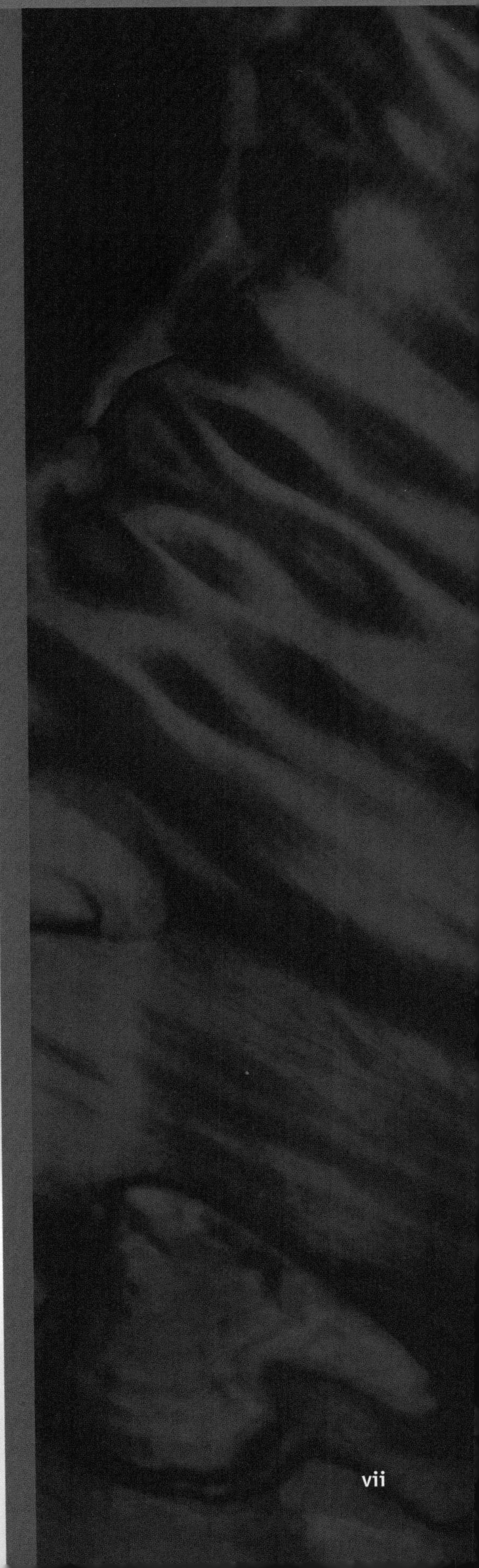

PART 1

ORIENTATION

1 CHANGES IN ESTHETICS 3

The Global Evolution of Spas and Spa Treatments . 6

Advanced Education and Employment Opportunities 8

Developing Critical-Thinking Skills 10

Clarify the Problem 10

Gather the Facts 10

Examine the Evidence 11

Define Solutions and Outcomes 11

Choose and Execute the Solution 11

SOAP Notes 11

Enhancing Soft Skills 11

The Power to Instigate Healing 12

Privacy Laws 13

Professional Organizations and Publications 13

Federal Links 13

State Links 14

Industry Links 14

Professional Publications 14

PART 2

GENERAL SCIENCES

2 INFECTION CONTROL 19

Rules and Regulations Governing Workplace Safety 21

How Do I Know If I Have to Follow OSHA Standards? 21

The Bloodborne Pathogens Standard 22

Hepatitis 23

Acute Hepatitis 24

Chronic Hepatitis 24

Hepatitis A 24

Hepatitis B 24

Hepatitis C 24

Hepatitis D 24

Hepatitis E 25

Hepatitis G 25

Hepatitis I (HIV) 25

Tuberculosis 25

The Principles of Infection Control 26
- Microbiology: The Study of Microorganisms 26
- Impact of Globalization on Infection Control 26
- Contamination vs. Infection 26
- Bacteria, Viruses, Fungi, and Parasites . . . 27
- Nosocomial Infections 27
- Breaking the Chain of Infection 28
- Asepsis 29
- Hand Washing 30
- Hand Washing at Work 30

Gloves 33
- Latex Sensitivity 33
- Allergic Contact Dermatitis (ACD) 34
- Glove Testing Methods 35
- Characteristics of Glove Breakdown 36
- Everyday Practices That May Affect the Glove Barrier 36

Body Hygiene and a Caring Attitude 36
- Body Hygiene 36
- A Caring Attitude 37

Disinfection and Sterilization 37
- Equipment Processing 37
- Cleaning Agents 38
- Disinfection 40
- Ultrasonic Cleaning 42
- Packaging 42
- Steam Sterilization 43
- Monitoring the Sterilization Process 43
- Storage 47

Potential Hazards for an Esthetician 47
- Sharps Sticks 47
- Other Hazards 47
- Airborne Infections 48
- Bloodborne Diseases 48
- Accidents, Fire, and Emergencies 48

Basic Safety Guidelines 48
- Clean Your Space Systematically and Routinely 48
- Follow Hand Washing Regulations 48
- Wear Gloves 48
- Dispose of Potential Infected Material . . . 49
- Use the Autoclave for Sterilization 49
- Use Disposables 49
- Read and Keep Material Safety Data Sheets . . 49
- Create a Room-Cleaning Checklist 49
- Understand and Use Eyewash Protocol 49

OSHA Inspections 49

3 ADVANCED HISTOLOGY OF THE CELL AND THE SKIN BY PETER T. PUGLIESE, M.D. 53

Cellular Structure and Function 57
- The Cellular Membrane 57
- Organelles 58
- Cellular Function 59

A Brief Overview of Skin Structure and Function 60

The Cells of the Epidermis 60
- Keratinocytes 60
- Keratinocytes and Skin Repair 61
- The Melanocyte 62
- The Langerhans Cell 62

Major Cells in the Dermis 63
- Fibroblasts 63
- The Mast Cells 63
- The Leukocytes 64

How Keratinocytes Replace the Stratum Corneum 65

Proteins of the Dermis—The Extracellular Matrix (ECM) 66
- Collagen 66
- Elastin 67
- Proteoglycans 67

The Cell Cycle 69

An Introduction to Embryology—The Stem Cell 70
- The Ectoderm Germ Layer's Three Parts . . . 70
- The Mesoderm 70
- Endoderm 71
- The Ectoderm, Mesoderm, and Endoderm Make Up True Stem Cells 71

The Major Tissues in the Body 71
- Epithelial Tissue 72
- Connective Tissue 72
- Nervous Tissue 72
- Muscle Tissue 72

The Basic Immune System 72
- The Two Immune Systems 72
- Other Components of the Immune System . 73

The Mechanism of Exfoliation—The Desmosomes 73
- Tight Junctions 73
- Adherens Junctions 73
- Gap Junctions 74
- Desmosomes 74
- The Stratum Corneum's Rate of Recovery . . 75

Skin Penetration and Permeation 75

Sensory Nerves and Perception in the Skin . . . 77
The Sensory Receptors in the Skin 77

4 HORMONES 87
What Are Hormones? 89
The Endocrine Glands 90
Hormones Produced by the Ovaries and Testes 92
The Hormonal Phases of Life 92
Puberty 92
The Menstrual Cycle 94
Pregnancy 95
Premenstrual Syndrome 97
Birth Control Pills 97
Menopause 98
Hirsutism 100
Obesity, Anorexia, and Hormones 100
Other Hormonal Disorders That Affect the Skin 100
Thyroid Hormones 100
Adrenal Glands 100

5 ANATOMY AND PHYSIOLOGY: MUSCLES AND NERVES 103
Muscle Types 105
Cardiac Muscles 105
Smooth Muscles 106
Skeletal Muscles 106
Function of Skeletal Muscles 106
Muscles of the Head and Face 108
Muscles of the Forehead 108
Muscles of the Eye 108
Muscles of the Mouth 109
Nasal Muscles 111
Muscles of the Neck 111
Sternocleidomastoids 111
Platysma 111
Muscles of the Trunk 111
Anterior Muscles of the Trunk 111
Posterior Muscles of the Trunk 112
Muscles of the Arms and Shoulders 112
The Deltoid 112
The Bicep Brachii 113
The Brachialis 113
The Tricep Brachii 114
Muscles of the Legs 114
Muscles Associated with the Hip 114
Muscles Associated with the Knee 116
Muscles Associated with the Ankle and Foot 116
Facial Nerve Patterns 117
Cranial Nerve VII, the Facial Nerve 117
Cranial Nerve V, the Trigeminal Nerve . . . 118

6 ANATOMY AND PHYSIOLOGY: THE CARDIOVASCULAR AND LYMPHATIC SYSTEMS 121
The Cardiovascular System 124
Blood 124
Blood Composition 124
Blood Disorders 125
The Heart 126
Heart Disease 128
The Arterial System 128
The Arteries 128
Arterioles 129
Capillaries 130
The Venous System 130
The Veins 130
Peripheral Venous Return 130
Diseased Veins 131
The Lymphatic System 132

7 CHEMISTRY AND BIOCHEMISTRY 137
Principles of Chemistry 139
Hydrogen 140
Oxygen 140
Carbon 142
Sodium 142
Chlorine 142
Chemical Reactions 142
Chemicals Found in the Skin and Body 143
Proteins 143
Carbohydrates 143
Lipids 144
pH, Acids, and Bases 144
Why pH Is Important in Cosmetics 145
Chemical Terms Estheticians Should Know 145
Botanical Chemistry 146
Metabolites 146
Plant Compounds in Skin Care 147
Essential Oil Chemistry 150
Terpene Compounds 150
Phenylpropanoid Compounds 152

8 LASER, LIGHT ENERGY, AND RADIOFREQUENCY THERAPY 155

The History of Light and Energy Devices . . . 158

Physics 158

Electromagnetic Spectrum of Radiation . . 158

Properties of Laser Light 160

Tissue Effects 160

Creation of Laser Light 162

Selective Photothermolysis 162

Safety Governmental Agencies 164

U.S. Food and Drug Administration (FDA) 164

American National Standard Institute . . . 164

Occupational Safety and Health Administration (OSHA) 165

State Licensure and Regulations 165

Safety 165

Procedural Controls 166

Engineering Controls 169

Administrative Controls 170

Laser Therapy 172

Photothermal Tissue Reactions 172

Photomechanical Tissue Response 173

Common Procedures 175

Intense Pulsed Light 176

Types of IPL Devices 176

Common Procedures 177

Radiofrequency Devices 178

Types of Monopolar RF Devices 178

Types of Bipolar RF Devices 178

Common Procedures 179

Light-Emitting Diodes (LED Devices) and Low-Level Light Therapy 180

Types of Devices 180

Common Procedures 180

Conclusion 181

PART 3

SKIN SCIENCES

9 NUTRITION AND STRESS MANAGEMENT 187

Nutrients and Diet 189

Metabolism and Aging 189

Free Radicals and Antioxidants 190

Poor Nutrition and How It Stresses the Body 190

Nutrition and Aging 193

Glycation 193

The Maillard Reaction 193

What We Can Do to Slow These Processes 194

Smoking 194

Effects of Stress on the Body 195

The Fight or Flight Response 195

Chronic Stress 197

Becoming Proactive in Stress Management . . 197

Recognizing Stress Triggers 197

Non-Food-Related Strategies for Dealing with Stress 197

10 ADVANCED SKIN DISORDERS: SKIN IN DISTRESS 200

The Inflammation Cascade 203

Wound Healing 204

Superficial Injuries 204

Deeper Wounds (Epidermis and Dermis) . . 204

Wound Repair Techniques 206

Aftercare Impacts 207

Silicone Patches 209

Injuries from Laser and Other Treatment Therapies 210

Pigmentation 210

Other Injuries from Light Therapy Treatments 210

Short-Term Sun Damage 211

Other Short-Term Sun-Related Problems 211

The Real Damage from the Sun 212

What You Do Not Know about Short-Term Sun Exposure 212

Long-Term Photoaging 212

Skin Cancers 213

Basal Cell Carcinomas 214

Squamous Cell Carcinomas 214

Skin Cancer Treatment 215

Other Sun-Related Skin Growths 216

Actinic Keratosis 216

Sebaceous Hyperplasias 217

Seborrheic Keratoses 217

Solar Freckles 217

Acne 218

Hereditary Factors in Acne 218

Noninflammatory and Inflammatory Acne Lesions 218
The Grades of Acne 220
Why Scars Form 221
Hormones 221
The Beginning of Teenage Acne 223
Environmental Factors That Influence Acne 224
Overcleaning 225
Self-Trauma Excoriations. 225
Nutrition and Diet. 225
Acne and Cosmetics. 226
Acne-Related Conditions. 226

Rosacea. 227
Causes of Rosacea. 228
Subtypes of Rosacea 229
Why Is There More Rosacea? 231
Medical Intervention 231

When to Refer for Medical Evaluation 232

11 SKIN TYPING AND AGING ANALYSIS 235

Fitzpatrick Skin Typing. 238
The Glogau Scale. 240
Rubin Classification. 240
Kligman Rosacea Classification 242
Oriental Reflex Zones of the Face 242
Internal Energetic Flow and Balance 242
Put "Energy" in Your Practice 242
The Body and the Five Elements of TCM . . 243
The Five Elements and Skin Conditions . . 243
Skin from the Oriental Perspective 243
Points of Acupuncture 243
Zones of the Face 244
Treatments. 244

Hormonal Balance for Skin Identification. . . 245
Estrogen Isotypes 245
Androgen Isotypes 246

Skin Categories. 247

12 SKIN CARE PRODUCTS: INGREDIENTS AND CHEMISTRY 249

Categories of Cosmetic Ingredients 252
Functional and Performance Ingredients . 252
Drug versus Cosmetic. 252
"Cosmeceutical" Ingredients 253

Types of Functional Ingredients 253
Vehicles 253
High-Tech Vehicles 260
Antimicrobials and Preservatives 261
Gellants and Thickening Agents 263
Coloring Agents 263
Fragrances 264

Performance Ingredients. 264
Cleansing Agents. 264
Performance Agents in Toners 266
Performance Ingredients for Dehydrated Skin 267
Plant Extracts. 272

Ingredients for Aging Skin 273
Free Radicals and Their Effect on the Skin 274
Antioxidants 275
Sunscreen Ingredients 276
Peptides and Collagen Stimulants. 276
More Performance Ingredients for Aging Skin. 277
Combining Anti-Aging Ingredients 277

Reading Ingredient Labels 277

13 BOTANICALS AND AROMATHERAPY 281

What Are Botanical Ingredients? 284
Plant Compounds and Extracts. 284
Methods of Botanical Extraction. 284
Tinctures. 284
Dried Herbs 284
Infusions. 284
Expeller Pressed Oils 285
Supercritical Carbon Dioxide 285
Solvent Extraction. 285

Eleven Botanicals for Skin Care 286
Aromatherapy and Essential Oils. 289
What Is Aromatherapy? 290
Essential Oils 290
Essential Oils and the Sense of Smell . . . 290

What Essential Oils Can Do 291
Antiseptic and Antimicrobial Properties 291
Anti-Inflammatory Properties 291
Sedative and Stress Relief Properties . . . 291
Antispasmodic Properties 292
Expectorant and Mucolytic Properties . . . 292
Cell Regenerative and Wound Healing Properties. 292

Essential Oil Chemistry. 292

Contraindications 294
Responsible Use of Oils 294
Quality of Essential Oils 294
Genuine and Authentic Oils. 294
Thirteen Essential Oils 295
Application of Essential Oils 298
Essential Oil Blends. 298
Essential Oil Synergy 299
Carrier Oils. 299
Dilution Amounts and Measurements. . . . 299
Calculation for a Basic Essential Oil Blend. 299
Recipes for Skin and Spa 301
The Aromatherapy and Botanical Practice. . . 301
Holistic Consultation 302
Legal Considerations 302

14 INGREDIENTS AND PRODUCTS FOR SKIN ISSUES 305
Cleansers. 308
Product Profile: Rinsable Cleanser for Oily and Combination Skin 308
Product Profile: Rinsable Cleanser for Dry and Combination Skin 308
Product Profile: Rinsable Cleanser for Very Oily Skin 309
Product Profile: Rinsable Medicated Cleanser for Acne 309
Product Profile: Milk Cleanser for Oily and Combination Skin 309
Product Profile: Cleansing Milk for Combination Skin 310
Product Profile: Cleansing Milk for Sensitive Skin 310
Product Profile: Cleansing Milk for Dry Skin 310
Toners. 311
Product Profile: Toner for Oily and Combination Skin 311
Product Profile: Toner for Extremely Oily Skin 311
Product Profile: Astringent for Acne-Prone Skin 312
Product Profile: Toner for Normal Skin. . . 312
Product Profile: Toner for Extra-Dry Skin . . 312
Day Creams and Treatments. 312
Product Profile: Day Sunscreen Protection Fluid for Oily and Combination Skin 313
Product Profile: Day Cream for Dry and Dehydrated Skin 313
Product Profile: Sunscreen Day Lotion for Sensitive Skin 314
Night Creams and Treatments. 314
Product Profile: Night Treatment Fluid for Oily-Combination Dehydrated Skin 314
Product Profile: Night Treatment for Oily, Clogged Adult Skin 314
Product Profile: Night Hydrating Cream for Combination Mature Skin 314
Product Profile: Night Moisturizing Lotion for Dehydrated Combination Dry Skin 315
Product Profile: Night Cream for Dry, Dehydrated Skin 315
Product Profile: Firming Night Cream for Mature Skin with Lack of Elasticity. 315
Ampoules and Serums 316
Product Profile: Firming Serum for Mature Skin with Lack of Elasticity. 316
Product Profile: Lipid Serum for Wrinkles and Dry Skin 316
Specialty Creams and Treatments 316
Product Profile: Alpha Hydroxy Treatment for Dry, Sun-Damaged Skin . . . 316
Product Profile: Alpha Hydroxy Treatment Gel for Oily-Combination, Clogged Skin 317
Product Profile: Lightening Treatment Gel for Hyperpigmented Skin. 317
Product Profile: Benzoyl Peroxide Gel for Acne-Prone Skin. 317
Eye Creams 317
Neck Creams. 318
Masks 318
Exfoliants 318
How Products Are Developed 318
Step 1: The Idea 318
Step 2: Product Characteristics and Client Type 319
Step 3: Choosing Ingredients and Budgeting 319
Step 4: The Prototype and Use Testing . . 319
Step 5: Independent Testing 319
Step 6: Production 319
Step 7: Marketing 320
Additional Acne Care Considerations 320
Care for Young Teens 320
Care for Adults 320
Additional Rosacea Product Selection Tips . . 320
Sunscreen Ingredients 321

Reducing Redness 321
Lifestyle Modifications 322

15 PHARMACOLOGY FOR ESTHETICIANS 323
Clients and Their Medications 326
The FDA and Drugs 326
Prescription Drugs 327
Definition of a Prescription 327
Common Prescription Drugs 327
Over-the-Counter (OTC) Drugs 328
Drug Categories 328
Drugs Used to Treat Hormonal Imbalances and Birth Control 328
Drugs Used to Treat Blood Conditions . . . 330
Drugs Used to Treat Heart Conditions . . . 331
Drugs Used to Treat Lung Disorders 333
Drugs Used to Treat Gastrointestinal Disorders 333
Drugs Used to Treat Mental Disorders . . . 335
Drugs Used to Treat Diabetes 337
Drugs Used to Treat Bacterial Infections . . 337
Drugs Used to Treat Viral Infections 338
Drugs Used to Treat Fungal Infections . . . 339
Drugs Used to Treat Skeletal Conditions . . 340
Corticosteroids 341
Drugs Used to Treat Pain 341

PART 4
ESTHETICS

16 ADVANCED FACIAL TECHNIQUES 349
Treatment Variations 351
The Building Blocks of Treatment 351
Treatment Arc and Theory 353
Thermotherapy and Pressure Therapy 354
Rosacea and Sensitive Skin Treatments 357
Treatment Concepts for Sensitive Skin . . . 357
Treatment Contraindications for Treating Sensitive Skin 357
Client Reactions in the Treatment Room . 361
Rules for the Retinoid Client 361
Clinic Exfoliation Treatments 362
Manual Microdermabrasion 362
Enzymes 367
Acids 367
Deeper Exfoliation (Superficial Peels) . . . 374
Stronger Exfoliating Treatments 381
Mask Therapies 381
Mask Theory 381
Basic Masks 382
Zone Therapy 383
Collagen Sheet Masks 383
Powder Masks 384
Rubber-Type Masks 387
Specialty Layered Masks 388

17 ADVANCED SKIN CARE MASSAGE 390
Advanced Facial Movements 393
Selecting and Incorporating Advanced Movements 393
Eye Express 394
Around We Go 394
Center Point 394
Sinus Relief 395
Paddlewheel 395
Feather Off 396
Forehead Press 396
Gallop 1-2-1 396
Full-Face Sweep 396
Advanced Neck and Décolleté Movements . . . 396
Rolling Along 396
Feels Good 396
Décolleté Sweep 397
Ski Up 399
Neck-Shoulder-Arm 399
Rock-a-Bye 400
Advanced Back Movements 400
Back Sweep 400
Spine Munch 401
Swim Up Back 401
Shiatsu Massage for the Face 402
Performing Shiatsu 402
Reflexology for the Face 407
Ear Reflexology 408
Stone Massage for Estheticians 410
Warm Stones 410
Cold Stones 410
Stone Handling 411
Stone Placement and Massage 411
Contraindications 411
Lymphatic Massage for the Face and Neck . . 417
Identifying Face and Neck Indications and Contraindications 417

Treating Chronically Swollen Lymph Nodes 418
Locating Lymph Nodes on the Face and Neck 418
Observing and Palpating Lymph Nodes on the Face and Neck 418
Establishing a Lymph Drainage Pattern on the Face and Neck 420
Extending Lymph Drainage Massage to the Face and Neck 420
Machine-Aided Lymphatic Massage Treatments 430
Pressotherapy 430
Machine-Aided Facial Lymphatic Massage . . 430

18 ADVANCED FACIAL DEVICES 435
The Purchasing Process 437
Analysis of Your Practice Needs 438
Equipment Options 438
New or Used Equipment Options 438
Financing Options 439
Company Stability 439
Legalities and Insurability 439
Disposables or Reusables 439
Education 439
Warranties and Service Contract 440
Device Labeling 440
Skin Analysis Devices 440
IPL Facial Rejuvenation 440
Indications for Treatment 441
The Consultation 441
Contraindications 443
Light-Emitting Diodes (LEDs) 448
Treatment Guidelines 449
Indications for Treatment 449
Contraindications to Treatment 449
Photodynamic Therapy (PDT) 452
Microdermabrasion 452
Crystal Devices 453
Non-Crystal Devices 453
Indications for Treatment 454
Contraindications to Treatment 454
Client Protocol 454
Ultrasonic Technology 460
Electrodessication Devices (Radiofrequency) 465
Indications for Treatment 466
Contraindications to Treatment 466
Microcurrent "Facial Toning" 469
Indications for Treatment 469
Contraindications to Treatment 469
Client Protocol 470
Management of Complications 472

19 HAIR REMOVAL 475
Safety and Disinfection First 477
Herpes Simplex Breakouts 477
Genital Warts 478
Pregnancy 478
Threading 478
The History of Threading 478
The Benefits of Threading 478
Preparation of Equipment and the Treatment Area 478
Preparation of the Client 478
Threading Technique 478
Sugaring 480
The History of Sugaring 481
The Benefits of Sugaring 482
Sugaring Paste 483
Application Techniques for Sugaring 484
Post-Treatment Care 486
Hard Wax 486
Soft Wax 487
Product Evaluation 488
Advanced Facial Waxing 488
Brow Design 488
The Sides of the Face 491
Speed Waxing and Body Techniques 491
Arms 492
Hands 493
Bikini Variations 493
Advanced Male Waxing 501
Eyebrows 501
Back 502
Chest 503
Ears 503
Male Brazilian 503
Laser and Pulsed Light Hair Removal 503
Monochromatic Light 503
Intense Pulsed Light 504
Safety in the Laser Treatment Room 504
Client Selection 505
Effects of Laser on Skin Type 507

The Consultation 507
Patch Testing 509
The Laser Hair Removal Treatment 509
Skin Preparation 509
Topical Anesthesia. 509
Laser/IPL Treatment Parameters. 510
Post-Treatment in the Clinic 514
At-Home Care 514
Spacing the Return Visit. 514
When to Stop Treating 514
Treatment Consequences. 515
Side Effects and Complications 515
Liability Concerns 515

20 ADVANCED MAKEUP 518
Semipermanent Eyelash Extensions. 521
Consultation 521
Preparation, Health, and Safety. 521
Client Comfort 522
Eyelash Growth. 522
Procedure Notes 522
Technique Variations 529
Application Variations 529
Lash Removal. 529
After the Procedure 531
Eyelash Perming 531
Mineral Makeup. 535
Typical Ingredients in Mineral Makeup. . . 536
Benefits of Mineral Makeup. 536
Application 537
Minerals for Camouflage 541
Covering Redness 542
Hiding Circles Under the Eyes 542
Hyperpigmentation and Vitiligo 545
Scarring 546
Bruising and Tattoos 546
Airbrush Makeup 546
The Foundation. 547
Airbrush Tools and Equipment 548
Airbrush Techniques 548
Cleaning Method 549
Airbrush Beauty Breakdown. 550
Maximum Coverage Makeup 550
Fantasy Makeup 554
Permanent Cosmetics 554
Regulations and Training 555
Training and Trainers 556
Common Modalities 556
Eyebrows 557
Eyeliner. 557
Lip Coloration 557
Areola Work 557
Client Care. 558

PART 5

SPA AND ALTERNATIVE THERAPIES

21 SPA TREATMENTS 563
Understanding Spas and Their Services 565
Spa Types 565
Body Treatments 566
Preparing the Client. 570
General Client Preparation Procedures . . . 570
Comfort. 571
Towel Techniques for Product Removal . . 572
Facial for the Body 573
The Popularity of Body Wraps and Masks . . . 576
Types of Body Wraps 578
Seaweed and Algae Wraps. 579
Herbal Wraps 584
Essential Oils and Wraps. 589
Cellophane, Space Blankets, or Foil Wrapping Agents. 590
Blanket Wraps 590
Dry Blanket Wraps or Cool Moist Blanket Wraps 591
Kneipp Body Wraps 591
Soothing Leg Treatment 591
Hydrotherapy and Other Specialty Treatments. 596
The Vichy Shower 596
Scotch Hose. 596
Baths 596
Raindrop Therapy 597
Music Therapy. 597

22 ALTERNATIVE THERAPIES 600
The History of Alternative Medicine 603
Energy Basics 604
Energy Management. 605
The Four Bodies 605
The Chakra System. 608

Reiki Hands-On Healing 608
The Origin of Reiki 611
The Benefits of Reiki 611
The Three Levels of Reiki 612
Choosing a Reiki Master Teacher 612
Energy Medicines. 613
Bach Flower Remedies 613
Gem Elixirs 613
Energy Infusions. 613
Crystals and Gemstones 613
Selecting Stones. 613
Getting to Know Your Stones. 614
Sanitizing and Clearing Your Stones 614
Color's Role in Healing. 615
The Laying of Gemstones 615
Introducing Energy-Balancing Treatments to Clients. 620

23 AYURVEDA THEORY AND TREATMENTS 627
What Are Ayurvedic Treatments?. 630
What Makes a Spa Treatment Ayurvedic? . . . 630
Five Vedic Principles to Apply to Treatments. 630
Principle and Application No. 1 630
Principle and Application No. 2 631
Principle and Application No. 3 631
Principle and Application No. 4 631
Principle and Application No. 5 631
The Doshas 631
Prakruti Is Your Personal Blueprint. 632
Vikruti Is Your Present State of Subtle Energy. 632
The Qualities of the Five Elements. 632
Dosha Overview 633
Vata Body-Mind Characteristics 633
What Unbalances the Vata Dosha? 633
Balancing the Vata Dosha 633
Treatment Tips for Balancing the Vata Dosha 635
Pitta Body-Mind Characteristics 635
What Unbalances the Pitta Dosha?. 635
Balancing the Pitta Dosha 635
Treatment Tips for Balancing the Pitta Dosha 635
Kapha Body-Mind Characteristics 636
What Unbalances the Kapha Dosha? 636
Balancing the Kapha Dosha. 636
Treatment Tips for Balancing Kapha Dosha 636
Ayurvedic Treatments. 637
Ayurvedic Skin Care. 637
Magical Marmas 639
Opening Sequence. 640
Shirodhara Treatment. 649
Other Ayurvedic Treatments. 654

PART 6

MEDICAL

24 WORKING IN A MEDICAL SETTING 661
Medical Aesthetics. 663
How Estheticians Work with Physicians 663
Common Misconceptions. 663
Esthetician Credentials. 663
Esthetician License in the Medical Practice 664
Scope of Practice 664
The Medical Aesthetic Practice. 665
Plastic Surgery 665
The Medi-Spa 665
Training and Education. 666
Esthetic Education Model 666
Medical Education Model 666
Nurse Training 667
Interfacing with Medical Professionals 667
The Scientific Method 668
Terminology. 669
Medical Record Keeping 669
Office Culture. 669
Human Resource Management 669
Nepotism. 669

25 MEDICAL TERMINOLOGY. 672
How Medical Terminology Works. 675
The History of Medical Terminology 675
Egyptian, Greek, and Roman Influences. . 675
The Middle Ages and Renaissance Period . .676
Contemporary Times 676
The Basics of Medical Terminology 676
Word Analysis. 676
Plurals 677

Root Words 678
Prefixes. 682
Suffixes. 683
Pronunciation. 685

26 MEDICAL INTERVENTION 688
Medical Intervention Defined. 691
The Esthetician's Role 691
General Information Estheticians Can Give Clients 692
An Introduction to Botox 693
Indications for Botox. 694
Complications and Side Effects of Botox 695
An Introduction to Dermal Fillers 696
Bovine Collagen 697
Human Collagen 698
Hyaluronic Acid 700
Complications and Side Effects of Dermal Fillers. 701
Combining Botox and Dermal Fillers 702
An Introduction to Sclerotherapy 702
Causes of Problem Veins. 702
Vein Therapy 703
The Esthetician's Role in Sclerotherapy . . 703
An Introduction to Medical Peels 704
Types of Peeling Agents 704
Glycolic and Lactic Acids 705
Other Solutions. 706
Benefits of Medical Peels 706
Contraindications, Complications, and Side Effects of Medical Peels 707

27 PLASTIC SURGERY PROCEDURES 709
Face-Lift (Rhytidectomy) 712
Indications 712
Mechanism of Action and Target Tissues . 712
Pre-Procedure Considerations. 712
Procedure Techniques. 712
Thread Lift. 713
Forehead-Lift (Brow-Lift) 713
Indications 713
Mechanism of Action and Target Tissues . .714
Pre-Procedure Considerations. 714
Procedure Techniques. 714
Eye Lift (Blepharoplasty) 715
Indications 715
Mechanism of Action and Target Tissues . .716
Pre-Procedure Considerations. 716
Procedure Techniques. 716
Post-Surgical Concerns 716
Nose Job (Rhinoplasty) 717
Indications 717
Mechanism of Action and Target Tissues . .717
Pre-Procedure Considerations. 717
Procedure Techniques. 718
Facial Implants. 718
Indications 718
Mechanism of Action and Target Tissues . .719
Pre-Procedure Considerations. 719
Procedure Techniques. 719
Breast Implants (Augmentation Mammaplasty) 720
Indications 720
Mechanism of Action and Target Tissues . . 720
Pre-Procedure Considerations. 720
Procedure Techniques. 720
Mammograms and Breast Implants 721
Breast-Lift (Mastopexy) 721
Indications 722
Mechanism of Action and Target Tissues . .722
Pre-Procedure Considerations. 723
Procedure Techniques. 723
Breast Reduction (Reduction Mammaplasty) 723
Indications 723
Mechanism of Action and Target Tissues . .723
Pre-Procedure Considerations. 724
Procedure Techniques. 724
Breast Reconstruction 724
Indications 724
Mechanism of Action and Target Issues . . 724
Pre-Procedure Considerations. 725
Procedure Techniques. 725
Surgical Options 725
Follow-Up Procedures. 726
Postoperative Considerations. 726
Tummy Tuck (Abdominoplasty). 727
Indications 727
Mechanism of Action and Target Tissues . 727
Pre-Procedure Considerations. 727
Procedure Techniques. 727
Liposuction (Suction-Assisted Lipoplasty) . . 728
Indications 728
Mechanism of Action and Target Tissues . 729

Pre-Procedure Considerations. 729
Procedure Techniques. 729

28 THE ESTHETICIAN'S ROLE IN PRE- AND POST-MEDICAL TREATMENTS 732
Pre-Medical or Laser Intervention Procedures 735
Superficial Chemical Peels. 736
Microdermabrasion 736
Enzyme Peels 737
Ultrasonic 737
Microcurrent Facial Toning 737
Lymph Drainage 737
Pre-Surgical Home Care 738
Pre-Laser Home Care 738
Preoperative Home Care 738
Post-Procedure Guidelines. 738
After CO_2/Erbium Nd:YAG Laser Resurfacing 739
Post-Surgical Procedures. 740
When to Refer Back to the Physician. 743

PART 7

BUSINESS SKILLS

29 FINANCIAL BUSINESS SKILLS 747
Calculating Business Risk 749
The Business Plan 749
Executive Summary 750
Marketing Plan 751
Strategic Design and Development Plan 751
Operations Plan 751
Financial Plan 751
Conclusion. 751
Financial Planning. 751
Financial Tools 752
Technology 752
The Balance Sheet. 752
The Income Statement 752
The Cash Flow Statement 752
Break-Even Analysis. 752
Protecting Business Assets 753
Insurance 754
Employee Compensation 754
Independent Contractors 755
Understanding the IRS 756
Tax Identification Numbers 756
Employee Tax Status 756
Filing Tax Returns 756
Business Taxes 757
Tax Penalties 761

30 MARKETING 764
The Definition of Marketing. 767
The Marketing Mix. 767
Product. 767
Price. 768
Promotion 768
Place 768
Customer Value. 768
Strategic Value 769
Customer Relationship Management 770
The Promotion Mix 771
Advertising 771
Public Relations 772
Publicity 772
Direct Marketing 772
Personal Selling 773
Sales Promotions. 773
The Marketing Plan 774
Establishing Goals. 774
The Marketing Budget 774
The Brochure, or Menu of Services 774
The Internet. 775
The Use of Technology 776
Analyzing Sales Promotions. 776
Tracking Sales, Client Information, and Employee Performance 776
Using the Computer as a Marketing Tool . 777
Marketing Responsibly 777

REFERENCES AND RESOURCES 781

GLOSSARY 787

INDEX 813

Procedures List

PROCEDURE 2–1: HAND WASHING TECHNIQUE

PROCEDURE 2–2: THE STERILIZATION PROCESS

PROCEDURE 2–3: POLICY AND PROCEDURE FOR OPERATING AUTOCLAVES

PROCEDURE 16–1: THERMOTHERAPY FOR CLOGGED PORES

PROCEDURE 16–2: TREATMENT FOR SENSITIVE SKIN

PROCEDURE 16–3: MANUAL MICRODERMABRASION

PROCEDURE 16–4: ALPHA HYDROXY TREATMENT (AHA)

PROCEDURE 16–5: JESSNER'S SOLUTION OR 20% BHA TREATMENT

PROCEDURE 16–6: APPLICATION AND REMOVAL OF POWDER MASK

PROCEDURE 17–1: SHIATSU MASSAGE FOR HEAD AND NECK

PROCEDURE 17–2: EAR REFLEXOLOGY MASSAGE

PROCEDURE 17–3: STONE MASSAGE FOR FACE

PROCEDURE 17–4: MANUAL LYMPHATIC DRAINAGE MASSAGE

PROCEDURE 17–5: MACHINE-AIDED LYMPHATIC DRAINAGE MASSAGE

PROCEDURE 18–1: IPL PHOTOREJUVENATION

PROCEDURE 18–2: LED SKIN TREATMENT

PROCEDURE 18–3: MACHINE-AIDED MICRODERMABRASION

PROCEDURE 18–4: ULTRASONIC FACIAL

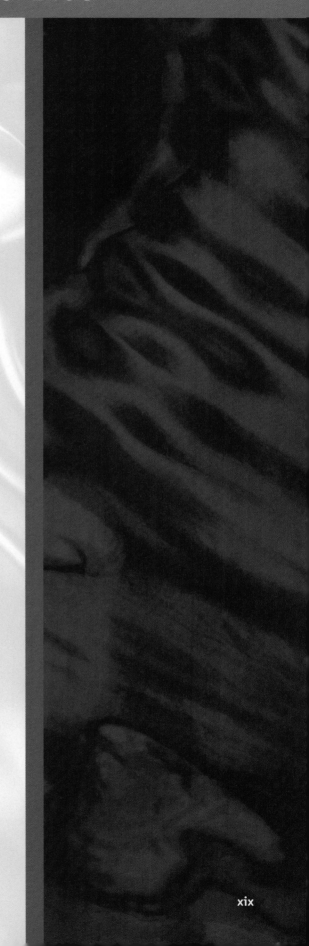

Procedures List (continued)

PROCEDURE 18–5: ELECTRODESSICATION TREATMENT FOR SKIN TAG

PROCEDURE 18–6: MICROCURRENT FOR OBICULARIS OCCULI

PROCEDURE 19–1: BRAZILIAN WAX

PROCEDURE 19–2: PERFORMING LASER OR IPL HAIR REMOVAL TREATMENTS

PROCEDURE 20–1: APPLYING SEMIPERMANENT EYELASH EXTENSIONS

PROCEDURE 20–2: LASH EXTENSION REMOVAL

PROCEDURE 20–3: EYELASH PERMING

PROCEDURE 20–4: APPLYING MINERAL MAKEUP

PROCEDURE 20–5: MAXIMUM COVERAGE AIRBRUSHING

PROCEDURE 21–1: STEPS FOR A BODY SCRUB WITH HYDRATING PACK/MASK

PROCEDURE 21–2: APPLYING AND REMOVING SEAWEED WRAP

PROCEDURE 21–3: HERBAL BODY WRAP

PROCEDURE 21–4: SOOTHING LEG TREATMENT

PROCEDURE 22–1: 30-MINUTE REJUVENATION PROCEDURE

PROCEDURE 23–1: OPENING SEQUENCE MASSAGE

PROCEDURE 23–2: BASIC MARMA POINT MASSAGE

PROCEDURE 23–3: SHIRODHARA TREATMENT

Preface

Now that you have the foundations of your esthetic training, you are ready to journey into all of the aspects open to those with more advanced education. It is a new frontier ripe with opportunity for success and personal satisfaction. The need for professional estheticians with advanced skills continues to grow in new and exciting ways, providing ample room for personal success in a variety of career paths.

As you move forward from your basic training, consider myriad options open to the highly skilled technician, and you will approach your course of study with a positive attitude, study skills and habits, and perseverance, even when the going gets tough. Stay focused on your goal—to become skilled far beyond a basic licensed esthetician and to create more options as you move forward in your career. Should any problems arise that might prevent you from reaching your goal, talk to your instructor or support team.

ORGANIZATION AND CHAPTERS

By learning and using the tools in this text together with your teachers' instruction, you will develop the abilities needed to build a loyal and satisfied clientele. To help you locate information more easily, the chapters are grouped into seven main parts:

Part One, Orientation, provides an in-depth look at the evolution of esthetics and its advancements and opportunities in today's world, in addition to learning problem solving and critical thinking and enhancing soft skills.

Part Two, General Sciences, presents scientific knowledge necessary for the safe practice of esthetics. Chapters include topics on state laws and organizations, infection control principles, bacteriology, anatomy and physiology, chemistry, and equipment safety tips and training.

Part Three, Skin Sciences, opens with the effects of proper nutrition and stress on the body and prepares students with the information to address and identify clients' skin issues and plan for the best treatment protocols through skin analysis, selection of ingredients and products, and even aromatherapy.

Part Four, Esthetics, begins with descriptions of the hands-on, step-by-by step procedures for employing both equipment and non-equipment techniques in the treatment room. Readers can gain a diverse repertoire of treatment variations and information on safely customizing treatments to meet an individual client's needs.

Part Five, Spas, discusses the wide array of specialty spa treatments that technicians can incorporate into their own signature services; products, such as body wraps and masks; and Ayurveda and other alternative healing techniques. Part Five also touches on the importance of client privacy and preparation.

Part Six, Medical, offers a glimpse into working in a medical setting, including surgical treatments; pre- and post-operative care; and medical intervention products, such as Botox, dermal fillers, and injection vein therapy.

Part Seven, Business Skills, provides an overview of operating your own business, from drafting a business and financial plan, calculating the risks, and complying with legal guidelines to marketing your salon or spa.

A FRESH DESIGN

Milady's Standard Esthetics: Advanced includes more than 1,200 full-color illustrations and photographs, along with a text design similar to the tenth edition of *Milady's Standard Esthetics: Fundamentals* for easy transition from the basic to the more advanced material. The procedures are formatted with clear, easy-to-understand directions and step-by-step photographs to help students visualize important techniques.

EDUCATIONAL ELEMENTS OF THIS EDITION

Many features are included to help you recognize and master key concepts and techniques.

Focus On...

Throughout the text are boxes in the outer column that draw attention to various skills and concepts that will help you obtain your goal. The "Focus On..." pieces target all aspects of personal and professional development. These topics are crucial to your success as a student and as a professional.

Activity

The "Activity" boxes offer engaging and timely classroom exercises that will help you understand first hand the concepts explained in the text.

Did You Know?

These features call attention to a special point and provide information that will enhance your understanding of what you are learning in the text.

Regulatory Agency Alert

Laws differ from region to region, so it is important to contact state boards and provincial regulatory agencies to learn what is allowed and not allowed where you are studying. The "Regulatory Agency Alert" icon appears in this text next to procedures or practices that are regulated differently from state to state, alerting you to refer to the laws in your region. Your instructor will provide you with contact information.

FYI

These features offer additional important information related to the content.

Chapter Glossary

At the beginning of each chapter is a list of key terms. The first time a key term is used and defined in the text, it will appear in boldface. All key terms and their definitions are included in the glossary at the end of the chapter as well as in the Glossary/Index at the end of the text. The glossary terms and definitions from *Milady's Standard Esthetics: Fundamentals, Tenth Edition,* also appear in the back-of-book Glossary and Index for easy reference.

Learning Objectives

At the beginning of each chapter is the list of learning objectives, which is the important information in the chapter you will be expected to know. Icons placed within the chapter indicate that a learning objective has been completed.

Caution!

Some information is so critical for your safety and the safety of your clients that it deserves special attention. The text directs you to this information in the "Caution!" features found in the margins.

Here's a Tip

These helpful hints draw attention to situations that might arise or give you quick ways of doing things. Look for these tips in procedures and throughout the text.

Review Questions

At the end of each chapter is a list of questions designed to test your understanding of the information just presented. Your instructor may ask you to write the answers to these questions as an assignment or to answer them orally in class. If you have trouble answering a question, go back to the chapter, review the material, and try again.

Resources

These features offer Web addresses and references for additional information and activities. You can find this information in the back of this textbook.

EXTENSIVE TEACHING/LEARNING PACKAGE

While *Milady's Standard Esthetics: Advanced* is the center of the curriculum, students and educators have a wide range of supplements from which to choose.

Student Supplements

All student supplements correlate to the content in the core textbook.

Milady's Standard Esthetics: Advanced Workbook

Designed to reinforce classroom and textbook learning, the *Student Workbook* contains chapter-by-chapter exercises. Included are fill-in-the-blank exercises, matching exercises, short-answer questions, crossword puzzles, word searches, and illustrations to label, all coordinated with material from the text.

Milady's Standard Esthetics: Advanced Exam Review

The *Exam Review* contains chapter-by-chapter questions in a multiple-choice format to help students prepare for the licensure exam. While not intended to be the only form of review offered to students, this book aids in overall classroom preparation. The *Exam Review* has been revised to meet the most stringent test-development guidelines. The questions in the *Exam Review* are for study purposes only and are not the exact questions students will see on the licensure exams.

Milady's Standard Esthetics: Advanced Student CD-ROM

Milady's Standard Esthetics: Advanced Student CD-ROM is an interactive product designed to reinforce classroom learning, stimulate the imagination, and aid in preparation for board exams. Featuring many helpful video clips and animations to demonstrate practices and procedures, this exciting educational tool also contains a test bank with approximately 1,000 chapter-by-chapter or randomly accessed multiple-choice questions to help students study for the exam. Other features include the game bank, which offers games to strengthen knowledge of terminology, and a glossary that pronounces and defines each term.

The content of the CD-ROM follows and enhances the *Milady's Standard Esthetics: Advanced* textbook. The technology of the program is designed to be interactive, allowing the learner to be surrounded or "pulled into" the content, and it tracks the student's progress through the program.

Milady's Online Licensing Preparation: Advanced Esthetics

Milady's Online Licensing Preparation: Advanced Esthetics provides students with an online alternative to better prepare for state board exams. A thousand multiple-choice questions, different from those in the *Exam Review*, appear with rationales for correct and incorrect choices; each correct answer links to the portion of *Milady's Standard Esthetics: Advanced* where the information is given. Students have the flexibility to study from any computer, whether at home or at school. Because exam review preparation is available to students at any time of day or night, class time can be used for other activities, and students gain familiarity with a computerized test environment as they prepare for licensure. This product is also offered in Spanish.

Educator Supplements

Milady offers a full range of products created especially for esthetics educators to make the classroom preparation and presentation simple, effective, and enjoyable.

Milady's Standard Esthetics: Advanced Course Management Guide

The *Advanced Course Management Guide* contains all the materials educators need in one package. This innovative, instructional guide is written with esthetics educators in mind and is designed to make exceptional teaching easy. With formatting that provides easy-to-use material for use in the classroom, it will transform classroom management and dramatically increase student interest and understanding. Included are comprehensive lesson plans, instructor support forms, handouts, and the answers to the review questions in the textbook and in *Milady's Standard Esthetics: Advanced Student Workbook.*

FEATURES YOU WILL FIND ON THE CD-ROM VERSION

- Every page from the *Advanced Course Management Guide* can be printed to appear exactly like the page from the print product.
- A computerized test bank contains multiple-choice questions that instructors can use to create random tests from a single chapter or create a more comprehensive exam from all of the material in the book. In this new edition, computerized test bank questions are not the same questions as in the *Exam Review.* Answer keys are automatically created. A gradebook feature to track students' progress is also included.
- An Image Library of *all* of the photos and illustrations from *Milady's Standard Esthetics: Advanced* can be easily imported to Microsoft® PowerPoint® presentations or printed onto paper or acetate to create overheads. They can even be imported into other documents to further enhance instruction.

Milady's Standard Esthetics: Advanced Instructor Support Slides (Microsoft® PowerPoint® Presentation)

The Microsoft® PowerPoint® presentation created to accompany the *Milady's Standard Esthetics: Advanced* makes lesson plans simple yet incredibly effective. Complete with photos and art, this chapter-by-chapter CD-ROM has ready-to-use presentations that will help engage students' attention and keep their interest through its varied color schemes and styles. Instructors can use it as is or adapt it to their own classrooms by importing photos they have taken, changing the graphics, or adding slides.

Milady's Standard Esthetics: Advanced DVD

This set of brand-new DVDs consists of approximately two hours of guided demonstrations of key procedures found in the *Milady's Standard Esthetics: Advanced* textbook. The DVDs provide instructional video on topics such as Jessner's peel, microdermabrasion, ultrasonic facial, LED skin treatment, IPL photorejuvenation, lymphatic drainage, ear reflexology massage, stone massage for the face, and Shirodhara treatment.

About the Authors

JUDITH CULP, EDITORIAL CONTRIBUTOR

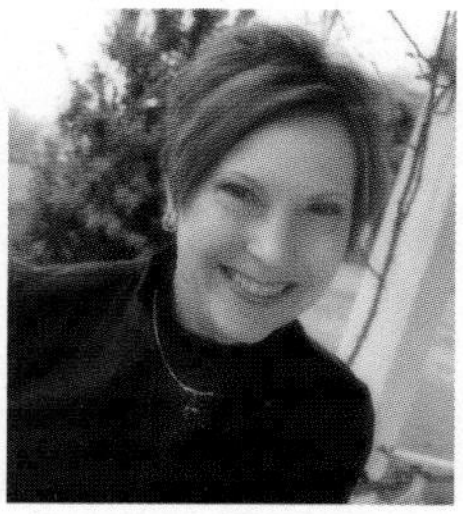

Judith Culp has spent nearly 30 years in the field of esthetics. A working professional, she has lectured at both state and national events, has contributed to trade publications, written a column for *Stylist* and *Salon* newspapers, is the editor for the Society of Permanent Cosmetic Professionals (SPCP) quarterly, and is also an educator. She holds certifications with CIDESCO, NCEA, and the SPCP. She has reviewed numerous books for Milady and was the subject matter expert with Pamela Hill's *Tips & Tricks for Permanent Cosmetics*. Her school is the first in the Northwest to offer both 600- and 1,200-hour esthetics programs. She can be reached through her Web site at http://www.estheticsnw.com.

EFRAIN ARROYAVE, M.D.

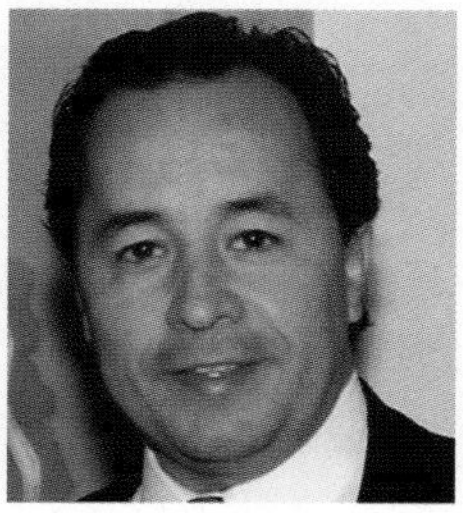

Efrain Arroyave, M.D., is a retired surgeon of plastic and reconstructive surgery with an emphasis in aesthetic surgery. He practiced in Miami Beach from 1988 to 1996. Along with several leading plastic surgeons in Beverly Hills, New York, and Miami Beach, he co-authored a book for skin care specialists titled *Understanding Cosmetic Procedures: Surgical & Nonsurgical* (Thomson Delmar Learning, 2006). Arroyave was the CEO and founder of MedicusMedia, the world's largest medical multimedia company for the global Latin Internet community. Arroyave was also the editor-in-chief for the medical section for *Nexos,* American Airlines' Spanish-Portuguese in-flight magazine. Arroyave now serves as the medical director for econoLABS.com, which provides anti-aging and other health screens and routine blood testing for uninsured patients across the United States.

LINDA BERTAUT

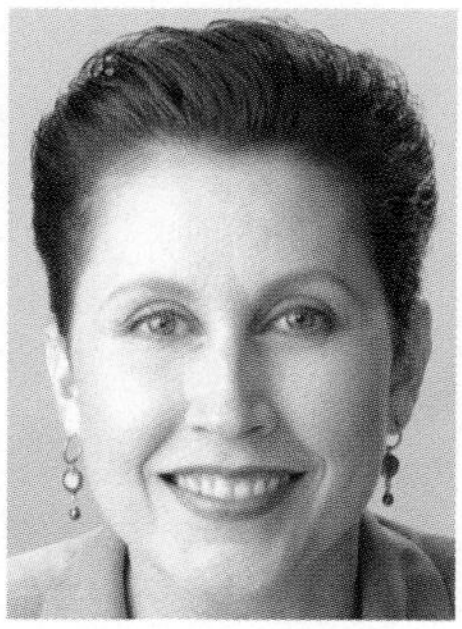

Esthetician, Reiki master teacher, and award-winning inner and outer beauty expert Linda Bertaut specializes in bringing inner beauty to the surface and inspiring others to do the same. Her lifetime passion for performing makeovers led her to the beauty industry more than 20 years ago. What started as makeup and image makeovers turned into wellness and "Energy Make-Overs" for body, mind, and spirit. Known as the beauty industry's Reiki master teacher, she founded Bertaut Beauty to help professionals add value to their services by training them in her signature wellness techniques and all-natural EnergyCeuticals products; Petal Potions mood-enhancing mists and elixirs; healing gemstone kits; and Face Options, "energy-infused" mineral cosmetics. Her products, seminars, and retreats are enabling beauty professionals and their clients to unlock their incredible potential, realize their true beauty, and live their best lives.

HELEN BICKMORE

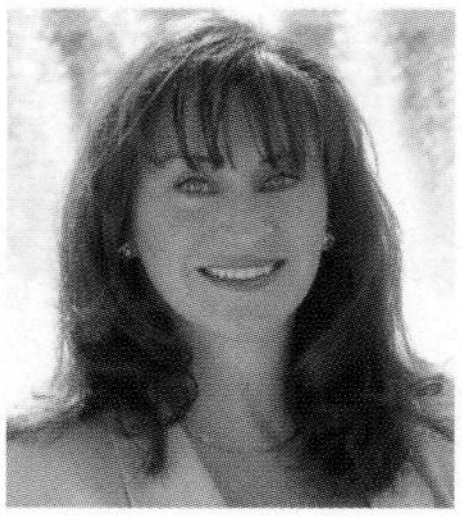

Helen Bickmore received her diplomas for beauty therapy (esthetics), body treatments, massage, and electrolysis in 1979 through both the London College of Fashion and the City and Guilds of London Institute (CGLI). She is a New York State Licensed Esthetician and Massage Therapist (LMT) and is a Certified Professional Electrologist (CPE) with the American Electrology Association (AEA).

Helen has taught esthetics at the Yorkshire Coast College—(the former) Scarborough Technical College—in England and over the years has worked in salons providing services and as a spa director as well as owning her own businesses in the United Kingdom and United States. She continues to provide services to a busy clientele.

In addition Helen has reviewed manuscripts, written articles, appeared on television news programs, given workshops, and served on a number of panels and boards. She currently serves as a board member of the New York Electrology Association. She is also the author of *Milady's Hair Removal Techniques: A Comprehensive Manual* and its companion *Course Management Guide* (both Thomson Delmar Learning, 2004) as well as the co-author (with Pamela Hill) of the *Aesthetician Series: Advanced Hair Removal* (Cengage Learning, 2008). She resides in Albany, New York, with her husband of 22 years and three children.

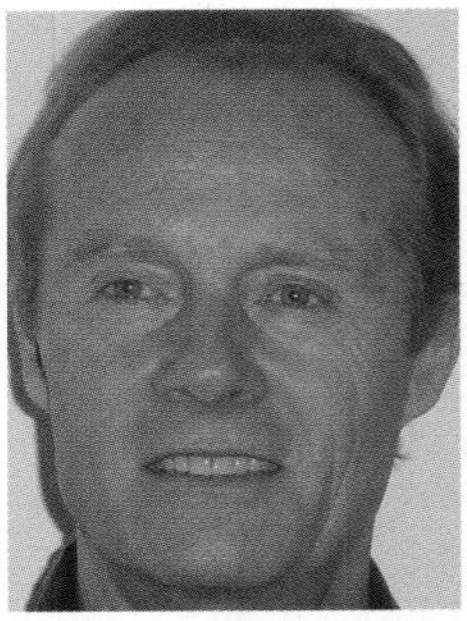

JON CANAS

Jon Canas is president of Laboratoire Gibro S.A., a Swiss company that makes the skin care line PHYTO 5™,which is based on the unique skin care and wellness method known as Phytobiodermie®. He is also the president of a Florida-based company distributing the products in the United States.

Originally from France, Jon went to Cornell, Northeastern, and Harvard universities. His first career was in the hotel industry. He has authored a number of articles for trade publications and spoken at trade shows and conferences regarding the benefits of traditional Chinese medicine for the beauty and spa industry. He authored *Beauty Is Health Made Visible: Naturally Energetic and Holistic Skincare and Wellness for Consumers and Professionals.* The segment on reflex zones of the face is extracted from this book. He can be contacted through his Web site, www.Phytobiodermie.com.

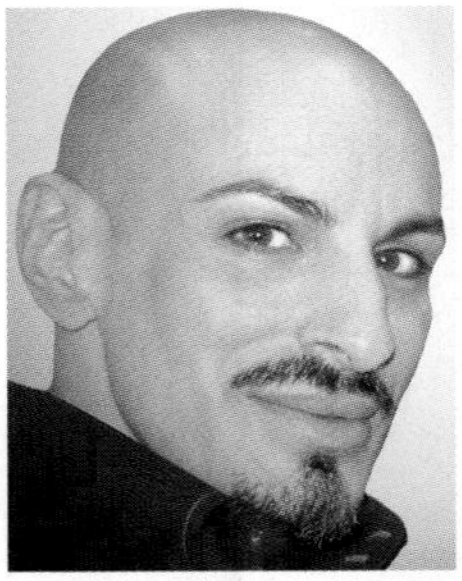

ROQUE COZZETTE

A connoisseur of beauty with more than 20 years of experience in print, television, fashion, cosmetic product development, and makeup instruction, Cozzette brings an extraordinary depth of scope and experience to his multifaceted role as the Director of Makeup for Kett Cosmetics. As a freelance artist, Roque brought airbrushing to the fashion forum, where it was seldom featured. He perfected the synergistic blend of traditional makeup techniques combined with airbrush makeup to create beauty, couture fashion, and chic-urban style. Celebrity clients, such as Anika Noni Rose, Christina Milian, and Heather Graham, appreciate his innovative approach to beauty.

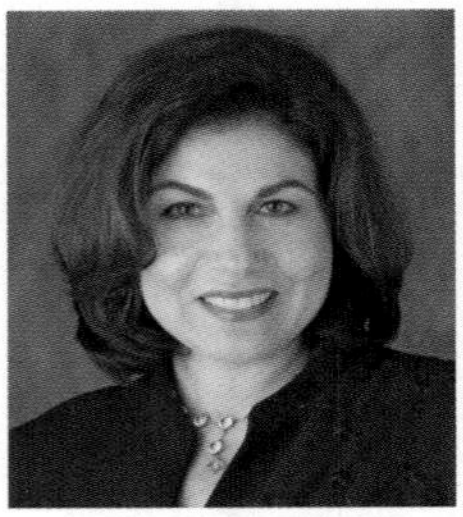

JANET M. D'ANGELO

Janet M. D'Angelo, M.Ed., is founder and president of J. Angel Communications, LLC, a marketing and public relations firm specializing in the health, beauty, and wellness industry. With more than 20 years of experience developing marketing and management strategies across all segments of the skin care market, Janet is a featured speaker at trade shows and conducts seminars and workshops on a wide range of business topics.

Janet began her career in the skin care industry in 1979 as one of the first separately licensed estheticians in Massachusetts. Since then she has worked tirelessly to raise industry awareness and promote professional standards. In addition to her work on this text, Janet is the author of *Spa Business Strategies: A Plan for Success* (Thomson Delmar Learning, 2006). She is also a contributing editor and author of the Business Communication Skills of

Milady's Standard Comprehensive Training for Estheticians (Thomson Delmar Learning, 2003) and *Milady's Standard Esthetics: Fundamentals* (Cengage Learning, 2009). She has written numerous articles for newspaper, consumer, and trade publications and is responsible for conducting the Day Spa Association's First Compensation & Benefits Survey.

Janet is a member of several professional organizations, including the American Marketing Association (AMA), the Day Spa Association (DSA), the International Spa Association (ISPA), and the National Coalition of Estheticians, Manufacturers, Distributors and Alliances (NCEA). She can be reached at janet@jangelcommunications.com.

SALLIE DEITZ

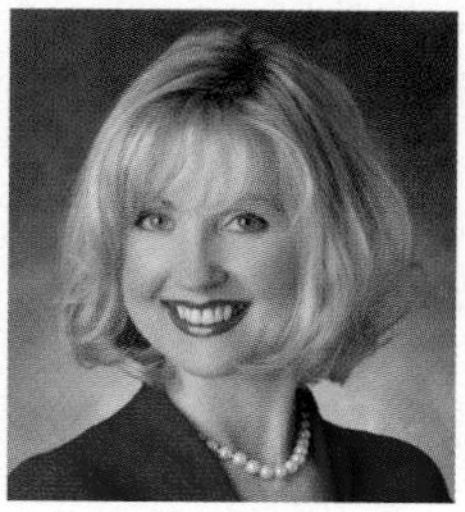

Sallie Deitz serves in education and product development with Bio Therapeutic, Inc., and the Bio Therapeutic Institute of Technology, in Seattle, Washington. Deitz has been a licensed esthetician for 25 years, has 12 years of clinical experience, and is the author of *The Clinical Esthetician: An Insider's Guide to Succeeding in a Medical Office* (Thomson Delmar Learning, 2004) and *Amazing Skin: A Girl's Guide to Naturally Beautiful Skin* (Drummond Publishing Group, 2005). Sallie Deitz is a contributing author on *Milady's Standard Comprehensive Training for Estheticians* (Thomson Delmar Learning, 2004) and *Milady's Standard Esthetics: Fundamentals, Tenth Edition* (Thomson Delmar Learning, 2009). Deitz is an editorial advisory board member for Plastic Surgery Products in Los Angeles, California, and serves as a committee member in test development for NIC (National Interstate Council of State Boards of Cosmetology, Esthetics Division).

MICHELLE ELDRIDGE

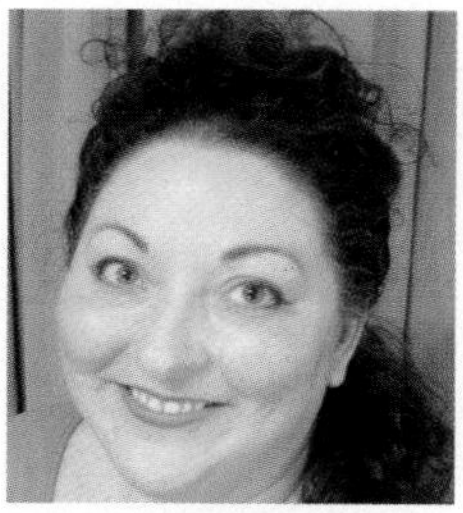

Michelle Eldridge has been involved in the esthetics industry for more than eight years and is the owner of Lucia Skincare in Eugene, Oregon. In addition to her practice, Michelle is an educator for Esthetics Northwest, where she plays an active role in curriculum design and recruitment. Michelle is NCEA certified and holds a B.A. in English and an M.A. in professional communication. She has also worked as freelance writer and editor.

RAMONA MOODY FRENCH

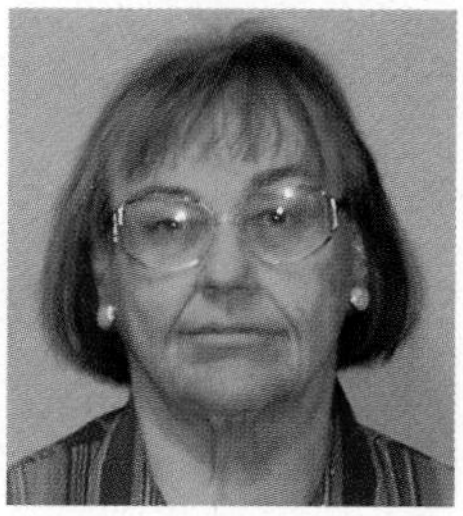

Ramona Moody French has been a massage therapist for 20 years. Her first exposure to lymph drainage massage (LDM) was in a workshop taught by a colleague. She began to use LDM techniques in her practice and to look for other teachers so she could learn more. She also began to observe different techniques for reducing swelling, whether they were LDM or not. French was fascinated by LDM, which has such profound effect with such subtle work. The more she learned and experienced, the more she wanted to know. In addition to seeking more training and practice, French began systematically surveying the medical literature on LDM. Because LDM is the most scientifically researched style of massage, a great deal of information is available. Ramona currently owns and operates the Desert Resorts School of Somatherapy and is part owner of Massage Rx in Rancho Mirage, California.

JUDY GARCIA

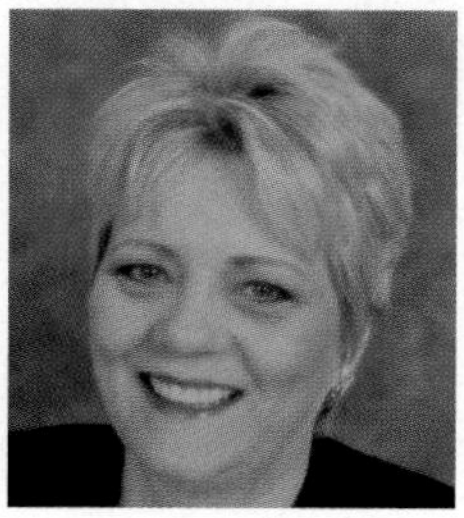

Judy Garcia is a freelance esthetics educator and skin care salon owner with more than 25 years of experience in the professional beauty business. Over these years she spent two-and-a-half years training and working with a noted dermatologist and acne care specialist and also traveled as an international educator for a prominent U.S. skin care company. She has traveled throughout the United States and Alaska, Hong Kong, Malaysia, Korea, and Canada teaching advanced esthetics classes to estheticians, cosmetologists, and medical professionals. Judy is a licensed esthetician, an AIE Certified Clinical Esthetician, and a CIDESCO Diplomaté.

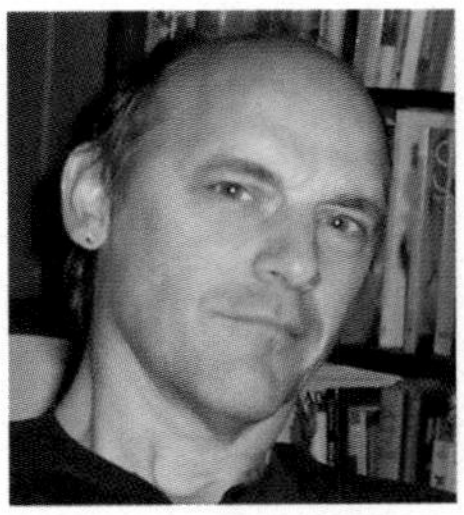

JIMM HARRISON

Jimm Harrison is an innovative educator and holistic health consultant with more than 25 years' experience in the beauty industry. His unique approach to beauty is the culmination of years of in-depth research on natural and nutritional beauty principles, apprenticing to some of world's leading educators and researchers in the fields of essential oils and plant-based medicines. He is a licensed cosmetologist, former salon owner, and Certified Master Aromatherapist.

Jimm founded the Phytotherapy Institute in 1995, conducting certification programs in essential oil therapy and natural skin care for accredited massage, spa therapy, cosmetology, and medical institutions. He is best known for his work on Global Healthy Aging, a unique beauty program that blends physiological, biological, psychological, and sociological principles.

Jimm has written numerous articles on the subjects of essential oil therapy, "green" skin care, holistic beauty, and cosmetic safety. He is the co-founder of Spirit of Beauty Nutritional Skin Care and OHA Bio-Active Skin Care and is the author of *Aromatherapy: Therapeutic Use of Essential Oils for Esthetics* (Thomson Delmar Learning, 2007).

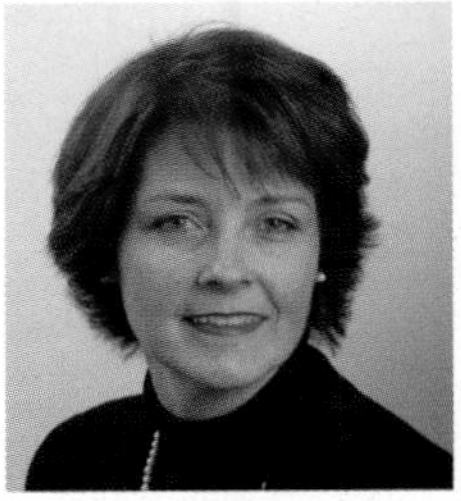

PATRICIA HEITZ

Patricia Heitz has a career that spans more than 30 years as an esthetics industry professional. She has earned the prestigious title of CIDESCO Diploma Holder as well as having served as an advisor and examiner to the New York State Department of State for the Esthetics Examination. Her roles have included esthetics school director, instructor, esthetician, and medical spa business consultant. She is currently a consultant in Patricia Heitz Consulting-Spa and School Training and Consulting, representative for a leading medical esthetics skin care products manufacturer, author/consultant for Milady-Cengage Learning, and a prestigious member of Gerson/Lehrman Financial Analysts Council of Advisors in New York. She has also written several articles in leading industry magazines.

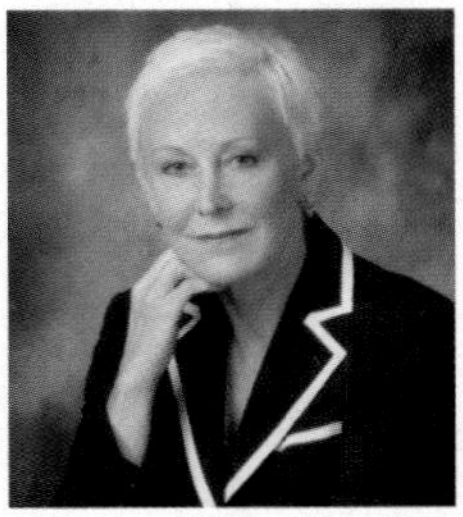

PAMELA HILL

Pamela Hill received her nursing diploma from Presbyterian Hospital and Colorado Women's College, Denver, Colorado, and has practiced as a registered nurse for more than 20 years. Her background includes 15 years of operational and leadership experience in the medical spa, medical skin care, and educational sector. Pamela has been instrumental in the growth and development of Facial Aesthetics, Inc. (FAI), a successful Colorado-based medical spa. An astute results-oriented leader with a proven track record of building and growing companies in the medical appearance sector, she has been actively involved in the evolution of the medical spa model as well as the research and development of the Pamela Hill Skin Care product line. Pamela has been active with patient care, the development of policy and procedure, and clinician education. Passionate about the education of aestheticians in medical spa settings, Pamela began a relationship with Milady, an imprint of Cengage

Learning, in 2003. This relationship launched Milady's Aesthetician Series, a 14-book series dedicated to the education of medical aestheticians and the must-have information for on-the-job success. Currently 13 of the books are in print.

JANE IREDALE

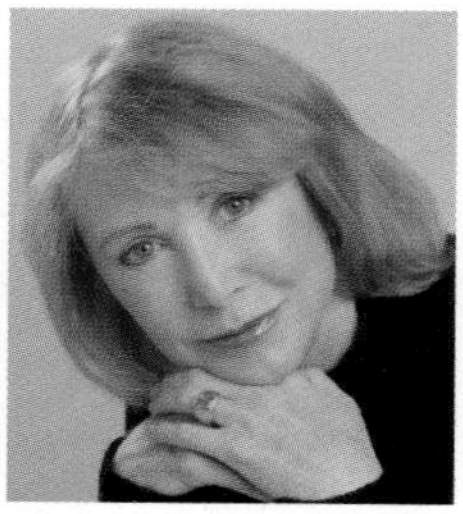

Jane Iredale is the president and founder of Iredale Mineral Cosmetics. She introduced her unique skin care makeup line in May 1994. It was the first full makeup line on the market to offer not just color enhancement but also benefits to the skin. The products are based on micronized minerals and are made without fillers and binders (such as talc and mineral oil) and without chemical dyes or preservatives. As a result, she was the first to supply the aesthetics industry with a full line of makeup based on minerals and the first to see the potential of offering physicians a makeup that was good for the skin. Before she formed her cosmetics company, Jane Iredale's background had been in film, theatre, and television. She started as a casting director working in television commercials with models such as Lauren Hutton, Jaclyn Smith, and Cybill Shepherd and then in film and television with actresses like Susan Sarandon, Glenn Close, and Sarah Jessica Parker.

She then formed her own production company and produced more than 50 programs for PBS and HBO. When she moved from film to theatre, she was nominated for a Tony Award for the Broadway musical *Wind in the Willows,* the show that brought fame to Vicki Lewis and Nathan Lane.

Throughout her career, she has worked with the best makeup artists in the field. She has seen firsthand that true makeup artistry comes not from trying to make a face conform to the latest fashion trends but from enhancing the wearer's natural beauty and, as a result, allowing her personality to shine.

Her experience in working with women whose careers depended on a clear complexion has allowed her to see how skin disorders and sensitivities not only threaten careers but can also destroy self-confidence. This is what led her to develop a makeup line with the influence of world-renowned plastic surgeons and dermatologists that could contribute to the lives of women by aiding the health of the skin.

The company still remains true to its original concept of bringing women a makeup that enhances the health of the skin. From its base as the leading mineral cosmetics company in North America, jane iredale has expanded into more than 35 countries, including the United Kingdom, Europe, Australia, and the Far East.

MARK LEES

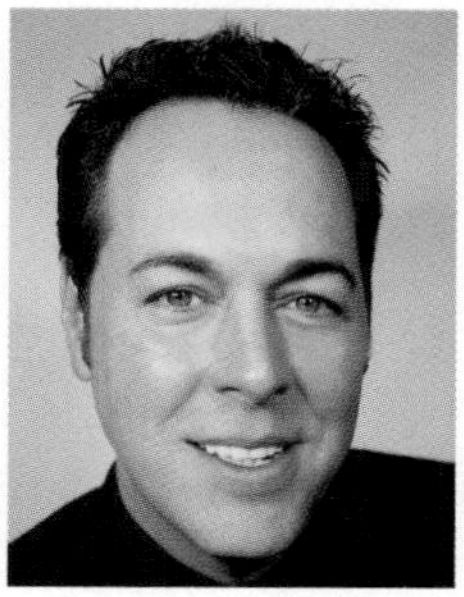

An award-winning speaker and product developer, Dr. Mark Lees is one of the country's most noted skin care specialists. He has been actively practicing clinical skin care for more than 20 years at his multi-award-winning CIDESCO-accredited Florida salon, which has won multiple awards for "Best Day Spa on the Coast" and "Best Skin Care Center on the Coast" from the *Independent Florida Sun.*

His professional awards are numerous and include American Salon Magazine Esthetician of the Year, the Les Nouvelles Esthetiques Crystal Award, the Dermascope Legends Award, the Rocco Bellino Award for outstanding education from the Chicago Cosmetology Association, and Best Educational Skin Care Classroom from the Long Beach International Beauty Expo. Dr. Lees has recently been inducted into the National Cosmetology Association's Hall of Renown.

Dr. Lees is former chairman of Esthetics America, the esthetics education division of the National Cosmetology Association. He currently serves on the Board of Directors of the National Cosmetology Association. He has also served as an affiliate officer for NCA and has served as a CIDESCO International Examiner.

Dr. Lees is former Chairman of the Board of the Esthetics Manufacturers and Distributors Alliance, and is a member of the Society of Cosmetic Chemists, and is author of the popular book, *Skin Care: Beyond the Basics,* now in its third edition, and contributing science author of *Milady's Comprehensive Training for Estheticians.* He holds a Ph.D. in Health Sciences, a Master of Science in Health, and a CIDESCO International Diploma. He is licensed to practice in both Florida and Washington State. His line of products for problem, sensitive, and sun-damaged skin is available at finer salons and clinics throughout the United States.

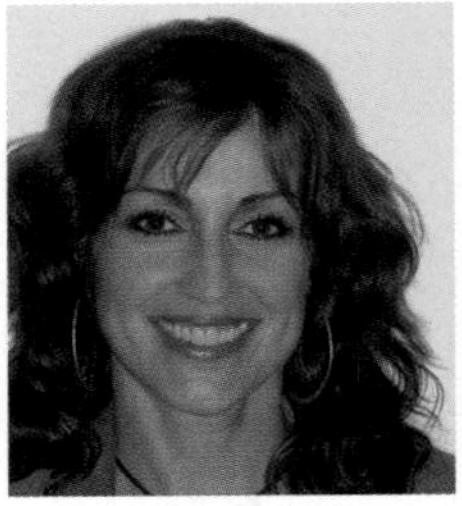

SHEILA MCKENNA

With more than 20 years experience in the fields of television, print, runway, and product development, Sheila is bridging the gap between makeup artist and airbrush enthusiast with airbrush makeup awareness and education to the world of professional makeup artistry. The new millennium brought technological advances in digital photography and hi-definition television, creating a need for changes in makeup design and application techniques. Sheila took advantage of this opportunity and created Kett Cosmetics… *makeup for the digital age.* Since its launch in 2003, Kett can now be found in numerous salons and spas, television networks, and hi-definition productions globally.

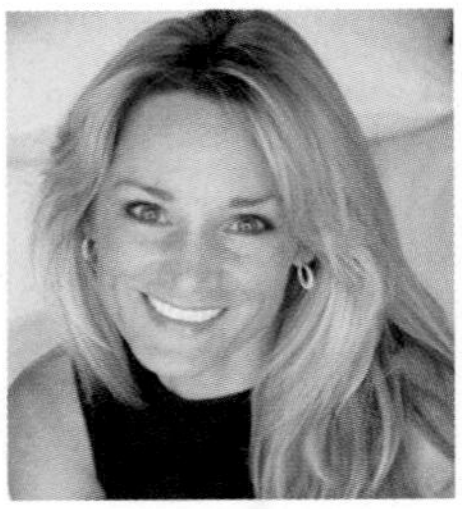

ANNE MILLER

Anne is the founder and president of E'lan Lashes Eyelash Extensions and one of the pioneers of eyelash extension certification training. Her strong desire to motivate and inspire women to reach their full potential is a major driving force in her success. Anne has spent the past 15 years as an entrepreneur in the salon and spa industry as well as retail, marketing, and publicity, while raising her daughters, Brianna and Brooke. She has been featured in several major trade publications.

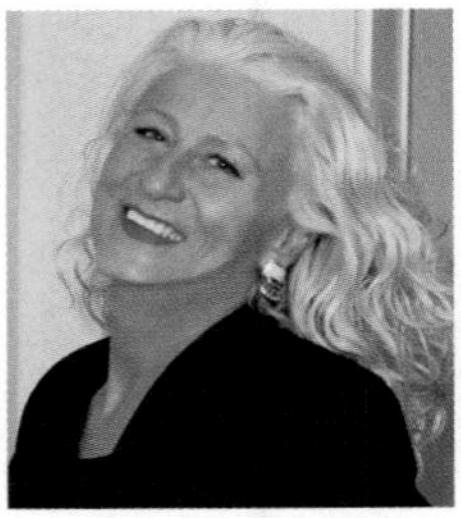

SANDRA ALEXCAE MOREN

Sandra Alexcae Moren, B.Ed., author and owner of Kyron Spa and Salon Consulting, a division of Chiron Marketing Inc. (www.kyron.ca), shares her 30-plus years of experience in the professional beauty industry. A member of the Cosmetology Association (www.ciabc.net), a member of the Technical Committee of Skills Canada, educator and business owner for years, Sandra has taken her in-depth, practical life experience, knowing, and knowledge and shared it in her books.

Sandra is the author of *Spa & Salon Alchemy: The Ultimate Guide to Spa & Salon Ownership* (Thomson Delmar Learning, 2005) and *Spa & Salon Alchemy: Step by Step Procedures* (Thomson Delmar Learning, 2006). Creating these books to guide individuals to build and manage their own spas and salons was a natural evolution for Sandra, who has an extensive background in writing articles for trade magazines, media promotional material, curriculum development, and corporate brochures. In her books, she applies her elaborate professional knowledge, array of experiences, wisdom, and whimsical insight. Her passion, enthusiasm for life, and a belief in actualizing the human spirit has also enabled Sandra to inspire and transform others and make heart connections on her journey. The creation of these books took a lot of passion, commitment, persistence, discipline, creativity, and good old-fashioned hard work to become reality.

PATRICIA OWENS

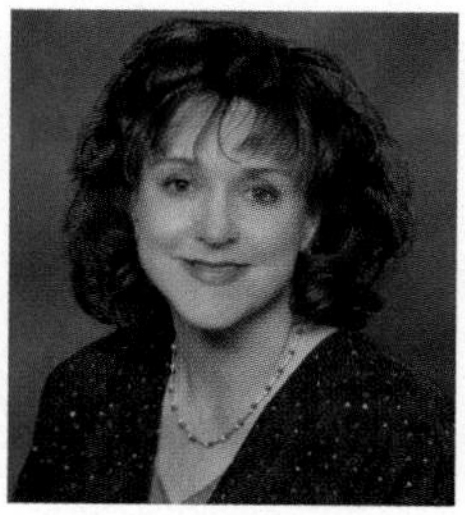

Patricia (Patti) Owens is presently working with dermatologist James Brazil, M.D., at the Olympic Dermatology and Laser Clinic in Olympia, Washington. She has managed the laser/aesthetic and marketing program along with performing cosmetic and aesthetic laser procedures under Dr. Brazil's direction. Patti is also involved with coordination of medical training workshops, preceptorships, and research on a national level. She has been a clinical investigator in the planning and initiation of various FDA studies. She is presently awaiting the publishing of her contributions in two textbooks for Milady, an imprint of Cengage Learning.

Patti established a consulting business, Northwest Laser Aesthetic, in 1999. She has coordinated regional and national laser education workshops along with hospital and office-based management programs. She has served on the Governing Council of AORN Advanced Technology Assembly for Nurse/Allied Health Personnel. She has been the Nursing/Allied Health Chairperson of the American Society of Laser Medicine and Surgery (ASLMS) and in 1999 received the Nurse Excellence Award. She is presently a national consultant for a variety of laser companies and national organizations including the ASLMS, Rockwell Laser Industries (RLI), Dermatologic Nurses Association (DNA), and Lumenis Laser Company. She has served on the ANSI Z136.3 subcommittee for the 2002 and 2007 revisions.

Patti Owens received her BSN from the University of Colorado in 1976 and graduated with her master's degree in health administration from Chapman University in 1996. Her past employment includes being laser manager at Providence St. Peter Hospital from almost 15 years. Her responsibilities included program development and supervision of 13 laser systems, implementation of the laser perioperative role, development of an aesthetic laser in-house and mobile program, and enforcement of safety policies as the facility's acting Laser Safety Officer.

PETER T. PUGLIESE, M.D.

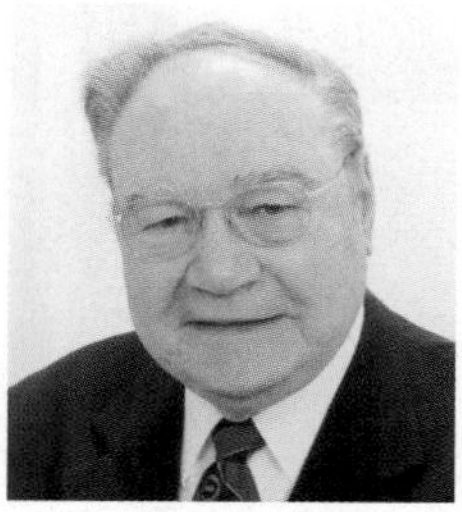

Dr. Peter T. Pugliese earned his M.D. in 1957 from the University of Pennsylvania in Philadelphia. The following year, he entered private practice in rural Berks County, Pennsylvania, where he practiced family medicine for 22 years. Since 1972, Dr. Pugliese has engaged in the study of skin physiology and has made discoveries that have influenced the course of professional skin care around the globe.

Dr. Pugliese did postgraduate research at the Johnson Foundation of Biophysics and held academic positions at the Hershey Medical School and at the University of Pennsylvania. He holds ten patents, including functional raw materials, bovine teat dip, and anticellulite hosiery. Dr. Pugliese is a member of the Society of Bioengineering and the Skin, the American Academy of Dermatology, and the Society of Investigative Dermatology and has given more than 125 presentations at scientific meetings worldwide.

Dr. Pugliese founded the Circadia Skin Care Institute in 2003, where he teaches advanced courses for the skin care professional in skin physiology, histology, biochemistry, cosmetic chemistry, and medical esthetics. His goal is to elevate the practice of esthetics to the status of a professional through higher standards of education in the United States.

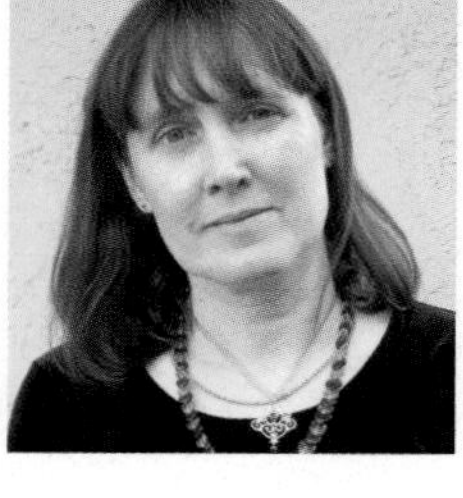

MELANIE SACHS

The pioneer of integrating Tibetan and Indian Ayurvedic wellness techniques into the spa and beauty industry, Melanie Sachs has worked steadily over the last 20 years to bring the deep benefits of this sacred healing art to her students and clients worldwide. Ayurveda is now listed as one of the top ten spa trends. It is fully accepted and respected as a precious gem that is capable of transforming the spa experience into a journey toward beauty through balance. Through her writing and teachings Melanie explains that it is by eating a healthy diet and participating in suitable exercise and regular spiritual practices together with a natural skin care regiment that we all can reach our goal and discover our own personal happiness and lasting radiance; this is a quality in Ayurveda beyond inner and outer beauty known as our secret beauty.

Melanie works closely with her husband, Robert Sachs, and in 1996, they founded Diamond Way Ayurveda together. There, they provide excellence in education and pure Ayurvedic products to complement their unique spa treatments. Melanie and Robert created *Ayurvedic Beauty Care1994, Ayurvedic Spa 2007* (both with Lotus Press), educational DVDs, and numerous articles for magazines. Melanie teaches worldwide, training individuals and spa teams in standard and signature Ayurvedic treatments using organic essential oil blends, powdered herbs, and specialized Ayurvedic spa equipment they designed personally. She is the main trainer in Ayurveda for the Buddha Bar Spa chain, the first group to fully embrace the full flavor and all the traditional Tibetan protocols in the Diamond Way system.

The name "Diamond Way" comes directly from the Tibetan tradition and means that our path to the highest joy is through helping others. It is this core belief that fuels the energy behind this determined, groundbreaking team.

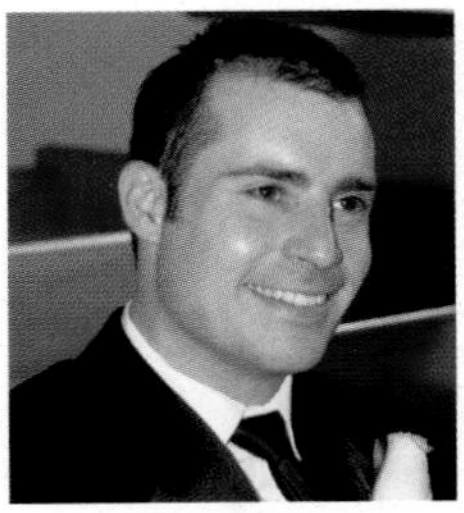

CHRISTIAN STERLING

Christian has been writing and editing esthetician educational materials since 2003. He attended the University of Colorado in Boulder, Colorado, and began working for Facial Aesthetics in Denver. There he met and subsequently began working with the Pamela Hill Institute, with the goal of unifying and improving esthetics educational standards. He currently resides in Florida, where he continues his pursuits.

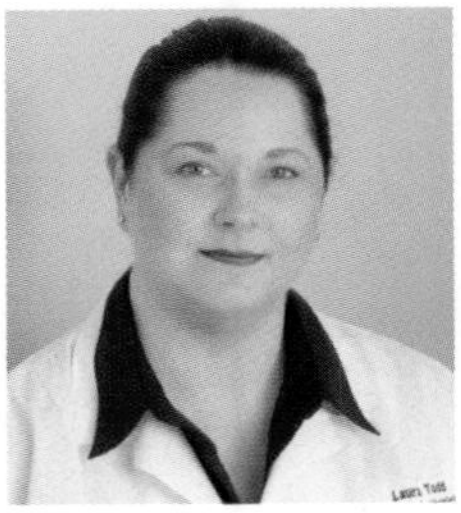

LAURA TODD

Laura Todd has been in the esthetics industry for more than 20 years, earning national attention and commendation. She holds a B.S. in science with a minor in biology and is a master's degree candidate. Currently, Laura is the president of the Institute of Advanced Medical Esthetics and the University of Professional Sciences in Richmond, Virginia. She is also a practicing medical esthetician at her medi-spa, Spa Rx. Laura has been an active participant in advocating for and implementing current legislation to establish licensure for estheticians in the state of Virginia. Laura holds Virginia's first full-term Esthetician Seat, appointed by the governor, and serves on the board that regulates esthetics in Virginia. She was an integral part of developing state regulations for esthetics education, which has influenced policy in other states as well as national legislation. Laura has also served as a subject matter expert, assisting in the development of Virginia's master esthetician examination and the national master esthetician examination for National-Interstate Council of State Boards of Cosmetology NIC.

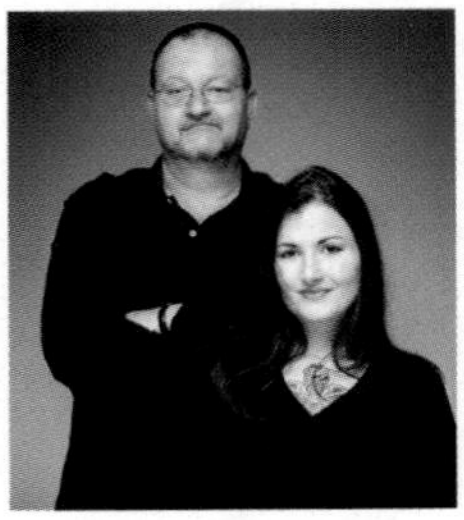

DAVID VIDRA

In 1996 David A. Vidra, CLPN, MA, founded Health Educators, Inc., an educational company in response to the lack of industry-specific health and safety information available to traditional tattoo artists, body piercers, and cosmetic tattoo practitioners (i.e., the modification industry). The goal of Health Educators, Inc., is to provide pertinent, up-to-date, industry-specific information to traditional and cosmetic tattoo artists, body piercers, studio and salon owners, public health officials, and medical professionals regarding the prevention of disease transmission and occupational health and safety issues that pertain specifically to the beauty and body modification industries. Health Educators, Inc., strongly believes that establishing a consistent standard of practice among each group of practitioners, as well as the implementation of responsible regulations and appropriate education, will assist in developing safe, quality environments for practitioners as well as clients. For further information, please visit www.hlthedu.com.

Acknowledgments

After receiving numerous requests over the years for more comprehensive educational materials for skin care, we conducted a focus group attended by 11 of the nation's skin care experts and educators to formulate a plan for this new product. We then surveyed educators from across the country, asking them what needed to be included, in what order, and to what depth of coverage. What you hold in your hands is the result of this extensive research and review process. The authors and editors at Milady recognize with respect and gratitude the following educators and professionals who have played a part in the development of this program:

FOCUS GROUP PARTICIPANTS

Isabelle Calleros, Southwest Institute of Natural Aesthetics, Mesa, AZ

Lisia Cooley-Walch, Lisia's Electrolysis & Laser Hair Removal, Big Rapids, MI

Maria Ferguson, Hudson Valley School of Advanced Aesthetic Skin Care, New Paltz, NY

Merna Hilliard, Institute of Cosmetology & Esthetics, Houston, TX

Ruth Ann Holloway, Dermal Dimensions Progressive Skin Therapy Clinic, Providence, UT

Sherry Parker, Steiner Education Group, Pompano Beach, FL

Natalie Parkin, Skin Works, Salt Lake City, UT

Darlene Purdy, Euphoria Institute of Beauty Arts & Sciences, Henderson, NV

Pamela Springer, The Skin & Makeup Institute of Arizona, Peoria, AZ

Karen Wackerman, Kar-Che' The Professional Career Center, Mesa, AZ

Amy Waldorf, Harmony Day Spa, Caldwell, NJ

REVIEWERS

Sheryl Baba, Spa Owner, Esthetician, Makeup Artist, Solstice Day Spa, Hyannis, MA

Deborah Beatty, Instructor of Health Sciences/ Cosmetology, Columbus Technical College, GA

Linda Burmeister, Undergraduate School Program Training Manager, The International Dermal Institute, Carson, CA

April Coleman, Yvonne de Vilar Scientific Skincare, Assistant Director, Clinton, MD

Therese Cunningham, Educational Supervisor, The Skin & Makeup Institute of Arizona, Peoria, AZ

Denise Dubois, Complexions Spa for Beauty & Wellness, Albany, NY

Chris Farber, Aesthetician, Pacific Shores Club, Redwood City, CA

Stacy Heatherly, Owner, Image Enhancers, Papillion, NE

Kathy Hernandez-McGowan, Esthetics Instructor/ Licensed Acupuncturist, San Bernadino, CA

Ruth Ann Holloway, PMAE, LMT, Dermal Dimensions Progressive Skin Therapy, Providence, UT

Kim Jarrett, Esthetics Instructor, College of Hair Design, Belton, MO

Irene Koufalis, European Body Concepts, NACCAS team Inspector, NCEA State Representative Chair, PA

Helen LeDonne, Chair, Cosmetology, Santa Monica College, Santa Monica, CA

Opal Mobbs, Cosmetology Instructor (Retired), Texas College of Cosmetology, Abilene, TX

Elizabeth Myron, Industry Specialist, Bethesda, MD

REVIEWERS *continued*

Nancy Owens, Cosmetology/Esthetics Instructor, Olympia, WA

Sherry Parker, National Director of Skin Care Education, Steiner Education Group, Pompano Beach, FL

Sandra Peoples, Career Counselor/Esthetician, Aurora, CO

Darlene Purdy, Advanced Aesthetics Instructor, Euphoria Institute of Beauty Arts and Sciences, Henderson, NV

Sharalyn Riley, Instructor, Hacienda La Puente Adult Education, La Puente, CA

Amy Fields Rumley, Owner/Esthetician, Merle Norman Cosmetics and Skin Care Services, Stokesdale, NC

Pamela Springer, Instructor, The Skin & Makeup Institute of Arizona, Peoria, AZ

Anelka Szaruga, Director of Esthetics, American Beauty Academy, Philadelphia, PA

Karen Wackerman, Owner, Kar-Che' The Professional Career Center, Mesa, AZ

Amy Waldorf, Harmony Day Spa, Caldwell, NJ

PHOTO SESSION ACKNOWLEDGMENTS

Special thanks to Judith Culp and her talented staff and students at Northwest Institute of Esthetics in Eugene, Oregon, who graciously participated as models and assisted with the photo shoot production. Many thanks and appreciation to Jeani Wright and Pamela Haskin for transporting and supplying equipment for the photo shoot.

Photographers

Rob Werfel Photography, Ashland, Oregon

Karen Maze Photography, Santa Monica, CA

Manufacturers and Suppliers

The following manufacturers and suppliers provided supplies, products, and equipment for use during the photo shoot. We are grateful for their generosity.

ATZEN® Lymphobiology®, © 2006 Universal Companies

Skin Blends, LLC, Nixa, Missouri (MO), http://www.skinblends.com

Iredale Mineral Cosmetics, Ltd.

Kett Cosmetics

Bio-Therapeutic, Bio-Synthesis™ light-activated rejuvenation system

Universal Companies provided the moist heater and hydroculator.

Models

José Alexander

Melissa Baer

Brad Boyer

Okhui Coleman

Shannon Coleman

Judith Culp

Theresa DeLay

Temenoujka Dobreva

Michelle Eldridge

Kim Gilbert

Bonita Good

Holly Gregg

Destiny Henderson

Kendra Johnson

Nicole Johnson

Sherri Johnson

Casey Jorgenson

Molly Lynch

Lindsay Moseman

RaShel Pelzel

Maygan Phillips

Devin Ruffatto

Cynthia Shaw

Tiffany Lippold

Sean Veeck

Brittney Welch

Jason Wiese

Jeani Wright

Photo Credits

Chapter 1: Fig.1-1 (female doctor and patient): © dasilva, 2008; used under license from Shutterstock.com. Fig. 1-2 (Chinese woman relaxing at the resort SPA: © Ximagination, 2008; used under license from Shutterstock.com. Fig. 1-3 (steam treatment during a facial at a beauty spa): © Tyler Olson, 2008; used under license from Shutterstock.com. Fig. 1-4 (man getting a full body mud wrap): © Yanik Chauvin; used under license from Shutterstock.com. Figs. 1-5, 1-8: Larry Hamill Photography. Fig. 1-6 (blond bride preparing for the wedding and make-up): © Pavitra, 2008; used under license from Shutterstock.com. Fig. 1-7 (cruise ship leaving Las Palmas in Spain): © criben, 2008; used under license from Shutterstock.com. Fig. 1-9: Rob Werfel Photography.

Chapter 3: Figs. 3-5 to 3-20: Courtesy of Peter T. Pugliese, MD and Associates.

Chapter 4: Figs. 4-4, 4-9: Courtesy Mark Lees Skin Care, Inc. Fig. 4-7: Courtesy Timothy G. Berger, M.D. Fig. 4-8: Courtesy George Fisher, M.D.

Chapter 6: Fig. 6-8: Larry Hamill Photography.

Chapter 8: Fig. 8-1, 8-2, 8-5, 8-6, 8-12, 8-15, 8-19, 8-20: Courtesy of Technology Concepts International-Penny Smalley RN. Fig. 8-7, 8-8, 8-9, 8-10, 8-17a, 8-21, 8-22, 8-23, 8-28, 8-29, 8-30, 8-31: Courtesy of Lumenis® Ltd. Fig. 8-11: Courtesy of Laser Institute of America, Orlando, FL. Fig. 8-13, 8-14, 8-16, 8-17b: Courtesy of Rockwell Laser Industries. Fig. 8-18: Buffalo Filter®. Fig. 8-24: Courtesy of Olympic Dermatology and Laser Clinic. Fig. 8-25, 8-26, 8-27: Courtesy of Medlite Hoya Con Bio. Fig 8-31: Courtesy of Mark Taylor, MD, and Lumenis® Ltd. Fig. 8-33: Courtesy of Thermage. Fig. 8-34: Courtesy of Light Bioscience. Fig. 8-35: Courtesy of Photo Therapeutics, Ltd.

Chapter 9: Fig. 9-1 (overhead food background): © MorganLane Photography, 2008; used under license from Shutterstock.com. Fig. 9-2 (orange vitamin pills with dose on white background): © Trykster, 2008; used under license from Shutterstock.com. Fig. 9-3 (fresh vegetables, fruits and other foodstuffs): © Kiselev Andrey Valerevich, 2008; used under license from Shutterstock.com. Fig. 9-4 (Nurse measuring the patient's blood pressure): © Zsolt Nyulaszi, 2008; used under license from Shutterstock.com. Fig. 9-5 (shot of a stressed and ill businesswoman): © Supri Suharjoto, 2008; used under license from Shutterstock.com. Fig. 9-6 (Grillin' and chillin'): © James A. Kost, 2008; used under license from Shutterstock.com. Fig. 9-7 (rosemary roasted salmon served with asparagus, cherry tomatoes, and red bell pepper topped by mustard rosemary sauce and glass of ice water for healthy style dinner): © Eugene Bochkarev, 2008; used under license from Shutterstock.com. Fig. 9-8 (killing habit): © Loke Yek Mang, 2008; used under license from Shutterstock.com. Fig. 9-9: RLCQ courtesy of Dr. Thomas Holmes and Dr. Richard H. Rahe. Fig. 9-10 (young women relaxing and doing yoga exercise): © Dallas Events Inc., 2008; used under license from Shutterstock.com. Fig. 9-11 (carefree woman in white dress on tropical beach): © Christian Wheatley, 2008; used under license from Shutterstock.com.

Chapter 10: Fig. 10-1: Courtesy of Rebecca James Gadberry and YG Labs. 10-14 & 10-15: Courtesy of Leon Prete, LMT, and Barbara Prete, CE, SafeLase Institute for Cosmetic Laser Training. Fig. 10-17, 10-19, 10-42: Rube J. Pardo, M.D., Ph.D. Fig. 10-20, 10-22, 10-24: Michael J. Bond, M.D. Fig. 10-21: Courtesy of The Skin Care Foundation, www.skincancer.org. Fig. 10-25, 10-26, 10-27, 10-28 Grades 1 and 2, 10-30, 10-31, 10-32, 10-34: Courtesy of Mark Lees Skin Care, Inc. Fig. 10-33: Reprinted with permission from the American Academy of Dermatology. All rights reserved. Fig. 10-37: Courtesy Mark Lees Skin Care, Inc. and National Rosacea Society. Fig. 10-38 and 10-39, 10-40, 10-41, 10-43, 10-44: Courtesy of National Rosacea Society.

Chapter 11: Fig. 11-1: Larry Hamill Photography. Fig. 11-2, 11-3: Rob Werfel Photography. Content on the reflex zones of the face provided by Jon Canas, President of Phytobiodermie.®

Chapter 12: Fig. 12-1 (glass Erlenmeyer flask in a research lab): © Olivier Le Queinic, 2008; used under license from Shutterstock.com. Fig. 12-2 (extra virgin olive oil reflected on white background): © Rafa Irusta, 2008; used under license from Shutterstock.com. Fig. 12-3 (washing hands in water with bar of soap): © Michal Mrozek, 2008; used under license from Shutterstock.com. Fig. 12-4 (Four bottles with different scented aromatic oils): © Margreet de Groot, 2008; used under license from Shutterstock.com.

Fig. 12-5 (beauty lotion close-up with rose petals.): © Tan Kian Khoon, 2008; used under license from Shutterstock.com. Fig. 12-6 (toner close-up): © Tan Kian Khoon, 2008; used under license from Shutterstock.com. Fig. 12-7 (jar of white moisturizer surrounded by fresh cucumber slices on bright orange background): © Diane Maire, 2008; used under license from Shutterstock.com. Fig. 12-8 (close-up of exfoliating cream): © Johanna Goodyear, 2008; used under license from Shutterstock.com. Fig. 12-9 (close-up stack of sliced aloe on the white background): © Sveta San, 2008; used under license from Shutterstock.com. Fig. 12-10 (green tea leaves): © Olga Ultyakova, 2008; used under license from Shutterstock.com.

Chapter 13: Fig. 13-1 (bouquet garni of fresh rosemary, flowering sage, and oregano): © Robyn Mackenzie, 2008; used under license from Shutterstock.com. Fig. 13-3 (aloe vera isolated on black background/medicine concept series): © Miodrag Gajic, 2008; used under license from Shutterstock.com. Fig. 13-4 (Arnica Rocky Mountain Wild Flower):© Kris Butler, 2008; used under license from Shutterstock.com. Fig. 13-5 (asia bamboo tree/background of bamboo tree): © kd2, 2008; used under license from Shutterstock.com. Fig. 13-6 (broken cacao bean): © TZajaczkowski, 2008; used under license from Shutterstock.com. Fig. 13-7 (purple comfrey flowers): © Forin C, 2008; used under license from Shutterstock.com. Fig. 13-8 (fresh red juicy currants with green leaves): © Cornel Achirei, 2008; used under license from Shutterstock.com. Fig. 13-9 (green tea leaves): © OHMAE Jun-ichi, 2008; used under license from Shutterstock.com. Fig. 13-10 (High Key image of seaweed or kelp on beach): © Renate Micallef, 2008; used under license from Shutterstock.com. Fig. 13-11 (marigolds): © Phillip Date, 2008; used under license from Shutterstock.com. Fig. 13-12 (sea buckthorn): © Sergey Chushkin, 2008; used under license from Shutterstock.com. Fig. 13-14: Courtesy of Pacific Institute of Aromatherapy. Fig. 13-16: Courtesy of Jimm Harrison. Fig. 13-17 (herb chamomiles on a green meadow): © Svetlana Privezentseva, 2008; used under license from Shutterstock.com. Fig. 13-18 (eucalyptus): © Yakovleva Zinaida Vasilevna, 2008; used under license from Shutterstock.com. Fig. 13-19 (pink geranium): © Raynard Lyudmyla, 2008; used under license from Shutterstock.com. Fig. 13-20 (close-up of a half-cut ruby grapefruit): © Massimiliano Pieraccini, 2008; used under license from Shutterstock.com. Fig. 13-21 (yellow and orange straw flowers): © Sherri R. Camp, 2008; used under license from Shutterstock.com. Fig. 13-22 (lavender): © iwka, 2008; used under license from Shutterstock.com. Fig. 13-23: Courtesy of Jimm Harrison. Fig. 13-26 (a fresh bunch of rosemary): © Damian Herde, 2008; used under license from Shutterstock.com. Fig. 13-27 (junk on shore): © Christa DeRidder, 2008; used under license from Shutterstock.com. Fig. 13-29 (bottle of essential oil, massage stones, candles, lavender and bath-salt): © Liv friis-larsen, 2008; used under license from Shutterstock.com. Fig. 13-30 (aromatherapy treatment bowl with flowers and perfumed water): © Ye, 2008; used under license from Shutterstock.com. Fig. 13-31 (aromatherapy essentials): © mypokcik, 2008; used under license from Shutterstock.com.

Chapter 14: Fig. 14-1, Larry Hamill Photography. Fig. 14-3 (beauty lotion close-up with rose petals): © Tan Kian Khoon, 2008; used under license from Shutterstock.com. Fig. 14-5 (toner close-up): © Tan Kian Khoon, 2008; used under license from Shutterstock.com. Fig. 14-6 (face cream with dried flower petals): © Ewa Walicka, 2008; used under license from Shutterstock.com. Fig. 14-8: Larry Hamill Photography.

Chapter 16: Fig. 16-1 (colorful blocks isolated on white): © anna karwowska, 2008; used under license from Shutterstock.com. Fig. 16-3, 16-4, 16-18, 16-19: Rob Werfel Photography. Fig. 16-6 a–d: Courtesy of Mark Lees Skin Care, Inc. Fig. 16-7 a–d: Courtesy of Mark Lees Skin Care, Inc. Fig. 16-8 a, b: Courtesy of Murad Skin Research Laboratories. Fig. 16-9 a, b: Courtesy of Murad Medical Group. Fig. 16-10 a, b: Courtesy of Murad Skin Research Laboratories, Inc. Fig. 16-11 a, b: Courtesy Murad Medical Group. Fig. 16-12 a, b: Courtesy of Murad Skin Research Laboratories, Inc. Fig. 16-13 a, b: Courtesy of Murad Medical Group. Fig. 16-14 a–d, Mark Lees Skin Care, Inc. Fig. 16-14 e, f: Courtesy Sothys, USA. Fig. 16-15 (beauty treatment at the health spa): © Robert Anthony, 2008; used under license from Shutterstock.com. Fig. 16-16, 16-17, 16-20 a–c: Skin Blends LLC, Nixa, MO. Fig. 16-21: Courtesy of Christine Valmy, Inc.

Chapter 17: Fig. 17-1 to 17-18, 17-25 to 17-27: Rob Werfel Photography. Fig. 17-19 to 17-23: Courtesy 3D-Beauty International, Inc. Fig. 17-28 to 17-31: Cengage Learning. Fig. 17-32 (beautiful young woman ready for pneumatic massage—pressotherapy, Isolated on white background): © Andrejs Pidjass, 2008; used under license from Shutterstock.com.

Chapter 18: Fig. 18-1, 18-2, 18-11 to 18-13, 18-15: Rob Werfel Photography. Fig. 18-3, 18-6, 18-10: Larry Hamill

Photography. Fig. 18-4: Courtesy of Technology Concepts International—Penny Smalley R.N. Fig 18-5: Courtesy Lumenis® Ltd. Figures 18-7 a, b: Courtesy of Lumenis® Ltd. and Robert A. Weiss, MD. Fig. 18-8: Courtesy of DUSA Pharmaceuticals, Inc. Fig. 18-14a: Skin Blends, LLC, Nixa, MO. Fig. 18-14b: Courtesy of Lam Probe (www.lamskin.com). Fig. 18-9 a–d: Photos provided courtesy of Michael H. Gold, M.D., Gold Skin Care Center, Nashville, TN USA.

Chapter 19: Fig. 19-32, 19-35, 19-36, 19-38 a, b, 19-39 a, b: Courtesy of Leon Prete, LMT, and Barbara Prete, CE, SafeLase Institute for Cosmetic Laser Training. Fig. 19-37: LightSheer® diode hair removal laser, courtesy of Lumenis®. All other photos owned by Cengage Learning.

Chapter 20: Fig. 20-1, 20-2, 20-4, 20-11: Courtesy Anne Miller, E'lan Lashes Eyelash Extensions. Fig. 20-5: Courtesy 3D-Beauty International, Inc. Fig. 20-6 to 20-10, 20-16, 20-17, 20-19: Rob Werfel Photography. Fig. 20-12 to 20-15, 20-18, 20-20: Photos used by permission of Iredale Mineral Cosmetics. Fig. 20-21 to 20-37: Kett Cosmetics. Fig. 20-38, 20-40, 20-41, 20-43: Courtesy of Judy Culp, NW Institute of Aesthetics and Permanent Cosmetics. Fig. 20-39: Reprinted with permission from Marjorie Grimm at Faces by Design. Fig. 20-42: Reprinted with permission from Liza Sims in Anchorage, Alaska.

Chapter 21: Fig. 17-32 (massage table with candle and orchids): © Jerko Grubisic, 2008; used under license from Shutterstock.com. Fig. 21-5, 21-15: Rob Werfel. Fig. 21-10 (cacao therapy applied to young woman in a spa): © Yanik Chauvin, 2008; used under license from Shutterstock.com. Fig. 21-13, 21-21: Randall Perry Photography. Fig. 21-19 (sea mud full body wrap at a luxury spa): © Tyler Olson, 2008; used under license from Shutterstock.com. Fig. 21-22 (cute girl with a towel on her head in bath): © Yanik Chauvin, 2008; used under license from Shutterstock.com. Fig. 21-23 (Woman on massage table with oils, essential oils, candles, scents.): © Leah-Anne Thompson, 2008; used under license from Shutterstock.com.

Chapter 22: All art supplied courtesy of Bertaut Beauty. Figures 22-5, 22-7b and all photos in Procedure 22-1: Copyright © Karen Maze.

Chapter 23: Fig. 23-1: Reproduced with permission from *Ayurvedic Spa* by Melanie and Robert Sachs. Lotus Press, a division of Lotus Brands, Inc., P.O. Box 325, Twin Lakes, WI 53181, USA, www.lotuspress.com © 2007 All Rights Reserved. Fig. 23-2, 23-3, 23-4, 23-5: Courtesy of treatments taught by Diamond Way Ayurveda. Fig. 23-6: Rob Werfel Photography.

Chapter 26: Fig. 26-3, 26-4, 26-5a, 26-10, 26-13, 26-14, 26-16, 26-22, 26-25, 26-27: Courtesy of Hill, Facial Aesthetics, Denver, CO. All other photos provided by Larry Hamill Photography.

Chapter 27: Figures 27-3 a, b: David Rappaport, M.D., Plastic Surgeon, Park Avenue, NY. Figures 27-4 a, b: Courtesy R. Emil Hecht, M.D.

Chapter 28: Fig. 28-1: Larry Hamill Photography. Fig. 28-2: © used under license from Shutterstock.com. Fig. 28-3: Rob Werfel Photography. Fig. 28-4, 28-5 a, b: Courtesy of Lumenis® Ltd. Fig. 28-5: Courtesy of Suzanne Kilmer M.D., © Lumenis®. Fig. 28-6 a, b: David Rappaport, M.D., Plastic Surgeon, Park Avenue, NY. Fig. 28-7: Reprinted with permission from Shippert Medical and Design Veronique. Fig. 28-8 a–d, 28-9: Courtesy of Facial Aesthetics, CO.

Chapter 29: The forms in Figs. 29-2 to 29-6 are located on the Internal Revenue Service Web site (www.irs.ustreas.gov).

Chapter 30: Fig. 30-1: Rob Werfel Photography. Fig. 30-4, 30-7: Paul Castle Photography.

Chapter Opener Photos: **Chapter 1**: 15561610) © Juriah Mosin, 2009; used under license from Shutterstock.com. **Chapter 2:** 181161 (Drying hands after washing): © Leah-Anne Thompson, 2009; used under license from Shutterstock.com. **Chapter 3:** 4020976 (human brain): © Sebastian Kaulitzki, 2009; used under license from Shutterstock.com. **Chapter 4:** 11761591 (test on pregnancy and thermometer and diary): © Sagasan, 2009; used under license from Shutterstock.com. **Chapter 5:** 1520122 (rear view of shoulder muscles on male, flexed): © Douglas R. Hess, 2009; used under license from Shutterstock.com. **Chapter 6:** 13643467 (cardiovascular system): © Sebastian Kaulitzki, 2009; used under license from Shutterstock.com. **Chapter 7:** 21405235 (test tubes and dropper): © Chepko Danil Vitalevich, 2009; used under license from Shutterstock.com. **Chapter 8:** Courtesy of Lumenis® Ltd, Lumenis One™ **Chapter 9:** 14071975 (A young woman doing yoga outside): © Phil Date, 2009; used under license from Shutterstock.com. **Chapter 10:** 17193709 (wellness concept with face care spa therapy session): © khz, 2009; used under license from Shutterstock.com. **Chapter 11:** 13041736 (Gracious senior lady portrait on white background): © Martina Ebel, 2009; used under license from

Shutterstock.com. **Chapter 12:** Rob Werfel Photography, Ashland, OR **Chapter 13:** 15162910 (pebbles flowers and towels - body care): © Matka Wariatka, 2009; used under license from Shutterstock.com. **Chapter 14:** 21200770 (Natural face cream or skincare with green leaf): © Elena Elisseeva, 2009; used under license from Shutterstock.com. **Chapter 15:** 17130433 (Prescription form and pills bottle. See more medical images in my portfolio.): © Sorin Alexadru, 2009; used under license from Shutterstock.com. **Chapter 16:** 10687999 (A young woman has a facial treatment at a spa): © Phil Date, 2009; used under license from Shutterstock. com. **Chapter 17:** 1174708 (A male receives a facial massage): © Leah-Anne Thompson, 2009; used under license from Shutterstock.com. **Chapter 18:** 11980501 (ultrasound skin cleaning at beauty salon): © Serghei Strarus, 2009; used under license from Shutterstock.com. **Chapter 19:** 51751 (Jar of sticky green hair remover. Shallow dof with focus on applicator and gel.): © Jaimie Duplass, 2009; used under license from Shutterstock.com. **Chapter 20:** 18827536 (Set of cosmetic brushes in a black leather case): © Tereza Dvorak, 2009; used under license from Shutterstock.com. **Chapter 21:** Larry Hamill Photography, Columbus, OH **Chapter 22:** Karen Maze Photography, CA **Chapter 23:** 3477101 (Some of the basic elements of Ayurveda: sesame, chili, tincture, tea ball, and herbs.): © Elena Ray, 2009; used under license from Shutterstock.com. **Chapter 24:** 18791089 (Female African American doctor or nurse with a stethoscope on white background): © David Davis, 2009; used under license from Shutterstock.com. **Chapter 25:** 1244160 (Stethoscope on an open medical book series): © Amy Walters, 2009; used under license from Shutterstock.com. **Chapter 26:** 13189039 (syringe close-up, focus on the drop): © Suto Norbert Zsolt, 2009; used under license from Shutterstock.com. **Chapter 27:** 13368673 (surgeons in operative room): © Brasiliao, 2009; used under license from Shutterstock.com. **Chapter 28:** 16302277 (Young caring doctor 4): © Alexander Sysolvatin, 2009; used under license from Shutterstock.com. **Chapter 29:** 20140324 (business concept of an office desk with charts, business plan form, pen): © khz, 2009; used under license from Shutterstock.com. **Chapter 30:** 12427252 (man doing shopping in a grocery store and paying by credit card): © Diego Cervo, 2009; used under license from Shutterstock.com.

Procedures: Procedure 18-5: Photos provided by Skin Blends, Inc. Procedure 20-1, 20-2: Photos courtesy of E'lan Lashes Eyelash Extensions. Procedure 20-5: Photos supplied by Kett Cosmetics. Procedure 22-1: Supplied by Bertaut Beauty and Karen Maze Photography. All other photos provided by Rob Werfel Photography.

PART 1

ORIENTATION

Chapter 1 Changes in Esthetics

CHAPTER OUTLINE

- THE GLOBAL EVOLUTION OF SPAS AND SPA TREATMENTS
- ADVANCED EDUCATION AND EMPLOYMENT OPPORTUNITIES
- DEVELOPING CRITICAL-THINKING SKILLS
- ENHANCING SOFT SKILLS
- PRIVACY LAWS
- PROFESSIONAL ORGANIZATIONS AND PUBLICATIONS

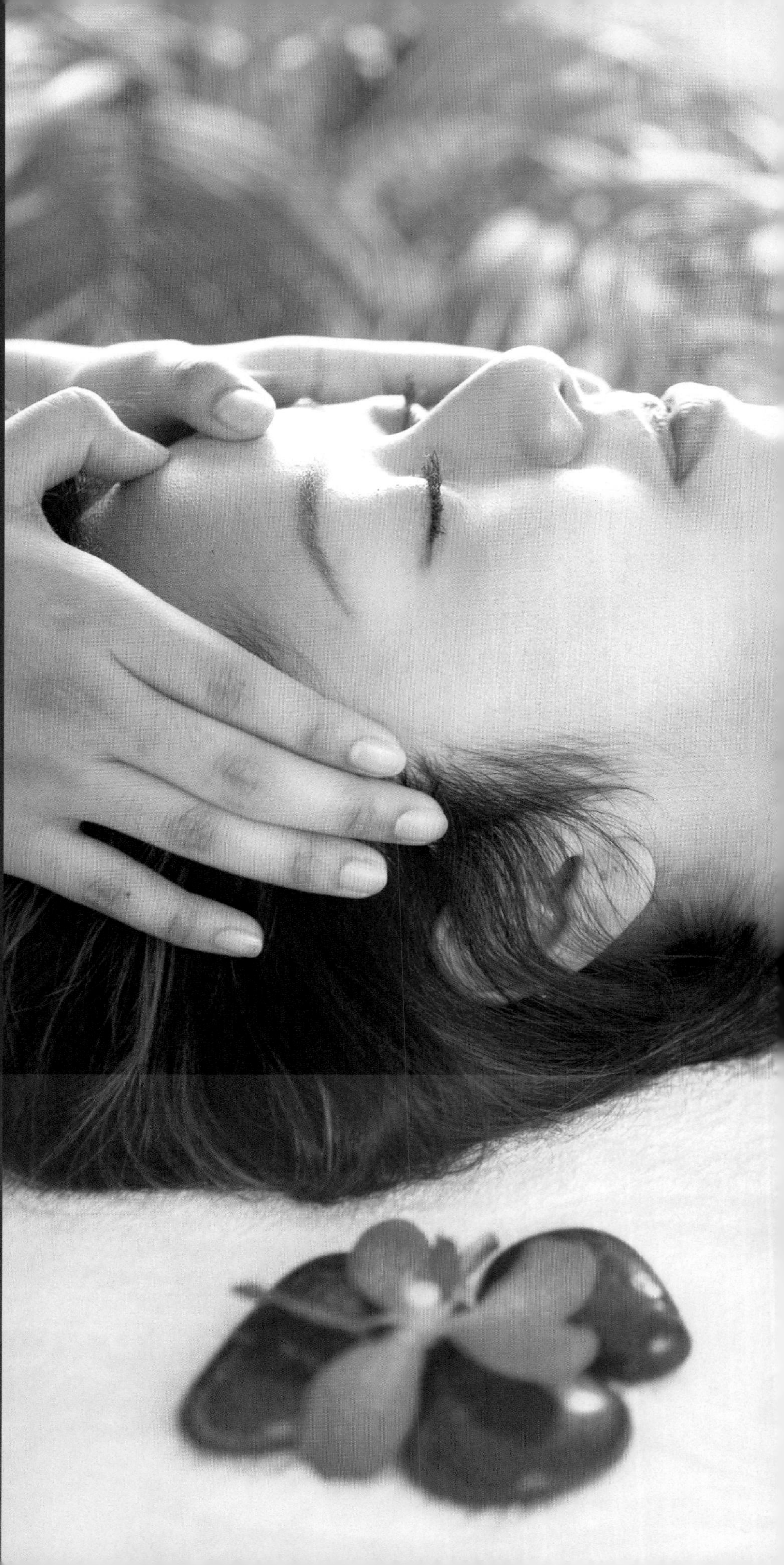

CHAPTER 1

CHANGES IN ESTHETICS

LEARNING OBJECTIVES

After completing this chapter, you should be able to:

- Describe the evolution of the esthetics industry.
- Discuss the need for advanced education and list a variety of employment opportunities.
- Identify and discuss the steps of critical thinking and problem solving.
- Explain soft skills and how to incorporate them into your work.
- Understand HIPAA and your legal obligations to your clients' privacy.
- Reference a broad range of resources to assist you in the industry.

KEY TERMS

Page numbers indicate where in the chapter the term is used.

balneotherapy 6

Health Insurance Portability and Accountability Act (HIPAA) 13

holistic 12

spa 6

spa therapy 6

E*sthetician*. The term has become a household word as awareness of skin treatments, hair removal, and myriad of other esthetic procedures has spread to the masses. No longer a Hollywood "beauty secret," estheticians are in great demand everywhere, and, thanks to advanced technology and education, the industry continues to experience exponential growth. Prior to the twentieth century, beauty techniques developed and transitioned at a snail's pace. In today's world, technology and unprecedented popular demand have brought the industry to an entirely new level of sophistication. New advances, products, and techniques are constantly popping up in the media. No doubt some of these are nothing more than smoke and mirrors, but many are legitimate and safe and offer significant rewards. People are leaving their old jobs and turning to esthetics as a way to earn their living. This includes people with advanced degrees in areas such as nursing, communication, chemistry, education, and marketing.

There is a perception among some people that estheticians are losing their footing to doctors who are licensed and insured to use powerful equipment and perform invasive procedures. But the opposite is true: As the medical profession has expanded into cosmetology, opportunities and demands for well-educated estheticians have grown and diversified. Similarly, as the public becomes more informed, estheticians are sought out. Baby Boomers' desire, willingness, and financial ability to do whatever is necessary to lengthen good health and youthfulness has had a huge effect on the industry. So each new technological advance offers the esthetician an opportunity to add to and improve upon his or her current skill set and to reach a broader audience. Most importantly, a solid knowledge of the supposed "latest and greatest" offers the chance to educate the public. A poorly trained or misinformed esthetician is a far greater threat to the industry than the medical profession. That said, if estheticians are to successfully meet challenges, they must constantly seek out education, encourage research, and take the time to root out the facts (Figure 1–1).

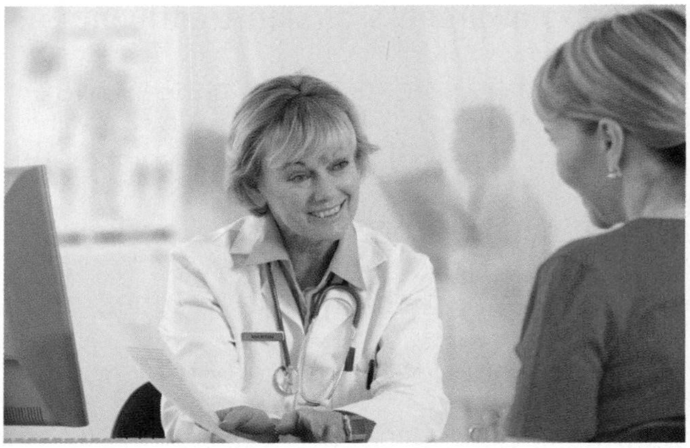

Figure 1–1 Forming positive doctor relationships.

THE GLOBAL EVOLUTION OF SPAS AND SPA TREATMENTS

Understanding the history of the **spa** and spa treatments helps the esthetician to know the purpose of a treatment and how the treatment evolved. The origin of the word *spa* has several possibilities. One theory is that the word *spa* may be derived from the Walloon (a dialect of the French language) word *espa,* which means "fountain" and originates from the name of the Belgian town Spa. Other possibilities are that *spa* is an acronym of the Latin phrase *sanitas per aquas* (health through water) or that it originates from the Latin word *spagere* (to scatter, sprinkle, moisten) (Figure 1–2). All origins communicate the process: the use of water and the implication for healing. The water treatments provided in the spa are defined as **balneotherapy, spa therapy,** and hydrotherapy and can be used interchangeably.

While many spa treatments seem new and never before tried, the reality is that most of the spa treatments provided today are derivations of ancient treatments. It is thought that spa treatments began in bathhouses in ancient Greece and in the Roman Empire. Originally, Roman bathing culture had a medicinal focus before evolving toward relaxation. There were three types of bathhouses in Rome: balnea (home), balnea private (private baths), and balnea public (public baths). Known for their vast aqueducts, the Romans created enormous bathhouses on their newly conquered lands, and they combined baths with other healthy endeavors, such as exercise and massage. The best-preserved of the ancient Roman spas is the famous Spa of Bath, England, which allows visitors to see how these baths functioned. Spa treatments highlighted the benefits of mud therapy, and elite Romans began to enjoy these luxuries.

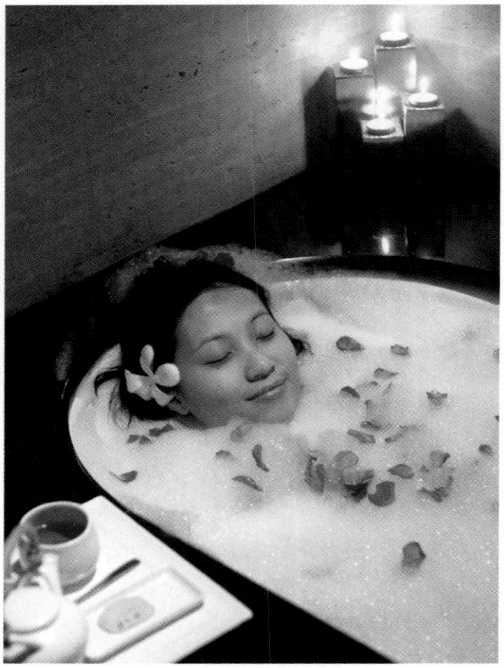

Figure 1–2 Spas originally developed as a means of healing via water.

Activity

Visit http://www.romanbaths.co.uk and explore the ancient Roman spa of Bath, England, to appreciate the engineering and advancements of this ancient civilization.

When the Roman Empire fell in A.D. 476, only a few of the original bathhouses escaped destruction. During this time, public bathing was prohibited by the religious culture; some people would avoid bathing for years. Most bathhouses were turned into churches since prayer was considered more important than relaxation.

There was not much advancement in spa culture from this time until the thirteenth century, when Moorish influence rose in southern Europe. A fastidious people, they contributed to resurgence in bathing and in public bath popularity. Again, bathing was primarily for the purpose of relaxation. But, medicinal processes, such as bloodletting, were also performed at the baths. (During

* Editor's Note: Please notice that the term *salon* is being used as a general term throughout the text to include full service salons, spas of all natures, clinics and other skin care facilities.

medieval times, bloodletting, also known as *phlebotomy,* was a popular treatment for a wide variety of ailments. Bloodletters believed that reducing excess blood from the body restored balance and good health.)

The sixteenth century and the Renaissance period saw another decline in the use of public baths. This was due to many factors, including the lack of firewood to heat the bathhouses and water and common public fear that the bathhouse was the cause of diseases such as syphilis and leprosy. Nevertheless, the wealthy continued to visit bathhouses, though they preferred natural sources, such as hot springs or mineral water.

During this time natural mineral springs gained popularity. An attempt was made to analyze the water's mineral content scientifically to establish if there actually was any therapeutic value in balneology, the study of bathing for health purposes. At this time, the philosophy of drinking the water as well as bathing in the water became commonplace. The general population did not drink a lot of water, and physicians recommended drinking large amounts of the mineral waters for potential curative effects. One early "bath" was used exclusively for drinking mineral water. Additional pools were built for bathing purposes.

During the seventeenth century, the French joined the movement with both hot and cold springs. They used cold springs for drinking therapies only and hot springs for drinking cures as well as bathing. The French took these therapies quite seriously, and it was at this time that physicians became an integral part of the spa experience.

As the popularity of bathing in springs grew, scientists attempted to replicate natural mineral springs' benefits for medicinal purposes. A nineteenth century Bavarian monk, Father Sebastian Kneipp, believed that using water to eliminate waste from the body could cure disease. He developed more than 100 different hydrotherapy treatments using water in solid, liquid, and vapor forms to treat individuals. His treatments included washings, wraps, packs, compresses, steam, and baths (Figure 1–3).

When Europeans began to immigrate to the U.S. they brought the spa concept with them. But it wasn't until the mid-1800s that hotels and guesthouses built near mineral springs started drawing guests to enjoy the waters. This movement led to what was known as *spa resorts*. These resorts, which also included theaters and casinos, became very popular with both the elite and middle classes over the next few decades.

When depression hit in the 1930s, development of spas halted in the United States, and many European spas that had catered to Americans closed. After World War II, with the worldwide economy on the rise, spas regained popularity, and new treatments, such as health and exercise regimens, mud therapy, balneology, and hydrotherapy, were added. Eventually, however, the focus of a preventive practice lost ground to the advances of modern medicine. Spas once again went on the decline.

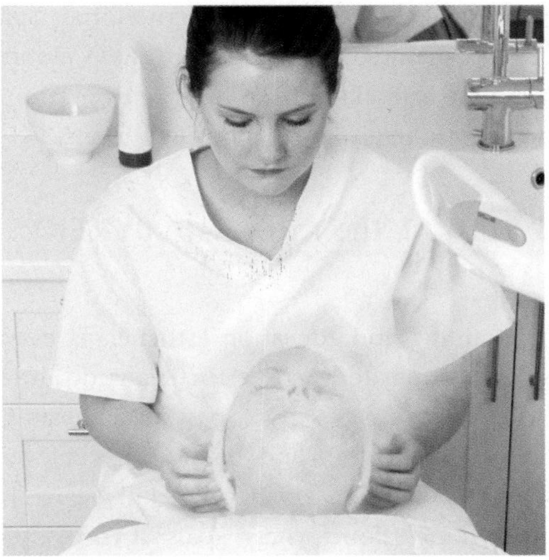

Figure 1–3 Steaming is just one of many hydrotherapy treatments.

Today, there is a worldwide spa revival that recognizes the benefits of preventative therapies (Figure 1–4). One of the fastest-growing industries in the United States, spas have become an important component of American life.

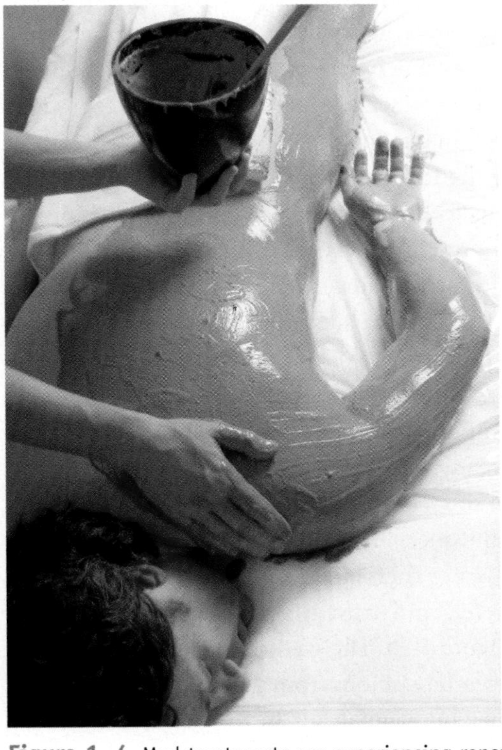

Figure 1–4 Mud treatments are experiencing renewed popularity.

According to statistics from ISPA (International Spa Association), spas generated $9.4 billion in 2006 alone. The American public is flocking to spas for rejuvenation, relaxation, therapeutic treatments, and much more.

ADVANCED EDUCATION AND EMPLOYMENT OPPORTUNITIES

The amount of training and education estheticians need has long been up for debate. Many estheticians do little more than attend cosmetology school, pass a state examination, find a job in a salon, and memorize whatever product lines are carried there. This level of knowledge is sufficient to meet some salon owners' goals: If the esthetician uses only those products, he or she may become proficient at selling them. Many skin care lines cater to this philosophy, offering pre-packaged products for four or five different types of skin. Sales are the bottom line, with actual skin treatments seemingly secondary to retail goals. No doubt, monetary gains are essential to continued success, but not at the expense of the client and her needs. These environments may always exist on some level, and sadly, there may always be estheticians willing to settle for them.

Fortunately, as the medical profession has embraced esthetics, the demand for solid, advanced esthetics education has skyrocketed. Today's successful esthetician holds many qualifications beyond a simple certificate to practice, such as problem-solving abilities, knowledge of research methods and available resources, and an understanding of the methodology and science behind a procedure, product, or piece of equipment. Equally important is the knowledge of what an esthetician cannot do—all of the restrictions and limitations to his or her practice. An individual with a deep and thorough education from which to draw will know where to turn whatever the circumstance.

Why is this model in such demand? The reasons are simple: A doctor trying to decide whom to hire is far more likely to choose the better-trained candidate. Less time is involved training the new employee because most of the training is already in place. Think of the lengths doctors must go to in order to practice—college, medical school, internships, and specialty programs—years of demanding education is part of their background. Naturally, they will recognize, prefer, and trust a similar demonstration of dedication (Figure 1–5). The well-trained esthetician now enjoys a wide variety of jobs from which to choose. Below are descriptions of occupations in this field, and the list is ever-expanding.

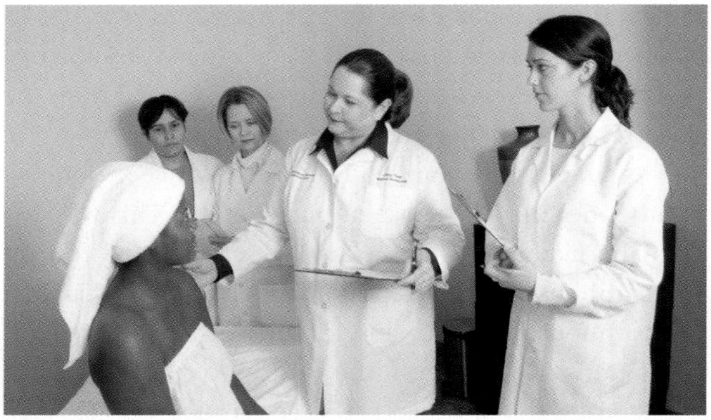

Figure 1–5 Estheticians with advanced education are in high demand.

Esthetician: Estheticians specialize in the care of the skin. They perform various facials and skin treatments and may also apply cosmetics. They also provide preventative care for the skin and offer treatments to keep skin healthy and attractive. Upon graduation and becoming licensed, many estheticians decide to work in a salon or day spa. Full-time and part-time opportunities are often available, and some estheticians choose to specialize in such areas as spa treatments, age management, acneic skins, or even waxing. Others decide to provide all services to their clients, and this is the most common type of employment new estheticians seek upon graduation.

Makeup Artist: Another area that an esthetician may choose to specialize in is as a makeup artist. Makeup artists are trained to embellish and enhance facial features through the skillful application of cosmetics. Many will choose to specialize even further by focusing on bridal makeup, theatrical makeup, or makeup for television and print ads or even fashion shows. Some makeup artists decide to work for themselves on a freelance basis,

? Did You Know

You will see the spelling of esthetician vary slightly depending on where you are working. In the medical realm, you will more often see the word spelled as aesthetician in reference to the original Greek word aesthetikos. Many cosmetic surgeons, nurses, and clinical estheticians prefer the original spelling. In recent history the initial letter a has been dropped in Western Europe and in the United States because the word esthetician relates more to the newer spa culture and has become a more modern term.

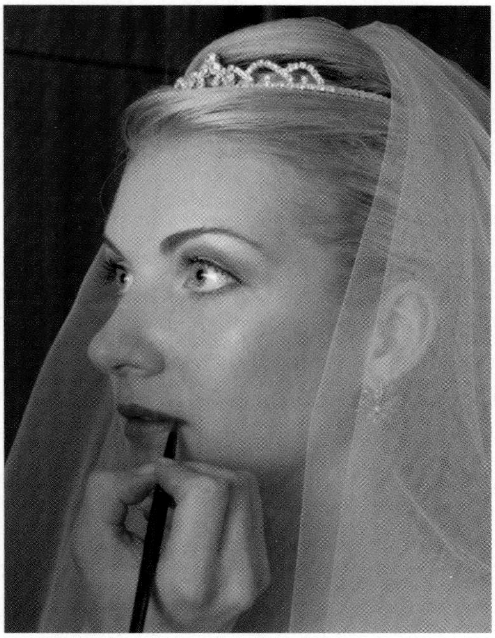

Figure 1–6 Bridal makeup is just one of many options in which an esthetician might specialize.

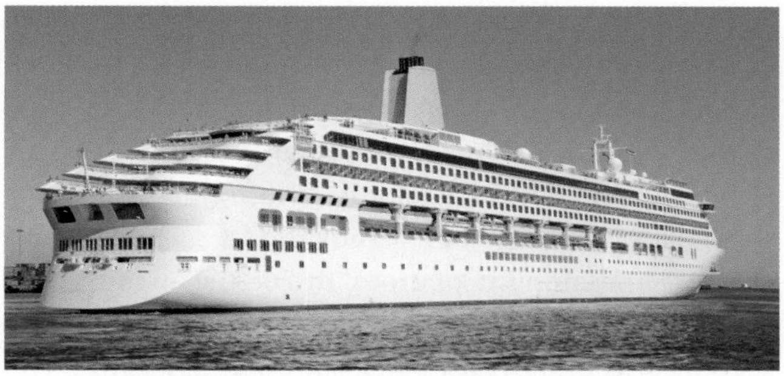

Figure 1–7 Cruise ships need estheticians to work in the spas on board.

and others choose to work at a salon or spa focusing only on makeup. Still others decide to work for a makeup line sold at a department store (Figure 1–6).

Permanent Makeup Artist: A technician trained in cosmetic tattooing is in increasing demand today. Eyebrows, eyeliner, and lipliner are the most common services offered. Permanent cosmetics requires specialized and ongoing training to stay informed of rapidly advancing technology in this field.

Medical Aesthetician: In this area, the aesthetician partners with a dermatologist or plastic surgeon and becomes part of a "team" whose goal is taking care of a patient's skin. A sound knowledge of advanced skin care combined with medical terminology is invaluable, as many patients seeking out the plastic surgeon's or dermatologist's services are interested in advanced age-management techniques. The medical aesthetician may help devise a skin care routine that fits any type of more invasive treatment that the doctor has planned for the patient. She or he should also be educated in corrective makeup techniques to properly assist the patient in makeup selection after a more invasive procedure.

Esthetician and Makeup Artist for Resorts and Cruise Ships: Resorts and cruise ships offer full-service salons that offer full- or part-time employment. Services often include facials, eyebrow shaping, waxing, and makeup application for special occasions, such as "formal nights." In addition to offering personal services, these estheticians also often offer special demonstrations in skin care and makeup techniques to interested groups (Figure 1–7).

Salon or Spa Owner: Many students entering the field of esthetics think of this position as their goal. Most successful salon and spa owners have worked in the field for a respectable amount of time before deciding to work for themselves. Some owners continue to work in the treatment room, providing services for their established clientele, while other owners decide to get away from the hands-on work and focus more on marketing, customer service, and training and development of staff.

Esthetics Instructor: Many private schools have a teacher-training program for promising graduates. Some states require an instructor to train in teaching all subjects, while others require instructors to specialize in one area. As an instructor, one must keep up with developments in the educational field as well as keep abreast of new beauty treatments and products entering the market. Most instructors attend workshops and conferences to keep their knowledge up to date.

Manufacturer/Sales Representative: Manufacturers of skin care products and equipment employ estheticians to explain, demonstrate, and ultimately sell the company's products. As a representative, the esthetician calls on salons, spas, doctor offices, hotels, and specialty businesses to build clientele and increase product sales. This position requires an outgoing personality, an impeccable appearance, and sales ability. Representatives often expect to travel a great deal—throughout his or her designated sales territory as well as to various trade shows and conventions.

Department Store Cosmetics Representative: Many cosmetic lines now pay higher wages to licensed estheticians as they have realized how much their clients benefit.

Cosmetic Buyer or Assistant Buyer: As a buyer of cosmetics in a department store, specialty store, or salon, you must keep up with the latest products advertised in the industry as well as present and future trends. Buyers travel frequently, visiting markets, trade shows, and manufacturer's showrooms. A buyer must estimate the amount of stock his or her organization will need for a determined period of time and must keep records of purchases and sales. The assistant buyer places orders, tracks inventory, and helps the buyer in any way possible to ensure that adequate product is purchased.

Manager or Salesperson: In this field, duties might include keeping records of sales and inventory on hand, demonstrating products, selling to clients, and cashiering. An esthetician in this position must have thorough product knowledge of all available products and be able to answer questions and help clients select products that suit their skin type and/or coloring. In some cases this person might answer the phone or schedule appointments. Good organizational skills, a neat appearance, and a friendly personality are a must for this position. A sales manager needs the same qualities as the salesperson but has more responsibility. The manager runs the entire department and trains the sales staff.

Beauty Editor or Columnist for a Newspaper, Magazine, or Journal: An esthetician with a talent and or training in writing or journalism may wish to pursue a career in this area. An esthetician in this position may write about manufacturers' products to stimulate readers' interest and boost product sales. He or she may be responsible for a weekly or monthly column, a "question and answer" column, feature articles, or educational books and brochures distributed to teachers, in addition to lecturing and making media appearances.

State Licensing Inspector or Examiner: Most states have laws governing esthetics and personal services and hold periodic examinations for esthetics licenses. A licensed, experienced esthetician may become a state inspector or examiner. A state examiner prepares and conducts examinations, announces and enforces rules and regulations, investigates complaints, and conducts hearings. To ensure that rules and regulations are enforced and ethical practices are maintained, each state employs a team of inspectors to cover specified territories throughout the year. These teams inspect salons and spas to see that owners, managers, and employees are conforming to all regulations and codes.

DEVELOPING CRITICAL-THINKING SKILLS

If there is one skill that separates the poor esthetician from the excellent esthetician, it is the ability to think critically. You no doubt know of one or two estheticians who rely only on what they learned in beauty school or product training. They have learned one basic facial and perhaps five product routines based on skin type. They plow through the service automatically and give little consideration to meeting client needs beyond the minimum requirement. Rest assured they will not succeed and will eventually find themselves squeezed out of the industry by well-trained, smart-thinking counterparts who do whatever is necessary to identify and solve their clients' problems. Solid critical-thinking, problem-solving, and decision-making skills are paramount to your success and credibility—not just in your career, but every aspect of your life. The good news is that they are learned abilities—anyone with the desire to do so can train himself or herself to think smart. Follow the steps below, and repeat, repeat, repeat.

Clarify the Problem

Identify what your client needs and wants. This does not apply just to an accurate skin assessment, which is critical, but also to areas such as the client's time frame. If a client has scheduled an aggressive peel three days before his or her wedding, you will want to know that so you can explain the consequences, reschedule the appointment, and keep the client. Ask questions. Interact. Be curious. Think. Do not proceed until the problem is identified and understood. Is there even a problem? Many cosmetic surgeons can no doubt tell you they have met a patient who is sure he or she needs plastic surgery when physically there is nothing wrong. The problem is in the client's self-image, and he or she needs a different kind of doctor entirely.

Gather the Facts

Once the problem is identified, you need to figure out not only how to solve it, but also how it may have been caused. You may have a client with rosacea, who loves to play outdoor tennis, drink wine, and eat spicy food. Certainly you can help to some small degree, but if the client wants real change, he or she needs to make some adjustments to lifestyle and diet. If you are not sure how to proceed, reschedule the appointment and do your homework. Be prepared with all the information you need.

Examine the Evidence

Now you have your problem and your evidence; it is time to examine them. Where did you get your evidence? Did you consider different points of view? Is the evidence based on opinion or fact? If your new waxing client says he or she has never used Accutane®, yet all the evidence points to that possibility, you had better have your facts straight before waxing him or her. Naturally, you would not accuse her of lying to you, but you are the expert, and if you do not feel that the waxing is safe based on the evidence, do not do it. (Of course, you would already have the client's signature agreeing to hold you harmless should damages result.)

Define Solutions and Outcomes

Now that you feel confident with the problem and the evidence, consider possible solutions, alternatives, and the results of each. Say your client wants a lot of extractions on her nose. She needs them, but her skin is quite dehydrated. You could work on her entire nose and remove everything possible. In doing so, you might cause unnecessary discomfort and permanent scarring, and you might end up with a client who is terrified of ever having another facial. Alternatively, you could prep the skin, be judicious in your extractions, and then explain what you have done and how a combination of at-home care and a series of facials over time will safely and effectively finish the job. Results here could include causing less discomfort and a smaller chance of scarring, allowing the skin to clear up a bit on its own, and gaining a satisfied and loyal client (Figure 1–8).

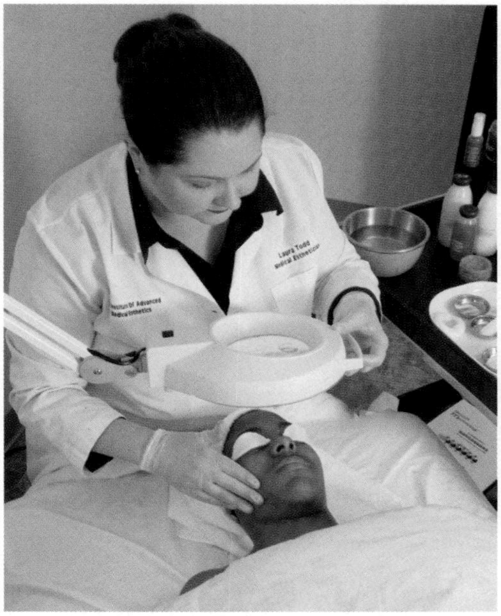

Figure 1–8 Critical thinking involves examining solutions and their possible outcomes.

Choose and Execute the Solution

After sufficient consideration, choose the best solution and act on it. Make sure to follow through, examine the results, and make adjustments as necessary. Make a habit of following these steps, and soon they will come naturally to you. As stated earlier, these are learned abilities—no one is born with them and anyone can incorporate them into his or her life with practice. You will find yourself better able to zero in on the real issues at hand and solve them efficiently and effectively. You will also find yourself in high demand and better able to obtain both professional and personal goals.

SOAP Notes

SOAP notes are a popular method of documenting the critical thinking process. Used by a wide variety of healthcare providers, SOAP notes not only ensure consistency, but thorough, effective analysis and communication. SOAP is an acronym for the four steps you should follow in evaluating the client:

SUBJECTIVE: What the client tells you
OBJECTIVE: What you see
ASSESSMENT: Details of what you observed
PROCEDURE: Steps to take for the desired outcome

You will learn about SOAP in more depth in a later chapter.

ENHANCING SOFT SKILLS

Now that you're on your way to developing critical thinking, here's a way to use it toward protecting and magnifying your greatest asset: you. As discussed earlier, today more than ever before, clients are flocking to spas to rejuvenate themselves. This desire is not rooted solely in improving and maintaining their exteriors but also in enhancing their interior selves—finding relief from the constant stresses of daily life through the healing power of touch. In these circumstances, you, the esthetician, play an important role by establishing an environment wherein healing can commence. This process is referred to as a *soft skill* because it is rather intuitive in nature, but it is also a matter of paying attention to details and each of the senses throughout a treatment. It also requires that you have your own head in the right place (Figure 1–9).

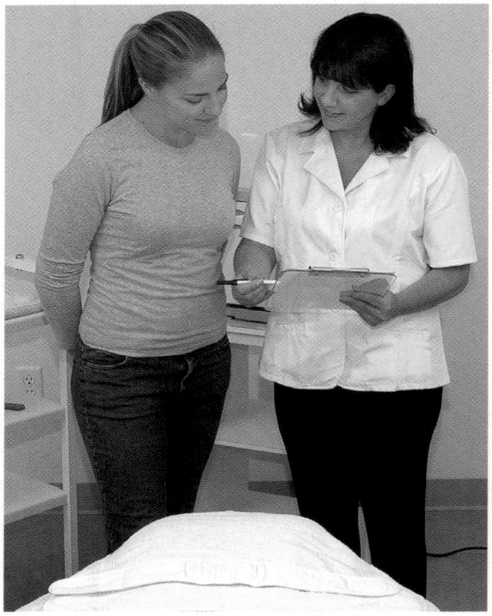

Figure 1–9 Mastering soft skills will take a treatment from good to fabulous.

The Power to Instigate Healing

You may be familiar with the term **holistic.** Holistic thought revolves around the idea of treating the person as a whole rather than focusing solely on a disease or disorder. Your client, whether he or she realizes it or not, not only wants you to provide an effective treatment but also to calm and soothe, make him or her feel rested and ready to dive back into a busy schedule. Your knowledge and implementation of holistic thought is what will turn a good treatment into a fabulous one. Say your client is trying to relax but your voice is too loud or too harsh. Each time you speak, you interrupt his process of relaxation. He may leave with beautiful skin, but he will not feel rejuvenated. You have not addressed his holistic, or whole, needs. Below is a list of considerations toward providing holistic treatments. It is not a complete list by any means, but it should help you better understand your goal.

- Do you greet your client with a warm and friendly handshake, eye contact, and a welcoming smile? Do you use his or her name when you speak? Do you show the client where to put his or her things and give directions to the bathroom?
- What is the client's mood? Does he or she seem shy and unsure or rushed and stressed? Is there anything you can do to change that? Is your voice soft and sure? Do you really listen to what the client is saying? Do you invite him or her to turn off the cell phone and step away from the world for the next hour? Do you invite him or her to remain silent and not feel obligated to converse with you? Do you encourage him or her to let go of stress, focus on breathing, and just enjoy time with you?
- Is your room temperature comfortable? Is the music volume too loud? Is the music soothing in nature? How does the room smell? Does the client need a pillow under his or her knees or an extra blanket? Do you have water and herbal teas to offer?
- How is your breathing? Are you providing an example of feeling calm? Are your hands warm? Is your touch confident and nurturing? Are you aware of the client's breathing? Are you working with the intention of providing peace? Are your thoughts focused solely on your client?
- Do you end the treatment quietly, allowing the client to come back to reality slowly? Do you step lightly, close doors carefully, and provide instruction on what to do next? Do you bring the client a glass of water? Do you let the client know you enjoyed meeting him or her and, again, use his or her name when you speak? Are you sincere in your recommendations for home care? Do you help the client with his or her coat and show him or her to the door? Do you smile and thank the client for coming in?

This might seem like a lot to consider, but what each question really refers to is your heightened awareness of your client on an intuitive, nearly spiritual level. You must begin each treatment with intention—have a goal in mind, such as maintaining peaceful thoughts throughout the service or filling the room with calming energy. Such talk may sound silly to a practical-minded person, but rest assured there is something to all of this. If you are wound up about personal problems or about getting out of work early or if you drank too much coffee at breakfast, how can you ever hope to relax your client?

Holistic thought can be challenging at first, and you may find your mind wandering. Bring it back to your original intention each time. Keep your goal in mind and work with the aim of meeting that goal. You will soon discover the effectiveness and simple beauty of this process.

While you are learning how to think holistically about your client, you must also pay attention to yourself. You may notice that you have a particular client who drains you—you feel exhausted when he or she is gone, yet you have not treated that client any differently than anyone else. This feeling is due to the energy he or she brings into the room, not you, and you need to learn how to protect yourself from

FOCUS ON: *The Eight Steps to Managing Negative Emotions*

1. Stop whatever you are doing and take a deep breath.
2. Think proactively rather than reactively. Try to remove yourself from the emotion and view the situation constructively.
3. Ask yourself what is really going on. Where does this emotion come from? What is behind it?
4. Consider whether you are meant to learn something from this feeling. Is your subconscious trying to tell you something?
5. Imagine that a good friend is feeling what you are feeling. What advice would you give him or her?
6. Consider the source of the negative emotion—does it really have anything to do with you? Is someone else's negativity rubbing off on you?
7. How can you best handle the situation? Think of someone you respect and admire and imagine how he or she might handle it.
8. Let it go—whether the emotion is yours or someone else's, learn what you can from it then let it go. It has served its purpose. Be forgiving and move on.

getting energy drained. Treating yourself holistically is the answer here, and doing so will not only provide you with the ability to set client boundaries; you will set an example for your client and enjoy benefits that are all your own.

You might try meditating, healing techniques, affirmations, or breathing exercises. Tape an inspiring quote to your refrigerator, stand up straight, and laugh out loud. Write your own mission statement. Imagine yourself as you wish to be. Visualizing a state of relaxation and happiness often leads to one. There are so many ways you can release yourself from negativity and distractedness. Just keep focusing on your intention.

PRIVACY LAWS

On April 14, 2003, the **Health Insurance Portability and Accountability Act (HIPAA)** of 1996 was put in place to protect patient privacy regarding medical records and health information provided to health plans, doctors, hospitals, and other health-care providers. The U.S. Department of Health and Human Services (HHS) developed this standard to provide patients with access to their medical records and help them gain more control over how their personal health information is used.

The ease with which computers and fax machines can proliferate private information has made some people reluctant to share critical information with their physicians or other health-care providers, including pharmacists. HIPAA was created to give the public confidence and encourage full disclosure of medical concerns without worry of privacy intrusions. Following are a few key standards of patient protection:

- **Access to Medical Records.** Patients are able to see and receive copies of their medical records.
- **Notice of Privacy Practices.** Health-care providers must provide a notice to their patients on how they may use their personal medical information.
- **Limits Use of Personal Medical Information.** This rule governs health-care providers sharing of information on a *need-to-know* basis.
- **Prohibits the Use of Patient Information for Marketing.** Permission must be obtained from the patient to use personal medical information.
- **Stronger State Laws.** All states must comply with privacy standards.
- **Confidential Communications.** Patients can request that health-care providers ensure that all communications are kept confidential.
- **Complaints.** Patients can file formal complaints regarding a breach of confidentiality.

In addition, all employees are required to take HIPAA training through their new employer, and these rules will be strictly enforced. A complete description of this standard is available at http://www.hhs.gov.

PROFESSIONAL ORGANIZATIONS AND PUBLICATIONS

The following list includes governmental and professional resources so you can stay current and informed on the industry and its regulations.

Federal Links

- Internal Revenue Service, http://www.irs.gov
- OSHA, http://www.osha.gov
- U.S. Food and Drug Administration, http://www.fda.gov

- National Accrediting Commission of Cosmetology Arts and Sciences, http://www.naccas.org
- National-Interstate Council of State Boards of Cosmetology, http://www.nictesting.org

State Links

- State Cosmetology Regulatory Agencies, http://www.ncacares.org
- National-Interstate Council of State Boards of Cosmetology (NIC), http://www.nictesting.org

Industry Links

This is a selection of the links you can find online for our industry:

- Aesthetics International Association, http://www.beautyworks.com
- National Cosmetology Association, http://www.ncacares.org
- National Coalition of Estheticians, Manufacturers/Distributors & Associations, http://www.ncea.tv
- CIDESCO International, http://www.cidesco.com
- International Therapy Examination Council, http://www.itec-usa.com or http://www.itecworld.co.uk
- Medical Spa Association, http://www.medicalspaassociation.org
- Spa Industry Associations, http://www.spatrade.com
- Day Spa Association, http://www.dayspaassociation.com
- Society of Permanent Cosmetic Professionals, http://www.spcp.org

Professional Publications

While these are commonly used publications, you may find more in an online search or at trade shows.

- Dermascope Magazine, http://www.dermascope.com
- Skin Inc. Magazine, http://www.skininc.com
- Les Nouvelles Esthetique Magazine, http://www.lneonline.com
- Milady/Cengage Learning, http://www.milady.com
- Day Spa Magazine, http://www.dayspamagazine.com
- Spa Magazine, http://www.spamagazine.com
- American Spa Magazine, http://www.americanspamag.com
- Medical Spa Report, http://www.medicalspareport.com

Learning to use all of the tools and resources available to you will help you continue to grow as an esthetician. Magazines, websites, networking groups and boards, webinars, trade shows, manufacturer classes, and a diversity of other advanced training options help estheticians keep a competitive edge in an industry with a huge diversity of options and opportunities.

REVIEW QUESTIONS

1. How has the medical community contributed to the esthetics community?
2. Why has advanced esthetics education become so important?
3. From what country is the term *spa* believed to have originated?
4. What is the meaning of the term *spa*?
5. List three terms for water treatments.
6. Who is credited with inventing hydrotherapy treatments such as wraps and steam baths?
7. List five different areas in which an esthetician might find employment.
8. List each step in developing critical-thinking skills.
9. List several ways you can tune in to your client's needs.
10. What is HIPAA and how does it affect you?

CHAPTER GLOSSARY

balneotherapy: body water treatments that use mud or fango, Dead Sea salt, seaweed, enzymes, or peat baths. Many of these treatments originated in ancient Greek and Roman bathhouses. While water treatments were originally used primarily for medicinal purposes, they eventually evolved into relaxation treatments as well.

Health Insurance Portability and Accountability Act (HIPAA): a federal act passed in 1996 outlining federal privacy standards for patients. The act covers access to medical records, notice of privacy practices, limitations of use regarding personal medical information, prohibitions on using patient information for marketing, stronger state laws, confidential communication, and complaint procedures.

holistic: the practice and/or philosophy of treating the person as a whole and remaining alert to all of a client's needs rather than focusing solely on a disease or disorder.

spa: term originally meaning "health through water." Today it most often refers to day spas or destination spas, where clients can find a wide range of treatments.

spa therapy: water treatments provided in a spa.

PART

2

GENERAL SCIENCES

Chapter 2 Infection Control

Chapter 3 Advanced Histology of the Cell and the Skin

Chapter 4 Hormones

Chapter 5 Anatomy and Physiology: Muscles and Nerves

Chapter 6 Anatomy and Physiology: The Cardiovascular and Lymphatic Systems

Chapter 7 Chemistry and Biochemistry

Chapter 8 Laser, Light Energy, and Radiofrequency Therapy

CHAPTER OUTLINE

- RULES AND REGULATIONS GOVERNING WORKPLACE SAFETY
- HEPATITIS
- TUBERCULOSIS
- THE PRINCIPLES OF INFECTION CONTROL
- GLOVES
- BODY HYGIENE AND A CARING ATTITUDE
- DISINFECTION AND STERILIZATION
- POTENTIAL HAZARDS FOR AN ESTHETICIAN
- BASIC SAFETY GUIDELINES
- OSHA INSPECTIONS

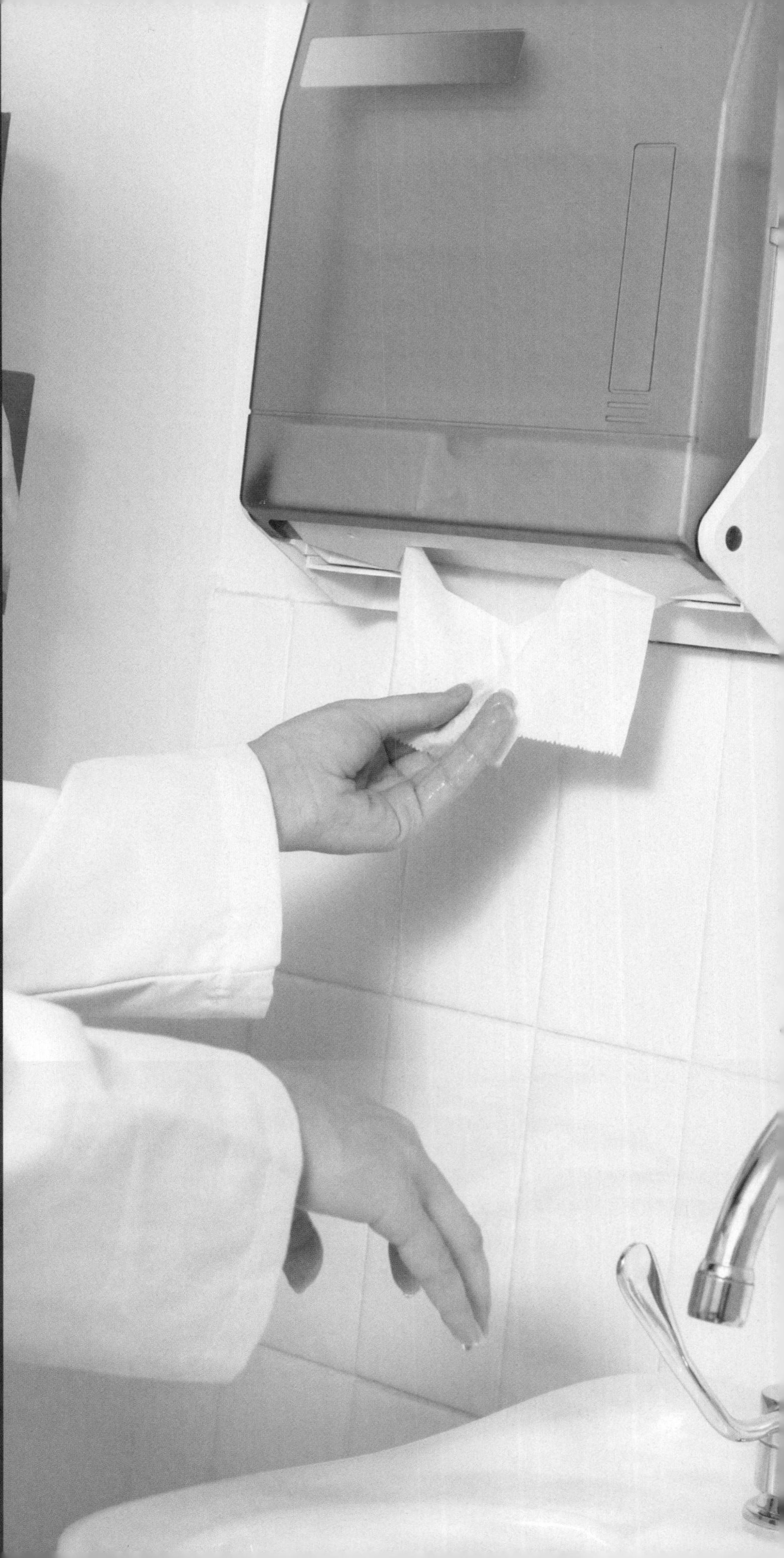

CHAPTER 2

INFECTION CONTROL

LEARNING OBJECTIVES

After completing this chapter, you should be able to:

- Understand the purposes and roles of the OSHA and the CDC.
- Know the Bloodborne Pathogens Standard.
- Discuss autoimmune disorders caused by bloodborne pathogens.
- Know the principles of infection control.
- Identify potential hazards an esthetician may encounter.
- Establish and use safety guidelines for estheticians.

KEY TERMS

Page numbers indicate where in the chapter the term is used.

Acquired Immune Deficiency Syndrome (AIDS) 25
acute 24
antibacterial 30
antibiotic 27
antimicrobial 30
asepsis 29
aseptic technique 29
autoclave 41
autoimmune disorders 21
bacteria 27
bloodborne 33
bloodborne pathogen 48
chronic 24
contaminated 29
decontaminate 22
disinfection 28
engineering controls 22
Human Immunodeficiency Virus (HIV) 25
immunization 24
mucous membrane 27
Occupational Safety and Health Administration (OSHA) 21
organisms 26
other potentially infectious material (OPIM) 22
pathogen 26
personal protective equipment (PPE) 28
safety plan 48
sharps 22
spores 27
standard precautions 22
sterilize 26
tuberculosis 25
U.S. Environmental Protection Agency (EPA) 41
U.S. Food and Drug Administration (FDA) 41

In today's world, what you can't see can kill you. **Autoimmune disorders,** such as hepatitis and HIV, can be spread by contact with potentially infectious body fluids. Hepatitis and HIV do not discriminate by age, race, gender, sexual preference, or financial status. The new breed of carriers are upper-middle-class adults who share needles at the local fitness center as they inject steroids in an effort to improve their bodies.

Standard precautions have become a fact of life, not only for those in the medical field but for teachers and playground assistants, tattooists, electrologists, and estheticians. Whether you are an independent contractor, a practitioner working alone, or a salon/clinic owner, your knowledge and understanding of state regulations, OSHA guidelines, and infection-control principles can help you protect yourself and your clients. Indeed, it can save your life.

RULES AND REGULATIONS GOVERNING WORKPLACE SAFETY

If you have been practicing for even a short time, you are aware that there are a number of regulatory agencies—both federal and state—that have issued rules and regulations for keeping workplaces safe. These regulations have been documented in the Occupational Safety and Health Act of 1970, the Chemical Right-to-Know Law of 1983, and the Bloodborne Pathogens Standard 29CFR 1910.1030, along with other health and safety regulations as recommended by the Centers for Disease Control and Prevention (CDC).

Probably best known of the agencies that issues and enforces the regulations is the **Occupational Safety and Health Administration,** or **OSHA,** which was created by the 1970 act. Originally called the Safety Bill of Rights, OSHA's guidelines were written as a response to hazards faced by employees in the workplace. Many states have chosen to administer the OSHA program as is; others have adapted the regulations and have created standards that go further than the federal regulations. States must at a minimum enforce and comply with OSHA's guidelines.

REGULATORY AGENCY ALERT

Check your state's OSHA guidelines and learn how they compare to the federal standards. If they exceed OSHA requirements, follow them.

How Do I Know If I Have to Follow OSHA Standards?

These regulations are enforceable under the law and were developed to protect your health and that of your coworkers and clients. However, if you are not an employee, you may question whether the OSHA guidelines apply to you.

- If you are an independent contractor renting space, these regulations apply to you. OSHA has determined that the leaseholder of a facility that rents work areas becomes the "host" employer and all within that facility must follow OSHA guidelines.
- If you are a contract worker, independent contractor, or temporary help, both the "host" employer (the worksite) and the employment service share the responsibility for training personnel and for ensuring their compliance to all provisions of the OSHA standards.

- If you work alone, the rules may not technically apply to you, but if you wish to live a long and healthy life, it is essential that you follow the regulations.

If you are still uncertain about your legal obligation to follow OSHA standards, here is another measure: OSHA looks at an IRS form called SS-8, which is used to determine the status of a worker for withholding income taxes. This form helps OSHA decide if an individual is an employee or employer. Besides the form, OSHA looks at four key factors:

1. Who determines the schedule of the worker, the daily routine, and requirements for how services are performed? Are there designated dress codes and days or hours that are required of the worker?
2. How is the worker compensated and what is his or her level of risk for financial gain?
3. What is the relationship between the worker and the firm, and does the worker perform similar services for others?
4. For service providers or salespersons, it ascertains how clients are provided and any reporting/documentation requirements.

CAUTION!

To protect your health and the health of those around you, follow OSHA regulations, regardless of your employment status.

The Bloodborne Pathogens Standard

In 1991 OSHA issued the Bloodborne Pathogens Standard in response to hazards that health-care workers face every day at work—among them, exposure to the hepatitis B and hepatitis C viruses and the human immunodeficiency virus (HIV). Created to minimize the transmission of these potentially deadly viruses, this standard covers all employees who can be "reasonably anticipated" to come into contact, in performing their duties, with blood and **other potentially infectious materials (OPIM).**

While compared to, say, surgical nurses, estheticians are at a fairly low exposure risk, the term *potential* resonates. Performing extractions, waxing, postoperative treatments, facials, peels, or microdermabrasion all increase the likelihood of exposure.

Following are the key elements of the Bloodborne Pathogens Standard.

1. **Standard Precautions.** OSHA's standards are based on the assumption that all body fluids are infectious and contact with all tissue is hazardous. Frequent hand washing, wearing gloves, appropriate body protection during treatment, and clean up are essential to following this rule.
2. **Engineering Controls and Work Practice Controls.** The employer must provide protection devices. These include antiseptic soap, splashguards, masks, eye-flush stations, **sharps** disposal containers for lancets and gloves, and appropriate labels for biohazardous materials.
3. **Personal Protective Equipment.** In addition to engineering and work practice controls, the standards require that workers wear lab coats, goggles, masks, and gloves and that the employer launder and clean this equipment.
4. **Cleanliness of Work Areas.** The employer is to ensure a work environment that is clean and sanitary. All surfaces must be **decontaminated** after procedures. In addition, gloves must be worn in all treatments and procedures where there is a potential exposure to blood or OPIM. All surfaces must be cleaned with a 10% bleach/water solution or the equivalent.
5. **Hepatitis B Vaccine.** Employers must make this vaccine available to employees within 10 days of the employee beginning work. It is given in three doses over a 6-month period. Estheticians working in a medical office are considered a Group One Classification, as they are exposed to bodily fluids while performing their job. Estheticians working outside the medical office may be considered to be at a slightly lower risk, but they still clearly risk potential exposure when performing their routine tasks.
6. **Follow-Up after Exposure.** If an employee is exposed to potentially hazardous bodily fluids, the employer must make a confidential medical evaluation detailing:
   - the circumstances surrounding the event.
   - the route of exposure.
   - the identification of person who was the source of the exposure.
   - immediate washing of the exposed area with soap and water or, in the case of eye exposure, a flushing of the eyes.

   In addition, after an employee's exposure, OSHA requires:
   - the exposed employee be tested for HBV, HCV, and HIV (providing consent is given).
   - the source individual's blood be tested for HBV, HCV, and HIV.

- the employee be offered prophylaxis, gamma globulin, or HB vaccine following a confidentiality guarantee.
- the employee be counseled regarding precautions to take to avoid transmission.
- an OSHA 200 form be filled out.
- a medical record of employee exposure be kept for 30 years and the employee's confidentiality guaranteed.

HEPATITIS

Hepatitis is an inflammation of the liver that is caused by a viral infection, which results in injury or destruction of liver cells and interferes with the liver's ability to function properly. Severe viral infection can cause liver failure, which is often fatal. There are a number of known viruses that cause hepatitis, including hepatitis A, B, C, D, E, F, G, GB, and H (Table 2–1). Many hepatitis viruses are extremely infectious, and the odds of becoming infected with one of them are much higher than the odds of being infected with HIV. The causes of hepatitis are sometimes unexplained, indicating the need for more studies and identification.

? Did You Know

Commonly, all strains of hepatitis either have no symptoms or have flu-like symptoms.

Table 2–1 Common Hepatitis Varieties

COMMON HEPATITIS			
Virus	**Transmission**	**Symptoms**	**Treatment**
Hepatitis A	By drinking water or eating food contaminated with fecal material that contains the virus.	Flu-like symptoms, such as fatigue, nausea, vomiting, abdominal discomfort, dark urine, and jaundice. Liver enzymes in the blood may be elevated much higher than normal.	Bed rest and avoidance of intimate contact. Can last between 3 weeks and 6 months. Two approved vaccines: immune globulin for short-term protection and for patients already exposed and hepatitis A vaccine for long-term protection.
Hepatitis B	Exposure to infected blood, unprotected sex with an infected person, the sharing of contaminated needles, and travel to countries with a high rate of infection. Infected mothers also may infect newborns.	Loss of appetite, nausea, vomiting, fever, fatigue, abdominal pain, dark urine, or jaundice. No symptoms in some people.	Interferon alpha. A vaccine is available that can provide immunity.
Hepatitis C	Direct contact with human blood, which can occur from being pricked accidentally by a contaminated needle, injecting illegal drugs, and sharing razors or toothbrushes with an infected person.	More than half have no symptoms. Others have appetite loss, fatigue, nausea, fever, dark-yellow urine, and jaundice. Liver tests may be elevated.	Interferon or a combination of interferon and the drug ribavirin. No vaccine.
Hepatitis D	Contact with infected blood. Requires the hepatitis B virus to replicate, so it infects either at the same time as hepatitis B or infects those who already have hepatitis B.	Same as for hepatitis B, but typically more severe: appetite loss, fatigue, nausea, vomiting, abdominal pain.	Interferon alpha for hepatitis B may have some effect.

Hepatitis varies in severity, with prognoses ranging from total recovery to long-term illness to death. Hepatitis is often defined as either **acute** (sudden onset, short-term) or **chronic** (prolonged, long-term). In some cases, acute hepatitis develops into a chronic condition, but chronic hepatitis can also occur independently. The degree of severity associated with either of these conditions can vary widely. In addition to these two classifications, hepatitis is also identified by the virus that caused it in an individual: A, B, C, D, E, F, G, GB, or HIV.

Acute Hepatitis

Acute hepatitis can develop suddenly or gradually, but it has a limited course and rarely lasts beyond 4 to 8 weeks. Usually there is only spotty liver cell damage and evidence of immune system activity, but on rare occasions, acute hepatitis can cause severe, even-life threatening, liver damage.

Chronic Hepatitis

The chronic forms of hepatitis persist for prolonged periods. Experts usually categorize chronic hepatitis as either *chronic persistent* or *chronic active* hepatitis. Chronic persistive is usually mild and nonprogressive or slowly progressive, causing limited damage to the liver. In some cases more extensive damage can occur. Chronic active hepatitis can occur if damage to the liver is extensive and cell injury widespread. Chronic active hepatitis develops in a liver with more extensive damage from other causes, such as alcohol or drug use.

Hepatitis A

Hepatitis A is generally contracted from eating food contaminated with the virus, usually through fecal material and poor sanitation. (Think of the restaurant worker who used the restroom but did not wash his or her hands before returning to prepare the next menu item.) It is also the type of hepatitis associated with eating raw shellfish. This form of hepatitis used to be called *infectious* hepatitis. Current studies do not indicate if or how the virus actually injures the liver, but this form is always acute. However, hepatitis A is the least dangerous form of the disease, and most people who contract the virus recover completely. There is a vaccine available, and it is recommended for those who depend heavily on fast-food restaurants or who travel to third-world countries.

Hepatitis B

Hepatitis B is a more serious infection and is often spread by body fluids or sexual contact. Its technical name is *serum hepatitis*. Unlike HIV, hepatitis B can be contracted through kissing. Symptoms may last for months or be nonexistent. Some hepatitis B patients can develop chronic hepatitis without an acute stage. Most people do recover from it, but some develop permanent liver damage, and about 10% become carriers. Liver cancer is known to occur in long-term carriers after 30 or more years of living with the virus.

A vaccine series is available for hepatitis B and **immunization** is highly recommended for those whose work may expose them to risk of infection, such as estheticians. For those who have the vaccine, about 87% will develop immunity after the second dose, and 96% will develop immunity after the third. Immunity is established by a serological test (blood test) which is administered after the vaccination series. If the test shows immunity, no further vaccines are necessary.

You should not receive the vaccine if you are allergic to yeast or any other component of the vaccine. Consult a physician if you have heart disease, fever, or illness at the time of the vaccination or are pregnant or breastfeeding. Although side effects are generally minimal, they may include localized swelling; pain; bruising; redness; or flu-like symptoms. If you are an employee and choose to decline the series, your employer will most likely ask you to sign a hepatitis B declination form, which your employer will keep on file.

Hepatitis C

Hepatitis C was identified only a few years ago. The symptoms are similar to those of hepatitis B, and it is sometimes associated with HIV infection. Hepatitis C is the major cause of all cases of hepatitis resulting from transfusions and intravenous drug use. Because of the efficiency of today's methods of blood screening, the risk from transfusions is 1 in 10,000. It can also be transmitted through injuries in the skin or may be transmitted sexually. Skin transmission, especially, is a risk for those working in esthetics. About 10% to 60% of acute hepatitis C patients develop the chronic form, which can occur without a preceding acute stage.

Hepatitis D

The hepatitis D virus (HDV) can develop in people who have the hepatitis B virus. This reinforces the need for immunization. This is a serious infection and permanent liver damage is much more likely to occur, making it all the more imperative that people at risk of hepatitis infection seek the vaccination series.

Hepatitis E

Hepatitis E (HEV) is similar to hepatitis A, but this form occurs mainly in underdeveloped countries. It too is transmitted via contact with contaminated food or water. It was thought to be rare, but experts now estimate that up to 20% of people in the United States may be infected.

Hepatitis F is a name given to a non-substantiated virus that wasn't hepatitis A, B or C.

Hepatitis G

Hepatitis G, or its variation GB, accounts for about 9% of cases that cannot be diagnosed with one of the other hepatitis viruses. It occurs in about 25% of patients with hepatitis A, 32% of those with hepatitis B, and 20% of those with hepatitis C. Hepatitis G always appears to be chronic, but indications are that it is mild and does not increase the severity of any accompanying hepatitis virus.

Hepatitis I (HIV)

Hepatitis I is the **Human Immunodeficiency Virus,** or **HIV,** which can be the precursor to an even more serious condition, **Acquired Immune Deficiency Syndrome,** or **AIDS.** By killing or impairing cells of the immune system, HIV progressively destroys the body's ability to fight infections and certain cancers, leading to the development of AIDS. Individuals diagnosed with AIDS are susceptible to opportunistic infections, which are caused by microbes that usually do not cause illness in healthy persons.

HIV is spread through contact with infected blood and semen, most likely during unprotected sex or the sharing of needles. Because HIV attacks white blood cells, it can spread very rapidly in the body, but an infected person may show no symptoms for months or years—perhaps even a decade after exposure. (The person is considered asymptomatic, infected but without exhibiting symptoms during this time.) Even when there are no symptoms, the HIV is multiplying, infecting and killing cells of the person's immune system. During this time, however, an infected person can transmit the disease to others. When the immune system is under attack from itself, it is called an autoimmune disorder.

When symptoms do develop, they may be subtle and can be either persistent or severe. Other effects, such as a decline in blood levels, slowly appear. As there is no way to identify a potential carrier, those who are at risk of infection should engage only in protected sex and use only single-use needles or sharps. Standard Precautions must be followed, treating every person as a carrier.

> **? Did You Know**
>
> 79% of all autoimmune disorder sufferers are women.

Tuberculosis

Tuberculosis is a highly infectious disease that most often affects the lungs but can occur in almost any part of the body. While at one time tuberculosis was nearly eliminated, the numbers of infected people have reached alarming proportions in recent years. More than one-third of the world's population now has this bacterium in their bodies and new infections are occurring at the rate of 360 every hour, or one every second.

While in some parts of the world, people have contracted bovine tuberculosis from consuming unpasteurized milk and other products from infected cattle, the most common mode of transmission of tuberculosis in the United States is inhalation of infected droplet nuclei from someone coughing or sneezing into the air. The bacteria have the ability to live in the air for 20 minutes and on surfaces up to 6 months.

Fortunately, most people that carry the bacteria that cause tuberculosis never develop the disease and are asymptomatic. In this primary phase they are not contagious; the only indicator that they are carriers is that they will commonly have a positive reaction to a skin test called a Mantaux. The best defense against contracting or transmitting this disease are excellent sanitation procedures. In addition, if you work with someone who has a cough, ask that he or she seek treatment and wear a protective mask. Last, if a client appears or sounds ill, ask that he or she reschedule an appointment until recovered.

> **? Did You Know**
>
> Because tuberculosis can live on a sidewalk for up to 6 months under certain circumstances, many cities have passed laws prohibiting spitting on sidewalks.

THE PRINCIPLES OF INFECTION CONTROL

Now that you know how easily serious diseases can be spread, it is also important to know the principles of infection control. These principles are based on an understanding of the cause of an infection, its transmission, and the steps necessary to avoid that transmission.

Microbiology: The Study of Microorganisms

Every practitioner needs an appreciation of basic microbiology and an understanding of what causes infections and disease. Microbiology is the study of microscopic **organisms**, some of which can be infectious. Organisms such as bacteria, viruses, fungi, and parasites are the "enemy"; since the "enemy" is not visible to the naked eye, it is important to remember that what can't be seen can, in fact, cause disease and even death. Following is a discussion of a few of the microorganisms that might be found in a workplace.

Resident Microorganisms

Resident microorganisms, also known as "normal flora," are constantly present on the human body. Examples of resident microorganisms include *Streptococci*, *Pseudomonas*, and *Staphylococci*. Most are found in the superficial layers of the skin. However, about 10% to 20% inhabit the deep epidermal layers. Since skin cannot be **sterilized**, no amount of scrubbing will remove these microorganisms completely. Resident microorganisms can become opportunistic, or infectious, when they are introduced into a wound site, such as a fresh or healing tattoo, scratch, abrasion, or other non-intact skin.

Transient Microorganisms

Transient microorganisms travel easily on hands, clothing, and other inanimate objects. Thorough washing removes them. Since waxing, some peels, improperly done microdermabrasion, or extraction procedures can cause an increased susceptibility to transient infections, hand washing, proper pre-procedure skin preparation, and post-procedure care are imperative.

Pathogens and Nonpathogens

Pathogens are organisms that cause disease. Both resident and transient microorganisms can be pathogenic. Resident microorganisms can become opportunistic when they are introduced into a fresh wound or other non-intact skin. (Consider the last time you had a hangnail that became irritated or red for no apparent reason.) This breach of the skin barrier can result in an infection or disease if proper pre-procedure skin preparation and post-procedure aftercare methods are inadequate or faulty.

Not all microorganisms are harmful to humans. Some microorganisms are beneficial, or nonpathogenic, such as those that synthesize vitamins in our digestive tract. However, other microorganisms that normally do not harm humans in a specific area of the body can become infectious if they are introduced to a different part of the body. For example, *E. coli* is normally found in the intestines, where it does not cause disease, but when it enters the bladder, it can cause a serious infection.

Impact of Globalization on Infection Control

Our world seems to be getting smaller as more people are traveling great distances more easily and quickly than ever before. Microorganisms like to hitch rides into new frontiers right along with us. Globalization has demonstrated dramatically that infectious diseases, such as Severe Acute Respiratory Syndrome (SARS), can travel quickly from China into Canada and then into the United States. In addition, we're seeing diseases such as polio, tuberculosis, and malaria, which were considered conquered years ago, reemerging in the United States; however, the Centers for Disease Control and Prevention (CDC) monitors outbreaks and issues alerts about the need to adjust infection control practices.

Contamination vs. Infection

Contamination happens when an organism enters a person's body through a fresh wound or non-intact skin. When the organism enters that person's cells, the person is infected. Once the infection begins to have harmful effects on the body, it is called a disease.

Humans have a complicated defense system called the **immune system.** This system is made up of many different cells that either fight off invading organisms or cause the body to react and kill invading germs. The components of the immune system learn to recognize specific germs and remember them if they enter the body again. A healthy immune system is effective at fighting off most germs.

KEEP IN MIND . . .

DISEASE IS CAUSED BY INFECTION.
Disinfect to prevent disease.

Bacteria, Viruses, Fungi, and Parasites

Bacteria, viruses, fungi, and parasites (infectious agents) have unique sizes, shapes, and functions that help microbiologists identify them. The three basic shapes are:

- Round (cocci)
- Rod (bacilli)
- Spiral (spirilla)

The functions that help reveal each infectious agent's identity include:

- The temperature at which they best grow and reproduce
- Their style or technique of reproduction
- Specific growth pattern(s)
- Rate of growth or reproduction
- Locations in which they are typically found
- Their ability (of lack of ability) to accept dyes as stains

Bacteria

Bacteria are specific types of small cells that come in many varieties. Bacteria can be found almost anywhere, including on hands, on environmental surfaces, and in food. Some bacteria are "good" and can assist in the digestion of food, the breakdown of garbage, and many other important processes. Other types of bacteria are "bad" and have the ability to infect living organisms and cause disease.

Many bacteria have a layer of slimy, mucoid substance surrounding each cell called a *capsule*. The presence of a capsule is associated with the virulence of certain pathogenic virus forms. Certain species of rod-shaped bacteria bacilli can develop a resting stage known as a **spore,** or endospore, a unicellular body that is resistant to its environment. The size, shape, and position of the spore within the cell are unique to a particular species. Bacterial spores are remarkably resistant to heat, drying, and the action of disinfectants.

Viruses

A virus is a microscopic particle much smaller than a cell. Like bacteria, some viruses are able to enter living organisms and infect them, causing disease. Viruses differ from bacteria in that they are much smaller and are not made up of cells. Viruses consist of genetic material and are separated by a covering of protein called a *capsid*. Viruses cause a variety of infectious diseases, including:

- The common cold
- Hepatitis B
- Hepatitis C
- Human Immunodeficiency Virus (HIV)
- Herpes
- The majority of upper respiratory infections

Fungi

Fungi are plantlike organisms that include molds and yeasts. They invade or grow on another organism and get their food from that organism. Fungi can grow either on or inside people, but only a few fungal infections cause disease in humans. Most usually affect the skin, nails, and subcutaneous tissue.

Parasites

A parasite is an organism made up of one or more cells, and it is larger and more complicated than bacteria or a virus. A parasite enters a person's body and gets nourishment from that person or animal. Parasites can cause symptoms and disease. Examples of parasites include:

PROTOZOA: Single-celled organisms transmitted via direct or indirect contact or by an infected carrier

ARTHROPODS: Include scabies (mites), lice, and fleas, all of which generally infest the skin, causing inflammation and itching

HELMINTHS: Include roundworms, tapeworms, and flukes. They infect humans principally through ingestion of fertilized eggs or when the larvae penetrate the skin or **mucous membranes**—the lining of portions of the body that come in contact with the internal organs and the exterior such as the nose, ear, or lips.

Nosocomial Infections

Nosocomial infections are usually acquired in a hospital or other health-care environment. These infections occur most commonly when a hospital patient acquires a new infection unrelated to their admitting illness but related to the hospital's environment. The number of nosocomial infections has increased because of the common use of **antibiotics.** Each year nearly two million hospital patients contract a nosocomial infection while being treated for another illness or injury. Close to 88,000 of these people die as a direct or indirect result of their infection.

Nosocomial infections can also occur in an esthetic or permanent cosmetic setting if proper infection control and sterilization methods are not followed. For example, a client can come in for a service and leave with an MRSA contamination, which results in an infection. MRSA is the abbreviation for Methicillin-resistant Staphylococcus Aureus. It is a type of bacteria that is resistant to certain antibiotics and therefore can be difficult to cure.

Breaking the Chain of Infection

The most important things to understand about infection are the different ways infection can be transmitted and how the "chain of infection" can be broken. The "chain of infection" includes six links. For infection to occur, all six must be present: 1) the infectious agent; 2) the reservoir where the agent resides; 3) the portal from which the agent moves into the body; 4) a means of transmission; 5) a portal of entry into the body; and 6) a host to infect.

FOCUS ON: *Breaking the "Chain of Infection"*

All six links of the "chain of infection" must be present for the spread of infection or disease to occur. The goal is to break at least one or more links in the chain.

The Chain of Infection

1. **Infectious Agent:** A microorganism with the ability to spread infection. Examples include:
   - Bacterium
   - Virus
   - Fungus
   - Parasite
2. **Reservoir:** A "hangout" where an infectious agent can survive. Examples include:
   - Yourself and co–workers
   - Clients
   - Equipment
   - Work surfaces
   - The environment

   Reservoirs are eliminated by following proper cleaning, **disinfection,** rinsing, drying, and storage techniques. Reservoirs are further reduced when work areas and the tools used to process contaminated items are cleaned and disinfected. The goal of the disinfection process is to kill as many microorganisms as possible.
3. **Portal of Exit:** A way for the infectious agent to get out of the reservoir. Examples include:
   - Acne lesions
   - Hangnails
   - Any non-intact skin
   - Mucous membranes (eyes, nose, mouth)
   - New tattoo or permanent cosmetics
   - Blood

   To eliminate all portals of exit, everyone would have to stop breathing, coughing, sneezing, and moving. Since this is not realistic, other tactics can be used to reduce the likelihood of transmission. These include:
   - Hand washing using proper technique
   - Covering wounds properly
   - Safe handling of sharps
   - Disposing of waste properly
4. **Mode of Transmission:** The method by which an infectious agent gets from the reservoir, or old "hangout" to a new "hangout." Examples include:

   DIRECT CONTACT: person-to-person contact, such as client-to-practitioner, practitioner-to-client, practitioner-to-practitioner, and client-to-client

   INDIRECT CONTACT: person-to-object contact, such as practitioner-to-work surface, client (or practitioner)-to-contaminated tools and equipment, and so on

   AIRBORNE: Airborne transmission occurs when the residue of evaporated droplets from an infected person remains in the air long enough to be transmitted (inhaled) into the respiratory tract of a susceptible host. Tuberculosis is one example of an organism that is transmitted through the air.

   VECTORBORNE: Contact with an animal, insect, or parasite that transports the pathogen from reservoir to host. Transmission takes place when the vector injects salivary fluid by biting the host or deposits feces or eggs in a break in the skin.

   Controlling the modes of transmission include:
   - Hand washing using proper technique
   - Appropriate use of barriers
   - Disinfection and sterilization of equipment
   - Environmental control measures
   - Engineering control measures
   - Work practice controls

   Consistently following Universal Precautions will help to prevent an infectious agent's mode of transmission. REMEMBER: Your hands provide a very mobile transport vehicle. Proper hand washing technique and consistent use and appropriate disposal of **personal protective equipment (PPE)** are among the most effective means to prevent the spread of infection
5. **Portal of Entry:** A way for the infectious agent to get into the new "hangout." Any break in the skin, intentional or unintentional, is an open invitation for pathogens. Examples include:
   - Acne lesions
   - Hangnails
   - A new or unhealed tattoo or permanent cosmetics
   - A new or unhealed body piercing

Any non-intact skin
Mucous membranes (eyes, nose, mouth)
Percutaneous injuries (i.e., needlesticks or lancet wounds)

6. **Susceptible Host:** This is the infectious agent's new "hangout." An example of a susceptible host is a person that is unable to resist infection by the infectious agent. A number of factors that can affect a host's susceptibility include but are not limited to:

   Age
   Gender
   Ethnicity
   Disease history
   Nutritional status
   Compromised immune system

   To prevent becoming a susceptible host, it is important to maintain a healthy diet, have good personal hygiene, take care of your skin, and get adequate rest—all of which help your immune system fight intruding microorganisms. The second line of defense is consistent use and appropriate disposal of personal protective equipment (PPE). Doing so helps break the portal of entry link in the "chain of infection."

Asepsis

Asepsis is defined as all measures taken to reduce the number of microorganisms to a miniscule number for the purpose of preventing infectious transmissions. These measures include hand washing, disinfection, and sterilization. The use of these procedures is called **aseptic technique.** There are two levels of aseptic technique most often used by estheticians: medical and surgical.

Medical asepsis, also called "clean technique," includes procedures and practices that reduce the number of microorganisms to minimize their spread. Examples of medical asepsis include proper hand washing technique, pre-procedure skin preparation, and the decontamination of equipment and tools used in esthetic procedures.

Surgical asepsis, or "sterile technique," includes procedures that eliminate the presence of *all* microorganisms and/or prevent the introduction of microorganisms into an area. Sterilization of tools and equipment are examples of surgical asepsis.

Following is a discussion of the five keys for using asepsis technique:

1. **Know what is clean.** The foundation of aseptic technique is cleanliness. Any item that has been thoroughly washed with a chemical disinfectant is considered clean and decontaminated. The task of physically washing removes soil and most microorganisms from the surface of an item. A disinfectant will kill or prevent the growth of any microorganisms that were not removed from the item by physical washing.
2. **Know what is contaminated.** All extraction procedures and waxing procedures have the inherent risk of creating **contaminated** waste. Any item used on a client or any item that is visibly soiled is considered contaminated. Items are either contaminated or not contaminated. *There is no difference between a "little contaminated" and "a lot contaminated."* All contaminated waste products generated from extraction or waxing must be disposed of properly. All sharps, including lancets or disposable razors, must be placed in a regulated sharps container. All other contaminated waste must be disposed of in accordance with your state law. Some states require double bagging in sealable bags; others require placing the material in a red biohazard bag and having it collected by a professional service.
3. **Know what is sterile.** Sterility is the absence of all microorganisms. It is important to note that you cannot tell by looking at an item if it is sterile. The tools and instruments utilized throughout procedures must be made sterile beforehand. Proper handling, opening, and storage of sterile equipment are essential. Sterilized items used in esthetic procedures include but are not limited to:
   - Lancets
   - Comedo extractors
   - Tweezers

FYI

The Five Keys of Asepsis

1. Know what is clean.
2. Know what is contaminated.
3. Know what is sterile.
4. Keep clean, contaminated, and sterile items separated.
5. Resolve contamination immediately.

REGULATORY AGENCY ALERT

Know the laws in your state for disposing of contaminated waste.

- Microdermabrasion tips
- Microcurrent tips
- Galvanic rollers and wands

4. **Keep clean, contaminated, and sterile items separated.** Dirty (or contaminated), clean, and sterile items must be kept completely separate from one another. Once a clean item comes into contact with a dirty item, it is considered "dirty" again. Sterile items must not have any contact with nonsterile items, or those items are no longer considered sterile.

   In addition, sterile items should never be stored near sinks, plumbing, or in any location where there is the risk of becoming wet or soiled. Moisture allows for the passage of microorganisms through packaging, resulting in contamination.
5. **Resolve contamination immediately.** Estheticians have a responsibility for maintaining proper aseptic technique throughout every procedure. If at any time clean technique is broken or cross-contamination occurs, the situation must be resolved immediately.

Hand Washing

According to the Centers for Disease Control and Prevention (CDC), *hand washing is the single most important means of preventing the spread of infection.* It is also a *critical* part of asepsis. Hand washing can be completed with plain soap or antimicrobial products. Hand washing with plain soap suspends microorganisms and allows them to be mechanically removed by rinsing under tepid running water. Hand washing with antimicrobial products kills or inhibits the growth of both resident and transient microorganisms. This process is also referred to as *antisepsis*. Antisepsis is defined as the *removal* of transient microorganisms from the skin with a *reduction* in resident microorganisms. Hand washing, cleaning, decontamination, disinfection, and sterilization are all important parts of antisepsis.

Your hands are your livelihood! Without healthy hands, you cannot perform procedures safely. Take extra care to avoid chapped, dry, or irritated hands, which might allow microorganisms a portal into your hands which could result in infection. Proper hand washing technique and the use of appropriate lotions can help prevent these symptoms. However, it is important to note that certain ingredients in lotions, particularly petroleum, can adversely affect glove integrity. Excess water from improperly dried hands can also affect glove integrity.

Hand Washing at Work

The skin can function as a reservoir for infectious agents and a vehicle for transmission of infectious agents. Clients are considered susceptible because procedures break the integrity of the skin (i.e., waxing = abrasion of the skin and extraction = possible breaking of the skin). In a salon setting, broken skin can also occur from a nick with hairdresser's scissors or manicure/pedicure implements. In a medical setting, the client may receive a procedure that leaves his or her skin non-intact.

Hand washing should be performed:

- Upon arriving at work
- Before gloving
- After removing gloves
- After contact with any potentially contaminated surface or item
- After working in common areas or performing housekeeping duties
- Between direct contact with different clients
- Before and after eating, drinking, or handling food
- After personal use of toilet facilities
- When hands are visibly soiled, including after sneezing, coughing, or blowing your nose
- Before leaving work
- Whenever necessary (use sensible judgment)

Hand Washing Products

Hand washing with plain soap for 20 seconds is effective in removing most transient microorganisms. Plain soaps may not remove resident microorganisms which are located within the deep epidermal layers of the skin. However, resident microorganisms can usually be killed or inhibited with **antimicrobial** products which may be sold with the label **antibacterial** as they kill bacteria.

Antiseptics

An antiseptic is an agent that inhibits the growth of some microorganisms on skin and/or tissue. Examples include para-chloro-meta-xylenol (PCMX) and Triclosan. These products should be used no more than four times per 8-hour shift or per the manufacturer's instructions. Most antiseptics used by estheticians are antimicrobial soaps (e.g., Provon® and Satin®) or skin preparations such as pre- and post-waxing toners.

Alcohol-Based Antiseptic Solutions

Though alcohol-based antiseptic solutions (e.g., Purell®) have gained popularity within the medical community,

FYI

Hand washing remains the single most important means of preventing the spread of infection.

estheticians should use them with caution as they can dry the skin, leaving it more prone to irritation or infection contraction.

Antimicrobial soaps have been used by estheticians with great success. However, improper or excessive use of the antimicrobial agents can cause destruction of the resident flora that lives on skin. In addition, a breakdown in skin integrity can increase the risk of acquiring allergic contact dermatitis (ACD) the reaction that can occur when skin develops an allergy to a product it comes in contact with. To avoid chapping and irritation of the skin, hand washing with antimicrobial soaps is not recommended more often than once every 6 to 8 hours.

Non-antimicrobial, or plain, soaps can be used in conjunction with antimicrobial products between hand washings. Plain soaps do not kill or inhibit the resident microorganisms of the skin. Alternating the use of plain and antimicrobial soaps helps preserve skin integrity and aids in the decrease of ACD occurrences.

FOCUS ON: *Hand Washing Solutions*

- **Antiseptic solutions should never replace hand washing.**
- **Antiseptic solutions are not to be used when hands are visibly soiled. Organic matter (blood, proteins, etc.) will inactivate their antimicrobial properties.**
- **Antiseptic solutions are acceptable for use at the front counter after casual contact with clientele.**
- **Antiseptic solutions are acceptable for use in a convention setting. A bottle of antiseptic gel cleanser located in each treatment room for the practitioner to use immediately after glove removal is ideal. Hands should be washed as soon as possible.**
- **Antiseptic products should be used according to the manufacturer's instructions.**

PROCEDURE 2–1 HAND WASHING TECHNIQUE

IMPLEMENTS AND MATERIALS

- Soap
- Paper towels
- Access to sink with hot and cold running water

FYI

Friction is the most important part of hand washing. Routine hand washing should take approximately 20 seconds.

Preparation

Assure that the materials are available. Disinfect the sink area before hand washing and on a routine scheduled basis.

Procedure

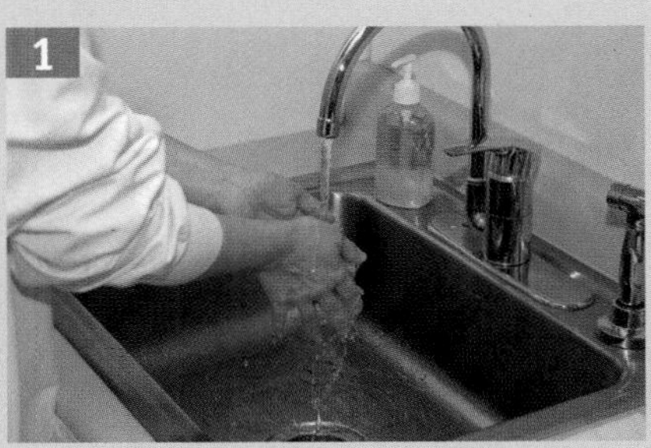

Wet your hands.

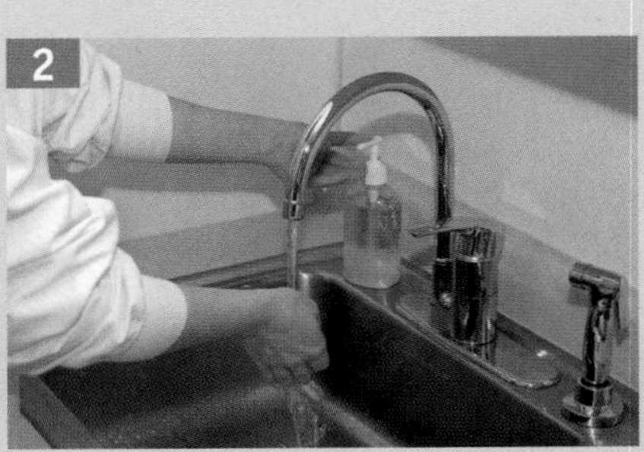

Apply soap.

1 Wet your hands with warm running water.

2 Apply soap (either antimicrobial or plain) as directed by the manufacturer and thoroughly distribute it over your hands.

continues on next page

PROCEDURE 2-1, CONT. HAND WASHING TECHNIQUE

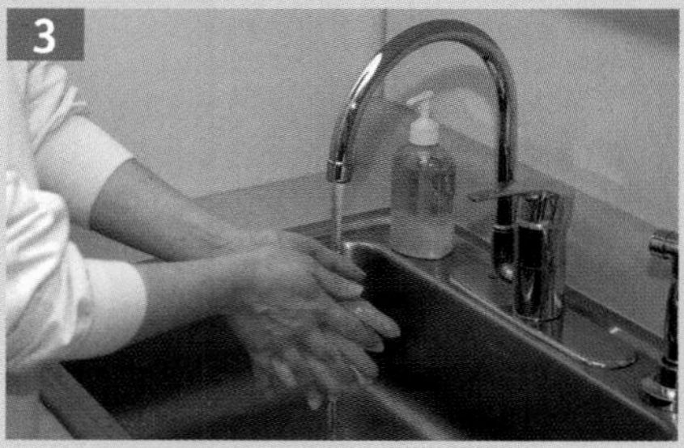

Lather between fingers.

3 Vigorously rub together all surfaces of your lathered hands for 20 seconds, including:

a. Between the fingers
b. Thumbs
c. Wrists
d. Nail beds
e. Beneath fingernails
f. Palms of hands

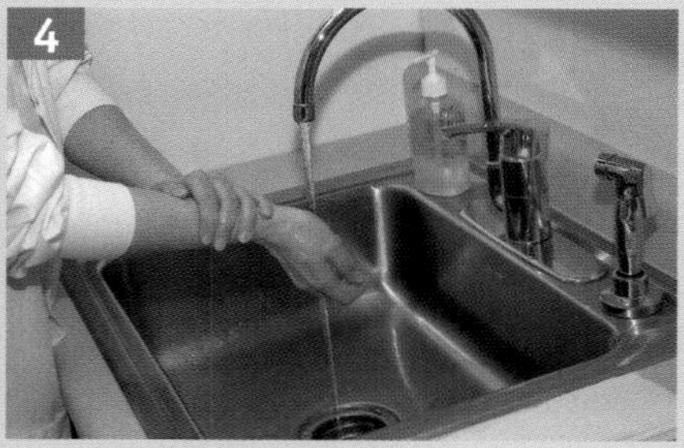

Rinse hands to remove soap.

4 Thoroughly rinse your hands, from the top of the wrists down to the fingertips, under warm running water to remove residual soap.

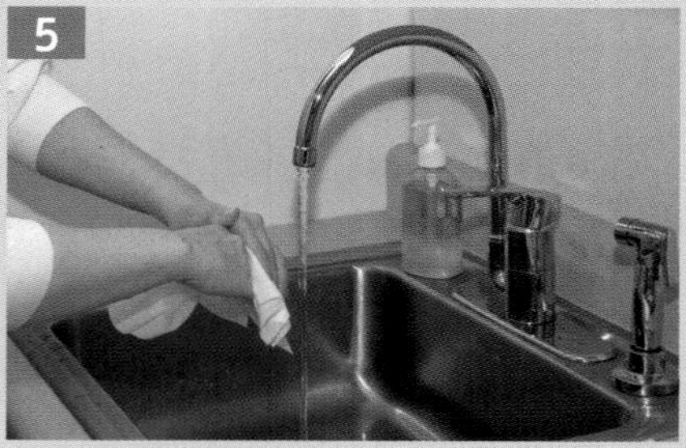

Pat hands dry.

5 Blot your hands dry with a disposable paper towel. Take the time to pat your hands dry. Do *not* rub hands together vigorously. This can cause tiny abrasions, which compromise the skin's integrity.

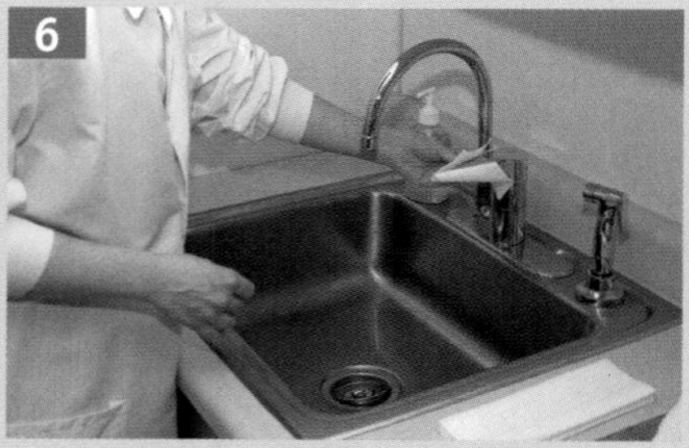

Avoid recontamination.

6 If the hand washing sink does not have foot controls or an automatic shutoff, use a clean paper towel to turn off the faucets and handle any doorknobs to avoid recontaminating your hands.

7 As an optional step, apply hand lotion as needed.

Post-procedure

Inspect your hands, including cuticles, for any visible abrasions. If you see any, wear gloves to prevent micro organisms from entering this portal.

Clean-up and Disinfection

8 Disinfect the sink area before hand washing and on a routine scheduled basis.

9 Take the paper towel you used to dry your hands and place it properly in a trash receptacle.

FOCUS ON: *Key Points of Hand Washing*

Always use warm water. Hot water is much harder on the skin; it strips the essential oils that protect the skin, thus causing excessive dryness and irritation. Also, washing hands in hot water for the recommended amount of time will likely be uncomfortable. On the flip side, cold water causes pores in the skin to constrict, thus trapping microorganisms in the superficial layers of the skin. Cold water also inhibits the proper lathering of soap.

Rinse properly to remove residual soap and take the time to thoroughly pat your hands dry to help prevent chapping and cracking of the skin.

Always pat hands dry gently with a disposable paper towel. Vigorous rubbing can cause microabrasions and remove the top layer of your protective skin.

Use hand lotion throughout the day. However, keep in mind that many lotions contain products which may compromise glove integrity. Check with your glove manufacturer or distributor to find a product that will not affect glove integrity.

Keep fingernails short and unpolished. Fingernails are a good source of infectious bacteria. Microorganisms can "hide" in the cracks of the polish and under long or false nails. *Natural or artificial nails should be no more than ¼ inch long.* Having long nails increases the risk of tearing gloves.

GLOVES

OSHA requires that gloves be worn whenever there is a "reasonable" likelihood that hands will be in contact with blood or other potentially infectious material (OPIM), mucous membranes, non-intact skin, contaminated items, or contaminated surfaces. Estheticians routinely wear single-use, medical-grade exam gloves as a safety barrier. However, while gloves offer important protection, constant use may cause irritant dermatitis due to mechanical irritation from the glove, glove powder, chemical processing agents, or from residual soap trapped between the glove and the skin. In addition, some people are allergic to the latex proteins in the gloves.

Gloves are made of many different materials (Table 2–2). Most are similar, if not better, choices than traditional latex gloves. You should determine which glove(s) to wear based on:

- The type of procedure
- Length of the procedure
- Stresses to which the gloves will be exposed throughout the procedure
- Your and your client's sensitivity
- Your preference, such as:
  - Powdered, powder-free, or synthetic
  - Latex versus non-latex
  - Low residual chemical levels (Colored gloves have a higher chemical level in order to produce the color of the glove than non-colored gloves do.)
- Quality assurance measures taken by the manufacturer and assurance that the gloves meet the ASTM F1671 standard for barrier protection against the penetration of **bloodborne** pathogens (**Note:** *Gloves are not completely resistant to pathogens.*)
- Availability of test data for the gloves' effectiveness in the handling of hazardous materials

Latex Sensitivity

Natural rubber latex (NRL) contains a variety of proteins that may cause allergic reactions. As the number of people exposed to NRL increases, the number of reported latex allergies continues to rise. *Anyone* can develop an allergy to NRL and it is important to have an understanding of the potential adverse reactions. Following are three distinct reactions that can be attributed to an NRL allergy.

- **Irritant dermatitis.** Irritant dermatitis is a nonallergenic response to NRL. Improper hand washing techniques, poor hand hygiene, soaps, lotions, disinfectants, and the wearing of latex gloves may cause it. Irritation has also been associated with processing chemicals and even the user's own perspiration inside the glove.
- **Type IV (delayed) hypersensitivity.** Type IV (delayed hypersensitivity) is an allergenic response caused by chemicals found within latex and other synthetic gloves. The delayed reaction can take place within minutes and up to several hours after contact. Some of the symptoms include itching, sores, and drying skin.
- **Type 1 (immediate) hypersensitivity.** Type I (immediate) hypersensitivity is an allergenic reaction to protein(s) within the latex gloves. The powders used to coat latex gloves may absorb the latex proteins and can come in contact with mucous membranes. Symptoms include itching, hives, asthma, and anaphylaxis.

Table 2–2 Common Glove Materials

COMMON GLOVE MATERIALS
Natural Rubber Latex (NRL) • Has long-standing barrier qualities • Is strong and durable • Has a reseal quality against puncture resistance • Is available in a low-powder version, which is preferred due to the allergic responses contained within the latex protein(s)
Polyvinyl Chloride (PVC/Vinyl) • Has good puncture resistance and is resistant to oxidation, acids, alkalis, fats, and some alcohols • Has poor resistance to most organic solvents • May have a different feel than latex gloves; however, does not have a reduced barrier performance • Does not contain the allergenic proteins or processing chemicals found in NRL that are associated with Type IV and Type I responses • Can contain additional chemicals that may cause a Type IV reaction
Nitrile • Is often resistant to many chemicals and oil-based products • Has good tensile strength and puncture resistance • Can be less elastic than NRL and thermoplastic elastomers • May contain the same processing chemicals as in NRL • Does not contain allergic NRL proteins, but can provoke ACD similar to NRL
Chloroprene (Neoprene) • Can contain processing chemicals similar to NRL and thus provoke ACD responses • Has good elastomer properties and exhibits good resistance to chemicals, oils, and fats
Thermoplastic Elastomers (Polyurethane and Styrene-based) • Is not vulcanized like NRL, but gains its final rubber-like properties during cooling or solvent evaporation • Has higher tensile strength, better stretch properties, and an increased soft feel over some other synthetics • Exhibits superior resistance to abrasion, cracking, and oxidation compared to NRL • Due to processing: Does contain some of the chemicals found in NRL • Due to processing: Is *not* considered solvent resistant • Due to processing: Has variations that can exhibit low resistance to heat, has moderate tear-strength and poor tacking properties

If you primarily use latex gloves and are aware of a client's latex sensitivity, take the appropriate precautions and follow proper procedures in order to keep the client safe. If you are not prepared ahead of time, reschedule the client for another day, preferably in the morning. This will give you the opportunity to remove all latex gloves from the room and then clean the room using EPA-registered disinfectant and synthetic (non-latex) gloves. Remember: It is not the client's fault that he or she has a latex allergy, so be courteous and understanding about the issue.

Allergic Contact Dermatitis (ACD)

Often mistaken for a "latex allergy," allergic contact dermatitis (ACD) is an immune-mediated inflammation of the skin that occurs when the skin comes into contact with a chemical allergen. ACD is a common response to the processing chemicals found in rubber products. Processing chemicals (i.e., thiurams, carbarnates, thioureas, and thiazoles) are used in the production of nitrile, neoprene, and NRL medical exam gloves. Other chemicals, such as antiseptics, adhesives, and disinfectants can also produce allergic reactions.

You may be at an increased risk of occupationally acquired ACD because of repeated exposure to chemicals in the workplace. Known as a Type IV (delayed) hypersensitivity, ACD is localized to the skin, unlike a Type I (immediate) hypersensitivity. Symptoms take time to develop—anywhere from minutes to days—and can persist for weeks or longer. While not life-threatening, if left mismanaged or untreated, ACD reactions can cause permanent damage to the skin.

Whether or not an individual develops ACD is dependent upon the following:

- Individual susceptibility
- Exposure history
- The allergenic potential of the chemical(s)

Accurate and complete diagnosis by a medical professional is essential. A diagnosis should begin with a detailed medical and occupational history to identify potential chemical sources, as well as previous allergic reactions.

Glove Testing Methods

Manufacturers have developed a variety of tests to ensure gloves meet the standards for which they are designed. Select gloves based on the type of chemicals and exposure to which they will be subjected.

Water Leak Test (ASTM D5151)

This test is performed by placing an unused glove over the end of a vertical cylinder and filling it with 1,000 milliliters of water. After a 2-minute period, the glove is observed for leaks. Values are stated as Acceptable Quality Levels (AQL), which is roughly the percentage failure rate allowed.

Relevance: Holes, rips, and/or very weak areas that rupture in the leak test indicate that barrier protection is compromised.

Thickness Test (ASTM D3767)

The thickness of a single layer of glove is measured in millimeters using a micrometer at specified locations on the upper finger, palm, and cuff.

Relevance: Thickness is an important component of barrier protection consistency for both durability and chemical permeation.

Tensile Strength Test (ASTM D412)

Strength is measured in megaPascals (MPa) to assess the amount of force applied to a glove until it breaks. The calculation is adjusted to normalize for thickness.

Relevance: The lower the tensile strength, the more easily materials of the same thickness can break when snagged or pressure is applied. For example, fingernails exert a tremendous amount of concentrated pressure at glove fingertips.

Ultimate Elongation Test (ASTM D412)

The ability to stretch is determined by extending a strip of glove until it breaks. The percentage the strip is stretched until the break is the ultimate elongation.

Relevance: The amount of stretch a glove has is very important at the microscopic level. Glove material must be able to give rather than break when stressed or snagged by instruments or fingernails or while the wearer is performing any task.

Modulus, Resistance to Movement or Stress at 50% Elongation (ASTM D412)

This test looks for the amount of force (effort) required to stretch the glove. The lower the modulus, the less effort required for movement.

Relevance: This measurement helps predict the effort wearers will exert to perform tasks. This has an indirect impact on barrier performance as hand fatigue may lead to accidents (e.g., puncture, tearing, and/or ripping glove material) during procedures. Since the physical properties of synthetic materials differ from each other and from natural rubber latex, one standard cannot be applied to all gloves. Manufacturers vary in the rigorousness of their internal requirements. For instance, some manufacturers have standards that are more stringent than ASTM requirements.

Viral Penetration Test (ASTM F1671–97b)

The viral penetration test is not required but is performed by some manufacturers. It is a standardized test method used to assess the ability of protective clothing to resist viral penetration. A single layer of glove is placed between two halves of a test chamber. A liquid suspension of the challenge virus, Phi X 174, is placed in one side of the chamber. The other half of the chamber is filled with receiving media. Samples are pulled from the receiving chamber at various times throughout the challenge period. Detection of any virus in the receiving media indicates breakthrough and thus failure of the glove material.

Chemical Barrier Test (ASTM F739)

The quality of chemical protection that a glove provides is essential since gloved hands are routinely exposed to numerous antiseptics, disinfectants, and/or other liquid chemicals. Although no requirements exist for gloves, some manufacturers choose to use this method to evaluate the resistance of their gloves to specific chemicals. Information regarding chemical resistance must be obtained directly from the manufacturer. Though use will vary among facilities, frequently used chemicals include disinfectants, antiseptics, petroleum, and isopropyl alcohol.

Characteristics of Glove Breakdown

There are several general characteristics that may indicate the breakdown in glove barrier integrity (Table 2–3). Recognizing these characteristics is important to help ensure optimal glove protection.

Table 2–3 Characteristics of Glove Breakdown

The characteristics of glove breakdown include:
• Hardening or embrittlement
• Softening (may see extending of fingertips)
• Tackiness
• Cracking
• Loss of strength
• Loss of tear resistance
• Loss of elasticity

Everyday Practices That May Affect the Glove Barrier

The barrier protection of any glove can be compromised by everyday practices, including:

Storage conditions

Skin care

Personal habits

Inability to rapidly identify type of glove base material

Are the Gloves Powdered?

Powdered gloves can:

Defeat the intent of barrier protection by transporting infectious microorganisms to where the powder is deposited.

Cause dermatitis with non-intact skin on the hands. This may enhance microbial access into the body, thus making you a "susceptible host."

Absorb and aerosolize disinfectants or other chemicals with which the powdered glove comes in contact.

Immediate Identification of Glove Base Material

When you reach for a glove, how do you identify the type of glove material? Are they labeled generically as "synthetic" or do they specify "vinyl" "nitrile" or other synthetic material? Are the gloves colored so that vinyl gloves, for instance, can be differentiated from natural rubber latex gloves? Understanding the differences in barrier capability among glove materials does little good if you cannot immediately identify what the glove is made of.

Mistaken identity can lead to the use of colored latex gloves when the barrier protection quality of a nitrile glove was needed. More importantly, an esthetician or client that is allergic to NRL may mistakenly come into contact with a latex glove.

Selection of Glove Size

A full range of glove sizes should be available to accommodate all staff. Glove length, width, finger contour, and thumb position are among the factors to consider when evaluating appropriate glove fit. Gloves should conform to the hands, yet allow ease of movement to minimize fatigue. Poor-fittings gloves can interfere with the optimal performances of procedures and can cause wearers to execute procedures awkwardly.

Adhesives on the Glove

If the glove is being used for tasks that require tape or adhesive label contact, check to see if the adhesive material adheres to the glove. Consider an alternate glove if adherence occurs, as forced removal may cause microscopic tears in the material.

Clumps and Debris

A "halo effect" may be seen around debris imbedded in glove material. The halo may indicate a weakened area that can fracture during use. This effect is occasionally seen at glove fingertips where a drop of the liquid glove material solidifies during the production process.

Donning Techniques

Poor donning techniques (putting gloves on) can result in glove rips and tears, as well as cross-contamination. Take care to don gloves correctly and avoid excessive stretching. Hands should be thoroughly dry before putting on gloves.

BODY HYGIENE AND A CARING ATTITUDE

Body Hygiene

Body hygiene is an extension of hand washing. Keeping clean and maintaining a professional appearance aids in the practice of infection control. Following is a list of good habits of personal hygiene.

Bathe or shower daily.

Keep your hair clean.

Cover or pull back long hair at work.
Keep nails trimmed and clean.
Wear clean clothes every day.
Keep jewelry and cologne at a minimum.
Wash your uniform (if applicable) separately from household laundry.

A Caring Attitude

A caring attitude is reflected within the work practices that surround the principles of infection control. It is impossible to protect ourselves and our clients without following appropriate infection control methods. Every staff member must care enough to consistently follow nationally recognized infection control guidelines in addition to clinic-specific policies and procedures.

Though safety measures have been implemented for our protection, it seems more and more people are in a hurry and believe an immediate task is more important than taking the time to put on appropriate personal protective equipment (PPE) or wash their hands properly. These tasks should be an automatic part of daily practice. Appropriately trained professionals should feel uncomfortable if they have not washed their hands or put on gloves.

DISINFECTION AND STERILIZATION

Equipment Processing

Cleaning and decontaminating equipment must be completed according to established principles and procedures to assure that sterilization will be effective. Failure to properly clean tools and equipment may allow foreign material located outside and inside of the equipment to interfere with the effectiveness of subsequent disinfection and/or sterilization. (For example, organic materials, including microorganisms, inorganic matter, and lubricants, may remain on the equipment.)

CAUTION!

You can clean without disinfecting, but you cannot disinfect without cleaning. You can clean without sterilizing, but you cannot sterilize without cleaning. The sterilization process cannot produce a sterile device that has not been cleaned first.

Cleaning Equipment

An important first step in the disinfection/sterilization process, cleaning involves removing all visible soil, debris, and foreign material from tools and equipment. Dead organisms in debris left on implements and equipment can cause fever-producing or foreign-body reactions. If the tool is later used where there is an entry portal or in a manner to create a portal, it can create a breeding place for infectious organisms. Residual debris can also affect an instrument's ability to function properly. (For example, scissors and other hinged instruments may not close properly.)

Thorough cleaning is absolutely essential before any item is subjected to sterilization. Effective cleaning is a multi-step process that relies on several interrelated factors, including:

- Water quality
- Detergent (quality and type)
- Acceptable washing method
- Proper rinsing and drying

Cleaning is normally accomplished by manual wiping, scrubbing, or brushing, along with the use of mechanical aids (for example, with water and detergents to remove foreign material). Gross debris are removed as soon as possible in order to

- reduce the number of microorganisms on the item.
- reduce the nutrient material that might support microbial growth.
- reduce the potential for environmental contamination by aerosolization or spillage.
- minimize damage to devices from such substances as blood.

Decontaminating Equipment

Decontamination involves the use of physical or chemical procedures to remove, inactivate, or destroy bloodborne pathogens on a surface or item. This is an important second step in rendering the surface or item safe for handling, use, or disposal. The level of decontamination required depends upon:

- What the item was last used for
- What the item will be used for next

For your safety, you must assume that every tool and piece of equipment poses a risk and is in need of decontamination. Decontamination is accomplished in multiple steps of cleaning, disinfecting, and then sterilizing as is appropriate for the item.

Cleaning Agents

Some cleaning agents commonly used by estheticians are water, detergents, and enzymatic detergents. Effective cleaning agents have several ideal properties, including the following:

- They are nonabrasive.
- They are low-foaming.
- They are free-rinsing.
- They are nontoxic.
- They are biodegradable.
- They allow for rapid soil dispersion.
- They are effective on all types of soil.
- They have a long shelf life.
- They are cost-effective.
- They are capable of being monitored for effective concentration and/or use life.

Water

The relevant measurable characteristics of water are pH level, hardness, temperature, and purity (microbial contamination). The pH level of water is important because the effectiveness of detergents and enzymatic cleaners is influenced by pH. Cleaning agents have optimal pH levels of performance, and there are levels where these cleaners are completely inactivated. Hard water ions such as calcium and magnesium can cause deposits or scale formation during the cleaning process because of their inverse solubility (lower solubility at higher temperatures). A final rinse with distilled or de-ionized water will remove mineral deposits.

Detergents

Detergents are substances that are capable of dislodging, removing, and dispersing solid and liquid soils from a surface being cleaned. Many detergents are formulated for specific applications (for example, in ultrasonic cleaners). Detergents should be compatible with the equipment on which they are being used and with the materials from which equipment and tools are constructed. Detergents should not be corrosive.

Detergents work by

- lowering surface tension so the cleaning liquid can penetrate the soil and the object being cleaned.
- removing soil and clumps of dirt and dissolving or suspending small particles in the cleaning fluid (usually water-containing detergent).
- keeping soils and dirt clumps in suspension or solution so they can be washed and rinsed away, rather than being re-deposited on the material or object being washed.

Traditionally soaps were made from animal fats combined with mineral alkali such as sodium or potassium hydroxide. These soap compounds should never be used for cleaning instruments.

The pH level of a detergent measures its acidity or alkalinity. A detergent with a low pH is acidic (for example, vinegar and lemon juice). A detergent with a high pH is alkaline (for example, soap). For most cleaning applications, a neutral pH or mildly alkaline detergent is preferred.

Enzymatic Detergents

Enzymatic detergents usually consist of a detergent base with a neutral pH, one or more enzymes, and a surfactant. A surfactant is a surface-acting agent that lowers the surface tension of the liquid so it can penetrate more deeply, thus preventing debris from being redeposited. After the organic material is broken down, the detergent removes the dissolved particles from the instrument's surface.

Enzymatic detergents are biodegradable and can be used in place of high alkaline or acidic products that may harm instruments. Always follow the manufacturer's recommendations regarding the proper amount of water and the correct water temperature. Temperatures above 104°F (40°C) can affect the detergent's chemical reaction. Temperatures that are too cool may fail to activate the enzyme.

Instrument Lubrication

An important part of maintaining hinged instruments is lubrication, which helps to maintain the integrity of the instruments and keep them in good working order. Instrument lubrication, which is performed after cleaning, involves dipping or spraying instruments with a lubrication solution resembling milk. It is important that the lubrication solution follows the equipment manufacturer's recommendations to assure proper contact time and dilution.

Cleaning Brushes

Cleaning brushes are an important part of the cleaning process. It is important that the correct size brush is used for the equipment being cleaned. If the brush is too large, it will not get into the openings of, say, a comedo extractor. If the brush is too small, it will not have complete contact with the edges of the implement and they will not be thoroughly clean.

Verifying the Cleaning Process

The most common method of verifying the cleaning process is a meticulous visual inspection of tools and equipment upon completion. If any visible residue is present, there is a clear indication the cleaning parameters were not achieved.

Sterilizing Equipment

To assure terminal sterilization, these steps must be followed in the exact order by everyone, every time, for all equipment processing.

PROCEDURE 2-2 THE STERILIZATION PROCESS

IMPLEMENTS AND MATERIALS

- Autoclave
- Brushes
- Soap
- EPA-registered disinfectant in tub
- Paper towels
- Autoclave packaging
- Pen

Preparation

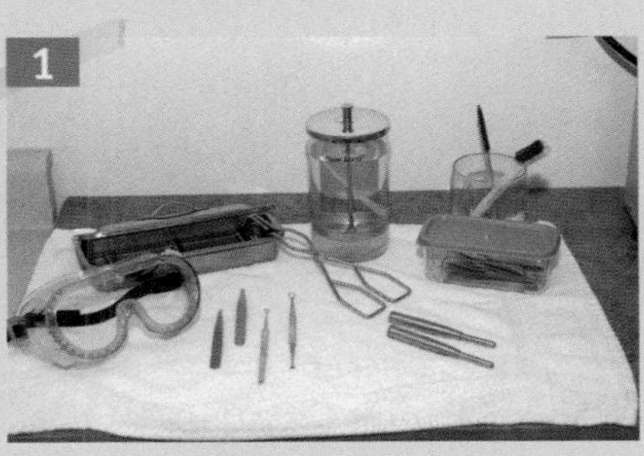

Gather supplies.

1 Gather supplies.

2 Gather equipment to be processed.

Procedure

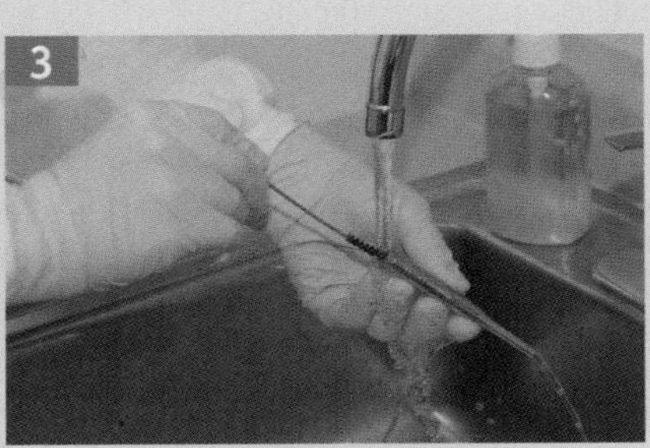

Rinse equipment.

3 Rinse equipment.

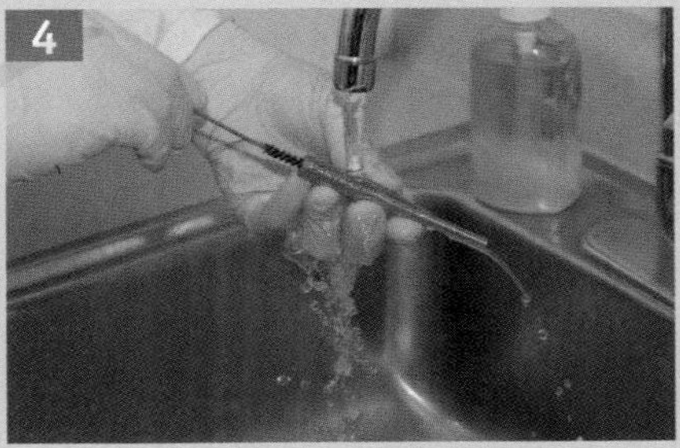

Scrub equipment under water.

4 Thoroughly scrub equipment under water to remove any visible gross debris (hair, blood, sebaceous material, etc.).

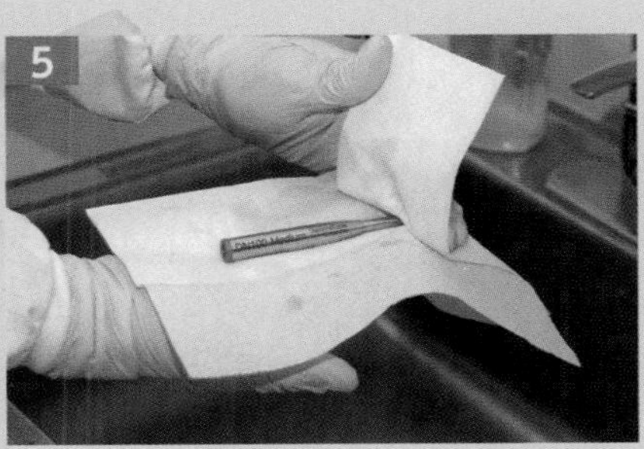

Pat equipment dry.

5 Rinse equipment and pat dry.

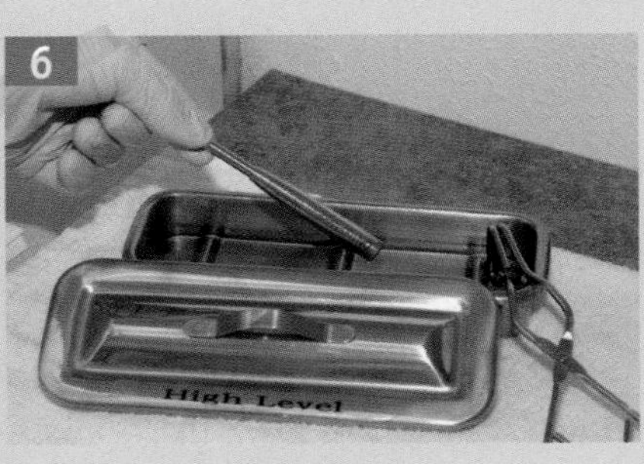

Disinfect equipment.

6 Place equipment in a disinfecting tub filled with an EPA-registered disinfectant.

Equipment should be fully submerged in disinfectant for 10 minutes or per the manufacturer's instructions. All hinged equipment (nippers, scissors, etc.) should be in the open position.

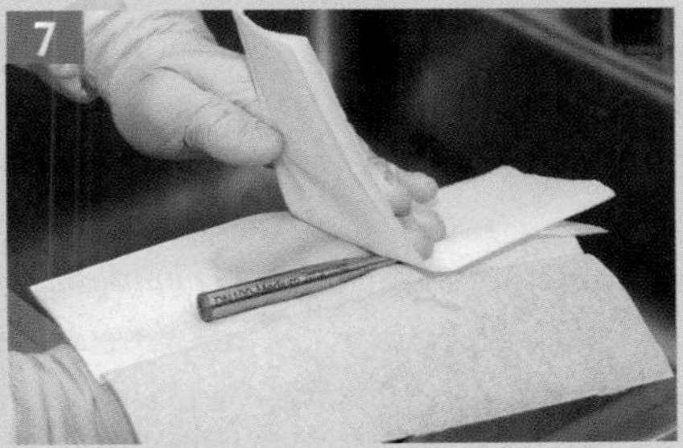

Rinse and pat dry equipment.

7 Rinse equipment and pat dry.

8 Inspect equipment for any residual debris.

continues on next page

PROCEDURE 2-2, CONT. THE STERILIZATION PROCESS

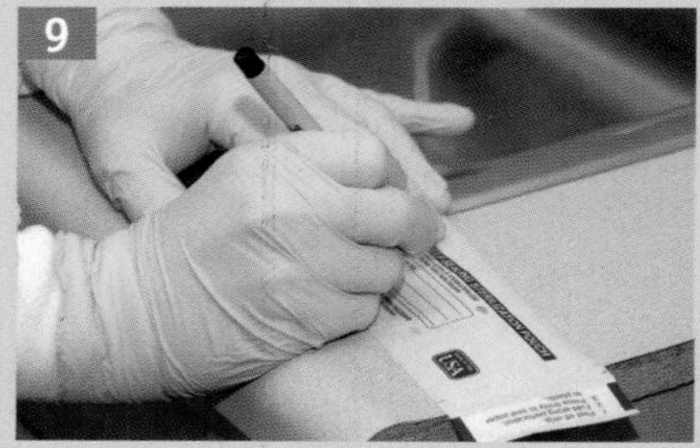

Label equipment properly.

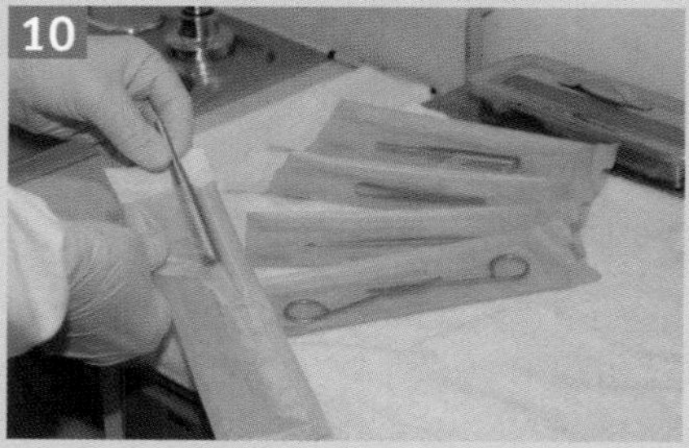

Package equipment.

9 Ensure that all equipment packages and indicators are properly marked with the equipment description, date, and your initials as the practitioner processing the equipment.

10 Package equipment with indicators dated for the day of autoclaving (within 24 hours of packaging). Place all hinged equipment in the package in the open position.

Post-procedure

Place packets ready for sterilization where they will be readily accessible for sterilization process, but not where they will become wet. Do not load autoclave if it will not be run within 24 hours.

Clean-up and Disinfection

Follow clean-up and disinfection procedures in accordance with state guidelines.

Disinfection

Chemical disinfectants are used for many tasks, including the disinfection of work surfaces and instruments. A disinfectant is a chemical used on inanimate objects to kill all organisms with the exception of spores. Disinfectants cannot make something sterile (free from all living organisms) nor are they antiseptics (chemicals used on living tissue).

Disinfection is an often misunderstood and misused process. It is critical that it be done correctly. This requires knowledge about numerous usage parameters such as contact time, dilution rate, water conditions, product use life, and temperature.

The Effectiveness of Disinfectants

The thorough cleaning of tools and instruments is the first and most important step in any disinfection or sterilization process. Organic matter such as lymph or blood can dilute or de-activate the active ingredient in the disinfectant. It can also hinder the contact of the disinfectant's ingredients with microorganisms on the surface of the equipment being processed.

Excessive moisture must be removed from tools and equipment before disinfection because the disinfectant solution can be diluted by water that remains on the surface or inside an item. This can lower the concentration of the disinfectant's active ingredient and render it unable to kill certain microorganisms in the recommended exposure time. The effectiveness of a disinfectant also depends on other factors, including:

- **The Type and Number of Microorganisms:** Some microorganisms are more resistant to liquid disinfectants that others. For example, the tubercule bacillus is more resistant than some common vegetative organisms.
- **Direct Contact with the Item:** For an item to be disinfected, all surfaces must come in direct contact with the disinfecting agent for a specified amount of time. That means that there can be nothing—including oils, protein, soil, or detergent films—between the disinfectant and the surface of the item being disinfected.
- **Time:** Direct contact with the disinfectant for a required amount of time is essential to achieve the desired bacteriocidal effect.
- **Temperature of the Disinfectant:** Some disinfectants are more effective when heated. *Always refer to the manufacturer's recommendations.*
- **pH Level:** Disinfectants are formulated over a range of pH values so they will be most effective. However,

some disinfectants work better in an alkaline pH (greater than 7), while others work best under acidic conditions (less than pH7).

- **Hardness of Water:** Minerals such as calcium and magnesium can affect the efficacy of a disinfectant by tying up its active ingredients. Most products are tested in hard water. Check the manufacturer's label for the disinfectant's claim of effectiveness in solution that is up to 400 parts per million.
- **Material Compatibility:** Tools and instruments are designed from many different types of materials. Check the manufacturer's label for the disinfectant's compatibility with the materials from which your tools and equipment are made.
- **Positioning of Instruments:** The position of tools and instruments is critical to ensure contact with all surfaces. All hinged instruments must be placed in the disinfectant in the "open" position. Do not overfill the disinfecting tub.

Risk Levels of Disinfectants

All chemical disinfectants in the United States are regulated by two federal agencies: the **U.S. Environmental Protection Agency (EPA)** and the **U.S. Food and Drug Administration (FDA).** The risk levels of chemical disinfectants are based upon the Spaulding Classification System, which has been adopted for use by the Centers for Disease Control and Prevention (CDC).

The selection of a disinfectant must be based upon the intended use of the tool or instrument being disinfected and the degree of disinfection required for that tool or instrument. Instruments used on clients are divided into three categories based on the degree of infection risk when the items were used on clients. Following are the three categories.

- **Critical Items:** Instruments or objects introduced directly into the bloodstream or into other normally sterile areas of the body, including any item that comes in direct contact with non-intact skin. Examples include tattoo needles, piercing needles, lancets, and comedo extractors. Sterilization is required for critical instruments.
- **Semi-Critical Items:** Inanimate objects and items that do not ordinarily penetrate body surfaces but have the potential to be exposed to blood, OPIM, or contaminated items. Examples include work surfaces and other inanimate objects in the work area. Though sterilization is preferred, it may not be feasible. In such case, cleaning, disinfection, and appropriate barrier protection are essential.
- **Noncritical Items:** Items that come into direct contact with unbroken skin only. Disinfection is preferred.

Activity Levels of Disinfectants

Disinfectants are classified into three levels of activity based upon the grouping of microorganisms according to their resistance to physical or chemical germicidal agents.

HIGH-LEVEL DISINFECTION is known as "cold sterilization," which is performed using glutaraldehyde-based disinfectants. High-level disinfection is used where sterilization is not possible. In some states it is still an accepted method for disinfecting implements between clients. It does not offer the level of sterilization available with the use of an **autoclave.**

INTERMEDIATE-LEVEL DISINFECTION is the preferred method of disinfection for tools, equipment, and work surfaces in the esthetics industry. Intermediate-level disinfectants kill vegetative microorganisms, *Mycobacterium tuberculosis,* fungi, and lipid and non-lipid medium-sized and small viruses, but not necessarily bacterial spores.

LOW-LEVEL DISINFECTION cannot be relied on to kill bacterial endospores, *Mycobacterium tuberculosis,* fungi, or viruses. However, it is appropriate for cleaning noncritical areas, such as a floor.

Selecting a Disinfectant

The selection and purchase of a disinfectant should be based upon the following factors:

- Level of disinfection required
- Limitations of the product
- The manner in which tools and equipment should be cleaned before exposing them to the disinfectant
- Whether or not the disinfectant is user-friendly
- Special preparations needed to prepare tools or equipment for the disinfection process
- Potential toxicity
- Specific instructions explaining how to avoid toxic conditions or reactions during use
- Storage conditions
- Whether the disinfectant leaves any residue on tools or equipment that could be potentially toxic to clients or staff
- Any potential physical hazards, such as fire or explosion

- Whether heat or environmental conditions cause chemical changes to the disinfectant

The effectiveness of a disinfectant depends upon several factors, each of which must be considered prior to use. These factors include the following:

- With what types of materials or devices can the disinfectant be used?
- Should items be partially or completely disassembled before exposure to the disinfectant?
- What are the manufacturer's recommended parameters to ensure effectiveness of the disinfectant? For example, how many times, or for what length of time can the disinfectant be reused?
- Is the positioning of tools and/or instruments in the disinfectant critical?
- Does the disinfectant have an expiration date (shelf life and use life)?
- Is mixing or other preparation required?
- What are the important factors in the reuse of the disinfectant, including dilution, time, temperature, organic soil, and bioburden?

Ultrasonic Cleaning

The word *ultrasonic* is made up of two parts: *ultra,* meaning "beyond," and *sonic,* meaning "sound." Ultrasonic cleaners, then, clean using sound frequencies as high as millions of vibrations per second. When an ultrasonic wave passes through a liquid, it makes the liquid vibrate very fast. Medical-grade ultrasonic cleaners produce from 20,000 to 38,000 vibrations per second. The vibrations are transmitted through the detergent bath and create cavitation: Ultrasonic waves pass through a cleaning solution, the molecules of the solution are set in very rapid motion, and small gas bubbles develop. As the bubbles become larger, they become unstable until they implode (not explode). This imploding creates a vacuum in the solution, which draws minute bits of foreign matter (including microorganisms) from cracks and crevices, such as hinges on instruments. This vacuum action results in thoroughly cleaning the instruments, including hard-to-reach areas.

Instruments being processed in this manner must first be cleaned manually to remove gross debris such as OPIM and then disinfected, reducing bio-burden and keeping the ultrasonic solution clean. In addition, bath temperatures should be between 80°F (27°C) and 110°F (43°C). Temperatures above 140°F (60°C) will coagulate protein, allowing it to absorb sound and making it more difficult to remove.

The lid of the ultrasonic cleaner should be closed at all times when the unit is operating. This prevents aerosols from being dispersed into the air. Instruments should always be placed into the ultrasonic cleaner in the open position. Stainless steel instruments should not be mixed with aluminum, brass, copper, or gold counterparts.

Packaging

Packaging is a generic term that includes all types of materials available that are designed to wrap, package, and contain reusable equipment and other single-use supplies for sterilization, storage, and aseptic presentation. Packaging reduces the risk of nosocomial infections by protecting sterile equipment and supplies from contamination.

The Food and Drug Administration (FDA) classifies sterilization packaging as a Class II medical device. There are three basic requirements for effective packaging materials. They must

- Allow effective penetration of heat and steam to all surfaces of the package and its contents.
- Be designed to maintain sterility of the contents up to the time of use.
- Be user-friendly (i.e., allowing easy removal of the contents without contamination).

To be considered appropriate for steam sterilization, packaging must also

- Be able to withstand the physical rigors of the steam sterilization process, such as high temperatures, moisture, and pressure.
- Allow for adequate air removal. A vacuum is created in some steam sterilization processes, and therefore, packaging material must allow for complete air removal without compromising the integrity of the package or its seal during the vacuum draw.
- Allow for proper drying of the packaging material and the enclosed contents.
- Provide a reliable barrier to microbial penetration and to the dust and moisture that can serve as vehicles for bacteria, fungi, and other microorganisms.
- Be flexible and conform to the contents.
- Be capable of being adequately sealed and labeled.
- Be durable and resistant to tears and punctures during handling and transport. The challenge to the packaging material will depend on the size, weight, and shape (for example edges, corners, pointed tips, and odd shapes) of the items being packaged.
- Be easy to open without contamination or shedding of fibers or particles.

- Not be resealable.
- Be economical.
- Be available as needed.

Paper–Plastic Combinations

Paper–plastic combinations are the most commonly used packaging in the esthetics industry. They are compatible with steam sterilization and ideal for the smaller-sized instruments that skin care practitioners use.

Pouches are manufactured with one open end to allow insertion of the contents and subsequent sealing using adhesive or heat seals. The opposite end is presealed during manufacturing and is designated for the opening and presentation of the sterilized contents of the package.

Packaging Procedures

Pouches must be sized properly to allow for adequate air removal, steam penetration, and drying. Since trapped air acts as a barrier to heat and moisture, it is important to remove as much air as possible from the pouch before sealing. Never fill a pouch too full. Overfilling may cause the paper to tear or seals to rupture during sterilization or handling. Leave about 1 inch of space between the items in the pouch and the sealed edges to allow space for package contraction and proper circulation. Pouches should not be too large for the contents, as excessive movement could break seals or puncture the paper side of the pouch.

Always check the inside of paper–plastic pouches for moisture after sterilization and again before storage. When steam comes in contact with metal instruments, it condenses on the surface as heat is transferred to the metal. The retained moisture forms water droplets on the contents and may compromise the integrity of the seal or the barrier protection of the pouch itself. To prevent condensation, the sterilizer must either have a dry cycle or the door must be vented open during the cooling process.

Labeling

It is essential to properly label packages before sterilization. Labeling is necessary not only for the practitioner, but also for quality assurance, stock rotation, and inventory control purposes. Label information should include the following:

- Description of the package contents
- Initials of the package assembler
- Lot control number (for example, the last four digits of the current spore test number)
- Date of sterilization

Standardized abbreviations and terms should be used to avoid confusion. Labeling should be documented on label-sensitive tape or adhesive labels, *not written directly on the packaging material.* For pouches, labels should not be placed on the paper side as they may inhibit steam penetration. Felt-tipped pens are generally used for marking, but they must be indelible, non-bleeding, non-fading, and nontoxic.

Whether sterilized in-house or purchased as "sterile-ready-to-use" products, ALL sterile packages should be inspected before storage *and* before use to ensure the packaging materials and/or seals have not been compromised.

Steam Sterilization

Steam under pressure is becoming a preferred method of sterilization for the esthetics industry. To attain sterilization, the proper combination of time, temperature, pressure, and moisture/saturation must be attained inside the autoclave. Following are explanations of these parameters for sterilization.

- **Temperature Gauge:** The temperature of the sterilizer must be maintained to ensure that all organisms are killed (usually 274°F). The amount of time that the machine takes to reach this temperature must be added to the actual processing time.
- **Pressure Gauge:** Pressure is necessary to raise the temperature of the water above the boiling point.
- **Timer:** The length of time necessary to complete the cycle depends on the item being processed and the type of packaging being used. Refer to the manufacturer's instructions to determine the appropriate cycle length. The "standard" is 274°F/15 minutes.
- **Moisture/Saturation:** The steam in the autoclave must reach 100% relative humidity.

Monitoring the Sterilization Process

Mechanical Monitoring

A mechanical indicator is a device that provides an assessment of cycle conditions, including time, temperature, and pressure. Temperature gauges, pressure gauges, timers, and printouts are all examples of mechanical monitoring. They must be checked with each load to ensure that the parameters are being met and as an additional measure to ensure that the autoclave is functioning properly.

Chemical Monitoring

Chemical indicators and integrators are used to monitor the actual physical conditions inside the autoclave.

They respond to the conditions via a characteristic color change. There are two distinct types of chemical indicators:

1. **Indicators** are devices that respond to steam, or moist heat. Often, the outside of the packaging will include an area that changes color. Special sterilization tape or chemical strips behave in a similar fashion. Indicator strips are designed for placement inside packages in order to show penetration of steam.
2. **Integrators** are process indicators. They behave similarly to steam indicators in that they react to physical conditions via a color change. However, integrators are designed to respond to more than one required parameter of sterilization. Although different brands will vary, integrators go one step further in terms of parameter monitoring. Integrators must be subjected to the same conditions (packaging, etc.) as the equipment being processed.

While indicators and integrators are useful in determining point-of-use process errors, it is important to note that *they do not prove sterilization.*

Biological Monitoring

Biological monitoring, commonly referred to as spore tests, are the only true method of determining the success of the sterilization process. A spore test is a control-based test in which a live sample of bacterial spores (commonly Bacillus stearothermopolis for steam autoclaves) are placed into an autoclave and processed. Manufacturer instructions will indicate proper use of the test. The processed spore sample is then cultured or incubated along with the control sample. Total destruction of spores indicates success of the sterilization process. Although guidelines will vary in terms of frequency, the most common recommendation is to spore test at a minimum of once a month. However, in medical settings where there is high volume testing may be done weekly. The spore test should be run in the same load as routinely used implements.

Countertop Steam Autoclaves

Countertop or transportable steam autoclaves all have fully automatic, predetermined cycles and generate steam internally by boiling water with electrical heaters. They also have a single manually operated door. The safe and efficient operation of these autoclaves is dependent on training and a sound knowledge of the autoclave and its function. Professional advice on the selection, purchase, and testing of autoclaves may be obtained from an "Authorized Sterilization Technician." This is the type of autoclave most commonly found in a clinical or private medical practice.

With steam autoclaves air is displaced by steam. New models are equipped with an active vacuum air removal system which operates prior to the sterilizing stage. This system removes trapped air from wrapped, porous and tubular devices. Vacuum countertop autoclaves also have a post-sterilization drying cycle and, although smaller, mimic the cycle parameters of the much larger autoclaves used in hospitals. The drying stage is included to reduce the moisture content of packages and porous materials, which may otherwise compromise the protective quality of the material from a bacteriological standpoint. Vacuum autoclaves are preferred because of their suitability for a much wider range of load items. In addition, the packaging can incorporate a process indicator and a label showing the contents. This will assist with tracking should an adverse incident occur.

Steam autoclaves must be installed and maintained appropriately and tested routinely. Sterilization cannot be confirmed by inspection of the load. Successful sterilization depends on the consistent reproduction of sterilizing conditions. Autoclaves have to be validated before use, their performance monitored routinely, and the equipment properly maintained. It is essential that wrapped instruments are not processed in "displacement" (non-vacuum) steam autoclaves. Vacuum-assisted air removal is recommended for all packaged loads.

Safety

All autoclaves are potentially dangerous as they include pressure vessels and therefore must comply with 'the pressure systems and transportable gas container regulations.' Under these regulations all steam autoclaves are subject to periodic inspection by an "Authorized Sterilization Technician." It is the responsibility of the owner of the autoclaves to ensure that it is not used until there is a written procedure for use, maintenance, and routine inspection. The "Authorized Sterilization Technician" will give advice on this if required.

The Medical Devices Agency now recommends that only autoclaves bearing the European Commission (EC) mark be purchased and used as they comply with European Safety and Medical Device Regulations (93/42 EEC 1998).

PROCEDURE 2-3 POLICY AND PROCEDURE FOR OPERATING AUTOCLAVES

To ensure proper sterilization of equipment and to preserve the longevity of the autoclave, *always follow the manufacturer's instructions for the specific make and model of autoclave you are using.*

IMPLEMENTS AND MATERIALS

- Gloves
- Hand soap
- Paper towels
- Distilled water (or as directed by autoclave manufacturer)
- Precleaned and prepackaged items to be autoclaved
- Integrator
- Autoclave

Preparation

1 Wash hands and pat dry.

2 Gather supplies and items to be autoclaved.

Procedure

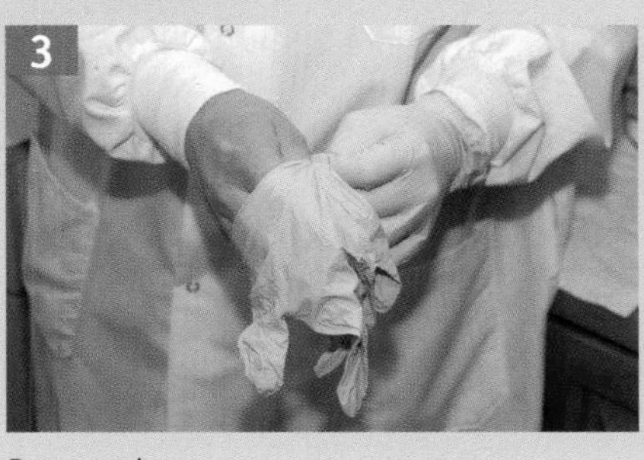

Put on gloves.

3 Put on gloves.

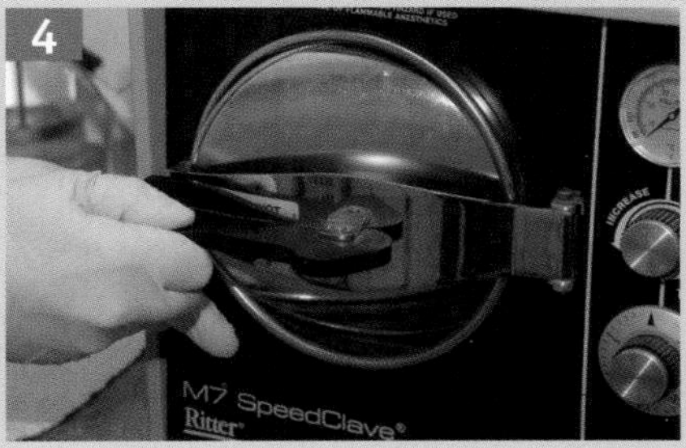

Remove reservoir cover.

4 Water level should be to the bottom of ring release valve. Check water storage per manufacturer's directions.

5 If the water level is not adequate, add water until the proper level is reached. Do not overfill the autoclave.

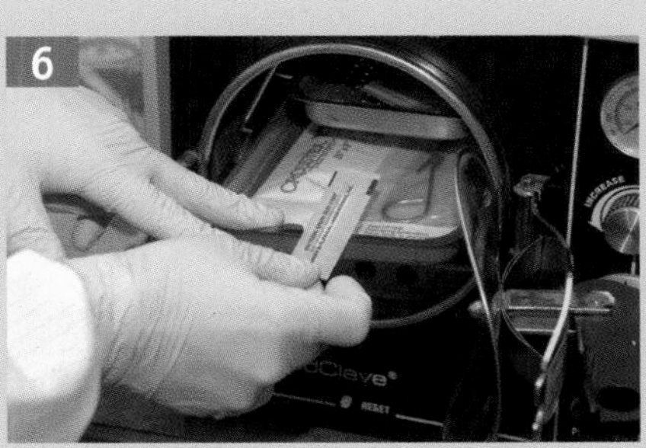

Place integrator on a mid-shelf.

6 Place integrator on a mid-shelf of the autoclave or as the manufacturer directs.

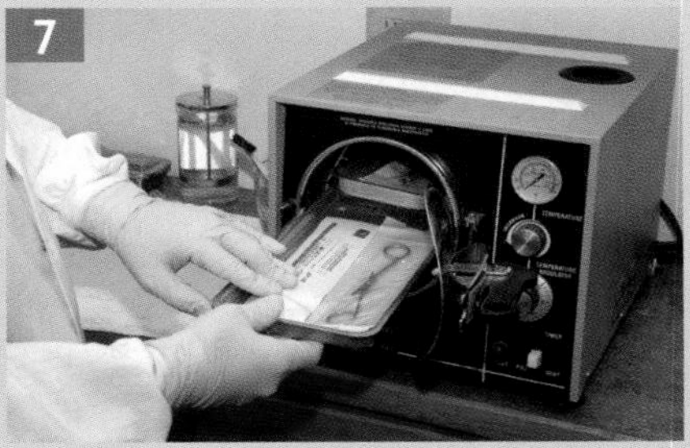

Load autoclave.

7 Document the autoclave load according to procedure.

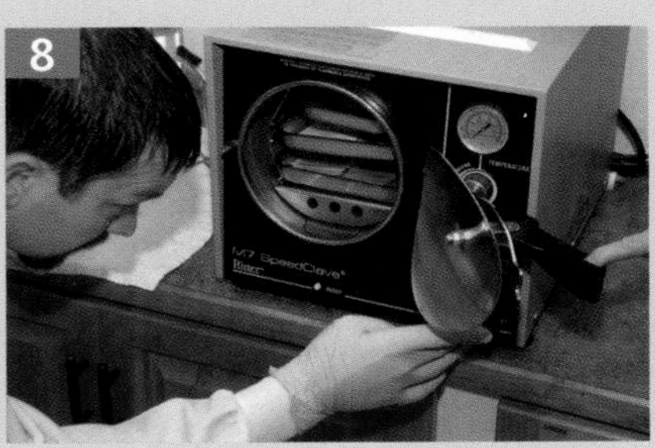

Do not overlap items.

8 Load the autoclave according to procedure. Place prepackaged items on autoclave shelves, but do not overlap or overload as this could compromise sterilization.

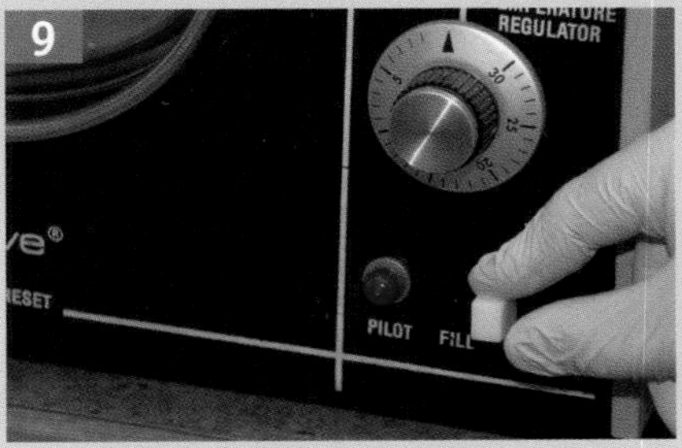

Turn dial to the Fill position.

9 Turn autoclave function select dial to the Fill position. Check storage water level per manufacturer's directions.

continues on next page

PROCEDURE 2–3, CONT. POLICY AND PROCEDURE FOR OPERATING AUTOCLAVES

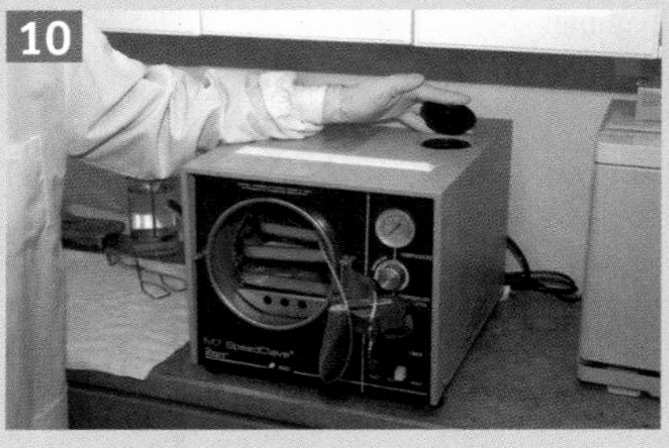

Fill until water reaches the indent marker.

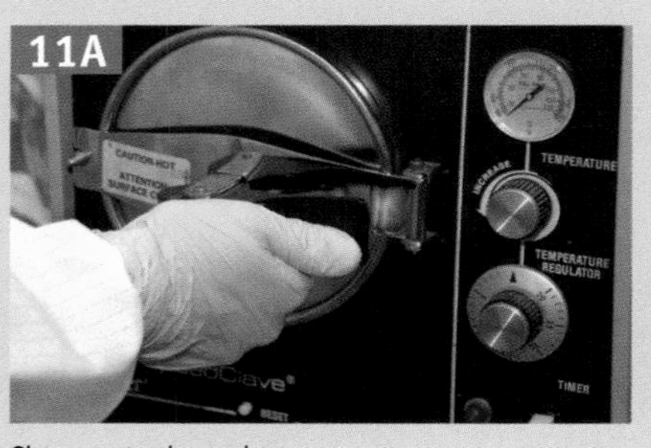

Close autoclave door.

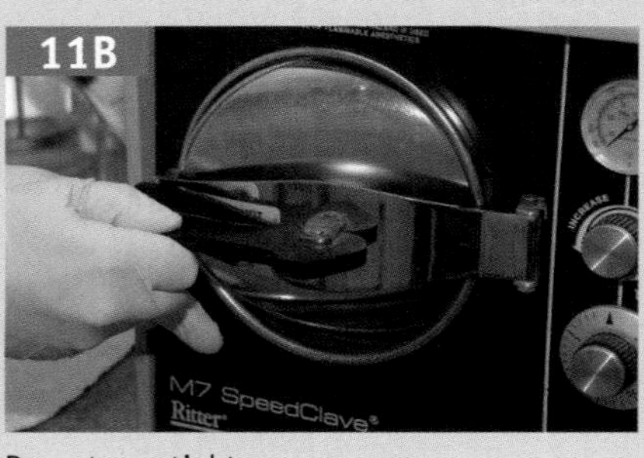

Do not overtighten.

10 Allow water to fill until it reaches the indent at the front of the chamber, following manufacturer guidelines.

11 Close and secure autoclave door. Do not overtighten.

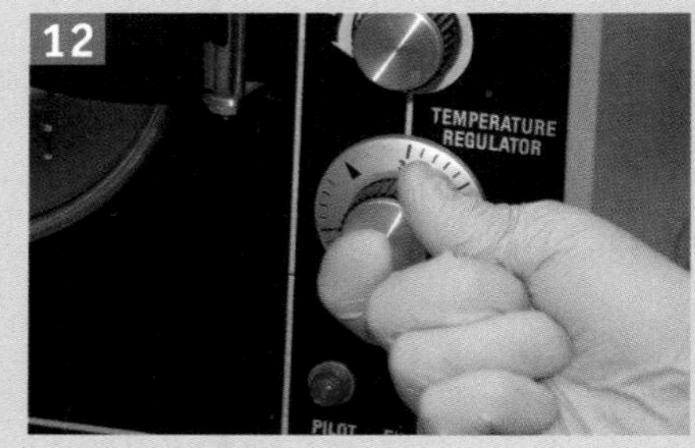

Turn autoclave timer dial.

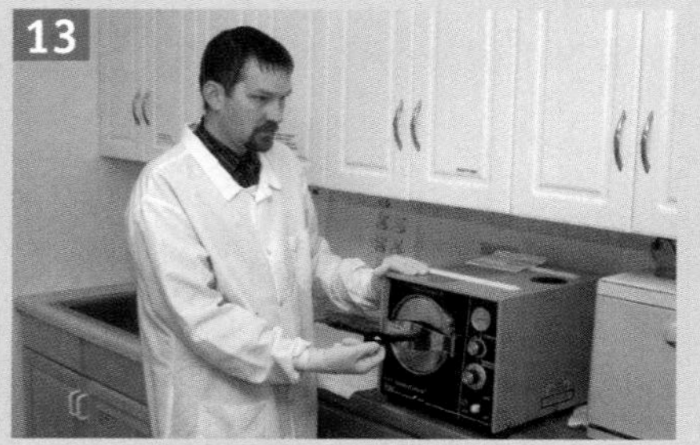

Monitor the autoclave dials.

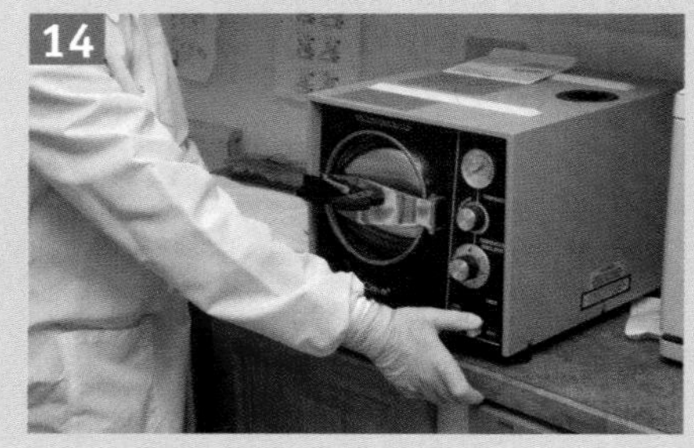

Vent autoclave.

12 Turn autoclave timer dial to start autoclave.

a. Turn timer dial to 40 minutes if running the first load of the day.

b. Turn timer dial to 30 minutes if running a load after autoclave is already warm.

13 Visually monitor the autoclave dials to ensure that the autoclave reaches the temperature required by the manufacturer.

14 At end of processing time, vent the autoclave per the manufacturer's directions, if required to do so manually.

CAUTION!

Always **refer to the manufacturer's instruction manual for the operating instructions specific to the make and model of your autoclave.**

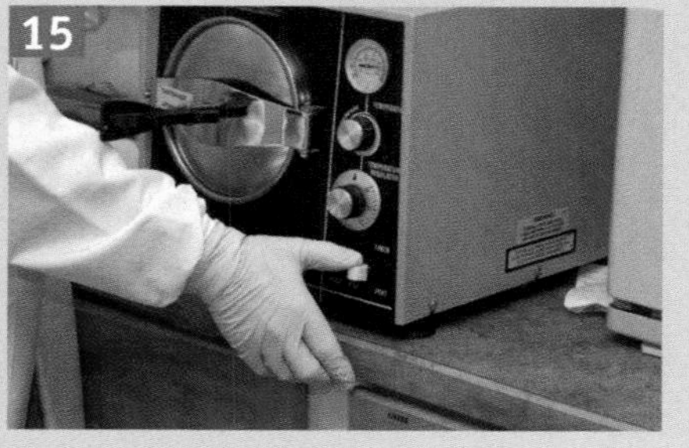

Allow autoclave to cool.

15 Allow the autoclave to cool completely before removing packages.

Post-procedure

16 Double-check to make sure no packages appear to be "wet."

17 If any appear wet, repackage and reprocessed them.

18 Place cooled packages in a designated clean, dry storage area.

Clean-up and Disinfection

Follow manufacturer's guidelines for cleaning of autoclave equipment both in outline and frequency.

Storage

Where, how, and why sterile instruments and supplies are stored is important in achieving the ultimate goal of maintaining sterility up to the time the items are used. Conditions that can adversely affect the ability of a package to maintain sterility until it is used include the following:

- Moisture and other liquid/fluid contamination
- Dirt, dust, and debris
- Physical damage to the package, such as tears, punctures, broken seals, or a breakdown of packaging

Storage environments should be clean, dry, and easily accessible. *Stored items should be arranged so that packages are not crushed, bent, or compressed.*

POTENTIAL HAZARDS FOR AN ESTHETICIAN

Estheticians in medical facilities may have a heightened awareness of potential hazards because they may be assisting medical personnel with procedures or performing postoperative care on fresh wounds. However, no matter where an esthetician works—whether it is a salon or a medical facility—he or she has to watch for the same potential hazards.

Sharps Sticks

Contact with a used lancet or other sharp stick may have serious consequences if a client has a communicable disease. A client may not be aware of a condition and may share an infection with you. Always assume transmission and follow these rules for needlestick response.

1. First, treat the wound:
   - **Bleed:** Allow the area to bleed.
   - **Wash:** Wash and irrigate the site vigorously.
   - **Cover:** Cover and protect the wound.
2. Then, screen exposure for:
   - **Severity.** Was there actual source blood contact with your non-intact skin or mucous membrane? If yes, check with the owner/administrator/physician and follow office protocol.
   - **Source.** The client reports to your Emergency Medical/Occupational Medicine Facility (or local medical services qualified to do this) for appropriate evaluation and screening according to OSHA and your state agency requirements.
   - **Employee.** You will be directed to the same facility for appropriate evaluation and screening according to the OSHA and state agency requirements.

Other Hazards

While a needle/lancet stick is the most prevalent risk, other services can generate a risk factor as well. Every day, you need to inspect your own skin for breaks in the stratum corneum. Check for hangnails, torn cuticles, and any form of dermatitis or chapping, as all of these create an entry portal for pathogens. Avoid overuse of antibacterial soaps as these can cause chapping of the hands. When you are handling harsh cleansers or chemicals, wear the appropriate gloves.

The area of the client's skin to be treated also needs a visual inspection before any treatment begins. Check carefully for any breaks in the skin surface or the presence of lesions.

Airborne Infections

Estheticians do not often work in an environment where they encounter patients with a known airborne illness. However, a client with influenza, measles, or tuberculosis may not know he or she has a disease. It can be transferred via a cough and the virus is very difficult to destroy. It is advisable to wear a mask while performing microdermabrasion, extractions, laser hair removal, or chemical peels due to vapor and/or other unknown airborne transmissions. *Always use standard precautions.*

CAUTION!

Always use standard precautions!

Bloodborne Diseases

Bloodborne pathogen transmission of diseases such as HBV, HCV, delta hepatitis, HIV/AIDS, syphilis, and malaria are potential risks for estheticians practicing anywhere in the world. These pathogens are undetectable to the naked eye, and some, such as HBV, can live dry on a surface for a week. In addition, these diseases can enter your body through any open cut or lesion. Standard precautions are always necessary.

Accidents, Fire, and Emergencies

Recurrent safety instruction is critical to your well-being and the well-being of those around you. Your employer will provide specific training on handling emergency situations and will assess your knowledge of such responses as fire drills, bacteriology/sanitation, eyewash protocol, evacuations/bomb threats, CPR, first aid, patient emergencies, domestic violence safety training, and self-defense instruction through routine written and oral examinations, which will be placed in your file. The key to handling an accident is in using your training, care, and tact. Your office manager or administrator will provide or delegate an individual to create a clinical emergency protocol, an evacuation policy, and other emergency procedure flowcharts.

Activity

Create a **safety plan** for your school or your proposed facility. How can you help yourself and colleagues be safer? Create daily, weekly, and monthly cleaning plans and weekly and monthly safety reviews.

BASIC SAFETY GUIDELINES

Avoiding the transmission of disease by using the established standards is the key to maintaining a safe working environment. Following is a review of the standards that will affect your daily work.

Clean Your Space Systematically and Routinely

Utilize approved cleaning solutions and perform cleaning after each client contact, treatment or procedure. Clean and disinfect all implements after each use. Place autoclave-ready implements in the autoclave, ready for the next run. You cannot be too compulsive about cleaning.

CAUTION!

***Every* esthetic establishment needs safety guidelines.**

Follow Hand Washing Regulations

Keep in mind that frequent hand washing is the first preventative measure to control the transmission of microorganisms. Follow the protocol outlined in Procedure 2–1.

Wear Gloves

Wearing gloves for all treatments, procedures, and applications, including makeup, reduces risks. Select gloves to use based on exposure risks and the type of products to which they will be exposed. In addition, wear them while cleaning and mixing solutions. Use the *inside-out* method to remove gloves immediately after use and avoid contaminating other surfaces. Then perform a thorough hand washing.

Glove Selection

Technicians not only need to select gloves based on propensity to allergic reaction but also to the protection offered by the glove. Key factors in your glove selection will be:

- Duration of the treatment
- Type of treatment

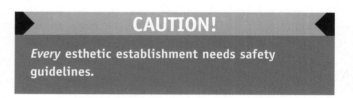

- Products to which the gloves are exposed
- Client/technician sensitivities
- Personal preferences

Dispose of Potential Infected Material

To prevent the risk of cross-contamination it is important to properly handle any other potentially infectious materials.

1. Place all sharps into an approved sharps container.
2. Place all cotton swabs, used gloves, and other questionable matter into an approved bag, and dispose of according to state or local regulatory protocol. If none exist follow OSHA bio-hazard protocols.

Activity

Where do you dispose of your biohazard container? Locate a local facility that will handle this or a service that will pick it up from your clinic.

Use the Autoclave for Sterilization

Use the autoclave for sterilizing whenever possible. Follow the protocols and guidelines for safe operation, testing, and achieving complete sterility.

Autoclaves, like other equipment, must be maintained. Follow the manufacturer's guidelines for recommended cleaning procedures. In addition, be sure to test the unit at appropriate intervals using spore strip testing. Normally, the spore strip testing unit is an envelope with two sides. You remove the test strip from one side, leaving the other in the envelope as a control or placebo. Once you have run the test strip in the autoclave, you return it to its side of the envelope. Fill out the front of the envelope and mail it to the testing firm. They will notify you if there are any concerns or issues with the test results. Often these results are available via the Internet within a brief period of time.

Use Disposables

The use of disposable items is the best way to ensure an aseptic procedure. These items are used once and discarded. Sharps (lancets or needles) are always single-use and should be placed in an approved sharps container after that use.

Read and Keep Material Safety Data Sheets

Read Material Safety Data Sheets. Create your own MSDS booklet by including these sheets for all of the professional products and supplies with which you work. This might include cleaning solutions, peels, and any other products. These sheets are provided by the manufacturer and many are available at their Web site for downloading. OSHA requires that this information be readily available and in a user-friendly format. Even an independent contractor or sole proprietor benefits from having an MSDS reference file.

Create a Room-Cleaning Checklist

This checklist is documentation necessary for use in the clinic. It shows the frequency of cleaning—daily, weekly, monthly, or quarterly—of the esthetic room. This includes all sinks, faucets, floors, treatment product bottles, equipment, vents, walls, ceilings, trash and biohazard units, and all other items used in the space.

Understand and Use Eyewash Protocol

Wear appropriate eye protection during treatments. If an accident does happen, be prepared by having every room equipped with single-use eyewash solutions and/or an eyewash station. In a medical facility, the eyewash station is standard. Flush the eye until comfortable or for 15 minutes. Refer to appropriate MSDS sheets on the product for further treatment and seek medical treatment as indicated.

OSHA INSPECTIONS

OSHA representatives conduct inspections without advance notice, and they cannot be rescheduled. OSHA inspectors have the right to enter and inspect *any* facility at their own choosing. The reasons for their visits are typically as follows:

- There is an immediate danger to employees.
- A fatality or accident has occurred in which three or more employees were injured.
- Someone filed a complaint.
- It is a random inspection assigned by OSHA's computer system.

An OSHA inspector will present credentials and ask to speak to the administrator or manager of your facility. The inspector will then tell the general scope, purpose, and nature of the inspection, as well as discuss the procedures to be followed. He or she will view your OSHA records, other records, charts, and treatment rooms and take a general walkaround of the facility. The inspector may interview employees. At the end of the inspection, he or she will discuss any violations with the clinic administrator or office manager.

To ensure your readiness for an inspection at any time, always post OSHA regulations in appropriate locations in the clinic, do your housekeeping, utilize all personal protective equipment when performing duties and procedures, and follow all rules set forth by standards and regulations, including medical documentations. If you are visited by an OSHA inspector:

- Do not panic.
- Wait to be asked for information.
- Answer questions truthfully.
- Write down the inspector's name and badge number, the time and date of each inspection, and the areas inspected.

REVIEW QUESTIONS

1. During a routine facial without extractions, should the esthetician wear gloves? Why or why not?
2. What does the esthetician do if there is an accidental needlestick while performing extractions?
3. What is OSHA?
4. What is the Bloodborne Pathogens Standard?
5. Discuss the difference between engineering controls and work practice controls.
6. How does the method of contracting hepatitis A differ from contracting hepatitis B or C?
7. How is tuberculosis transmitted?
8. Explain Universal Precautions.
9. What is the number one method of personal protection?
10. Name three guidelines for an esthetician to employ to protect themselves in his or her workplace.

CHAPTER GLOSSARY

Acquired Immune Deficiency Syndrome (AIDS): disease caused by the HIV virus that breaks down the body's immune system.

acute: the rapid-onset, short-term initial stage of disease. Contrast with *chronic*.

antibacterial: 1. destroying or stopping the growth of bacteria. 2. agent that destroys or prevents the growth of bacteria.

antibiotic: any variety of natural or synthetic substances that inhibit growth of or destroy microorganisms. Used extensively in treatment of infectious diseases.

antimicrobial: 1. destructive to or preventing the development of microorganisms. 2. agent that destroys or prevents the development of microorganisms.

asepsis: sterile; a condition free from germs and any form of life.

aseptic technique: the process of properly handling sterilized and disinfected equipment and implements to prevent contamination.

autoclave: apparatus for sterilization by steam pressure usually at 250° F (121° C) for a specified length of time.

autoimmune disorders: disorders or diseases in which the body produces disordered immunological response against itself. Normally the body's immune mechanisms are able to distinguish clearly between what is a normal substance and what is foreign. In autoimmune diseases this system becomes defective and produces antibodies against normal parts of the body to such an extent as to cause tissue injury.

bacteria: one-celled microorganisms with both plant and animal characteristics; also known as *microbes*. Capable of surviving on living and nonliving matter. Bacteria may be either pathogenic or nonpathogenic.

bloodborne: described transmission through direct blood-to-blood contact, such as sharing needles or through blood transfusion.

bloodborne pathogens: pathogenic microorganisms present in human blood that can cause disease in humans. These pathogens include, but are not limited to, hepatitis B virus (HBV), hepatitis C virus (HCV), and the human immunodeficiency virus (HIV).

chronic: long-term or persistent disease. Contrast with *acute*.

contaminated: the presence or reasonably anticipated presence of blood or other potentially infectious material (OPIM) on an item or surface.

decontaminate: the use of physical or chemical means to remove, inactivate, or destroy bloodborne pathogens on a surface or item to the point where they are no longer capable of transmitting infectious particles. The surface or item is rendered safe for handling, use, or disposal.

disinfection: the second-highest level of decontamination; nearly as effective as sterilization but does not kill bacterial spores; used on hard, nonporous surfaces.

engineering controls: controls that isolate or remove bloodborne pathogens from the workplace; examples include sharps containers, handwashing facilities, eyewash stations, and labels.

Human Immunodeficiency Virus (HIV): virus that causes AIDS.

immunization: becoming immune or the process of rendering a person immune.

mucous membrane: Membrane-lining passages and cavities communicating with the air. Consists of a surface layer of epithelium, a basement membrane, and an underlying layer of connective tissue. Mucus-secreting cells or glands usually are present in the epithelium but may be absent.

Occupational Safety and Health Administration (OSHA): an agency responsible for workplace safety and health.

organisms: any living thing, plant, or animal. May be unicellular (bacteria, yeasts, protozoa) or multicellular (all complex organisms including man).

other potentially infectious material (OPIM): human body fluids including, but not limited to, semen, vaginal secretions, cerebrospinal fluid, synovial fluid, pleural fluid, pericardial fluid, amniotic fluid, and all body fluids in situations where it is difficult or impossible to differentiate between body fluids.

pathogen: a microorganism or substance capable of producing disease.

personal protective equipment (PPE): specialized clothing or equipment designed for use by an employee in order to minimize, reduce, or eliminate the risk of exposure to bloodborne pathogens and other hazards. Examples include, but are not limited to, disposable latex or nitrile exam gloves, disposable sleeves, disposable aprons, and face and eye protection.

safety plan: a plan for avoiding potential exposure to contaminated fluids and for dealing with it should exposure occur.

sharps: any object that can penetrate the skin, including, but not limited to, needles, razors, scissors, and broken glass.

spores: reproductive cells, usually unicellular, produced by plants and some protozoa. Bacterial spores are difficult to destroy because high temperatures are required to destroy them, and they are very resistant to heat.

standard precautions: a widely recognized and utilized method of infection control. Under Standard Precautions all blood, other body fluids, secretions, excretions (except sweat), non-intact skin, mucous membranes, dried blood, saliva, and any other body substance are considered contaminated and/or infectious.

sterilize: the act of using a physical or chemical procedure to

CHAPTER GLOSSARY

destroy all forms of microbial life, including highly resistant bacterial spores.

tuberculosis: an infectious disease, chronic in nature and capable of affecting the lungs, although it may occur in almost any part of the body. The causative agent is mycobacterium tuberculosis (the tubercle bacillus). The most common mode of transmission is the inhalation of infected droplet nuclei.

U.S. Environmental Protection Agency (EPA): an agency charged with protecting human health as well as air, water, and land.

U.S. Food and Drug Administration (FDA): an agency responsible for safety regulation of foods, dietary supplements, medical related items, veterinary items and cosmetics.

CHAPTER OUTLINE

- CELLULAR STRUCTURE AND FUNCTION
- A BRIEF OVERVIEW OF SKIN STRUCTURE AND FUNCTION
- THE CELLS OF THE EPIDERMIS
- MAJOR CELLS IN THE DERMIS
- HOW KERATINOCYTES REPLACE THE STRATUM CORNEUM
- PROTEINS OF THE DERMIS—THE EXTRACELLULAR MATRIX (ECM)
- THE CELL CYCLE
- AN INTRODUCTION TO EMBRYOLOGY—THE STEM CELL
- THE MAJOR TISSUES IN THE BODY
- THE BASIC IMMUNE SYSTEM
- MECHANISM OF EXFOLIATION—THE DESMOSOMES
- SKIN PENETRATION AND PERMEATION
- SENSORY NERVES AND PERCEPTION IN THE SKIN

CHAPTER 3

ADVANCED HISTOLOGY OF THE CELL AND THE SKIN

By Peter T. Pugliese, M.D.

LEARNING OBJECTIVES

After completing this chapter, you should be able to:

- Recognize cellular components and their functions.
- Discuss the cellular membrane structure.
- Understand cellular receptors and their purpose.
- Understand internal cellular structure and function.
- Define cellular differentiation.
- Name the major functions of the skin.
- Recognize key cells of the epidermis of the skin: the keratinocyte, the melanocyte, and the Langerhans cell.
- Name key cells of the dermis of the skin: the fibroblast, the mast cell, and the leukocytes.
- Explain how keratinocytes replace the stratum corneum.
- Name the major proteins of the dermis, the ECM.
- Understand cell growth control mechanisms.
- Recognize stem cells: mesoderm, ectoderm, and endoderm.
- Discuss major types of tissues in the body.
- Understand immune system cells and reactions.
- Describe the mechanism of exfoliation—the desmosomes.
- Understand penetration and permeability.
- Discuss sensory nerves and perception in the skin.

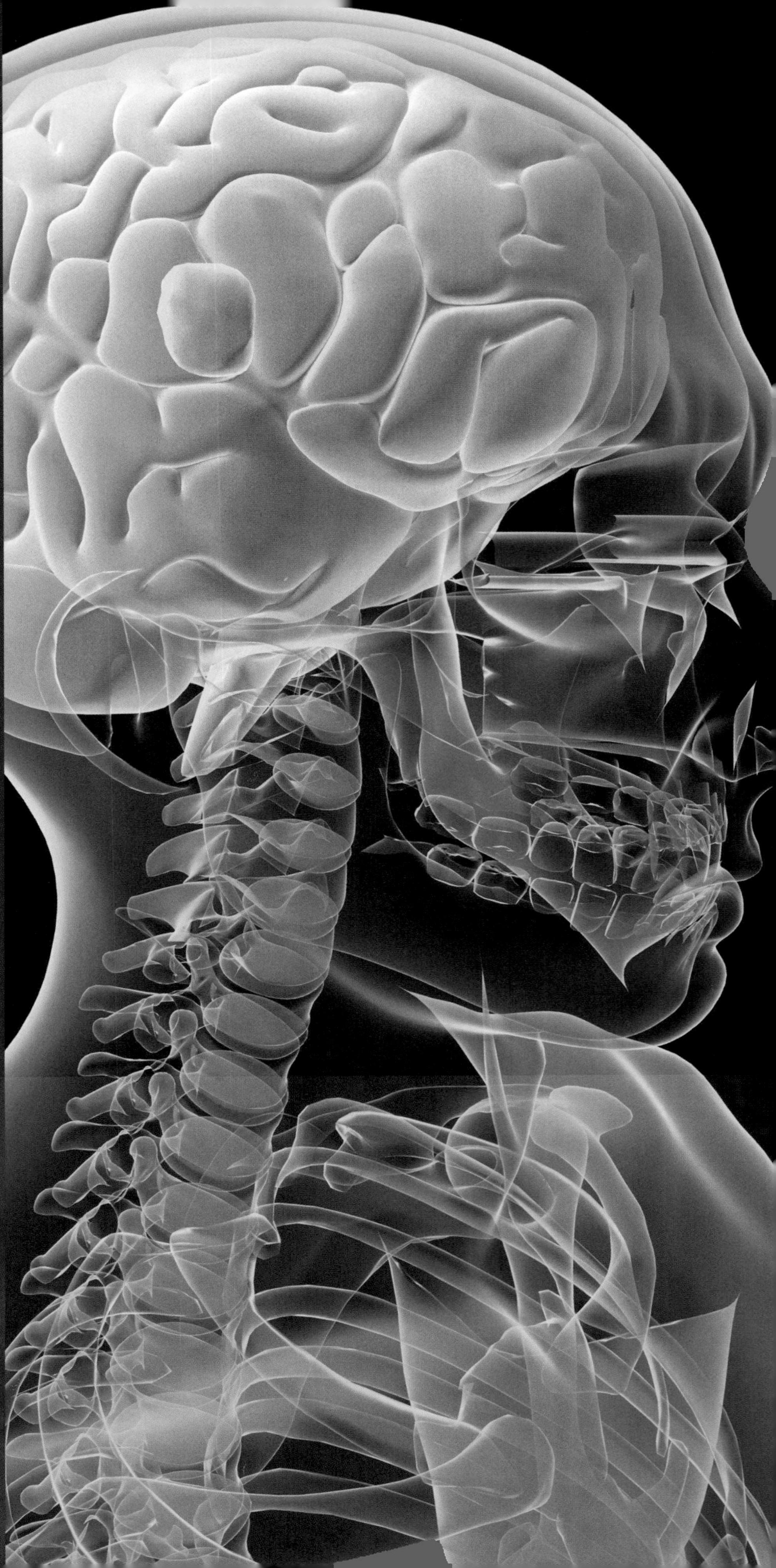

KEY TERMS

Page numbers indicate where in the chapter the term is used.

acidophilic normoblasts 71
actin 60
actin filaments 73
active transport 73
adenosine triphosphate (ATP) 58
adherens junctions 73
afferent 77
Akt 70
amino acids 58
anchoring system 74
antibodies 72
antigen 72
apoptosis 69
autonomic nervous system (ANS) 77
B cell 72
B lymphocyte 72
basophil 64
basophilic normoblast 71
blastocoel 70
blastoderm 70
blastula 70
cadherins 73
catenin 73
CdK 69
cell cycle 69
cell-mediated immunity 72
cellular membrane 57
cell wall 73
ceramides 75
cholesterol 75
chondroitin sulfate 67
cleavage 70
cluster of differentiation (CD) 73
complement system 73
connective tissue 72
connexins 74
corium 78
corneocyte 60
cornified envelope 75
corpuscles of Ruffini 78
cutaneous 63
cycle 59
cyclin 69
cyclin-dependent kinase (CdK) 69
cytokines 61
cytoplasm 57
cytoskeleton 60
cytotoxic (killer) T cell 73
daughter cell 60
dendrite 62
dendritic cell 62
dermatan sulfate 67
dermis 60
desmocollins 74
desmogleins 74
desmoplakin 74
desmosome 66
DNA synthesis 69
ectoderm 71
efferent 77
elaunin 67
embryo 70
end-bulbs of Krause 78
endoderm 71
endoplasmic reticulum (ER) 58
eosinophil 64
epidermal growth factor (EFG) 61
epidermis 60
epidermolysis bullosa 66
epithelial tissue 72
epithelium 72
erythrocyte 71
external ectoderm 70
fibril 66
fibroblast 63
fibroblast growth factor (FGF) 70
fibrocyte 63
fourth germ layer 70
free fatty acid 75
free nerve terminals 77
G_0 69
G_1 69
G_2 69
gap junctions 74
gastrula 70
gastrulation 70
germ layer 70
glial cells 72
glycosaminoglycans (GAGs) 66
Golgi apparatus 59
granulocytes 64
helper T cells 73
hemidesmosomes 74
hemocytoblast 71
heparan sulfate 67
heparin 67
homeostasis 76
humoral 72
hyaluronic acid 67
hypochlorous acid 64
immune system 72
insulin-like growth factor (IGF-I) 70
integrin 75
interleukin-1 61
intermediate filaments 61
islet of Langerhans cells in the pancreas 63

KEY TERMS, CONT.

JNK 70
keratin 61
keratin proteins 60
keratin sulfate 67
keratinocyte 60
keratinocytoblasts 66
keratinohyaline granules 66
Langerhans cell 63
leukocyte 64
lipase 64
lipid bilayer 57
lymphocytes 61
lymphokine 73
lymphotoxins 73
lysosome 59
lysozyme 73
macrophage 73
mandibular nerve 77
MAPK 70
mast cell 63
maturation promoting factor (MPF) 69
maxillary nerve 77
Meissner's corpuscles 78
melanocyte 62
melanocyte-stimulating hormone (MSH) 62
melanogenesis 62
melanosomes 62
membrane 57
memory T cells 73
Merkel's discs 78
mesenchymal tissue 63
mesoderm 70
microfilaments 60
microtubules 60
mitochondria 58
mitosis 69
monocyte 65
mother cell 60
motor (efferent) neuron or nerve 77
muscle tissue 72
myelin 72
myeloperoxidase 64
myosin 60
nervous tissue 72
neural crest 62
neural tube 70
neurofilament 61
neuroglia 72
neuron 70
neutrophils 64
nuclear membrane 59
nucleolus 59
nucleus 59
ophthalmic nerve 77
organelle 58
oxytalan 67
p27 protein 69
p53 protein 69
Pacinian corpuscle 78
parasympathetic divisions 77
phagocyte 64
phospholipids 57
plakoglobin 74
plaques 74
plasma membrane 74
platelet-derived growth factor (PDGF) 70
pluripotential stem cell 71
polychromatic normoblasts 71
polymorphonuclear cells 64
pro-enzyme 75
pronormoblast 71
protein 57
protein-tyrosine kinase activity 70
proteoglycans 67
proteolysis 75
receptor 58
receptor sites 58
reflex arc 77
respiratory burst 64
reticulocyte 71
ribosomes 58
selective permeability 57
senescent cell 69
sensory (afferent) neuron or nerve 77
stem cell 60
superoxide 64
suppressor T cells 73
sympathetic divisions 77
T cell 72
thymidine dinucleotide fragments 62
tight junction 73
transit time 61
trigeminal nerve 77
tubulin 60
vacuoles 59
versican sulfate 67
vimentin 61
white blood cell (leukocyte) 61
zygote 70

Estheticians' area of specialty is the skin, a living, breathing organism. To understand the skin, its functions, and its treatment, an esthetician must first understand the functions and activities of the body and, specifically, of the cell. This complex, nearly self-contained unit is the basis of the body and all bodily functions. An understanding of the histology of cellular function helps an esthetician better appreciate a cell's ability to work cooperatively with other cells in specialized cellular tissue, such as skeletal tissue, or in an organ, such as the heart, liver, or skin. Understanding the histology and the physiology of the skin provides the esthetician with a powerhouse of knowledge, which forms the basis of a successful skin care practice.

CELLULAR STRUCTURE AND FUNCTION

A cell is the basic unit of life, and all life functions go back to the cell. Every cell is composed of a nucleus, organelles, and a semipermeable cellular membrane (also called the plasma membrane). It is a miniature city with all the necessary parts for reproduction and for many other functions as well (Figure 3–1).

Although all cells have the same components, they fulfill different functions. Shortly after conception, the process of **cellular differentiation** starts to occur and each basic cell starts to specialize. Cells voluntarily gather together to form different tissues and perform different functions. They communicate with each other using electrical impulses and enzymes in a manner that dates to prehistory. They combine a limited number of "words" into a multitude of different commands in much the same way humans take the 26 characters of the alphabet and form them into millions of words. Cellular function and communication triggers growth and maintenance, resists aging, and is in a constant battle with external elements. To be able to treat skin conditions effectively, it is important to understand cell structure and functions.

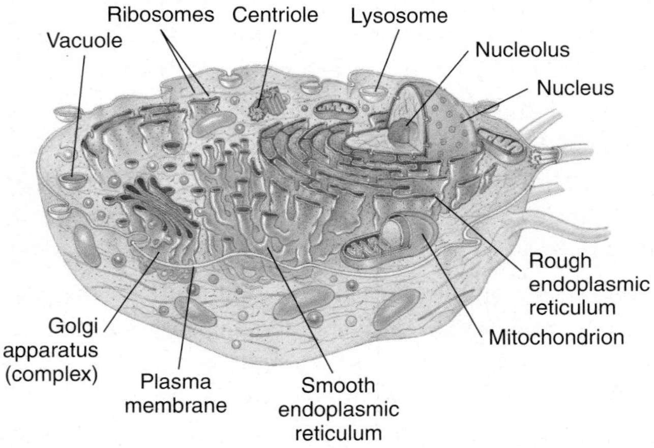

Figure 3–1 Structure of the cell.

The Cellular Membrane

The **cellular membrane** is made up of a network of lipids (fatty material) and **protein.** The **membrane** possesses a quality known as **selective permeability,** which gives it the ability to let substances into and out of the cell. The cell is furnished with food, water, and oxygen by the blood (which is itself made up of cells). Blood also carries waste materials and carbon dioxide away from the cell membrane and, eventually, out of the body.

The cellular membrane is not a single thickness but rather a **lipid bilayer**—two layers of lipid with water sandwiched in between. Figure 3–2 shows the **phospholipids** that make up this layer and give the cell its globe-like three-dimensional form. Each ball shape represents the lipid polar head, which is hydrophilic (water-loving) and carries a polar charge. The wavy lines represent the lipid tail, which is hydrophobic (water-hating) and nonpolar. The double-layer composition makes a very effective barrier to outside substances while retaining the **cytoplasm,** the fluid that fills the cell.

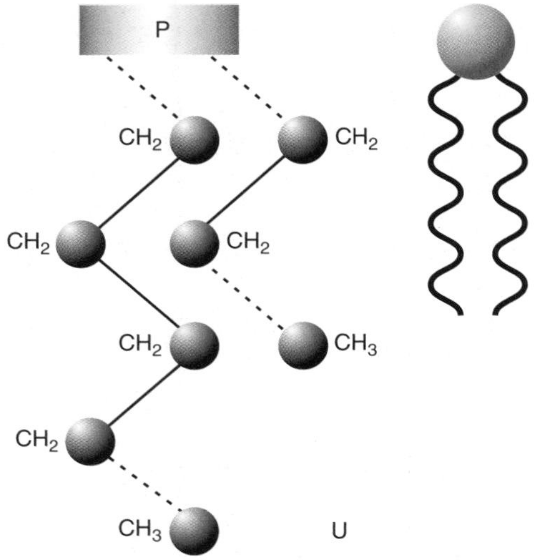

Figure 3–2 Phospholipids.

Located on the cell membrane are special structures called **receptor sites**. **Receptors** are the communication system between different cells, tissues, organs, and parts of the body. Each tissue has cells with unique receptor sites that carry out the activity of a particular type of cell. Receptors receive messages from hormones and other chemical messengers made by other cells. A chemical messenger must go to its correct receptor or it cannot communicate with the cell. Receptor sites work with these chemical messengers in a "lock and key" system (Figure 3–3). When a chemical—"the key"—comes in contact with its specific special receptor—"the lock"—a message is sent to the cell, which carries out specific functions. An example of this is sebaceous gland activity. Production of sebum in the sebaceous gland is stimulated by androgen hormones received by the receptor sites in the cells of the sebaceous gland. The sites are like switches that are turned on when androgen stimulates the receptor site. Any chemical messenger must go to its correct receptor or it is not allowed to communicate with the cell.

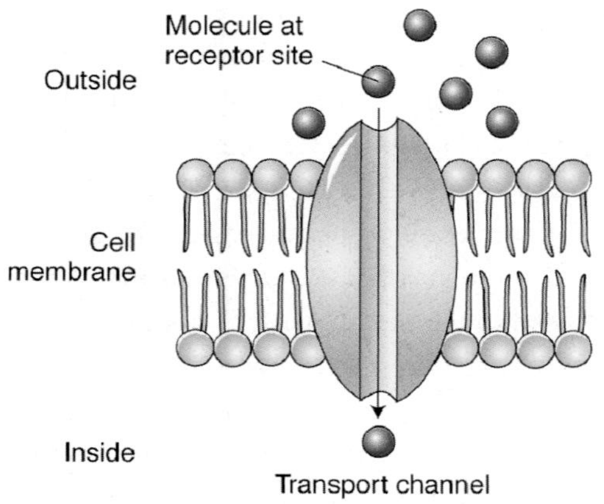

Figure 3–3 Cell receptor site.

Organelles

Organelles are small structures within a cell that each have their own function. Think of organelles as miniature body organs. For many years scientists did not know about the existence of organelles, but as science and microscopes progressed, these microscopically small structures were discovered. Following is a discussion of some of these organelles and their functions.

Endoplasmic Reticulum (ER)

Inside the cell cytoplasm, there is a structure that is formed like a maze, sort of like a house of mirrors at a carnival. This is called the **endoplasmic reticulum**, or **ER**. This network of material forms little canals with the cytoplasm that allow substances and other organelles to move around. Think of the ER as blood vessels within the body. When viewed through an electron microscope, ER can have two appearances, one rough and one smooth. The rough ER has ribosomes attached to it while the smooth does not.

Ribosomes

Ribosomes are very small organelles that are the protein "construction division" of the cell. They help build protein structures from a set of genetic instructions when needed by the cell. Ribosomes can float freely within the cytoplasm or attach to either the ER (endoplasmic rerticulum, a cell organelle) or the nuclear membrane.

Mitochondria

Mitochondria are the cell's lungs and digestive system, converting oxygen and nutrients so that they can be used as energy by the cell. The mitochondria are also responsible for converting oxygen to carbon dioxide, which is an essential part of the oxygen usage system within the body. The mitochondria also have "departments" that control the amount of water and other substances that are allowed into the cytoplasm at particular times. In their job as the digestive system, mitochondria help to break down simple sugars, fats, and parts of proteins called **amino acids**. Mitochondria take other nutrients, such as proteins, fats, and carbohydrates, and manufacture a substance called **adenosine triphosphate**, better known as **ATP**. ATP is a ready-to-use energy packet that can be used by any organelle in the cell.

The production of ATP happens in a **cycle** sequence known as the citric acid cycle or Krebs cycle, a complex sequence of enzymatic steps in which lactic acid is converted to energy. In the absence of oxygen all glucose in the skin is metabolized to lactic acid, which produces two energy molecules called ATP or adenosine in the process is known as anaerobic metabolism. Some skin treatments have been known to increase the production of ATP, making skin healthier.

The Golgi Apparatus

The **Golgi apparatus** is a packaging and processing apparatus for large proteins that prepares them for secretion.

Lysosomes

Lysosomes can be thought of as the cell's garbage disposal system or recycling center. They digest waste material and food within the cell. They manufacture enzymes that help break apart large molecules entering the cell so that they can be more easily converted to other necessary chemicals and substances. Lysosomes are also the "self-destruct" mechanism for the cell. When a cell dies, the lysosome releases enzymes that help destroy the cell membrane.

Vacuoles

Vacuoles are often the largest of the organelles. They are the cell's "storage vats" for molecules of waste and excess food supplies. They can be used to isolate materials that may be harmful to the cell. Their presence helps maintain the correct pH of the cell and gives it shape.

The Nuclear Membrane 25

The **nuclear membrane** surrounds and contains the nucleus which houses the DNA, the master molecule of the cell. Like the cellular membrane, the nuclear membrane is selectively permeable, allowing for transfer of chemical messages into the nucleus, where those messages can trigger actions (Figure 3–4). This membrane also has receptor sites that function in the same manner as those on the cellular membrane do.

The Nucleus 26

The **nucleus** is the brain of the cell. Like the central processing unit on a computer, the nucleus controls a multitude of functions quickly and efficiently. This large organelle is composed mainly of protein and is responsible for building certain proteins. Chromatin fibers within the nucleus—which are made up of nucleic acids, including DNA—are responsible for cellular division.

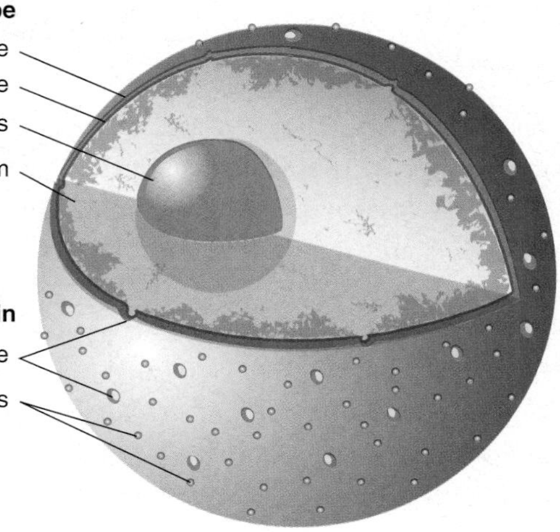

Figure 3–4 The nucleus and nucleolus.

The Nucleoleus

The main function of the **nucleolus,** which is a sub-organelle of the nucleus, is the creation of ribosome components. No membrane separates it from the nucleus. Scientists suspect that the nucleolus has some additional roles in cellular function, but these have not yet been identified.

Cellular Function

Once familiar with the components of a cell, it is easier to understand how that cell works. First, after food is broken down by a person's digestive system, absorbed through the intestinal wall, and absorbed by the blood, blood delivers food to the cells while other blood cells deliver fresh oxygen from the lungs. The cell membrane acts as a guard, allowing certain substances into the cytoplasm. Once inside, those substances may be guided to their destination by the canals of the ER. The lysosomes then start breaking down the large protein molecules. The ribosomes are building or "rebuilding" the proteins that the cell needs at the time. The mitochondria serve as a "power plant," making usable energy for the cell from the variety of proteins, sugars, oxygen, and fats that have arrived. Excess food and waste from production are stored in the vacuoles. The Golgi apparatus stores proteins to use later for manufacturing enzymes and hormones. 3 After the production process is over, the cell membrane releases waste materials and carbon dioxide into the blood, which takes the waste away to the lungs, where the carbon dioxide is breathed out, and to the kidneys, which filter out the other waste.

A BRIEF OVERVIEW OF SKIN STRUCTURE AND FUNCTION

The skin is the largest organ of the body—1.8 square meters in size. That is just about the size of a 4 feet by 8 feet piece of plywood! The two major layers of skin, the epidermis and the dermis, vary a great deal in size, cell structure, and function.

The **epidermis** is the outer, actively growing layer of the skin (Figure 3–5). The thickness of the epidermis varies on different parts of the body. The thinnest area ranges from 0.05 millimeters (mm) to 0.1 mm at the eyelids to the thickest area of 1 mm to 1.5 mm on the palms and soles. (A millimeter is a small measurement. In one inch, there are 25.4 millimeters.) The epidermis is made up mostly of a type of cell called a keratinocyte, but it also contains other types of cells—melanocytes, Langerhans cells, and Merkel cells.

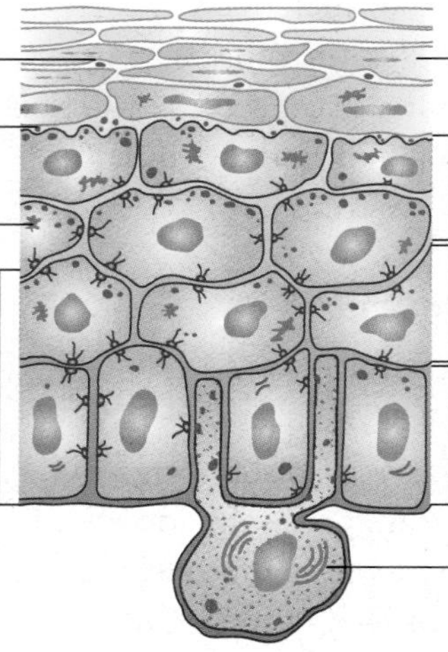

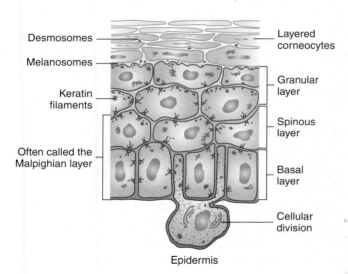

Figure 3–5 The epidermis.

The **dermis**, or underlayer, is much thicker. On the palms and soles and back it is 3 mm thick or more, but on the eyelids and the penis it is only 0.3 mm thick. The dermis contains some cells, but not as many as the epidermis does. These include cells called fibroblasts, mononuclear phagocytes, lymphocytes, Langerhans cells, mast cells, and histiocytes (many of which are covered in more detail later in this chapter).

Together, these layers of skin serve a number of purposes:

- Serve as a physical and chemical barrier, including against ultraviolet light, and prevent moisture loss from the body
- Provide body temperature control
- Enhance sexual attraction
- Metabolize many chemicals
- Protect the body against bacteria and other infectious organisms
- Produce vitamin D Converts—precursor to actual vitamin D
- Provide immune functions

THE CELLS OF THE EPIDERMIS

Keratinocytes

The majority of cells in the skin are **keratinocytes**, which have many functions and go through several stages of differentiation before they reach the skin's surface. Starting at the bottom, or basal layer, of the epidermis, the keratinocyte starts its journey to the top, beginning as a **stem cell**, known also as a **mother cell**. This cell is capable of dividing many times and forming new cells called **daughter cells**. After cell division, the mother cell rests until it is ready to divide again. Meanwhile, each new daughter keratinocyte starts its one-way journey, passing through four stages to the top of the epidermis. During the process, which is controlled by the cell nucleus, the cell is taken apart and provided with a protein-like armor that serves as a protective stratum corneum cell, also called the "horny layer." From a living viable cell, the daughter cell is transformed into a tiny slab of protein and lipid, a **corneocyte**.

The process starts by **keratin proteins** forming in the cell. This process is the differentiation of keratinocytes cytoskeleton, which is the support structure in the cell. The **cytoskeleton** is a fine network of protein fibers in the cytoplasm of the cell that provides shape and support for the cell; moves the organelles of the cell, such as the nucleus and mitochondria; and moves the cell. Three main fibers make up the cytoskeleton:

- **Microfilaments** are protein strands called **actin** (which is the most abundant protein in the cell). The microfilaments are responsible for cell movement and cell shape. Actin works with a second protein called **myosin** to contract muscles. These strands are 3 to 6 nanometers (nm) in diameter.
- **Microtubules** are tiny, cylindrical-shaped tubes composed of a protein called **tubulin**. Microtubules form the scaffold around which the shape of the cell is built and provide tracks (such as trains use) for cellular organelles to move on. A major function of microtubules is to separate chromosomes during

cellular division (often called "spindle fibers"). The microtubules are comparatively large at 20 to 25 nm in diameter.

- **Intermediate filaments** are complex fibers made up of eight subunits and long strands. They help to maintain cell shape, but they also add strength to cells and hold cells together. Some special intermediate filaments are **keratin**, which is found in the skin and hair and makes up most of the corneocyte; **vimentin**, which is an intermediate filament found in fibroblasts; and **neurofilaments**, which are found in nerve cells (Figure 3–6).

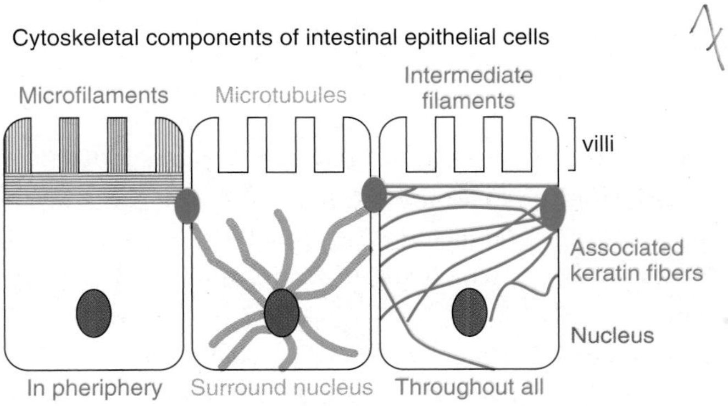

Figure 3–6 The cytoskeleton.

Keratinocytes and Skin Repair

Keratinocytes can either differentiate to become corneocytes or activate to repair the skin. The critical step is the activation that occurs when skin is injured, which sets in motion the process that repairs the injury to the skin. Many substances are involved in skin repair. Chief among these are **epidermal growth factors** (EGF), a hormone that stimulated kerartinocytes to proliferate. and **cytokines, proteins,** or **peptides** that are special messengers that trigger specific action by other cells (Figure 3–7). After an injury, the first signal that triggers the repair process is the cytoplasmic release of cytokines known as **interleukin-1**, or IL-1. The release of IL-I activates endothelial cells (the lining of blood vessels) of the capillaries, which brings fibroblasts and **lymphocytes,** or **white blood cells,** to the wound site. Simultaneously IL-I activates the keratinocytes to divide and grow by a process called **hyperproliferation.** These cells become migratory and deposit a provisional fibronectin-rich basement membrane. The IL-I causes the keratinocyte to produce certain keratins, such as express K6 and Kl6, and then to produce additional growth factors and cytokines, two of which are TGF-β and members of the EGF family. It is these growth factors and the cytokines that keep the keratinocytes activated.

While the activation process is going on, lymphocytes migrate to the wound site to fight infection. They also produce a signal to the keratinocytes to slow down the cell proliferation when the wound is healed. At this stage, fibroblasts also migrate to the wound site, producing a new cytokine called TGF-β, which activates the fibroblasts but also shuts off the activation process of the keratinocytes. When the wound is healed and the system returns to normal, the keratinocyte produces normal keratins. While the process of skin repair is very complicated, it illustrates the complexity of the skin and how much there is yet to learn.

? Did You Know

Keratinocytes need 14 days to grow from the basal layer to the granular-horny layer of the epidermis and 14 more days to reach the top of the horny layer, where they are shed. This is an average time, as younger individuals grow skin faster and older individuals move cells more slowly through the epidermis. This movement of skin cells is called **transit time.** Infections and allergic reactions can speed cell transit time to less than 24 hours! Compare this growth rate to scalp hair, which grows very fast at 0.37 mm/day, or fingernails, which grow at a rate of 0.1 mm/day or about 1 centimeter (cm) in 3 months.

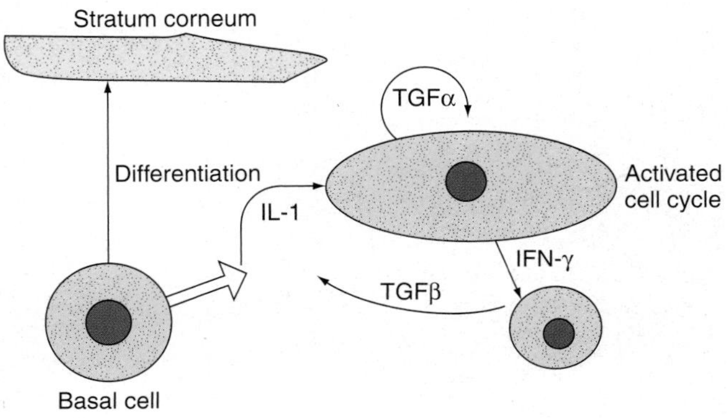

Figure 3–7 Repair cycle of a cell.

The Melanocyte

The **melanocyte** is a cell in the basal layer of the epidermis that produces melanin. The melanocyte is one of the most important cells in the body (Figure 3–8). Melanocytes average 7 micrometers in length. In the epidermis, there are about 1,000 to 2,000 melanocytes per square millimeter of skin. They make up about 5% to 10% of the cells in the basal layer of the epidermis, with a ratio of about 1 melanocyte per 10 keratinocytes.

Melanocytes originate in the **neural crest,** which is an early nerve tissue in the embryo. The early melanocytes migrate widely in the embryo and retain this ability to migrate when they are in the skin. It appears that the number of melanocytes is controlled by keratinocytes secreting growth factors and inhibitors. While a great deal is known about melanocyte growth control, there is still much to learn. Cancer of a melanocyte, known as melanoma, has the tendency to spread readily. Called *metastasis,* this spreading process is the single most important reason that melanomas are so dangerous and life-threatening.

Melanin production is a complicated process known as **melanogenesis.** It can be initiated by several factors: **melanocyte-stimulating hormone (MSH),** adrenal corticotrophic hormone, exposure to ultraviolet light, and inflammation. Exposure to ultraviolet rays causes damage to DNA, which then produces **thymidine dinucleotide fragments.** These fragments trigger release of the MSH, which can then bind to melanocytes to produce melanin. Normally, melanin is first produced in the melanocyte organelles, such as the ER, and passes to the cytoplasm for transport to the **dendrites,** or extensions of neurons. On the way to the dendrites, the melanin is formed into spheres called **melanosomes,** which are then transferred to the keratinocytes (Figure 3–9).

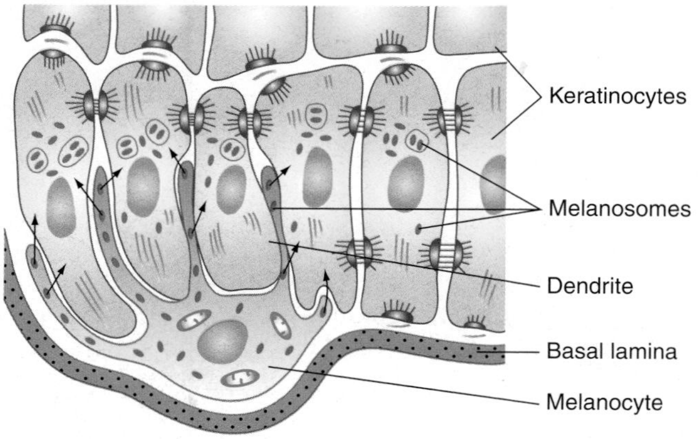

Figure 3–8 Melanocyte.

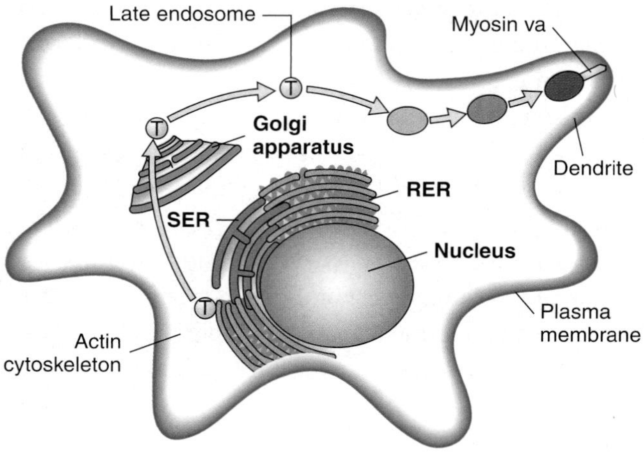

Figure 3–9 The formation of a melanosome.

The melanosomes provide the skin's color. White-skinned individuals have only about 20 small melanosomes per keratinocyte; black-skinned individuals have 200 or more large melanosomes per keratinocyte. True melanin is called *eumelanin* and is dark brown to black. Pheomelanin, which is chemically not identical to eumelanin, can be red or yellow.

Melanin is produced from the amino acid tyrosine by an enzymatic process that uses an enzyme called *tyrosinase.* Almost all skin-lightening agents are designed to block tyrosinase and prevent melanin from being formed. Hydroquinone, which was widely used as skin lightener, has now been moved to prescription drug status because of its side effects. Some safe agents for skin lightening are ascorbic acid, mandelic acid, phytic acid, mulberry extract, licorice root extract, arbutin, and many others.

The Langerhans Cell

In 1868 and 1869 a medical student at the University of Berlin, Dr. Paul Langerhans, made two remarkable discoveries. The first was the presence of a **dendritic cell** (a type of immune-system cell) in the epidermis and the second was the presence of some special cells in the tail of the pancreas. While Dr. Langerhans was not able to appreciate the magnitude of his discovery, his name remains forever linked to two cell types. The first is the Langerhans dendritic cell in the epidermis (which Langerhans thought was a nerve cell). The second cell is known as the **islet of Langerhans cells in the pancreas.** This cell makes insulin and is responsible for diabetes when the cell fails to function.

Langerhans cells reside in all parts of the epidermis, but more are seen in the upper spinosum layer. These young dendritic cells have a dark nucleus and a pale or clear cytoplasm, along with vesicles, multivesicular bodies, and lysosomes, but a Langerhans cell's most distinguishing feature is the Birbeck granules, which look like tiny tennis rackets. These are rod-shaped, 15 to 50 nm long by 4 nm wide, and dark in the center, and they have faint striations radiating from the center to the containing membrane.

In an area of infected or inflamed skin, the local Langerhans cells take up and process the antigens (proteins or other complex molecules that can produce an immune response)—they can be either bacterial, viral, or from plants—and they will travel to the T cell areas of a nearby lymph node (T cells are a component of the body's immune system discussed later in this chapter.) and mature to become fully functional antigen-presenting cells. When arriving in lymphoid tissue, these dendritic cells lose the ability to take up antigens but gain the ability to interact with native T cells.

The cell is free of desmosomes so it is not attached to neighboring cells and there are no tonofilament bundles and no melanosomes. These cells participate in the **cutaneous** immune response and migrate from the skin to the lymph nodes. They possess surface receptors common to macrophages and function as antigen-presenting cells to T or B lymphocytes. Remember that Langerhans cells serve to fix and process cutaneous antigens.

? Did You Know

Langerhans cells are critical for the functioning of the skin's immune system. Just one sunburn will wipe out all of the Langerhans cells in the burned skin for up to six weeks. Fever blisters appear after sun exposure for this reason.

MAJOR CELLS IN THE DERMIS

The dermis, or lower layer of the skin, comprises a number of types of cells, including fibroblasts, mast cells, and leukocytes (white blood cells). Each has its own specialized function within the dermis.

Fibroblasts

Many books could be written on the fibroblast, yet very little is known about this magnificent and versatile cell. It has been called a fibroblast and a **fibrocyte.** It is known that **fibroblasts** make collagen, the most abundant protein in the body, as well as elastin, reticulin, and the glycosaminoglycans, which will be discussed later. It is also known that a fibroblast is not fully differentiated, for it can go both forward and backward in life—that is, it can become a chondroblast or a myoblast or an osteoblast and make cartilage, muscle cells, or bone cells, respectively, or it can become a muscle cell and stay a muscle cell.

Fibroblasts originate in the embryo from **mesenchymal tissue** (stem cells), which is the subject of a section later in this chapter. Fibroblasts are found throughout the body in many tissues and are always associated with connective tissues such as collagen and reticulin. In the skin, the number of fibroblasts differs, but 2,100 to 4,100 per cubic millimeter (mm^3) is a representative range. (This means that 1 cubic centimeter of skin would contain more than a million fibroblasts.)

These are delicate cells, thin and flattened, and found near the fibers they have made. At times they show little cytoplasm, which stains lightly. Fibroblasts appear as spindle-shaped cells when seen on the side, but from the top, the oval nucleus and some thin cytoplasm around it are visible. They are often star-shaped with many long cytoplasmic projections. They are hard to see in dense connective tissue but much easier to see in loose connective tissue.

The Mast Cells

Mast cells can be found anywhere and in almost any connective tissue. Next to the fibroblast, they are the most frequently found cell in the dermis of normal skin. They are very difficult to see in standard skin slides known as H&E preparations. Mast cells have a single nucleus and many large granules in the cytoplasm. The mast cell's functions are not really understood, but they seem to be involved in allergic reactions. The coarse granules in the mast cells are their main identity characteristic. These granules contain heparin, histamine, and sometimes serotonin. In an allergic reaction the mast cells degranulate—that is, they release the contents of the granules into the dermal space.

The Leukocytes

The word **leukocyte** means "white cell." The **white blood cells** may be considered the shock troops of the body's defense forces. Perhaps they were so named because they were first isolated from pus. There are two major types of white cells: granulocytes and lymphocytes. Within those groups, there are three types of granulocytes—neutrophils, eosinophils, and basophils—and two types of lymphocytes—monocytes and macrophages.

The Granulocytes

Granulocytes are so named because they all contain granular particles within the cytoplasm of the cell. They are also called **polymorphonuclear cells,** or PMNs. Wright's stain is the standard stain used to identify the three types of granulocytes: neutrophils, basophils, and eosinphils. Neutrophilic components stain neutral pink, eosinophilic components stain bright red, and basophils stain a dark blue color. We are only speaking about granulocytes here.

NEUTROPHILS

Neutrophilic granulocytes, generally referred to as **neutrophils,** are the most abundant type of white blood cells, comprising 70% of all white blood cells, and are an important part of the immune system. All of the neutrophils are **phagocytes** that live in the blood and in times of infection migrate to the wound site. They are found mainly in the acute phase of inflammation, mostly when a bacterial infection is present. The process of migrating to the infected site is called *chemotaxis*. Neutrophils contain enzymes to digest and kill bacteria. They have a very short life span: If activated, they have an average half-life of about 4 to 10 hours; when activated and in an area of infection, they can survive from 1 to 2 days.

Neutrophils kill infected cells with oxygen in a process called a **respiratory burst** (Figure 3–10). This system requires an oxidative enzyme, which produces large quantities of **superoxide,** which is a free radical. Superoxide is changed to hydrogen peroxide, which in turn is converted to **hypochlorous acid** (HOCl, also known as chlorine bleach) by a second enzyme known as **myeloperoxidase.**

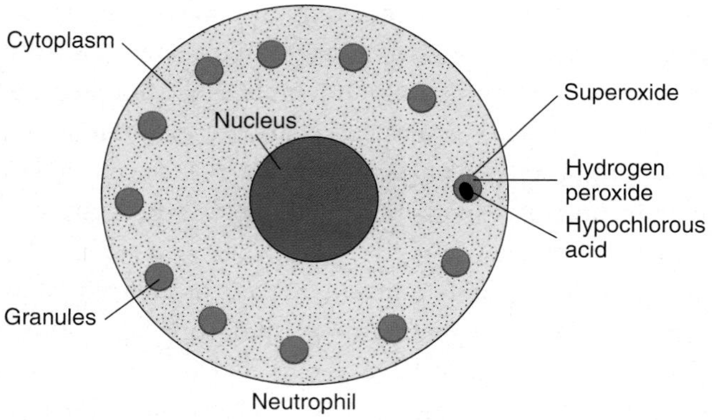

Figure 3–10 The killing action of neutrophils.

EOSINOPHILS

Eosinophilic granulocytes, commonly referred to as **eosinophils,** are white blood cells that specifically attack parasitic infections in the body. This is not their only function; they are also active in immunological reactions, including those to allergies and asthma. The granules in these cells contain many enzymes, including histaminase, peroxidase, Rnase, Dnases, **lipase,** plasminogen, and other enzymes and chemicals that are toxic to parasites. Eosinophils stay in the bloodstream for 6 to 12 hours but can survive for 2 to 3 days. They are a little smaller than neutrophils—10 to 12 micrometers—and comprise about 1% to 5% of a body's white blood cells. Eosinophils do not usually appear in the skin; if they do, it is a sign that a disease is present.

BASOPHILS

The function of **basophils** has only recently been understood, and they are still the subject of much research. They are the least common of the granulocytes, representing 0.5% to 1% of circulating white blood cells. When needed, basophils leave the bloodstream and go to a site of injury, infection, or allergy. They are powerful chemical factories, secreting histamine, leukotrienes, proteoglycans, and several cytokines (all chemicals important to the immune system, which will be discussed later). Interleukin-4 is considered one of the critical cytokines in the development of allergies and the production of IgE antibody by the immune system. Other plant or animals substances can activate basophils to secrete defense chemicals, suggesting that these cells have other roles in combating inflammation.

Lymphocytic Cells

The lymphocytic cells consists of the lymphocytes and the monocytes.

The lymphocytes are small cells with a dark blue nucleus and small amounts a pale blue cytoplasm. You will soon see that the two major types of lymphocytes, the B Cells and the T Cells make up a major part of the immune system.

Monocytes are large cells with a dark bean-shaped nucleus and pale cytoplasm with small red granules dispersed in the cytoplasm. When activated by certain cytokine they become a macrophage, one of the most poweful cells in the body.

HOW KERATINOCYTES REPLACE THE STRATUM CORNEUM

Keratinocytes provide a barrier between an individual and the environment. Remember that these cells must prevent the entry of toxic substances from outside the body and then keep the good things inside. To do this, the keratinocytes must differentiate, or undergo changes, as they move up from the basal layer to the skin's surface. Once they reach the top of the epidermis, they replace the stratum corneum in an ongoing process that protects the body.

The stratum corneum is 15 to 20 layers thick in most areas of the skin. Sunburn, abrasion, or just plain rubbing will cause the basal layer to proliferate—meaning stratum corneum cells are lost and must be replaced. Treatments such as alpha and beta hydroxy acids, enzyme peels, and microdermabrasion initiate repair of the stratum corneum. The turnover time for the stratum corneum is normally between 28 and 30 days, but this process can be slowed by infection or proliferative diseases such as psoriasis.

The study of this replacement process, or keratinocyte proliferation and regulation (control), is a rapidly advancing science with new findings almost every day. Because keratinocyte differentiation is critical to most of an esthetician's procedures, it is important to have a thorough understanding of this process (Figure 3–11).

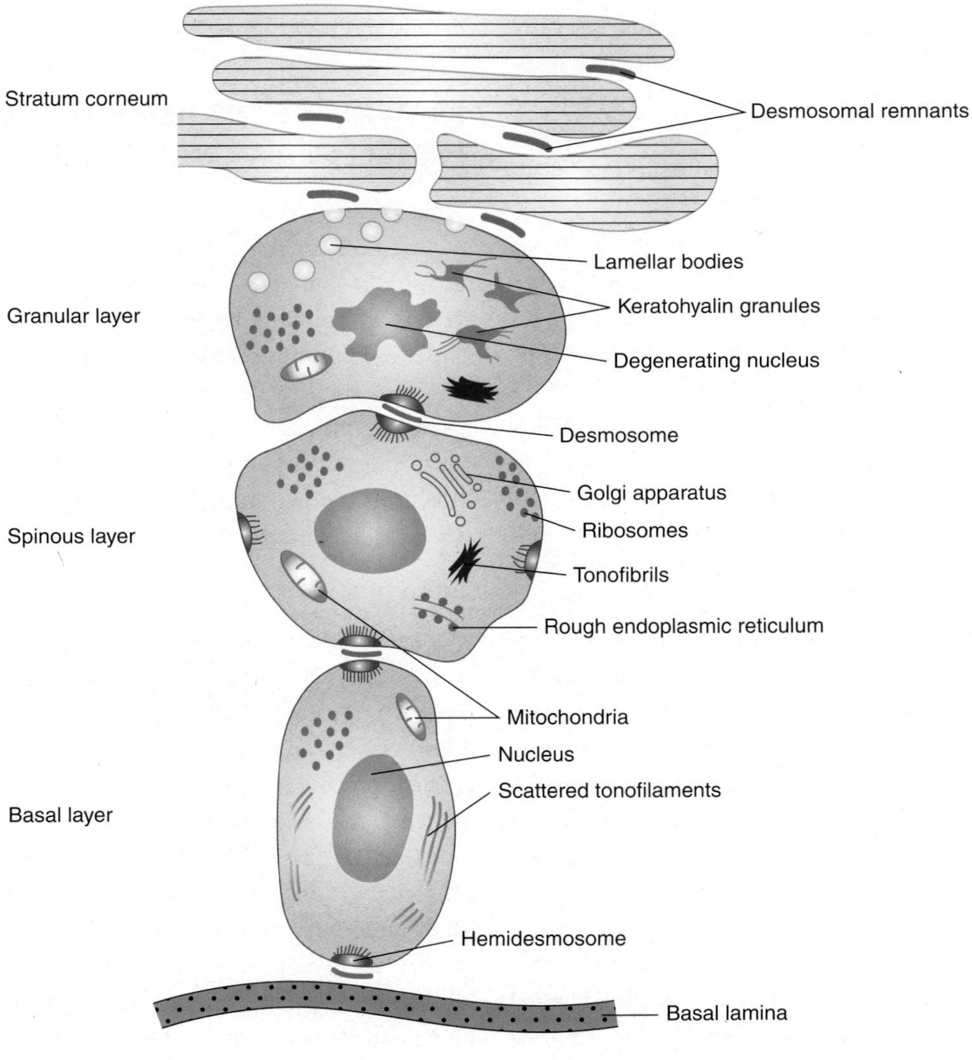

Figure 3–11 This is differentiation.

Once the replacement process is triggered, the keratinocytes arise from keratinocyte stem cells in the basal layer of the epidermis. These stem cells, known as **keratinocytoblasts,** do not have a high rate of mitosis (cell division) but do produce a type of cell known as a *transient amplifying cell,* or TA cell, which divide a limited number of times, then differentiate, and then move up in the epidermis to become stratum corneum cells.

Above the basal layer is the spinous layer, where little bridge-like structures resembling spines between the keratinocytes form intercellular adhesion complexes that are called **desmosomes.** The cells move upward to the granular layer and continue to differentiate, synthesizing **keratohyaline granules,** which are distinguishing features of the cells in that layer. Proteins are synthesized in the granular layer for use in the final cells, the corneocytes, which reside in the top layer, the stratum corneum. Some of these proteins include profilagrin, loricrin, involucrin, and cornifin.

The major proteins formed within keratinocytes, however, are keratins. As discussed earlier, keratins are intermediate filament proteins that form the cytoskeleton of keratinocytes. There are two families of keratins: Type I (acidic keratins) and Type II (basic keratins). These unite in assembly, forming an acidic and basic keratin pair to form units that unite to form keratin filaments. As the keratinocyte differentiates on the pathway to becoming a corneocyte, the types of keratins change.

While it is not important to remember all of these keratins, it *is* important to be aware that the various layers of the epidermis are composed of different keratins. Keratins 5 and 14 reside in the basal cells. As keratinocytes leave the basal layer, they become larger and synthesize keratins 1 and 10. In palmar skin there are keratins 1 and 9. In the granular layer keratins 2e and 10 are found. Certain disease states, such as the hyperproliferative disorders of psoriasis and atopic dermatitis, can be identified by keratins 6 and 16. A blistering congenital disease known as **epidermolysis bullosa** is caused by defects in keratins 5 and 14 in the basal layer. These kerartins are numbered so they can be easily recognized. The numbers are related to the structure of the keratin and where they appear in the epidermis. This disease affects mainly children and is very painful; even the pressure of a belt is enough trauma to raise ugly blisters.

Overall, in any understanding of the function of the skin and its complexity, it is important to remember that the epidermis is controlled by hormones called epidermal growth factors, or EGF; fibroblast growth factors, or FGF; and many other biochemicals. In addition, it is important to understand the relationship between the dermis and the epidermis and between the epidermis and the environment.

> **FYI**
>
> There is some evidence that differentiating transient cells are capable of undergoing a process called *dedifferentiation* to regain stem-cell characteristics. This is a rather startling observation for it implies that TA cells can have a new cell fate or even go back to being stem cells. Could this be the result of intrinsic factors within the cell or some effect from the external environment? What this means is that the TA cells that have left the stem-cell status and were believed to be committed to full differentiation are capable of responding to changing circumstances and inductive signals by reversing their differentiation and adopting new fates.

PROTEINS OF THE DERMIS—THE EXTRACELLULAR MATRIX (ECM)

The **extracellular matrix (ECM)** is a composite material having both solid and liquid protein structures that serve as support materials and monitoring systems in the skin. The ECM contains three major classes of biomolecules: structural proteins such as collagen and elastin; specialized proteins, such as fibrillin, fibronectin, and laminin; and proteoglycans, very large molecules having a protein core with long chains of carbohydrates, specifically disaccharide units, known as **glycosaminoglycans (GAGs)** that are attached at right angles to the protein core.

Collagen

Collagen is the most abundant protein in the body. There are at least 12 types and perhaps as many as 20 types of collagen (see Table 3–1). The making of collagen by fibroblasts is both an internal cellular process and an external cellular process (Figure 3–12). This section looks at Type I, which is the most common collagen in the body and the one that comprises the bulk of the skin. Collagen starts as a single **fibril,** or small fiber, called a pro-α-chain; this fibril then undergoes the addition of hydroxylation to certain proline and lysine amino acids in the fibril. (Vitamin C is critical at this stage. Hydroxylation is the addition of an OH group to a molecule.) Next, certain complex glucose molecules are added to the fibril by a process known as

Table 3–1 Eleven types of collagen

ELEVEN TYPES OF COLLAGEN		
Type	**Location**	**Source cell**
I	Skin, bone tendon	fribroblast
II	Cartilage, vitreous humor	chondrocytes
III	Skin and muscle, wounds	Heptocytes, fibroblast
IV	Basal lamina	All epithelial cells
V	Interstitial tissue	Fibroblasts
VI	Interstitial tissue	Fibroblasts
VII	Epithelial tissues	Epithelial cells
VIII	Endothelial cells, short collagens	Fibroblasts
IX	Cartilage, hypertrophic	Chondrocytes
X	Cartilage, fibrilar	Chondrocytes
XI	Associated with types I, III	Unknown

glycosylation. At this stage, three fibers come together and form a triple-helix structure that is then excreted into the extracellular matrix. That is the end of the cell stage.

In the extracellular space, the terminal peptide ends of the collagen fibrils are cut off and discarded. The fibrils are now assembled into a microfibril and cross-linked. Finally, the cross-linked microfibrils are aggregated into a large and tough collagen fiber.

Elastin

Elastin is a very important protein, not just for the skin but also for the lungs, elastic ligaments, bladder, arteries, and elastic cartilage. It is composed of the amino acids glycine, valine, alanine, and proline but contains two additional peptide structures called desmosine and isodesmosine, which are only found in elastin. Elastin starts as a soluble smaller tropoelastin protein molecule and is formed as a very large, highly insoluble protein. This reaction is carried out by an enzyme called lysyl oxidase, which cross-links the smaller strands.

Dermal tissue contains other elastin-like fibers of which there are three types of fibers—oxytalan, elaunin, and elastic—which are believed to differ in their relative contents of microfibrils and elastin. **Oxytalan** fibers contain only microfibrils and are 10 to 12 nm in diameter, **elaunin** fibers contain small quantities of amorphous elastin, and elastic fibers are predominantly elastin. It is believed that the oxytalan fiber forms a sort of scaffold onto which the elastic fibers are built. Some scientists think elaunin is an intermediate form of elastin. The elasticity is due to the highly crossed-linked elastin protein. There is a microfibrillar component to elastin called fibrillin 1, which is a very large glycoprotein. (Glycoproteins are molecules that contain both a sugar and protein, and the sugar is usually glucose.)

Proteoglycans

Within the dermis the ECM surrounds the cells and bathes the fibers with a thin syrup-like liquid that is highly responsive to external and internal stimulation. With a little pressure the liquid phase rapidly becomes a solid or gel phase and just as quickly returns to a liquid phase. This action occurs with water binding to large molecules (macromolecules) called **proteoglycans**. Proteoglycans consist of a protein and a complex sugar called a *polysaccharide,* which is also called a *glycosaminoglycan*. One of these glycosaminoglycans is **hyaluronic acid** (which has no protein component); another one is called **dermatan sulfate**, and between them they account for most of the proteoglycans. The proteoglycan content in the skin is only 0.1% to 0.3% (dry weight of the skin). The other five glycosaminoglycans are **chondroitin sulfate**, **keratin sulfate**, **heparan sulfate**, and **heparin**, but the most important one in this group is a newly identified one called **versican sulfate.** Versican is produced by fibroblasts, smooth muscle cells, and epithelial cells (Figure 3–13). Part of the reason it is so versatile is its ability to bind to various sites. The major function of versican is to provide turgor or tautness to the skin by interacting with the elastin and the hyaluronic acid.

The proteoglycans maintain water levels in the dermis, provide support for other dermal components, and

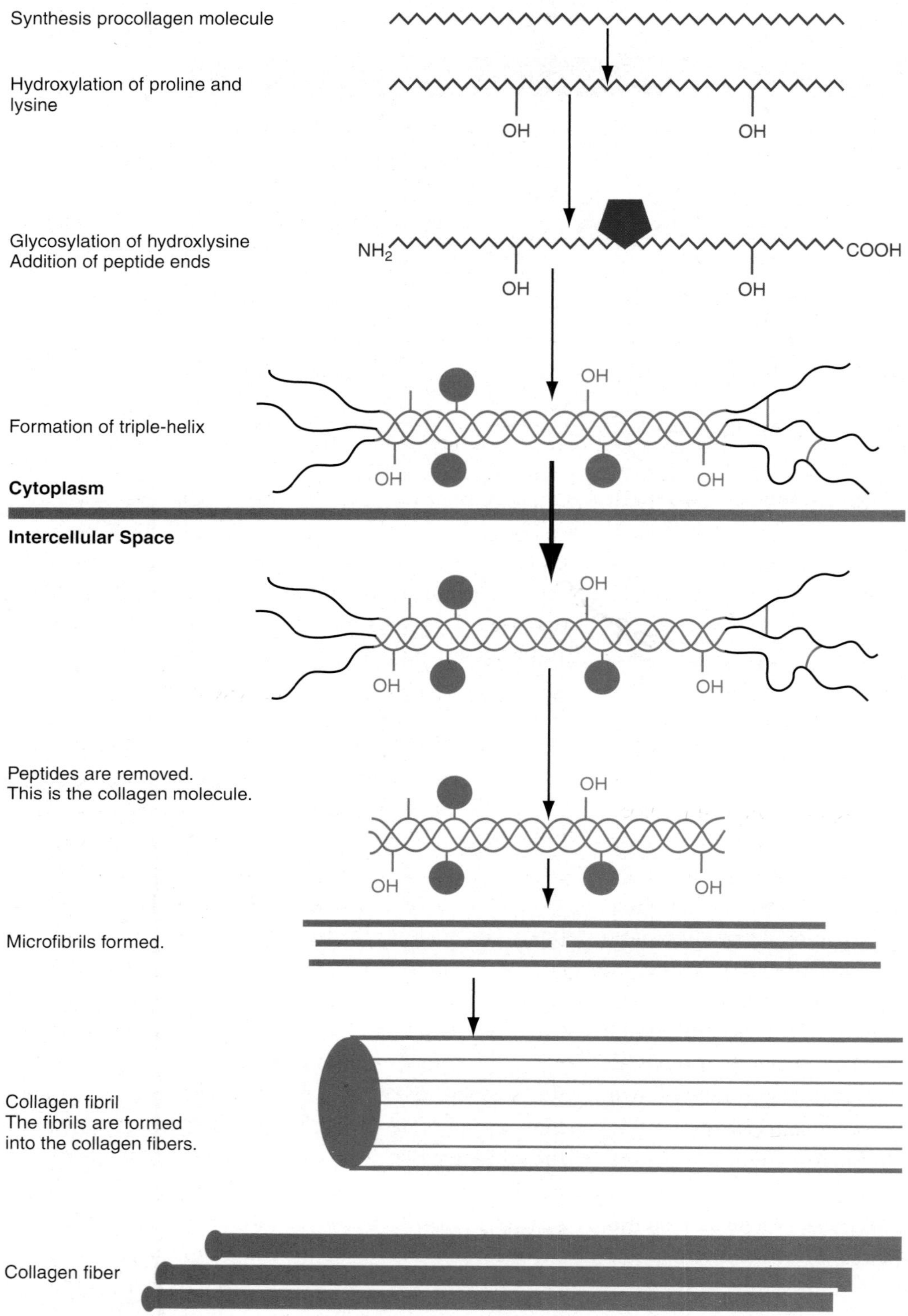

Figure 3–12 The many steps of making collagen.

function as a matrix for cell migration, metabolism, and growth. There are other smaller glycoprotein molecules in the ECM, such as laminins, fibronectin, vitronectin, matrilins, and tenascins, which all have functions in cell communication, cell adhesion, and intercellular communications. While support for the skin is one function of the ECM, the macromolecules provide exquiste regulation of cellular function.

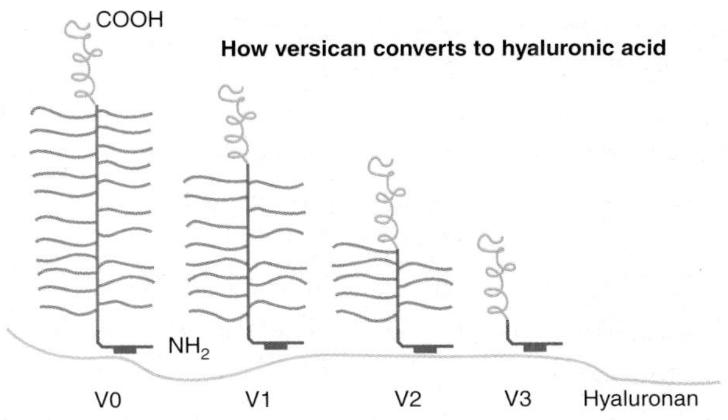

Figure 3–13 How versican converts to hyaluronic acid.

? Did You Know

DNA is a long sequence of chemicals called *bases* that make up about 35,000 pairs of genes. The genes are a precisely coded sequence of bases that have a specific function, from causing enzyme activation to making cells divide.

THE CELL CYCLE

For a cell to grow, it must keep all of the original DNA and make new DNA for the daughter cell. The purpose of this **cell cycle** is making new DNA. DNA, or deoxyribonucleic acid, is a large molecule made up of chains of repeating units of the sugar deoxyribose (which is simply the sugar ribose less one oxygen molecule) and phosphate linked to four different bases. The bases are abbreviated: A for adenine, T for thymine, G for guanine, and C for cytosine. These four bases contain all of the information DNA needs for specifying the proteins that allow life. Unless exact copies of the DNA in chromosomes are passed onto daughter cells, all life would cease!

The cell cycle starts with a resting cell at a stage called **G_0**. Something happens to cause the cell to divide, and then a whole series of events cause the cell to enter a new stage called **G_1**. At this stage *all* of the DNA must be checked before moving to the next stage—that means billions of base pairs! After these are checked, the cell enters a third stage in which the DNA is replicated—that is, a whole new set of chromosomes are made. This stage is called **S** (S is for synthesis). At the end of the synthesis stage, the DNA must be checked again to make sure it is exactly the same. This stage is called **G_2**. Again the billions of base pairs are checked,

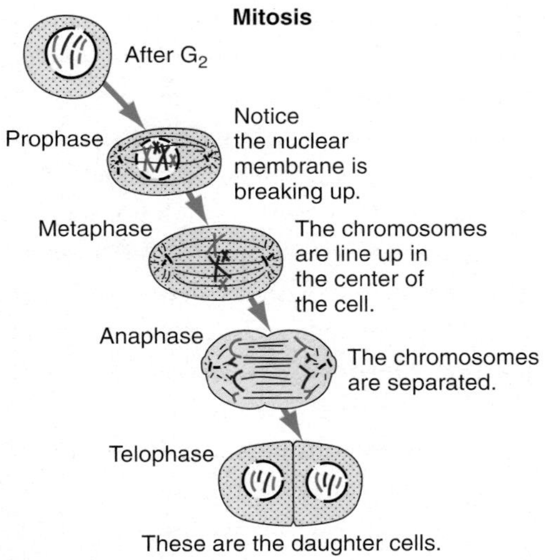

Figure 3–14 Mitosis.

but this time two sets of chromosomes must be checked! If all is well, the cell enters the final stage of growth, which is cell division. This stage is called **M** or **mitosis** (Figure 3–14).

Mitosis yields two new cells—not one young one and one old one, but two new ones. The next step is for the cell to receive a signal to go back into G_0 or to go into G_1 and divide again. What regulates the unbelievably complicated process of **DNA synthesis?** Put simply, **cyclin-dependent kinase**, or **CdK**, along with a series of enzymes called **cyclins**, are major control switches for the cell cycle, causing the cell to move from G_1 to S or G_2 to M. **Maturation promoting factor (MPF)** includes CdK and cyclins that trigger cell-cycle progression. **P53** is a protein that blocks the cell cycle if the DNA is damaged. If the damage is severe, this protein can cause **apoptosis** (cell death). **P27** is a protein that binds to cyclin and CdK, blocking entry into S phase. Clearly, the process of cellular division requires permission from these control chemicals to advance to the next stage, but if there is damage to the DNA that cannot be repaired, either the p53 gene or p27 gene will stop the process or destroy the cell.

FOCUS ON: *Senescent Cells and Cellular Change Associated with Aging*

If a cell is arrested in G_1, it cannot advance or go backward, and in some cases it cannot be destroyed. This is called a **senescent cell** and is a major cause of aging.

The epidermis and the dermis are regulated to a large extent by the same hormone that initiates cell growth. Two of these are epidermal growth factor (EGF) and fibroblast growth factor (FGF). A number of cytokines can also initiate cell division. Cellular proliferation in mammalian cells is associated with a highly organized series of events involving expression of growth-related genes. These genes produce growth regulatory cytokines such as **platelet-derived growth factor (PDGF), fibroblast growth factor (FGF),** epidermal growth factor (EGF), and **insulin-like growth factor (IGF-I)** which are thought to be responsible for initiating proliferation of fibroblasts and other connective tissue cells. Put simply, the process goes like this: Starting with an initiator such as a wound, the damaged tissue releases EGF, which binds to the receptor on the cell surface of a basal keratinocyte called EGFR, or epidermal growth factor receptor. This stimulates intracellular **protein-tyrosine kinase activity.** This action causes a cascade of events that ends by signaling several other proteins into action. These proteins are actually a series of signals within the cytoplasm of the function between the initiating signals and the actual target which is the DNA. Some of these downstream-signaling proteins—including **MAPK,** or **mitosis activating protein,** which stimulates additional intermediate signals such as **Akt** and **JNK** pathways—eventually lead to DNA synthesis and cell proliferation. One reason for all the complexity is possibly fine control of cellular activity which evolved over millions of years.

AN INTRODUCTION TO EMBRYOLOGY—THE STEM CELL

The term *stem cell* has become a household phrase in recent years, but most people could not define the term. Many people argue on one side or the other of stem-cell research but know nothing about stem cells. Because stem cells may eventually figure into skin care (in the remote future), estheticians should be familiar with the term. Understanding stem cells requires a basic knowledge of embryology, which is the study of the very early stages of development, after fertilization, of any living organism, including humans.

The word **embryo** is derived from a Greek word that means "full to bursting." (Actually, the word in current use is more related to medieval Latin, but originally it came from a Greek word.) The embryo starts with fertilization of a woman's egg (ovum) by a male sperm. The fertilized egg is called a **zygote** (from the Greek *zugotos,* yoke, from *zugoun,* to yoke). Through a series of rapid cell divisions, the zygote produces a cluster of cells that is actually the same size as the original zygote. This is called the **cleavage** stage. After 100 cells have been produced, the embryo is called a **blastula.** The blastula is a ball-shaped layer of cells (the **blastoderm**) surrounding a fluid-filled or yolk-filled cavity (the **blastocoel**). At this stage all the cells in the blastula are the same as the first cell—the zygote.

After the blastula is formed, a process called **gastrulation** begins. During this process, cells migrate to the interior of the blastula and form three **germ layers.** The embryo is now called a **gastrula,** and the germ layers are referred to as the *ectoderm, mesoderm,* and *endoderm.* These three germ layers are the stem cells from which all other cells of the body are derived. They are the most important words to learn in embryology. Each of these germ layers produce special cells, tissues, and organs. Here is a list of each type and the cells they produce.

The Ectoderm Germ Layer's Three Parts

The External Ectoderm

The **external ectoderm** is one of the three types of stem cells that derive from the embryo. The ectoderm differentiates into special tissues that supply the skin, along with glands, hair, nails, epithelium of the mouth and nasal cavity, and the lens and cornea of the eye.

The Neural Crest

The neural crest, another component of the ectoderm, is often called the **fourth germ layer** because it is so important. The neural crest makes many types of cells and tissues, such as the **neurons** and glia of the peripheral nervous system (PNS), skeletal and smooth muscle, chondrocytes, osteocytes, melanocytes, supporting cells, hormone-producing cells in certain organs, pigment cells in the skin, facial cartilage, and dentin (in teeth).

The Neural Tube

The **neural tube** provides cells to most of the central nervous system, such as the brain, spinal cord, and motor neurons (nerves), along with the retina and the posterior pituitary gland.

The Mesoderm

Mesoderm stem cells eventually become bones; almost all of the circulatory system, including the heart and major blood vessels and blood cells; the connective tissues of the gut and related covering of organs and gastrointestinal tract; muscles; the peritoneum, which lines the intestines; reproductive system; and urinary system, including the kidneys. Fibroblasts are of mesodermal origin, as are many cells of the immune system (which is discussed later).

Endoderm

The **endoderm** is also a very versatile germ layer. It forms the epithelial lining of the digestive tube, except part of the mouth and pharynx, and the terminal part of the rectum. It also forms lining cells of all glands that open into the digestive tube, which include the liver and pancreas, the epithelium of the auditory tube and tympanic cavity (both in the ear) of the trachea, bronchi, air cells of the lungs, the urinary bladder and part of the urethra, and the cells that line the follicles of the thyroid gland and thymus.

The Ectoderm, Mesoderm, and Endoderm Make Up True Stem Cells

The cells of the **ectoderm**, mesoderm, and endoderm make up the true stem cells. To illustrate the levels of stem-cell capability, start with the blood cell line (Figure 3–15). A **pluripotential stem cell** from the mesoderm is programmed to form all the cells in the bloodstream. In the first stage of this process, that cell becomes a **hemocytoblast.** This cell is now multipotential because it can form white blood cells and red blood cells and any other cells in the blood. In its

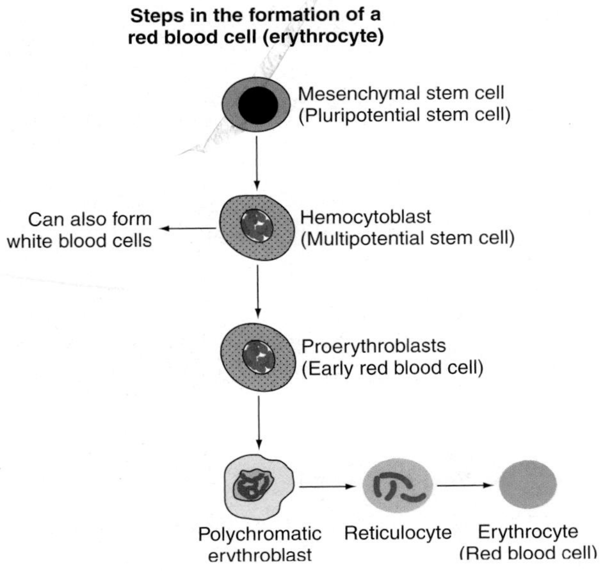

Figure 3–15 Formation of stem cells in the blood.

course of becoming the oxygen-carrying cell in the blood—the **erythrocyte**—the hemocytoblast divides and forms a **pronormoblast,** which is a big cell (20 microns). The pronormoblast continues to divide and form **basophilic normoblasts,** cells that are about 6 to 18 microns in diameter that go on to produce **polychromatic normoblasts,** which are 9 to 12 microns in diameter. The cells start to make hemoglobin at this stage but can no longer divide. The polychromatic normoblast develops into an **acidophilic normoblast,** which is smaller at about 8 to 9 microns in diameter.

At this stage, the cell loses its nucleus, an important diagnostic event. The cell enters the next stage as a **reticulocyte,** which is about 8 microns in diameter and shows a type of stippling in the cytoplasm that is blue in color. The cell contains mitochondria, but there is no nucleus. In the end stage, the erythrocyte appears. It is a small cell, 7 to 8 microns in diameter, with a biconcave appearance. There is no nucleus, but the cell is filled with hemoglobin.

A diagnostic event is a major change in a cell that tells the physician that the cell is either normal or abnormal. A red cell with a nucleus is an immature cell and its presence in the blood stream is diagnostic of severe anemia.

A hemocytoblast is a stem cell that is destined to become a producer of blood cells. It can only produce blood cells, all the types of blood cells. It is programmed to be a hemocytoblast. We do not know why, or how, some mesodermal stems cells become blood cells and others become muscle cells. Mesochymal means any mesodermal cell line, of which blood cells are only one type.

Knowledge of each of these steps is important, especially in situations when a diagnosis is needed. For example, a doctor with an anemic patient can look at a smear of the patient's blood and determine a course of treatment. If the doctor sees reticulocytes, he or she knows the patient is losing blood and trying to form more. If the doctor finds polychromatic normoblasts, he or she knows the patient has severe anemia.

THE MAJOR TISSUES IN THE BODY

All of the organs in the human body are built from four basic tissue types, and each tissue type has specific functions and features. Understanding these basic tissue types is a basis for the study of histology. The four basic tissues are: epithelial tissue, connective tissue, nervous tissue, and muscle tissue.

Epithelial Tissue

Epithelial tissue, which covers the body surfaces, is made up of cells attached to one another, forming an uninterrupted layer of cells that separates the underlying organs or tissues from the external environment. The **epithelium** covers the surfaces, as does the epidermis of the skin, while at the same time penetrating into deep organs such as the bladder. The key functions of epithelial tissue are protection, body fluids containment, and transport of material in and out of the body. Embryonically, most epithelial tissues arise from the ectoderm and a few from the endoderm, such as the lining of the trachea and the lungs.

Connective Tissue

Connective tissue supports other tissues. It consists of several cell types, along with extracellular products that provide functions of mechanical reinforcement, transport, and diffusion of nutrients and wastes, as well as energy storage in fat cells. Connective tissues derive from mesoderm. Collagen, elastin, and fibroblasts are examples of components of connective tissue.

Nervous Tissue

Nervous tissue is a highly specialized tissue that transports signals to other organs. Certain types of nerve cells—particularly **glial cells**—also act as support tissue. Glial cells, also called **neuroglia,** are not actually neuronal cells, though while they provide support and nutrition, they also form **myelin** and participate in signal transmission in the nervous system. Anatomically they lack dendrites and axons, which are the hallmark of neurons. Nerve tissue comes from the neuroectoderm and neural crest.

Muscle Tissue

Muscle tissue, which derives from mesoderm, provides movement for the body. There are three types of muscle tissue: skeletal, cardiac, and smooth. All of the muscles are contractile tissue, meaning they can move things by contraction. The contraction of the heart (cardiac muscle) and peristalsis (smooth muscle) in the bowel are involuntary. Voluntary muscle (skeletal) contraction is used mainly to move the body, or parts of it, while smooth muscle is involuntary and is mainly in the blood vessels and bowel.

THE BASIC IMMUNE SYSTEM

The human **immune system** is an extremely elaborate defense mechanism that the body uses to determine self from non-self; that is, it must recognize its own biological identity from any other object, both living or inert. Any material that elicits an immune response is called an **antigen.** The body's defense against antigens is to develop **antibodies** against them. Within the body every cell displays a marker, based on the major histocompatibility complex (MHC), to identify the cell as self. This marker says, basically, "I am part of you, do not attack me." Any cell not displaying this marker is treated as non-self and attacked. This is a fundamental concept of immunology. Sometimes the system does not function and the body attacks its own tissues, causing autoimmune diseases such as lupus erythematosis or multiple sclerosis.

The Two Immune Systems

The immune system has two major cell types that provide the two major functions. One is the B cell that makes antibodies and is know as the **humoral** immune system. The T cell forms the basis of the cellular immune system, also known as the cell-mediated immune system. While both of these cells are lymphocytes they are quite specific in their functions with no overlap.

The Humoral System—The B Cell

The first of two major parts of the human immune system is **humoral immunity.** In this system, an immature **B lymphocyte** (also known just as a **B cell**) is stimulated to maturity whenever an antigen binds to its surface receptors and there is a T helper cell to help the reaction. This primes the B lymphocyte and it undergoes a process called *clonal selection* and starts to divide and produce many new cells known as *clones*. Most of the new family of clones become **plasma cells,** which produce antibodies specific for the antigen that is binding to its surface. These cells can produce a great deal of antibody—as much as 2,000 molecules per second for up to five days. After this period, they slow down production, but some of the cells become memory cells to respond again should the same antigen reappear. This is the basis of all immunization techniques.

Cell-mediated Immunity—The T Cell

The second major part of the immune system is **cell-mediated immunity** in which the **T cell** (T stands for thymus) plays a large role. T cells are formed in the bone marrow and pass to the thymus gland, where they undergo two selection processes. The first is called the *positive* selection process, which is designed to weed out T cells with the correct set of receptors that can recognize the MHC molecules responsible for self-recognition. The next selection, called the *negative* selection process, finds T cells that can recognize MHC molecules that are complexed with foreign peptides. These T cells are allowed to pass out of the thymus and into circulation.

In the first step of cell-mediated immunity, a cell called a **macrophage** takes in antigens and then processes them internally. The second step is to display pieces of the antigen on the macrophage surface along with some of the protein from the macrophage to the T cell. This sensitizes the T cells so it can recognize the antigens. The problem is that all the cells are coated with various antigenic substances. There are more than 160 clusters (called **cluster of differentiation,** or **CD**), and each is a different chemical molecule that coats the surface. Every T cell and B cell has about 10^5 or 100,000 molecules on its surface.

The large number of molecules on the surfaces of lymphocytes allows huge variability in the forms of the receptors. There are some 10^{18} structurally different receptors in random configurations. Essentially, an antigen may find a near-perfect fit with a very small number of lymphocytes, perhaps as few as one.

There are several different types of T cells, and each have their own role to play in the immune system. **Cytotoxic** or **killer T cells** do their work by releasing **lymphotoxins,** which cause cell lysis. **Helper T cells** serve as managers, directing the immune response. They secrete chemicals called **lymphokines** that stimulate cytotoxic T cells and B cells to grow and divide, attract neutrophils, and enhance the ability of macrophages to engulf and destroy microbes. **Suppressor T cells** inhibit the production of cytotoxic T cells once they are unneeded, lest they cause more damage than necessary. **Memory T cells** are programmed to recognize and respond to a pathogen once it has invaded and been repelled. Cell death is defined as the dissolution of a cell so that no parts of it remain.

Other Components of the Immune System

Human beings are born with an innate immunity system that contains nonspecific antibodies. In addition, there are barriers to invaders, and the skin is one of the best barriers. It cannot be penetrated unless it has a scratch or cut that provides an entrance point. In addition, the low pH of skin is not favorable to bacteria. Should bacteria actually enter the skin, the **lysozymes,** or enzymes in skin cells, destroy bacteria by rupturing their **cell walls.**

Another component of the immune system is the **complement system,** a first line of defense that functions quickly to attack infections. This system is actually a complex series of enzymes in the blood that coats microbes with special molecules, making them more susceptible to phagocytosis. These enzymes also increase vascular permeability of the capillaries, which calls more plasma and complement fluid to flow to an infection site.

THE MECHANISM OF EXFOLIATION—THE DESMOSOMES

Recently there has been increasing interest in light skin-peeling techniques, both chemical and mechanical, associated with various skin care treatments, particularly in facial rejuvenation. All peeling techniques, regardless of the type, require breaking the protein bonds that hold the corneocytes together. Within the epidermis there are at least four types of cellular bonds.

Tight Junctions

Tight junctions occur at the top of the cell and possibly serve some cell communication function, but more likely they provide a barrier function. They prevent proteins from entering a cell unless there is **active transport** for a particular kind of protein. They also help to control the movement of other proteins on the cell membrane. It is only recently that these junctions have been identified in the epidermis.

Adherens Junctions

Adherens junctions provide strong mechanical attachments between adjacent cells. In the heart they hold cardiac muscle cells tightly together as the heart beats. In the skin they hold the cells together along with other proteins. Adherens junctions are complex structures made up of several proteins such as **cadherins**—transmembrane proteins that go from cell to cell and bind to each other. Another protein is known as a **catenin.** Catenins, connected to **actin filaments,** are important in stabilizing cell adherence to avoid the abnormal spread of cells.

Gap Junctions

Passageways are needed between cells to allow the free flow of small molecules that carry messages and signals. **Gap junctions** serve this purpose by forming intercellular channels that allow free passage between the cells of ions and small molecules (up to a molecular weight of about 1,000). The channels are only 1.5 to 2.0 nm in diameter and are constructed of six transmembrane proteins called **connexins.** They permit the flow of ions that cause the contraction of heart muscle and provide strong contraction of the uterus during labor. The control of cell-to-cell communication through gap junctions is thought to be crucial in normal tissue function and during various stages of abnormal growth. Scientists are just beginning to investigate the control of gap junction activity.

Desmosomes

The role that the above three binding proteins play in exfoliation is not fully known, but the role of the desmosome has been well studied and is of critical importance in daily exfoliation and therapeutic exfoliation. The desmosome is the major structure that holds the epidermal cells together, especially the cells of the stratum corneum. It looks much like a spot weld between cells, but its structure is made up of many proteins. First, visualize the two plates or **plaques** located in the cell membrane. This plaque is made up of two proteins:

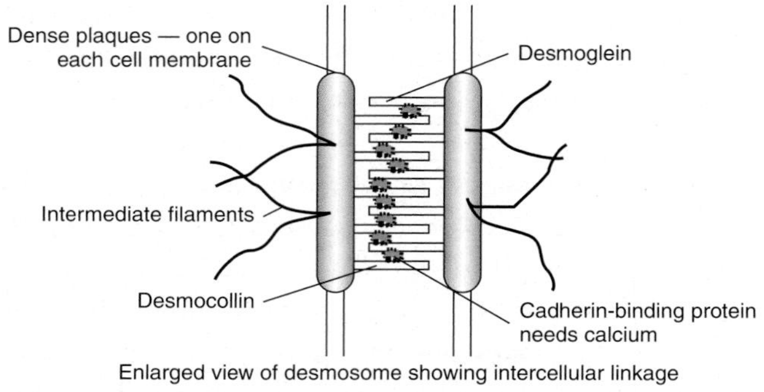

Figure 3–16 Desmosome.

desmoplakin and **plakoglobin.** Extending from the two plaques are projections composed of cadherin proteins called **desmogleins** and **desmocollins.** These proteins interlock with identical proteins from the adjacent cell (Figure 3–16). Inside the cell behind the plasma membrane is the **anchoring system.** The anchoring system ties the plaque to the cytoplasm through the cytoskeleton. First, the plakoglobin and plakophilin bind to the desmoglein and desmocollin proteins that run through the **plasma membrane** into the intercellular space between the cells. Desmoglobin then binds to these proteins and connects to the intermediate filaments in the cytoskeleton. This holds the cells together.

The **hemidesmosomes** bind the basal layer to the basement membrane through different types of proteins (Figure 3–17). The plaque is only on one side of the cell

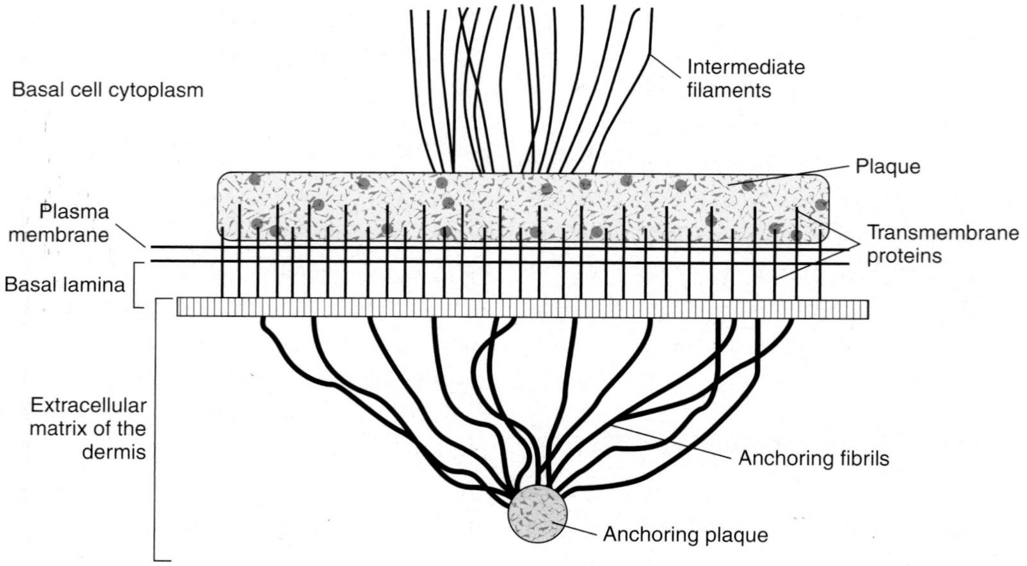

Figure 3–17 Hemidesmosome.

and is composed of plectin protein plus BPAG1. The plaque is held to the basement membrane, called the *basal lamina,* by proteins called **integrins.** The basal lamina is held to the dermis by collagen type IV fibrils.

In the natural process of exfoliation, called *desquamation,* humans lose about a layer of stratum corneum every day. Corneocytes are released one at a time from the skin's surface by breaking the desmosomal proteins that hold them together. This dissolution of the corneocytes is achieved through an enzyme known as *chymotryptic enzyme* (SCCE) in a process called **proteolysis.** This enzyme is packaged in the lamellar bodies of the stratum granulosum in an inactive form called a **pro-enzyme.** The pro-enzyme must be activated in order to hydrolyze the structure to initiate desquamation. (Hydrolysis adds water to the protein and breaks the peptide bond.)

When an esthetician wants to exfoliate the stratum corneum, he or she must use a peptide bond-breaking agent. Many acids do this, though some will only partially coagulate the protein and not actually destroy the peptide bond completely. While coagulation sounds simple, it is really devilishly complicated. There are at least three distinct processes that are closely related. One is the molecular conformational changes, the second is the solution demixing, and the third is intermolecular cross-linking. The body uses enzymes, which is the best method because it is specific; however, at this stage there are no chymotryptic enzymes available for clinical use.

The Stratum Corneum's Rate of Recovery

Generally, a superficial peel that is about 10 cell layers deep in the stratum corneum takes less than two weeks to heal. A good rule to follow is to do chemical peels at intervals of four weeks. The initial peel may be followed by a second peel in two weeks, but this is a one-time-only exception. Keep in mind the time it takes to heal—one layer per day. Healing of the stratum corneum is critical to the control of water loss in the epidermis. The transepidermal water loss is the signal the skin uses to regulate epidermal lipid synthesis, which first restores the lipids of the stratum corneum and then restructures the stratum corneum barrier function. The barrier function of the skin is linked to exfoliation; too much exfoliation can damage the barrier and allow abnormal materials to cross the barrier.

> **? Did You Know**
>
> When an esthetician exfoliates a client, he or she not only releases stratum corneum cells but the process also sends a signal to the basal layer to make more keratinocytes. At the same time, a second signal is sent to the dermis to make more collagen and elastin.

SKIN PENETRATION AND PERMEATION

The barrier of the skin controls the passage of everything that goes into the skin and prevents essential fluids and nutrients from getting out. The mechanical and chemical composition of the stratum corneum forms the skin's barrier. The esthetician needs a clear understanding of the physical and chemical properties of the stratum corneum (SC) and how it functions (Figure 3–18). The corneocytes represent the final stage of epidermal keratinocyte differentiation. At the end of that stage, the SC cells have a highly cross-linked layer of proteins called the **cornified envelope.**

The special construction of the SC involves a cellular arrangement that has been termed a "brick and mortar" construction. The corneocytes are the bricks and the intercellular matrix is the mortar. Visualize the corneocytes as flattened cells (only 1 micron thick) that are packed with keratin filaments and embedded within a protein/lipid matrix of fillagrin and are joined together by junctions called *corneo-desmosomes.* The cornified envelope contains a complex of lipids that surrounds individual corneocytes. The lipid layer is arranged in what is termed a *lamellar bilayer,* which is formed from the fusion of lipid granules called *lamellar bodies* secreted by the corneocytes. There are aqueous pores that open the hydrophilic barrier and allow certain water-soluble compounds to pass into the epidermis.

The lipid components of the SC consist of equimolar (a mole is the molecular weight of a substance in grams) amounts of **ceramides, cholesterol,** and **free fatty acids.** The ceramides are waxy lipids; cholesterol is now well known as a sticky, artery-clogging agent; and fatty acids are break-down products of triglycerides (which are pure fats). If there is any change in the

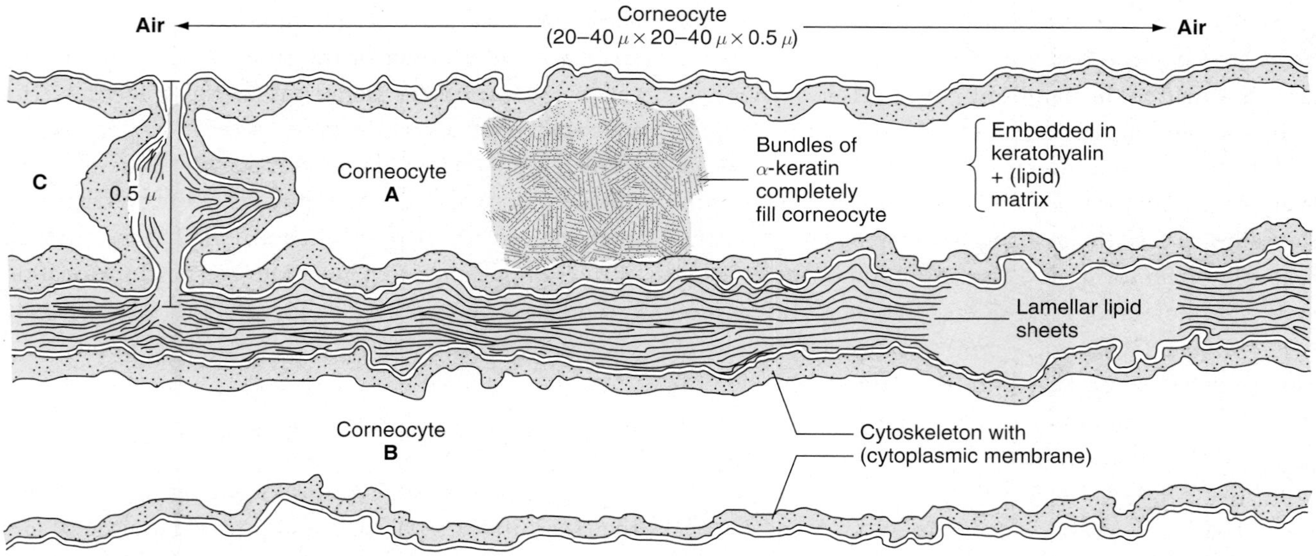

Figure 3–18 Stratum corneum cross section (shown at a magnification of 102,000x).

relative concentrations of any of these lipids, it will have an adverse effect on the barrier quality. For example, in aged and photo-aged skin there will be a barrier with high cholesterol content, while psoriasis is associated with an excess of free fatty acids. Ceramides make up about 50% of the total lipids in the stratum corneum, while cholesterol and free fatty acids make up the remainder.

Maintaining and repairing the barrier is a tough task. When damaged, the barrier's repair can be initiated by loss of these ions of potassium (K) and calcium (Ca) ions during water passing into the damaged area of the epidermis. The pH of the skin is important for barrier **homeostasis.** Scientists believe that the pH functions to keep the enzymes functioning at the proper level of acidity. While it is not known exactly how the pH is maintained, some believe it is due to the lactic acid in sweat and free fatty acids in sebum. Proper acid pH at about 5.5 is needed to maintain micrococci on the skin, which are nonpathogenic. Staphylococcus, which is a pathogen, tends to prefer neutral/basic conditions of pH.

Since an intact SC limits skin penetration, a damaged SC will allow many substances to pass into the epidermis. Soap and detergents are bad for the skin, and while alcohol can remove lipids, it is not as harsh as soaps and detergents. Acetone is a good remover of skin lipids, as is ethyl lactate. To increase penetration of a substance, first treat the skin with an agent to remove the lipids. This can be a physical or chemical agent and will be discussed at length in a later chapter.

The process by which substances penetrate the skin is very complex and not everything is known about it. However, here are a few facts:

- **Charged compounds** do not enter the skin easily; they need helpers such as chemical penetrators.
- **Water** is one of the best penetration helpers. Use of a steamer prior to applying an active ingredient will get more of the active agent into the skin.
- **Soap** and **detergent** used daily on the face is not good for the skin barrier.
- **Lipid compounds** penetrate faster than water-soluble compounds.
- **Hairy areas** of the body are sites for skin penetration.
- **Shaving skin** is a great way to get things into the skin.
- **By applying product via massage,** more product will be delivered into the skin. The mechanical action of massage will stimulate circulation and force more product into the skin.
- **Little molecules** (those under 10,000 molecular weight) get in skin easier than big ones do. In penetration, molecular size does matter.
- **Keep in mind that the effect is always related to the time and dosage.** How much gets into the skin and how long does it stay?

SENSORY NERVES AND PERCEPTION IN THE SKIN

It is important that the esthetician understand that nerves carry sensation to the spinal cord or brain, that message is acted upon by the brain, and a message is sent out. (Although the main facial nerves and the sensory system are discussed below, they will be dealt with in more depth in a later chapter.)

The seventh cranial nerve is the facial nerve. This is a very large nerve that supplies all of the muscles of expression in the face. Its purpose is to move muscles, so it is known as a **motor nerve**. The facial nerve has only a small sensory, or feeling, part, which carries the taste sensation in from the back of the tongue.

The main sensory nerve in the face is the fifth cranial nerve, known as the **trigeminal nerve**. The trigeminal nerve is a large and very complex nerve that supplies sensory feeling to almost all parts of the face. It is divided into three main divisions: the **ophthalmic nerve**, the **maxillary nerve**, and **the mandibular nerve**. The trigeminal nerve has only a small motor part for the chewing muscles, which are the buccinators, masseter, and myohyoid. The trigeminal nerve and its three branches can be remembered as "one up and two down"—that is, the eye branch, the upper jaw branch, and the lower jaw branch.

One other part of the nervous system that affects the face is the **autonomic nervous system** or **ANS**. The ANS is the part of the nervous system that is known as the peripheral nervous system (separate from the central nervous system, which comprises the brain and spinal cord). The ANS maintains all of the body's automatic, unconscious activities, controlling the cardiovascular, digestive, and respiratory systems. A truly autonomous system, the ANS is responsible for functions such as making saliva, perspiration, controlling the pupils, urination, and sexual arousal. It is impossible to separate it anatomically and functionally from the rest of the nervous system.

The **reflex arc** (Figure 3–19) is critical to understanding the ANS. There are two parts to the reflex arcs, a **sensory (afferent) neuron**, and a **motor (efferent or effector) neuron. Afferent** means "toward," as in carrying messages toward the brain or spinal cord. **Efferent** is just the opposite; it means to carry signals away from the brain or spinal cord to the organ, effecting an action. The two major functional divisions of the ANS are the **sympathetic** and **parasympathetic divisions.**

The sympathetic and parasympathetic divisions typically function in a complementary manner. The sympathetic division may be considered the "go" part and the parasympathetic division as the "stop." The sympathetic division functions when quick action is required, commonly called the "fight or flight" response. The parasympathetic division functions when actions do not require immediate reaction. The parasympathetic system is a human being's "friendly, laid-back," and rest system.

The Sensory Receptors in the Skin

The sensory system has a variety of receptors in the skin to detect and sort out sensations of heat, cold, pressure, pain, and itching. The vast majority of these endings are **free nerve terminals** that do not have a specialized ending. They are associated with pain and itching sensations, and their endings are closely situated in the epidermal tissue in the hairy areas of the skin. The skin must not only be able to sense pain, temperature,

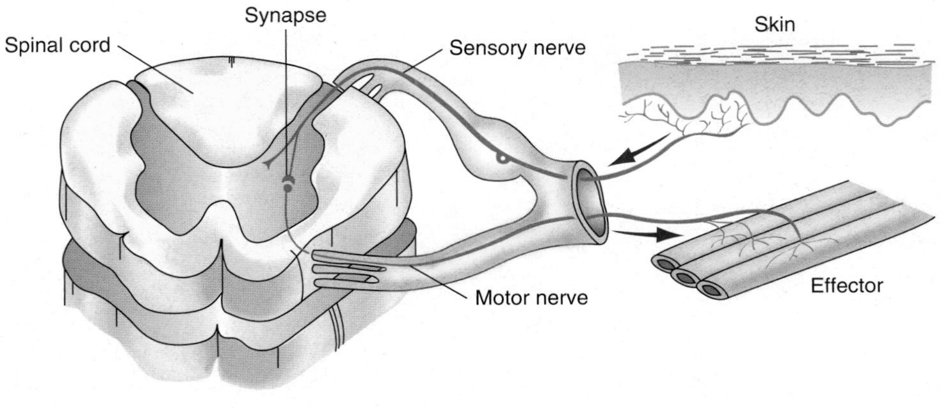

Figure 3–19 Reflex arc.

pressure, or vibration but also be able to distinguish degrees of these sensations—that is light or heavy, slow or fast. The main sensors are not all found in the face, but the following sections give a general idea of how sensation is received and perceived by the body (Figure 3–20).

Hair Follicle Endings

Hair follicle endings are single fibers joined at the hair bulb and wrapped around the end of the hair in fine body hair. In other hairs, the nerve is above the hair bulb, encircling the external root sheath.

Hederiform Endings

Not a great deal is known about **hederiform endings.** *Hederiform* means "ivy shaped" and refers to a nerve that occurs in glabrous, or hairless, skin. They also are called **Merkel's discs** by some anatomists since they were first described by Friedrich Sigmund Merkel. As the nerve ending approaches the base of the epidermis, it expands into flattened leaves that lie close to specialized cells near the epidermal/dermal junction. Each of the receptors consists of a modified epidermal cell, or Merkel cell, and its disc-shaped terminal. They are attached to the local keratinocytes by desmosomes. These receptors are thought to be mechanoreceptors for touch and other internal functions.

Meissner's Corpuscle

The **Meissner's corpuscle** is found in frictional areas of the skin: the hands, fingers, soles of the foot, and the glabrous skin of the toes. They are circular or ovoid structures with a distinct connective tissue capsule. They are supplied by myelinated nerves and are fairly large, 20 to $40 \times 150\mu$ in size. They transmit touch, pressure, and cold. They are grouped on the skin of the fingertips, lips, and orifices of the body and on the nipples. When touched, Meissner's corpuscles inform the brain about the shape and feel of an object in the hand, or a casual touch, or a kiss.

Pacinian Corpuscle

The **Pacinian corpuscle** is very large, between 0.5×3 mm and 0.5×4 mm in size. They are found in the deep part of the dermis of the palms and fingers near the bones, specifically, in the fingertips, palms, and soles, as well as the lips, tongue, and face. They also are found in the external genitalia and the breast and are sensitive to light touch. Many internal organs also contain these corpuscles. Pacinian corpuscles share the mechanoreceptor responsibility with the three other skin organelles. They have a special sensitivity to deep-pressure touch and high-frequency vibration, and they relay change of position of the arms and legs to the brain.

Thermoreceptors

Thermoreceptors detect both heat and cold. Besides the free nerve endings, there are two main types. The first type, the **end-bulbs of Krause,** are found in the skin, the conjunctiva of the eye, the mucous membrane of the lips and tongue, the penis and the clitoris, and the fingertips. They are true thermoreceptors and detect cold. The second type, the **corpuscles of Ruffini,** which are nerve endings in the subcutaneous tissue of the human finger, detect heat. They are principally located at the junction of the **corium** with the subcutaneous tissue. They detect stretches of connective tissue and send slow, continuous signals when stimulated. The receptors nearest to the epidermal-dermal junction are Merkel's disc and Meissner's corpuscles. The Pacinian corpuscles and the Ruffini corpuscles are in the dermis.

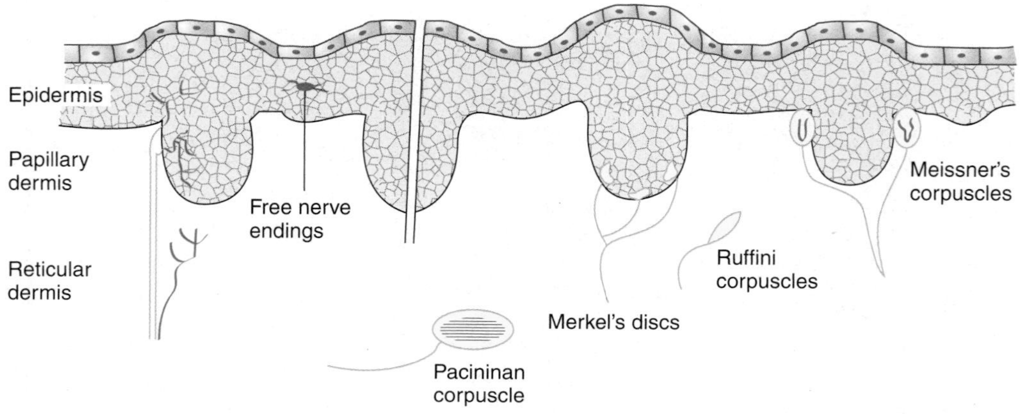

Figure 3–20 Sensory receptors.

REVIEW QUESTIONS

1. Discuss the components of cellular structure.
2. What are cellular receptors and how do they work?
3. What is cellular differentiation?
4. What does differentiation mean and why is cellular differentiation important in skin physiology?
5. How thick is the epidermis?
6. What are the three major cell types in the epidermis?
7. What is the turnover time of the epidermis?
8. What are the major functions of the skin?
9. Describe a stem cell.
10. Explain the cytoskeleton and the major fibers.
11. Describe melanogenesis.
12. What is a Langerhans cell?
13. Name two cells in the dermis.
14. Name five blood cells.
15. What is the extracellular matrix?
16. What is the difference between collagen and elastin?
17. Describe the cell cycle.
18. What is a gene?
19. What is embryology?
20. Define the terms *endoderm, mesoderm,* and *ectoderm.*
21. Name the four major tissues of the body.
22. Explain how desmosomes function.
23. Name the three lipids in the stratum corneum.
24. Name the principle sensory receptors of the skin.

CHAPTER GLOSSARY

acidophilic normoblasts: part of the blood cell line and formed from the polychromatic normoblast, this cell (8 to 10 microns diameter) loses its nucleus at this stage.

actin: a protein in a muscle fiber that, together with myosin, is responsible for contraction and relaxation.

actin filaments: connected to the catenins, they help stabilize cell adherence.

active transport: a process that requires expenditure of ATP energy to move molecules across a cell membrane; also called *facilitated transport*.

adenosine triphosphate (ATP): a multifunctional nucleotide that transports chemical energy within cells for metabolism and converts oxygen to carbon dioxide.

adherens junctions: provides strong mechanical attachments between adjacent cells.

afferent: (L. *ad*, "to lead"+*ferre*, "to bear") adjective meaning leading or bearing toward some organ, such as nerves conducting impulses toward the brain or blood vessels carrying blood toward an organ; contrast with *efferent*.

Akt: a pathway used as an intermediate signal as part of the DNA signaling cascade.

amino acids: organic acids that form the building blocks of proteins. There are 20 amino acids utilized within the human body. Nine of these are essential amino acids and must be supplied by the diet.

anchoring system: ties the plaque to the cytoplasm through the cytoskeleton; located inside the cell behind the plasma membrane.

antibodies: components of the immune system that neutralize antigens.

antigen: 1. a modified type of serum globulin synthesized by lymphoid tissue in response to antigenic stimulus. 2. any material that elicits an immune response.

apoptosis: (Gr., *apo*, "away from"+*ptosis*, "a falling") Genetically determined cell death; "programmed" cell death.

autonomic nervous system (ANS): the system that controls involuntary functions of the circulatory, respiratory, endocrine, and digestive systems and controls the actions of involuntary muscles, such as the heart.

B cell: a type of lymphocyte derived from bone marrow stem cells that matures into an immunologically competent cell (under the influence of the bursa of fabricius in the chicken, and the bone marrow in nonavian species); following interaction with antigen, it becomes a plasma cell, which synthesizes and secretes antibody molecules involved in humoral immunity. Also called *B lymphocyte*.

B lymphocyte: cell that manufactures antibodies involved in immunity.

basophil: white blood cell characterized by the presence of blue cytoplasmic granules that become stained by a basophilic dye.

basophilic normoblast: a blue colored cell formed from the division of the pronormoblast this cell (6 to 18 microns diameter) produces polychromatic normoblasts.

blastocoel: a fluid-filled or yolk-filled cavity surrounded by a blastoderm.

blastoderm: primary epithelium formed in early embryonic development of many arthropods when the nuclei migrate to the periphery and undergo superficial cleavage; usually encloses the central yolk mass.

blastula: (Gr., *blastos*, "germ"+ L. *ula*, "dim") An early stage in the development of an embryo; it consists of a sphere of cells enclosing a fluid-filled cavity (blastocoel).

cadherins: transmembrane proteins that go from cell to cell and bind to each other.

catenin: a protein important in stabilizing cell adherence to avoid abnormal spread of cells.

CdK: cyclin dependent kinase adds phosphate to a protein along with cyclins and is a major control switch for the cell cycle.

cell cycle: the regular sequence of events in the life of a cell, during which the cell grows, prepares for division, duplicates its contents and divides to form two daughter cells.

cell-mediated immunity: a part of the immune system that does not involve antibodies and the function of which is carried out mainly by T-cells

cellular membrane: also called plasma membrane. a semipermeable lipid bi-layer common to all living things.

cell wall: the rigid outermost layer of the cells found in plants, some protests (type of single-cell organism), and most bacteria. Found in plants composed principally of cellulose. Not found in animal cells.

ceramides: a lipid component of the intercellular cement within the stratum corneum layer.

cholesterol: a lipid component of the stratum corneum.

chondroitin sulfate: a proteoglycan found in the dermis.

cleavage: the early mitotic and cytoplasmic divisions of an embryo.

cluster of differentiation (CD): all cells are coated with antigenic substances; each of the more than 160 clusters has a different chemical molecule that coats the surface. Every T and B cell has about 10^5 molecules on its surface.

complement system: a complex series of enzymes in the blood that coats microbes with special molecules making them more susceptible to phagocytosis.

connective tissue: fibrous tissue that binds together, protects, and supports the various parts of the body; examples are bone, cartilage and tendons.

connexins: transmembrane proteins that permit the flow of ions that cause contraction of the heart muscle and strong contraction of the uterus during labor.

corium: (L. *corium*, "leather") The deep layer of the skin; dermis.

corneocyte: another name for a stratum corneum cell.

cornified envelope: a highly cross-linked layer of proteins found in the stratum corneum.

corpuscles of Ruffini: nerve endings in the subcutaneous tissue of the human finger that detect stretch of connective tissue and send slow continuous signals when stimulated, heat detectors; also known as *organ of Ruffini*

cutaneous: pertaining to the skin (e.g., a skin infection).

cycle: repeating unit that makes up the pattern of biological rhythms.

cyclin: a protein important in the control of the cell division cycle and mitosis.

cyclin-dependent kinase (CdK): see CdK.

cytokine: (Gr., *kytos*, "hollow vessel" + *kinein*, "to move") a molecule secreted by an activated or stimulated cell (for example, macrophages) that causes chemical immune responses in certain other cells.

cytoplasm: the watery fluid of the cell, including the protoplasm, containing food material necessary for growth, reproduction, and self-repair.

cytoskeleton: in the cytoplasm of eukaryotic cells, an internal framework of microtubules, microfilaments, and intermediate filaments that anchor, organize, and moves organelles and other structures.

cytotoxic (killer) T cell: (Gr., *kytos*, "hollow vessel") A special type of T cell activated during cell-mediated immune responses, that recognizes and destroys virus-infected cells.

daughter cell: a cell that results after a division of a stem cell. The original cell is called the mother cell/division.

dendrite: tree-like branching of nerve fibers extending from a nerve cell; short nerve fibers that carry impulses toward the cell.

dendritic cell: cells that serve to fix and process cutaneous antigens; they contain large granules named Birbeck granules. Also known as Langerhans cells.

dermatan sulfate: a glycosaminoglycan; a complex carbohydrate in the dermis.

dermis: 1. Live layer of connective tissue below the epiderms. 2. Contains the collagen and elastin fibers and acts as the main support structure of the skin.

desmocollins: a member of the desmosome family; projects proteins; is calcium dependent, and extends from the plaques that interlock with identical proteins from the adjacent cell.

desmogleins: a member of the demosome family; projects cadherin proteins, is calcium binding and extends from the plaques that interlock with identical proteins from the adjacent cell.

desmoplakin: one of the two proteins that make up the plaques in the cell membrane.

desmosome: (Gr., *desmos*, "bond" + *soma*, "body"). 1. Structures that assist in holding cells together. 2. Buttonlike plaque serving as an intercellular connection containing many complex proteins; can be affected by autoimmune disorders.

DNA synthesis: a complex process that reproduces the critical information in each cell for proper functioning and reproduction.

ectoderm: (Gr., *ektos*, "outside" + *derma*, "skin") Outer layer of cells of an early embryo (gastrula stage); one of the germ layers, also sometimes used to include tissues derived from the ectoderm.

efferent: (L. *ex*, "out" + *ferre*, "to bear") Leading or conveying away from some organ, for example, nerve impulses conducted away from the brain, or blood conveyed

CHAPTER GLOSSARY

away from an organ; contrasts with *afferent*.

elaunin: elastin-type fiber found in the dermis believed to be an intermediate form of elastin.

embryo: (Gr., "full to bursting") The first stage of human life; starts with fertilization of a women's egg (ovum) by a male's sperm.

end-bulbs of Krause: thermoreceptors that detect cold; found in the skin, conjunctiva of the eye, mucus membranes of lips and tongue, the penis and clitoris, and the fingertips.

endoderm: (Gr., "inner") Deep primary germ layer of the embryo; gives rise to the linings of the pharynx, respiratory tree, digestive tract, urinary bladder, and urethra.

endoplasmic reticulum (ER): cytoplasmic organelle composed of a system of interconnected membranous tubules and vesicles; rough ER has ribosomes attached to the side of the membrane facing the cytoplasm and smooth ER does not. Rough ER functions in protein synthesis while smooth ER functions in lipid synthesis.

eosinophil: white blood cells characterized by the presence of cytoplasmic granules that become stained by an acid (eosin) dye.

epidermal growth factor (EGF): involved in the skin repair process.

epidermis: 1. the outermost layer of skin: a thin, protective layer with many nerve endings. 2. Consists of four layers: the basal layer, the spiny layer, the granular layer and the stratum corneum.

epidermolysis bullosa: a blistering congenital disease caused by defects in the keratins 5 and 14 in the basal layer.

epithelial tissue: 1. Protective covering on body surfaces, such as the skin, mucous membranes, and lining of the heart; digestive and respiratory organs; and glands. 2. Capable of constant reproduction which lines other tissue.

epithelium: (Gr., *epi*, "on, upon" + *thele*, "nipple") A cellular tissue covering a free surface (internal and external) or lining a tube or cavity; consists of cells joined by small amounts of cementing substances. Epithelial tissue is classified into types based on how many layers deep it is and the shape of the superficial cells.

erythrocyte: (Gr., erythros, "red" + *kytos*, "hollow vessel") Red blood cell that has hemoglobin to carry oxygen from lungs (or gills) to tissues; during their formation in mammals, erythrocytes lose their nuclei, but erythrocytes of other vertebrates retain their nuclei.

external ectoderm: a layer of the ectoderm germ layer that supplies the skin.

fibril: (L. *fibra*, "thread") a strand of protoplasm produced by a cell and lying within the cell.

fibroblast: a cell that produces protein in the body, such as amino acids and collagen, and originates from the mesechymal tissue. Also known as fibrocyte.

fibroblast growth factor (FGF): a peptide that stimulates fibroblast to grow fibrocyte.

fibrocyte: A cell that is not fully differentiated for it can go forward or backward in life, makes the most abundant protein in the body called collagen, and originates from the mesechymal tissue, also known as fibroblast.

fourth germ layer: Component of the ectoderm known as the *neural crest*.

free fatty acid: a lipid component of the stratum corneum.

free nerve terminals: nerve endings in the skin without myelin sheaths.

G_0: a stage of DNA synthesis, the resting cell.

G_1: part of interphase that is the time of active metabolism in the cell cycle; also known as *Gap 1*.

G_2: part of interphase after the synthesis of DNA and before the start of nuclear division; also known as *Gap 2*.

gap junctions: intercellular channels that allow free passage between the cells of ions and small molecules to pass between cells.

gastrula: the name for an embryo during the gastrulation process.

gastrulation: a process during which the cells migrate to the interior of the blastula and form three germ layers.

germ layer: in the animal embryo, one of three basic layers (ectoderm, endoderm, mesoderm) from which the various organs and tissues arise in the multicellular animal.

glial cells: supportive cells closely associated with neurons.

glycosaminoglycans: A water-binding substance such as a polysaccharide (protein and complex sugar) found between the fibers of the dermis with water-binding properties.

Golgi apparatus: organelle of membranous, hollow sacs arranged in a stack; functions in modification, storage, and packaging of secretion materials; may be called *dictyosome* in plants. Also known as the *Golgi apparatus* or *Golgi complex*.

granulocytes: (L. *granulus*, "small grain" + Gr., *kytos*, "hollow vessel") White blood cells (neutrophils, eosinophils, and basophils) bearing granules (vacuoles) in their cytoplasm that stain deeply.

helper T cells: cells that serve as managers and direct the immune response; they also secrete lymphokines.

hemidesmosomes: binds the basal layer to the basement membrane through different types of proteins.

hemocytoblast: part of the blood cell line, this multipotential cell can form the white cell series and the red cells and any other cells in the blood.

heparan sulfate: a proteoglycan found in the dermis.

heparin: a proteoglycan found in the dermis.

homeostasis: the process of feedback and regulation that keeps the body in a state of equilibrium within its environment.

humoral: (L. *humor*, "a fluid") Pertaining to an endocrine secretion.

hyaluronic acid: a glycosaminoglycan that has no protein component that can hold up to 400 times its own weight in water. A hydrating fluid found in the skin; hydrophilic agent with water-binding properties. Also known as *sodium hyalurnat*.

hypochlorous acid: chlorine bleach, HOCl.

immune system: a bodily system made up of lymph, lymph nodes, the thymus gland, the spleen, and lymph vessels; protects the body from disease by developing immunities and destroying disease-causing microorganisms as well as draining the tissues of excess interstitial fluids to the blood. This system carries waste and impurities away from the cells.

insulin-like growth factor (IGF-I): growth regulatory cytokines thought to be responsible for initiating proliferation of fibroblasts and other connective tissue cells.

integrin: proteins that hold the plaque to the basal lamina.

interleukin: cytokines produced by white blood cells and mediating their own activities or those of other white blood cells.

interleukin–1: a cytokine produced by macrophages that stimulates T helper lymphocytes.

intermediate filaments: complex fibers that help to maintain cell shape, but also add strength to cells and holds them together.

islet of Langerhans cells in the pancreas: cell that makes insulin and is responsible for diabetes when it fails to function.

JNK: a pathway used as an intermediate signal as part of the DNA signaling cascade.

keratin: The major protein made in the epidermis.

keratin proteins: proteins that are made in the skin and hair that resist water and frictions.

keratin sulfate: a proteoglycan found in the dermis.

keratinocyte: cells composed of keratin; the dominate cell in the epidermis. It is multifunctional but makes proteins and lipids.

keratinocytoblasts: stem cells that do not have a high rate of mitosis but do produce a transient amplifying cell.

keratinohyaline granules: both horny and hyaline, a distinguishing feature of the cells in the granular layer.

langerhans cell: cell that fixes and processes cutaneous antigens; contains large granules named Birbeck granules. Also known as *dendritic cells*.

leukocyte: (Gr., *leukos*, "white" + *kytos*, "hollow vessel") 1. Any of several kinds of white blood cells (for example, granulocytes, lymphocytes, and monocytes), so-called because they bear no hemoglobin, unlike red blood cells. 2. Specialized cells that work with the immune system to combat disease and infection.

lipase: (Gr., *lipos*, "fat") An enzyme that accelerates the hydrolysis, or synthesis of fats.

lipid bilayer: A molecular structure composed of hydrophilic and hydrophobic components.

lymphocytes: (L. *lympha*, "water, goddess of water" + Gr., *kytos*, "hollow vessel") A type of white blood cell; a component of the immune system produced by stem cells in the bone marrow. 2. Type of white blood cell which is important to the immune system for its ability to digest foreign invaders.

lymphokine: (L. *lympha* + Gr., *kinein*, "to move") A molecule secreted by an activated or stimulated lymphocyte that causes physiological changes in certain other cells.

lymphotoxins: substances that, when released by cytotoxic or killer T cells, cause cell lysis.

CHAPTER GLOSSARY

lysosome: 1. cytoplasmic, membrane-bounded organelle that contains digestive and hydrolytic enzymes, which are typically most active at the acid pH found in the lumen of lysosomes. 2. cell organelle that digests foreign matter considered potentially threatening to the body.

lysozyme: an enzyme capable of dissolving and digesting many types of biochemicals.

macrophage: (Gr., *makros*, "long, large"+*phago*, "to eat") a phagocytic cell type in vertebrates that performs crucial functions in the immune response and inflammation, such as presenting antigenic epitopes to T cells and producing several cytokines.

mandibular nerve: a branch of the trigeminal nerve (fifth cranial nerve) that supplies the muscles and skin of the lower part of the face; also, nerve that affects the muscles of the chin and lower lip; carries sensory data from the mandible.

MAPK: a pathway used as an intermediate signal as part of the DNA signaling cascade.

mast cell: type of cell in various tissues that releases pharmacologically active substances with a role in inflammation.

maturation promoting factor (MPF): a protein that initiates part of the cellular division known as mitosis. Specifically, it initiates the prophase of mitosis and also functions in the process of mitosis by activating other proteins through the mechanism of phosphorylation, that is, it adds phosphorus to the protein, thereby making it an active protein.

maxillary nerve: a branch of the trigeminal nerve (fifth cranial nerve) the carries sensory data from the maxilla; supplies the upper part of the face.

Meissner's corpuscles: circular or ovoid structures with a distinct connective tissue capsule that transmit touch, pressure, and cold.

melanocyte: cells that produce pigment granules/melanin in the basal layer of the epidermis.

melanocyte-stimulating hormone (MSH): a hormone that stimulates melanocytes to make melanin.

melanogenesis: the process of making the pigment melanin inside the melanocyte.

melanosomes: pigment granules of melanocyte cells that produce melanin in the basal layer; provides skin's colors.

membrane: in living organisms, a phospholipid bilayer impregnated with protein and certain other compounds that is differentially permeable.

memory T cells: programmed to recognize and respond to a pathogen once it has been invaded and been repelled.

Merkel's discs: *see* hederi; form endings.

mesenchymal tissue: embryonic connective tissue

mesoderm: (Gr., *mesos*, "middle"+*derma*, "skin") the third germ layer, formed in the gastrula between the ectoderm and endoderm; gives rise to connective tissues, muscle, urogenital and vascular systems, and the peritoneum. This tissue from the mesoderm is called *mesochymal tissue*.

microfilaments: protein strands made of actin; responsible for cell movement and cell shape.

microtubules: tiny, cylindrical-shaped tubes composed of a protein called *tubulin*; its major function is to separate chromosomes during cellular division.

mitochondria: in eucaryotes, subcellular organelles that conduct cellular respiration and produce most of the ATP in aerobic respiration (oxidative phosphorylation).

mitosis: nuclear cells dividing of a cell into two new cells called *daughter cells*; the usual process of cell production of human tissues.

monocyte: large white blood cells or leukocytes, which travel the bloodstream neutralizing pathogens; become phagocytic cells (macrophages) after moving into tissues.

mother cell: a cell capable of multiple divisions, also known as a *stem cell*.

motor (efferent or effector) neuron or nerve: a neuron or nerve that carries an impulse away from the brain or spinal cord to the muscles and organs.

muscle tissue: tissue that is able to contract and conduct electrical impulses.

myelin: (Gr., *myelos*, "marrow") Fatty material forming the medullary sheath of nerve fibers.

myeloperoxidase: enzyme used in the killing action of neutrophiles.

myosin: (Gr., *mys*, "muscle"+*in*, suffix meaning "belonging to") a large protein of contractile tissue that forms the thick myofilaments of striated muscle. During contraction, it combines with actin to form actomyosin.

nervous tissue: a highly specialized tissue used to transport signals to other organs and coordinate all bodily functions.

neural crest: early nerve tissue in the embryo; site of origin for melanocytes; a layer of the ectoderm germ layer.

neural tube: a layer of the ectoderm germ layer; provides most of the central nervous system.

neurofilament: an intermediate filament found in nerve cells.

neuroglia: glial cells provide support and nutrition to the tissues.

neuron: a nerve cell; basic unit of the nervous system, consisting of a cell body, nucleus, dendrites, and axon.

neutrophils: 1. most abundant of polymorphonuclear leukocytes; an important phagocyte; so-called because it stains with both acidic and basic. 2. phagocytic white blood cells.

nuclear membrane: membrane surrounding the nucleus of eucaryotic cells.

nucleolus: (diminutive of L. *nucleus*, "kernel") a deeply staining body within the nucleus of a cell and containing RNA; nucleoli (plural) are specialized portions of certain chromosomes that carry multiple copies of the information to synthesize ribosomal RNA.

nucleus: the dense, active protoplasm found in the center of a eukaryotic cell that acts as the genetic control center; plays an important role in cell reproduction and metabolism.

ophthalmic nerve: a branch of the trigeminal nerve that carries only sensory fibers; supplies the skin of the forehead, upper eyelids, and interior portion of the scalp, orbit, eyeball, and nasal passage.

organelle: a body within the cytoplasm of eukaryotic cells. There are several different types of organelles, each with a specialized function, such as the chloroplast, which functions in photosynthesis.

oxytalan: elastin-type fiber found in the dermis that contains only microfibrils and is 10–12 nm in diameter.

p27 protein: a protein that binds to cyclin and CdK blocking entry into the S phase.

p53 protein: a tumor-suppressor protein with critical functions in normal cells. A mutation in the gene that encodes it, p53, can result in loss of control over cell division and, thus, cancer.

Pacinian corpuscle: a sensory receptor in skin, muscles, body joints, body organs, and tendons that is involved with the vibratory sense and firm pressure on the skin; also called a *lamellated corpuscle*.

parasympathetic divisions: a major functional division of the autonomic nervous system. It operates under normal nonstressful situations, such as resting, and helps to restore calm and balance to the body after a stressful event.

phagocyte: (G. *phagein*, "to eat" + *kytos*, "hollow vessel") Any cell that engulfs and devours microorganisms or other particles (process known as phagocytosis).

phospholipids: compounds that contain fatty acid and phosphoric acid groups.

plakoglobin: one of the two proteins that make up the plaques in the cell membrane.

plaques: located in the cell membrane; made up of two proteins: desmoplakin and plakoglobin.

plasma membrane: *see* cellular membrane.

platelet-derived growth factor (PDGF): growth regulatory cytokines thought to be responsible for initiating proliferation of fibroblasts and other connective tissue cells.

pluripotential stem cell: at the start of the blood cell line, this cell is programmed to form all the other cells in the blood stream.

polychromatic normoblasts: part of the blood cell line and formed from the basophilic normoblast, this cell (9 to 12 microns diameter) starts to make hemoglobin, but can no longer divide.

polymorphonuclear cells: Granulocytes.

pro-enzyme: an inactive form of chymotropic enzyme found in the lamellar bodies of the stratum granulosum.

pronormoblast: part of the blood cell line, formed from the division of the hemocytoblast, this cell (20 microns) continues to divide and forms the basophilic normoblasts.

protein: (Gr., from *proteios*, "primary") chains of amino acid molecules used in cell functions and body growth; a macromolecule of carbon, hydrogen, oxygen, and nitrogen, and at times, sulfur and phosphorus.

protein-tyrosine kinase activity: a complex enzyme that catalyze the phosphorylation of tyrosine residues. There are 91 of identified PTK enzymes which are involved in cellular signaling pathways, regulate key cell functions such as proliferation, differentiation, anti-apoptotic signaling and neurite outgrowth. Unregulated activation of these enzymes, through mechanisms such as point mutations

CHAPTER GLOSSARY

or over-expression, can lead to various forms of cancer as well as benign proliferative conditions. The importance of PTKs in health and disease is further underscored by the existence of aberrations in PTK signaling occurring in inflammatory diseases and diabetes. In short, this is a very important enzyme that activates other enzymes.

proteoglycans: a special class of glycoprotiens found in the extracellular substance. They vary in size depending on the glycosaminoglycan chains attached to them.

proteolysis: the act of breaking the desmosomal bonds of connecting proteins.

receptor: a special protein on a cells surface or within the cell that binds to specific ligands.

receptor sites: a protein on the cell membrane or within the cytoplasm or cell nucleus that binds to a specific molecule (a ligand), such as a neurotransmitter, hormone, or other substance, and initiates the cellular response.

reflex arc: critical to the autonomic nervous system (ANS), there are two parts of the reflex arc: the sensory (afferent) arm and the motor (efferent or effector) arm.

respiratory burst: process that uses oxygen in the killing action of neutrophils.

reticulocyte: part of the blood cell line, formed from the acidophilic normoblast,this cell (8 microns in diameter) contains mitochondria.

ribosomes: small dense organelles that assemble proteins in cells.

selective permeability: the ability of the plasma membrane to let some substances in and keep others out; permeable to small molecules, usually H_2O, O_2, and CO_2, but not permeable to larger molecules or ions.

senescent cell: a cell arrested in G_1 that cannot advance or go backward and in some cases is destroyed; a major cause of aging.

sensory (afferent) neuron or nerve: nerve that carries impulses or messages from the sense organs to the brain, where sensations of touch, cold, heat, sight, hearing, taste, smell, pain, and pressure are experienced.

stem cell: a cell capable of multiple divisions, also known as the mother cell.

superoxide: an unstable, reactive single oxygen atom.

suppressor T cells: inhibits the production of cytotoxic cells once they are no longer needed so they do not cause more damage than necessary.

sympathetic divisions: the part of the autonomic nervous system which is stimulated by activity and prepares the body for stressful situations, such as running from a dangerous situation or competing in a sports event.

T cell: type of lymphocyte with a vital regulatory role in immune response; so called because they are processed through the thymus. Subsets of T cells may be stimulatory or inhibitory. They communicate with other cells by protein hormones called cytokines.

thymidine dinucleotide fragments: fragments produced by damaged DNA, triggering release of MSH, which can then bind to melanocytes to produce melanin.

tight junction: region of actual fusion of cell membranes between two adjacent cells.

transit time: the time it takes for cells to move through the epidermal stages of growth.

trigeminal nerve: the main sensory nerve of the face having three major branches.

tubulin: a protein that forms parts of the microtubules.

vacuoles: membrane-bound compartments within some eukaryotic cells that can serve a variety of secretory, excretory, and storage functions.

versican sulfate: a proteoglycan found in the dermis, provides the turgor and tautness to the skin by interacting with the elastin and the hyaluronic acid.

vimentin: an intermediate filament found in fibroblasts.

white blood cell: (leukocyte) Blood cells responsible for the body's defense mechanisms. They act by destroying disease-causing germs. Also called *white corpuscles* or *leukocytes.*

zygote: diploid cell produced by the fusion of an egg and sperm; fertilized egg cell.

CHAPTER OUTLINE

- WHAT ARE HORMONES?
- THE ENDOCRINE GLANDS
- HORMONES PRODUCED BY THE OVARIES AND TESTES
- THE HORMONAL PHASES OF LIFE
- HIRSUTISM
- OBESITY, ANOREXIA, AND HORMONES
- OTHER HORMONAL DISORDERS THAT AFFECT THE SKIN

CHAPTER 4

HORMONES

LEARNING OBJECTIVES

After completing this chapter, you should be able to:

- Identify the endocrine glands.
- Understand hormone production.
- Discuss the hormonal phases of life.
- Demonstrate a knowledge of pregnancy and its impact on the skin.
- Be able to recognize PMS flare-ups.
- Understand the impact of birth control pills.
- Be able to discuss menopause.
- Know the conditions that can accompany menopause.
- Be able to recommend recourse for hirsutism.
- Understand other hormonal impacts on the skin.

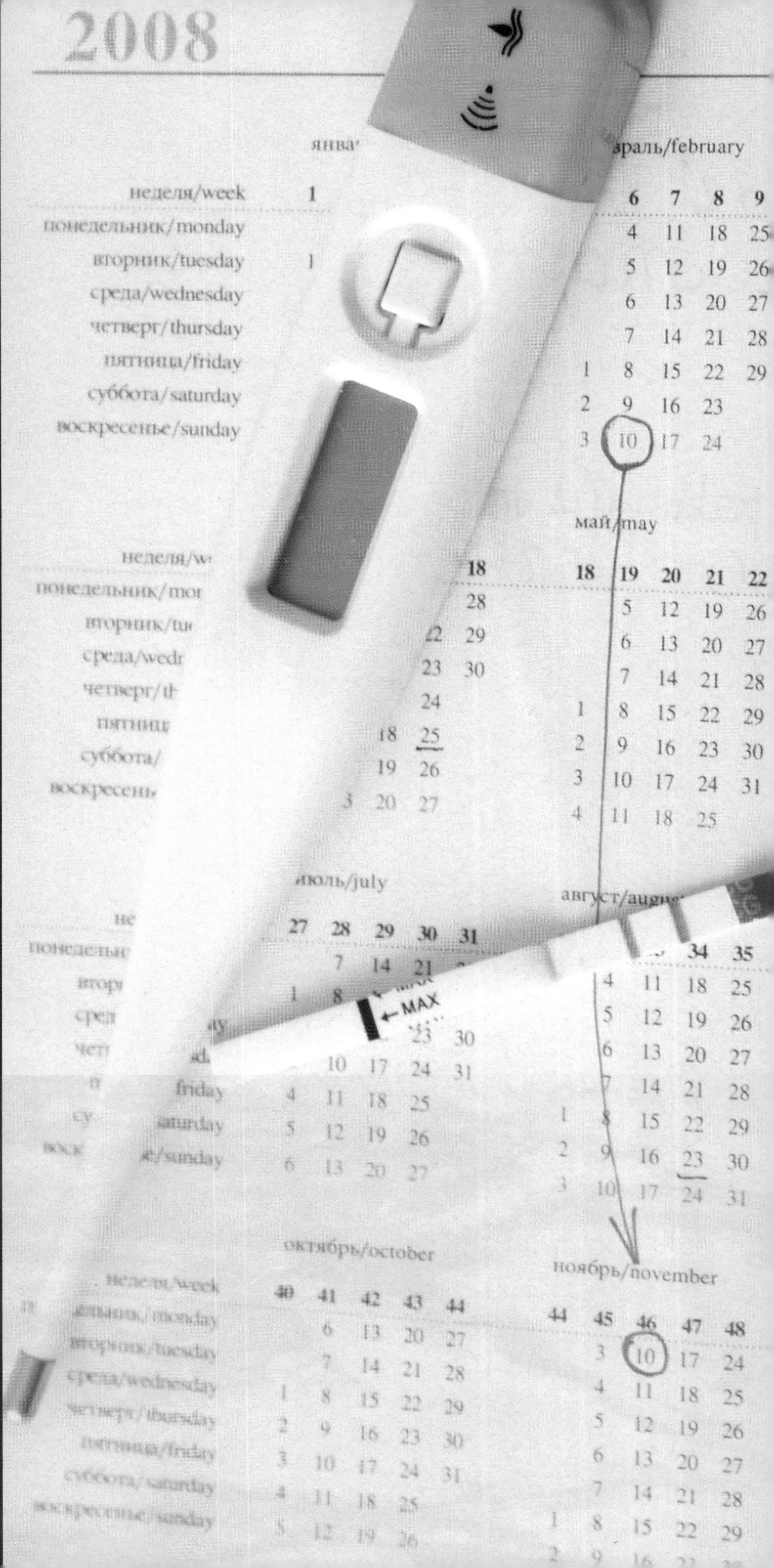

KEY TERMS

Page numbers indicate where in the chapter the term is used.

adrenal glands 91
adrenaline 91
androgens 92
apocrine glands 89
corpus luteum 94
diabetes 91
endocrine glands 89
endometrium 94
estradiol 92
estriol 92
estrogen 92
estrone 92
exocrine (duct) glands 89
follicle-stimulating hormone (FSH) 92
formication 99
hirsutism 100
hormone replacement therapy (HRT) 98
hormones 89
hyperthyroidism 100
hypothalamus 90
hypothalamus gland 90
hypothyroidism 100
keratosis pilaris 93
lutenizing hormone (LH) 92
menarche 94
menopause 98
menstruation 94
osteoporosis 98
ovaries 91
pancreas 91
parathyroid gland 90
perimenopause 98
pineal gland 91
pituitary gland 90
premenstrual syndrome (PMS) 97
progesterone 92
puberty 92
relaxin 92
secreted 89
striae distensae 96
testes 91
testosterone 92
thymus gland 91
thyroid gland 90
thyroxine 90
trophic hormones 90

Hormones have very definite effects on the skin, and their functioning is directly related to many skin problems. These skin problems change as the body undergoes hormonal changes due to medication or the natural aging process. This chapter will familiarize you with the major glands of the endocrine system and their function. You will also learn about the menstrual cycle, pregnancy, menopause, and diseases and disorders of the endocrine system, along with the affect of hormones on the skin.

WHAT ARE HORMONES?

Hormones are chemical messengers that are manufactured or **secreted** by glands within the body. Although most people think of hormones only in terms of sex hormones, sex hormones are only a few of the hormones that the endocrine system produces. Each endocrine gland produces different hormones, and each hormone affects specific cells in different ways. Hormones have special "keys" that fit the "locks" on the cell membranes that they are intended to affect. The key fitting the lock causes the cell membrane to produce enzymes that stimulate other chemical reactions within the cell. The "locks" on the cells are called *receptors* or *receptor sites*.

The system of glands is called the *endocrine system*. Among the glands in the human body are **exocrine glands,** such as the sebaceous glands and the sudoriferous glands, which have ducts through which chemicals move. **Apocrine glands** are present in the groin and armpit. The **endocrine glands,** which are discussed in the next section, empty hormones directly into the bloodstream.

THE ENDOCRINE GLANDS

There are eight major endocrine glands in the human body (Figure 4–1).

The **pituitary gland** is in the center of the head. It serves as the "brain" of the endocrine system. The pituitary gland secretes **trophic hormones,** which are "signal hormones." They cause other glands to make other hormones. Trophic hormones secreted by the pituitary gland include follicle-stimulating hormone (FSH), which causes production of sex hormones in the glands present in the sex organs. The pituitary gland also produces special hormones that cause regulation of the amount of fluid retained by the body, hormones that control growth, and hormones that cause the female breast to produce milk.

The pituitary gland is connected to the brain by another gland, the **hypothalamus gland,** which controls some involuntary muscles, such as the muscles in the intestines that help move food through the gastrointestinal system. The hypothalamus also manufactures a variety of hormones that cause stimulation of the pituitary gland to make other hormones. You might say that the **hypothalamus** is the "interpreter" between the brain and the pituitary gland. The hypothalamus is able to detect needs of various parts of the body by chemically monitoring the blood that flows through it.

The **thyroid gland** is located in the neck. It regulates both cellular and body metabolism and produces hormones that stimulate growth. One of the hormones secreted by the thyroid gland is called **thyroxine.** (Children born without thyroxine have a condition called *dwarfism*.) The thyroid gland uses a lot of iodine in its manufacture of hormones. This is why it is important to have some iodine in the diet. Iodine is present in fish, meat, and some vegetables.

Behind the thyroid gland lies a related glandular structure called the **parathyroid gland.** This is actually a set of multiple glands, most commonly four, that are generally attached to the thyroid gland. The parathyroids are

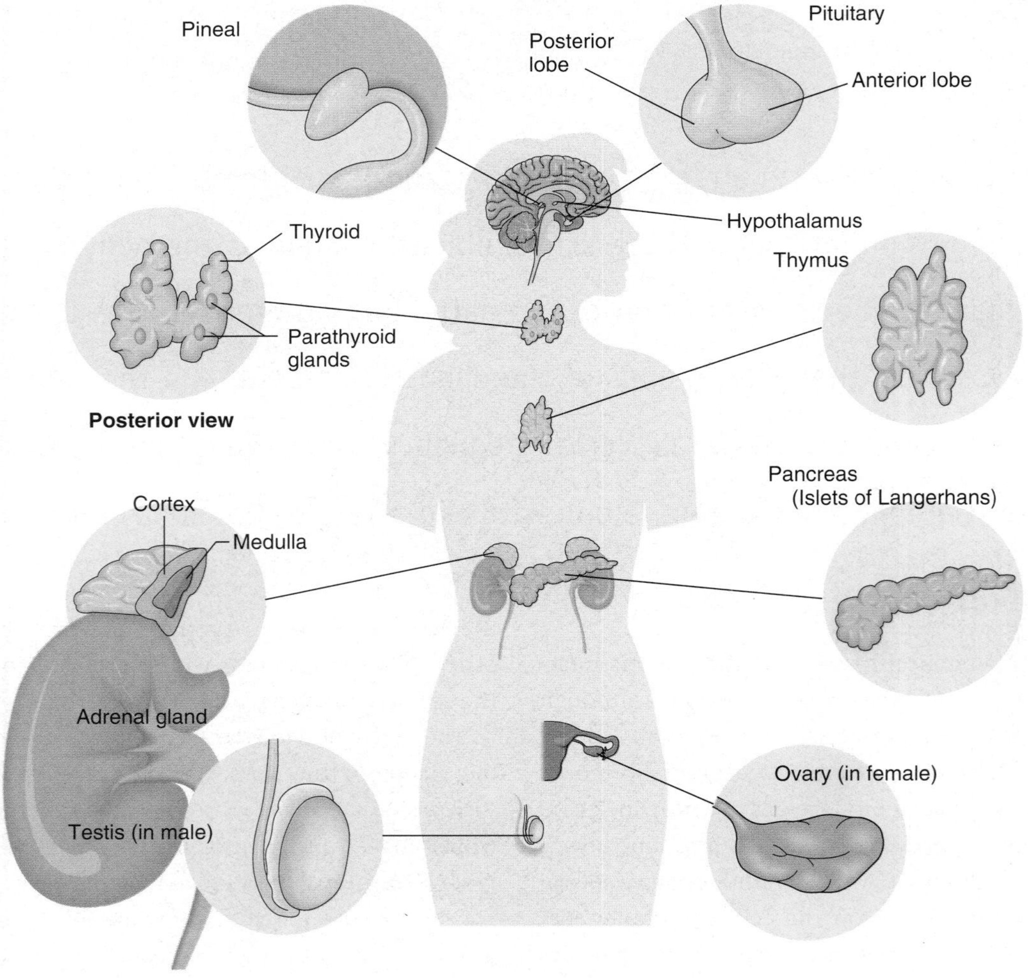

Figure 4–1 The endocrine system.

responsible for regulating calcium and phosphates in the bloodstream, which are necessary for proper bone growth.

The **adrenal glands** are located just above the kidneys. These glands have an inner part called the *medulla* and an outer core called the *cortex*. The medulla makes two main hormones, **adrenaline** and noradrenaline, which the nervous system needs for transporting nerve impulses. Adrenaline is also secreted when the body experiences stress. If you have ever had a close call when driving a car—a time when you just missed having an accident—you most likely experienced a rush of adrenaline, which is the feeling you had right after the incident. In addition, you have probably heard stories of people having almost superhuman strength during emergencies. This is also caused by the adrenal hormones. When a large amount of adrenaline is secreted suddenly into the bloodstream, the body responds by preparing for an emergency. The heartbeat increases, the pupils of the eyes dilate, the bronchi in the lungs expand, and the body generally focuses all of its attention on the impending emergency.

The cortex of the adrenal glands manufactures steroids, which are very small hormone molecules that penetrate cell membranes and enter cells for specific reasons. The steroid hormones produced by the adrenal cortex are called *corticoids*. The corticoids help regulate the metabolism and the body's use of carbohydrates, proteins, and fats. They also help to maintain water balance in the body and regulate sodium and potassium levels.

Like the pituitary gland, the **pineal gland** is located in the brain. Very small and funnel shaped, this gland's function is not well understood, but scientists have theorized that it is related to the sex hormones.

The **pancreas** is located in the abdomen. It has several functions. It secretes pancreatic enzymes that are delivered into the intestine. These enzymes help digest foods taken into the body. Within the pancreas are a group of specialized cells called the *islets of Langerhans*. These cells manufacture a hormone called *insulin,* which regulates blood sugar or glucose levels. If the pancreas does not secrete enough insulin, the body delvelops **diabetes.** People with diabetes must take synthetically produced insulin.

The **thymus gland** is part of the immune system. It produces specialized lymphocytes to help the body fight disease. The thymus gland grows during childhood and begins shrinking in later years.

The last, but not least, of the major endocrine glands are the sex glands. These are the **ovaries** in females and the **testes** in males. The ovaries are located above the uterus and are connected to the uterus by two hollow tubes called the *fallopian tubes* (Figure 4–2). The ovaries contain eggs that will eventually be released into the fallopian tubes for possible fertilization by sperm. The testes are present within the scrotum. The testes are connected to another tube called the *vas deferens*. The vas deferens leads to a holding sac called *the seminal vesicle,* which holds sperm manufactured by the testes. This series of tubules continues and eventually joins the urethra, which is the tube that leads to the outside of the penis (Figure 4–3).

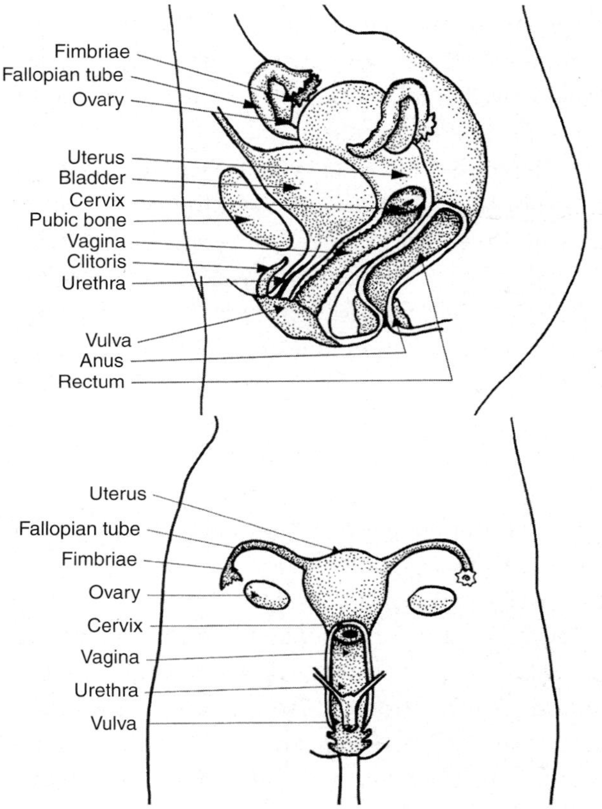

Figure 4–2 The female reproductive organs.

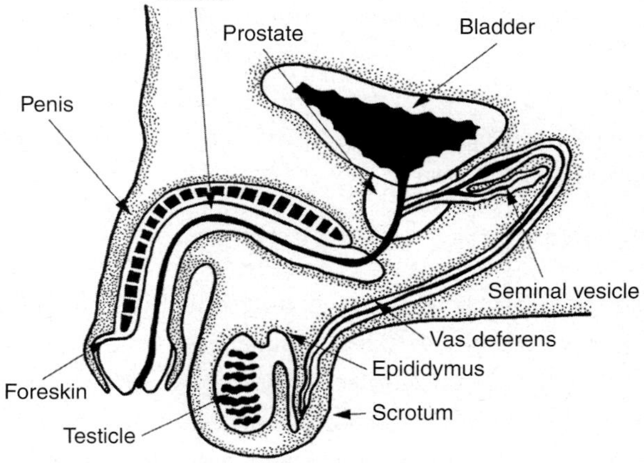

Figure 4–3 The male reproductive organs.

HORMONES PRODUCED BY THE OVARIES AND TESTES

The sex glands of both men and women produce hormones. The testes secrete **testosterone,** which is the hormone responsible for development of typical male characteristics, such as a deep voice, broad shoulders, body hair, and other male characteristics. Male hormones are called **androgens.**

Estrogen is the hormone that gives a woman female characteristics, such as breasts, and also helps with the development of the menstrual cycle. The ovaries produce three estrogenic hormones—estriol, estradiol, and estrone—as well as other hormones, such as progesterone and relaxin. The estrogenic hormones are all produced from androgens through enzymatic action. **Estradiol** is the strongest of the hormones and the most plentiful until menopause, when more **estrone** is present. **Estriol** is the weakest of the estrogens. **Progesterone** is a steroid hormone that helps prepare the uterus for pregnancy and is an important hormone in the menstrual cycle. Through a series of chemical conversions, progesterone converts to the androgen estrogens: testosterone, estrone, and estradiol. Another hormone manufactured by the ovaries is relaxin. **Relaxin** rises and falls with the monthly hormonal cycle. During childbirth it helps enlarge the pelvic opening.

Both male and female sex glands receive many of their "cues" for hormone production from the pituitary gland and the hypothalamus. The pituitary gland makes a hormone called **follicle-stimulating hormone,** referred to as **FSH.** FSH from the pituitary gland causes the testes to produce sperm. Another pituitary hormone called **luteinizing hormone,** or **LH,** causes the testes to manufacture testosterone.

The same types of pituitary hormones cause production of female hormones in the ovaries. The FSH produced by the pituitary gland causes the development of the ovum, or egg. Luteinizing hormone (LH) causes the actual process of ovulation or the release of the egg (ovum) from the ovary.

THE HORMONAL PHASES OF LIFE

Although human beings produce hormones throughout life, there are several phases that are dramatically influenced and caused by the presence or lack of hormones. These include puberty for both males and females and the onset of menstruation, pregnancy, and menopause for females.

Puberty

Puberty is the stage of life when physical changes occur in both sexes and when the sex glands begin to function, making sexual reproduction physically possible. At the beginning of puberty, which is usually at about 12 to 14 years of age (females may experience puberty earlier than males do), the hypothalamus begins producing luteinizing hormone, which in turn stimulates the pituitary gland to manufacture much larger amounts of both FSH and LH.

The FSH and LH are trophic hormones. They cause the ovaries and testes to secrete more hormones—specifically, estrogens and androgens. The sudden production of these hormones starts a number of drastic changes in physical appearance. Girls begin developing breasts, fat deposits form around the hips to provide feminine curvature, and the sweat glands begin producing body odor. Androgen production in females gives rise to pubic, leg, and underarm hair. In males, these changes in appearance include muscle development, development of the masculine form, broader shoulders, deeper voice, body and facial hair, and general physical growth. Puberty, of course, also triggers sexual attraction to the opposite sex.

Skin and Appearance Changes at the Onset of Puberty

It is interesting to note that just when sexual attraction begins, maintaining an attractive appearance becomes more difficult! This is because many of the hormone changes that start at the onset of puberty have an effect on the skin. The biggest change is the production of androgen, the male hormone, in both males and females. Androgen stimulates the sebaceous glands to produce sebum, which causes the follicles to dilate and the scalp to become oilier.

This is the age when "pores" are first easily visible. You may notice that small children have no easily visible pore structure on the skin's surface. In pre-teens and young teenagers, the pores become dilated due to increased sebum production. As the sebum fills the follicle, it begins pushing against the follicle walls, stretching them and making the pores on the surface appear larger. The nose is usually the first to develop visible pores. This development of the pore structure continues into the bridge of the nose, then the forehead, and then the chin. A 12-year-old client may have visible follicles only in these areas. This is the beginning of what many refer to as the "T-zone," so named because of its pattern on the face (Figure 4–4).

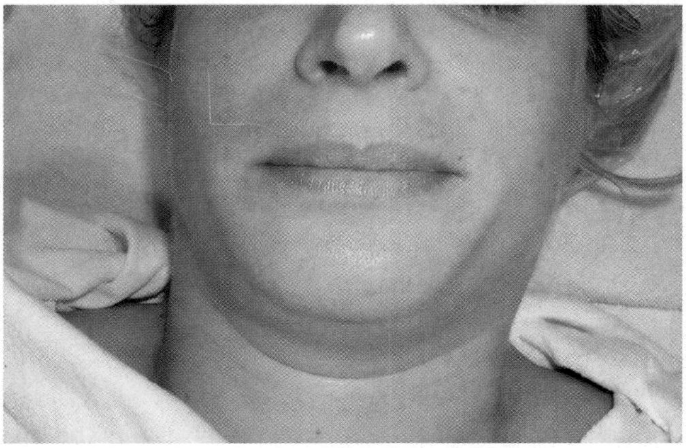

Figure 4–4 Combination skin recognized by the T-zone.

Puberty is also the time when many teenagers experience the beginning of acne. You may see a young client with large comedones in the nose, chin, and forehead areas or, occasionally, very small comedones on the nose only. The smallness of the comedones on this client's face indicates that the follicle walls have yet to stretch out, and the androgens have not yet had their full effect on the sebaceous glands.

Skin Care for Young Teenagers

If a mother brings in a young client with skin problems, advise the young person of proper home care, but keep it simple. Children of this age are often not used to daily skin care. Be thorough in your explanation of home care procedures, but remember that this young teenager cannot be expected to perform a seven-step regimen twice a day. Instruct him or her to use a washable, foaming cleanser twice a day followed by a gentle, low pH toner. He or she should use a mild anti-acne product—most likely a 2% salicylic or a 2.5% benzoyl peroxide gel—at night, if necessary.

In addition, it is important to convince young clients to start using sunscreen on a daily basis. This is the best way to prevent future sun damage. Teaching young people good health habits will help them maintain good skin for a lifetime. Emphasize the dangers of excess sun and give helpful hints about using sunscreens at the beach. Moisturizers are rarely needed by pubescent teenagers, except in very cold climates. Make sure you always recommend products that are noncomedogenic.

If you will be treating the teenager's skin in the salon, keep in mind that his or her first facial treatment should be an educational experience rather than a "feel-good" treatment. Help the young client understand, in simple terms, about acne and what is happening to the skin, along with the need for consistent hygiene. Explain the use of non-comedogenic cosmetics and the need for professional advice in choosing the right products. If this client already experiences acne flare-ups, you should make the proper treatment recommendations, which will be discussed in a later chapter. Treatment for most pubescent teens is only necessary bimonthly until further development of the pore structure or the beginning of acne flare-ups. As the teenager gets older, he or she will usually experience more problems with acne. Salon treatments should then be administered on at least a monthly basis, except in cases of more severe acne, when they should be more frequent.

When treating a young client's skin, follow these guidelines:

1. Cleanse the face well with a cleansing milk for oily or combination skin. Do not use toner or astringent at this point in treatment—the follicles are usually already tight and small. Using toner on this skin at the beginning of treatment will only make extractions more difficult.
2. Presoften the clogged areas by using a desincrustant solution or pre-mask. Steam with this solution on the face for about eight minutes. It is very important that the skin is hydrated for this type of treatment.
3. Remove the pre-mask or desincrustant solution. Gently pat the skin dry.
4. Begin extraction, being careful to explain to the young client what you are doing. Explain that extraction should always be performed by a professional. You may have difficulty extracting these tightly packed comedones. Be gentle, and take your time. Remember, this is the young client's first experience with extraction! Slow, gentle pressure applied in small areas is most effective.
5. After extraction is complete, apply a toner or antiseptic astringent.
6. Apply a light hydrating fluid and use high frequency.
7. Apply a clay-based drying mask for oily skin.

Keratosis Pilaris

Another problem associated with puberty is the development of a condition called **keratosis pilaris**. Keratosis pilaris appears as small pinpoint bumps, usually on the cheeks, accompanied by generalized redness. This condition is often seen in "rosy-cheeked" children. In this condition, the androgens have affected the growth of either terminal or lanugo hairs, which have started growing but are not strong enough to push through the follicle opening. The hairs remain trapped inside the follicle and, as a result, irritate the follicle and the surrounding skin. Although this condition is usually treated by a dermatologist, who uses mild retinoids or other exfoliating agents, it is sometimes treated in the salon. You can help the client resolve this condition by using mildly abrasive scrubs and light extraction. The client's routine use of a mild abrasive, such as granular scrubs that are not excessively drying, will help open the follicle and allow the hair to come out, cutting down on irritation. Advise him or her to apply a 10% glycolic lotion with a pH of 3.5 or higher once or twice a day.

The Menstrual Cycle

With puberty and adolescence comes **menarche,** the beginning of the menstrual cycle in females. The menstrual cycle is a 27- to 30-day cycle in which a female's ovaries manufacture an ovum, or egg, and hormonal changes take place that prepare the uterus for pregnancy in case the ovum is fertilized by sperm. When the ovum is not fertilized, the uterus sheds the lining, or **endometrium.** This process, called **menstruation,** has four phases (Figure 4–5):

Phase 1 occurs during the first 5 days of the cycle. The hypothalamus senses low levels of estrogen and progesterone and signals the pituitary gland to secrete FSH and LH. The ovaries then begin producing larger amounts of estrogen and progesterone, which prepare and release the ovum, or egg.

In **Phase 2**, days 6 to 12 of the cycle, the hypothalamus detects that the ovaries are secreting the right amount of estrogen necessary for ovulation, shuts down the pituitary gland's large production of FSH, and begins producing more LH.

In **Phase 3,** on days 12 and 13, the hormone levels of estrogen and progesterone are adjusted again. The estrogen level reaches a high point, which signals the pituitary gland to release a very large amount of LH, which then causes the release of the egg from the ovary.

Phase 4 is on day 14, when the egg (ovum) is released from the ovaries and begins its journey down the fallopian tube to the uterus. What is left of the follicle from which the egg was released turns into a hormone-producing structure called the **corpus luteum,** which produces large amounts of progesterone. The progesterone in turn produces the uterine lining, or endometrium, which is the "nest" that the uterus builds for a fetus. This fourteenth day is when a sperm can fertilize an egg and the woman can become pregnant.

Phase 5 is essentially the last two weeks of the 28-day cycle. If fertilization of the egg has not occurred, the pituitary hormones FSH and LH drop substantially. The corpus luteum shrinks, lowering its production of

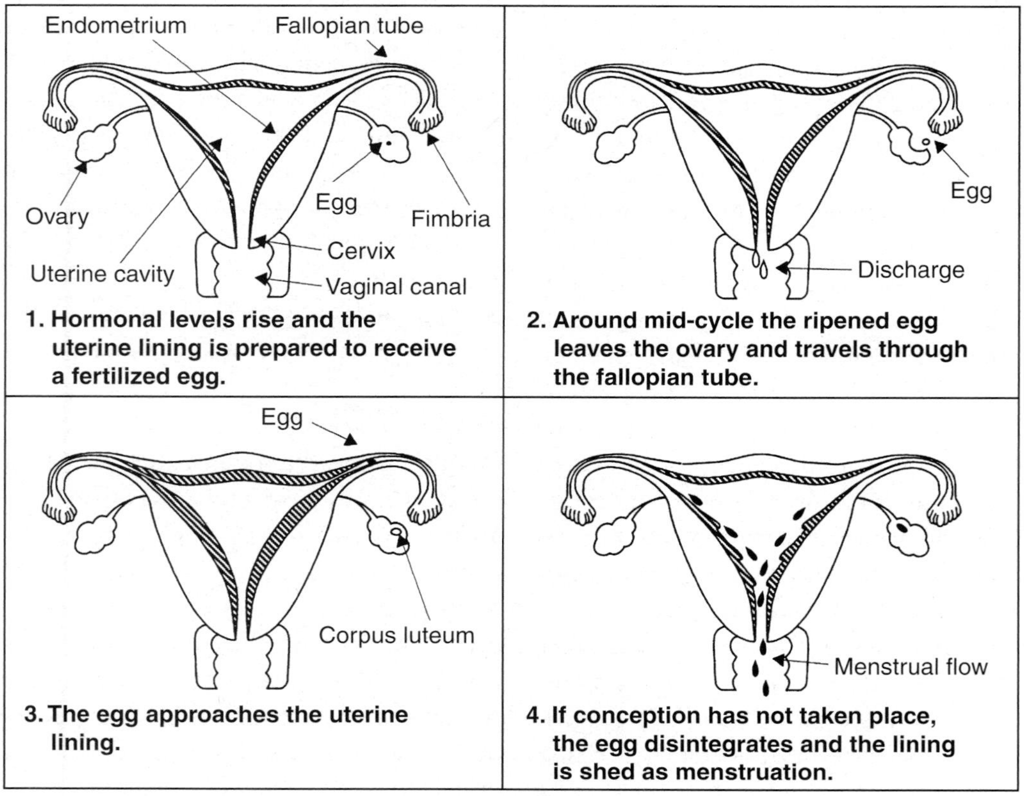

Figure 4–5 The menstrual cycle.

progesterone. This decrease in progesterone causes the breakdown of the endometrium.

Phase 6 begins menstruation, or the "period." The whole cycle begins again on day 28. Many women experience differences in the actual days on which different phases of the menstrual cycle take place (Figure 4–6). Stress, obesity, anorexia, and other endocrine system disorders can all affect the cycle.

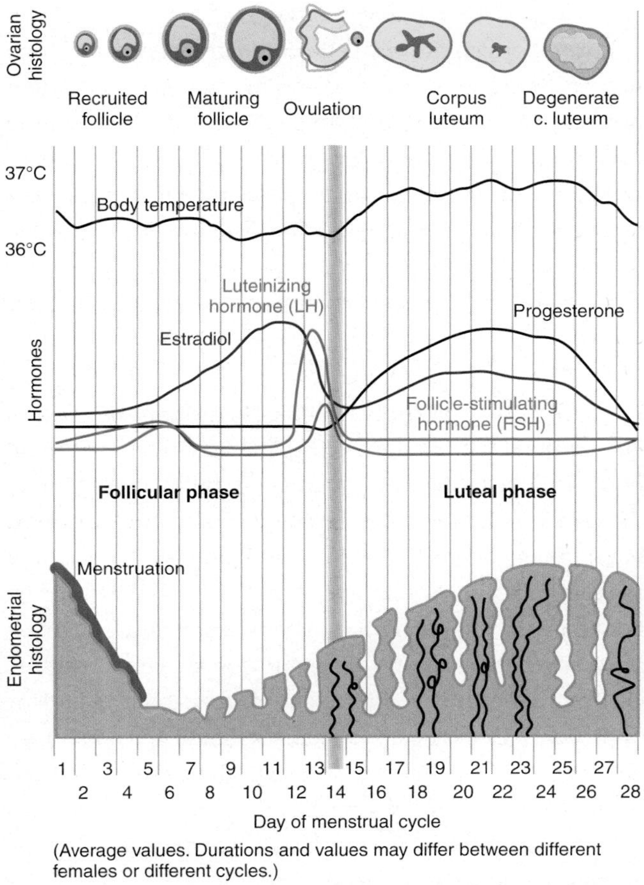

Figure 4–6 Hormonal changes during the menstrual cycle.

Pregnancy

If the ovum is fertilized by a sperm on the fourteenth day of the cycle, the female becomes pregnant. The corpus luteum continues to produce progesterone, and the endometrium becomes much thicker. The fertilized egg goes through a series of transformations, begins mitotic division, and forms a mass of cells. The embryo begins to form, surrounded by a capsule-like structure called a *trophoblast*. In simple terms, the trophoblast provides nutrition for the embryo. The membrane of the trophoblast eventually evolves into the placenta, which is a thick layer of hormone-producing cells that serves as the nutrient, oxygen, and waste exchange system between the growing embryo and the blood system of the mother. The placenta manufactures many hormones, including those that affect the corpus luteum, the growth of the embryo, and the production of milk in the mother's breasts.

Skin and Appearance Changes During Pregnancy

A vast number of obvious changes take place in the human body during pregnancy, and many of these changes affect the skin. The first is hyperpigmentation, a condition in which the skin darkens. Hyperpigmentation is caused by a hormone secreted by the placenta. This hormone stimulates the melanocytes in the skin. Pregnant women may also experience pregnancy mask, or melasma, a condition in which the face develops significant hyperpigmentation and resembles a dark facial mask (Figures 4–7 and 4–8). Light areas surround the eye areas, and the rest of the face is dark with pigment.

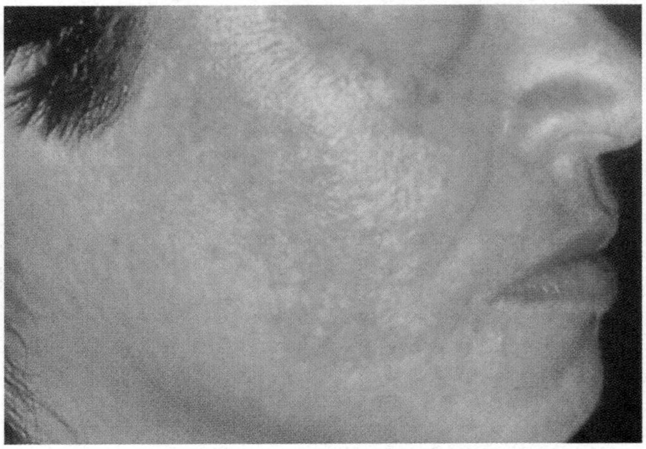

Figure 4–7 Mask of pregnancy with hyperpigmentation.

Tanning enhances the condition, so avoiding sun exposure helps cut down on the amount of pigment produced during pregnancy. Normally, hyperpigmentation subsides after the birth of the child, but sometimes the condition needs to be treated in the salon after childbirth. Treating hyperpigmentation during pregnancy is not advisable: Even if the skin returns to its normal color after use of melanin suppressants such as hydroquinone, the placenta continues production of the melanin-producing hormone, only to result in more hyperpigmentation. It is best to wait until the pregnancy is over. If the hyperpigmentation does not fade within several months, it can then be treated.

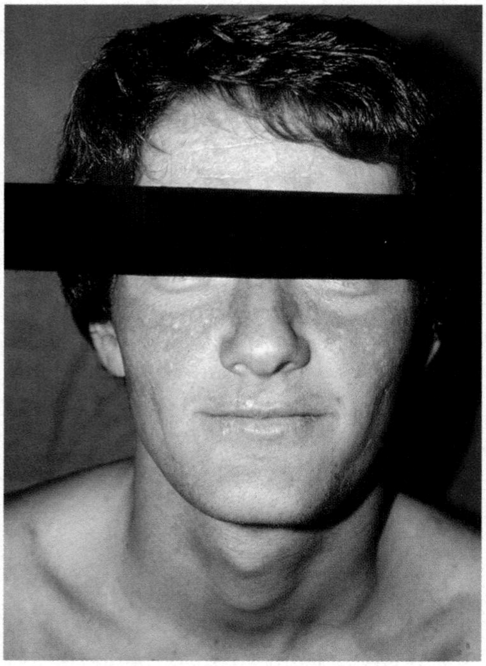

Figure 4–8 Melasma in a male patient is very uncommon.

Pregnant women may also experience stretch marks, or **striae distensae,** which are the result of rapid weight gain during pregnancy. The skin simply stretches quickly, and these strip-like red or tan-brown lines may appear on the abdomen, breasts, buttocks, and legs. Unfortunately, little can be done for stretch marks, many of which fade after childbirth. The use of good, hydrating body creams and lubricants during the pregnancy seems to help some women avoid stretch marks or at least reduces the severity of those that develop. For best results, the creams must be applied on a consistent, daily basis. However, in some women creams seem to have no effect. Some theories indicate that the development of stretch marks may be influenced by heredity. Research is currently being conducted using retinoids, electrical stimulation, and other methods to treat post-pregnancy stretch marks.

An increase in blood flow and blood pressure during pregnancy may lead to the development of telangiectasias, or small, red, enlarged capillaries on the face and other areas of the body. (Some European estheticians call these *couperose*.) Avoiding sun and hot temperatures helps reduce the possibility of telangiectatic development. Telangiectasias usually fade rapidly after childbirth. If there are still obvious red lines several months later, they may be treated by a dermatologist or plastic surgeon using an electric needle called a hyfrecator, Intense Pulsed Light (IPL Treatments) or laser.

Pregnant women may also develop varicose veins on the legs due to weight and pressure on the legs. Resting with the legs elevated helps to prevent their occurrence. Use of support hose is also helpful. Waterproof leg makeup may be used to conceal varicose veins (and can also be used to conceal telangiectasias). Most varicose veins fade after pregnancy, but those that do not can be treated by a dermatologist, plastic surgeon, or vascular surgeon.

Pregnant women may also have problems with their facial skin. Fluctuations in hormones may make problem skin worse or significantly better. In many cases, acne-prone skin becomes worse at the beginning of a pregnancy, then becomes much better in the third or fourth month, resulting in clear skin for the rest of the pregnancy. This is the result of the abundant female hormones present in the bloodstream during pregnancy. Acne will often flare up again after the baby is born, or just after the mother stops nursing, a result of a dramatic drop in female hormones in the bloodstream.

Precautions for Treating the Pregnant Woman

Pregnant women need lots of esthetic help during pregnancy. During the first trimester a pregnant client may have more breakouts due to increased androgen activity in her system. (For some women this happens during an entire pregnancy, but for many others the skin will clear and become glowing as their bodies shifts to higher estrogen levels that become dominant in the later months.) When treating acne or other skin conditions in a pregnant woman, check with the client's physician if you have any doubts about treatment or products. Under no circumstances should you administer any type of electrical therapy, specifically galvanic or high-frequency therapies, to a pregnant woman, without written permission from her physician. Physicians will often approve of electrolysis treatment, but for legal reasons it is important to obtain a written note from a client's doctor and keep it on file with the client's record.

Many topical preparations, including alphahydroxy acids, have never been extensively evaluated as to their safety for pregnant women. Although there is no currently available cosmetic agent known to affect a fetus, it is best to be conservative when using topical treatments and products, particularly newer functional agents. If you are in doubt about recommending a particular treatment to a pregnant client, check with her physician before administering that treatment or any questionable product for home use.

Most routine procedures may be performed on pregnant women. Special courses in body massage therapy for pregnant women are available from certified massage therapy schools. Make sure you have taken such a course before performing body massage on a pregnant woman.

Pregnant women may sometimes develop strange reactions to treatments they have tolerated well in the past. For example, waxing may suddenly be very irritating to a client's skin. The only way to predict these reactions is to start slowly and patch-test areas for treatment. A woman's physician should supervise any internal or external drugs she takes during pregnancy.

Overall, it is important to remember that pregnancy is a wonderful, but sometimes emotional, time for women. As the pregnancy progresses, your client may simply seek comfort. For example, because of changes in the nails, pedicures may become a necessity, rather than a luxury service. Especially during the third trimester, it is critical to make sure the client does not lay flat for any extended period of time. If she complains of light-headedness, immediately help her to a sitting position. Simply be sensitive to a pregnant client's needs.

Premenstrual Syndrome

Premenstrual syndrome (PMS) is a condition in which some women experience uncomfortable physical changes before menstruation. These changes are caused by the fluctuating levels of hormones in the bloodstream. Increased estrogen levels may lead to water retention that can cause bloating, swelling of the breasts, swelling of the hands and feet, and general heaviness. The increase in hormones can also cause mood swings and may make a woman more susceptible to stress.

Controlling stress is one of the best ways to deal with PMS. Stress-reducing techniques, such as deep-breathing exercises, aerobic workouts, massage, or general relaxation techniques, may help reduce the symptoms. Wearing looser clothes may help reduce feelings of constriction associated with water retention and increase overall comfort.

Esthetic care plays an important role in helping women with PMS feel better, both physically and psychologically. However, in severe cases, physician-administered hormones and other therapy may be warranted. Physicians may use medications for high blood pressure or hormone-suppressing drugs to treat women with severe PMS.

Women frequently experience acne flare-ups 7 to 10 days before menstruation. The specific days in the cycle associated with acne flare-ups may vary in some women. The cause of premenstrual acne is not completely understood. It is theorized that large levels of progesterone, present in the bloodstream during the cycle days normally associated with premenstrual acne, switch on the sebaceous glands, which quickly fill the follicles with sebum. This sudden surge of sebum inflames the follicle walls, causing acne papules to erupt.

Often, these flares occur in the chin and jawline areas. This is referred to as *chin acne*, which are large, sore papules (Figure 4–9). Many times they do not develop into pustules but clear up after a few days. Treatment at home with 2.5% benzoyl peroxide gel or a sulfur-resorcinol drying lotion may dry them faster. Women who experience constant, recurrent breakouts during premenstrual times should be referred to a dermatologist, gynecologist, or endocrinologist (hormone specialist) for treatment. Ortho Tri-Cyclen® is a birth control pill that can help clear up chin acne during premenstrual periods.

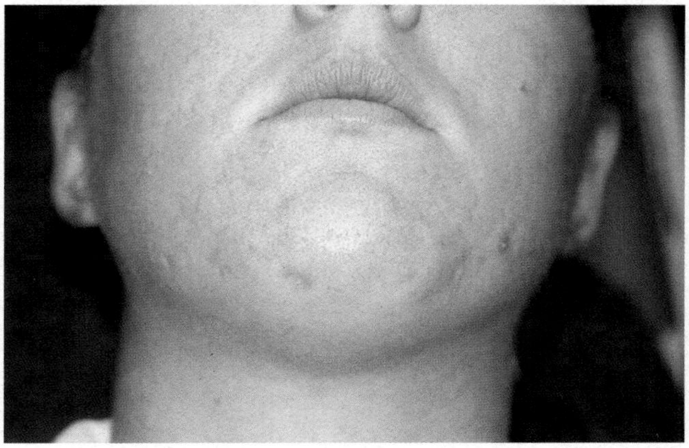

Figure 4–9 Chin acne.

In the salon, you can treat premenstrual acne in the same manner as any acne flare-up. Administer a good deep-cleansing facial treatment one week before the normal monthly breakout, which seems to help many women reduce or eliminate flare-ups. Use of noncomedogenic products also can help control the breakouts (as can other therapies that will be discussed in a later chapter). Increased stress during PMS can also cause breakouts or sudden acne flare-ups. Help your client choose some stress-reducing techniques or suggest that she treat herself to a body massage or other special pampering salon service to reduce stress and make herself feel better.

Birth Control Pills

Birth control pills work by regulating hormones normally associated with the menstrual cycle. They interfere with the normal development of the ovum by preventing or obstructing ovulation. There are two basic types of birth control pills. One type contains both estrogen and progesterone and works by preventing the egg from maturing, therefore preventing ovulation. The other type, often called the "mini-pill," is mainly made of progesterone. Mini-pills work by exposing the bloodstream to extra amounts of progesterone, which causes thickening of the uterine fluids, keeping an egg from becoming fertile.

Skin Problems Associated with Birth Control Pills

A skin problem often associated with the use of birth control pills is the tendency to have acne flares. This does not occur in all women using birth control pills, but it does occur in a substantial number. It is common that estheticians see clients with acne flares who have just started using a new type of birth control pill. The hormones in the pills change normal hormone levels, affecting sebum production.

Birth control pills that contain little or no estrogen tend to be more aggravating to acne conditions. Estrogen-dominant pills tend to improve acne-prone skin.

In the past, birth control pills with high levels of hormones often caused very frequent acne flares. More modern birth control pills contain smaller amounts of hormones and do not cause as many problems with acne flares.

Starting and stopping birth control pills may have a dramatic effect on acne. Starting an androgen-dominant or progesterone-dominant pill may make acne immediately worse, whereas starting an estrogen-dominant pill may make acne-prone skin immediately better.

Stopping the pill may have like effects. Because the pill has a tendency to suppress natural hormone levels, discontinuing the pill may throw off natural hormone levels, making acne worse. It may take some time for the body to adjust to not having the hormone "supplement" present in the birth control pills.

Hyperpigmentation and the Birth Control Pill

The other appearance problem related to birth control pills is that of hyperpigmentation, or melasma. Splotchy, pigmented complexions may be present after use of birth control pills. This hyperpigmentation usually is located in the forehead and cheeks. The upper lip is also often affected by melasma. Some women can develop a full-scale pregnancy mask associated with birth control pills.

Sunlight, especially during deliberate prolonged exposure, such as sunbathing, can make melasma much worse. Advise a client with melasma to stay out of the sun and, if she must go in the sun, to use a product with a high SPF. Sometimes a doctor can adjust the dosage or the type of the client's pill to reduce the possibility of melasma resulting from its use.

You should treat hyperpigmentation with skin-brightening agents and acids. (These are discussed in later chapters.) Paramedical camouflage cosmetics or other concealing agents can also be used.

Menopause

Menopause is the time in a woman's life when the ovaries stop releasing ova. A female is born with 700,000 to 2 million eggs, which are contained in the follicles within the ovaries. Many die or atrophy, but at puberty about 400,000 remain. The pituitary gland secretes FSH and LH, but the ovaries stop responding. When no follicles are left to respond to follicle-stimulating hormone, no estrogen is produced in the ovary, and the preparation of the uterus does not occur.

Menopause normally occurs when a woman is in her late 40s or early 50s. The time before and around menopause is called **perimenopause.** The drop in hormone levels in the bloodstream as perimenopause progresses to menopause causes a variety of physical symptoms, including hot flashes, rapid heartbeat, decreases in vaginal secretions, emotional irritability, and bloating.

A young woman who has had a complete hysterectomy may experience these same symptoms as early menopause. To keep that from happening, gynecologists try to leave the ovaries and remove only the uterus. The ovaries help secure hormone levels in the bloodstream, at least until true menopause takes place. Medical science has discovered that women who lose their ovaries early in life are more likely to develop **osteoporosis,** a weakening of the bones, which is a condition associated with aging that is predominant in women.

Hormone Therapy

Many women have **hormone replacement therapy (HRT)** after menopause or after a hysterectomy. Use of synthetic estrogen and progesterone, taken in the sequence of the normal menstrual cycle hormone secretions, helps prevent many of the symptoms associated with menopause. It, of course, will not make women ovulate again. Estrogen is believed to reduce the chances of osteoporosis development, offer a decreased chance of cardiac problems, and may help prevent rheumatoid arthritis.

Some recent studies indicate that there may be an increased risk of breast cancer in women who use HRT longer than five years. If there is a family history of breast cancer in the immediate family (sister, mother), there may be a greater risk. The use of HRT should be an individual and personal decision based on personal and family history; menopausal symptoms and their severity; and, most importantly, a thorough consultation with a doctor. There are many more HRT options available today than only a few years ago, so if your client is experiencing problems, encourage her to seek a knowledgeable specialist for an evaluation.

Skin Conditions Associated with Menopause

In the next two decades 40 million women will go through menopause. Esthetically, a woman may have any number of symptoms associated with perimenopause. This may include thinning hair, excess hair growth on the face or other body areas, or even increased oiliness or dryness of the skin.

Recent research indicates that the presence of estrogen has a strong influence on collagen formation. As menopause occurs, estrogen levels drop dramatically and may have an obvious effect on the appearance of wrinkles and lack of elasticity. Use of HRT may improve and reduce the loss of collagen, therefore causing skin to regain more of its previous elasticity and suppleness.

Lack of estrogen may significantly affect barrier function, increasing sensitivity of the skin, dehydration, possible hyperpigmentation, and fluctuations in blood flow. Estrogen is responsible for sending many hormonal messages to the skin, and a decrease can affect many functions of the skin and, therefore, its appearance.

Many aging problems associated with menopause may actually be the result of cumulative sun exposure earlier in life. It is coincidental that the damage of years of sun exposure happen to surface about the same time as menopause in some women. Having both sun damage and menopausal effects on the skin can cause real esthetic problems and is even more reason why your client needs lots of care at this important time.

Hot Flashes and Flushing

Hot flashes are caused by a fluctuation in blood flow resulting from decreased estrogen, which normally helps with smooth blood flow. Without estrogen, there are sudden "spurts" in blood flow, resulting in redness and the feeling of heat in the skin. Flushing and hot flashes can be reduced or eliminated with hormone replacement therapy.

Rarely, women experience a condition called **formication,** which feels like continuous tingling and itching. Some women have described it as feeling like "bugs crawling on the skin." Again, this can be treated with HRT.

Use of nonfragranced creams with lipid replacement ingredients such as sphingolipids or ceramides may help with dryness and itching. The skin may be more sensitive to any stimulating product, so be careful with these, especially stimulating aromatherapy products.

Moodiness

Women may experience moodiness during menopause. Although some of this may be caused by hormonal fluctuations, it may also be stress-related or may be complicated by depression. It is important that you understand your client's needs and offer stress-reducing services such as massages or aromatherapy.

Perimenopausal Acne

Clients may experience a sudden flare of acne during or just after menopause. This is again caused by a decrease of estrogen in the bloodstream, which, in turn, increases the percentage of the male hormone androgen that turns on the sebaceous glands. This results in increased oiliness, hirsutism, and acne lesions. Treat this as you would any other acne case, but remember that the client may more readily experience dehydration and be concerned about aging skin. Be careful not to overdry the skin.

Esthetic Management of Menopausal Skin

You can play a significant role in helping your menopausal client with skin problems. You may actually notice small symptoms in the client's skin before she is even fully aware that she is beginning menopause. Some symptoms include the following:

1. Dryness and itchy skin on the face and body
2. Increased sensitivity
3. Sudden flares of acne
4. Sudden hair growth on the face
5. Mood swings
6. Client complains of "suddenly aging" skin
7. Hot flashes and flushing
8. A "tired" look to the skin, with increased elastosis

Keep a client's age in mind when noticing some of the symptoms discussed here. Adjusting a client's home care and treatment schedule may help a great deal. For clients experiencing aging symptoms, recommend lipid-based creams, which can help improve barrier function. Soothing antioxidants can help reduce redness and discomfort. Alphahydroxy acids or the use of vitamin A products may also relieve various symptoms. More frequent salon treatments may help esthetic symptoms as well as help with stress management.

HIRSUTISM

Women who have hormonal fluctuations may experience **hirsutism,** or excess hair growth, primarily on the face. This may happen at any time in a woman's life, but it happens especially after menopause, caused primarily by the dominance of the androgenic hormones.

Hirsutism may be treated by waxing, electrolysis, LASER, or IPL hair removal. Excessive facial hair growth is often best treated by electrolysis or laser-type devices because the result is more long-lasting or eventually frees the client from unwanted hair. Waxing may provide temporary relief in minor cases. Stiffer hairs in the chin and lip areas are best treated by electrolysis. Estheticians and electrologists should be aware of other symptoms that may require referral to a physician. Although most excessive hair is mainly a cosmetic nuisance, accompanying symptoms such as thinning of the hair, deepening of the voice, and loss of menstruation should be referred to a gynecologist or endocrinologist.

OBESITY, ANOREXIA, AND HORMONES

Women who are extremely obese may experience a loss of hormone activity, resulting in menstrual irregularity, hirsutism, and acne. Women who are anorexic may have hormonal fluctuations and irregular menstrual cycles.

Women athletes who have a very low body fat percentage may also experience similar hormonal problems. Many estheticians have observed a correlation between avid female athletes and low body fat, hirsutism, and acne.

OTHER HORMONAL DISORDERS THAT AFFECT THE SKIN

Although it is not the esthetician's job to diagnose illness, you should be aware of some symptoms that you may connect with certain skin problems or be able to discuss a client's skin symptoms that are related to an endocrine illness. If you have a client who has multiple symptoms of any kind of illness, always refer the client to a doctor.

Thyroid Hormones

Hyperthyroidism is a condition in which the thyroid gland secretes too much thyroid hormone. Physical symptoms may include heart palpitations, weight loss, and fatigue. Esthetic symptoms include thinning of the skin, hair loss, and rapidly growing nails. In **hypothyroidism,** the opposite of hyperthyroidism, the thyroid gland does not produce enough hormone. Puffy eyelids, facial swelling, and coarse skin that is very dehydrated are esthetic symptoms of hypothyroidism. Hypothyroidism is also associated with weight gain, poor balance, and hearing problems.

Adrenal Glands

Adrenal gland disorders can also result in skin symptoms. Persons with Cushing's Syndrome, a disease of the adrenal glands, secrete too much hydrocortisone. Too much medicinal hydrocortisone can also cause the disease. Symptoms are thinning of the skin and bruises that occur easily. Addison's Disease is the exact opposite of Cushing's Syndrome: The adrenal glands do not produce adrenal hormones. Skin symptoms include severe hyperpigmentation on the face, dark freckles on the torso, and hyperpigmentation on the palms of the hands. Addison's Disease is easily treated with hormone therapy.

REVIEW QUESTIONS

1. What are the major endocrine glands?
2. What is puberty, and what hormonal changes take place with puberty?
3. What skin changes take place during puberty?
4. Discuss the menstrual cycle and its hormonal fluctuations.
5. What precautions should the esthetician take when treating a pregnant woman?

6. What are some esthetic side effects of birth control pills?
7. What is HRT and for whom is it beneficial?
8. What are some esthetic problems associated with menopause?
9. What are some skin symptoms of menopause?
10. Name several endocrine disorders and discuss their effects on the skin.

CHAPTER GLOSSARY

adrenal glands: endocrine glands, located just above the kidneys, that produce hormones needed by the nervous system to transport nerve impulses.

adrenaline: a hormone secreted by the adrenal glands during an emergency response, such as stress. Elevates the heartrate, increases blood pressure, and triggers the release of cortisol.

androgens: male hormones.

apocrine glands: coiled structures attached to hair follicles found in the underarm and genital areas. They produce a thicker form of sweat and are responsible for producing the substance that, when in contact with bacteria, produces body odor.

corpus luteum: a temporary endocrine structure that develops from the ovarian follicle during the menstrual cycle; esstential to establishing and maintaining pregnancy.

diabetes: disease that results when the pancreas does not secrete enough insulin.

endocrine glands: 1. ductless glands that release hormonal secretions directly into the bloodstream. 2. a group of specialized glands that affect the growth, development, sexual activities, and health of the entire body.

endometrium: the inner membrane of the uterus.

estradiol: a steroid made from the hormone estrogen that gives women female characteristics.

estriol: The third estrogen produced by the human body. It is only present in significant amounts during pregnancy. Other than at this time, levels of estriol do not change considerably during a person's life.

estrogen: the hormone that gives women female characteristics.

estrone: an estrogentic hormone secreted by the ovary and the least prevalent of the estrogen hormones. It can be converted by the body to estradiol.

exocrine (duct) glands: duct glands that produce a substance that travels through small tubelike ducts, such as the sudoriferous (sweat) glands and the sebaceous (oil) glands.

follicle-stimulating hormone (FSH): hormone secreted by the pituitary gland that causes the development of the egg, or ovum.

formication: itching and tingling feeling of the skin experienced by some women during menopause.

hirsutism: excessive growth of an unusual amount of hair on parts of the body normally bearing only downy hair, such as the face, arms, and legs of women or the backs of men.

hormone replacement therapy (HRT): oral, topical, implanted or injection methods used to administer female hormones to control or prevent symptoms of menopause. HRT may also help prevent skin changes or osteoporosis in women.

hormones: secretions produced by one of the endocrine glands and carried by the bloodstream or body fluid to another part of the body, or a body organ, to stimulate functional activity or secretion; the internal messengers for most of the body's systems.

hyperthyroidism: a condition in which the thyroid gland secretes too much thyroid hormone.

hypothalamus: 1. manufactures hormones that stimulate the pituitary gland to make

CHAPTER GLOSSARY

other hormones. It is also able to detect needs of various parts of the body by chemically monitoring the blood. 2. Regulator of important metabolic functions, hormone release and autonomic function.

hypothalamus gland: controls movement of some involuntary muscles, such as the muscles of the intestines that help move food through the gastrointestinal system.

hypothyroidism: a condition in which the thyroid glands secretes too little thyroid hormone.

keratosis pilaris: redness and bumpiness common on the cheeks or upper arms caused by blocked hair follicles. The patches of irritation are accompanied by a rough texture and small pinpoint white papules that look like very small milia.

luteinizing hormone (LH): hormone that causes the actual process of ovulation or the release of the egg from the ovary. It also causes the testes to manufacture testosterone.

menarche: the first menstrual period.

menopause: the time in a woman's life when the ovaries stop producing ova.

menstruation: process by which the female body rids itself of an unused ovum and accompanying endometrium.

osteoporosis: a thinning of the bones, leaving them fragile and prone to fractures; caused by the reabsorption of calcium into the blood.

ovaries: organs in the female reproductive system located just above the uterus and connected to the uterus by two hollow tubes called fallopian tubes.

pancreas: organ located in the abdomen; secretes pancreatic enzymes that are delivered into the intestine.

parathyroid gland: gland responsible for regulating calcium and phosphates in the bloodstream.

perimenopause: the time before and around menopause.

pineal gland: gland located in the brain. Its function is not well understood, but it is thought to be related to the sex hormones.

pituitary gland: gland found in the center of the head; serves as the "brain" of the endocrine system.

premenstrual syndrome (PMS): a condition in which some women experience uncomfortable physical changes before menstruation.

progesterone: hormone that helps prepare the uterus for pregnancy and is an important hormone in the menstrual cycle.

puberty: stage of life when physical changes occur in both sexes and when sexual function of the sex glands begins to take place.

relaxin: hormone manufactured by the ovaries that helps enlarge the pelvic opening during childbirth.

secreted: synthesized or released by various cells or organs.

striae distensae: stretch marks commonly occurring during pregnancy.

testes: organs of the male reproductive system; reside in the scrotum and produce sperm.

testosterone: male hormone responsible for development of typical male characteristics.

thymus gland: gland located under the breastbone in the chest; secretes hormones and helps to trigger synthesis of more lymph tissue.

thyroid gland: gland located in the neck; regulates both cellular and body metabolism and produces hormones that stimulate growth.

thyroxine: one of the hormones secreted by the thyroid gland.

trophic hormones: chemicals that cause glands to make hormones.

CHAPTER OUTLINE

- MUSCLE TYPES
- FUNCTION OF SKELETAL MUSCLES
- MUSCLES OF THE HEAD AND FACE
- MUSCLES OF THE NECK
- MUSCLES OF THE TRUNK
- MUSCLES OF THE ARMS AND SHOULDERS
- MUSCLES OF THE LEGS
- FACIAL NERVE PATTERNS

CHAPTER 5

ANATOMY AND PHYSIOLOGY: MUSCLES AND NERVES

LEARNING OBJECTIVES

After completing this chapter, you should be able to:

- Identify the facial muscles.
- Understand the functions of facial nerves.
- Demonstrate a knowledge of the body muscles.
- Identify the different types of muscles.
- Explain the types and functions of the skeletal muscles.
- Explain the various types of muscle movement.
- Identify the purpose of these muscles.
- Identify the facial nerves and their innervation.

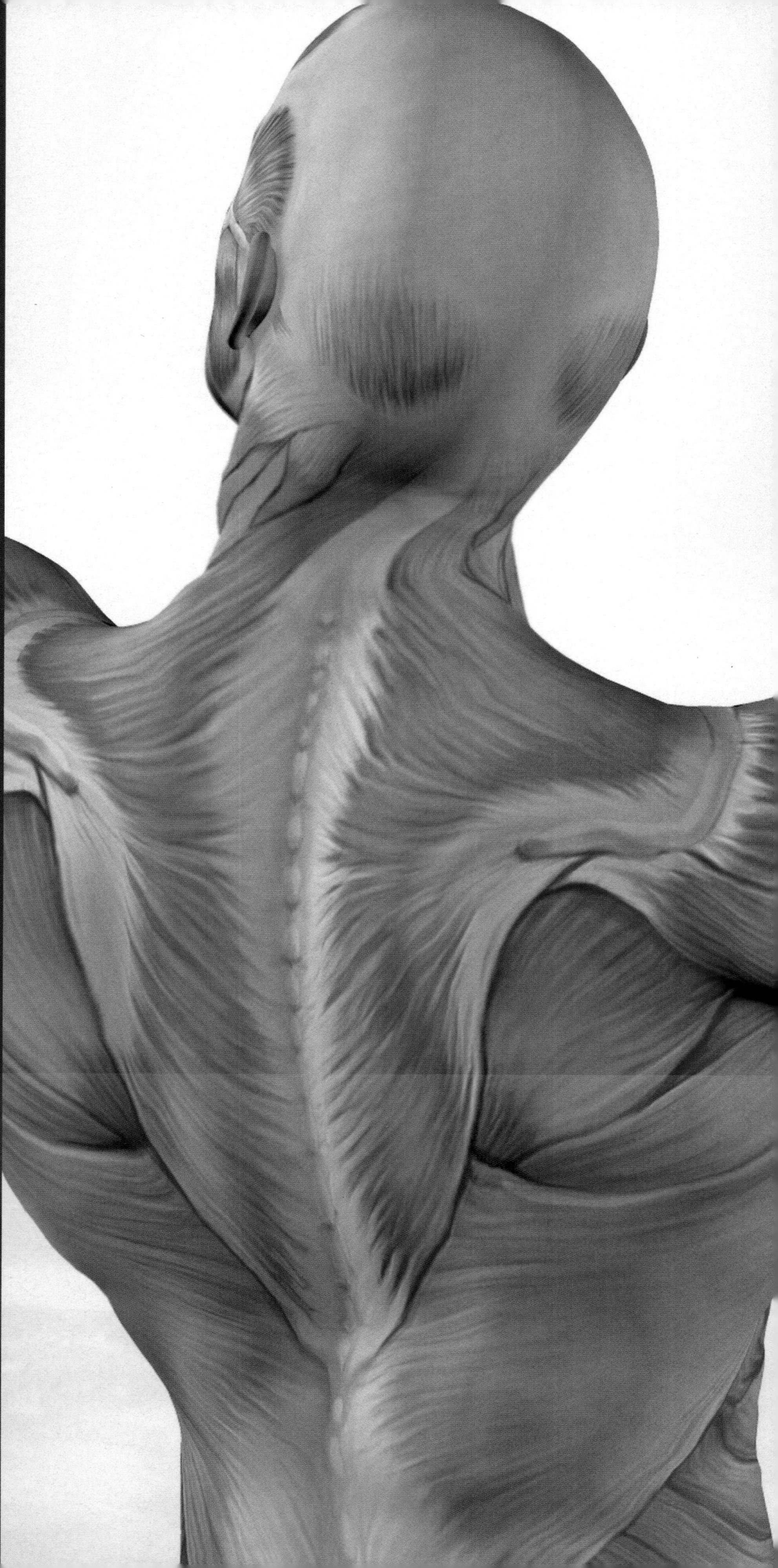

KEY TERMS

Page numbers indicate where in the chapter the term is used.

acetylcholine 106
adduction 111
adductor group of muscles 115
ala 111
antagonist 110
aponeurosis 108
bicep brachii 112
brachialis 112
cardiac fibers 105
depression 112
endomysium 106
epimysium 106
erector spinae 112
extensor digitorium longus 117
external obliques 112
fibularis muscle group 117
flexation 111
frenulum 110
gastrocnemius 117
gluteus group of muscles 115
hamstrings 116
hyperextension 112
insertion 107
intercostal muscles 111
internal obliques 112
lateral 109
latissimus dorsal 112
muscle fibers 105
myofilaments 105
nare 111
neuromuscular junction 106
neurotransmitter 106
obliquely 109
orifice 109
palpebra 109
perimysium 106
quadriceps 116
rectus abdominis 112
soleus 117
supination 113
synapse 106
tendons 106
tibialis anterior 117
trapezius 112
traverse abdominals 112
tricep brachii 112

It is important to have a rich understanding of what is under the skin on which you work. Whether your career goals lean toward spa or medical, this knowledge will help you offer the best and safest treatments to your clients and to be able to communicate in a more informed manner with specialists or medical practitioners with whom you may work. This chapter builds on the terms and basic knowledge you already have and moves into a more in-depth study of the facial nerves and the muscles of face and body.

MUSCLE TYPES

What makes muscle tissue unique compared to other types of tissue in the body is its ability to contract and shorten. **Myofilaments** aid this process. Muscle cells are uniquely elongated, cylindrical in shape, and multinucleate. Muscle cells (except cardiac muscle cells) are referred to as **muscle fibers.** Cumulatively, muscle cells make up three different types of specialized muscle tissue: cardiac muscles, smooth muscles, and—most significant to estheticians—skeletal muscles (Figure 5–1).

Cardiac Muscles

As the name implies, cardiac muscles reside in the heart. **Cardiac fibers** (the name for muscle cells in the heart) are unlike any other type of muscle tissue. They are striated

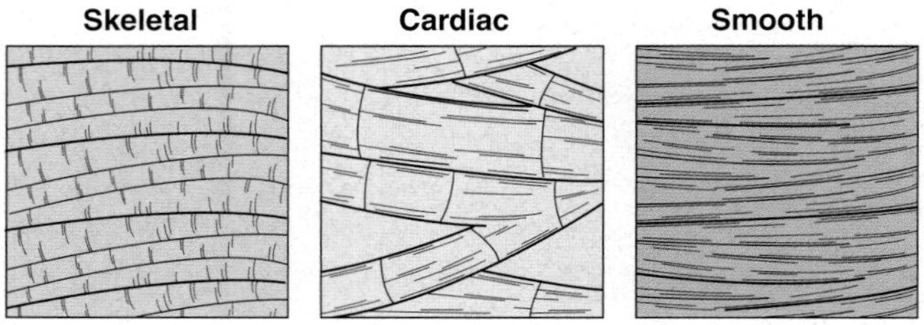

Figure 5–1 Muscle types.

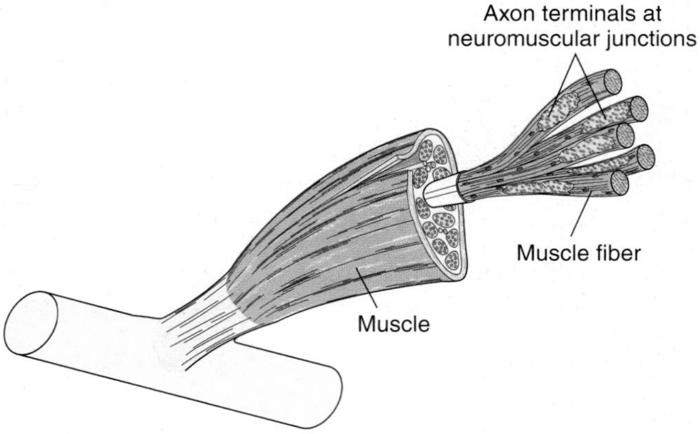

Figure 5–2 Cross section of skeletal muscle.

and contract involuntarily, meaning a person cannot consciously control his or her movements. The regulation of these contractions is determined by an internal pacemaker and can also be determined by the central nervous system. (See Chapter 6 for a larger discussion of the heart.)

Smooth Muscles

Smooth muscles are found in hollow internal organs, most often in passages where substances need a push to get through (such as the stomach and the digestive tract). These muscle fibers have a single nucleus and lack striations. Like cardiac fibers, the muscle fibers of smooth muscles are involuntary in their movements.

Skeletal Muscles

As their name implies, skeletal muscles are attached to the skeletal system. They are the largest muscles in the body and are often visible to the naked eye. Located just below the skin, skeletal muscles are a key contributor to the shape of the human form.

Skeletal muscle fibers are long and cylindrical with noticeable striations. What makes skeletal muscles unique is that they operate voluntarily. This means that a person's conscious decision to turn his or her head will result in the head turning. Skeletal muscle can also move involuntarily as well (for example, blinking). Both voluntarily and involuntary movements of skeletal muscle are regulated by the brain. (See the following section for more information.)

Skeletal muscles can exert a great deal of force with very little effort. Their inherent design allows for this. Individual muscle fibers are protected by connective tissue known as an **endomysium.** Several muscle fibers are bunched together and wrapped in a fibrous sheathing called a **perimysium.** In between these bunches, blood vessels supply nutrients and oxygen and remove waste buildup. These bunches are further supported by a tough outer sheathing known as the **epimysium.** The epimysium connects to strong connective tissue, called **tendons,** which attach the muscle to the bone.

Skeletal Muscles and the Nervous System

As already mentioned, skeletal muscles (Figure 5–2) move voluntarily. For example, when the brain makes a conscious decision to turn the head, the muscles in the neck respond. But how is this accomplished?

In simple terms, human muscles have the ability to respond to a stimulus (usually an electrical impulse sent from the brain) by contracting. Littered throughout muscle tissue are neurons (nerve cells). These neurons branch out and meet muscle cells at a point called the **neuromuscular junction.** In the neuromuscular junction the nerve endings and the muscle fibers never quite touch one another (Figure 5–3). In between is the **synapse.** A **neurotransmitter** called **acetylcholine** (ACh) crosses the synapse and is received on the other end. Once ACh reaches its port of reception, a chemical reaction produces an electrical current that travels the length of the muscle cell. Because muscle fibers have the ability to respond to a stimulus, a property known as *irritability,* the response is the contraction of the muscle fiber. Cumulatively, the response is the shortening of the muscle, and hence, the desired motion intended by the original conscious decision.

FUNCTION OF SKELETAL MUSCLES

Human muscles don't just serve the singular purpose of movement. In fact, they are multifunctional. Muscles help maintain upright posture, stabilize joints, generate heat, and hold internal organs in place.

Movement is necessary, but what is truly splendid about movement is instinctual motion. Instinctual motion saves people from hurting themselves. Consider touching something that is hot. Before the pain truly

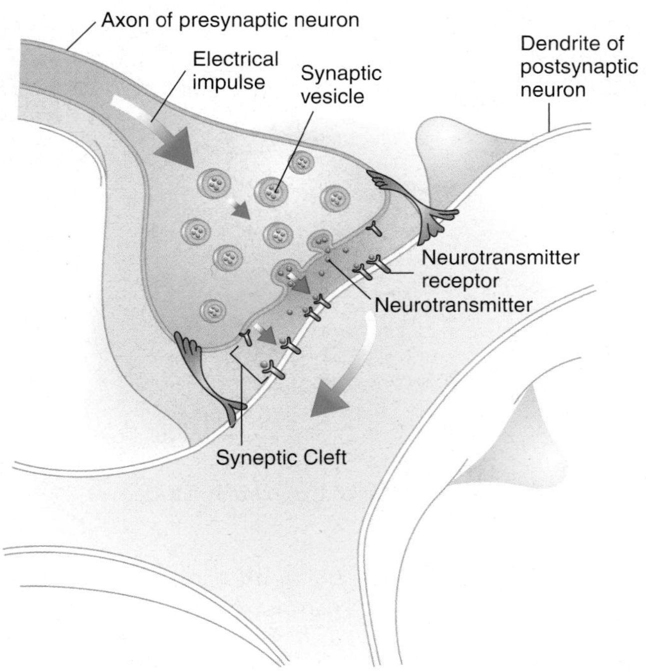

Figure 5–3a Synapse structure.

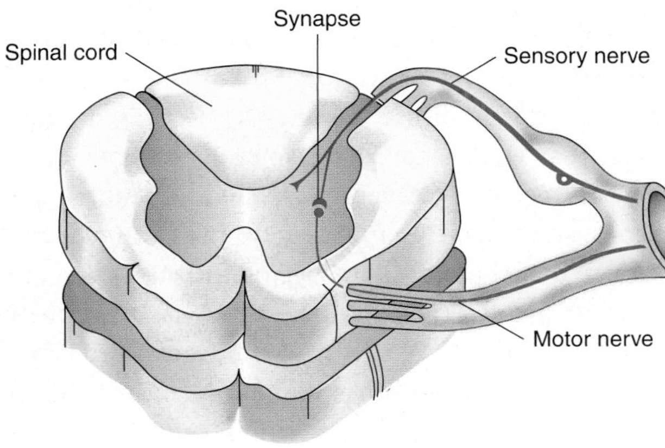

Figure 5–3b The path of a nerve impulse.

registers, you unconsciously pull your hand away from the heat. While your conscious mind realizes the pain and you remove your hand entirely, this instinctive motion means the difference between a superficial burn and a deep thermal injury.

Movement is something that usually comes easily and is often taken for granted. Without the ability to move, humans couldn't eat, breathe, talk, walk, or even smile. The ability to "do" is thanks to muscles (Table 5–1).

People owe upright posture to muscles. While gravity is constantly trying to pull the body down, muscles are actively resisting. This allows people to stand up, jump, walk, and sit down at will. Even the mere act of standing requires muscles to perform complex tasks in conjunction with the brain. Repeated exposure to poor ergonomic conditions causes muscles to overcompensate and become strained and tense over time.

Table 5–1 Types of Body Movement

TYPES OF BODY MOVEMENT	
Flexation	to move a joint in such a way as to decrease the angle of the joint
Extension	to move a joint in such a way as to increase the angle of the joint
Hyperextension	to extend beyond the normal range of motion, commonly beyond 180°
Rotation	to turn on an axis as in ball and socket joints
Abduction	to move a limb away from the center of the body
Adduction	to move a limb toward the center of the body
Circumduction	the combination of many movements to describe a cone or circle in space
Dorsiflexion	moving up and down as in the foot
Inversion	related to the foot; turning the sole to the center of the body
Eversion	the opposite of inversion
Supination	to turn backward
Pronation	to turn forward
Opposition	to touch the thumb to the fingers

Muscles also work very closely with the skeletal system—and joints in particular. The strength of muscles and tendons compensate for some inherent design flaws in the joints, which allows the joints to function over longer periods of time.

Mentioned less often but still a vital duty of the muscles is the production of heat. Remember that energy is neither created nor destroyed, and the same is true for the body. The energy that creates the kinetic energy of movements is mostly converted to heat. This heat, in turn, is important to maintain ideal body temperature.

All muscles have a beginning point, which is called the origin. Similarly, all muscles have an end point, which is called the **insertion**. These terms will be used throughout this chapter. Also, muscles control movements, and each of these movements has a name. See Table 5–1 for a detailed list of these movements.

MUSCLES OF THE HEAD AND FACE

Faces are wrought with expression. These expressions have their origins in the muscles that lie beneath the skin.

Muscles of the Forehead

The skin of the scalp is among the thickest of the body. Hair follicles cover much of it, along with a few sebaceous glands. The scalp adheres closely to fascia and underlying muscle, and those muscles move our skin. There are no muscles underneath the scalp proper. Muscles of the forehead and temple fan out into fascia in the direction of the crown.

The forehead musculature is simple: There is only one muscle, the frontalis (Figure 5–4). While the frontalis is a single muscle, it can behave as if it were two muscles or at least bifurcated, but it is not. You no doubt have seen expressions where only half of the forehead was used, such as a lift of one eyebrow. The frontalis lies directly beneath the skin of the forehead, stretching from temple to temple and from the eyebrows to approximately the hairline (Figure 5–5). At the hairline, the frontalis shades off into an **aponeurosis** with the thick fascia of the vertex of the skull.

As you might expect, the frontalis is responsible for lifting the eyebrows. At the same time it works to draw the scalp forward, producing transverse or horizontal wrinkles. Although as a muscle it stands alone, the frontalis is still a team player. In its lower middle it blends into the procerus, a muscle of the nose; to each side it blends with the upper eye muscles, the corrugator and orbicularis oculi. The nerve powering the frontalis muscle is a branch of the facial nerve aptly called the *frontal branch.*

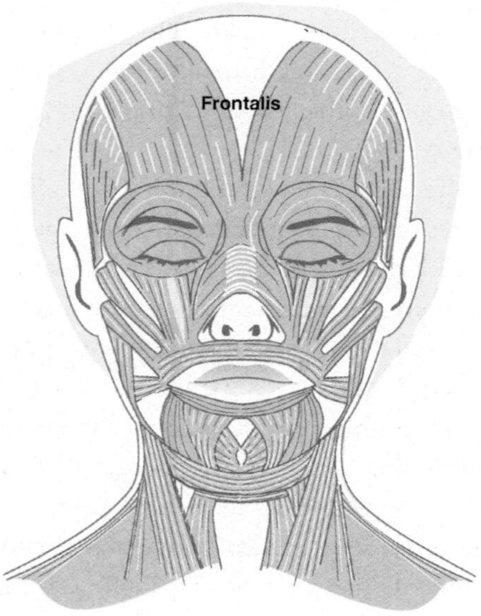

Figure 5–4 The frontalis muscle.

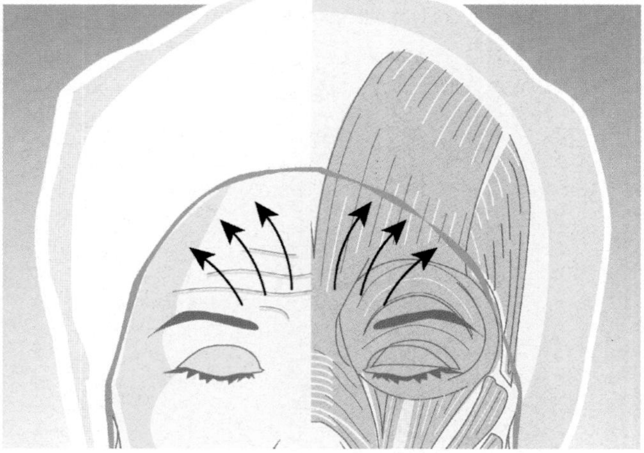

Figure 5–5 The movement of the frontalis muscle.

Muscles of the Eye

The periocular area, the area around the eyes, including two muscles lying beneath the eyebrows and over the eyes, have a lot to do with facial expressions. As time dances on, habitual expressions tend to become rather well tracked into the face (Figure 5–6).

Eyelids and eyebrows are mobile because of these muscles that work together for smooth movement: the orbicularis oculi, the levator palpebrae superioris, and the corrugator supercilii. If you know any Latin, you will recognize that the orbicularis begins with the word *orb,* so it must involve the eye; the levator has to do with lifting. *Super-* means "above" and the Latin word *cilium* means "eyelash"; *supercilii* is plural and means "above the eyelashes." As to *corrugator*—think cardboard which though quite thin has great strength.

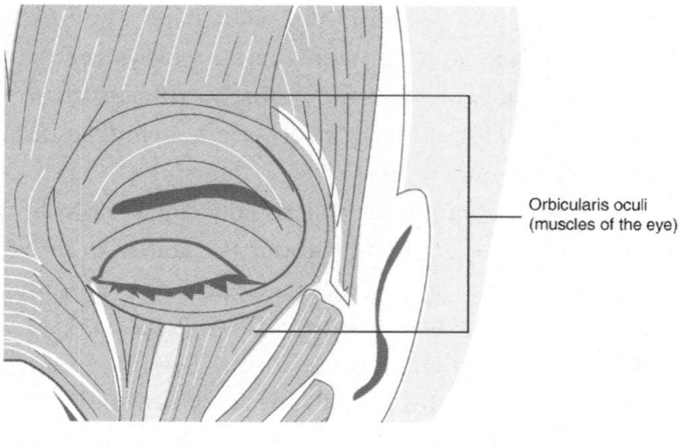

Figure 5–6 Muscles of the eye.

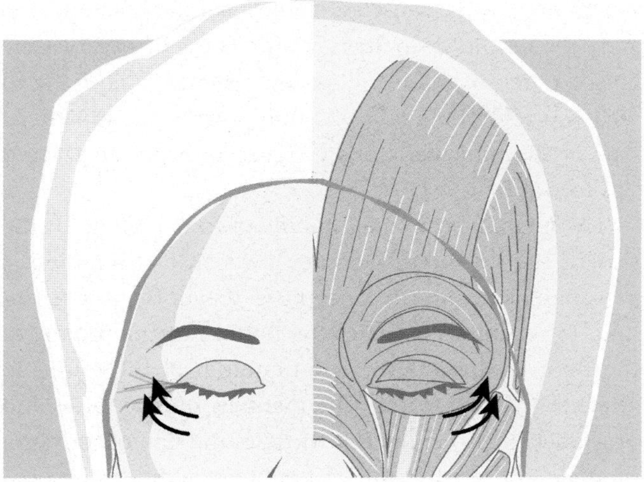

Figure 5–7 Muscle movement that causes crow's feet.

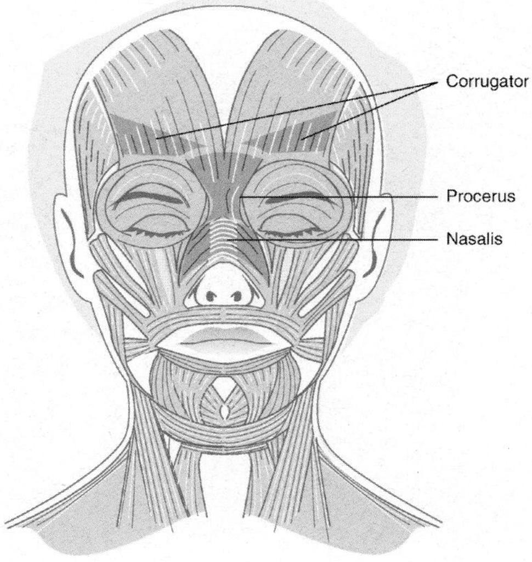

Figure 5–8 Glabellar, corrugator, procerus, and pyramidalis nasi.

The orbicularis oculi starts from the nose and wraps over the orb of the eye to form the eyelid, or **palpebra,** and finally fans out toward the temple. It is a *sphincter* muscle, meaning that it contracts to close an **orifice,** the eye. The muscle acts involuntarily to close the eye, as in sleep or blinking, and it can also be moved voluntarily. When the entire muscle is worked, as when a person shuts the eyes tightly, the skin of the forehead, temple, and cheek is pulled together, causing folds to radiate from the outside or **lateral** angle of the eyelid. As a person ages, these folds become permanent and are called *crow's feet* (Figure 5–7).

The levator palpebrae superioris antagonizes, or works against, the orbicularis oculi as it raises the upper eyelid to expose the orb of the eye. And the corrugator—this aptly named muscle is the "frowning" muscle, drawing the eyebrow down and toward the middle and producing those vertical wrinkles everyone knows so well (Figure 5–8).

Muscles of the Mouth

Many muscles are involved in the movement of the mouth and cheek areas. Table 5–2 lists those that produce characteristic expressions and their consequent lines.

The quadratus labii superioris is a broad sheet of muscle extending from the side of the nose and the upper lip to the zygomatic, or cheek, bone. This muscle elevates the upper lip, at the same time pushing it a little bit forward. Parts of this muscle help to form the *nasolabial* furrow, sometimes known not so fondly as "marionette lines," the lines passing from the side of the nose to the upper lip, imparting an expression of sadness. When the whole muscle works, pushing the lip out farther, it causes and expression of contempt or distain.

The muscles of the upper lip—the levator labii superioris and levator anguli oris—raise the angle of the mouth. Their combined efforts assist in forming the nasolabial ridge, that pesky line passing from the side of the nose to the upper lip. This line can be an indication of age based on its depth and surrounding tissue laxity (Figure 5–9). The levator labii inferioris controls the lower lip, raising the lower lip and making it protrude. That causes the skin of the chin to wrinkle in a pout.

The zygomaticus attaches to the front of the zygomatic bone—hence its name—and descends **obliquely** until it

Table 5–2 Major Muscles of the Mouth

ABOVE THE MOUTH	BELOW THE MOUTH	AROUND THE MOUTH
Quadratus labii superioris	Levator labii inferioris	Orbicularis oris
Levator labii superioris	Depressor anguli oris	Mentalis
Levator anguli oris	Depressor labii inferior	Quadratus labii inferioris
Zygomaticus		Risorius Buccinator

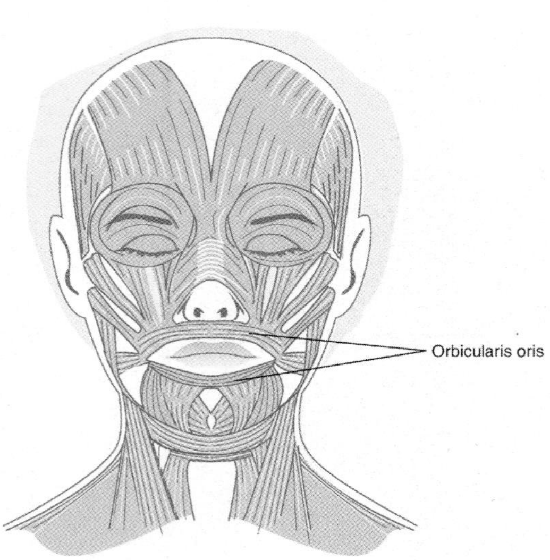

Figure 5–9 The muscles of the mouth.

inserts into the angle of the mouth. It draws the angle of the mouth back and upward during a laugh.

The muscles of the lower jaw and lower lip—the depressor anguli oris and depressor labii inferioris—give further expression to movements of the lower lip. The depressor labii inferioris draws the lower lip down and a little out, giving an expression of irony. The depressor anguli oris is the **antagonist** to the levator anguli oris; instead of pushing the lower lip forward it draws it down and back, as if to draw away from a bitter taste.

The orbicularis oris encircles the mouth but is not a simple sphincter muscle. It consists of many layers, or strata, of muscular tissue surrounding the mouth but having opposing actions. It also attaches and blends into neighboring facial muscles. Its most common action is to close the lips; its deep fibers compress the lips against the alveolar arch of the teeth, as when someone is trying to feed you something that you don't want. The superficial part of the orbicularis oris can also protrude the closed lips forward.

The mentalis is a small bundle of muscle fibers at the side of the **frenulum** of the lower lip. A frenulum is a tissue that connects one thing to another—a frenulum, for example, attaches the bottom of the tongue to the floor of the mouth. The frenulum of the lower lip attaches it to the gums. The mentalis muscle raises and protrudes the lower lip as it wrinkles the skin of the chin, producing an expression of doubt or disdain. The quadratus labii inferioris, arising from the mandible to insert into the lower lip, draws that lip down and somewhat to the side, producing an expression of irony.

The risorius begins over the masseter, the muscle used in chewing, and passes horizontally forward to insert into the angle of the mouth. It retracts the angle of the mouth downward, producing an unpleasant grinning expression.

The name *buccinator* comes from the Latin *buccina,* meaning "trumpet." The buccinator muscle is formed at the outer surfaces of the maxilla and mandible at about the level of the three molar teeth. Its fibers converge into the angle of the mouth, and it compresses the cheek so that, during chewing, food is kept at the mercy of the teeth. After distending the cheek with air, the buccinator muscle can expel it from between the lips in a whistle or a trumpet blow.

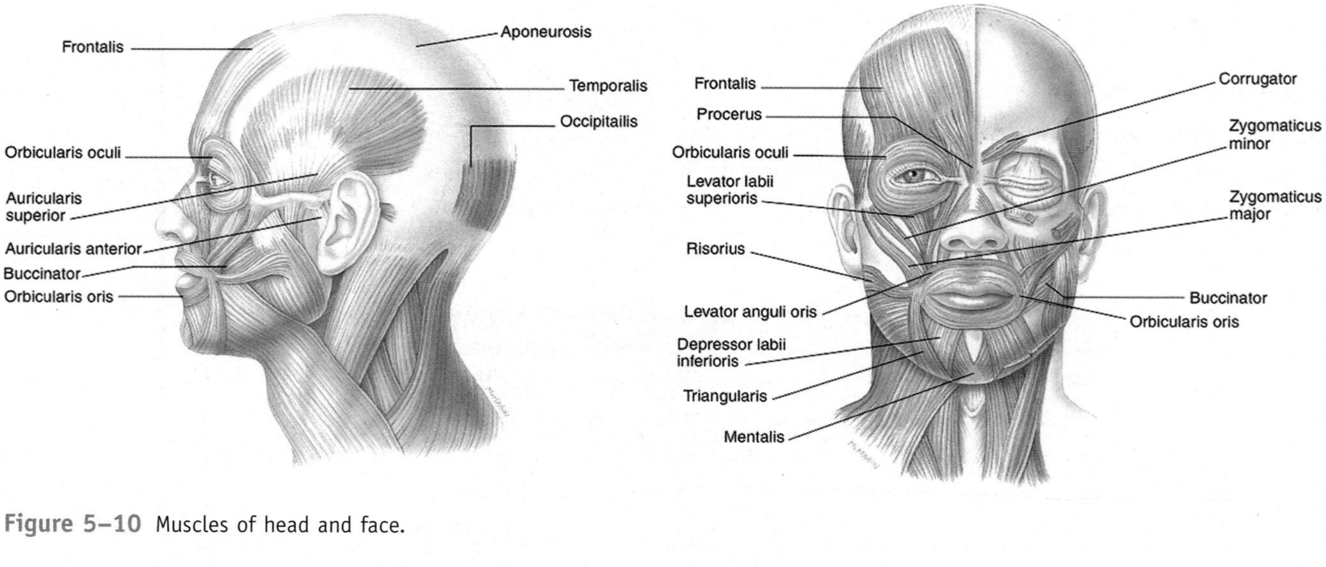

Figure 5–10 Muscles of head and face.

Nasal Muscles

The procerus, a muscle of the nose, draws the nose up and the central brow area down. Just below is the pyramidalis nasi, which, as you might imagine, is shaped like a pyramid over the nasal bone. It draws down the inner angle of the eyelids to make transverse "squinting" wrinkles across the nose. Just below that, on the side of the nose and extending between the inner margin of the eye and the upper lip, lies a small triangular muscle with a truly impressive name, the levator labii superioris alaeque nasi. This little muscle pushes upward the upper lip and **ala,** the flaring expansion on the side of each **nare,** or nostril. This causes a noticeable dilation of the nose and a wrinkling upon its ridge, the effect of which is a marked expression of contempt or disdain.

MUSCLES OF THE NECK

The muscles of the neck have a heavy load to carry. They support the head and all the valuable contents contained within. They provide rotational movement of the head, an act without which our safety would be compromised on many levels. There are, in fact, many muscles that work the neck; however, only two, the sternocleidomastoid and the platsyma, are relevant to the scope of this text.

Sternocleidomastoids

The sternocleidomastoids are found on either side of the neck. They act to flex and rotate the head. Sometimes referred to as "prayer muscles," they are charged with lowering the head when they act together or, when acting alone, rotating the head in either direction. The sternocleidomastiods are considered "dual headed" muscles, meaning they are broad at their points of origin (the sternum on one side and the clavicle on the other) and destination (the temporal bone) and tapered in the middle. These muscles contain a lot of stress and are often the source of stress headaches due to their proximity to major blood vessels that supply blood to the brain.

Platysma

The platysma is a superficial muscle that originates in the chest area and ends just below the chin (Figure 5–11). Its sheath-like form is responsible for the external contours of our neck. This muscle crisscrosses both the trapezius and the sternocleidomastoid. It pulls the corners of the mouth downward and supports and balances the upright head.

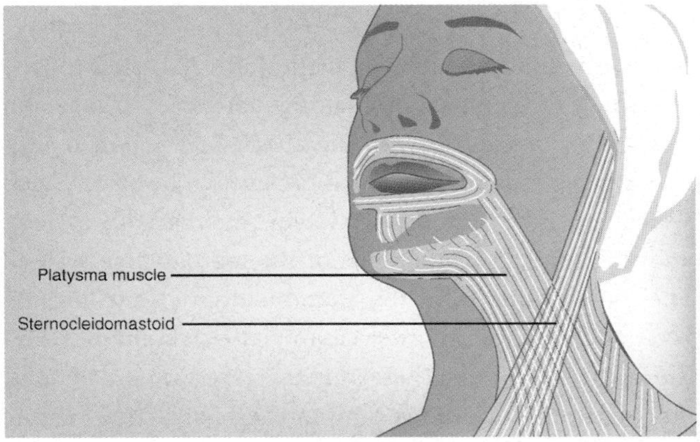

Figure 5–11 Platysma.

MUSCLES OF THE TRUNK

The trunk of the body, or the thorax, houses the vital organs of the body and provides many more essential functions, including balance. Within the trunk there are several muscle groups that provide balance and upright posture and fight gravity. These muscles are subcategorized into their position on the body—anterior or posterior.

Anterior Muscles of the Trunk

Anterior muscles are those on the front of the body. They provide balance, contribute to the operation of the limbs, and provide support for vital organ systems contained within.

Pectoral Muscles

The main muscle of the upper chest is the pectoralis major. This large convergent muscle resembles a fan, and its point of origin is broad. It begins at the sternum, clavicle, and ribs. Their destination point is much more narrow and inserts into the crest of the greater tubercle of the humerus (the bone that runs shoulder to elbow). These muscles are primarily responsible for the upward **(flexation)** and side-to-side **(adduction)** movement of the upper limbs.

Intercostal Muscles

Intercostal muscles are found between the ribs, and there are two kinds: the *internal* and *external* intercostals. The internal intercostal muscles (on the inside of the ribcase) extend from the front of the ribs and go around back, past the bend in the ribs. The external intercostal muscles (on the outside of the ribcase) wrap around from the back of the rib almost to the end of the bony part of the rib in front. The intercostal muscles are comparatively small but play a vital role in providing movement of the ribcage to allow breathing.

Abdominal Muscles

The abdominal muscles sit on the front and sides of the lower half of the torso, originating along the rib cage and attaching along the pelvis. The abdominal region houses major organ systems that the muscles hold in place. These systems include the urinary system, the digestive system, and the internal components of the reproductive system. The muscles that form the abdominal group include traverse abdominals, the internal and external obliques, and the rectus abdominis. These muscles serve a variety of tasks, ranging from forced breathing to excretion. They lay one on top of each other and run in different directions, allowing for the most support for the internal organs within.

The **traverse abdominals** are the deepest of the abdominal muscles. Their side-to-side striations compress the internal organs. They originate at the lower ribs and end at the pelvis.

The next abdominal layer is the **internal obliques.** They run at obtuse angles to the traverse abdominal muscles. Along with the **external obliques** above, the major function of these muscles is movement of the vertebrae and rotation of the trunk.

The outermost layer is the **rectus abdominis.** They are paired side by side, with vertical striations. These are the muscles that comprise the sought-after "six pack." They are responsible for vertebrae movement, forced breathing, and the specialized tasks of childbirth.

Posterior Muscles of the Trunk

Posterior muscles are those that are located on the back of the body. They provide balance, contribute to the operation of the limbs, and provide support for vital organ systems contained within.

Trapezius

The **trapezius** is a diamond-shaped coupling of superficial muscles that make up the majority of our upper backs. They originate at the occipital bone of the skull and run down through the thoracic vertebrae. Their insertion point is on the scapula, shoulderblade. They are responsible for a wide range of motion of the back and shoulders. This includes scapular *elevation* (shrugging up), scapular adduction (drawing the shoulder blades together), and scapular **depression** (pulling the shoulder blades down).

Latissimus Dorsal

If the trapezius comprises the majority of muscle tissue on the upper back, the **latissimus dorsal** comprises most of the muscle tissue on the lower back. Like the pectoralis major on the anterior side, the latissimus dorsal is fan-shaped with a broad origin and relatively small insertion point. The latissimus dorsal originates along the lower spine and finds its destination along the posterior side of the humerus. Theses muscles are especially useful for rotational movement of the arms.

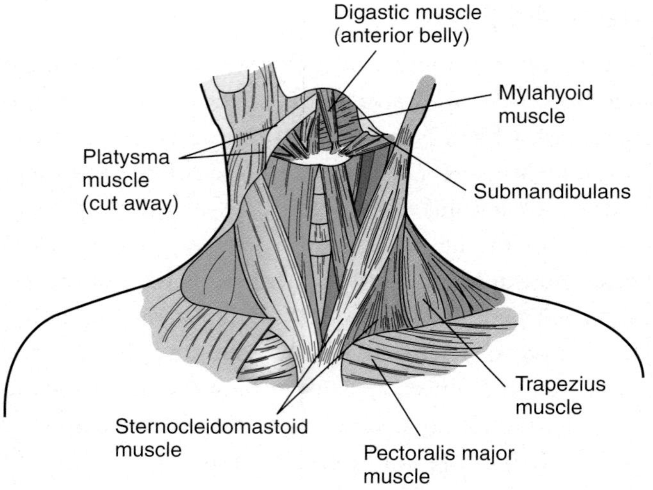

Figure 5–12 Muscles of the neck and chest.

Erector Spinae

Those who suffer from back pain are acutely aware of the **erector spinae** muscle group. This set of three muscles run along either side of the spinal column. Their chief responsibility is to protect upright positioning and to act as the antagonist muscle for the action of bending from the waist.

MUSCLES OF THE ARMS AND SHOULDERS

The muscles of the arms and shoulders are both powerful and resourceful. After all, without these muscles, humans could not do most of the things that separate them from other animals. Anatomically speaking, the arm is the region of the body from the shoulder joint to the elbow joint. The forearm is the section from the elbow to the wrist. However, collectively, they are commonly referred to as *the arm*. The major muscles found in the collective arm are the deltoid, the **bicep brachii**, the **brachialis**, and the **tricep brachii.**

The Deltoid

The deltoid is a triangle-shaped muscle that forms the rounded contour of the shoulder. It is an extremely fleshy muscle and serves to protect and aid the shoulder joint, as well as arm abduction and shoulder **hyperextension.** It originates at the clavicle and is inserted at the humerus. Because of the fleshy nature of this muscle, it is a preferred location to inject intramuscular medications.

The Bicep Brachii

As far as muscles go, none are more recognizable than the bicep brachii, or just bicep. In fact, it has become a symbol for fitness and musculature. The name *bicep* literally means "two heads," because it originates from two heads attached to the scapula (collar bone) and the humerus. The main duties of this muscle are flexation and **supination** (rotation of the arm). When it contracts, it works to flex the forearm at the elbow. Because of the iconic nature of the muscle, those who lift weights work this muscle hard. It is also a muscle that responds well to such workouts. In fact, it can grow up to 30 inches in height!

The Brachialis

Below the bicep is the brachialis. While the bicep gets all the attention, the brachialis is equally important for the arm's ability to flex at the elbow. Its origin is at the deltoid muscle and it inserts at the lower half of the humerus (Figure 5–13 and Table 5–3).

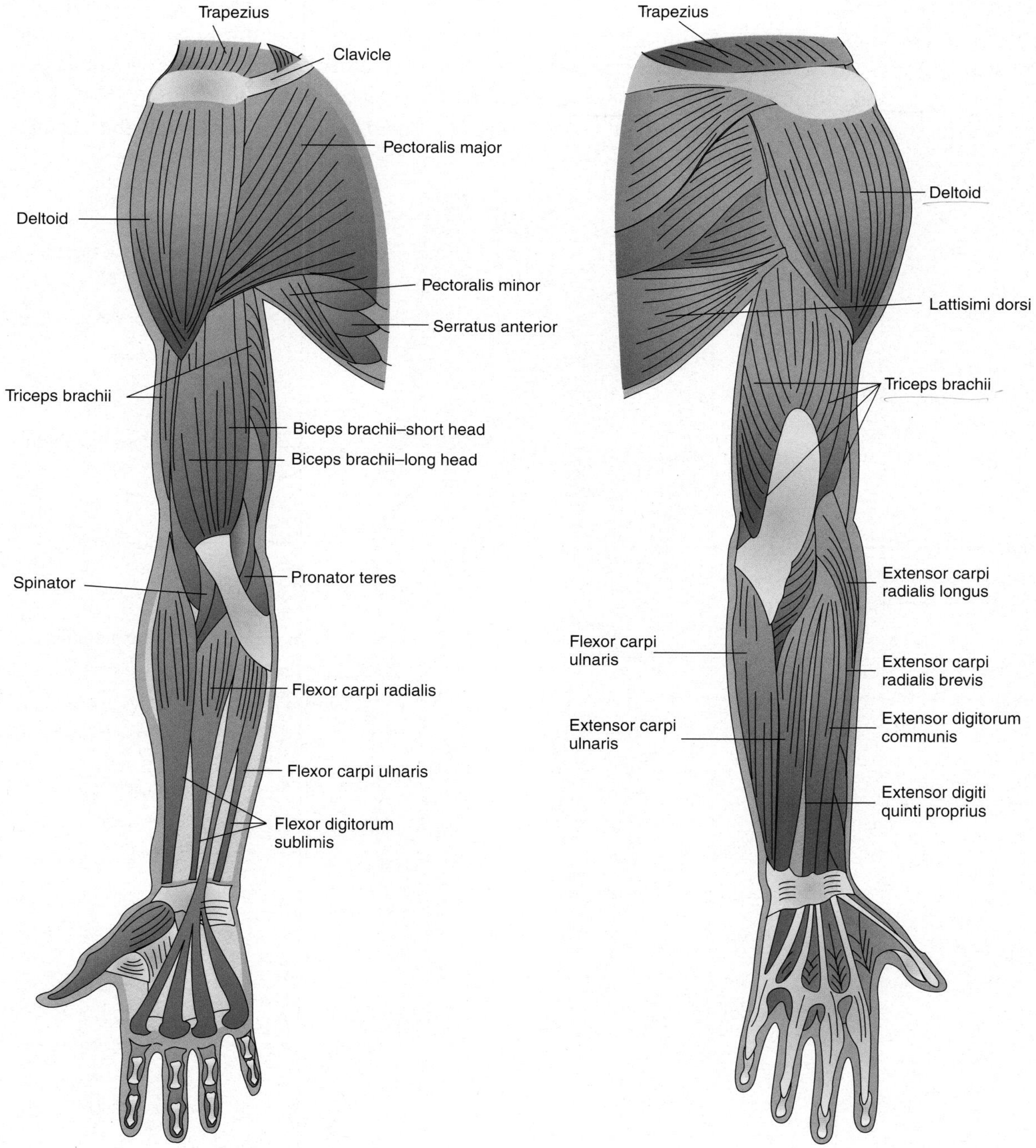

Figure 5–13 Muscles of the arm.

Table 5–3 Muscles of the Arms and Their Movement

MUSCLES OF THE ARMS AND THEIR MOVEMENT	
Deltoid	Arm abduction and shoulder hyperextension
Bicep brachii	Flexation and supination of the arm
Brachialis	Flexes the elbow
Tricep brachii	Extension of the arm and elbow

The Tricep Brachii

Just as the bicep has two heads, the triceps have three heads, as the name implies. They originate from the shoulder and the humerus, inserting in the ulna. The tricep is a superficial muscle that is tasked with extension of the arm and elbow. This muscle allows holding arms out in front.

MUSCLES OF THE LEGS

The legs are tasked with moving and carrying the entire body, so the legs have some of largest, densest muscle tissue in the body. These muscles move the legs in coordination with three joints: the hip, knees, and the ankle (Figure 5–14).

Muscles Associated with the Hip

The hip is a remarkable joint. It holds the body upright and allows for biped posture. While it is not as flexible as other joints, its sturdiness is necessary and impressive. The limited movement is powerful, nonetheless. Walking, standing upright, and balancing on one leg are accomplished thanks to subtle contractions of muscles that regulate the hip. There are five muscle groups that regulate

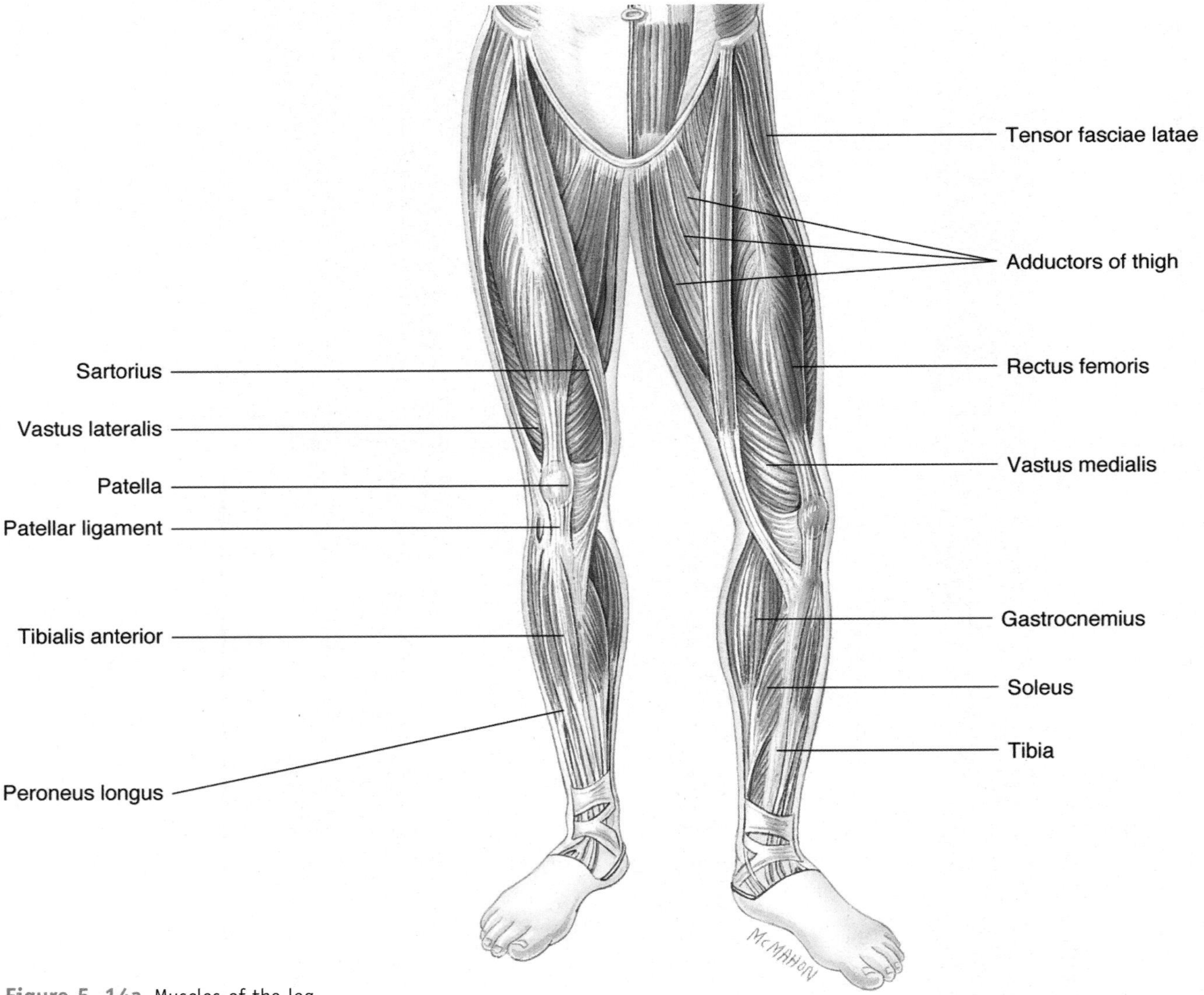

Figure 5–14a Muscles of the leg.

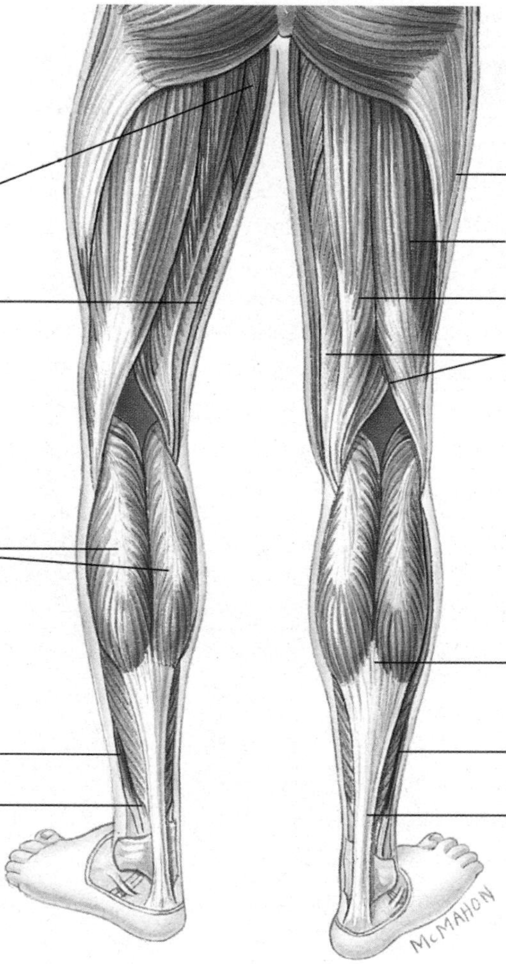

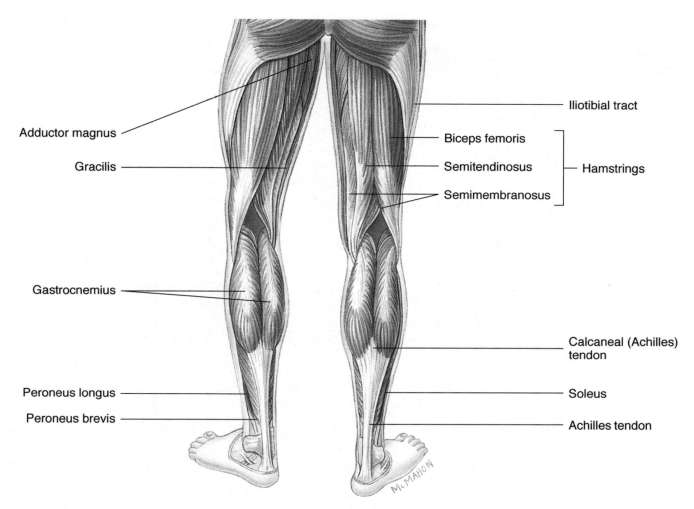

Figure 5–14b Muscles of the leg.

hip movement: rotators, adductors, abductors, flexors, and extensors. Following is a discussion of the larger, more superficial muscles.

Gluteus Group of Muscles

Probably the most well-known of the muscle groups in the lower limbs, the **gluteus group of muscles** together form the exterior contours of the buttocks. Aside from the important movements they allow, they also provide cushioning that protects the hips and spine while sitting or laying down. These fleshy muscles are named according to their size and all have varying duties.

The largest one, the gluteus maximus, has its origin at the hip and connects to the femur. Its major task is to maintain a safe alignment with the femur. This is important for activities such as climbing. The gluteus maximus is considered part of the hip extensors.

Next is the gluteus medius. This muscle is located below the gluteus maxiumus, connecting at the ilium and inserting in the femur on either side of the leg. The gluteus medius is considered to be both a rotator and an abductor. It functions to provide support for this hip while walking or running and also during hip rotation. Due in part to its frequent use, this muscle is often subject to stress build-up.

Finally, the brevis are a coupling of muscles that work in conjunction with the gluteus medius, primarily for hip rotation. A small muscle (as the name implies), its origin is found in the ilium, and its insertion is in the upper femur.

Adductor Group of Muscles

The **adductor group of muscles** are smaller muscles that work to keep the legs together during most physical activity. The adductor magnus, longus, brevis, and pectineus make up the adductor group. Their origin is at the hip or pelvic bone and the insertion point is at the knee joint. Groin pulls are a strain at the attachment of the adductors to the pubic bone (Table 5–4).

Table 5–4 Muscles of the Legs and Their Function

MUSCLES OF THE LEGS AND THEIR FUNCTION	
Gluteus maxiumus	Hip extensor
Gluteus medius	Hip rotator
Gluteus minimus	Hip rotator
Adductor magnus	Leg abduction
Adductor longus	
Adductor brevis	
Adductor pectineus	

Muscles Associated with the Knee

The main movements of the knee are flexation and extension. Several groups of muscles make this possible. Obviously, the knee is one of the most used joints and is subject to much strain over time. Also in the knee, there are some vital ligaments that affect movement. Athletes are particularly subject to tears in these ligaments, which can be extremely painful. While the ligaments are crucial to the flexation and extension performed by the knee, the muscles do all the heavy lifting. While there are many muscles that participate in knee movement, following is a discussion of a few superficial muscles and muscle groups.

The Posterior Thigh (Hamstrings)

On the top or posterior side of the thigh is a muscle group called the **hamstrings.** These three muscles, the biceps femoris, the semitendinosus, and the semimembranosus, control the pull on the knee joint, or flexation of the knee. They originate at the ischial tuberosity on the lower pelvis, and insert at the tibia, the shinbone. This muscle group consists of large and strong muscles that are responsible for the external contours of the front of the thigh.

The Anterior Thigh (Quadraceps)

Whereas the hamstrings regulate flexation of the knee, the **quadriceps,** located on the anterior, or rear, of the thigh regulate extension. As the name implies, there are four muscles in this muscle group: the rectus femoris, the vastus medialis, the vastus lateralis, and the vastus intermedius. The most superficial of these muscles is the rectus feoris, which originates at the pelvis. The vastus muscles, which lay below and to either side, originate from the femur. All four muscles in this group insert in the knee by way of the patellar ligament. The rectus femoris acts as a flexor muscle for the hip and all four act to extend the knee. This is a very powerful group of muscles, even on persons who are less athletic.

Muscles Associated with the Ankle and Foot

No place in the body has as many bones as the foot and ankle. This network of many tiny bones works in conjunction with several ligaments and small muscles to perform a variety of motions for the foot. Since the feet act as the contact with the ground, there is a lot of emphasis on shock absorption in this region (Figure 5–15 and Table 5–5).

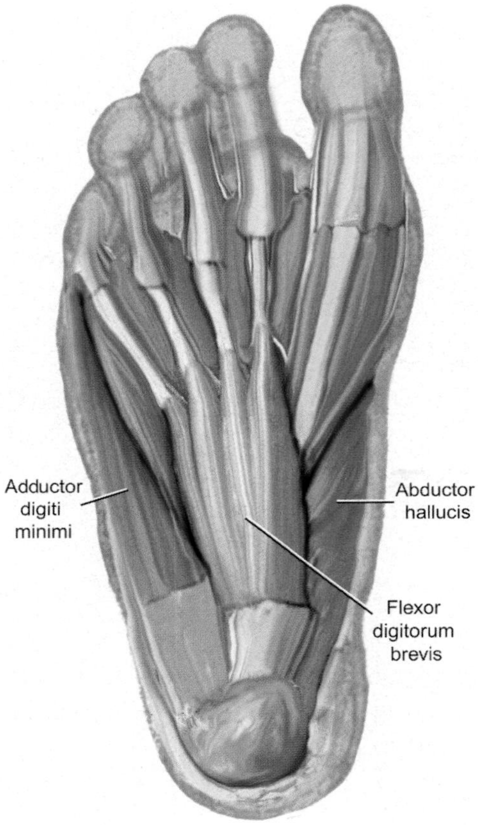

Figure 5–15 Muscles of the feet.

Table 5–5 Muscles of the Feet and Their Function

MUSCLES OF THE FEET AND THEIR FUNCTION	
Tibialis anterior	Dorsiflexion of the foot
Extensor digitorum longus	Dorsiflexion of the ankle
Tertius peronaeus	Dorsiflexion of the ankle
Peronaeus longus	Dorsiflexion of the ankle
Peronaeus brevis	Dorsiflexion of the ankle
Gastrocnemius	Plantar flex of the foot
	Flexation of the knee
Soleus	Plantar flex of the foot

The Tibialis Anterior

Situated on the length of the inside of the tibia bone, the **tibialis anterior** is a vital muscle for controlling dorsiflexion of the foot. It originates just below the knee and inserts at the base of the first metatarsal bone of the foot. At its point of origination, the tibialis anterior muscle is fleshy and thins out toward its end, becoming tendonous.

The Extensor Digitorum Longus

The **extensor digitorium longus** is a long, thin muscle that runs the length of the side of the tibialis anterior muscle. Between the two muscles are a few vital nerves. It originates just below the knee and inserts between the third and fourth toes. It is responsible for lifting the second through fifth toes as well as dorsiflexion of the ankle.

The Fibularis Muscle Group

The **fibularis muscle group,** also called the peronaeus muscle group, consists of three muscles, the tertius peronaeus, peronaeus longus, and the peronaeus brevis. The first one, the tertius peronaeus, is a small muscle that is considered to be part of the extensor digitorium longus. Interestingly, not all individuals have this muscle. It begins below the outside of the knee and inserts into the little toe. The second one, the peronaeus longus, is a superficial muscle that runs along the side of the fibula. The third muscle of this group, the peronaeus brevis, lies below the peronaeus longus. It originates around the same place as the peronaeus longus, just below the knee, and inserts at the ankle. Collectively, this group of muscles moves the ankle.

The Gastrocnemius

Most people are familiar with the **gastrocnemius,** even though they may not know it. That is because most people know it as the *calf muscle*. It originates from two heads, just above the rear of the knee and inserts along with the soleus into the calcaneus tendon, or *Achilles Heel*. These powerful muscles are critical to the function of walking. The calf muscle acts to plantar flex (curling the toes downward toward the sole) the foot and also plays a secondary role in flexation of the knee. Since there are several major blood vessels within the calf, this muscle plays a major role in peripheral venous return (see Chapter 6) when in the upright position.

The Soleus

Some professionals consider the **soleus** to be part of the calf. However, this powerful muscle is vital to the functions of standing and walking, so therefore, it deserves due credit. Located on the back of the leg, this fleshy superficial muscle originates at the fibula and inserts at the calcaneus tendon at the heel. Like the gastrocnemius, the soleus acts to plantar flex the foot. Different from the gastrocnemius, the soleus plays an important role in posture, supporting the ankle and the leg as a whole.

FACIAL NERVE PATTERNS

The cranial nerves consist of 12 pairs of nerves, one for each side of the body, that arise from the bottom of the brain and branch out to serve the head and upper neck area (Figure 5–16). Some of these nerves bring information from senses to the brain (sensory nerves), some control muscles (motor nerves), and others affect glands and internal organs. (Spinal nerves arise at points along the spinal canal and control sensory and motor input from the neck down.)

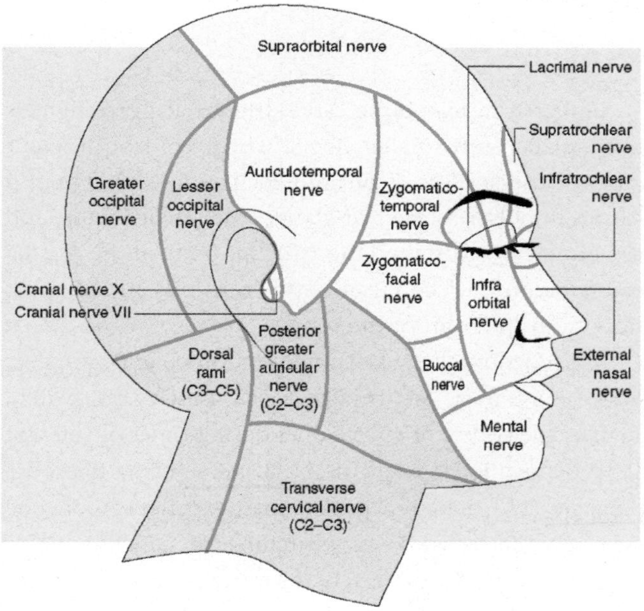

Figure 5–16 The cranial nerves.

Cranial Nerve VII, the Facial Nerve

Estheticians, especially, need to be familiar with the function of the cranial nerve VII—or, as it is known, *the facial nerve*—and its branches, which are important because they are responsible for all facial expressions. The facial nerve passes through the base of the skull and enters the bone of the ear through the internal auditory canal, the bony tube that also carries nerves concerned with hearing and balance. (This connection is the reason inner ear infections can affect balance.) From the ear, the facial nerve fans out to span the face from the outer and inner orbit of the eye, to the cheek and mouth, and down to the lower jaw (Figure 5–17).

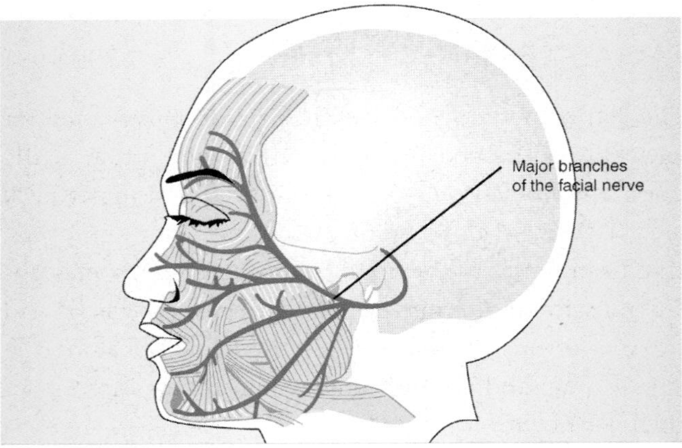

Figure 5–17 The seventh cranial nerve and its branches.

Similar to a telephone cable, the facial nerve divides into smaller and smaller fibers, which control different parts of the specific facial muscle. The facial nerve also carries impulses to the tear glands, the saliva glands, and the muscle of the stapes, the "stirrup" bone in the middle ear. In addition, the facial nerve transmits the sense of taste from the front of the tongue.

The function of the facial nerve is varied and complex. When these fibers are irritated, facial muscles can twitch, such as the corner of an eye does during times of stress or sleep deprivation. When the facial nerve or its fibers are damaged or irritated, a person may experience—on one side only—facial weakness, twitching, or paralysis; he or she may also notice dryness of the mouth or eye or a disturbance in taste. As a clinician, you may have an opportunity to see a patient with Bell's palsy, a disease that damages (sometimes temporally and sometimes permanently) the facial nerve; it is also the nerve that becomes paralyzed when a dental block is administered for facial surgery, dental surgery, or dermal fillers. You may notice that the patient will have been not only anesthetized from the block, but also paralyzed, affecting the motor function.

Cranial Nerve V, the Trigeminal Nerve

The cranial nerve V is called the *trigeminal nerve* (Figure 5–18). This nerve, too, is important to estheticians and cosmetic nurses because it is intimately associated with the face. The cranial nerve V has three major branches: the ophthalmic nerve, which goes to the eye; the maxillary nerve, which goes to the upper jaw; and the mandibular nerve, which goes to the lower jaw. All of these branches are sensory nerves, carrying the perceptions of touch and feeling to the areas they *innervate*. The trigeminal nerve innervates the cheek, side of the face, conjuctiva, skin of lower eyelid, side of the nose, nasal vestibule, teeth, tympanic membrane, and anterior two-thirds of the tongue. The motor root of the trigeminal nerve is smaller, extending to innervate muscles in the lower jaw and floor of the mouth.

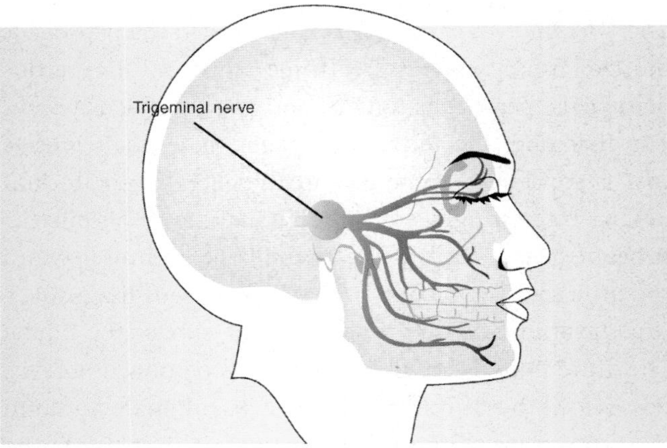

Figure 5–18 The fifth cranial nerve.

As opposed to the cranial nerve VII, which is a motor nerve, the cranial nerve V, or trigeminal nerve, is a mixed nerve that serves sensory impulses. It conducts sensory information such as touch and pain from the face, and it is the principal motor nerve controlling the muscles of mastication (chewing). Notably, those muscles are also used for speaking.

The sensory branches of the cranial nerve V, which extend to eyes, nose, lips, and both jaws, respond to touch, temperature, and pain in the face. These sensory branches are the ones that are numbed with a dental block. If this nerve is damaged, a person may not be able to feel the air temperature or pain in the cheek, lips, and nose, or in parts of them.

REVIEW QUESTIONS

1. What are muscle fibers?
2. What types of muscle tissue are found in humans?
3. Do cardiac muscles move voluntarily or involuntarily? What about skeletal muscles?
4. What functions do skeletal muscles serve?
5. What is the point where muscles begin? End?
6. What purposes do neck muscles serve?
7. What is adduction? Flexation?
8. What purposes do trunk muscles serve?
9. What do trapezius muscles do?
10. What major muscles are found in the arm? What do they do?
11. Which muscles assist in hip movement/ support?
12. Where are adductor muscles?
13. What are the key nerves of the face and neck?

CHAPTER GLOSSARY

acetylcholine: enzyme found in various tissues and organs, associated with muscle movement.

adduction: side-to-side movement.

adductor group of muscles: smaller muscles that work to keep the legs together during most physical activity.

ala: Flaring cartilaginous expansion on the side of each nare.

antagonist: something that opposes the action of another.

aponeurosis: any of the deep and thick facia, resembling flattened tendons, that attach muscles to bones.

bicep brachii: muscle of the upper arm; name literally means "two heads," because it originates from two heads attached to the scapula (collar bone) and the humerus.

brachialis: important muscle for the arm's ability to flex at the elbow.

cardiac fibers: muscle cells in the heart.

depression: pulling down of muscle.

endomysium: individual muscle fibers protected by connective tissue.

epimysium: the connective tissue sheath that surrounds skeletal muscle.

erector spinae: set of three muscles that run along either side of the spinal column.

extensor digitorium longus: thin long muscle that runs the length of the side of the tibialis anterior muscle.

external obliques: muscles responsible for the movement of the vertebrae and rotation of the trunk.

fibularis muscle group: muscle group consisting of three muscles—the tertius peronaeus, peronaeus longus, and the peronaeus brevis; also called the peronaeus muscle group.

flexation: upward movement.

frenulum: tissue that connects one thing to another.

gastrocnemius: the "calf muscle."

gluteus group of muscles: form the exterior contours of the buttocks.

CHAPTER GLOSSARY

hamstrings: muscle group on the top or posterior side of the thigh.

hyperextension: extension of a muscle beyond normal limits.

insertion: the point where the skeletal muscle is attached to a bone or other more movable body part.

intercostal muscles: muscles situated between the ribs.

internal obliques: middle layer of abdominal muscles.

lateral: to the side.

latissimus dorsal: broad, flat muscle covering the back of the neck and upper and middle region of the back: controls the shoulder blade and the swinging movements of the arm.

muscle fibers: describes muscle cells.

myofilaments: cells that help muscles contract and shorten.

nare: nostril.

neuromuscular junction: point at which nerves and muscles connect.

neurotransmitter: 1. substances that travel across synapses to act on or inhibit a target cell. 2. chemical messengers, synthesized from food nutrients, transmit instructions from the brain to the nervous system. The health of neurotransmitters is dependent on the quality of nutrients in food.

obliquely: slanting or inclined.

orifice: opening or aperture, such as the mouth or entry to a tube.

palpebra: the upper or lower eyelid.

perimysium: 1. several muscle fibers are bunched together and wrapped in a fibrous sheathing. 2. thin membrane covering a muscle.

quadriceps: muscles located on the anterior, or rear, of the thigh that regulate extension.

rectus abdominis: outermost layer of the abdominal muscle.

soleus: located on the back of the leg, this fleshy superficial muscle originates at the fibula, and inserts at the calcaneus tendon at the heel.

supination: rotation of the arm.

synapse: junction by which a nerve impulse travels.

tendons: strong connective tissue which attaches muscle to bone.

tibialis anterior: muscle vital to the control of dorsiflexion of the foot.

trapezius: 1. diamond shaped coupling of superficial muscles that make up the majority of our upper backs. 2. muscle that covers the back of the neck and upper and middle region of the back; stabilizes the scapula and shrugs the shoulders.

traverse abdominals: deepest of the abdominal muscles.

tricep brachii: muscles causing extension of the arm and elbow.

CHAPTER OUTLINE

- THE CARDIOVASCULAR SYSTEM
- BLOOD
- THE HEART
- HEART DISEASE
- THE ARTERIAL SYSTEM
- THE VENOUS SYSTEM
- DISEASED VEINS
- THE LYMPHATIC SYSTEM

CHAPTER 6

ANATOMY AND PHYSIOLOGY: THE CARDIOVASCULAR AND LYMPHATIC SYSTEMS

LEARNING OBJECTIVES

After completing this chapter, you should be able to:

- Discuss the cardiovascular system.
- Understand components and function of the blood.
- Understand the function of the heart.
- Know the diseases and disorders of the heart.
- Discuss the components of the arterial system.
- Identify the components, function, and disorders of the venous system.
- Identify the components and function of the lymphatic system.

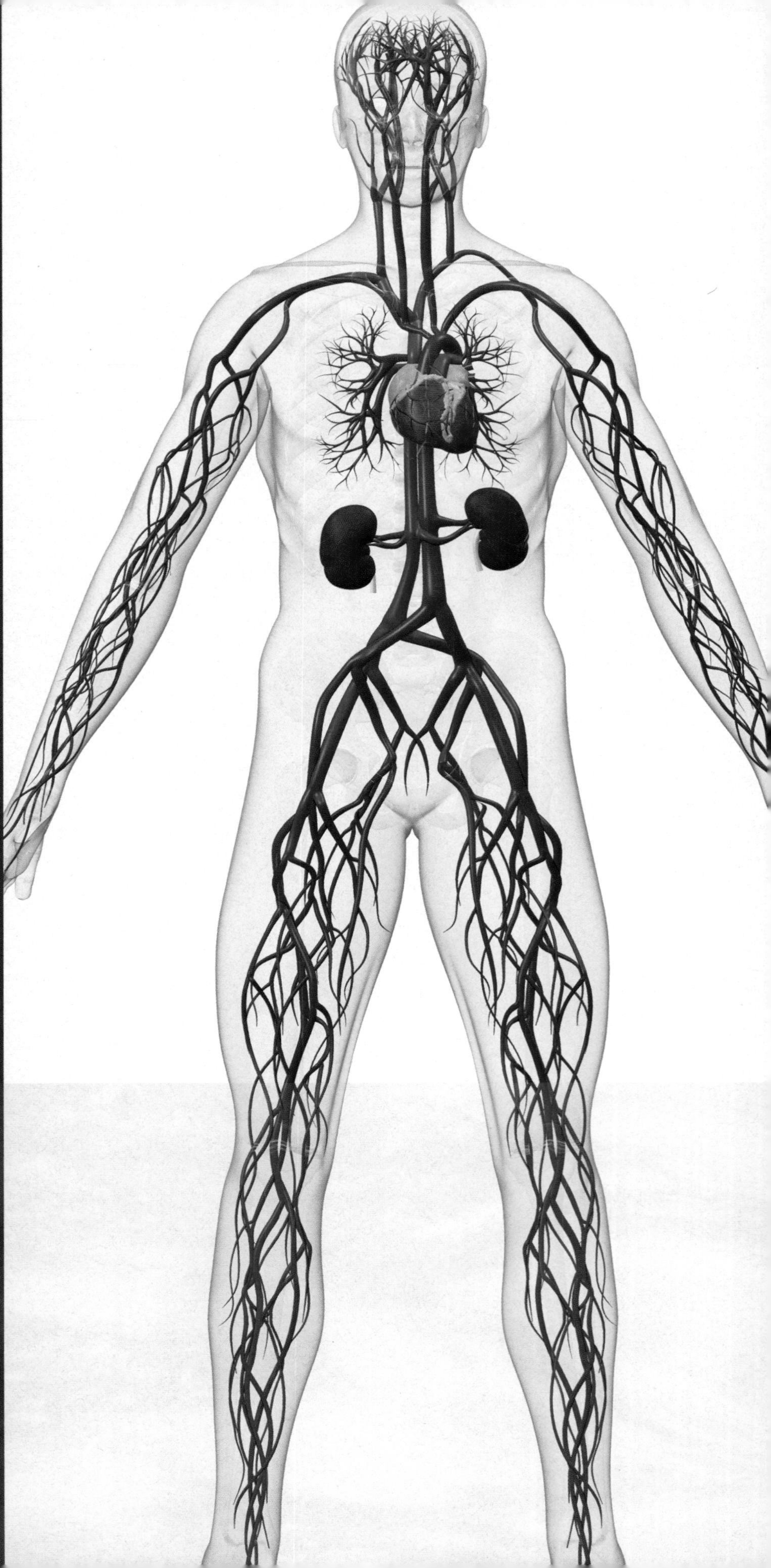

KEY TERMS

Page numbers indicate where in the chapter the term is used.

agranulocytes 125
albumin 124
anastomosis 128
anemia 125
antibodies 124
aorta 128
aortic semilunar valve 128
arterioles 124
atria 127
atrioventricular valves 128
basophils 125
bicuspid valve 127
blood pressure 127
cardiovascular system 124
clotting factors 124
collateral circulation 129
deoxygenated 124
diastole 127
electrolytes 124
eosinophils 125
epicardium 126
erythrocytes 125
formed elements 125
granulocytes 125
heart disease 128
hemophilia 126
hydrostatic pressure 131
hypoxia 125
leukemia 126
leukocytes 125
ligature 129
lymph 132
lymph nodes 132
lymphatic vessels 132
monocytes 125
myocardium 126
neutrophils 125
oxygenated 127
peripheral edema 131
phagocytes 125
plexuses 130
pulmonary circulation 127
pulmonary valve 128
semilunar valve 128
stethoscope 127
systemic circulation 127
systole 127
thalassemia 126
tortuous 129
tricuspid valve 127
varicose veins 132
ventricles 127

While it is important that all of the body's systems work in harmony, each is important in its own way. This chapter explores the components of the circulatory system and, in particular, the veins and arteries. Other topics include the diseases and injuries that might befall the circulatory system. Diseases of the circulatory system that readily come to mind are heart disease or heart attacks. This chapter focuses on one particular condition that affects nearly 50% of the population, varicose veins. In fact, half of the women reading this book will experience some variation of varicose veins—either spider veins in some form or large-scale varicosities. Before beginning a discussion of varicose veins, however, it is important to look at the normal anatomy and physiology of veins and arteries and how they relate to the overall circulatory system. The chapter ends with a discussion of another important body system, the lymphatic system.

THE CARDIOVASCULAR SYSTEM

At the center of the **cardiovascular system**—also known as the circulatory system—sits the heart, a hollow muscle that really does not sit at all. It pumps blood constantly, through contraction and relaxation movements, sending oxygen and nutrients to all parts of the body through a sinuous series of tubes called *arteries*. Arteries branch out into smaller and smaller vessels, finally ending in **arterioles**, which in turn open into a sieve of microscopic vessels called *capillaries*. After the blood passes through the capillaries, it begins its homeward route by entering venules, the smallest branches of veins, the vessels that return blood to the heart, carrying **deoxygenated** blood—blood that has distributed its load of oxygen—and metabolic waste. The importance of blood to the body cannot be overstated; therefore, it is the logical place to begin a tour of the circulatory system.

BLOOD

While the sight of blood is repellant to some, it is an unmistakable necessity to every cell, tissue, organ, and system of the human body. Blood is of such fantastic and life-sustaining value that it has become a cultural symbol representing life and death, pain and healing, horror and beauty, and everything in between. Almost every form of spirituality possesses its own representations of blood and its value.

Blood is just as significant from a scientific standpoint. It transports the requisite components to where they are needed, while redistributing the useless and harmful components to where they can be properly disposed. In addition to nutrient supply, gas exchange, and waste disposal, the blood is actively engaged in almost every function of the body, including thermoregulation, wound healing, and immunologic responses. With so much to accomplish, it is easy to see why blood is considered the fluid of life (Table 6–1).

Blood Composition

As mentioned above, blood is considered a fluid tissue. While it appears to the naked eye as a liquid, it also has solid and gaseous properties. This versatility allows blood to accomplish its varied tasks as needed. The liquid component, *plasma,* is a yellowish fluid that accounts for about a little more than half of the blood's volume. Plasma is 90% to 95% water and the remaining 5% to 10% consists of proteins and trace minerals, including **albumin, clotting factors, antibodies,** and **electrolytes** (Table 6–2).

Table 6–1 Facts about Blood

FACTS ABOUT BLOOD
Blood is considered to have solid, liquid, and gaseous properties.
The human body produces 17 million red blood cells per second to replace the ones destroyed.
The human body has about 6 quarts of blood, which travels through the body three times every minute. In one day, the blood travels four times the distance from one coast of the continental United States to the other.
The weight of a person's complete blood supply is roughly 10% of total body weight.
The heart pumps about one million barrels of blood during an average lifetime—that's enough to fill more than three supertankers.
Blood is classified as a circulating connective tissue.
Oxygenated blood is a brighter and purer red compared to the duller deoxygenated load carried by the veins.
Blood temperature and flow is regulated by a delicate balance called *homeostasis*. Blood temperature is maintained at 100.4°F, slightly warmer than overall body temperature.
White blood cells are bigger than and different in appearance from red blood cells. White cells circulate in the blood, but they can also change their shape to squeeze through a capillary and digest germs.
When blood becomes too cold, the body enters a condition called *hypothermia*. When blood flow is temporarily cut off and then releases, the action of the blood is called *restriction*. If blood gets too warm, the body enters *hyperthermia*. All of these conditions have severe consequences, ranging from tissue necrosis to death.
Flow restriction, hypothermia, and hyperthermia are also used as therapies for massage, cancer, and brain injuries, respectively.

Table 6–2 Plasma Contents Carried in Blood

SUBSTANCE	FUNCTION
Water	Transports minerals and formed elements; retains heat
Albumin	Transports fatty acids, hormones, and drugs; maintains osmotic pressure; and buffers pH
Clotting factors	Are essential to wound healing and tissue continuity
Antibodies	Proteins dispatched by the immune system to identify and neutralize foreign bodies
Electrolytes	Trace minerals that assist osmotic pressure and aid hydration of muscles and nerves
Nutrients	Vitamins, amino acids, and fatty acids essential to tissues and organs
Waste products	Lactic acid, urea, uric acid
Respiratory gases	Oxygen and carbon dioxide
Hormones	Chemical messengers that are vital to intercellular communication

Table 6–3 Formed Elements Found in Blood

FORMED ELEMENTS FOUND IN BLOOD		
Erythrocytes (red blood cells): Anucleate cells that transport oxygen to other cells by way of hemoglobin		
Leukocytes (white blood cells): Specialized cells that work with the immune system to combat disease and infection. Less numerous than erythrocytes.		
Granulocytes	**Neutrophils**	Phagoctic cells that multiply at times of acute infection
	Eosinophils	Antiparasitic phagocytes
	Basophils	Provide histamine at inflammatory sites
Agranulocytes	**Lymphocytes**	Produce antibodies and fight viral infections
	Monocytes	Phagocytes that become macrophages to aid overall systemic waste removal
Platelets: Required for blood clotting		

The second component of blood is the **formed elements,** specialized blood cells suspended in the liquid (plasma) vehicle that make up just under half of blood's total volume (Table 6–3). The vast majority of these are **erythrocytes,** commonly referred to as *red blood cells.* Vast numbers of red blood cells perform the oxygen exchange with other cells in the body. They are anucleate (without a nucleus) and much leaner than other cells in the sense that they lack many of the organelles found in other cells. They accomplish the gas transfer with the assistance of *hemoglobin,* an iron-rich protein.

Less numerous, but equally important are **leukocytes,** or white blood cells, which are the only complete cells found in the blood (each has a nucleus, mitochondria, and other common organelles). White blood cells play an important role in protecting the body against disease and infection. Unlike red blood cells, white blood cells can exit and re-enter the bloodstream at will. They use the flow of blood as a transport mechanism to go wherever in the body they are needed. At the first sign of infection, the body increases leukocyte production and dispatches white blood cells for damage control.

There are two subcategories of leukocytes, **granulocytes,** and **agranulocytes.** Granulocytes have granules, and they are highly specialized **phagocytes,** or waste collecting cells. Agranulocytes are more general phagocytes and play an important role in the cellular clean-up. They work directly with the immune system as well as with the lymphatic system.

Blood Disorders

With all that the blood must accomplish in a quick trip throughout the body, any disturbance in its delicate balance can rapidly progress to a dire situation. With so many components, there are an equal number of disorders.

Anemia

Anemia is a common blood disorder that occurs when there are fewer red blood cells than normal or there is a low concentration of hemoglobin in the blood. Most symptoms of anemia are a result of the decrease of oxygen in the cells or **hypoxia.** Because red blood cells carry oxygen via hemoglobin, a decreased production or number of these cells results in hypoxia. Many of the symptoms are not present in a case of mild anemia, as the body can often compensate for gradual changes in hemoglobin. There are several different subtypes of anemia, including sickle cell anemia, aplastic anemia, and hemolytic anemia (Table 6–4).

Table 6–4 Symptoms of Anemia

SYMPTOMS OF ANEMIA
• Abnormal paleness or lack of color of the skin
• Increased heart rate (tachycardia)
• Breathlessness or difficulty catching a breath (dyspnea)
• Lack of energy or tiring easily (fatigue)
• Dizziness or vertigo especially when standing
• Headache
• Irritability
• Irregular menstrual cycles
• Absent or delayed menstruation (amenorrhea)
• Sore or swollen tongue (glossitis)
• Jaundice or yellowing of skin, eyes, and mouth
• Enlarged spleen or liver (splenomegaly, hepatomegaly)
• Slow or delayed growth and development
• Impaired wound and tissue healing

Here's a Tip

Lack of energy can be a sign of anemia.

Thalassemia

Thalassemia is an inherited disorder that affects the production of normal hemoglobin, which causes anemia. The severity and type of anemia depends upon an individual's genetic makeup. This disorder is common in populations around the Mediterranean Sea, Africa, and Southeast Asia.

Hemophilia

Hemophilia is an inherited bleeding disorder, more common in males than females, characterized by a reduced number or complete absence of clotting factors. The result is an inability to stop bleeding at the site of a wound, easy bruising, and bleeding from joints. There are a number of types of hemophilia, and each is determined by the specific clotting factor that is absent.

Leukemia

Leukemia is cancer of the blood that develops in the bone marrow. The bone marrow is the soft, spongy center of the long bones that produces the three major blood cells: white blood cells to fight infection, red blood cells that carry oxygen, and platelets that help with blood clotting and stop bleeding. Normal, healthy cells reproduce only when there is enough space for them to fit. The body can regulate the production of cells by sending signals to stop reproduction. In a person with leukemia, the bone marrow, for an unknown reason, begins to make white blood cells that do not mature correctly but continue to reproduce themselves. These cells do not respond to the signals to stop and thus reproduce, regardless of available space.

THE HEART

The central organ of the circulatory system is the heart, which is roughly the size of a clenched fist. It is hard to believe that something so small can handle such copious responsibilities, yet, starting just weeks after conception, the heart manages its responsibilities with clocklike diligence. Literally, the heart pumps sustenance to every cell in the body (Figure 6–1).

Located just left of center of the middle thorax cavity, the heart is surrounded by the lungs on each side and the diaphragm below. The exterior of the heart is surrounded by a thin fibrous sheath called the *pericardium* and is attached to surrounding organs by the **epicardium**. The pericardium blends in with the walls of the heart and actually forms the outermost layer of three. The second layer, the **myocardium**, is

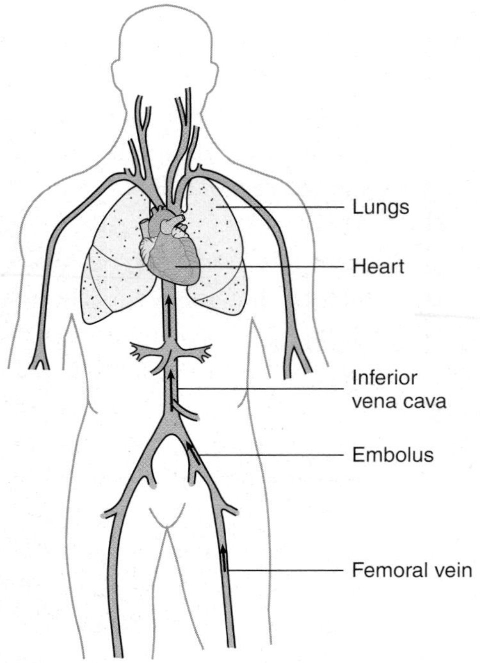

Figure 6–1 The heart is about the size of a clenched fist.

muscle tissue that contracts, which results in "pumping" blood through the chambers and throughout the body. The innermost layer of the heart, the endocardium, is made up of serous epithelial tissue. This tissue blends in with the connecting blood vessels, enabling critical fluid transfers.

Although the heart is basically hollow, it contains divided sections called *chambers*. There are four chambers, two on the top and two on the bottom. The top chambers are called **atria** (singular, *atrium*), and they receive blood. The two bottom chambers are called **ventricles,** and they pump blood out of the heart.

This heart's division into chambers prevents the blood that has been **oxygenated** from interacting with blood that has lost its oxygen load. During the cardiac cycle, the right atrium receives blood that is deoxygenated from the body and sends it to the right ventricle, which pumps the blood to the lungs to pick up another load of oxygen. This is referred to as **pulmonary circulation.** The left atrium receives oxygenated blood from the lungs and sends it to the left ventricle, from which it is pumped into the body. This is referred to as **systemic circulation.** Because the oxygen-rich blood pumped out to the body from the left ventricle has to travel such a great distance, the left ventricle's walls are much thicker than the walls of the right ventricle.

The heart's contractions occur independently of the nervous system. This means that unlike most muscles, which move in response to cues from the nerves connected to the brain, the heart contracts automatically. The cells within the heart contract on their own with the help of specialized tissue that is a hybrid of muscle and nervous tissue. This hybrid tissue is not found anywhere else in the body. The heart's contractions form what is known as the *heartbeat*. That is the sound made by the actions of the left ventricle, which does the majority of the pumping, when heard through a **stethoscope.** A person's **blood pressure** is decided by the contraction (**systole**) and relaxation (**diastole**) of the heart. The cardiac cycle is the process of both atria relaxing and contracting. Typically, this occurs 75 times a minute in a healthy adult (Figure 6–2).

Aiding the pumping processes of the heart are valves, which prevent the backflow of blood between chambers. On the left side, the valve preventing backflow is called the **bicuspid valve.** It is comprised of a dual layer of endocardium tissue. Likewise, separating the right chambers is the **tricuspid valve.** The

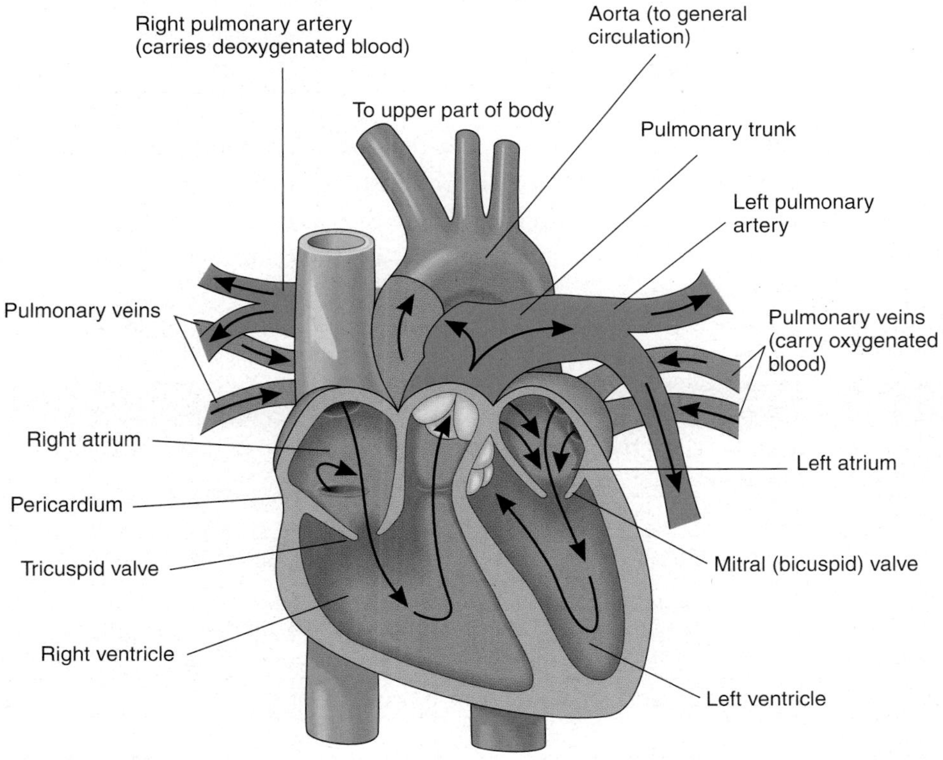

Figure 6–2 Inside of the heart.

tricuspid valve is comprised of three layers of endocardium tissue. Collectively, these two valves are referred to as *AV valves,* or **atrioventricular valves.** The second set of valves is called the **semilunar valves.** These valves regulate the flow of blood between the ventricles and the major blood vessel to which they connect. On the right side is the **pulmonary valve,** and on the left side is the **aortic semilunar valve.** Without the work of these valves, the heart would not function optimally.

HEART DISEASE

Heart disease is the broad term used to describe any condition that affects the performance of the heart or the cardiovascular system. As a whole, heart disease is the leading cause of death among both men and women in the United States.

As we age, normal wear and tear occurs in the cardiovascular system. In particular, the arteries lose elasticity with time. However, the cardiovascular system is resilient and reliable. Most of the conditions that qualify as heart disease (barring congenital conditions) have a manageable environmental component. Medical professionals agree that diet, exercise, and elimination of excesses (such as smoking and drinking) can reduce heart disease (Table 6–5).

THE ARTERIAL SYSTEM

As mentioned earlier, arteries supply the body with oxygenated blood pumped out from the left ventricle (Figure 6–3). While this sounds simple, the actual process is quite complicated. In fact, the breadth of this discussion is much greater than the scope of this book. However, for the treatments that you, as an esthetician, will be performing, it is important to have a working knowledge of the arterial system.

The arterial system is the higher-pressure portion of the circulatory system. Once the heart pumps the blood through the aorta and the greater arteries, the blood branches out through the lesser arterial structures—including arterioles and capillaries—and feeds oxygen to cells and organs.

The Arteries

The arteries of the body are like a tree that starts from a trunk and divides into branches, continuing to divide into ever smaller twigs. The trunk, or **aorta,** starts from the left ventricle, which pumps oxygenated blood. The branches and twigs forming the arterial system reach to every part of the body and its organs, with the exceptions of the hair, nails, epidermis (top layer of skin), cartilage, and corneas. The larger trunks of the arterial system tend to be in places more protected from harm, running in the limbs through the *flexor* or contractile surfaces. This protects the body from fatal injury if a laceration or wound occurs.

Arteries are tubular and, as they distribute themselves, they communicate with each other in what are called *anastomoses* (singular, **anastomosis**), which look like intertwined fingers. Anastomoses enable blood to reach areas that need it, such as the brain, in great concentration. Another area that needs a lot of oxygenated blood is the abdomen for digestion. The intestinal arteries have numerous anastomoses between and among their larger arterial branches. In the limbs, the largest and most

Table 6–5 Diseases of the Heart

CONDITION	DESCRIPTION
Coronary artery disease (CAD)	Plaque caused by fat clogs the arteries, restricting oxygen and nutrients needed by the heart. Often results in a heart attack.
Arrhythmia	Irregular heart beat or loss of rhythm.
Heart failure	Reduction in the pumping ability of the heart, resulting in limited flow (congestion).
Heart valve disease	Inefficacy of valves in the heart, resulting in backflow or limited flow. Often congenital.
Congenital heart conditions	A defect in one of the heart's structures, which occurs prior to birth
Cardiomyopathy	Gradual enlarging of heart tissues, resulting in heart failure
Pericarditis	Inflammation of the pericardium
Aortic aneurism	Weakened pocket of lining in the aorta

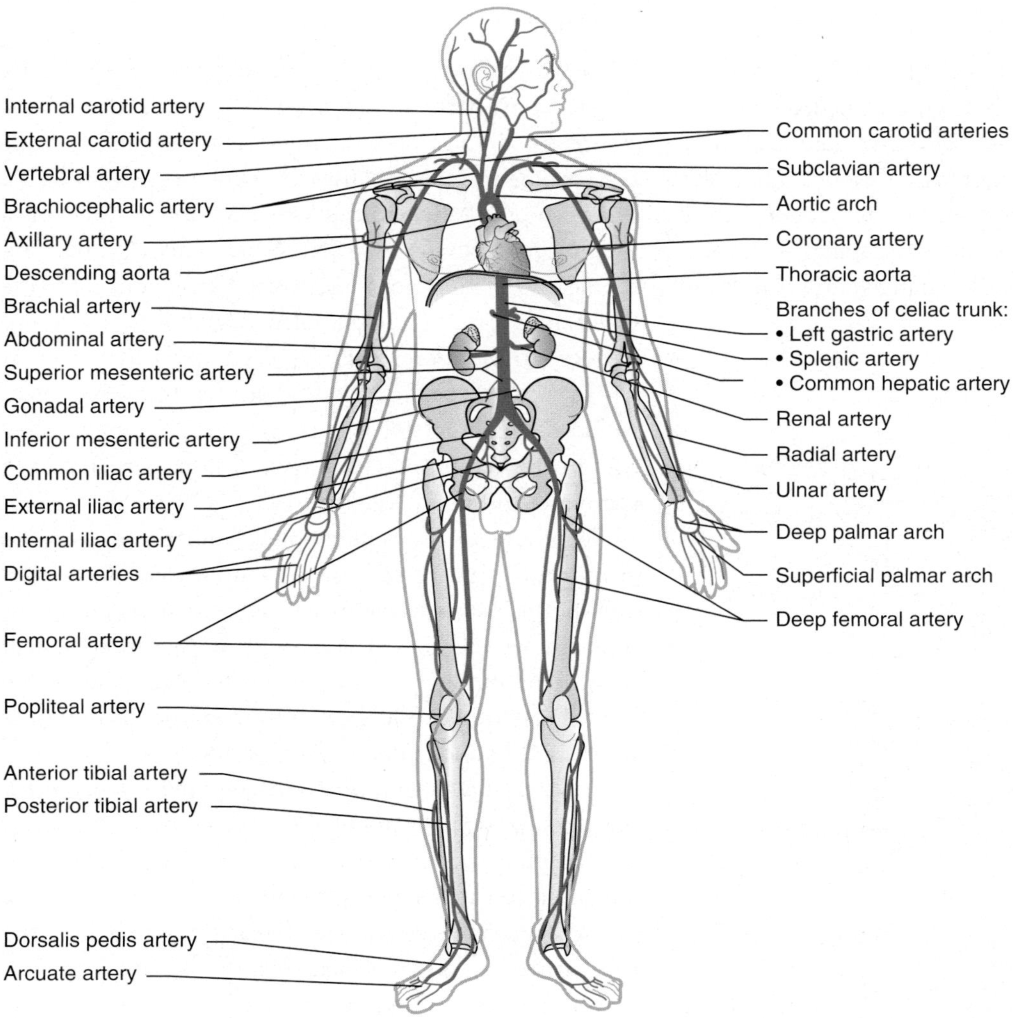

Figure 6–3 The arterial system.

numerous anastomoses occur around the joints, where branches of an artery above may unite with branches of an artery below. Anastomoses around joints are of interest to surgeons. This is because when a **ligature,** the tying or binding of a vessel occurs in a surgical procedure, the anastomoses may enlarge to produce extra circulaton called **collateral circulation** around the tied-off place.

The arteries' duty is to deliver blood quickly, and in most places the vessels flow in fairly straight lines. There are occasions, however, when it is to their benefit for them to become **tortuous,** or highly curved and bent. This happens with the external maxillary artery, which serves much of the face, and with the labial arteries of the lips; these arteries become quite tortuous to accommodate the variety of facial movements of which primates, including humans, are capable. The uterine arteries are tortuous as well, because during pregnancy they need to accommodate a growing fetus.

Arterioles

If arteries are the trunk of the tree, then arterioles are the branches. These smaller arterial routes connect to organs and other tissues and eventually feed the capillaries. Arterioles have the greatest collective influence on both local blood flow and on overall blood pressure. They are the primary "adjustable nozzles" in the blood system, across which the greatest pressure drop occurs. The combination of heart output (cardiac output) and total peripheral resistance, which refers to the collective resistance of all of the body's arterioles, are the principal determinants of arterial blood pressure at any given moment.

? Did You Know

Arteries branch out into smaller and smaller vessels, called arterioles.

Capillaries

If arteries are the trunk and arterioles are the branches, then capillaries are the leaves (Figure 6–4). They are the smallest part of the network, and it is here that they connect with the venous system so blood can begin its journey back to the heart. All the true action of the circulatory system occurs within the capillaries. This is where gases and nutrients are exchanged and wastes are eliminated.

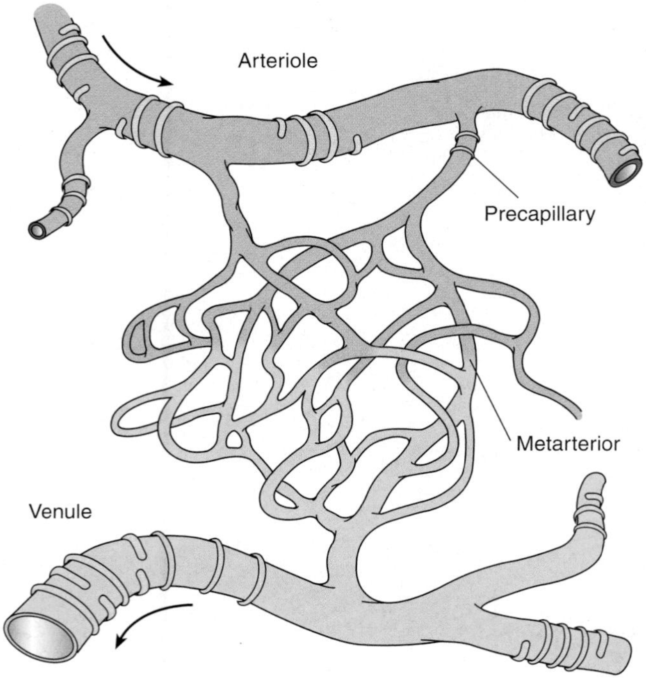

Figure 6–4 The capillary bed.

THE VENOUS SYSTEM

The venous system picks up where the arterial system leaves off, in the capillaries. The venous system is a complex network of veins and venules, tiny veins through which blood returns to the heart and lungs for a recharge of oxygen (Figure 6–5). This is not done via a direct connection but rather an area of interchange where the systems seem to "communicate" with each other.

> **FYI**
>
> Capillaries connect arterioles to venules.

The Veins

Veins convey deoxygenated blood from various parts of the body back to the heart. Veins arise from tiny **plexuses,** or networks, of intersecting venules, which receive blood from capillaries, tiny branches of arterioles. These venous branches unite with each other into trunks, then meet at tributaries or join other veins. Approaching the heart, the veins increase in size to the point of being larger than corresponding arteries (Figure 6–6). Large and frequent anastomoses exist between veins in the neck, where a blockage of blood returning from the brain would be unacceptable. Veins also compose many plexuses in the abdominal and pelvic region, particularly in spermatic and uterine regions.

Veins and arteries share some similarities: Both are cylindrical in shape and they communicate freely with one another. However, veins are larger and more numerous than arteries; therefore, the capacity of the venous system to hold its product—blood—is greater than that of the arterial system. Veins also differ from arteries in that their walls are thin and collapse when empty.

Another difference in the veins are their valves, which open and close, allowing blood to move toward the heart and keeping it from flowing backward. When blood is returning to the heart, it generally flows upward against gravity. The valves reduce the pressure of blood below by supporting it at different places on its way up.

Valves are more numerous in deep veins than in superficial veins, and, because humans are upright creatures, valves are also more common in veins of the lower limb than in those of the upper. Unlike deep veins, veins near the surface of the skin are not supported by muscles and so they get no assistance in the task of keeping blood flowing upward.

Peripheral Venous Return

The circulatory system is a closed circuit system, which means that the blood flow leaving the extremities via the veins must equal that being pumped in via the arteries

> **FOCUS ON:** *Major Components of the Circulatory System*
>
> **The veins carry deoxygenated blood.**
> **The arteries carry oxygenated blood.**
> **The heart is the center of the circulatory system.**

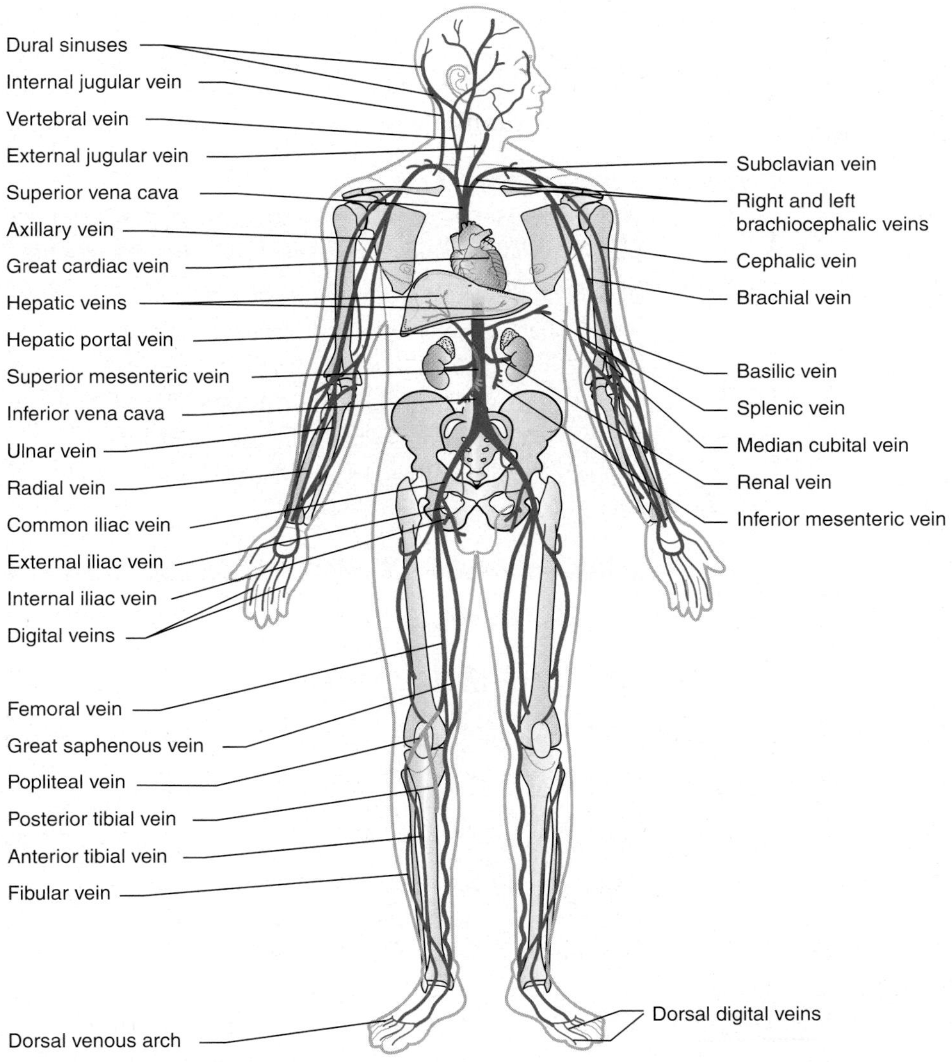

Figure 6–5 The venous system.

(Figure 6–7). The flow is variable and depends on such factors as temperature, degree of activity, and the body's position.

When a healthy individual is standing or sitting, as most people are during most of a day, the circulatory system is forced to work against the forces of gravity. To accomplish as much, deep veins use the muscles and tendons surrounding them to act as a pump to assist the blood's return to the heart, known as *peripheral venous return*. This is accomplished mostly by the calves with the help of the valves. However, the feet and ankles contribute to this work, which explains why walking is so good for the circulation of blood. Sometimes this system of the blood returning to the heart does not work as well as it should, resulting in a backup of blood in the veins and swelling of tissue. This swelling, known as **peripheral edema,** can indicate other diseases and conditions, including congestive heart failure, kidney failure, stasis dermatitis, and varicose veins.

CAUTION!

Peripheral edema can be a sign of a serious disease.

DISEASED VEINS

When valves in the legs get "leaky" and no longer do their job of preventing backflow, they are said to have become "incompetent." Incompetent valves allow gravity to pull blood back down into ever-widening pools in the veins, creating **hydrostatic pressure.** The veins

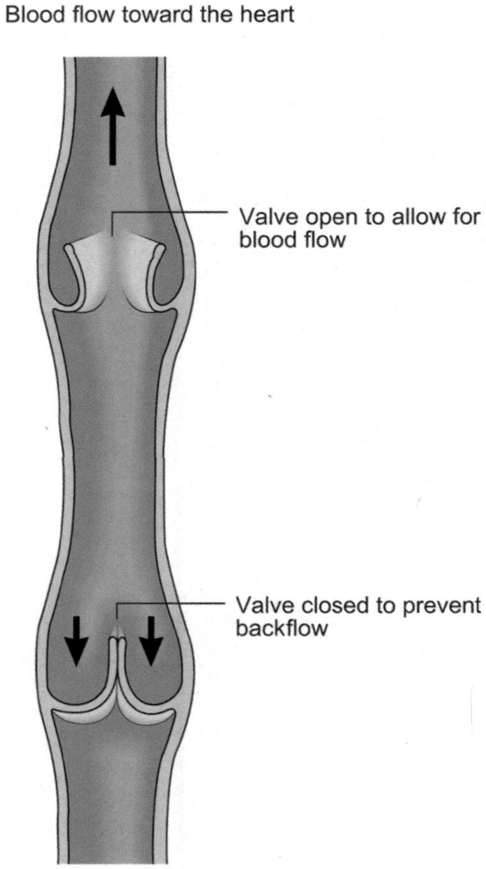

Figure 6–6 Veins open and close.

begin to bulge and stretch, and the results are **varicose veins** and spider veins (Figure 6–8). The differences between varicose veins and spider veins are primarily size and depth. Varicose veins are larger and generally deeper than spider veins. Varicose veins can also be found in internal organs, and hemorrhoids are varicose veins around the anus.

What causes varicose veins and spider veins is hard to say with certainty, but they can be associated with pregnancy, hormonal shifts, weight gain, standing occupations, and certain medications as well as other conditions. Pregnancy is a particular culprit; not only does it increase hormone levels and blood volume, which causes veins to enlarge, but the enlarged uterus also increases pressure on the veins. Successive pregnancies may make the problem worse. Certain medical conditions such as diabetes affect blood flow and may predispose a person to varicose veins. Finally, heredity cannot be discounted; indeed, it may be the chief contributor to spider and varicose veins.

Varicose veins in the legs may measure more than a ¼-inch across and tend to bulge as blood backs up behind incompetent valves. When blood congestion is ongoing, the veins enlarge and distend, causing them to be not only more prominent but, in some cases, uncomfortable. Simple sclerotherapy is sufficient to deal with varicose veins, but other options are also available.

FYI

Although the vast majority of varicose and incompetent veins are merely inconvenient, many are painful and some may indicate the presence of disease. If you have a client who complains of pain but has not had his or her condition evaluated by a physician, advise the client to be evaluated as soon as possible.

THE LYMPHATIC SYSTEM

The lymphatic system is a vital component to both the circulatory system and the immune system. The main purpose of the lymphatic system is that of clean-up for the circulatory system. As arteries and veins make their fluid, gas, and nutrient exchanges by way of capillaries and venules, excess fluid, called **lymph,** seeps out and must be reabsorbed in order for blood to remain at acceptable levels and perform its various duties. This is where the lymphatic system comes in (Figure 6–9).

Without **lymphatic vessels** and organs, fluid would accumulate, resulting in swelling and redness, a condition known as *edema*. Lymphatic vessels reabsorb the lymph, store it in the lymphatic collecting vessels and lymph nodes, and return it to the heart. Unlike capillaries and venules, lymphatic vessels are highly permeable. To this effect, bacteria, viruses, and cell debris can easily find their way inside. If not for the lymph nodes, this means of entry could be catastrophic. Scattered throughout the body, the **lymph nodes** remove all of the excess debris while checking the remaining fluid with the help of the immune system. Once cleared for reentry, lymph returns to the bloodstream by way of the thoracic duct. There, it connects to the subclavian vein, where it returns to the heart for a re-uptake of nutrients.

As vital as the lymphatic system is, it is prone to fatigue overtime. The result of this fatigue is fluid stagnation. This stagnation results in edema and has consequences for the circulatory system, immune system, and nervous

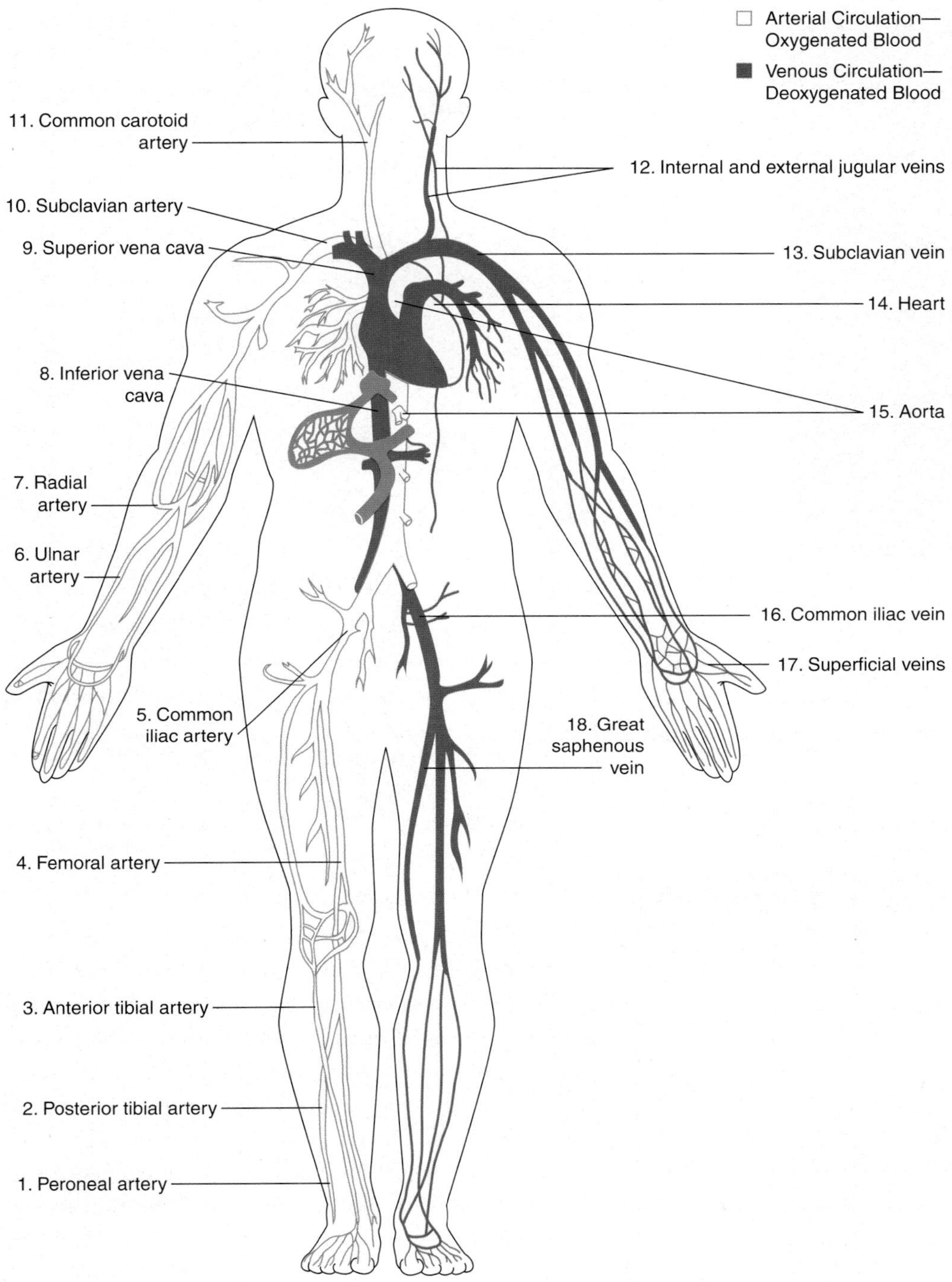

Figure 6–7 The circulatory system.

system. To combat this, lymphatic drainage is often used to rouse the system to a greater level of efficacy.

Lymphatic drainage was first employed by a European doctor, Dr. E. Vodder, in the 1930s. More recently, Dr. Bruno Chikly has used scientific methods to build upon Dr. Vodder's work. Using precise anatomy and specific manual processes, practitioners detect the direction and quality of lymphatic flow and manually encourage optimal flow by means of alternate pathways. In doing

Here's a Tip

Lymphatic drainage can be beneficial to a post-surgical patient.

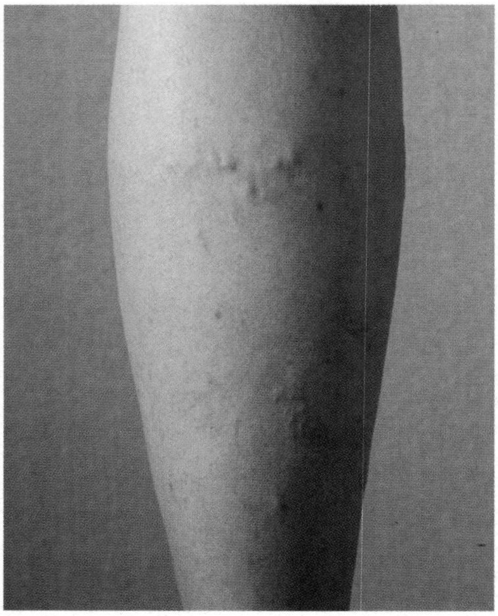

Figure 6–8 Varicose veins.

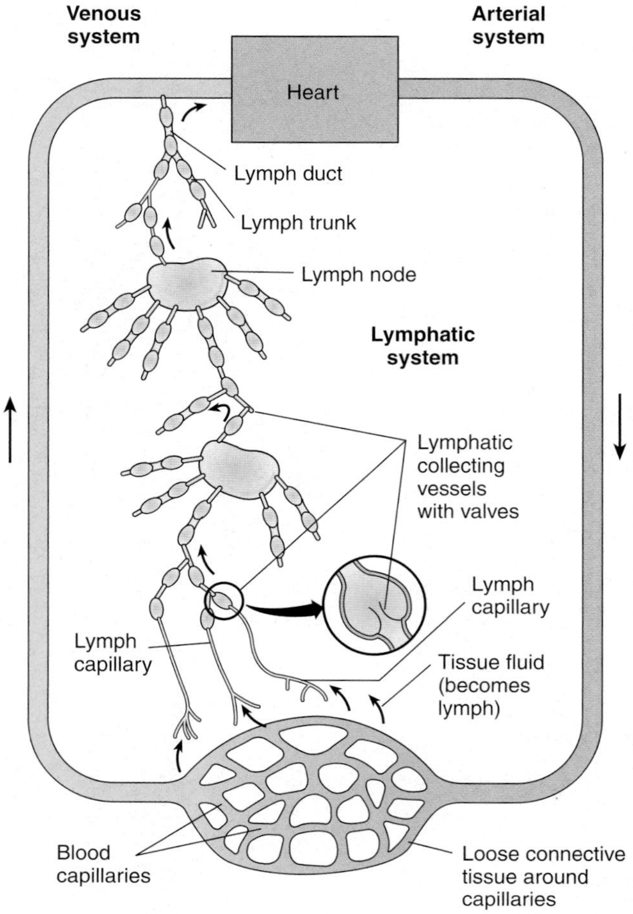

Figure 6–9 The lymphatic system.

do, researchers believe that the resulting optimal flow stimulates the overall circulation and immunologic protection and promotes optimal nervous system function (Table 6–6).

Table 6–6 Benefits from Lymphatic Drainage

BENEFITS FROM LYMPHATIC DRAINAGE
Reduces edema
Detoxifies
Enhances tissue regeneration
Combats aging
Combats fatigue
Relieves certain inflammations
Relieves pain
Relieves constipation
Promotes relaxation

At the center of the circulatory system is the heart. But, as we have learned the heart alone is not responsible for the cardiovascular system. The arteries, veins, and lymph system work with the heart to transport blood to the tissues. Any disease that affects a part of the system may in fact affect the functioning of the entire system. It is important to counsel clients to sustain healthy cardiac health, including attention to diet and exercise.

REVIEW QUESTIONS

1. Name the parts of the circulatory system.
2. Discuss the components of blood.
3. Name three facts about blood.

4. What are some blood disorders?
5. How are veins different from arteries?
6. How are veins and arteries similar?
7. How do varicose veins occur?
8. Name two heart diseases.
9. Describe the operation of the heart.
10. How does the lymphatic system differ from veins and arteries?
11. What is lymphatic drainage?
12. What are some benefits of lymphatic drainage?

CHAPTER GLOSSARY

agranulocytes: nongranular white blood cells.

albumin: a grouping of certain water-soluble proteins as those found in blood or egg whites; the most abundant blood plasma protein.

anastomosis: the connection point of different parts of branching network.

anemia: condition characterized by a deficiency in iron.

antibodies: components of the immune system that neutralize antigens.

aorta: arterial trunk that carries blood from the heart to be distributed by branch arteries through the body.

aortic semilunar valve: valves that prevent blood from flowing back into the heart.

arterioles: smallest component of the arteries; connects with capillary beds.

atria: two upper chambers of the heart that receive blood (singular atrium).

artioventricular valves: valves that prevent blood from flowing back into the ventricles of the heart.

basophils: white blood cell characterized by the presence of blue cytoplasmic granules that become stained by basophilic dye.

bicuspid valve: heart valve located between the left atrium and ventrical that regulates blood backflow between the two chambers.

blood pressure: force exerted by circulation of blood on the walls of blood vessels.

cardiovascular system: system that controls the steady circulation of the blood through the body by means of the heart and blood vessels. Also known as the circulatory system.

clotting factors: specific proteins that act together in clotting; defects in specific protein changes result in clotting conditions such as hemophelia.

collateral circulation: blood vessels that supply blood and nutrients to the body.

deoxygenated: formerly oxygen-rich blood routed back to the heart, via the veins, after its nutrient load has been distributed.

diastole: part of the normal rhythm of the heart during which the heart chambers fill with blood.

electrolytes: ions required by cells to regulate the electric charge and flow of water molecules across the cell membrane.

eosinophils: white blood cells characterized by the presence of cytoplasmic granules that become stained by an acid (eosin) dye.

epicardium: inner layer of the pericardium, which has direct contact with the heart.

CHAPTER GLOSSARY

erythrocytes: (Gr., *erythros*, "red" + *kytos*, "hollow vessel") red blood cell that has hemoglobin to carry oxygen from lungs (or gills) to tissues; during their formation in mammals, erythrocytes lose their nuclei, but erythrocytes of other vertebrates retain their nuclei.

formed elements: red or white blood cells or platelets separated from the fluid part of the blood.

granulocytes: (L., *granulus*, "small grain" + Gr., *Kytos*, "hollow vessel") white blood cells (neutrophils, eosinophils, and basophils) bearing granules (vacuoles) in their cytoplasm that stain deeply.

heart disease: any condition that affects the performance of the heart or the cardiovascular system.

hemophilia: 1.) disorder characterized by deficiencies of clotting factors reducing the blood's ability to clot. 2.) a recessive genetic disorder occurring almost exclusively in men and boys in which the blood clots much more slowly than normal, resulting in extensive bleeding from even minor injuries.

hydrostatic pressure: means of devising fluid pressure by measuring the pressure imposed by an external force.

hypoxia: deficiency in the blood's ability to transport oxygen.

leukemia: disease of the bone marrow characterized by excessive and unwanted white blood cell proliferation.

leukocytes: (Gr., *leukos*, "white" + *Kytos*, "hollow vessel") 1.) Any of several kinds of white blood cells (for example, granulocytes, lymphocytes, and monocytes), so-called because they bear no hemogloblin, unlike red blood cells. 2.) specialized cells that work with the immune system to combat disease and infection.

ligature: a tying or other binding mechanism.

lymph: clear, yellowish fluid that circulates in the lymph spaces (lymphatic) of the body; carries waste and impurities away from the cells.

lymph nodes: special structures found in the lymphatic vessels that filter lymph products.

lymphatic vessels: reabsorb the lymph, store it in the lymphatic collecting vessels and lymph nodes, and return it to the heart.

monocytes: large white blood cells or leukocytes, which travel the bloodstream neutralizing pathogens; become phagocytic cells (macrophages) after moving into tissues.

myocardium: muscular tissue around the heart.

neutrophils: 1.) most abundant of polymorphonuclear leukocytes; an important phagocyte; so-called because it stains with both acidic and basic 2.) phagocytic white blood cells.

oxygenated: rich in oxygen.

peripheral edema: swelling resulting from fluid accumulation in the lower limbs.

phagocytes: (Gr. *phagein*, "to eat" + *kytos*, "hollow vessel") any cell that engulfs and devours microorganisms or other particles (process known as phagocytosis).

plexuses: network of nerves that branch and rejoin. There are nearly 100 in the body.

pulmonary circulation: the path deoxygenated blood travels to become oxygenated; through the right ventricle, into the lungs through the pulmonary artery, and into the left atrium via the pulmonary vein.

pulmonary valve: one of the two valves that regulates the flow of blood between the ventricles and the major blood vessel to which it connects.

semilunar valve: valves of the arteries, preventing backflow from arteries into the ventricles.

stethoscope: device used to magnify the sound of a beating heart.

systemic circulation: blood and lymph circulation from the heart, through the arteries, to tissue and cells, and back to the heart by way of the veins; also called *general circulation*.

systole: contraction of the heart (as opposed to diastole).

thalassemia: condition characterized by defective hemoglobin cells, resulting in oxygen difficiency.

tortuous: taking a twisting, nonlinear path.

tricuspid valve: heart valve which prevents backflow between the right atrium and right ventricle.

varicose veins: condition characterized by incompetent values in the veins, most commonly in the legs.

ventricles: the lower, thick-walled chambers of the heart, which force blood to the lungs for oxygenation or throughout the body.

CHAPTER OUTLINE

- PRINCIPLES OF CHEMISTRY
- CHEMICAL REACTIONS
- CHEMICALS FOUND IN THE SKIN AND BODY
- CHEMICAL TERMS ESTHETICIANS SHOULD KNOW
- BOTANICAL CHEMISTRY
- ESSENTIAL OIL CHEMISTRY

CHAPTER 7

CHEMISTRY AND BIOCHEMISTRY

LEARNING OBJECTIVES

After completing this chapter, you should be able to:

- Demonstrate a knowledge of chemistry and its principles.
- Define biochemistry and its importance to esthetics.
- Understand chemical reactions and their importance to estheticians.
- Identify chemicals found in the body.
- Discuss important chemical terminology.
- Demonstrate a knowledge of botanical chemistry.

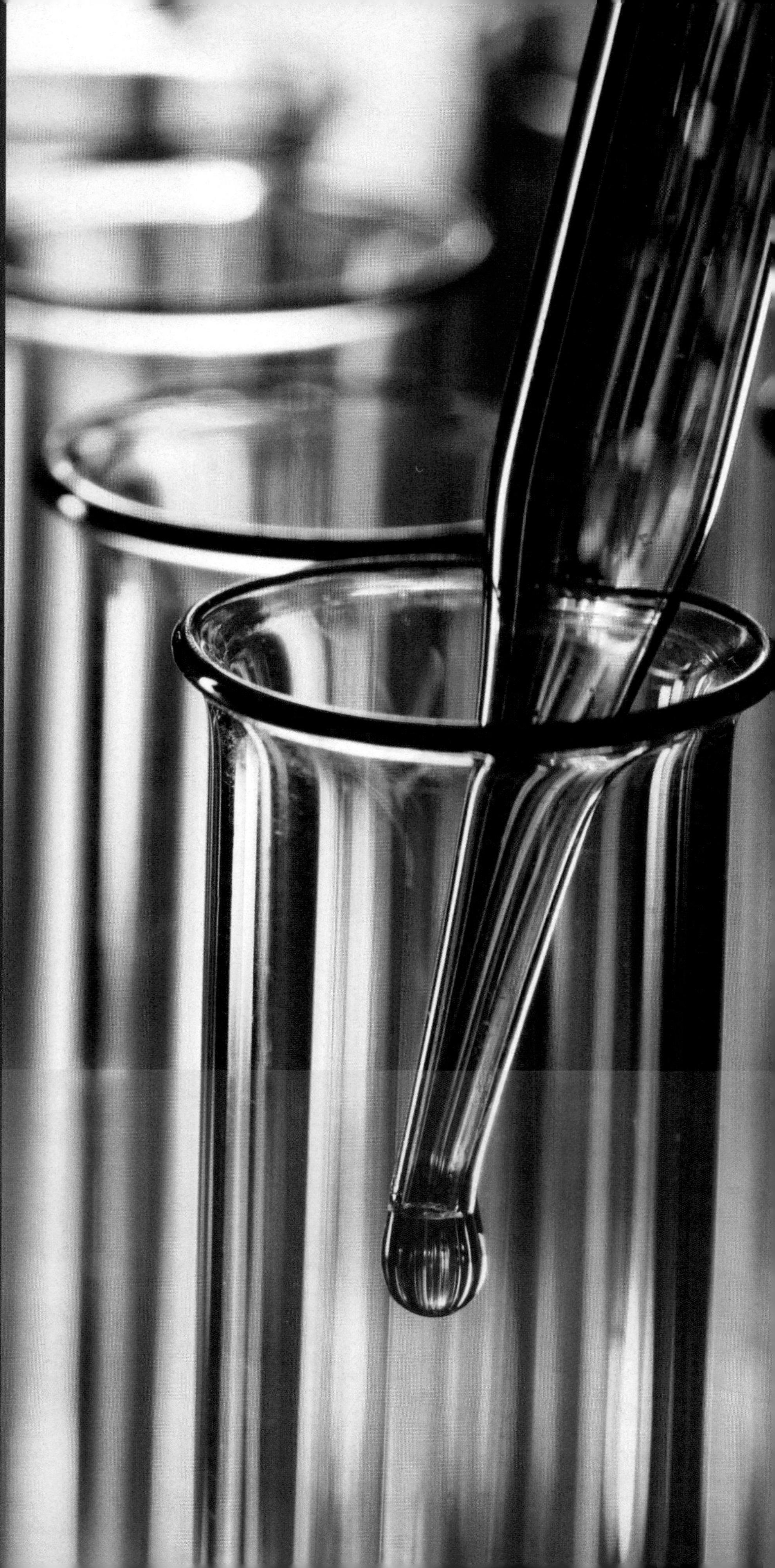

KEY TERMS

Page numbers indicate where in the chapter the term is used.

alkaloids 148
amino acids 143
analgesic 148
bases 145
benzene ring structure 152
biochemistry 143
carboxylic acid 149
carotenoids 148
catalyst 143
chemical reactions 142
co-enzymes 147
disaccharide 144
enzymes 147
equation 143
ester 149
fatty acids 148
fatty waxes 149
flavonoids 148
functional group 150
isoprene units 150
metabolism 146
metabolites 146
monosaccharide 144
monounsaturated fatty acids 148
organic compound 140
peptide bond 143
periodic table 140
phenylpropanoids 152
polysaccharide 144
polyunsaturated fatty acids 148
primary metabolites 146
protein 143
rancidity 149
saccharide 144
saturated fatty acids 148
secondary metabolites 146
terpenoid compounds 150
unsaturated fatty acids 148

An esthetician specializes in applying cosmetic chemicals and teaching clients about their uses. While not really a chemist, an esthetician must have a working knowledge of basic chemistry to better understand the biochemical functions of both the skin's cells and the cosmetics and products used in the practice of esthetics. This chapter revisits basic chemistry and introduces a more in-depth look at the common elements in the esthetic realm. It also takes a look at botanical chemistry as an important base to better understanding the ingredients so common to skin care products and aromatherapy.

PRINCIPLES OF CHEMISTRY

Chemistry is the science that deals with the composition, structure, and properties of matter, and how matter changes under different conditions. There are two branches of chemistry–organic and inorganic. Matter is anything that takes up space and has substance. You are matter. This text is matter. Essentially, everything is matter. All matter is made from about 110 known elements. Remember that an element is a substance (matter) in its simplest form; it cannot be broken down any further. Everything on earth is made up of matter except light and electricity. Examples of elements include oxygen, silver, and gold. Elements interact, through chemical reactions, creating chemical substances.

Practicing esthetics, you handle chemicals every day. For example, when you use galvanic current or clean a steamer with vinegar, you are dealing with chemistry and chemical reactions. In esthetics your career depends on chemicals and chemical reactions.

? Did You Know

Water is a chemical, air is a chemical. People are made up of chemicals. The only things that are not chemicals are light and electricity.

The smallest measurable unit of an element is an atom. An atom is made up of a nucleus, which is the center of the atom, and electrons, negatively charged particles that orbit the nucleus, just as planets orbit the sun. The nucleus of an atom is made up of protons and neutrons. Protons are tiny, positively charged particles, whereas neutrons are tiny particles with no charge.

Remember how positive and negative charges are attracted? This principle is what keeps electrons orbiting the nucleus. The electrons, which are extremely light (it takes about 1,800 electrons to equal the mass of one proton), are attracted to the nucleus because it has a positive charge (thanks to the protons) and they are negative. Electrons orbit the nucleus in circular patterns called *electron shells* or *energy levels*. The number of shells depends on what kind of atom it is.

All atoms of the same element are the same size, weigh the same, and have the same number of protons. The number of protons in one atom's nucleus gives that element what is called its *atomic number*. An atom with the same number of electrons as protons has a neutral charge and is called *stable*. However, sometimes an atom loses an electron, leaving the atom with more positively charged particles than negatively charged particles. The atom is then called an *ion*. It is now unstable and will most likely react with other atoms in an effort to garner another electron and become stable. Chemical reactions are described in more detail later in this chapter.

FYI

Atoms are described as stable or unstable. A stable atom might have 2 electrons in the first energy ring, 8 electrons in the second ring (if the atom has one), 8 electrons in the third ring, and so on. If an element does not have this number naturally, it is unstable and will react with other atoms in an effort to become stable.

The **periodic table** of the elements shows the known elements arranged by atomic number (Figure 7–1). Each element's atomic weight—the total weight of one atom's protons and neutrons—is also shown. Last, each element is shown by its symbol, one or two letters that stand for the element's name. Elements are divided into gases, liquids, and solids. The following sections discuss some of the basic elements of human life.

Here's a Tip

The weight of a single element is called its atomic weight.

The weight of a chemical made of a combination of elements is called molecular weight.

Hydrogen

Hydrogen is represented by the letter H and has an atomic weight of 1. It is an odorless, tasteless, colorless, highly flammable gas, the lightest and most abundant of the elements in the universe. Elemental hydrogen is relatively rare here on Earth. Hydrogen can form compounds with most elements and is present in water and most **organic compounds**. It plays a particularly important role in acid-base chemistry and the reactions between acid and alkaline chemicals. These reactions occur in electrolysis and in many other product and skin interactions.

Oxygen

Oxygen is represented by the letter O and has an atomic weight of 8. On Earth oxygen is usually bonded to other elements either covalently or ionically. (These terms will be discussed later in the chapter.) A colorless gas, oxygen is one of two major components in the air humans breathe and is a product of photosynthesis. At standard air pressure oxygen molecules exist as a two-molecule couplet called a *diatomic molecule* with the formula O_2. This molecule has the electron configuration of what is called a *triplet oxygen molecule,* sometimes referred to as double bond. This form of oxygen is the least reactive state of oxygen or other radicals. A single oxygen molecule, O, is very unstable and readily forms compounds with many other elements creating, among other things, the "oxides" which can affect skin care and the body.

Periodic Table of the Elements

Color Legend

- Alkali metals
- Alkaline earth metals
- Transition metals
- Lanthanides
- Actinides
- Other metals
- Semi-metals
- Nonmetals
- Noble gases

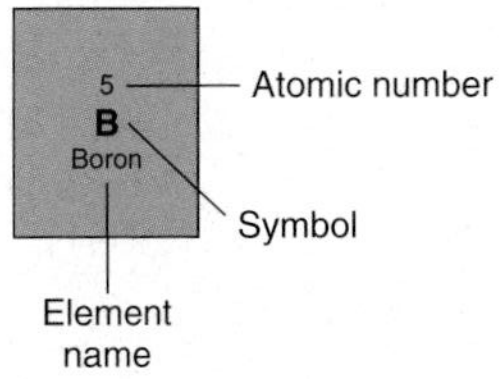

1 **H** Hydrogen																	2 **He** Helium
3 **Li** Lithium	4 **Be** Beryllium											5 **B** Boron	6 **C** Carbon	7 **N** Nitrogen	8 **O** Oxygen	9 **F** Fluorine	10 **Ne** Neon
11 **Na** Sodium	12 **Mg** Magnesium											13 **Al** Aluminium	14 **Si** Silicon	15 **P** Phosphorus	16 **S** Sulphur	17 **Cl** Chlorine	18 **Ar** Argon
19 **K** Potassium	20 **Ca** Calcium	21 **Sc** Scandium	22 **Ti** Titanium	23 **V** Vanadium	24 **Cr** Chromium	25 **Mn** Manganese	26 **Fe** Iron	27 **Co** Cobalt	28 **Ni** Nickel	29 **Cu** Copper	30 **Zn** Zinc	31 **Ga** Gallium	32 **Ge** Germanium	33 **As** Arsenic	34 **Se** Selenium	35 **Br** Bromine	36 **Kr** Krypton
37 **Rb** Rubidium	38 **Sr** Strontium	39 **Y** Yttrium	40 **Zr** Zirconium	41 **Nb** Niobium	42 **Mo** Molybdenum	43 **Tc** Technetium	44 **Ru** Ruthenium	45 **Rh** Rhodium	46 **Pd** Palladium	47 **Ag** Silver	48 **Cd** Cadmium	49 **In** Indium	50 **Sn** Tin	51 **Sb** Antimony	52 **Te** Tellurium	53 **I** Iodine	54 **Xe** Xenon
55 **Cs** Cesium	56 **Ba** Barium	57–71 Lanthanides see below	72 **Hf** Hafnium	73 **Ta** Tantalum	74 **W** Tungsten	75 **Re** Rhenium	76 **Os** Osmium	77 **Ir** Iridium	78 **Pt** Platinum	79 **Au** Gold	80 **Hg** Mercury	81 **Tl** Thallium	82 **Pb** Lead	83 **Bi** Bismuth	84 **Po** Polonium	85 **At** Astatine	86 **Rn** Radon
87 **Fr** Francium	88 **Ra** Radium	89–103 Actinides see below	104 **Rf** Rutherfordium	105 **Db** Dubenium	106 **Sg** Seaborgium	107 **Bh** Bohrium	108 **Hs** Hassium	109 **Mt** Meitnerium	110 **Uum** Ununnilium								

Lanthanides	57 **La** Lanthanum	58 **Ce** Cerium	59 **Pr** Praseodymium	60 **Nd** Neodymium	61 **Pm** Promethium	62 **Sm** Samarium	63 **Eu** Europium	64 **Gd** Gadolinium	65 **Td** Terbium	66 **Dy** Dysprosium	67 **Ho** Holmium	68 **Er** Erbium	69 **Tm** Thulium	70 **Yb** Ytterbium	71 **Lu** Lutetium
Actinides	89 **Ac** Actinium	90 **Th** Thorium	91 **Pa** Protactiniuim	92 **U** Uranium	93 **Np** Neptunium	94 **Pu** Plutonium	95 **Am** Americium	96 **Cm** Curium	97 **Bk** Berkelium	98 **Cf** Californium	99 **Es** Einsteinium	100 **Fm** Fermium	101 **Md** Mendelevium	102 **No** Nobelium	103 **Lr** Lawrencium

Figure 7–1 Periodic table of the elements.

Carbon

Carbon is identified by the letter C and has an atomic weight of 6. Black in color, it is an abundant nonmetallic element that can be found in a variety of configurations. Carbon-based compounds have the ability to form polymers, long carbon-based chains that are found in the body and elsewhere. (DNA is a polymer.) This ability, in addition to its abundance, make carbon the element that is the basis of chemistry for all known life. Graphite, diamonds, and coal are all variations of carbon configurations. Carbon can bond with itself or other elements to form nearly 10 million known bonds. Carbon occurs in all organic life and is the basis of organic chemistry.

When carbon combines with oxygen, it forms carbon dioxide, which is the basis for plant growth. When it combines with hydrogen, it forms flammable hydrocarbons, which are essential to industry in the form of fossil fuels. When carbon combines with both oxygen and hydrogen, it forms many important biological compounds, including sugars, celluloses, alcohols, and fats. When carbon combines with nitrogen and sulfur, it forms antibiotics, amino acids, and proteins. When phosphorous joins the blend, it forms DNA and RNA.

Sodium

Sodium's letters are Na and it has an atomic weight of 11. It is a soft, silvery white, highly reactive element that belongs to the metals group. Sodium is present in great quantities in the Earth's oceans as sodium chloride. It is also a component of many minerals, and it is an essential element for animal life. Because it is so highly reactive, it is only found in nature as a compound, not as a free element.

Sodium is important to the body for numerous functions. While it is needed by all animals, it is not needed by plant life and is not found there. Those eating only a plant-based diet must supplement their sodium needs from another source.

Chlorine

Chlorine, or Cl, has an atomic weight of 17. In nature chlorine is most commonly found as the chloride ion, part of salt. In this state it forms about 1.9% of the mass of seawater. It is abundant in nature and essential to human life. In its elemental state it is a poisonous pale green gas. It is a powerful oxidant and is often used in disinfecting, as in chlorine bleach or as a cleaning agent for swimming pools.

Activity

Look up the Periodic Table of the Elements on the Internet and explore the different aspects of the elements.

CHEMICAL REACTIONS

Reactions between two elements or two compounds that result in chemical changes are called **chemical reactions.** There are two types of bonds that take place in chemical reactions: In a *covalent bond*, atoms share pairs of electrons. For example, carbon's atomic number is six, so it has six protons and should have six electrons. A carbon atom with four electrons requires two more electrons to become complete, or stable. Hydrogen has two protons, so a hydrogen atom with one electron requires one electron to become stable (Figure 7–2). When atoms steal or give away electrons to become balanced in their electron shells, the resulting atoms are called ions. In an *ionic bond*, two atoms—one metal and one nonmetal—with opposite charges are attracted to each other An example is when sodium which has one electron in its outermost shell gives away that electron to a chlorine atom which has only 7 electrons in its valance. The result is an ionic bond between the two different atoms.

Reactions between two elements or two compounds that result in chemical changes are called chemical reactions. During the chemical reaction, electrons of the elements or compounds involved begin to either share energy levels in a covalent bond, or form ionic bonds. Some chemical reactions take place by mixing others and require more stimulus.

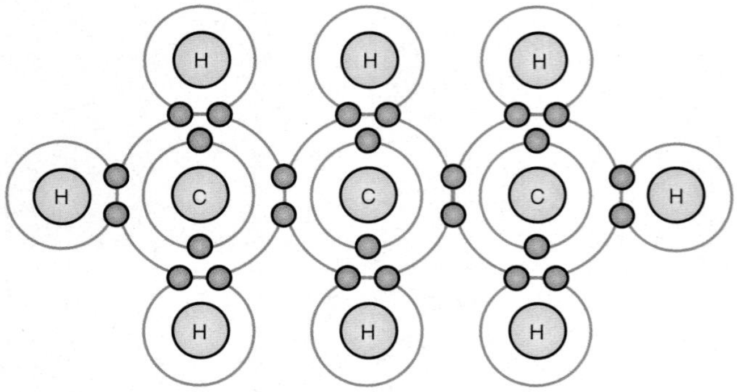

Figure 7–2 Polymer molecule "sharing" electrons between hydrogen and carbon atoms.

Chemical reactions are described using **equations.** For example, the following equation shows a reaction between two molecules of sodium and two water molecules:

$$2Na + 2H_2O = 2NaOH + H_2 + \text{energy (heat)}$$

Remember that Na is the symbol for sodium; O is for oxygen; and H is for hydrogen. The number in front of each chemical stands for the number of molecules of each chemical present in the reaction. Numbers below a chemical symbol stand for the number of atoms of that element in a particular molecule. So, 2Na stands for two atoms of sodium, and $2H_2O$ stands for two molecules of water (a bond formed between two atoms of hydrogen and one of oxygen), which equals 2NaOH, or two molecules of sodium hydroxide.

This reaction uses everything on the left side of the equation to produce the sodium hydroxide plus one molecule of hydrogen, H_2, on the right side. Note that because this is an equation, both sides are equal, so the same number of atoms are present before and after the reaction. Before the reaction, there were two sodium atoms, four hydrogen atoms, and two oxygen atoms, $2Na + 2H_2O$. After the reaction, there are the same number of atoms, only with a different chemical structure. Because of the electron changeovers, we now have two totally new chemicals, lye and hydrogen. 2NaOH, or two molecules of sodium hydroxide, have two atoms of sodium, two atoms of oxygen, and two atoms of hydrogen. The other two hydrogen atoms are given off as H_2 (hydrogen gas). Heat is required for some chemical reactions. Some reactions require exposure to ultraviolet light or pressure to take place.

Some reactions such as the one discussed here occur very naturally, by simply combining two chemicals. Other reactions do not happen as naturally. These types of chemical reactions require what is called a **catalyst,** a substance that helps to cause or speed up the reaction without its atoms becoming a direct part of the reaction's products.

CHEMICALS FOUND IN THE SKIN AND BODY

As discussed in previous chapters, almost every body function involves chemical reactions. The hormones that tell cells what to do are chemicals that react with receptor sites. The pituitary hormones signal other glands to manufacture compounds containing carbon atoms.

The chemicals that the body uses most are oxygen, carbon, hydrogen, and nitrogen. Carbon and hydrogen frequently bond together in chains. These chains of carbon-carbon and carbon-hydrogen bonds are known as polymers. Polymers are found in many of the body's chemicals. Proteins, DNA, sugars, and carbohydrates are just a few of the examples of polymers in the body's chemistry. The study of chemicals and chemical reactions within the body is known as **biochemistry.**

> ***FYI***
>
> The chemicals that the body uses most are oxygen, carbon, hydrogen, and nitrogen.

Proteins

An important substance in the human body is **protein,** which is made of carbon, oxygen, nitrogen, hydrogen, and sulfur. The basic unit of a protein molecule is called an **amino acid.** Think of amino acids as modules or cars of a toy train. When many different modules are placed together, a protein molecule results. Simple proteins are groups of amino acids linked together. Sometimes the amino acids will have another chemical linked that is not an amino acid. These proteins with a non-amino-acid group are called *conjugated proteins.* Glycoproteins are amino acid chains with a carbohydrate group attached to the chain. Lipoproteins are amino acid chains with lipids or fats attached to the chain. Phosphoroproteins have a phosphorus or phosphate group attached to the protein chain.

The bond between amino acid groups is called a **peptide bond.** When many amino acids are in long chains, there are obviously many bonds. A chain of amino acid molecules is known as a polypeptide.

Simple proteins make up basic material for the body's tissues. The skin, hair, and connective tissue are made up of *scleroprotein.* The protein that makes up the blood and lymph is called *globulin.* Albumin is another type of simple protein used in the blood. Nucleic acids with protein DNA structures are another type of simple protein product.

Carbohydrates

The carbohydrate groups include sugars and other compounds. Carbohydrates are formed by a chain of carbon atoms united with oxygen and hydrogen. They form units similar to protein and amino acid units. A simple unit of a carbohydrate is called a **saccharide** (Figure 7–3). A single saccharide is called a **monosaccharide.** Two saccharides together form a **disaccharide.** Many saccharides bonded together form a **polysaccharide.** Monosaccharides are simple sugars like glucose (blood sugar). Disaccharides include sucrose, or table sugar, and malatose, the sugar used to make malted milk. Polysaccharides are more complex carbohydrates. They include the sugars in starch and the carbohydrates that make up vegetables and cellulose-type substances.

Lipids

Lipids are basically fats. They are a third major chemical group within the body. Lipids, comprising carbon, oxygen, and hydrogen, do not form units like proteins and carbohydrates. They are more complex. Triglycerides are the best-known type of lipid, and other lipids include waxes, fats, and steroids.

Lipids are important to skin care. They can bind with proteins to form proteolipids, which are a major part of the intercellular cement. Phospholipids and glycolipids are two examples of lipid-protein compounds found in the intercellular cement.

pH, Acids, and Bases

When water is added to certain compounds such as acids, the water (H_2O) breaks up and restructures, with some atoms joining the acid chemicals. For example, when mixed with water, hydrogen chloride (HCl) becomes hydrochloric acid. The hydrogen ions float separately in the acid. The measurement of these hydrogen ions is known as the *pH* of the substance. pH is an abbreviation for the negative logarithm of hydrions (positively charged

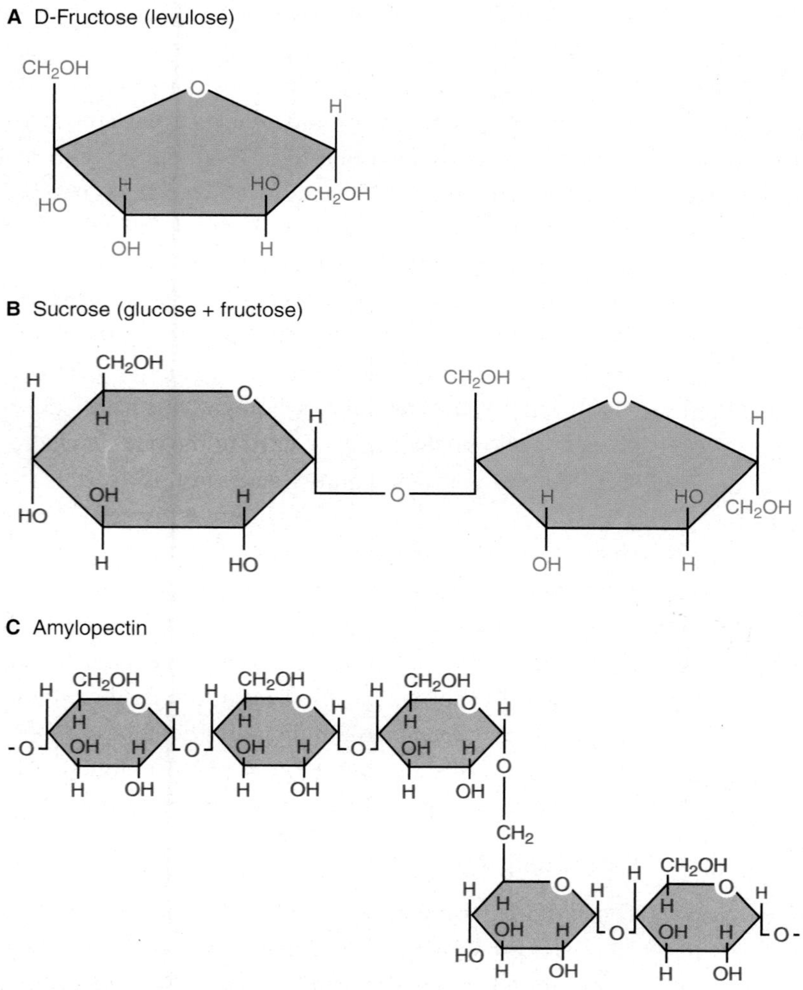

Figure 7–3 Examples of saccharides.

hydrogen ions). Acids have a low pH, which actually means that they have a large number of hydrogen ions. Alkaline substances, or **bases,** have a low concentration of hydrogen ions. They have high pH values. The pH scale ranges from 0 to 14. The lower the pH, the more acidic the substance. The higher the pH, the more alkaline the substance. Figure 7–4 give examples of various substances and their pH values.

Why pH Is Important in Cosmetics

Anyone involved in skin care needs a thorough knowledge of pH. On its surface the skin has an acid mantle, which is made of a mixture of lipids, sebum, and sweat. This acid mantle has a pH of about 5.5, which is a slightly acidic pH. Cosmetics should also have a slightly acidic pH. Higher pH values tend to swell the skin and make it more permeable. This can be good or bad, depending on the circumstances. For example, desincrustation solutions and "pre-masks" used for treating clogged pores and oily areas need to have a slightly alkaline pH to slightly dilate the pores for easier extraction. They also help to conduct electricity (galvanic current) better for desincrustation.

Cleansers for oily skin may also have a slightly higher pH than that of the acid mantle. They can then perform a more efficient job of cutting the subaceous secretions of oily or problem skin. Most of the high pH cleansers are followed by low pH toners. A cleanser with a pH of 6.5 or 7.0 is often followed by a toner with a pH of 4.0 or 4.5. High pH values, however, can be harmful to the skin, particularly if they are not controlled. High pH increases the permeability of the skin, making it easier for bacteria, microorganisms, and other harmful substances to enter the body. Harsh, high pH products such as soaps can be very irritating and can severely overdry the skin.

The other exception to the acidic pH guideline is products with new high-tech ingredients, some of which are not stable at acidic pH levels. Products containing these ingredients, such as peptide proteins, may need to be at a more neutral pH for stability purposes. The skin will normalize the pH of these products in a short period of time, a small tradeoff for the ability to incorporate the next generation of antioxidant or age-fighting ingredients.

Being aware of pH values is especially important in chemical exfoliation and peeling procedures. Alpha hydroxy acid (AHA) and beta hydroxy acid (BHA), professional esthetic exfoliation treatments, have lower pHs. The lower the pH, the more acidic the product. The ideal pH for AHA professional esthetic treatments is 3.0, with an AHA concentration not greater than 30%. When the pH is less than 3.0, the irritation potential of exfoliation treatments increases dramatically. Likewise, concentrations greater than 30% also increase irritation potential.

CHEMICAL TERMS ESTHETICIANS SHOULD KNOW

There are a variety of additional terms that you should know to better interpret ingredient labels and understand more about cosmetic chemicals. Some of these words are actually suffixes or prefixes that you will see attached to different chemical names. Most of these are derived from Latin.

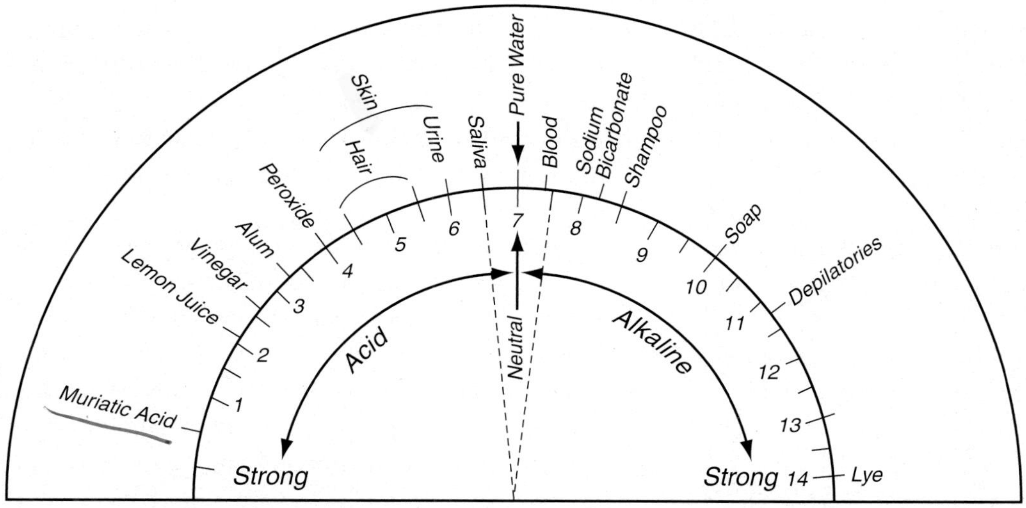

Figure 7–4 Various substances and their pH values.

AEROBIC: Refers to a reaction that takes place in the presence of oxygen. *Anaerobic* means "without oxygen."

ALCOHOL: Molecule that has a hydroxyl (OH) group bonded to it. The molecule must be a hydrocarbon—made of carbon and hydrogen atoms.

ALDEHYDE: A compound made of carbon and hydrogen, with a carbon, hydrogen, and oxygen group on the end of the molecule.

AMINO: (prefix) Refers to compounds that have an amino acid group attached; may also indicate protein derivation.

AQUEOUS: Water-based, as in an *aqueous solution.*

CARBO: (prefix) Has carbon as a base in the molecule, such as a carbohydrate.

CYCLO: (prefix) Means that the molecule is in a ring structure. The carbon atoms are joined in a ring formation.

DI: (prefix) Means "two." *Disodium* means two sodium atoms are included in a molecular structure.

DISTILLED: Heated to remove one chemical from another. For example, water is distilled by boiling it and allowing the gas to condense back into liquid, separating the water from impurities and other contaminant chemicals.

ENZYME: Protein that is involved as a catalyst in a chemical reaction. Enzymes in cosmetics are often used to break down substances, as a proteolytic enzyme breaks down keratin protein in dead cells. The chemical names of enzymes generally end in the suffix *-ase.* Examples are *lipase* (fat-dissolving enzyme) and *maltase,* which breaks maltose, a disaccharide, into two simple glucose (sugar) molecules.

HYDRATION: Water is added.

HOMOGENOUS: A mixture that is even. The solute is evenly dispersed throughout the solvent.

IONIZED: Substance has been charged by changing atoms to ions. *Deionized* means that ions have been neutralized and do not have a charge.

LIPO: (prefix) Refers to fats, lipids, or waxes. Examples are lipoproteins, found in the intercellular cement, or liposuction, the surgical procedure used to remove fat.

MONO: (prefix) Means "one." For example, monosaccharide is a simple sugar with one saccharide group.

POLY: (prefix) Means "many." Examples: *polymer, polysaccharide.*

PROTEO: (prefix) Refers to protein. *Proteolytic,* as in proteolytic enzyme peelings, means protein-dissolving.

SACCHARIDES: Can refer to any carbohydrate group. For example, mucopolysaccharide is a popular moisturizing ingredient.

SATURATED: Can either mean that a solution has absorbed as much solute as possible or that a molecule has taken on as many hydrogen atoms as it can hold, as in saturated fat.

SUSPENSION: The solute is suspended throughout a solvent. Suspension is usually not homogenous. A separating makeup foundation is an example of a suspension.

TRI: (prefix) Means "three." For example: *tridecyl trimellitate,* an emollient.

BOTANICAL CHEMISTRY

Over the past decades there has been an increase of information regarding the wide range of health-giving properties offered by such botanicals as food, supplements, and in-skin care. Science has reduced the botanicals and their extracts to individual components with known biological activity. Continued research of these chemical substances has clarified the potential in creating balance to all skin types and alleviating many skin conditions. A basic knowledge of these plant compounds can enhance any esthetician's work.

Metabolites

The active chemical components found in foods and botanical extracts play a part in the metabolism of a plant. **Metabolism** involves the chemical and physical changes that occur within all living organisms as well as the energy and chemical transformations that happen in the cells. **Metabolites** are the products used by living organisms in the process of metabolism. The same metabolites used by and contained in a plant are the vitamins and other nutrients that humans use in metabolic processes.

Metabolites are classified in two groups: primary and secondary. **Primary metabolites** are required for the growth, structure, and reproduction of a plant. Examples of primary metabolites are amino acids, enzymes and co-enzymes, lipids, and polysaccharides, such as cellulose (Table 7–1). Primary metabolites have a common and broad distribution among living things. The **secondary metabolites** are the products generated within the plant that are not required for the

Table 7–1 Primary Metabolites

PRIMARY METABOLITES
Amino acids
Enzymes and co-enzymes
Fatty acids and lipids
Carbohydrates

most basic, life-sustaining needs. Secondary metabolites have important functions, especially in the protection of the plant from the environment and herbivores. Unlike primary metabolites, the compounds that make up secondary metabolites are found mainly in plants. The individual secondary compounds are not common among all plants and, instead, tend to be unique to specific plant species or families. The compounds produced as secondary metabolites have a wide range of activity and, just like their function within the plant, are used for the health and protection of the body and the skin (Tables 7–2 and 7–3).

Plant Compounds in Skin Care

Both primary and secondary compounds find their use in skin care. These compounds can be utilized as a whole plant extract, such as the starches in whole kelp, or as extracts, like the fatty acid oils from olives. Compounds, such as amino acids and enzymes, may also be isolated from the plant material. There are many diverse and complex molecular compounds that have beneficial properties for the skin. Following is a discussion of some of the more important, more common, and most available groups of compounds used in skin care and cosmetics.

Table 7–2 Some Important Functions of Secondary Metabolites in Plants

SOME IMPORTANT FUNCTIONS OF SECONDARY METABOLITES IN PLANTS
Protection from environmental damage
Protection from herbivores: insects and animals
Protection from microorganisms, such as parasitic bacteria, viruses, and fungi
Promotion of seeding and pollination through attraction of animals and insects

Table 7–3 Common Uses of Secondary Metabolites by Humans

USE	EXAMPLES
Drugs	Hallucinogenics, sedatives, stimulants
Medicines	Antibiotics, cholesterol regulation, pain relief
Poisons	Insecticides, rat poisons
Dyes	Clothing, food, and hair coloring
Dietary supplements	Antioxidants, anti-inflammatories, detoxifiers
Skin care	Antioxidants, anti-inflammatories, cell regeneration, detoxifiers, skin conditioning, wound healing
Reproduction	Aphrodisiacs, perfumes

Amino Acids

Amino acids are primary metabolic compounds that are naturally present in the skin. To utilize amino acids in skin care, they must be isolated from a plant source or synthetically processed. Manufacturers claim that topical application of amino acids helps maintain moisture content or may trigger a response within the skin that will synthesize collagen peptides.

Enzymes and Co-Enzymes

Enzymes and **co-enzymes** are responsible for metabolic functions in the plant and the body. They are necessary in the breakdown of foods and other changes that are made to chemical components so they can be reformed and used by the organism for vital functions. Research has demonstrated that enzymes already present on the skin may be activated by topical substances and may assist in their absorption and utilization. Some studies have shown how specific enzymes applied topically may react with DNA to reduce or prevent skin cancers and other skin disease.

Polysaccharides

Polysaccharides are made up of a large number of glucose-containing monosaccharide units. Plants produce polysaccharides for structural support, to metabolize for energy, and to store as food. The carbohydrates, gums, and mucilages (slimy semisolids that provide moisture and calm irritation) used in skin care are derived from oats, seaweeds, plants, and fruits. Gums are often used as thickening agents, such as guar gum and gum tragacanth.

Alkaloids

The **alkaloids** are the most notorious group of secondary metabolites found in plants. Caffeine, nicotine, and cocaine are all alkaloids, as are many compounds recognized as poisons, hallucinogenics, sedatives, and others having similar physiological effects in the human body. It would be uncommon to find isolated alkaloids used in skin care. They are a component within a botanical extract, especially the herbal extracts, and may provide an **analgesic,** or pain killing, effect.

Carotenoids and Flavonoids

Deep-colored purple and blue berries, green tea, chocolate, red vegetables, and several of the foods that are highly recommended in a healthy diet contain high amounts of **flavonoids** and/or **carotenoids.** Both carotenoids and flavonoids are subcategories of a group of secondary metabolites called *glycosides.* These compounds contain several double bonds, making them more reactive and therapeutically active. Carotenoids and flavonoids are extremely valuable for the overall health of the body and skin due to their powerful antioxidant properties. They may also contribute anti-inflammatory and anti-spasmodic effects and are often documented for their anticancer effects. Color is one of the main features of these compounds, so skin care products claiming to contain fruit and vegetable extracts are off-white to deeper shades of yellow, brown, green, or orange. See Table 7–4 for a list of flavonoids and carotenoids valued for their skin-nourishing benefits.

Fatty Acids

Fruit and vegetable oils are composed of hydrocarbon chain structures called **fatty acids.** There are several important groups of fatty acids used in skin care, and each is classified by the amount of double bonds it contains. **Saturated fatty acids** contain no double bonds, meaning that all the carbon atoms in the chain are complete and bonded to a hydrogen atom or another carbon and do not have to share electrons with other carbon atoms (Figure 7–5). Saturated fats are stable and are solid at cooler temperatures. Coconut oil, cocoa butter, and shea butter all contain high amounts of saturated fatty acids, giving them their solid, "buttery" texture.

Table 7–4 Flavinoids & Carotenoids

FLAVONOIDS	BOTANICAL SOURCE
Anthocyanidins	Dark blue, red, purple and black berries; plums; red potatoes
Flavan-3-ols	Cocoa, grapes, tea
Flavanones	Citrus fruits
Flavones	Beets, bell peppers, celery, spinach, thyme
Flavonols	Apples, berries, broccoli, grapes
Proanthocyanidins	Cocoa, berries, grapes, French pine (*Pinus pinaster* ssp. *atlantica*)
CAROTENOIDS	
Carotenes	Carrots, palm oil, and many other deep-colored green, orange, red, and yellow fruits and vegetables
Xanthophylls	Algae, corn, bacteria, fungus, kale, tomato

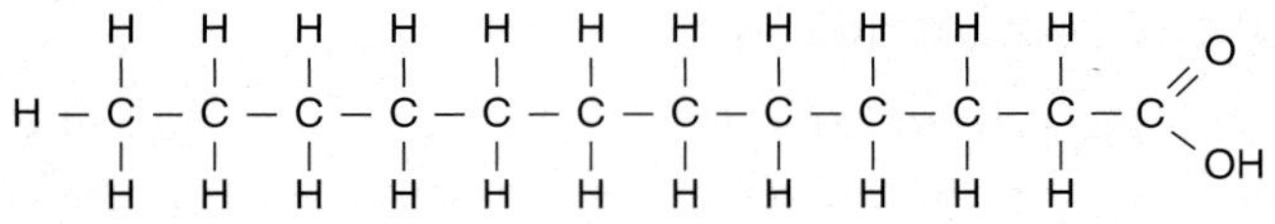

Figure 7–5 Lauric acid.

Double bonds within the hydrocarbon chain indicate an **unsaturated fatty acid.** Unsaturated fats have a lower melting point than saturated fats and are liquid at room temperature. **Monounsaturated fatty acids** contain one double bond in the carbon chain (Figure 7–6). The **polyunsaturated fatty acids** contain two or more double bonds, giving them their status as having a superior therapeutic benefit in skin care (Table 7–5 and Figure 7–7).

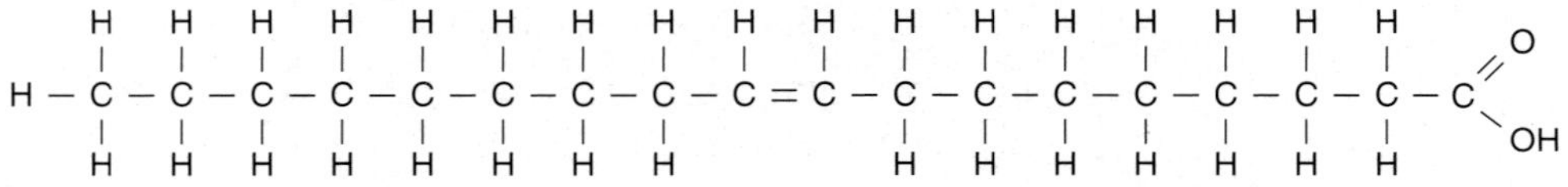

Figure 7–6 Oleic acid.

Table 7–5 Saturated and Unsaturated Fatty Acids

SATURATED FATS	BOTANICAL SOURCE	PROPERTIES
Lauric acid	Coconut, palm	Moisturizing, protective
Palmitic acid	Avocado, palm	Moisturizing, protective
Stearic acid	Cashew, neem	Moisturizing, protective
MONOUNSATURATED FATS		
Oleic acid	Avocado, olive, sunflower	Anti-inflammatory, moisturizing
Palmitoleic acid	Almond, avocado, macadamia	Anti-inflammatory, moisturizing
POLYUNSATURATED FATS		
Linoleic acid (Omega-6)	Borage, black currant, cranberry seed, evening primrose, hemp, raspberry seed	Anti-inflammatory, antioxidant, moisturizing
Alpha-linolenic acid (Omega-3)	Blackberry seed, cranberry seed, flax seed, hemp seed, raspberry seed	Anti-inflammatory, antioxidant, immunostimulant, moisturizing

Polyunsaturated fatty acids are the least stable and tend to go rancid more quickly than monounsaturated oils. **Rancidity** occurs when oxygen reacts at the unsaturated sites, causing a decomposition of the oil and the disagreeable odor associated with it.

FYI

Sebum, jojoba oil, and beeswax are composed of **fatty waxes.** They contain a fatty acid chain and an alcohol chain with an ester between them. An **ester** is a compound structure that is formed through the reaction of an acid with an alcohol. Nature utilizes fatty waxes to protect and coat the skin and in animal furs, feathers, and plant leaves.

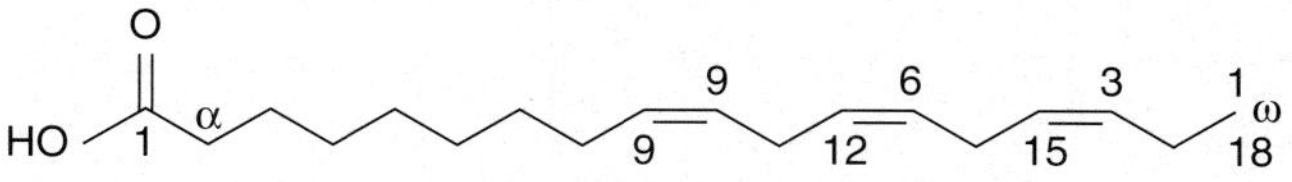

Figure 7–7 Alpha-linolenic acid.

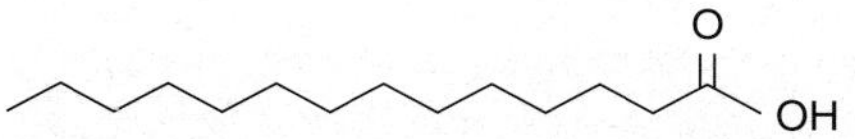

Figure 7–8A Saturated fatty acid (myristic acid).

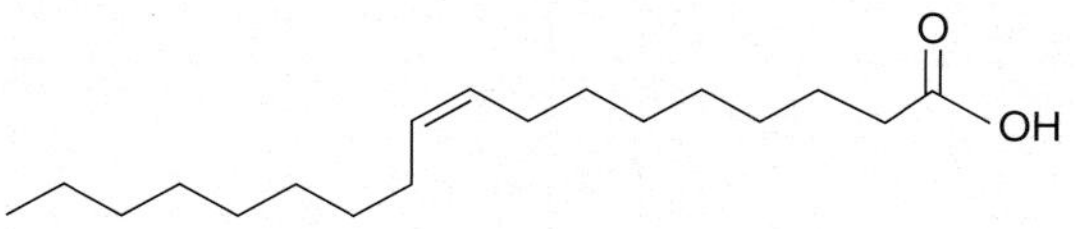

Figure 7–8B Oleic acid.

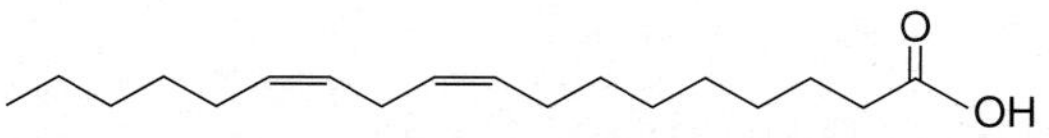

Figure 7–8C A polyunsaturated fatty acid (the omega-6 linoleic acid).

Atoms bond to other atoms to become stable, thus forming molecular structures. A hydrocarbon, composed of just carbon and hydrogen, is a very stable structure and a very good building block for life. The hydrocarbon is the skeleton structure of lipids and fatty acids. When the carbon atoms are completely filled with electrons, bonding to either a hydrogen atom or another carbon, the chain is saturated (Figure 7–8A). When a hydrocarbon is unsaturated, it means there is a missing hydrogen atom. At this site the carbon shares a second electron with a neighboring carbon, creating a double bond (Figures 7–8B and C).

You will notice at one end of all three compounds there is a carbon atom with double-bonded oxygen. This is not a double bond that defines a saturated or unsaturated fatty acid. This double bond, along with a single bond of the same carbon atom to an oxygen and hydrogen pair is a **carboxylic acid.** A carboxylic acid attached to a hydrocarbon chain is what defines, or creates, a fatty acid. The opposite side of the fatty acid is called the methyl end.

Also of interest is the naming of a polyunsaturated fatty acid based on the position of the first double bond. For example, alpha-linolenic fatty acid (Figure 7–7) is also called an Omega-3 fatty acid because the first double bond appears on the third carbon-to-carbon bond starting from the methyl end of the chain.

ESSENTIAL OIL CHEMISTRY

Essential oils, which have various uses in the work of esthetics, are composed mainly of **terpenoid compounds**, which are lipids made up of **isoprene units**—hydrocarbon chains with five carbon atoms. The terpenoid compounds are defined by the number of isoprene units in their structure (Table 7–6).

The properties associated with the essential oils are related to their chemical composition. Essential oils can be fairly simple, with just a few known active compounds, or very complex, with hundreds of compounds that combine to give an oil its overall healing potential. Understanding the chemical structure and the properties of the chemical compounds allows you to more accurately choose essential oils.

The compounds found in essential oils are categorized by a chemical family. Each family is known for specific properties that are useful in the health and balance of the body and emotions. There are numerous compounds that belong to each chemical group, and each essential oil may contain compounds from two or many more of the chemical groupings.

Table 7–6 The Prefix Identifies the Isoprene Composition of the Terpenoid Compound

PREFIX	NUMBER OF ISOPRENE UNITS (NUMBER OF CARBON ATOMS)
Mono-	2 (10 carbon atoms)
Sesqui-	3 (15 carbon atoms)
Di-	4 (20 carbon atoms)
Tri-	6 (30 carbon atoms)

Terpene Compounds

The most basic compound found in essential oils is the monoterpene hydrocarbon. The prefix *mono-* tells you this is a terpenoid compound that consists of 10 carbon atoms. The sesquiterpene hydrocarbons in essential oils are made up of 15 carbon atoms. A hydrogen atom in a hydrocarbon chain can be replaced by another atom, or group of atoms, called a **functional group**. The functional group on the terpene chain is now an area that becomes more reactive and gives a new characteristic to the terpene compound. The compounds are categorized according to the functional group that has bonded to the terpenoid hydrocarbon. As an example, when an alcohol group (Figure 7–9) attaches to a monoterpene, the compound is a monoterpene alcohol. See Table 7–7 for a list of the chemical families, their properties, and the essential oils that contain them. Keep in mind that essential oils contain other compounds that are not included under the chemical groupings.

—OH

Figure 7–9 Alcohol functional group.

Table 7–7 The Essential Oil Chemical Families

TERPENOID HYDROCARBONS
Monoterpene Hydrocarbon
These molecules are the most abundant in essential oils.
Essential oils: needle trees, such as cypress, pine, spruce; citrus oils such as grapefruit, lemon, orange; frankincense
Properties: antiviral, diuretic, stimulating, tonic
Compounds within the family: camphene, limonene, pinene.
Contraindications: possible skin irritant due to peroxidation; kidney irritant at high, prolonged dosages.
Sesquiterpene Hydrocarbon
Essential oils: German chamomile, *Helichrysum italicum* (everlasting)
Properties: anti-inflammatory, anti-allergic, cooling
Compounds within the family: chamazulene, caryophyllene
FUNCTIONAL GROUPS
Monoterpene Alcohol
These are considered the most beneficial and safest of the aromatic molecules.

Essential oils: lavender, MQV (*Melaleuca quinquenervia viridiflora*), palmarosa, peppermint, rosemary, tea tree, ylang ylang
Properties: almost zero toxicity, antimicrobial, antiseptic, energizing (except linalool, a sedative in lavender and others), immune stimulant
Compounds within the family: geraniol, linalool, menthol, terpenin-4-ol
Sesquiterpene Alcohol
Essential oils: cedarwood, ginger, patchouli, sandalwood
Properties: properties vary according to oil; overall they are similar to the monoterpene alcohols
Compounds within the family: cedrol, patchoulol, santalol
Aldehyde
Essential oils: citronella, *Eucalyptus citriodora*, lemon verbena, lemongrass, melissa
Properties: anti-inflammatory, antiseptic, antiviral, hypotensors, sedative
Compounds within the family: citral, citronellal, gernial, neral
Contraindications: can be skin irritant when used undiluted
Ester
Essential oils: bergamot, clary sage, geranium, lavender, Roman chamomile
Properties: anti-inflammatory, anti-spasmodic, balancing to central nervous system, calming, fungicidal, stress relieving
Compounds within the family: butyl angelate, geranyl acetate, linalyl acetate, neryl butyrate
Ketone
Essential oils: Eucalyptus dives, helicrysum, mugwort, peppermint, rosemary (verbenone type)
Properties: promotes tissue and cell formation, mucolytic.
Compounds within the family: camphor, damascone, dione, menthone, verbenone
Contraindications: neurotoxic, abortive
Lactone
Essential oils: inula graveolens
Properties: strong mucolytic
Contraindications: used with caution
Compounds within the family: alantolactone
Oxide
Essentail oils: eucalyptus oils (especially globulus and radiata), MQV, ravensare, tea tree
Properties: antiviral, expectorant
Compounds within the family: 1,8 Cineole (eucalyptol), rose oxide
Phenol
Essential oils: oregano, savory, thyme (thymol type)
Properties: antifungal, anti-parasitic, heart tonic, immune stimulant, strong bactericidal, warming
Compounds within the family: carvacrol, thymol
Contraindications: skin irritant; toxic to the liver with prolonged use and high dosages
PHENYLPROPANOIDS
Phenylpropane
Essential oils: Cinnamon, clove
Properties: Similar to phenols; analgesic (clove)
Compounds within the family: cinnamic aldehyde, eugenol
Contraindications: similar to phenols

Table 7–7 *continued*

PHENYLPROPANOIDS
Phenylpropane Ether
Essential oils: Anise seed, basil, fennel, tarragon
Properties: anti-spasmodic, digestive imbalance (fennel, anise), mental stimulant (basil, tarragon)
Compounds within the family: anethol, methyl chavicol
Contraindications: toxic to the nervous system at high dosages

Phenylpropanoid Compounds

Another class of compounds important to aromatherapy are the **phenylpropanoids.** These are the highly active compounds that contain the aromatic ring structure (see the FYI sidebar on this page) and include the flavonoids. The phenylpropanoids are a by-product of amino acid or fatty acid metabolism in the plant. There are two essential oil chemical families classified as phenylpropanoid compounds: One is simply called *phenylpropanoids,* or *phenylpropanes,* and the other are the *ethers,* or *phenylpropane ethers.*

Having a good foundational knowledge and understanding of the compounds and properties found in botanicals and essential oils will deeply enhance your practice as an esthetician. This knowledge will help you better understand the products, and the ingredients, you work with and will assist you in intelligently answering the questions asked by today's educated consumers. The study of botanical chemistry will help you fine tune treatments, increase your therapeutic potential and, as your proficiency grows, become aware of potential contraindications and sensitivities that may otherwise be hidden.

FYI

In chemistry, the occurrence of a benzene ring structure is pictured as a circle within a hexagonal shape (Figure 7–10). The **benzene ring structure** is responsible for some of the most antibacterial and antimicrobial compounds found in essential oils. It is a hydrocarbon containing six carbon atoms and six hydrogen atoms. It was at first believed to have three double bonds but now it is known to be more stable and does not react typically to other unsaturated hydrocarbons. The stability of this structure appears to be due to an unusual distribution of the electrons within the cyclic ring of the carbons.

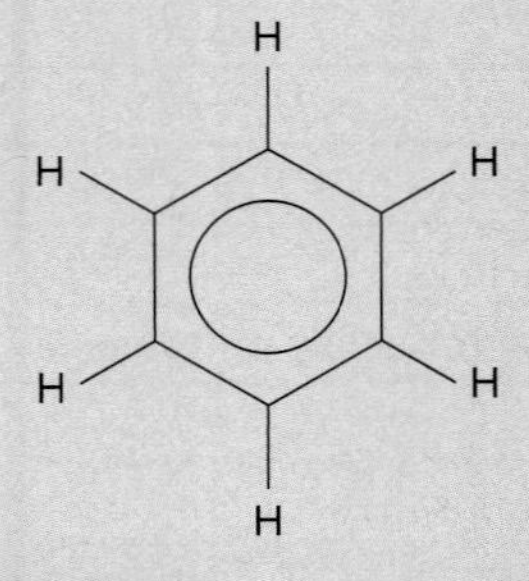

Figure 7–10 Benzene ring.

Due to the fragrant odors of compounds containing a benzene ring, early chemists referred to them as *aromatic compounds.* This name has nothing to do with aromatherapy or with other compounds found in essential oils. Members of the aromatherapy trade may refer to all essential oil compounds, inaccurately, as aromatic compounds.

The benzene ring is a structure found in the chemical family phenols and the phenylpropanoids. Most essential oil compounds containing a benzene ring are hot and irritating to the skin. The exceptions are the phenylpropane ethers, which are mild with a more soothing activity.

REVIEW QUESTIONS

1. What is an element?
2. Give examples of three elements.
3. Give some examples of the pH for various substances.
4. What is biochemistry?
5. What are polymers, proteins, and peptides and what is their impact on skin?
6. What is botanical chemistry?
7. Discuss metabolites: What are they and what is their function?
8. Discuss fatty acids and fatty waxes.
9. What is essential oil chemistry?
10. What are some of the essential oil chemical families?

CHAPTER GLOSSARY

alkaloids: secondary metabolites found in plants. They are nitrogen-containing organic compounds, such as caffeine, morphine, nicotine, and quinine, which are very physiologically active in the human body.

amino acids: organic acids that form the building blocks of proteins. There are 20 amino acids utilized within the human body. Nine of these are essential amino acids and must be supplied by the diet.

analgesic: a pain killing effect.

bases: alkaline substances; substances with a pH above 7.

benzene ring structure (aromatic ring): hydrocarbon containing 6 carbon atoms and 6 hydrogen atoms; is responsible for some of the most effective antibacterial and antimicrobial compounds found in essential oils.

biochemistry: the study of chemicals and chemical reactions in the body.

carboxylic acid: organic compounds containing the carboxyl functional group, a carbon with a double-bonded oxygen and an alcohol group attached.

carotenoids: terpenoid compounds with 40 carbon atoms (tetraterpenoids). Those that contain oxygen are called *xanthophylls*—such as lutien found in tomatoes; those without oxygen are subcategorized as *carotenes*—beta-carotene being the most popular of those. These deeply pigmented compounds have a wide range of powerful health-giving properties.

catalyst: something that triggers a change.

chemical reactions: reactions between two elements or two compounds that result in chemical changes.

co-enzymes: a vitamin or hormone that assists in an enzyme's activity, or acts as a co-factor.

disaccharide: two saccharides together; sugar made up of two simple sugars such as lactose and sucrose.

enzymes: proteins that regulate and catalyze biological reactions in living organisms; they break down complex food molecules to utilize extracted energy.

equation: a chemical reaction such that equal numbers of the same atom are on either side of the reaction.

ester: a compound structure that is formed through the reaction of an acid with an alcohol.

fatty acids: lubricant ingredients derived from plant oils or animal fats. Fatty acids are defined by a carboxylic acid group attached to a hydrocarbon chain (an organic aliphatic compound). They are vital factors in the function of the nervous, cardiovascular, immune, and other body systems and hold

CHAPTER GLOSSARY

important roles in the health and protection of the skin. Fatty acids are used as emollients, both as functional spreading agents and texture softeners for creams.

fatty waxes: a fatty acid chain and an alcohol chain with an ester between them.

flavonoids: active phenylpropanoid compounds with extremely beneficial properties for maintaining health and reversing disease. Foods rich in flavonoids are citrus fruits, grape skins, and tea.

functional group: an atom or group of atoms that bond to a reactive area of an organic compound, giving the compound its overall characteristics.

isoprene units: hydrocarbon chains with 5 carbon atoms.

metabolism: 1.) chemical process taking place in living organisms whereby the cells are nourished and carry out their activities. 2.) the process of changing food into forms the body can use as energy. Metabolism consists of two parts: Anabolism and Catabolism.

metabolites: the products used by living organisms in the process of metabolism.

monosaccharide: a family of saccharides (carbohydrates) made of a single sugar unit that cannot be converted into smaller saccharide molecules.

monounsaturated fatty acids: unsaturated fatty acids that contain one double bond in the carbon chain.

organic compound: compounds that contain the element carbon.

peptide bond: the primary linkage between all proteins. It occurs when the carboxyl molecule of one peptide reacts with the amino group of another peptide.

periodic table: chart of all the chemical elements.

phenylpropanoids: physiologically active organic compounds containing an aromatic ring and a 3-carbon chain.

polysaccharides: carbohydrates that contain three or more simple carbohydrate molecules.

polyunsaturated fatty acids: unsaturated fatty acids that contain two or more double bonds.

primary metabolites: the metabolites required for the growth, structure and reproduction of a plant.

protein: (Gr. from *proteios*, "primary") chains of amino acid molecules used in cell functions and body growth; a macromolecule of carbon, hydrogen, oxygen, and nitrogen, and at times, sulfer and phosphorus.

rancidity: condition that is the result of an oxygen reaction at the unsaturated site of a fatty acid, causing a decomposition of the oil and the disagreeable odor associated with it.

saccharide: any of a various group of organic compounds that contain carbon, hydrogen, and oxygen and includes cellulose, gums, sugars, and starches; also referred to as *carbohydrates*.

saturated fatty acids: fatty acids that contain no double bonds.

secondary metabolites: metabolites that are not required for the most basic, life sustaining needs. Most secondary metabolites have to do with protection and reproduction.

terpenoid compounds: lipids made up of multiples of isoprene units.

unsaturated fatty acids: fatty acids that contain at least one double bond.

CHAPTER OUTLINE

- THE HISTORY OF LIGHT AND ENERGY DEVICES
- PHYSICS
- SAFETY GOVERNMENTAL AGENCIES
- SAFETY
- LASER THERAPY
- INTENSE PULSED LIGHT
- RADIOFREQUENCY DEVICES
- LIGHT-EMITTING DIODES (LED DEVICES) AND LOW-LEVEL LIGHT THERAPY

CHAPTER 8

LASER, LIGHT ENERGY, AND RADIO-FREQUENCY THERAPY

LEARNING OBJECTIVES

After completing this chapter you should be able to:

- Describe how laser light is created.
- List three regulatory agencies that govern laser and light therapy usage.
- Review the role of the Laser Safety Officer.
- Identify common lasers used in the cosmetic field.
- Identify common lasers/light therapies for facial rejuvenation.
- List the required safety control measures when using a laser system.
- Discuss common uses of LEDs.

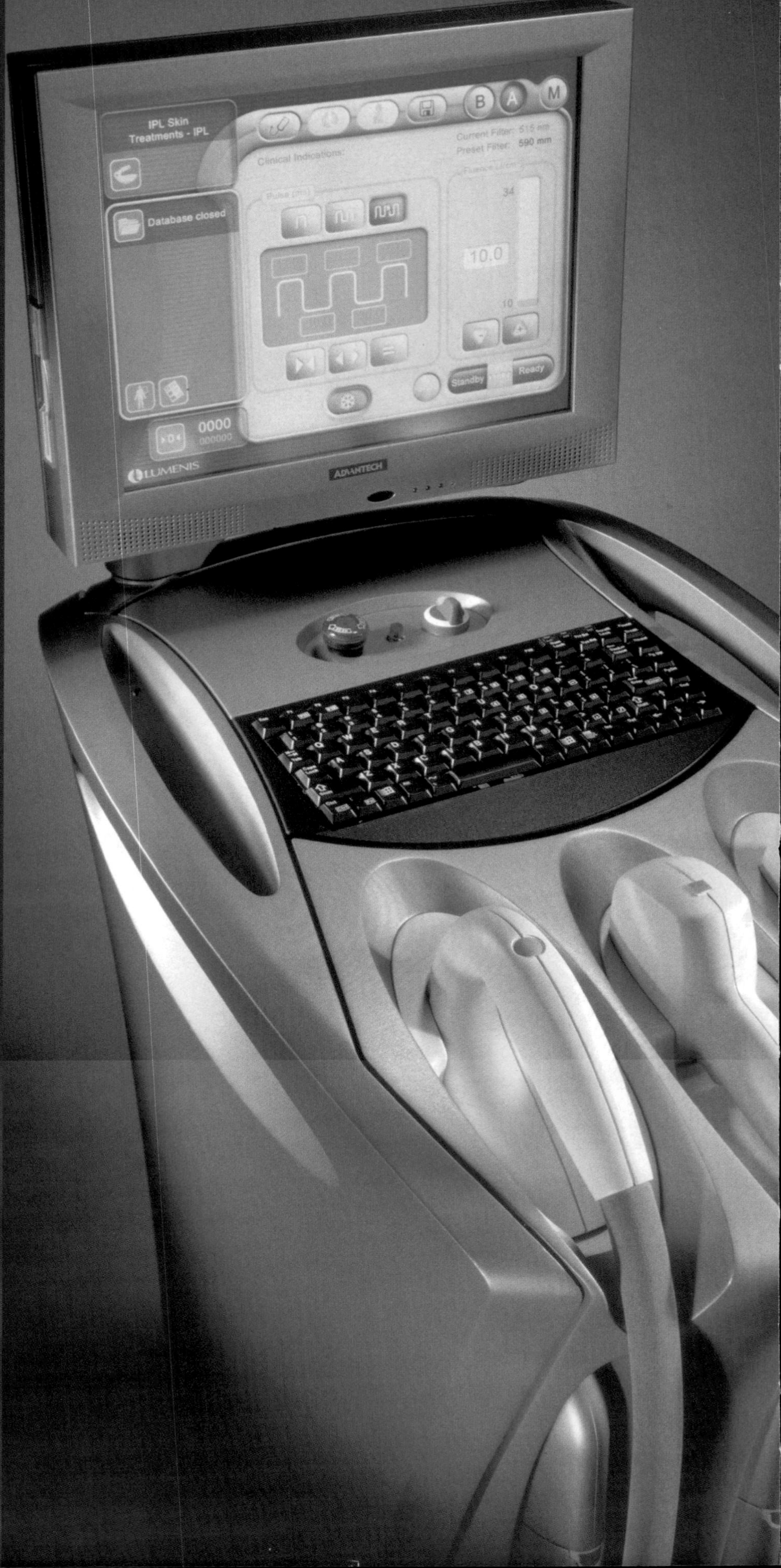

KEY TERMS

Page numbers indicate where in the chapter the term is used.

ablation 158
ablative 172
absorption 161
attenuation 167
bipolar radiofrequency (RF) energy 178
chromophore 161
coherent light 160
cryogen 163
cytochromes 180
dispersing electrode 178
electromagnetic spectrum (EM) 159
fluence 162
impedance 178
infrared 159
intense pulsed light (IPL) 176
irradiance 163
joules 163
laser-generated air contaminates (LGAC) 168
laser safety officer (LSO) 165
light-emitting diode (LED) 180
lipolysis 175
maximum permissible exposure (MPE) 165
micrometer 159
micro thermal zone (MTZ) 173
microwave amplification by stimulation emission of radiation (MASER) 158
modulate 180
monochromatic 160
monopolar radiofrequency (RF) energy 178
nanometer 159
Nevus of Ota 175
nominal hazard zone (NHZ) 166
optical density (OD) 167
optical resonator cavity 162
oxyhemoglobin 161
photomodulation 180
photons 159
power density 163
pulse duration 162
pulse width 163
radiant energy 163
scatter 162
selective photothermolysis 162
spot sizes 160
thermal relaxation time (TRT) 162
ultraviolet 159

The use of lasers, energy, and light sources is intensifying in the field of esthetic procedures. This is an advanced specialty, so a comprehensive understanding of the technology, client safety, national and state regulations, and user techniques is paramount. Your knowledge of the skin, coupled with your skill to provide the appropriate treatment parameters, will allow you to become a highly trained professional and produce predictable outcomes for a client. Whether you practice in a small medi-spa or you wish to work in a large medical/cosmetic clinic, this theoretical knowledge is essential.

> **Did You Know**
>
> The NCEA (National Coalition of Estheticians, Manufacturer/Distributors and Associations) guideline for the 1,200-hour esthetics programs includes *theoretical* training in light and energy devices. With more technicians completing school and finding employment in medical settings, this knowledge becomes more and more important. Due to state regulations, the variation between devices, and insurance issues, all estheticians should find hands-on training with the specific device with which they will work.

THE HISTORY OF LIGHT AND ENERGY DEVICES

The creation of medical light sources began with Albert Einstein in 1916. Einstein was able to understand the concept of how sunlight was emitted and, theoretically, how humans could create and harness a brilliant form of light energy. However, it was not until 1958 that Arthur Schawlow and Charles Townes were able to translate Einstein's mathematical equation into the creation of a **MASER (Microwave Amplification by Stimulation Emission of Radiation)** at Bell Laboratories. This first type of man-made light was microwave-driven but never proved to be very popular. In 1960 the first visible LASER (which stands for light amplification by stimulation emission of radiation) was created by Theodore Maiman of the Hughes Research Laboratories from a ruby crystal (Figure 8–1). This pure form of light was used initially in dermatology and ophthalmology and ignited the technological explosion still happening today. There are more than 150 different types of laser light and energy devices sold in today's cosmetic market.

> **Did You Know**
>
> Laser is an acronym which means Light Amplification by the Stimulated Emission of Radiation, now commonly written as *laser*.

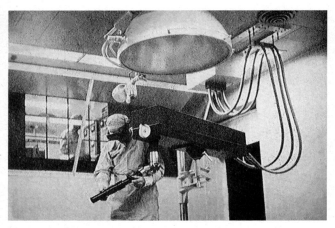

Figure 8–1 Early laser.

PHYSICS

Most lasers and light sources are devices that, when applied appropriately, will produce positive results for a client's skin. But how is this light created? What are the tissue effects? What differentiates one type of laser from another? What are the advantages of these light devices compared to conventional equipment? These are questions that are frequently asked at the outset of a study of laser and light technology. Before commencing this study, it is critical to review a key term: **ablation,** the vaporization, cutting, or removal of a portion (or all) of the epidermis and or dermis. In general, neither estheticians nor nurses are allowed to ablate tissue.

Electromagnetic Spectrum of Radiation

Laser light is really a sophisticated method of converting a flashlight into a high-powered medical device. Sunlight is a beam or a ray of light that is made up of a variety of invisible and visible forms of energy. There are different types of

> **REGULATORY AGENCY ALERT**
>
> Presently, most states do not allow nurses and estheticians to ablate tissue.

> **Did You Know**
>
> The term *radiation* refers to all visible, invisible, infrared, and ultraviolet forms of energy. Only long-term exposure to ultraviolet wavelengths can be considered to be potentially hazardous to living tissue.

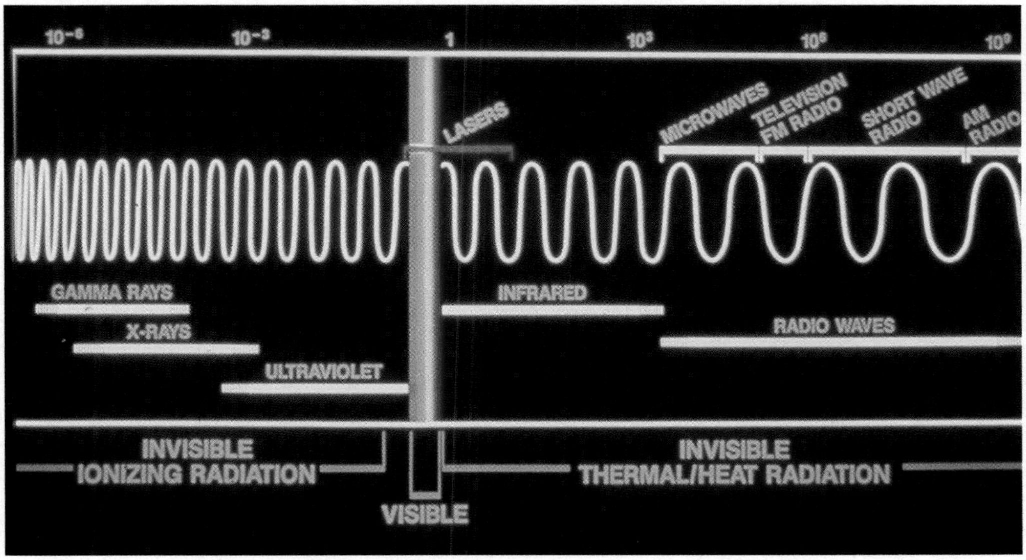

Figure 8–2 Electromagnetic spectrum of radiation.

energy: visible light, invisible **infrared** light, and invisible **ultraviolet** light. They make up the **electromagnetic spectrum (EM)** of radiation (Figure 8–2).

These forms of light are composed of small particles of energy called **photons.** Photons travel at the speed of light in a form of a wave. Each type of light, whether it is visible or invisible, generates a different type of waveform. A wavelength is measured from the distance of the top of one wave (amplitude) to the next (Figure 8–3). The wavelength distances can be measured in a **nanometer,** a billionth of a meter (nm), or a **micrometer,** a millionth of a meter (µm).

Laser light can be visible, as seen with the particular color properties of the rainbow's spectrum of light (Figure 8–4). Clients may ask if exposure to laser light will be harmful or potentially cause a type of cancer. You can assure the client that the visible spectrum of cosmetic lasers have presently not been shown to have the capablility to cause any long-term mutagenic effects. Short-term side effects will result only from using the device on an inappropriate client, such as one with epilepsy, or from using it in a manner that could cause skin trauma. Indications and contraindications will be discussed relative to specific device types.

Near infrared to far infrared lasers ranging from 800 nm to 10,600 nm are invisible to the eye but are still safe and very therapeutic, like the visible lasers, in the cosmetic industry. However, ultraviolet radiation can have enough energy per photon over time, to potentially cause a harmful response. These types of energy are not commonly used in an esthetic clinic and are most likely seen in the forms of X-ray and nuclear ultraviolet radiation. Therefore, you can work around lasers during your entire

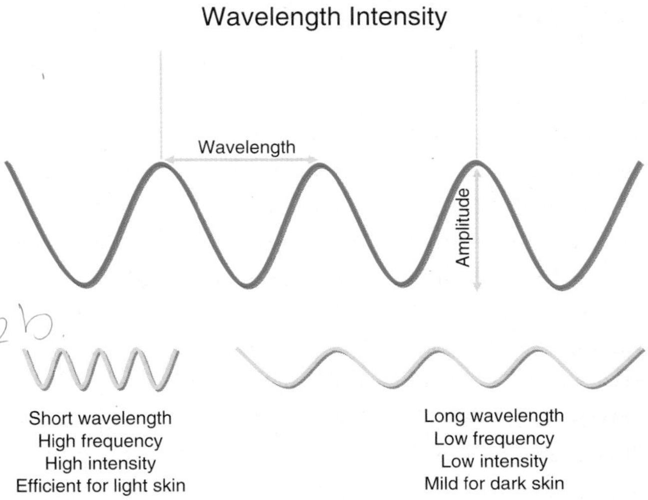

Figure 8–3 A waveform.

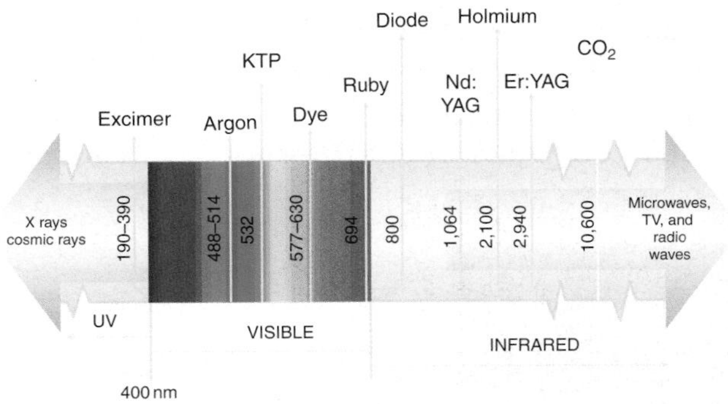

Figure 8–4 Common lasers seen throughout the visible and invisible spectrum.

> **? Did You Know**
>
> Wavelengths are described in nanometers (nm). The wavelength of most cosmetic lasers is on a spectrum, ranging from 400 to 10,600 nm. In most cases, the longer the wavelength, the deeper it will penetrate. The wavelength is specific to the type of light source used. For example, a diode laser (hair removal lasers that use diode semi-conductor technology) has a wavelength of 800 nm, whereas an Nd: YAG laser (a vascular and hair removal laser that uses a YAG crystal doped with neodymium electrons) has a wavelength of 1,064 nm.

career and successfully treat your clients without any fears from the wavelength's effects.

Properties of Laser Light

Lasers have unique properties that are not seen in any other type of energy form, which allow them to be harnessed for esthetic treatments. Normal white light is made up of a multitude of visible and invisible infrared wavelengths of light. Once formed together, they make up white light that is diffuse in nature and can quickly disperse in space within a very short distance.

Coherent Light

The photons from normal white light seen from a flashlight or lightbulb can quickly disperse in all different directions. Laser light is coherent. **Coherent light** is light energy that is "in phase." This means that all of the light waves are traveling in the same direction and in unison with each other, much as a military division on parade travels in perfect precision (Figure 8–5). Photons traveling in such a way work as a single unit of energy. Therefore, they can be focused with a focusing lens to produce a variety of different **spot sizes** and tissue effects. The degree of precision and the ability to manipulate the light make lasers almost impossible to replicate.

Laser photons are in phase in both time and space and act together as single units of energy.

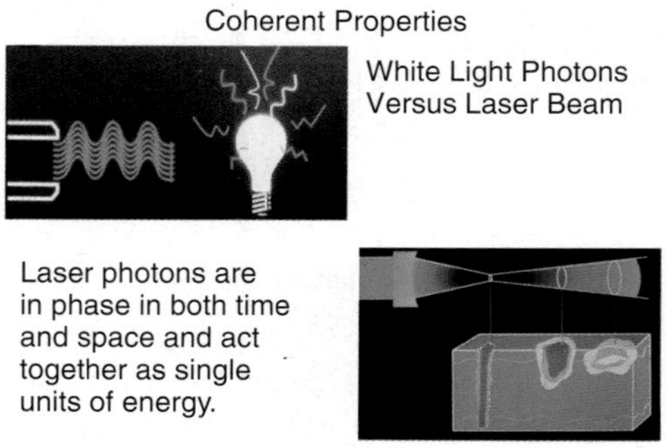
Coherent Properties
White Light Photons
Versus Laser Beam
Laser photons are
in phase in both time
and space and act
together as single
units of energy.

Figure 8–5 Coherent light.

Monochromatic Light

Normal light contains all of the visible colors of light and is white in appearance. When shown through a prism or water droplet, one actually sees the full spectrum of light in a "rainbow." Laser light differs as it is **monochromatic** and made up solely of one wavelength and one color, whether visible or not. This light's color is important because the color determines the type of chromophore in the body tissue with which the light will react. Each different color of light acts differently when exposed to tissue and creates a unique clinical effect.

Collimated Light

The photons from a flashlight or lightbulb are composed of multiwavelengths in the visible and invisible spectrum of light (Figure 8–6). They can travel only short distances before the energy diffuses and disappears. However, laser photons are parallel to each other and can travel very long distances before terminating. Because of this unique property, laser light is used diversely throughout the aerospace, military, engineering, entertainment, and medical fields. Conversely, the laser light that exits from a device's handpiece can fire across a room or even a clinic, which is why safety protection controls need to be in place.

Tissue Effects

During a laser treatment, the amazing properties of laser light can cause four different tissue effects to skin (Figure 8–7).

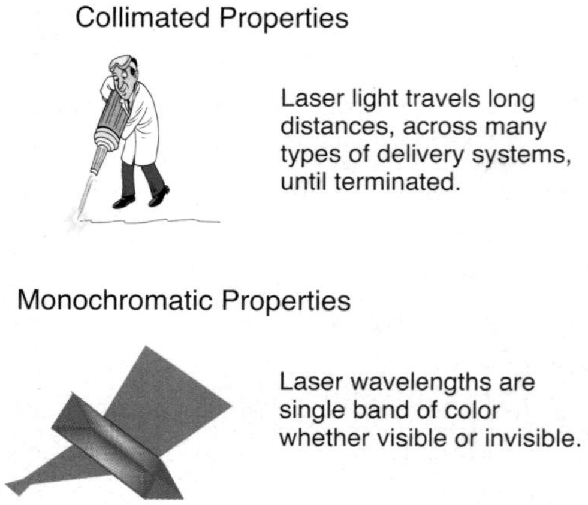
Collimated Properties
Laser light travels long
distances, across many
types of delivery systems,
until terminated.
Monochromatic Properties
Laser wavelengths are
single band of color
whether visible or invisible.

Figure 8–6 Collimated light.

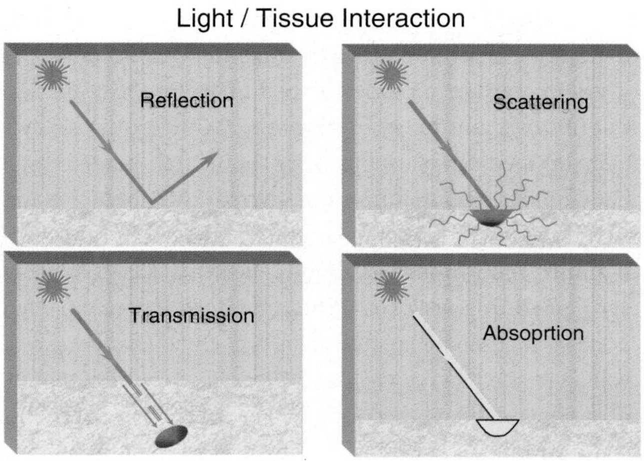

Figure 8–7 The four properties of lasers.

Absorption

If there were no absorption of light by a tissue, there would be no reaction. When a specific wavelength of light comes in contact with tissue, the photon of light loses its heat energy to the target, or **chromophore**; this is called **absorption.** More specifically, a chromophore is the target in the epidermis or dermis that absorbs the laser beam's thermal energy, causing the desired injury or destruction of the material. Common chromophores in the body are water, blood, collagen, protein, and pigment. All lasers react to different chromophores, depending on the wavelength. A substance may be a chromophore to one wavelength and not to another. This is what allows laser light to be target-specific. There are so many different laser systems, each with a different purpose. When selecting a laser system, work closely with your supervising physician to select an effective device that targets the correct chromophore.

FYI

Different cosmetic lasers are absorbed by different chromophores:

- Hair removal lasers are absorbed by dark pigment or melanin.
- Vascular lasers seek out blood or **oxyhemoglobin** as their chromophore.
- Lasers that produce new collagen and rejuvenation tend to be water or collagen absorbers.
- Lasers used for clearance of pigmented lesions or lentigos target melanin in the epidermis and dermis.
- Tattoo lasers target specific dyes or tattoo pigment.

The absorption spectrum of light illustrated how hemoglobin, melanin, and water are absorbed at different wavelengths of light (Figure 8–8).

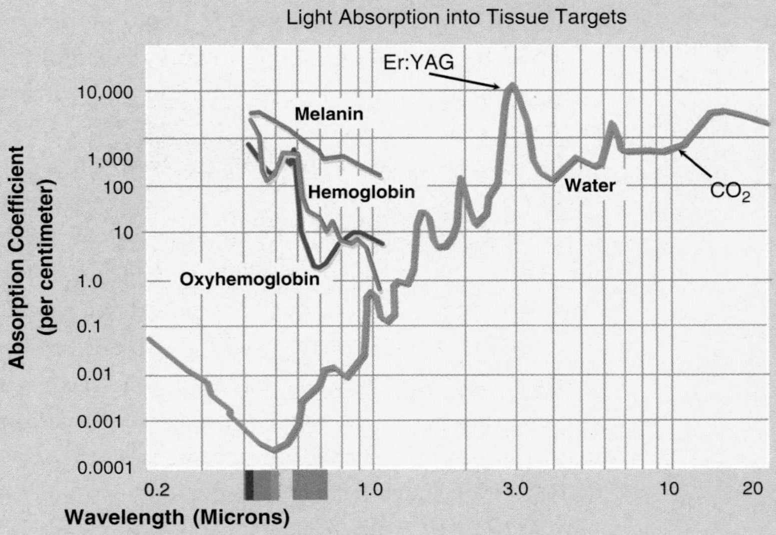

Figure 8–8 Absorption curve.

Reflection

A laser beam can also reflect off a shiny surface, such as a mirror, jewelry, or instrumentation. The flatter or smoother the surface, the greater the potential safety hazard for you and your client. Once reflected, the thermal properties of the laser light could possibly cause a surface skin burn, a fire, or even eye damage.

Transmission

Some laser light can also be transmitted through tissue, fluid, and even glass. Visible light lasers and some in the near infrared zones can easily pass through the epidermis and dermis until the light finds its targeted chromophore. Lasers that are absorbed by water, however, do not possess these characteristics and their effects are more superficial.

Scatter

With some visible and invisible wavelengths, like the Nd:YAG (1,064 nm), there is deep forward and backward **scatter**, or diffusion, of the light. The deeper the light is able to transmit through the skin, the more scatter that is possible. Laser energies can therefore cause thermal destruction at greater depths but also backscatter toward the client's and operator's eyes. For this reason, it is mandatory to place eye protection on the client undergoing laser treatment. It is also important to remember that ocular injuries are the most common reported hazard for those working with laser devices. To avoid injuries, be aware of all potential hazards of a particular device and the control measures need to be in place.

Creation of Laser Light

The secret to the creation of laser light lies within a machine's general design, computer software, cooling system, and optics. Within every laser device, there is a laser tube or **optical resonator cavity** (Figure 8–9). The optical resonator contains some type of medium which is responsible for the creation of light—usually a gas, solid, or liquid. For example, a gas medium can be made up of argon, carbon dioxide, or helium-neon gas particles. A liquid medium refers to tubes of organic liquid or dye. A crystal medium is usually a synthetic man-made crystal made up of yttrium aluminum garnet (YAG) particles and then doped with certain elements such as holmium, neodymium, and thulium or erbium electrons. Lasers are usually named in reference to their medium. There are even diode lasers that are created electronically by a diode array display in the head of the laser. Diode lasers tend to be the most dependable and economical and have longevity due to the simplicity and stability of the components.

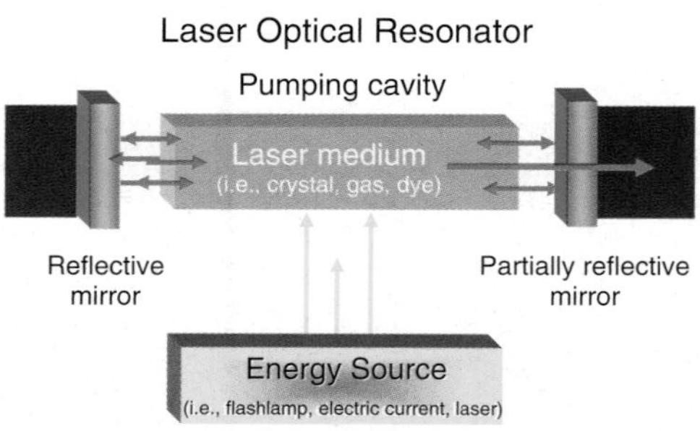

Figure 8–9 The optical resonator.

Turning on a laser machine creates either high-voltage electricity or stimulates an intense light source from a flashlamp within the machine. The electrons in the laser medium become stimulated by this energy and spontaneously create identical photons as they collide into mirrors placed on opposite ends of the laser tube. As a result, all of the photons travel at the same frequency, parallel to each other and in phase in a collimated, coherent, and monochromatic beam of light.

Selective Photothermolysis

Modern lasers used in today's esthetics operate on the theory of selective photothermolysis. **Selective photothermolysis** is a theory created by Drs. Rox Anderson and J. A. Parrish in the 1980s to describe the selective absorption of a specific light by a targeted chromophore. This light, or photo, delivers "thermal" energy that is engineered to cause selective destruction, or lysis, of the designated target. Selective photothermolysis is achieved by selecting an appropriate wavelength at the right exposure time and pulse duration and with sufficient energy or **fluence.**

To achieve selective photothermolysis, an operator needs to be aware of the **thermal relaxation time (TRT)** of the target. TRT is the amount of time necessary for a chromophore, blood vessel, or hair follicle to lose over 50% of its heat, produced by the targeted laser system. By limiting the exposure of the laser light to a time shorter than the TRT, the energy is contained in the selected target and does not produce collateral damage to the surrounding tissue. Thermal relaxation time varies on the size and density of the target. A coarse 200-micron hair follicle may have the TRT of 40 ms while a large .4 mm vessel's TRT is 80 ms. Therefore, the larger the target, the longer the TRT, and subsequently requiring a longer **pulse duration** (or

FYI

If the target is sufficiently heated with a pulse duration shorter than the thermal relaxation time of the tissue, little damage will result in the adjacent tissue. However, if a pulse duration is longer than the thermal relaxation time, significant amounts of heat will be conducted to adjacent tissue with risk of damage.

FYI

Used in pulsed lasers, energy fluence is measured in joules per square centimeter (j/cm^2). The pulse should also be longer than the thermal relaxation time of the epidermal tissue but shorter than the thermal relaxation time of the target.

pulse width). The longer pulse width is needed for the larger object to slowly absorb the heat and then slowly cool down through diffusion. The opposite is also true: Small objects with short TRT need shorter pulse durations in order to destroy the object while sparing the epidermis. This theory is essential in producing the desired therapeutic response without causing excessive surrounding epidermal heating and undesirable side effects of blistering, hyper- or hypopigmentation or scarring.

Cooling the Skin

Skin cooling is a necessary and integral part of laser therapy used for photothermal reactions (Figure 8–10). Selectively cooling the skin allows for a higher and more effective fluence while sparing the epidermis. There are different modes of cooling the skin during treatment. They are engineered for either pre-cooling, parallel cooling, or post-cooling. Among the different types of cooling are **cryogen** *spray,* which can be used before and after each laser pulse; *forced air cooling* with high-flow, subzero air to the treatment area; *chilled gel* applied to the skin for pre-cooling; *contact parallel cooling,* which circulates cold water through a window on the laser head; and a *chilled tip* which uses a cold sapphire window on the handpiece to cool the epidermis throughout each laser pulse. The cooling not only helps prevent epidermal tissue damage; it reduces the discomfort of the treatment. Lowering the skin temperature allows safe application of more energy to the target without excessive trauma to the epidermis.

FOCUS ON: *Laser Terms*

- **Power density is the rate of energy being delivered and termed irradiance. A unit of power is referred to as a watt. This measurement is usually seen with continuous wave lasers and expressed in watts/cm^2. The size of the area where the laser is concentrated makes a great difference on the impact of the power delivered. The more concentrated the light, the greater its impact. The smaller the laser's beam size, the more power per unit area and the higher the irradiance.**
- ***Fluence* refers to the energy of the pulsed laser beam or radiant energy—it is expressed in joules /cm^2 (j/cm^2) and refers to the energy x time. Fluence can be increased by increasing the energy output of the laser, by decreasing the pulse duration, or by decreasing the diameter of the beam.**
- ***Pulse duration* (or *pulse width*), which is measured in nanoseconds (ns) or milliseconds (ms), is the timing of light energy, or how long the laser is actually on the skin and determines the clinical effect of the light energy. The light energy must be maintained long enough to destroy the target but not so long as to burn the skin.**
- ***Spot size,* usually measured in millimeters, is the size or width of the beam affecting treatment. The larger the laser beam's spot size, the less fluence is affecting the tissue. By decreasing the spot size in half, one increases the energy or fluence x 4. Technicians must exercise extreme care and understand this to avoid using too much energy and creating burns.**

? Did You Know

Cooling the epidermis allows for a higher fluence and a better result possible. However, if you cool the skin too much, you can interfere with the thermal relaxation time of the skin.

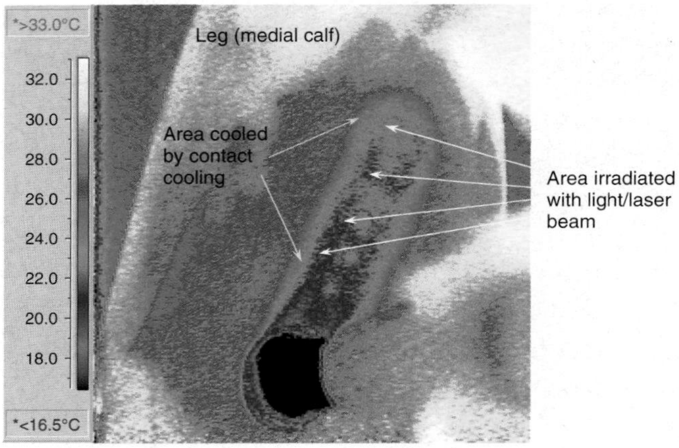

Figure 8–10 Laser with cooling device.

SAFETY GOVERNMENTAL AGENCIES

Traditionally, lasers have been used only in a hospital setting. Today, lasers and other types of light and energy are being utilized in a multitude of settings, ranging from clinics, medi-spas, shopping malls, and mobile laser services. As laser devices and other types of energy/light sources have become increasingly available to consumers, there has also been an increase of reported injuries and even deaths. These tragic incidences can be attributed to a lack of training and supervision. Before being mesmerized by the excitement of working with these cosmetic devices, you need to gain an in-depth understanding of potential hazards, national and state standards, and state licensure. There are a number of agencies that regulate the standards of practice in the use of lasers and light/energy devices, including the FDA, OSHA, and state agencies.

U.S. Food and Drug Administration (FDA)

The U.S. Food and Drug Administration, or FDA, is a government agency that has specific authority to regulate the design, testing, manufacturing, and distribution of medical devices. The FDA classifies equipment as to its potential degree of hazard and specifies the level of training needed to operate each device. Many light and energy devices that are used by estheticians have a Class I medical device labeling and are under an esthetician's scope of practice. Class I esthetic devices include esthetic use ultrasonic and microdermabrasion machines. However, most lasers, Intense Pulsed Light (IPL) devices, and some radiofrequency devices are Class II medical devices requiring extensive education and training for safe operation. There is confusion as to whom these devices may be sold to. A Class II medical device may be listed by the FDA as prescriptive and to be used by medical professionals only. Very similar devices may be listed as prescriptive or non-prescriptive, in large part dependent on the manufacturer's intended use statement. Therefore, based on state regulations, estheticians' use of many of these devices may be regulated or may be subject to supervision by a licensed medical practitioner. FDA Class III medical devices are very restricted and are for medical practitioner use only. Class III devices usually support or sustain human life, and are of substantial importance in preventing illness and health disdorders.

> **REGULATORY ALERT**
>
> Some states are using the manufacturer's intended use statement for determining scope of practice and use by estheticians. I.e., is the device intended for services that are within the scope of practice of an esthetician?

American National Standard Institute

The American National Standard Institute (ANSI) is a nonregulatory, nonprofit, professional organization that has established more than 100,000 national safety standards. The organization attempts to base its standards of practice on those of the International Electrotechnical Commission (IEC). This committee establishes international regulations for a variety of products including laser related technologies. The Z136.3 2005 edition of ANSI standards is a document that pertains specifically to safe laser use in a variety of clinical practices, including hospitals, clinics, offices, spas, and mobile laser services (Figure 8–11). Even though this document is not regulatory, it is viewed as a legal document and the benchmark for all practices in the medical/cosmetic field. Other types of light sources, including intense pulsed light (IPL) devices, are not presently included in this document. However, future revisions will most likely include these forms of cosmetic technology. All estheticians need to be aware of the ANSI Z136.3 document, as courts often use it to evaluate safe levels of practice in cases of malpractice.

The ANSI document describes, on an administrative, engineering, and procedural level, which policies and procedures must be in place to establish a safe laser program. Sometimes it is the esthetician's role to conduct

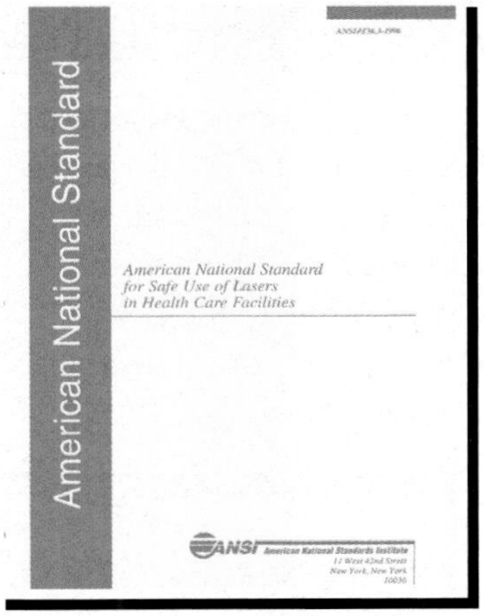

Figure 8–11 The ANSI standards.

FYI

The ANSI Z136.3 document contains:

- Scope
- Definitions
- Hazard evaluation and classification
- Control measures
- Laser Safety Program
- Non-beam hazards
- Exposure criteria for the eyes and skin
- Measurements
- Appendices

FYI

The role of the Laser Safety Officer includes:

- Hazard classification of all laser systems
- Hazard evaluation of the degree of hazard to eyes, skin, and respiratory tract
- Hazard response in emergency situations
- Control measures to reduce the risk of injury
- Procedural and policy controls
- Approving protective laser equipment for staff and clients
- Approving all laser signs and labels
- Overseeing facilities and servicing of the laser equipment
- Training of staff
- Medical surveillance of possibly injured staff or client

a risk assessment of potential laser hazards, draft safety policies, and become the **Laser Safety Officer (LSO)** of the facility. The LSO has advanced training and knowledge of the facility's laser equipment and potential hazards, and it is this person who monitors and enforces all safety policies and procedures.

Occupational Safety and Health Administration (OSHA)

OSHA is an agency of the U.S. Department of Labor that oversees the safety of employees in the workplace. OSHA investigators are aware of ANSI guidelines and expect all facilities and medi-spas to comply with ANSI Z136.3. An employer who is found to be negligent can be cited under the General Duty Clause 29CRF1910. Both the employer and employee share equal responsibility in providing a safe environment for the client. If a facility is found to be negligent, then both employer and employee may face heavy fines or other penalties, including the revocation of a professional and/or business license.

State Licensure and Regulations

Nationally and internationally, there is a diversity of practitioners performing cosmetic procedures, including nurses, technicians, electrologists, estheticians, and nonmedical personnel. Each state differs regarding the requirements for training, levels of practice, on-site or off-site physician supervision, and esthetician responsibility. As an esthetician, you need to check with your licensing board before performing any laser or light/energy treatment. In addition, you should obtain individual malpractice insurance, making sure your carrier knows your level of practice so it can protect you. If you are not honest with your insurance carrier about your use of laser devices, you may not be legally protected in the event of an accident or injury.

SAFETY

As described in the ANSI Z136.3 2005 document, there are different levels of safety controls that need to be established and enforced at one's facility. Based on the ANSI standards, lasers are classified as to the degree of skin and eye hazards. This system is different than the FDA classifications of medical devices. ANSI classification is based on the **Maximum Permissible Exposure (MPE)** one might receive from an accidental exposure to

OPTICAL GAIN OF THE EYE

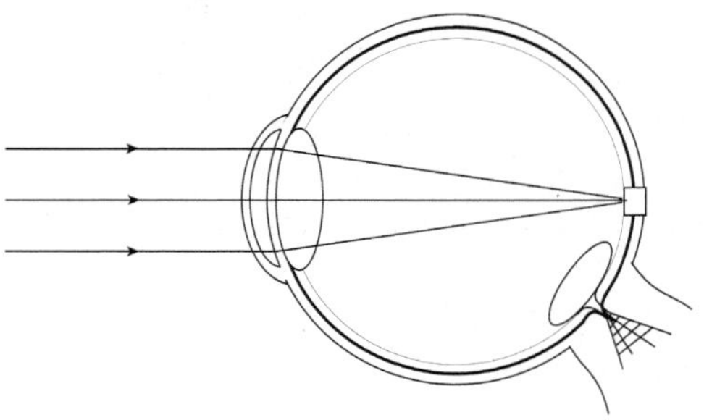

- Wavelengths that focus on retina (400 to 1400 nm), optical gain is 100,000 times
- Irradiance entering is 1 mW/cm^2, at retina will be 100 W/cm^2

Figure 8–12 Laser light coming in contact with skin/eye.

the eye or skin (Figure 8–12). In order to assess the degree of potential hazard at a facility, all who work there need to be aware of the specific ANSI classification.

FYI

Know the machine you are working with and follow all safety guidelines associated with the device.

CLASS I: These devices are completely safe to view and pose no ocular or skin risk if exposure occurs. These devices are exempt from labeling requirements. Common examples include laser compact disc players or laser printers.

CLASS II: These devices are those types of lasers that do not pose any hazard under normal viewing conditions. They are low power visible lasers (400 to 700 nm) that could only cause damage if viewed directly over a 15-minute time period. Examples include laser pointers and grocery food scanners.

CLASS III: These devices are potentially hazardous if viewed directly. These lasers, which require special training to operate and suitable safety eye protection, include ophthalmic eye lasers or scanners.

CLASS IV: These are the most hazardous of all laser systems and can cause injury from a direct, scattered, or reflected laser beam to the eyes or skin. Strict controls need to be in place. Some states even require Class IV lasers be registered with the Bureau of Radiation Control. Most cosmetic laser systems are Class IV laser devices, including CO_2 and Erbium lasers.

FYI

You cannot associate wavelength with the classification of lasers. Laser classification is determined by a variety of parameters: beam diameter, shutter speed, beam divergence, energy output, and so on. All of these combine to create the intensity of the emitted beam and its potential risk to cause injury. This risk factor is what is used to establish classification.

Procedural Controls

Procedural controls are those outlined in ANSI Z136.3 to include all work practices that are enforced at a facility in order to reduce any potential risks or hazards associated with laser use. Lasers are a high-powered, collimated form of thermal energy that can be dangerous if used carelessly or inappropriately. Hazards to you, a client, and other staff members can result from direct or indirect exposure to a laser beam. The following controls are mandatory for ensuring a safe laser environment and preventing injury.

Controlled Access

ANSI describes the treatment area where a laser is used as the **nominal hazard zone (NHZ)**. It is the space in which the level of a direct, reflected, or scattered laser light exceeds the MPE for that laser. Simply stated, it is the entire procedure room where an injury to the skin or eye can occur. The LSO should consider each treatment room as the space where the following controls need to be rigidly enforced.

Policies should state that every door to the laser room needs to be closed during treatments but never locked. The appropriate signage must be hung on each door, at each access point, but only when the laser is actually being used (Figure 8–13). A pair of laser goggles with the

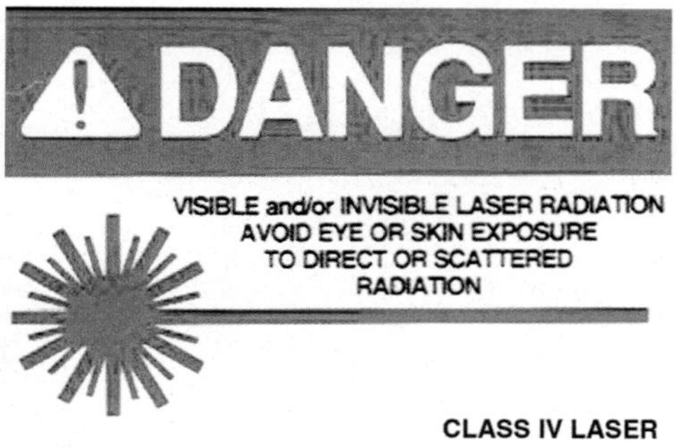

Figure 8–13 Laser sign on the treatment door.

correct wavelength and **optical density (OD)** needs to be readily available outside of the door. Optical density is the amount of **attenuation** or reduction of radiant laser energy as it passes through the filter material in the laser eyewear. When the laser treatment is completed, the operator must remove the control key and store it in a location with limited access. All windows need to be covered with occlusive, nonflammable barriers for laser systems that can transmit through water or glass for they tend to have a long NHZ (Figure 8–14). (When in doubt, contact the laser manufacturer for specifics on window barriers.)

Occular Protection

The eyes are most vulnerable to exposure to a direct, scattered, or reflected beam of light. Visible wavelengths from 400 nm to 1,400 nm and near-infrared wavelengths are the most hazardous due to their melanin or oxyhemoglobin absorption in the retina, producing a disastrous retinal burn. These lasers can be transmitted through clear liquids, eye fluids, and even windows. Permanent eye injuries and blindness are the most common accident reported in the cosmetic laser field (Figure 8–15). Conversely, lasers that are absorbed by water (CO_2 and Erbium lasers) tend to cause more superficial burns or corneal injuries during accidental exposure. Damage to the cornea can be painful, can cause clouding, or, if the injury is severe, may require a corneal transplant.

Eye protection is mandatory for everyone in the NHZ treatment room—operator or client. The client's eyes are completely protected with occlusive eyewear if a cosmetic procedure is performed on the face (Figure 8–16).

The cornea is the superficial protective covering of the eye that is the essential focusing mechanism. The lens in the eye can act as a magnifying glass and can magnify a laser's energy 100,000 times as directed to the back of the retina.

FYI

During an OSHA inspection, if an inspector finds a laser key in the machine, you can be fined $5,000 per occurence.

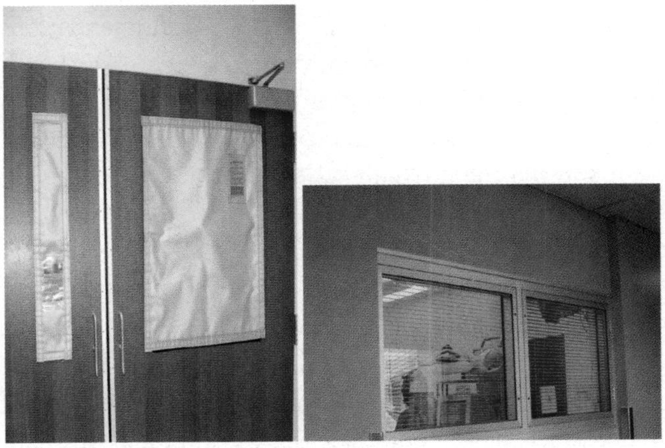

Figure 8–14 Laser window coverings.

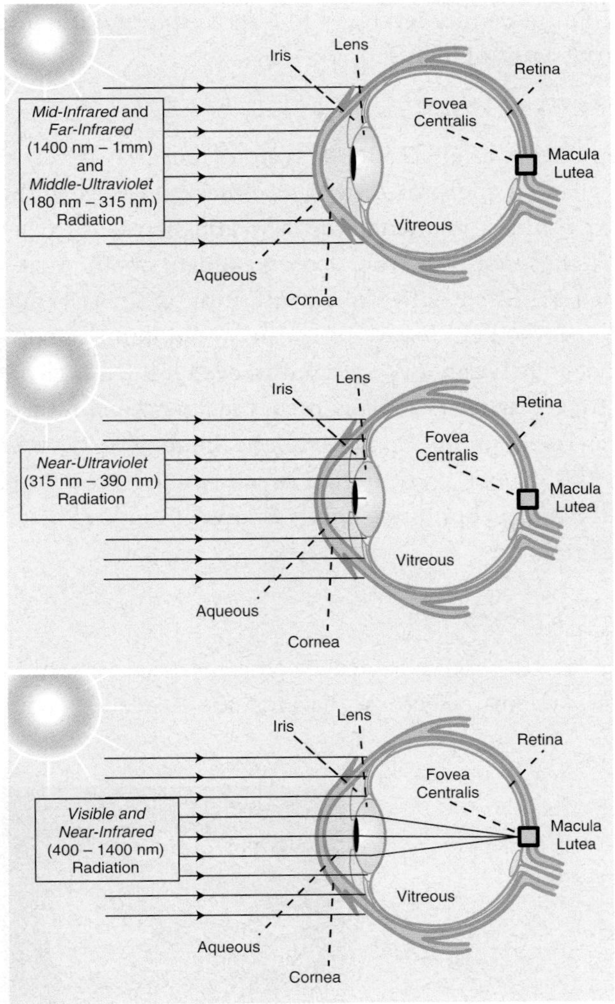

Figure 8–15 The laser light through the eye.

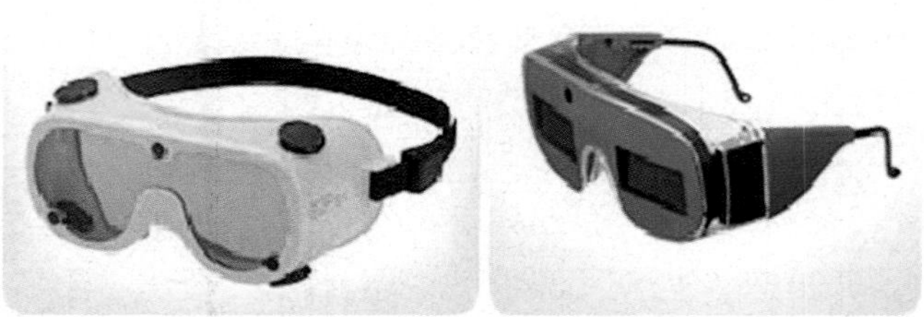

Figure 8–16 Laser goggles.

Whether disposable laser eyeshields or metal devices are used, they need to be approved by the LSO and show documentation of testing by the manufacturer (Figure 8–17). Procedures performed on the eyelids or inside the periorbital areas need the application of metal corneal shields. These should only be applied under the supervision of a physician. For below-the-neck procedures, the client should wear protective eyewear, provided by the technician—with the appropriate laser wavelength and optical density marked on the glasses or goggles. One will find most laser eyewear to possess an optical density level of 4 to 8 for visible and infrared wavelengths of light.

Controlled Laser Usage

The laser is a potentially dangerous tool that needs to be guarded and protected at all times. Never leave the laser running unattended in a treatment room. Never lock the door(s) to your laser treatment room. When you are finished with a treatment, turn off the laser and remove the key. Always place the machine on standby mode in between uses. In standby, even if the foot pedal or trigger switch is actually fired, the laser remains inactive. Furthermore, *never* place the handpiece or fiber on the client's body during breaks in the procedure. Burns and eye injuries have occurred from accidental misfiring.

Electrical Controls

Due to the high-powered electrical capacitors within laser systems, electrical hazards are a reality; both electrocutions and deaths have been reported. Follow these simple rules:

1. Do not place fluids or liquids on top of the device. These could accidentally spill into the unit.
2. Do not use a laser with frayed cords or extension cords.
3. Do not turn on a system if coolant or water is pooling underneath the laser.
4. Document, in your service records, all problems with the device and any corrective actions.

Inhalation Controls

The creation of smoke and plume generated by laser devices can be a serious respiratory hazard to staff. Publications that recognize the inhalation dangers include those by OSHA, NIOSH, the CDC (Document Number 96–128), and the ANSI standards. It has been researched and documented that certain lasers which are absorbed by water, CO_2 and erbium: YAG vaporize cells upon impact, generating smoke at the tissue site. This plume can possess the same airborne contaminants that are released with the use of electrosurgical cautery units (ESU). Laser plume is contaminated with potentially viable particles of virus, bacteria, and aerosolized blood, along with 80 types of noxious gases. In the ANSI document, laser smoke is referred to as **laser-generated air contaminates (LGAC).** Control of this occupational hazard is essential to reducing risks of lung damage and/or disease with long-term exposure. ANSI dictates that laser operators will employ the following control measures (Table 8–1).

Most hair-removal lasers and IPL systems generate odor during client treatment. What about this noxious odor—is it a hazard? Analysis has revealed released air particles resulting from the heat ablating melanin, chemical dyes, and/or drugs that may be permeated throughout the follicle. Presently, there are no national standard control measures. However, general recommendations include the use of a smoke evacuation system, use of high filtration (laser) masks, and/or frequent room ventilation to provide a safe and pleasant environment for both the staff and the client (Figure 8–19).

Fire and Explosion Controls

Lasers are intense thermal devices that can ignite flammable substances, including hair, nail polish, paper, hair spray, alcohol-based cleansing solutions, oxygen, methane gas, clothing, plastic, and cotton sponges. To prevent these hazards, the area should be cleansed of all makeup, skin preparations, and anesthetic gels prior to a treatment.

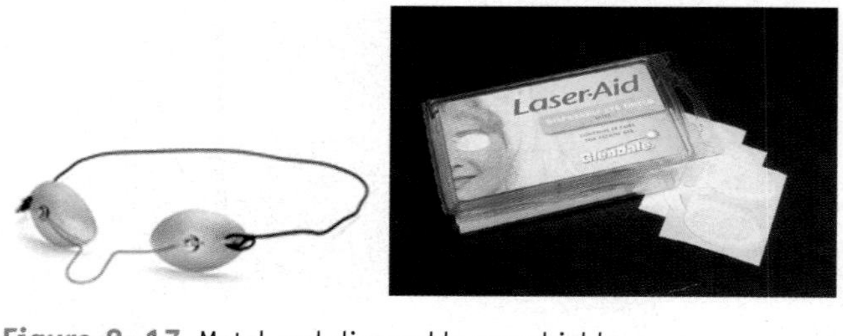

Figure 8–17 Metal and disposable eye shields.

FOCUS ON: *ANSI Control Measures*

- ***Airborne contaminants shall be controlled by the use of ventilation and respiratory protection.*** **Smoke evacuation systems should be used with ULPA (Ultra Low Particulate Air) filters, which occlude particulate matter down to a .1 micron level. The collecting hose shall be held no further away than 2 cm from the ignition source in order to capture at least 50% of the emitted plume (Figure 8–18).**
- ***High filtration masks (laser masks) can filter down to a .1 micron level but are not the first line of protection against this occupational hazard.*** **The uses of laser masks are required, however, for all smoke-producing procedures.**
- ***Filters are considered biohazard and users shall use control measures, such as standard precautions covered by the Bloodborne Pathogens Standard.*** **Gloves shall be worn when handling and disposing of potentially biohazardous tubing, collecting canisters, and filters. These disposable items need to be red-bagged with other contaminated waste and disposed of appropriately using EPA guidelines.**

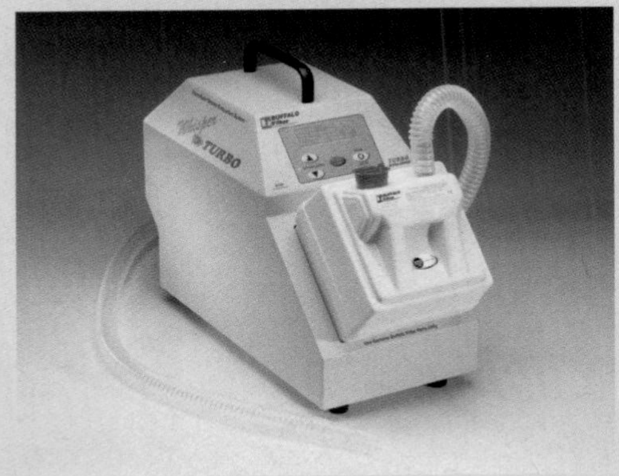

Figure 8–18 Smoke evacuator.

Also, water should be available in the procedure room to immediately suppress and contain a fire. The facility should have a fire extinguisher outside the treatment room, along with a fire evacuation plan (Figure 8–20). Also, because of the inherent reflection properties of laser light, all shiny jewelry, body piercings, mirrors, and instrumentation needs to be removed from the client and the surrounding area. Never treat a client using free flowing oxygen via a nasal cannula or mask. Nothing should be in the beam path between the end of the laser fiber/handpiece and the client's area of treatment.

.1micronFiltration Masks

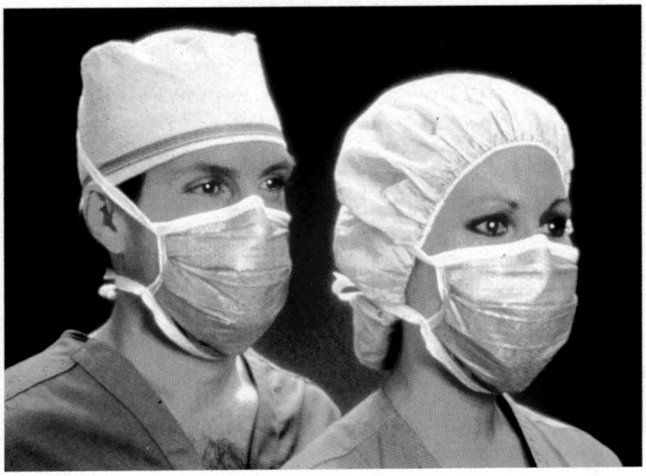

Figure 8–19 Laser filtration mask.

Engineering Controls

Engineering controls refer to safety features on each laser device that are required by the FDA's Center for Devices and Radiological Health (CDRH). Safety requirements include appropriate labeling of the device classification, safety interlocks, beam housing, and a guarded footswitch to prevent accidental exposure to a laser beam. Other features include a key lock or password to turn on the laser, audible and visible laser emission indicators, and an emergency stop button to turn off the machine in case of

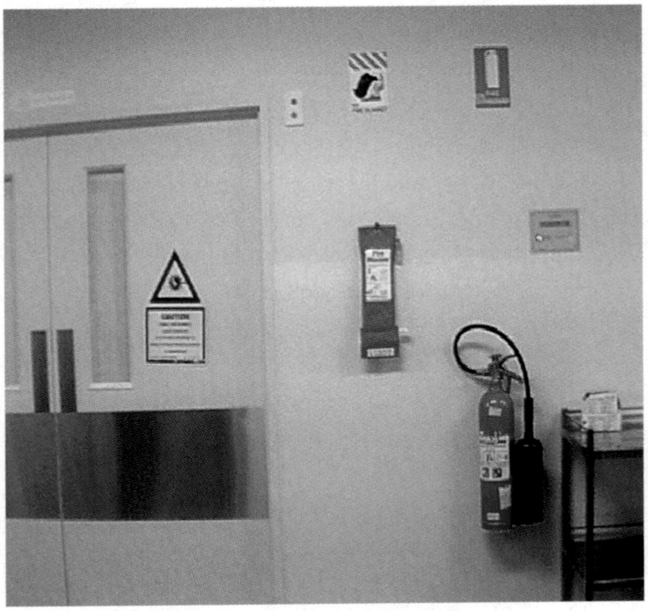

Figure 8–20 Fire extinguisher outside the laser room.

malfunction. These engineering controls provide safety and should never be removed, altered, or tampered with.

Lasers are very complex machines that can produce amazing results. However, they are designed with electrical capacitors, computer software, sophisticated optics, and, in short, components that can malfunction or become inoperable. Laser equipment, like all devices, needs to be inspected, maintained, and serviced by manufacturer-trained and qualified laser technicians. All preventive maintenance, system upgrades, and service calls to correct fault codes or malfunctions need to be documented in the laser's service manual. This is an important step in guaranteeing a device's excellent performance for a client and risk management for a business.

Administrative Controls

ANSI document mandates the need for controls on an administrative level in order to establish a laser safety program at a facility. This includes the establishment of a Laser Safety Operator (LSO), laser training and education for the operator, development of facility safety policies and procedures, and yearly competency skills checks of the laser-trained staff.

Policies and Procedures

Policies and procedures that are based on ANSI Z136.3 standards need to be established and enforced at a facility, approved by the LSO, and updated on an annual basis. Even though IPL devices and radiofrequency energy are not incorporated in the ANSI document, numerous state licensing boards and professional organizations include them in their standards of practice (Table 8–1).

Quality Assurance (Q-A) and Audits

ANSI and OSHA dictate that a laser safety audit of the facility and personnel safety equipment shall be conducted for all Class III-B and IV devices with annual documentation under the supervision of the LSO. Due to the rise in the number of injuries and deaths from cosmetic laser/light-based technologies, state licensing boards in Texas and Washington have recently required that a quality assurance (Q-A)/risk management program be implemented. As a result, an esthetician will become increasingly involved in the Q-A program, laser audits, and documentation of compliance to office policies. A quality assurance program is essential to the documentation of a facility's efforts to uphold the highest standards of care in case of an accident, incident, or occurrence.

FOCUS ON: *Quality Assurance Programs*

Washington state and Texas Q-A mandate for the use of Laser and Light Devices with suggestions for compliance:

- ***A mechanism to review the adherence of supervised professionals to written protocols***
  - Create and update policies/protocols/procedures to assess whether or not they are current, enforced, applicable, and practiced.
  - Empower a Laser Safety Officer.
  - Conduct an office audit.
  - Interview staff.
  - Observe practice and document findings.
- ***A mechanism to monitor quality of treatments***
  - Patient satisfaction questionnaires
  - Chart/laser record audit
  - Peer review of outcomes
  - Observe patient consultations and procedures
- ***A mechanism to identify complications and untoward effects of treatment and to determine their cause***
  - Analyze treatment records
  - Review incident reports
  - Examine patient complaints
- ***A mechanism by which the findings of the quality assurance program are reviewed and incorporated into future protocols***
  - Hold mandatory staff meetings.
  - Review and revise the laser safety policies and protocols.
  - Order safety equipment if needed.
  - Obtain additional reference materials.
  - Allocate additional resources.
  - Secure additional training.
- ***Ongoing training to maintain and improve the quality of treatment and performance of treating professionals***
  - Seminars and workshops
  - Professional conferences
  - New equipment training
  - Updates and education during staff meetings
  - Webinars
  - Professional journals
  - Professional societies

Table 8–1 Laser, RF, and IPL Safety Policy and Procedure

PURPOSE:
1. Provide for client and personnel safety during all treatments
2. Provide for proper care of the laser, RF, and IPL system
3. Provide for the optimum usage of laser, RF, and IPL system
PROCEDURE:
1. Physician will be ultimately responsible for selecting the appropriate delivery system, basic parameters, and mode for each type of treatment. Standing orders are in place for parameters and delivery systems if a laser/IPL/RF procedure is delegated to the other credentialed licensed professionals within our office.
2. Only the doctor or credentialed laser operator will exclusively operate the laser/IPL/RF foot pedal.
3. All Class 4 and 3B lasers and IPL procedures will be operated in a closed room where windows are covered with the appropriate Ocular Density material. No one will be allowed in the room during treatments unless authorized and protected.
4. The laser operator will test the laser/RF/IPL system prior to use, using a standard checklist.
5. Facility-authorized personnel trained in the system will perform all service and maintenance of the laser/RF/IPL systems. Preventative maintenance will be conducted per manufacturer recommendations. Records will be maintained.
6. When the unit is not in use, operator will place the unit in standby. Devices will not be left unattended or with the doors open when activated. Device will be turned off when not in use.
7. ANSI-approved laser warning signs will be posted on doors prior to use. The sign shall list the type of laser/IPL system, eye protection, and classification of laser used. A pair of designated laser safety eyewear shall be hung on the entryway door.
8. Client's eyes will be protected either with appropriate manufacturer's designated eyewear marked with the laser wavelength and OD or laser/IPL approved occlusive eye shields. Occlusive eyewear shall be worn for all procedures involving treatment of the face.
9. All personnel working in areas with potential of direct, indirect, or scattered laser exposure shall wear appropriate laser eyewear marked with the laser wavelength and designated OD. Protective glasses will be utilized during IPL treatments.
10. Procedure records shall be used to document client selection, treatment parameters, and safety measures utilized during the treatment.
11. Only qualified trained personnel shall have access to the laser keys. This key will be removed and secured when the laser is not in use.
12. A fire extinguisher is to be kept available in the office, near the treatment rooms, during procedures.
13. A water source will be available in the rooms during laser treatments.
14. No flammable prepping solutions will be used prior to treatments. Clients should be cautioned not to use hair spray.
15. Shiny, reflective jewelry shall be removed prior to treatments, if deemed appropriate.
16. Electrical safety measures are to be utilized during laser/IPL and RF treatments.
– Foot pedal and equipment shall be used in a dry environment.
– Electrical cords shall be routinely inspected, frayed ones repaired.
– Grounding pads should be used during monopolar RF procedures.
– Extension cords are not to be used during device operation.
17. During procedures in which a laser plume is generated, a smoke evacuation system shall be used along with laser safety masks. All tubing, filters, adapters, and wands shall be utilized appropriately and disposed of per manufacturer's and biohazard recommendations.
18. During laser hair removal, room ventilation systems, smoke evacuation system plus laser masks shall be available to reduce the noxious odor.
19. Oxygen or flammable anesthetic gases shall not be used during laser/IPL/RF treatments.
20. Safety reviews and updates are to be conducted annually for office personnel.
21. Laser safety audits will be conducted by the LSO annually or semi-annually as deemed appropriate.

LASER THERAPY

The present cosmetic laser field comprises a myriad of technological advances ranging from facial rejuvenation, tightening of skin laxity, hair removal, and lightening of tattoos. There are so many decisions to make, so much information to process, and so much variability between laser and light systems. The best way to understand the cosmetic laser field is to grasp an understanding of which lasers are used for which procedures. Today's lasers used in the cosmetic arena are a result of biological interactions between tissue and laser energy.

Photothermal Tissue Reactions

Traditionally, most therapeutic effects are seen as a result of cells' reactions to thermal laser energy. As the laser-radiant energy comes in contact with tissue, the light is absorbed by its target chromophore and transformed to heat. As the cells' internal temperature reaches between 50°C and 100°C, most tissue undergoes irreversible destruction and coagulation of cellular proteins. In other words, the intracellular content begins to boil and the cellular membrane explodes, leading to vaporization or the creation of laser plume (Figure 8–21). The CO_2 and Er:YAG lasers are classic examples of an **ablative** skin reaction that is utilized solely by physicians for facial laser resurfacing.

Vascular Lesions Response

Other types of photothermal reactions can occur and produce nonablative treatments of telangectasias and/or erythema as seen with rosacea. Vascular lasers target blood vessels by utilizing a pulse duration synchronized close to the TRT of oxyhemoglobin, or the targeted chromophore. Pulse durations and fluence need to be adjusted to the size of the targeted vessel. Upon exposure, the blood coagulates and conducts heat to the vessel wall, which becomes damaged. The immediate response is either darkening or coagulation of the vessel; vasospasm, in which the vessel blanches and then can disappear; or vasoconstriction in which the vessel wall collapses. Clearance of the vascular lesion is seen slowly over the next three to six weeks as blood clots and wall debris are eliminated by the immune system (Figure 8–22). Noting the absorption spectrum of oxyhemoglobin coupled with the depth of epidermal and dermal vessels, lasers ranging from 532 nm to 1,064 nm are the most appropriate for vascular lesions.

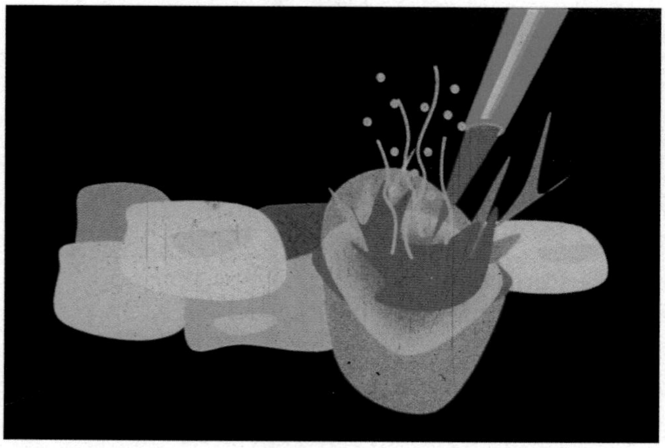

Figure 8–21 Cell being vaporized by a CO_2 laser.

Pigmented Lesions Response

Photothermal nonablative devices can also be used successfully for the treatment of pigmented lesions. With melanin being the chromophore, 532nm, Q-switched 532nm lasers and some alexandrite lasers appear to be the most effective. Once the laser beam comes in contact with the targeted lentigo, or age spot, melanin absorbs

> **FYI**
>
> Remember, the longer the wavelength, the deeper the penetration. That is why the 532-nm wavelength is more appropriate for superficial facial vessels and the 1,064-nm light is used primarily for deep leg veins and more vascular abnormalities.

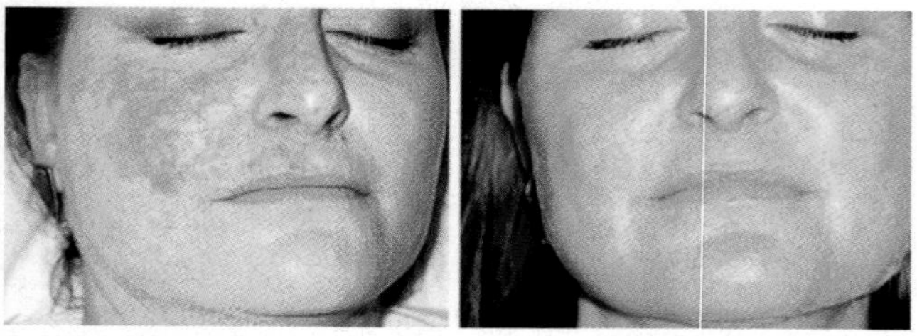

Laser-resistant facial telangectasias caused by estrogen therapy.
Courtesy of Melody Dwyer DO, Boise, Idaho.

Figure 8–22 a) Before and b) 2 years after a vascular light treatment.

the light, which is transformed to heat. Melanin is broken into small particles and melanin-containing cells (melanocytes/keratinocytes) are damaged. The immediate response is seen as either darkening, which occurs with melanin break-up, or erythema due to local inflammation. Within 24 hours one can see a crusting or darkening over the lentigo, which either lightens or flakes off within 7 to 10 days (Figure 8–23). Clearance is achieved when the immune system eliminates melanin particles and cell debris.

Collagen Stimulation Response

Traditionally, ablative lasers such as the CO_2 and Er:YAG lasers were the gold standard for improvement of mild to moderate rhytids, acne scarring, and sun-damaged skin. Since the targeted chromophore is water, these lasers can be engineered to remove microns of tissue with minimal adjacent thermal injury. With a series of passes, the photothermal energy causes vaporization of the epidermis and portions of the dermis, followed by weeks of wound healing and re-epithelialization. However, as a result, the client experiences collagen shrinkage, remodeling, and improvement in tone, texture, facial wrinkles, and scarring. The benefits from this procedure, however, were not without the reported risks of hypopigmentation, scarring, and infection.

More and more physicians are now embracing nonablative technologies, as the benefit of epidermal preservation is achieved. Nonablative collagen remodeling has been associated with infrared lasers that are selectively absorbed by water (1064 nm, 1,320 nm, 1,450 nm, 1,540 nm). With these different wavelengths, the common tissue reaction is for laser energy to cause thermal injury, which results in fibroblast stimulation and the production of new collagen. Recently, there has been an explosion of new technology in the field of "fractional resurfacing." In 2004 Reliant Technologies developed the Fraxel™ laser, a 1,550-nm wavelength that is absorbed by water but could be delivered microscopically in a pixel-type matrix. These columns of thermal energy **(micro thermal zones, MTZ)** could be adjusted for more superficial penetration to treat pigmented lesions and melasma along with deeper dermal penetration for photoaging and acne scarring improvement (Figure 8–24). Through a series of treatments, gradual improvement is seen with an average of around 20% surface coverage per treatment. Since the arrival of this technology, there are now 18 different "fractional" non-ablative and ablative technologies with a variety of wavelengths, including the 10,600nm CO_2 laser, 2940nm Er:YAG laser, and 2790nm Er:YSGG.

Photomechanical Tissue Response

Photomechanical reactions occur when lasers are mechanically engineered to deliver a beam of light that is pulsed in a nanosecond duration. With an extremely short pulse the energy is delivered in megawatts, or high peak power, to the tissue. These Q-switched shutter devices allow common laser wavelengths to produce photoacoustic shock waves which raise the tissue temperature by 300 °C in nanoseconds, fast enough to explode particles of tattoo ink or pigment granules. They can also be referred to as *photoacoustic* responses. Clinically, there is whitening of the impact site due to vacuolization of the impact site without necrosis to the underlying tissue. However, the pigment fragments are

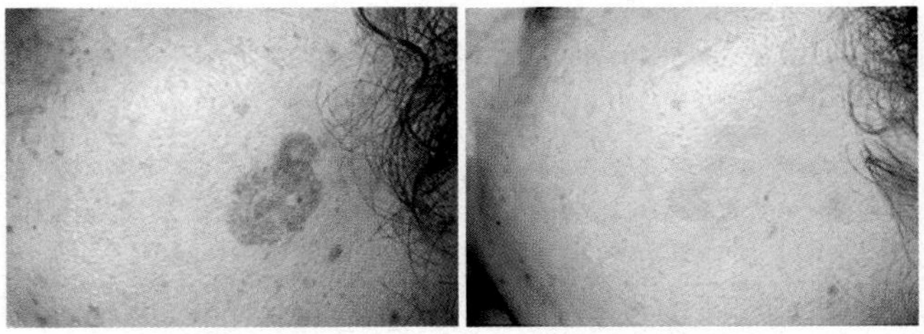

Before and 2 months after 2 IPL treatments

Courtesy of William Merkel, MD, Grand Junction, Colorado

Figure 8–23 a) Before and b) after pigmented lesion treatments.

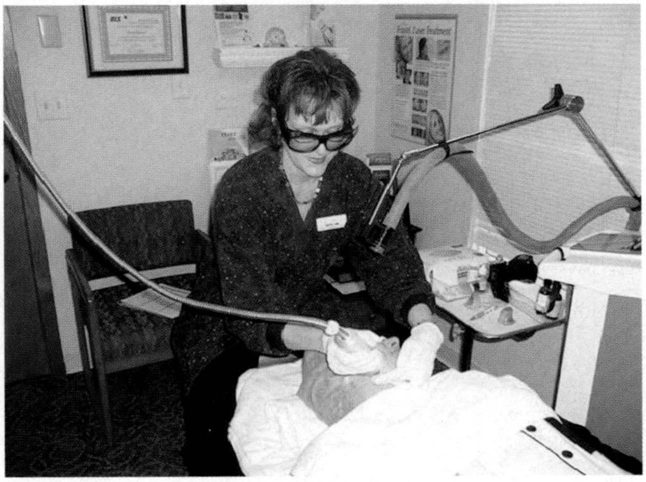

Figure 8–24 MTZ and fractional resurfacing.

fractured microscopically in the surrounding tissue. It takes more than three weeks for healing and clearance of the fragmented particles by the body's immune system (macrophages).

Photomechanical lasers are used primarily for tattoo removal and treatment of pigmented lesions. Tattoos are prevalent—36% of all Americans 25 to 29 years old have a tattoo. Many incorporate names or lettering, and later some wish to have those particular tattoos removed. Due to the absorption curve of lasers versus color of tattoo ink, each color may need a different laser system for clearance (Figure 8–25). That is why it can be a very long process, with multiple treatments using different laser wavelengths in order to remove a multicolored tattoo. In the end there can be evidence of nonpigmented skin, incomplete removal of tattoo dye, or skin texture changes (Figure 8–26 and Table 8–2).

Q-switched lasers are commonly used for the treatment of pigmented lesions. A client should be assessed, and an appropriate treatment and device chosen, under the watchful eye of a physician or advanced practitioner. The client's skin type, tendency for wound healing, and hyperpigmentation response are all factors in this decision-making process.

The Q-switched 532 nm, the Q-switched 755 nm alexandrite, and the Q-switched 694 nm ruby lasers are

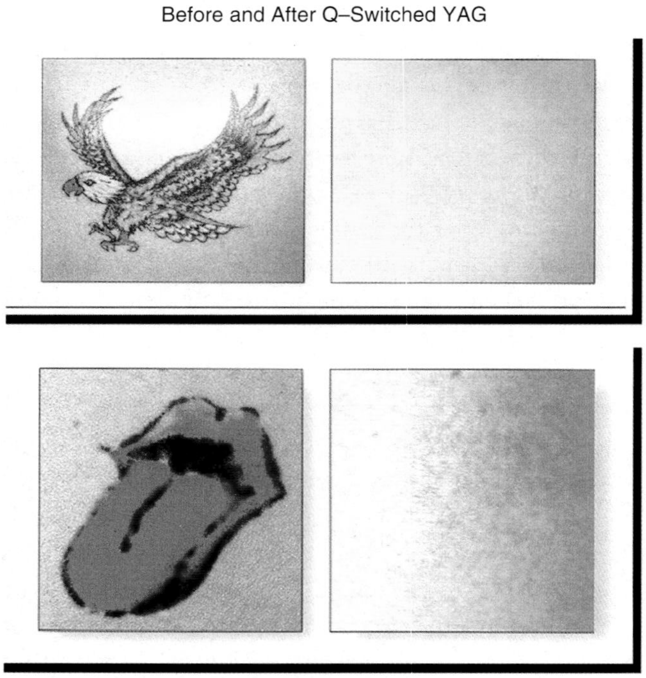

Figure 8–26 Tattoo laser treatments a) before and b) after.

commonly used for the treatment of lentigos, age spots, melasma, seborrheic keratosis, and some birthmarks. Immediately after laser exposure, the lesion exhibits visible whitening, and wound healing usually takes 7 to 10 days (Figure 8–27). Several treatments with a Q-switched laser may be indicated and there is always a possibility of repigmentation, depending on the type of lesion and whether appropriate sun protection is utilized.

> **CAUTION!**
>
> **Even though the same wavelengths may be used for a photothermal response to tissue, these tattoo removal devices are completely different laser systems. One *cannot* use a thermal laser or IPL device on a tattoo! When this has been attempted, the client experienced scarring and hypopigmentation, with resulting litigation.**

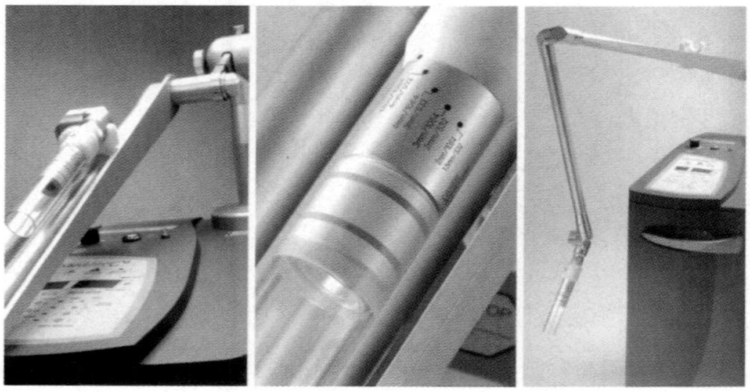

Figure 8–25 Tattoo laser.

> **CAUTION!**
>
> **Whenever treating melanin-containing lesions, you must have a physician verify that the lesions are noncancerous or precancerous.**

Table 8–2 Different Wavelengths of Light versus Tattoo Dye Absorption

LASER WAVELENGTHS	DYE ABSORPTION
Q-switched 532 nm	Red pigment
Q-switched 1,064 nm—Nd:YAG	Blue, black pigment
Q-switched 755 nm—Alexandrite	Green, black, blue pigment
Q-switched 694 nm—Ruby	Green, black, blue pigment

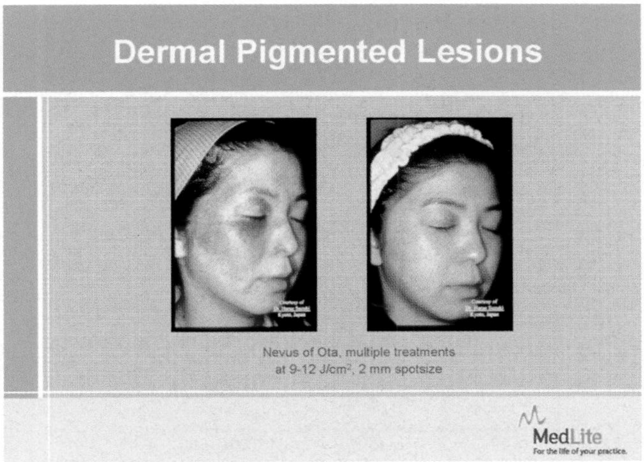
Dermal Pigmented Lesions
Nevus of Ota, multiple treatments
at 9-12 J/cm², 2 mm spotsize
MedLite
For the life of your practice.

Figure 8–27 a) Before and b) after Q-switched treatment of pigmented lesion.

Common Procedures

The ever-increasing use of lasers for cosmetic procedures is a constantly changing, dynamic trend (Table 8–3). Lasers have unique properties but are usually limited to only a few specialized applications per system. Basically, in spite of what a sales representative may say, one laser does not do everything. However, lasers that are absorbed by oxyhemoglobin have a multitude of applications in the treatment of vascular lesions, including diffuse erythema, telangectasias, hemangiomas, leg veins, and port-wine stains. Lasers absorbed by melanin are indicated for treatment of superficial epidermal lentigos and melasma to deep pigmented birthmarks, such as a **Nevus of Ota.** Lasers have become the gold standard for hair removal for all skin types and body sites. Laser technology has expanded in the field of acne treatments with and without the use of topical prescription agents. Furthermore, lasers are constantly being modified and upgraded for treatment of sun-damaged skin, wrinkle reduction, and collagen stimulation for facial rejuvenation. As Americans' body mass index increases, a new focus on fat and cellulite is emerging. Lasers that perform **lipolysis** for fat removal, cellulite reduction, and body sculpting are just now leaving the research labs and entering into clinics and medi-spas. Given the rapidly advancing technology, an esthetician who stays informed and educated will provide the most effective modalities for his or her clients.

Table 8–3 Common Cosmetic Lasers*

LASER	WAVELENGTH	TISSUE EFFECT	CLINICAL APPLICATIONS
Diode	800 nm 900 nm 980 nm	Photothermal Photothermal Photothermal	Hair removal Leg veins, vascular lesions Endovenous fibers
Ruby Q-switched	694 nm 694 nm	Photothermal Photomechanical	Hair removal Tattoo removal
Nd:YAG Q-switched	1,064 nm 1,064 nm	Photothermal Photomechanical	Leg veins, vascular lesions, collagen stimulation, hair removal Tattoo removal and Nevus of Ota
CO_2	10,600 nm	Photothermal	Ablative laser resurfacing
Er:YAG	2,940 nm	Photothermal	Ablative laser resurfacing
Pulsed dye	585,595 nm	Photothermal	Vascular and pigmented lesions
Alexandrite Q-switched	755 nm 755 nm	Photothermal Photomechanical	Vascular and pigmented lesions, hair removal Tattoo removal
Erbium glass	1,540 nm	Photothermal	Collagen stimulation, acne scarring
Frequency doubled Nd:YAG	1,450 nm	Photothermal	Collagen stimulation, acne scarring, wrinkle reduction
Q-switched	532 nm 532 nm	Photothermal Photomechanical	Vascular and pigmented lesions Pigmented lesions, red tattoo ink
Fractional Erbium glass	1,550 nm	Photothermal	Collagen stimulation, melasma, wrinkle reduction, photodamage, non-ablative fractional resurfacing
Nd:YAG	1,320 nm	Photothermal	Collagen stimulation, acne scarring, wrinkle reduction, endovenous fibers

*All are Class IV devices and require physician supervision.

INTENSE PULSED LIGHT

In 1995 the first noncoherent, filtered flashlamp marketed as **Intense Pulsed Light (IPL)** became available. Since its initial development, IPL devices have emerged as the gold standard of treatment of photodamaged skin and are making significant inroads in hair removal (Figure 8–28). Due to technological advances, IPLs are increasingly thought of as equivalent to cosmetic laser systems. With the variety of skin chromophores, it makes sense to use a broadband light to treat the variety of skin abnormalities seen with photodamaged skin. Intense pulsed light can act like a laser from the perspective of photothermolysis. Lasers treat one chromophore with one monochromatic light while intense pulsed light can target multiple chromophores. IPLs are different as they cover both the superficial melanin absorption area (green wavelengths) and the hemoglobin absorption area (yellow wavelengths). In addition, IPLs can emit red wavelengths, which provides deeper penetration into the tissue along with infrared wavelengths for collagen stimulation. The interaction of the multiple wavelengths with the skin is sufficiently selective to treat a variety of conditions.

The IPL device consists of a flashlamp housed in a treatment head with filter systems that can select a specific spectrum of visible and invisible wavelengths. These filters are referred to as "cut-off" filters (Figure 8–29) for they exclude lower wavelengths and selectively emit only the broad band of visible and infrared light stated on the filter or handpiece. For example, with some systems, a 515 nm filter can emit a bandwidth of 515 nm to 1200 nm of light. A 695-nm filter will only emit wavelengths from 695 nm to 1200 nm. When pulsed, a bright white light is visible, different from laser light, for it is polychromatic, non-coherent, and non-collimated (Figure 8–29). Forward, backward and lateral scattering does occur.

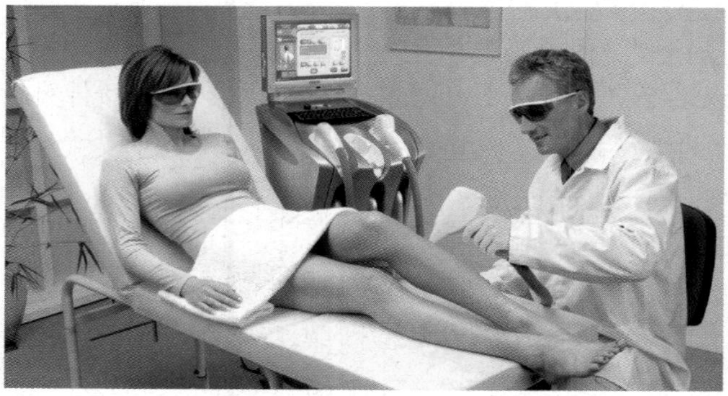

Figure 8–28 The Lume 1 IPL device.

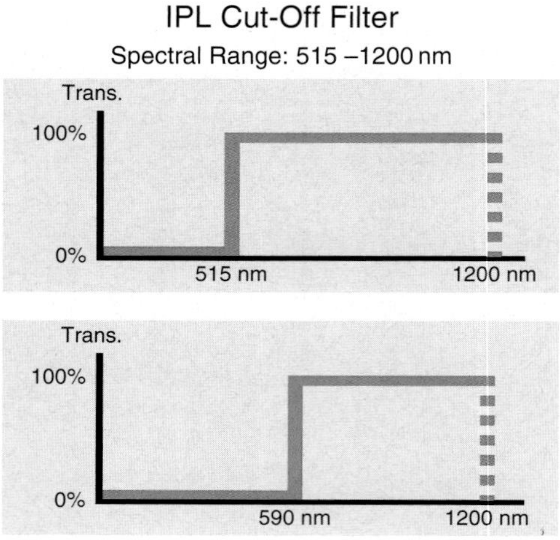

Figure 8–29 IPL cut-off filter.

Types of IPL Devices

IPL systems can be confusing to the novice for there can be a high degree of variability in the selection of parameters within each device and each company.

- **Broad Spectrum (500 nm to 1400 nm)**: Filter selection is based on the targeted chromophores and desired outcomes. For vascular lesions, one usually selects a 515-, 550-, 560-, 570-, or 590-nm filter or inserts a handpiece with the yellow filter (about 578 nm) installed. For superficial pigment lesions the green filter (about 500 nm to 515 nm) is selected as this is the level at which melanin absorption is the highest. Longer wavelength filters, such as the red (about 700 nm) but possibly ranging from 615 nm to 755 nm, are used for darker skin types, hair removal, and collagen stimulation.
- **Pulsed (1 to 3 pulses)**: Each IPL system has the capability to emit a single, double, or triple pulse. The

> **FYI**
>
> Filter selection is based on the desired chromophore interaction. Each device has a different type of filter options.
>
> Hair shaft: longer wavelength needed = red filter (600 to 755 nm)
>
> Epidermal age spots: superficial tissue = green filter (505 to 575 nm)
>
> Vascular lesions: medium depth = yellow/amber filter (about 570 to 590 nm)

Did You Know

IPL devices do not have an established nominal hazard zone because of their polychromatic rather than monochromatic characteristics.

attempt is to match the number of pulses with the targeted chromophore's TRT. A single pulse is appropriate for smaller vessels, superficial aged spots, and finer hair due to the shorter TRT. Double and triple pulses are more appropriate for treatment of larger vessels, darker skin types, and pigmented lesions.

- **Variable Pulse Duration**: Pulse widths can be adjusted to shorter or longer millisecond durations, depending on the target and the client's skin condition.
- **Variable Inter-Pulse Delay**: Cooling times between pulses can also be manipulated to prevent elevation of epidermal temperatures. Larger lesions and darker skin types need more inter-pulse cooling time as compared to that needed for smaller lesions and lighter skin types.
- **Variable Fluence**: Energy levels can be adjusted depending on the size of the target, the skin type of the client, and the depth of the lesion.
- **Large versus Small Spot Size**: Usually IPL devices come with two different sizes of filters, one for small spot treatments and a larger one for quick and efficient treatments of large areas.
- **Skin Cooling**: Most devises employ the use of a clear, water-soluble medium-grade viscosity gel that cools the skin and transmits the light into the epidermis. Some IPL devices also have a built-in "chilled crystal tip" technology, which offers more effective cooling of the epidermis, enhances efficacy, and reduces side effects. Another alternative is a recessed head with an air-cooling mechanism, which means the light face never comes directly in contact with the skin, thus reducing heat generation.
- **IPL with Radiofrequency**: Some device companies have coupled IPL with bipolar radiofrequency energy. The near simultaneous emission of the IPL light and RF current has been researched and proposed to demonstrate better outcomes in hair removal and facial rejuvenation. Clinical studies are still being reviewed and compared to the documented outcomes with the more traditional IPL systems.

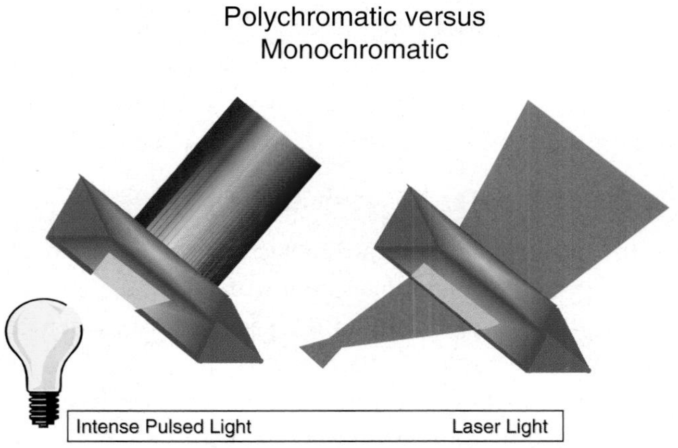

Figure 8–30 IPL properties.

CAUTION!

These are Class II medical devices, and numerous injuries have been reported. Before administering patient treatments, you need education, hands-on training, and certification demonstrating competency. Indeed, some insurance firms require 30 hours of training before offering coverage.

Common Procedures

Since 1996, IPL systems have produced documented significant, reproducible, and sustained facial rejuvenation effects. Different filters or handpieces can produce a broadband of light that selectively targets different skin structures: hair, pigment, or vessels. A series of facial rejuvenation treatments can produce a significant reduction of facial telangectasias, lentigos, diffuse ruddiness or erythema, and Poikiloderma of Civatte. Poikiloderma of Civatte is a common photoaging condition that is usually seen on sun-exposed necks and chests and consists primarily of vascular lesions and pigmentation. The IPL can also be an effective tool in the treatment of a variety of skin types and different body sites, including sun damage on hands, forearms, legs, and backs. Various research studies by David Goldberg and Brian Zelickson demonstrated that with a series of treatments spaced three to four weeks apart, fibroblasts can be stimulated to produce collagen. Facial rejuvenation clients will experience the benefits of collagen production with improvement of skin tone and texture and shrinkage of pores. IPL systems have also been used quite successfully for long-term reduction of hair on a variety of skin types and body sites (Figure 8–31).

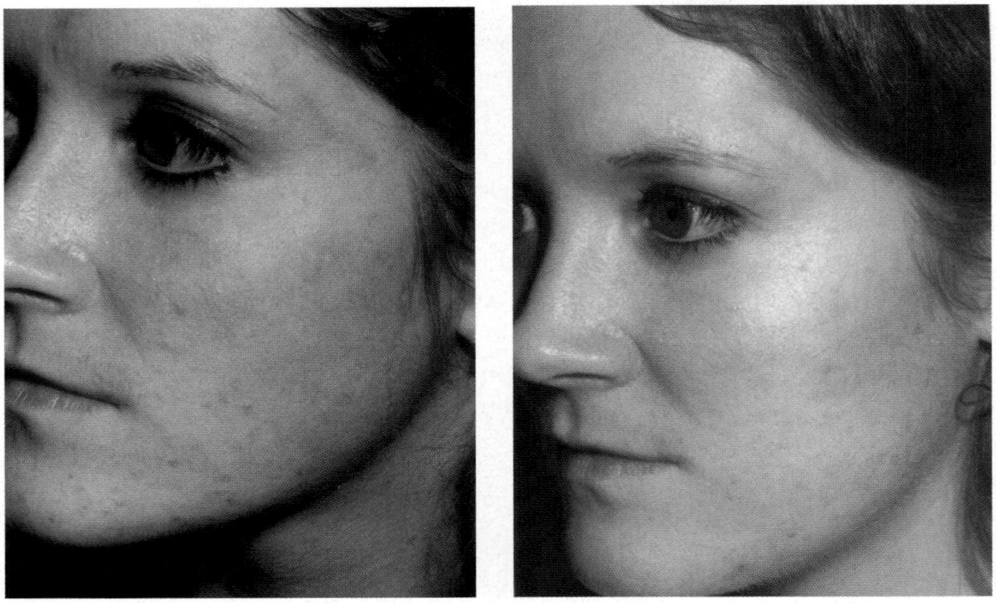

Figure 8–31 a) Before and b) after IPL treatments for rosacea.

RADIOFREQUENCY DEVICES

Radiofrequency energy is a form of energy that differs from light or optical energy. It is based on alternating energy waveforms that produce localized, nonspecific heat into the epidermis and dermis.

Types of Monopolar RF Devices

Radiofrequency devices have commonly been used in the surgical arena for the last 50 years for cauterizing bleeding vessels and reducing blood loss during surgery. This type of device is referred to as **monopolar radiofrequency (RF)** energy (Figure 8–32). With most monopolar systems, rapidly alternating electrical energy gives **impedance** or resistance at the epidermis, which then converts to heat. Upon heating the area, the current travels the path of least resistance and seeks an exit from the body. A **dispersing electrode**, a grounding pad, is usually placed on the client's thigh or back, at a point distant from the area being treated. The electrical current then exits the body via the grounding pad and returns to the machine. Electrical current has also been used during facial procedures to increase blood circulation, aid in healing, and increase cellular metabolism.

The first nonablative monopolar device used for facial tightening and rejuvenation was brought to market in 2001. This unit presently uses a large (3 cm) tip that delivers the current uniformly into the tissue, creating deep volumetric heating (Figure 8–33). A cryogen gas spray cools the epidermis before, during, and after the pulse to reduce the chances of epidermal injury and post-treatment side effects. Studies have indicated that tissue tightening occurs with immediate collagen tightening, contraction of the fibrous septae, and new collagen synthesis during a four- to six-month process. Other devices are presently being marketed for skin tightening. Before choosing a device, always ask for clinical studies to determine equivalent effectiveness.

CAUTION!

Use ablative RF devices to treat skin lesions only under direct medical supervision. Never attempt to treat any form of skin lesion, whether raised or flat, without medical supervision.

Types of Bipolar RF Devices

If the positive and negative electrodes are placed at opposite ends of a handpiece or treatment head, then the current flows superficially in the path of least resistance from one electrode to another. This is referred to as **bipolar radiofrequency (RF)** energy, because the current is contained within the treatment head and does not require a dispersing electrode.

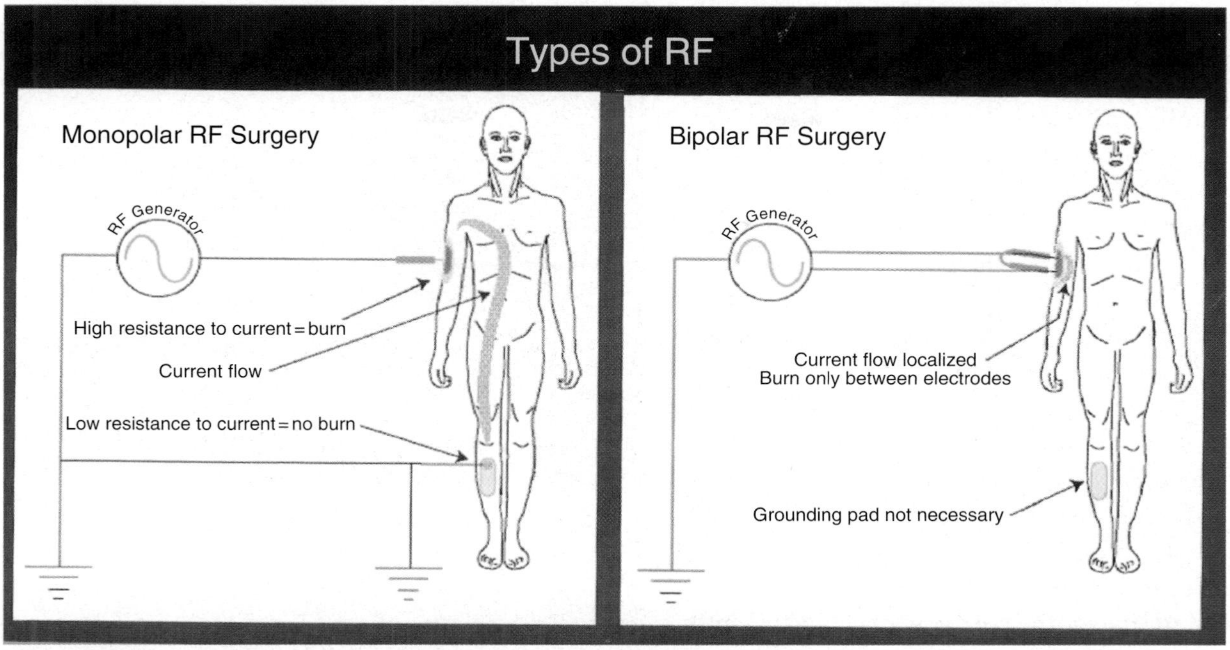

Figure 8–32 Monopolar versus bipolar

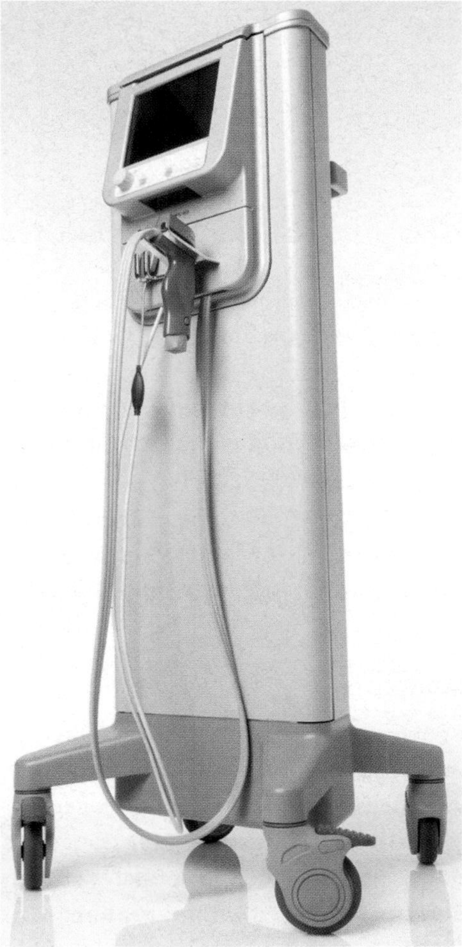

Figure 8–33 Thermage unit.

Within the last five years, several companies have developed a variety of rejuvenating and tightening devices that involves coupling RF bipolar energy with an intense pulsed light or 800 nm to 900 nm diode laser. In theory, the addition of radiofrequency energy allows for the reduction of the IPL or laser energy output while increasing the efficacy of the treatment. Bipolar RF energy is also being combined with a vacuum-assisted handpiece for skin tightening and wrinkle improvement.

Common Procedures

As technology advances, esthetics will see more coupling of nonablative radiofrequency energies with different types of light sources for tightening all body sites. Depending on your scope of practice, this technology may become part of your treatment portfolio. These tightening procedures do not replace face-lifts, tummy tucks, or thigh lifts. To begin, you must evaluate a client's skin tone and degree of laxity with your physician or advanced practitioner. You need to inform the client that changes will be subtle, several treatments may be needed, and the result will not be as dramatic as a surgical tightening procedure. In that way, your client will have realistic expectations of the procedure and results. In return, the recovery period is minimal, the tightening effect is more natural, there are no surgical scars, and the client can return to a daily routine the following day.

LIGHT-EMITTING DIODES (LED DEVICES) AND LOW-LEVEL LIGHT THERAPY

In contrast to thermal laser and diffuse light source devices, there is an exciting new field of nonthermal, nonablative cellular stimulation called **photomodulation.** Unlike other laser/light-based procedures that rely on heat and thermal injury to improve the skin's appearance, **light-emitting diodes (LEDs)** trigger a photobiochemical response. The process involves using low-level light energy to **modulate** or activate cellular metabolism by interacting with **cytochromes,** color-coded proteins that exist within the cytoplasm of the cell. These proteins assist in electron transport. LED devices include panels of tiny diodes that are pulsed at an exclusive array sequence. This makes it critical to understand the sequence any specific company offers in a device. When your client undergoes a treatment, the cell's energy-producing mitochondria are stimulated to reduce melanocyte production, reduce inflammatory response, enhance wound healing, or increase collagen. LED photomodulation can also simultaneously suppress collagenase, a collagen-degrading enzyme that can the accelerate the skin's aging process. With four to eight repeated treatment sessions, LED can minimize fine lines and pores, reduce skin redness, and increase circulation.

Low-level laser light can also have beneficial effects on cellular function, stimulation of the immune system, and tissue regeneration. Literature in the field describes a variety of visible wavelengths that can be used to improve the treatment of decubitis ulcers (bed sores), fibrous tissue in arthritis, herpetic lesions, joint pain, scars, body aches, and lymphoedema. In the future, estheticians may see some of these devices enter their cosmetic practices.

Types of Devices

There are a variety of devices marketed for photomodulation using different wavelengths in the visible and infrared spectrums of light (Figures 8–34 and 8–35). The most common LED color wavelengths include blue, 470 nm +/– 10 nm, for acneic skins; green, 525 nm +/– 10 nm, for hyperpigmentation; yellow, 590 nm +/– 10 nm, for sensitive skin and to reduce inflammation and edema; and red, 640 nm +/– 10 nm, for maturing skins, repairing the effects of photodamage, and enhancing circulation and production of collagen and elastin.

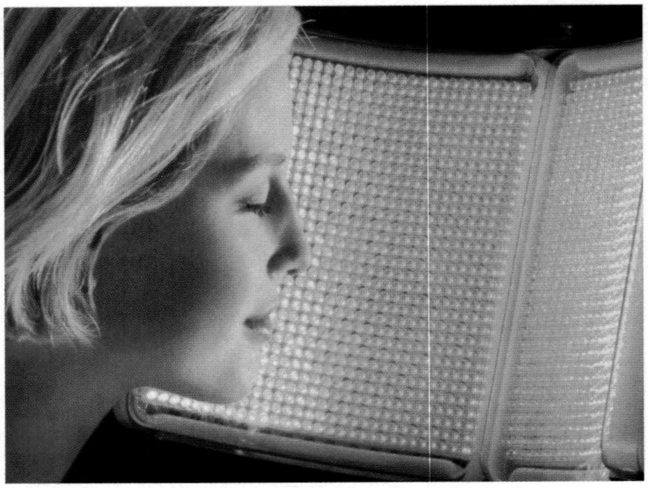

Figure 8–34 GentleWaves device.

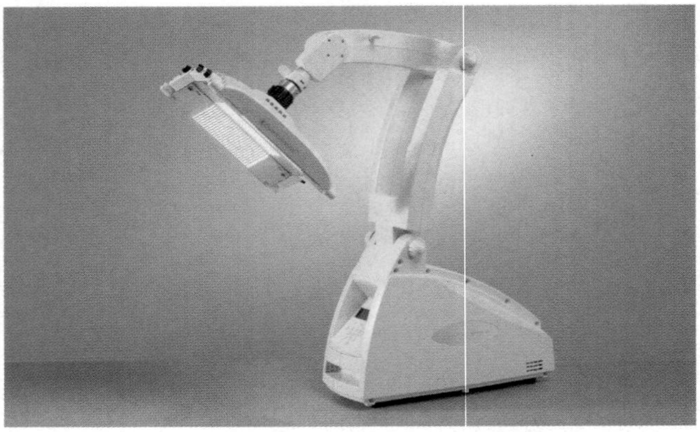

Figure 8–35 Omnilux device.

Recent studies have found the following benefits for LED rejuvenation:

1. Increased blood circulation in skin tissue
2. Collagen and elastin production enhancement
3. Enhanced synthesis and release of ATP
4. Reduction of inflammation
5. Enhancement of lymphatic circulation
6. Tissue regeneration and enhanced wound healing
7. Pain reduction

Common Procedures

LED devices are commonly used to treat sun-damaged skin, mild to moderate acne, erythema from laser/light therapies, and sunburns and to promote collagen for improvement of skin tone and texture. LED therapy is also being used clinically for reduction of pain, stretch marks, and eczema and enhanced wound healing, with a variety of reported successes.

Conclusion

Amidst the myriad cosmetic advancements, you as an esthetician will be challenged to stay up to date on the latest technology. Just when you think you have an understanding of the field of lasers, light sources, and Intense Pulsed Light, there will be new devices and treatments to learn: combination therapies, diffuse broadband light, and plasma-generated energy sources. Lasers are now being engineered with two wavelengths that are fired almost simultaneously for more enhanced clearance of vascular lesions or promotion of skin tightening. There are now companies selling multiwavelength laser equipment that houses two to four different lasers, along with Intense Pulsed Light options. Each company is in competition to create the newest and best device both for estheticians and for medical practitioners. Only careful scrutiny will allow you to make a careful, profitable purchase. The options are endless but exhilarating.

REVIEW QUESTIONS

1. List the three properties of lasers that are not shared by Intense Pulsed Light.
2. Describe four tissue interactions of lasers in the skin.
3. Discuss how laser light is made.
4. What is the role of OSHA?
5. What is a Class II medical device as classified by the FDA?
6. Is ANSI Z136.3 a regulatory agency?
7. Describe the role of the Laser Safety Officer.
8. Discuss procedural safety controls for the use of lasers in a clinic setting.
9. What are the ocular effects of a visible light laser?
10. Describe the difference between an IPL device and a laser.
11. List four common lasers used in the cosmetic field.
12. What devices are commonly used for facial rejuvenation?
13. Describe the tissue reaction seen when a vascular laser or IPL device is used.
14. Describe Q-switched laser technology.
15. List the required safety measures when using a laser system.
16. What are LED treatments used for?

CHAPTER GLOSSARY

ablation: the removal of surface material from the body. Ablative devices refer to those that vaporize, cut, or remove all or part of the epidermis and or dermis.

ablative: in surgical uses it refers to the ability to surgically cut or remove using a laser.

absorption: attraction of energy particles, liquid, or gas to a particular chromophore or target in the skin. The uptake of one substance into another.

attenuation: the act of removing light energy from a beam before it exits a second medium; a method of blocking laser energy.

bipolar radiofrequency (RF) energy: a current that flows on a path of least resistance between positive and negative electrodes that are placed at opposite ends of treatment forceps or device head. No dispersive electrode is needed.

chromophore: responsible for molecular color. Elements that laser light is attracted to; melanin, hemoglobin, or dye particles.

coherent light: parallel rays of light that travel spatially and temporally in phase with each other.

cryogen: liquified gas that is cooled below room temperature to −150 degrees C.

cytochromes: color-coded proteins that exist in the cytoplasm of a cell and are involved in the cellular transport system.

dispersing electrode: "grounding pad" placed on the individual's thigh or area of large tissue mass that receives the radiofrequency energy and returns it back to the RF unit.

electromagnetic spectrum (EM): spectrum that displays all the frequencies of electromagnetic radiation. The wavelengths of energy range from thousands of kilometers down to a fraction of the size of an atom.

fluence: irradiance multiplied by the exposure time, measured in joules/cm^2.

impedance: resistance or obstruction of electrical flow; commonly occurs when radiofrequency energy comes in contact with tissue.

infrared: electromagnetic radiation found in the invisible spectrum of light.

intense pulsed light (IPL): a polychromatic, noncoherent, dispersive band of light commonly utilizing wavelengths from 500 to 1200 nm; a common photoepilation hair-reduction method.

irradiance: referred to as Power Density or wtts/cm^2.

joules: units of energy or work. In thermodynamics, joules are defined as a unit of heat energy used to measure the energy change in an object as it warms or cools from temperature T1 to temperature T2. 1 joule = 1 watt per second.

laser-generated air contaminates (LGAC): plume or smoke that is generated from an ablative laser device.

laser safety officer (LSO): the person responsible for the laser safety program at the facility. The LSO is authorized to monitor, enforce controls, and oversee hazards associated with laser usage.

light-emitting diode (LED): a device that is made up of panels of tiny diodes that are pulsed at an exclusive array sequence to trigger a photobiochemical response.

lipolysis: the splitting up or destruction of fat cells.

maximum permissible exposure (MPE): the level of laser radiation to which a person may be exposed without hazardous ocular or tissue effects.

micrometer: a unit of length equal to a millionth of a meter or a micron.

micro thermal zone (MTZ): a column of tissue that is heated up from a fractional laser device.

MASER: microwave amplification by the stimulated emission of radiation.

modulate: the ability to stimulate or change the cellular function.

monochromatic: light consisting of one wavelength that is typically found emitted from a laser system.

monopolar radiofrequency (RF) energy: radiofrequency electrical current that utilizes a dispersive electrode to return the energy back to the generator device.

nanometer: metric measurement indicating a billionth of a meter.

Nevus of Ota: a deep dermal pigmented lesion usually found on the face in populations of darker-skinned Asians.

nominal hazard zone (NHZ): the direct, reflected, or scattered radiation, during normal operation, exceeds the MPE levels of exposure.

optical density (OD): the amount of attenuation or a reduction of radiant laser energy as it passes through the filter material in the laser eyewear.

optical resonator cavity: a cavity containing a laser rod or tube made up of two reflective mirrors at each end. The mirrors reflect light back and forth to build up amplification of the laser light under external stimulus.

oxyhemoglobin: hemoglobin in red blood cells that has been oxygenated; a protein in red blood cells.

photomodulation: LED technology that uses energy-producing packets of light to enhance fibroblast collagen synthesis.

photons: in quantum theory, the element unit of light; a particle of energy that has motion and travels in waves.

power density: the rate of energy that is being delivered to tissue by a laser light source.

pulse duration: the duration of an individual pulse of laser light; usually measured in milliseconds. *See* pulse width.

pulse width: the period of time in which a pulse of light is emitted. *See* pulse duration.

radiant energy (fluence): the energy level of a laser. It is calculated by integrating power with respect to time (joules).

scatter: a general physical process involving moving particles that are dispersed through a medium in a non-uniform manner.

selective photothermolysis: treatment utilizing an appropriate wavelength, exposure time, and pulse duration with sufficient energy fluence to absorb light into a specific area; allows damage to targeted tissue without involving the surrounding area.

spot sizes: the diameter of the optical or laser light. Beam diameter.

thermal relaxation time (TRT): the time it takes for the target tissue to dissipate one-half of the heat attained by a laser pulse.

ultraviolet: invisible rays that have short wavelengths, are the least penetrating rays, produce chemical effects, and kill germs; also called cold rays or actinic rays.

PART 3

SKIN SCIENCES

Chapter 9 Nutrition and Stress Management
Chapter 10 Advanced Skin Disorders: Skin in Distress
Chapter 11 Skin Typing and Aging Analysis
Chapter 12 Skin Care Products: Ingredients and Chemistry
Chapter 13 Botanicals and Aromatherapy
Chapter 14 Ingredients and Products for Skin Issues
Chapter 15 Pharmacology for Estheticians

CHAPTER OUTLINE

- NUTRIENTS AND DIET
- NUTRITION AND AGING
- EFFECTS OF STRESS ON THE BODY
- BECOMING PROACTIVE IN STRESS MANAGEMENT

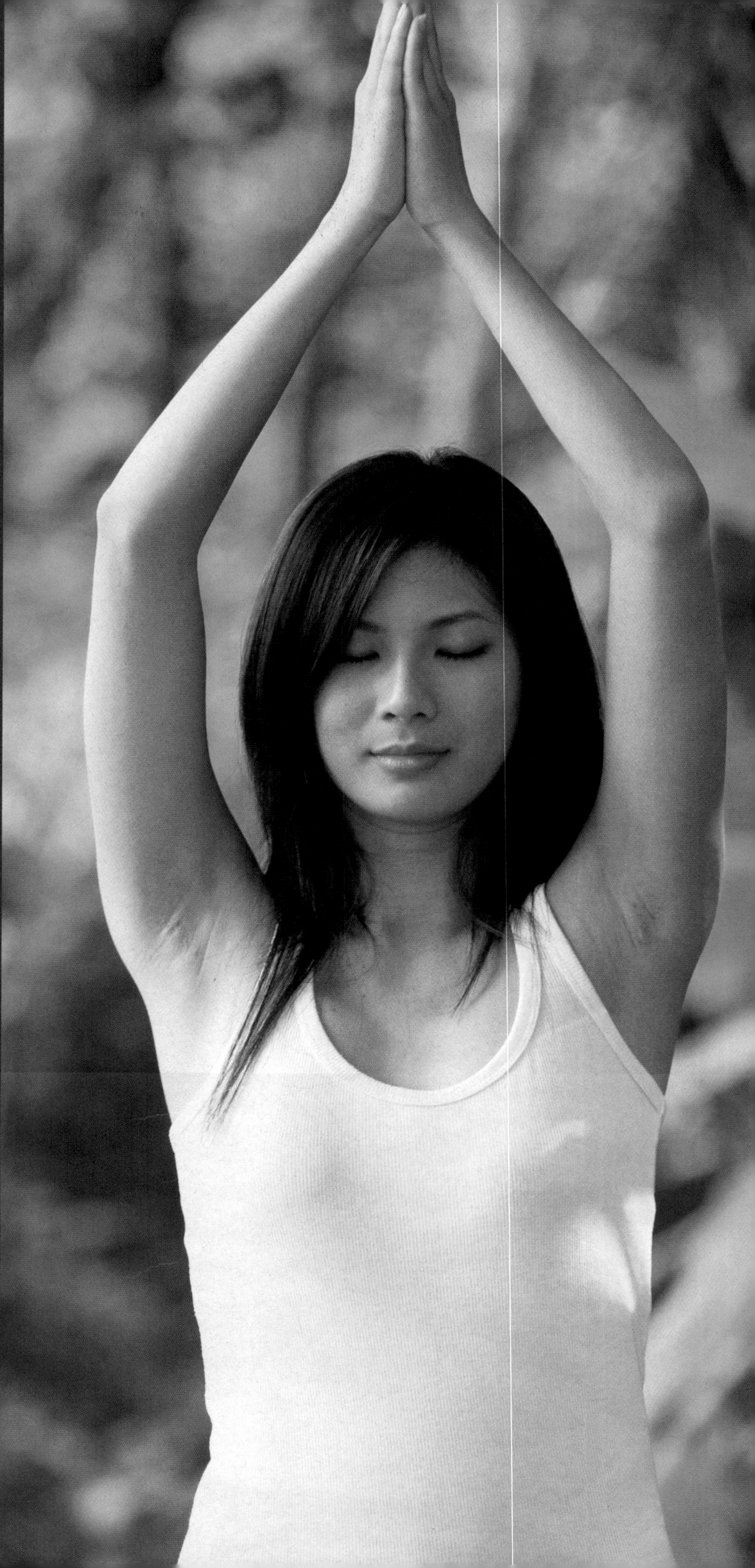

CHAPTER 9

NUTRITION AND STRESS MANAGEMENT

LEARNING OBJECTIVES

After completing this chapter, you should be able to:

- Identify the relationship between nutrition and stress.
- Understand how poor nutrition causes aging.
- Explain the effects of stress on the body.
- Discuss nutritional and non-food methods of managing stress.

KEY TERMS

Page numbers indicate where in the chapter the term is used.

adrenaline 197
AGE products 193
anabolism 189
antioxidants 190
catabolism 189
chronic stress 197
cortisol 197
energy nutrients 189
fight or flight response 192
food sensitivities 192
free radicals 190
glycation 193
Maillard Reaction 193
metabolism 189
neurotransmitters 192
stress triggers 197

At this point in your education and training, you should have a good working knowledge of basic nutrition: how the proper balance and digestion of nutrients can result in good health while imbalances, deficiencies, or the body's inability to process nutrients can stress the body and lead directly to disease and even death. The study of this correlation is called *nutrition science*, and its community has produced significant and sound information regarding the effect of nutrients on physical, mental, and emotional well-being. Many of these effects, including stress, are evidenced in the skin.

But a distinction is necessary: While nutritionists and dieticians study the science of nutrition, estheticians study the science of skin, and each must remain within their scope of practice. Estheticians are not trained nor qualified to dispense nutritional advice. However, a practical understanding of how food affects the body is beneficial for anyone desiring a high quality of life.

This chapter discusses poor nutrition and stress and how they affect one another and accelerate the aging process. You'll understand how to minimize stress and attain a balanced and healthy life. As an esthetician, you are in a role to set an example for your clients—after all, they come to you not only to improve their looks, but to relieve their stress as well.

NUTRIENTS AND DIET

No doubt you've heard the comparison of the body and its need for food to a car and its need for fuel. Not only does a car need fuel to run, it needs quality fuel to get good gas mileage and protect the engine. Likewise, the body takes in food to provide energy, which is essential in enabling the body to function and fight against disease. The components of food, or **energy nutrients** (Figure 9–1), are carbohydrates, fats, and proteins. The energy they provide is identified in their caloric content. Calories are often mistakenly identified as a part of food, but just as an inch is a measure of length and an ounce is a measure of weight, a calorie simply measures the amount of energy stored in the nutrients.

Metabolism and Aging

As soon as you put a morsel of food in your mouth, your body begins to metabolize, or change the food into forms it can use to provide energy. The process of **metabolism** is complicated, but it generally consists of two processes: catabolism and anabolism. In **catabolism**, which includes the digestive process, the body breaks down large units of living matter into smaller units that are then released as either energy or waste. Digestion uses both physical and chemical means to break down food so the body can absorb the nutrients contained therein. **Anabolism**, on the other hand, consists of building up tissue rather than breaking it down. This conversion process includes building muscle and other cellular growth.

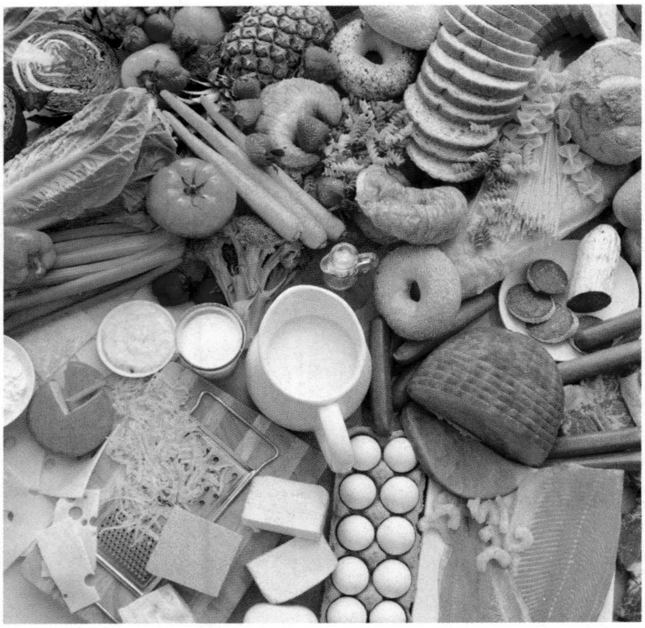

Figure 9–1 Energy nutrients: Fuel for the body.

When the body is receiving quality nutrients in a sufficient amount, it responds by releasing energy and growing stronger, providing the ability to think clearly, work more effectively, handle stress properly, and enjoy life in general. You've no doubt seen people with that "healthy glow" that radiates from their skin, eyes, and hair. This is most likely due to good nutrition and metabolism.

With aging, however, metabolism slows down. Muscle and bone mass begin to decrease while body fat increases. The major organs do not require as many calories as they used to, yet most people eat the same amount as they always have, resulting in excess energy that gets stored in fat cells. Fat continues to increase because, often, physical activity declines as well. But the situation isn't a hopeless one. Numerous medical reports endorse exercise—both aerobic and resistance training—to offset these changes and possibly even boost metabolism.

Basic esthetics introduced us to nutrients and their benefits, but a review of how nutritional components can impact ourselves and our clients is beneficial (Figure 9–2).

Free Radicals and Antioxidants

A major nutritionally based contributor to aging is the creation and culmination of free radicals. **Free radicals** are created from weak molecules that have split for one reason or another. Since they are unstable, they immediately attempt to remedy that by stealing an electron from the nearest stable molecule, which is then rendered unstable. It weakens, splits, and creates more free radicals on the lookout for electrons, and the process multiplies exponentially. Soon the overabundance of free radicals leads to tissue damage. The aging process is accelerated and the body becomes vulnerable to disease.

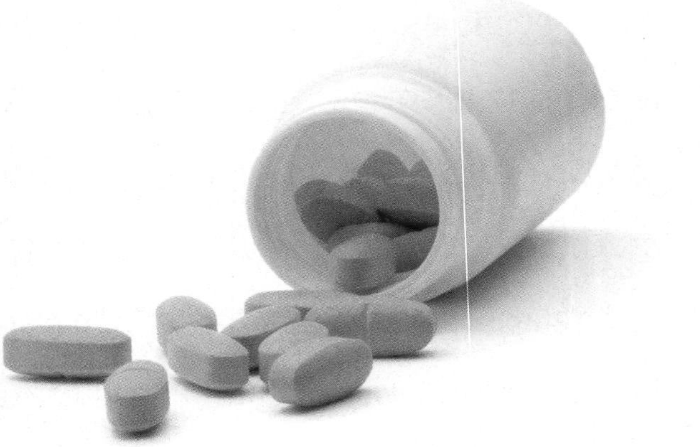

Figure 9–2 Vitamins provide esthetic benefits.

Antioxidants (Figure 9–3) neutralize free radicals because they are able to give the necessary electrons without becoming unstable themselves. Doing so interrupts the cycle; tissues and cells remain healthy and are able to function properly. Antioxidants, then, are a powerful deterrent to disease and aging. Foods high in Vitamins C and E, beta-carotene, and selenium are excellent antioxidants. This list includes nuts, legumes, leafy-green vegetables, fruits, and whole grains. Even red wine and dark chocolate offer antioxidants, but be sure to moderate your intake.

Poor Nutrition and How It Stresses the Body

While malnutrition or starvation can be the causes of poor nutrition, in today's affluent society it is not the lack of food but, rather, the wrong foods that put stress

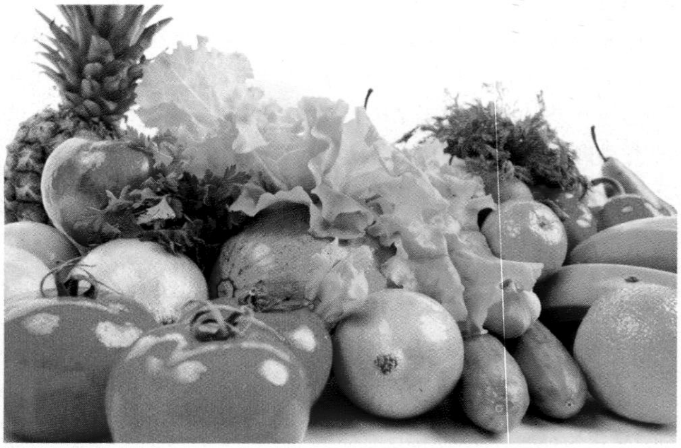

Figure 9–3 Good source of antioxidants.

FOCUS ON: *The Esthetic Benefits of Vitamins*

VITAMIN A

Helps hair, skin, and nails stay supple and glowing. A deficiency of Vitamin A can cause dry, cracked skin and brittle hair and nails.

VITAMIN B1 (THIAMINE)

When taken with other nutrients, thiamine reportedly helps accelerate hair growth after the noticeable thinning that often follows an illness or emotional upset.

VITAMIN B2 (RIBOFLAVIN)

Improves skin's ability to take in oxygen and helps keep oil production at an appropriate level. A deficiency of riboflavin can cause excessive oiliness.

VITAMIN B3 (NIACIN)

Necessary for the proper functioning of skin, including normal sun tolerance and a smooth, slightly moist surface. A niacin deficiency can cause skin infections and mouth sores.

VITAMIN B5 (PANTOTHENIC ACID)

Essential for maintaining the depth of natural skin color and relieving common skin inflammation. Also an anti-stress vitamin.

VITAMIN B6 (PYRIDOXINE)

Improves some facial pigment conditions and protects against sun damage. Deficiencies result in skin sores and inflammation as well as numbness and pricking.

VITAMIN B7 (BIOTIN)

Helps maintain skin's oil balance and has documented success in treating skin disorders related to the oil glands. Deficiencies result in hair loss, skin disorders, and dermatitis.

VITAMIN B9 (FOLIC ACID)

Plays an active role in maintaining and restoring the natural color of hair. Animal testing shows a deficiency in folic acid causes alterations in hair growth and dermatitis.

VITAMIN B12 (COBALAMIN)

Reportedly helps control the flow of oil from the sebaceous glands. Working in partnership with folic acid, cobalamin controls hyperpigmentation.

VITAMIN C

Essential in the formation of collagen protein, which gives skin its stretching properties. Vitamin C is also necessary for the effective functioning of the two amino acids responsible for developing the color of hair and skin (phenylalanine and tyrosine).

VITAMIN D

Greatly aids in skin respiration, resulting in a vitalized appearance. Also helps with healthy cell division.

VITAMIN E

Reportedly slows down skin aging, protects cells, and acts as an antioxidant.

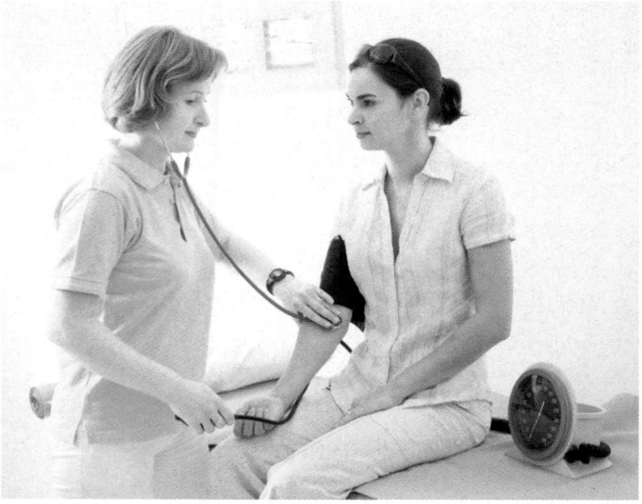

Figure 9–4 Stimulation of the fight or flight syndrome occurs when we are put under some form of stress.

84 on the body. For example, caffeine can trigger the sympathetic nervous system, resulting in the **fight or flight response** (Figure 9–4). Alcohol and diets high in fat can suppress the immune system. Too much sodium leads to fluid retention and a rise in blood pressure. Sugar-rich diets deplete the body of B vitamins, which are known to assist in moderating stress. Sugar is also responsible for allowing an overgrowth of yeast cells in the body and throwing the digestive system off-balance. Hydrogenated foods contribute to free radical damage that, over time, decreases the functionality of cells and is a direct cause of aging. Even chocolate can cause migraines in some people. This means that not only do the wrong foods fail to give the body what it needs; they can actually *cause* additional problems.

Have you ever noticed that after you've had a bit too much caffeine, you feel irritable? Or have you ever eaten a bowl of pasta and felt tired afterward? These are both examples of chemical reactions that take place in the brain. Think of the brain as the body's command center. The brain sends out instructions to the body by way of **neurotransmitters** such as serotonin and norepinephrine. Since they are synthesized from nutrients in food, the types of foods ingested have a large effect on the neurotransmitters' behavior. Serotonin comes from tryptophan, an essential amino acid. A dietary lack of tryptophan results in too little serotonin, which results in agitation, restlessness, and heightened sensitivity to pain. This is just one example of how foods can actually create stress in the body. And just as food can create stress, stress can lead us right back to food.

The lack of serotonin results in a bad mood. Meanwhile, the brain cleverly responds to this deficit by sending out cravings for foods that facilitate serotonin production, whether you are hungry or not. High-carbohydrate foods such as pastries facilitate serotonin and, in the process, provide a calming effect and relief from pain. Sugar foods are simple carbohydrates and provide the strongest, although briefest, relief. It is obvious why some people consider food a drug and how poor nutrition and stress can combine into an ever-worsening cycle (Figure 9–5).

Acne can sometimes be an indicator of poor nutrition. When the body is not getting a balanced diet, it cannot regulate stress responses, creating hormonal reactions, which increase the likelihood of breakouts. But sensitivities to certain foods can also cause acne. Some women are sensitive to dairy. Other people are sensitive to iodides. **Food sensitivities** are different from food allergies, as sensitivities do not involve the immune system and allergies do. Sensitivities occur when the body cannot properly digest particular foods. If your body cannot break down lactose, an enzyme found in ice cream, but you indulge in a double scoop anyway, you will soon feel the consequences due to digestive upset. And while the digestive system tries to eliminate it, the skin will try to eliminate it, too. This release of toxins via the skin may manifest itself in acne breakouts. A sluggish digestive system that is not keeping up with regular elimination can also contribute.

To at least manage the problem, try writing down everything you eat for a certain time period. A food diary allows you to identify possible food triggers by recording what you eat and when you break out. Examine not only what foods you are eating but also what foods you may not be eating enough of.

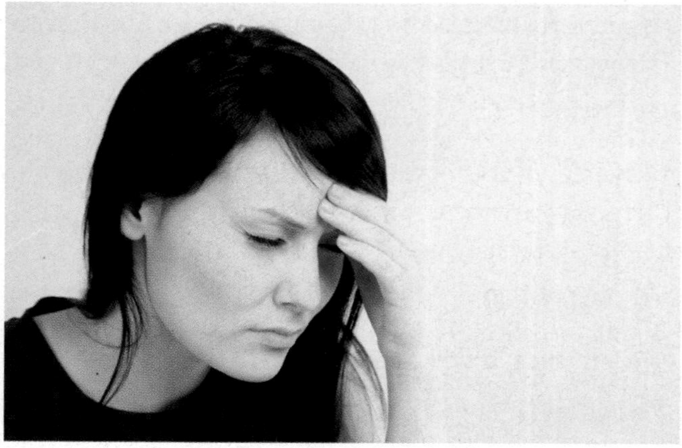

Figure 9–5 The fight or flight response can lead to chronic stress.

> **? Did You Know**
>
> The following foods may cause or contribute to stress:
>
> **Caffeine** A stimulant known to release stress hormones and create a state of agitation.
>
> **Fats** Create sluggishness and lead to weight gain, causing more stress and breakouts.
>
> **Salt** Dehydrates and increases water retention, leading to high blood pressure.
>
> **Sugar** Depletes B vitamins, resulting in anxiety, fatigue, headaches, and irritability.

Realize that sometimes neither diet nor your greatest esthetic skills can fix a problem. If you aren't seeing results, suggest that your client see a doctor. Other factors beyond your scope of practice and knowledge could be involved.

NUTRITION AND AGING

One of the cornerstones of an esthetician's job is helping clients retain youthful-looking skin. Nutrition, good or bad, has a significant impact on the skin's appearance, and no one can hide poor dieting and stress-management habits for long. A solid grasp on this topic will aid you in developing healthy habits of your own, and your clients will no doubt want to know the secret to your radiant appearance. However, you must be careful to remain within your scope of practice and be judicious about how you dispense advice. Consider investigating dieticians in your area to find one you can confidently recommend to clients who want more information.

Glycation

Glycation is a destructive biological process that causes the body to age. When carbohydrates (sugar and starch) react with proteins under high temperatures, little bonds are created that alter how the body handles the food and results in the formation of particles called **advanced glycation endproducts (AGE).** They cross-link with other proteins and lipids and render them inactive and deformed. As more and more of these mutations are stored, organs that need to be pliable and stretchy become stiff and unyielding. The results are extremely damaging to the heart, kidneys, and muscles. Skin loses its elasticity and begins to sag and wrinkle. Hyperpigmentation is another result. Glycation aids in formation of a glue-like substance that constricts and stiffens blood vessels, which is often referred to as "hardening of the arteries." It leads to inflammation and negatively affects fats, (hardening them as in hardening of the arteries or heightened cholesterol) DNA, and other biological materials, as it is cumulative and erosive in nature. Glycation is a known contributor to the following diseases:

- Alzheimer's disease
- Cataract formation
- Diabetes (Type II)
- Heart disease
- Obesity
- Premature aging of the skin

Amazingly, glycation is the number one cause of aging, with cigarette smoking coming in second!

Naturally, some glycation is unavoidable, but everyone can reduce its effects by avoiding foods high in AGE content. What foods contain the most AGE products? The answers are not surprising. They include high-fat dairy items, such as butter, oils, mayonnaise, and cream cheese; high-protein foods, like sausage and bacon; carbohydrate-dense foods, like pastries and French fries; and skins of fowl exposed to high temperatures during cooking, especially when they have been treated with fats to enhance the process. Processed foods are also high in AGE content.

The Maillard Reaction

Glycation doesn't simply apply to an individual food source but also to how food is prepared. The **Maillard Reaction** refers to what happens to food when cooked using particular methods, such as frying and broiling. When a reducing sugar interacts with an amino acid, a chemical reaction occurs that results in browning the

> ***FYI***
>
> Small changes make big differences: A fried egg has 100 times the AGE content of a hard-boiled egg. Other AGE content levels include the following:
>
> - **Orange juice = 600**
> - **Tea = 2,025**
> - **Coffee = 2,200**
> - **Diet soda = 9,500**
> - **Cereals = 193,400**
> - **Cakes = 838,000**
>
> The numbers show the levels of AGE within each product. Consider them as relative and comparisons to each other.

product. This reaction produces hundreds of different flavors depending on which amino acid is used, and because of this, it is hugely popular in the food flavoring industry. Food that is steamed or cooked in a crockpot, on the other hand, has less glycation factors than a fried or grilled item. This information is not meant to scare or overwhelm you, but to give you as much information as possible in choosing the right foods and preparation methods. (Figure 9–6).

What We Can Do to Slow These Processes

At this time no one knows how to reverse the effects of AGE products, but you can reduce the potential for further damage by limiting and/or avoiding high-AGE content foods and use less heat in cooking. If possible, keep temperatures under 110 degrees, and instead of cooking by searing, broiling, or barbecuing, try boiling, poaching, or stewing methods.

There is a great deal of research in process regarding the efficacy of supplements to fight AGE, but there are few hard facts. Supplements that look promising include l-carnosine, alpha-lipoic acid, n-acetylcysteine, and benfotiamine.

While these dietary changes may seem overwhelming, they are similar to dietary guidelines for both heart disease and diabetes. They will also slow the aging process both inside and out, so you will not only look great but feel great, too. Low AGE foods include (Figure 9–7):

- Dairy products (low fat)
- Fish (except fried or breaded)
- Fruit (in small quantities; eat dried fruit and honey sparingly)
- Grains
- Legumes
- Nuts
- Vegetables

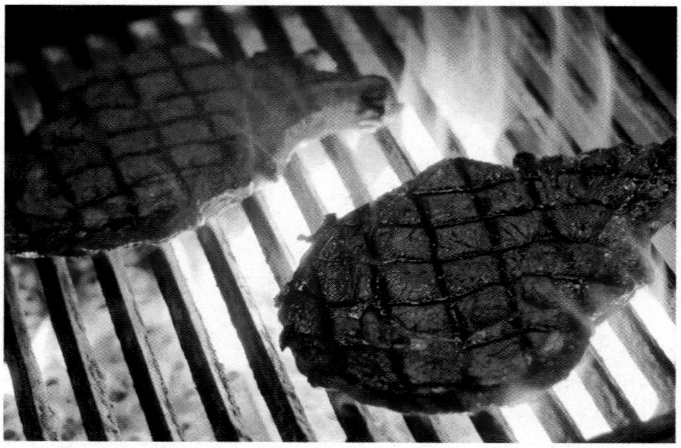

Figure 9–6 Barbecued foods contain high levels of AGE products due to the Maillard Reaction.

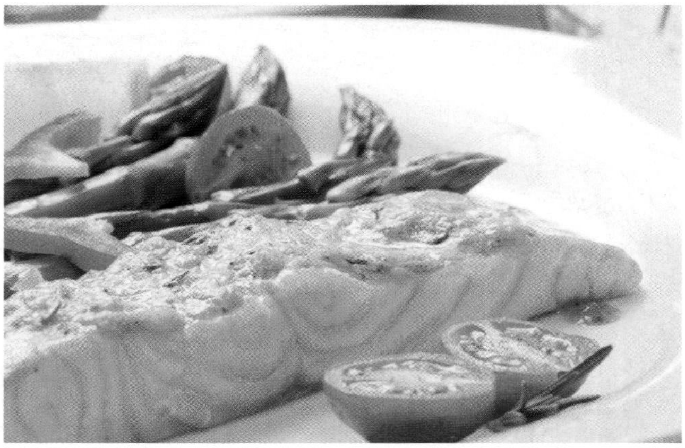

Figure 9–7 Low AGE foods.

Smoking

The skin of a smoker is on the fast track of aging. It is dry, leathery, dehydrated, and wrinkled beyond its years. Changes that occur to the skin include narrowing of the capillaries and, after just ten years of smoking, those

? Did You Know

While it is not a popular subject with smokers, there are mountains of evidence as to the detrimental side effects of smoking. Often a smoker uses cigarettes as a way to control eating and smokes to avoid ingesting calories. This means the skin is not only subjected to massive amounts of chemicals but is malnourished at the same time.

In the UK in 2003, the Chief Medical Officer highlighted the link between those who smoked and skin that is wrinkled and damaged. The report noted that smokers' skin can be prematurely aged by between 10 and 20 years of age and, although the damaging effects of cigarette smoke on the skin are irreversible, further deterioration can be avoided by stopping smoking.

The human body is composed of billions of cells, but there are more chemical oxidants in one puff on a cigarette than there are cells in the body. Studies have shown tobacco smoke contains thousands of chemicals. According to the American Lung Association, 69 of these are known to cause cancer. A detailed explanation of each of the chemicals found in, or converted from, smoke are detailed at the Web site of the Centers for Disease Control and numerous other research Web sites. To read them is chilling.

Activity

Go to the Internet and research five chemicals found in smoke and their effects on the human body.

changes are irreversible. Anyone who has cleaned a window in a room where there were smokers will tell you that the glass was coated with a yellow-tinged film. This film has also been accumulating in and on the smokers' skin. The smoke itself has a drying effect on the skin's surface.

Smokers are at risk for more skin disorders. They are three times more apt to develop psoriasis and at heightened risk for squamous cell carcinomas, basal cell carcinomas, and melanomas.

EFFECTS OF STRESS ON THE BODY

Everyone experiences stress. It is what has kept people alive for thousands of years and it can serve us well in certain situations. Humans also have the ability, to a large degree, to choose the level of stress experienced—for some, it comes and goes, for others it never seems to let up, and the numbers of people experiencing the latter are growing exponentially. The statistics on the effects of modern-day stress are alarming: Many scientifically sound public health studies show an alarmingly high percentage of diseases and illnesses that are related to stress.

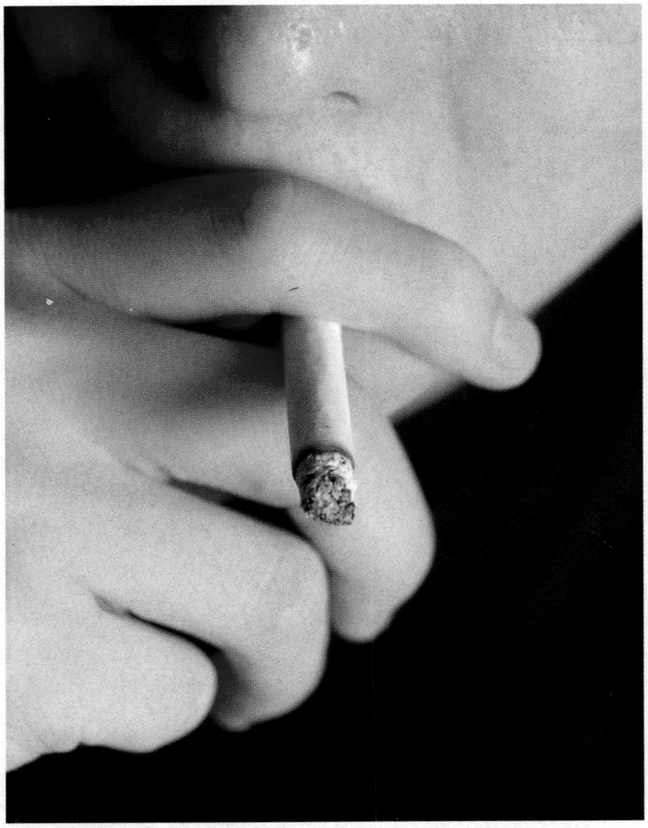

Figure 9–8 Smoking ages all skin, not just the face.

With figures like these, it is important to recognize, understand, and manage stress to stay healthy and live a long life (Figure 9–9). You should also be aware of your clients' stress levels as they often view you and your skills as stress management tools. Clients who exhibit signs of stress may simply need encouragement to take some quiet time, while others may want you to lend an ear to their worries. Some clients have difficulty relaxing at all and may be completely unaware of their tension. Your knowledge of this topic is essential as it will not only enable you to meet each situation appropriately, but it will also help you protect yourself from clients who thrive on stress and choose to let it control their lives.

The Fight or Flight Response

Modern-day humans still have something in common with cavepeople: If chased by a large, threatening animal, today's humans all run. Unfortunately, the types of stress experienced today have evolved in enormous ways that do not involve intense physical responses, and bodies haven't quite kept up. The "fight or flight" response still has its place, but it has also resulted in huge populations suffering from chronic stress.

FOCUS ON: *Symptoms of Stress as Exhibited on the Skin*

- ***Dullness:*** **Cell turnover is essential to fresh-looking skin, but stress slows the process, resulting in dull, sallow skin.**
- ***Congestion:*** **Because stress makes muscles stiff and tense, blood flow is restricted. Nutrients and oxygen cannot travel freely and wastes back up in the body. Skin becomes congested and looks lifeless.**
- ***Breakouts:*** **When you are upset, anxious, or frustrated, these emotions stimulate sebaceous gland activity. Pores are blocked with excess sebum, encouraging pimples.**
- ***Sensitivities and/or Irritation:*** **Because increased cortisone secretions suppress the immune system, the body's defenses begin to crack. Chemicals and pollutants can then attack the skin, which is unable to fend them off, resulting in redness, irritation, and allergic reactions.**

The Holmes-Rahe Life Stress Inventory
The Social Readjustment Rating Scale
INSTRUCTIONS: Mark down the point value of each of these life events that has happened to you during the previous year. Total these associated points.

Life Event	Mean Value
1. Death of spouse	100
2. Divorce	73
3. Marital Separation from mate	65
4. Detention in jail or other institution	63
5. Death of a close family member	63
6. Major personal injury or illness	53
7. Marriage	50
8. Being fired at work	47
9. Marital reconciliation with mate	45
10. Retirement from work	45
11. Major change in the health or behavior of a family member	44
12. Pregnancy	40
13. Sexual Difficulties	39
14. Gaining a new family member (i.e. birth, adoption, older adult moving in, etc)	39
15. Major business readjustment	39
16. Major change in financial state (i.e. a lot worse or better off than usual)	38
17. Death of a close friend	37
18. Changing to a different line of work	36
19. Major change in the number of arguments w/spouse (i.e. either a lot more or a lot less than usual regarding child rearing, personal habits, etc.)	35
20. Taking on a mortgage (for home, business, etc.)	31
21. Foreclosure on a mortgage or loan	30
22. Major change in responsibilities at work (i.e. promotion, demotion, etc.)	29
23. Son or daughter leaving home (marriage, attending college, joined mil.)	29
24. In-law troubles	29
25. Outstanding personal achievement	28
26. Spouse beginning or ceasing work outside the home	26
27. Beginning or ceasing formal schooling	26
28. Major change in living condition (new home, remodeling, deterioration of neighborhood or home etc.)	25
29. Revision of personal habits (dress manners, associations, quitting smoking)	24
30. Troubles with the boss	23
31. Major changes in working hours or conditions	20
32. Changes in residence	20
33. Changing to a new school	20
34. Major change in usual type and/or amount of recreation	19
35. Major change in church activity(i.e. a lot more or less than usual)	19
36. Major change in social activities (clubs, movies, visiting, etc.)	18
37. Taking on a loan (car, tv, freezer, etc)	17
38. Major change in sleeping habits (a lot more or a lot less than usual)	16
39. Major change in number of family get-togethers(" ")	15
40. Major change in eating habits (a lot more or less food intake, or very different meal hours or surroundings)	15
41. Vacation	13
42. Major holidays	12
43. Minor violations of the law (traffic tickets, jaywalking, disturbing the peace, etc)	11

Now, add up all the points you have to find your score.

150pts or less means a relatively low amount of life change and a low susceptibility to stress-induced health breakdown.

150 to 300pts implies about a 50% chance of a major health breakdown in the next 2 years.

300pts or more raises the odds to about 80%, according to the Holmes-Rahe statistical prediction model.

Sources: Adapted from Thomas Holmes and Richard Rahe. Homes-Rahe Social Readjustment Rating Scale, Journal of Psychosomatic Research. Vol II, 1967.

Figure 9–9 Holmes-Rahe Life Stress Inventory.

A threat creates a domino effect: The brain alerts the hypothalamus, which triggers the pituitary gland, which in turn triggers the adrenal glands to secret a hormone called **adrenaline.** Adrenaline then prepares the body for an emergency response, elevating the heart rate and raising blood pressure and triggering the adrenal glands to release **cortisol,** another hormone. Cortisol allows the body to address a threatening situation, be it fight or flight, by releasing energy from fat cells for use in the muscles. Now the threatened person has all of the body's reserves at hand to fend off the threat, and that is where the problem of chronic stress arises.

Chronic Stress

Chronic stress indicates that the stress response is long-term rather than immediate, with no apparent end in sight. You have heard of people who, in extremely stressful situations, can perform things they would never be able to do under normal circumstances: For example, a woman whose child is trapped in a life-threatening situation somehow finds abnormal physical strength, just enough to rescue him, and in the process she uses up all of the energy her body made available to her. But in the case of chronic stress, no real fight or flight is necessary, and all that triggered energy is left unused. A woman who is stressed due to a demanding job, children, financial worries, or other obligations does not get the same chance to release all of those hormones. Adrenaline and cortisol start to build up in her body, wearing down her natural defense mechanism. Soon she has no energy—she's tired but can't sleep, she gains weight and develops anxiety, digestive problems, and high cholesterol. Her body hurts and her head aches. Her memory and ability to concentrate begin to suffer and she's more prone to make mistakes. Her coping mechanisms begin to fail. Depression sets in, she loses any interest in sex, and she gets sick easily because her immune system is compromised. She may develop skin irritation or hives. Her nutrient and energy reserves are depleted and, if she isn't careful, she may end up with diabetes and/or heart problems, or even resort to suicide.

BECOMING PROACTIVE IN STRESS MANAGEMENT

How do you fight stress? There are many answers, but all require you to be willing and committed to incorporating them into your life. Some are simple, some require discipline and diligence, but all will help you balance out your life as you strive for good mental, emotional, and physical health. Recognizing what triggers stress is the first place to start.

Recognizing Stress Triggers

Stress triggers, or situations that bring on a stress response, are countless and different for everyone. They may be internal, such as fear of being laid off from your job or anxiety about an upcoming final exam. Some internal triggers are simply part of a personality, such as perfectionism or cynicism. External triggers range from financial problems to toxic relationships to losing a loved one. You may be nervous about a new job, pleasing your boss, speaking in public, or flying cross-country. A move to a new area can cause stress, as can a new relationship. Certain foods can bring on stress, as well as drugs and alcohol. Physical conditions can bring on stress, such as small spaces, a room that is too warm, heavy traffic, uncomfortable shoes, or loud music. Health is certainly a factor; you may be hungry or tired, suffer from premenstrual symptoms, feel ill, or be in pain. Take a moment to consider some of your own triggers.

Non-Food-Related Strategies for Dealing with Stress

While it may be tempting and quick to grab a chocolate bar to deal with stress, other techniques may offer more long-term benefits (Figure 9–10).

Breathing

Learning to take those slow, deep cleansing breaths is a great way to mitigate stress. Mimic the slow in-and-out breaths of a sleeping child and feel the body start to relax. This is great to do before you enter what you know will be a stressful situation.

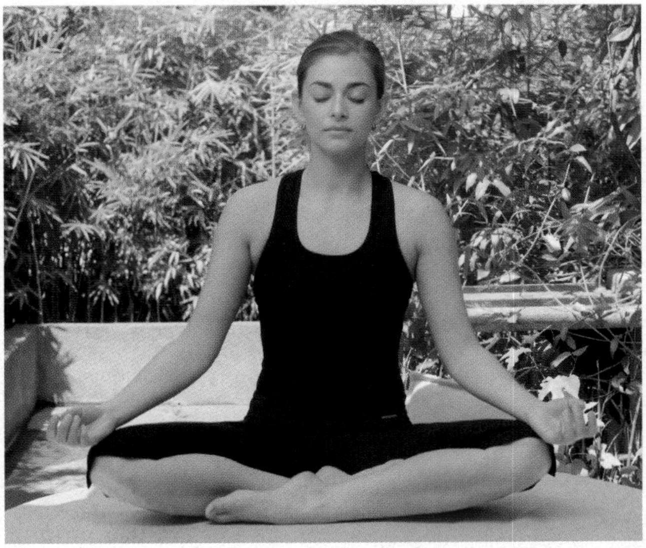

Figure 9–10 Non-food-related strategies for dealing with stress.

Put on the Brakes

When under stress, you have a tendency to speed up your body movements, speech, and breathing, so slow down. Deliberately speak more slowly. Allow yourself time to calm down.

Practice Anger Control

Anger triggers more stress and is a known energy waster. Make a deliberate choice to avoid getting angry or upset.

Go for a Walk

There is nothing like a walk in the fresh air to help the body relax and make stress melt away regardless of the weather (Figure 9–11). Even a five-minute walk will make you feel better able to handle the next event of the day.

Choose What You Do Next

Completing a simple nagging task or choosing to take the evening and relax can make you feel more in charge of your stress level. Of course, doing one to the exclusion of the other repeatedly may not be the best answer either.

Aging is presently an inevitable and intrinsic life process, and there are many ways to speed the decline—poor nutrition, unprotected sun exposure, smoking, alcohol, chronic stress, and even cooking methods. The mere knowledge of all of them can cause stress! But science has uncovered many ways to protect and avoid premature aging, and there is little doubt researchers will discover even more methods that may not only slow, but reverse and possibly halt this process. As a successful esthetician, your obligation is to stay abreast of the latest technology and separate the hype from the facts. Incorporate sound habits into your lifestyle. Not only will you stay youthful and healthy longer, you'll present a beautiful example to the world and naturally attract clients who are also eager to hold off aging for as long as possible. It is a win-win situation!

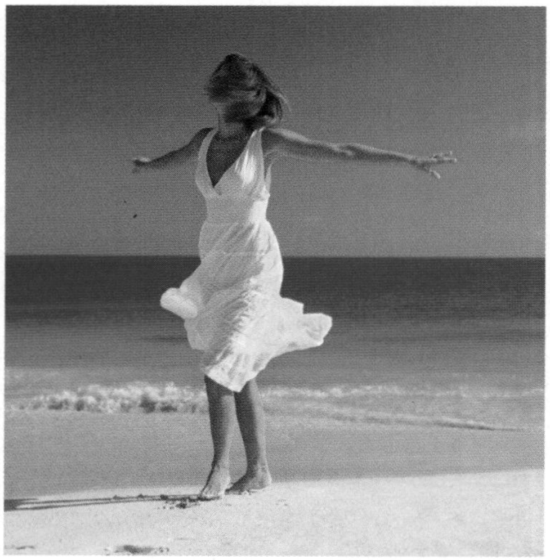

Figure 9–11 Get some fresh air.

REVIEW QUESTIONS

1. What are energy nutrients?
2. What is a calorie?
3. Biotin is also known as which vitamin?
4. A deficiency in which vitamin causes wiry hair texture?
5. List three items that can contribute to poor nutrition.
6. Describe how brain chemistry is involved in nutrition.
7. Which vitamin becomes depleted with the intake of sugar?
8. Salt can dehydrate the body. What else can it do?
9. Describe the two main processes in metabolism.
10. Describe the process of glycation and list three of its results.
11. Describe the Maillard Reaction and list three of the cooking methods involved.

12. Why has the "fight or flight" response caused such problems in the modern world?

13. Name five skin problems that are stress-related.

14. What are the physical effects of chronic stress?

15. List five things that trigger stress in you and five things you can do to alleviate stress.

CHAPTER GLOSSARY

adrenaline: elevates the heart rate, increases blood pressure, and triggers the release of cortisol.

AGE products: AGE stands for advanced glycation end products, which are particles created in glycation that cross-link with proteins and lipids, resulting in tissue damage.

anabolism: part of the metabolic process wherein larger molecules are built up from smaller molecules.

antioxidants: substances that neutralize free radicals, thereby decelerating the aging process and leaving tissues and cells healthy and able to function properly.

catabolism: part of the metabolic process wherein larger molecules within cells are broken down into smaller molecules which are then used for energy or waste.

chronic stress: Long-term stress that occurs when the body's fight or flight response doesn't shut off; which can lead to a wide variety of health problems.

cortisol: a hormone that allows the body to address a threatening situation by releasing energy from fat cells for use in the muscles.

energy nutrients: components of food: carbohydrates, fats, and proteins.

fight or flight response: a brain-stimulated response to stress that prepares the body for trauma.

food sensitivities: A non-allergic, yet negative response to food. Food sensitivities occur when the body cannot properly digest particular foods, but they differ from allergies as the immune system is not involved

free radicals: a major contributor to aging, free radicals are unstable molecules that have broken away from weak molecules. In an attempt to stabilize themselves, they steal electrons from stable molecules, creating more and more unstable molecules. The result is tissue damage, accelerated aging, and vulnerability to disease.

glycation: a destructive biological process that is the number one cause of premature aging. Under high temperatures, the carbohydrates sugar and starch react to protiens and alter how the body handles food, resulting in the formation of AGE products.

Maillard Reaction: a term used to describe the chemical reaction produced by browning foods or cooking them at high temperatures, thereby creating AGE products.

metabolism: 1.) chemical process taking place in living organisms whereby the cells are nourished and caring out their activities. 2.) The process of changing food into forms the body can use as energy. Metabolism consists of two parts: anabolism and catabolism.

neurotransmitters: 1.) substances that travel across synapses to act on or inhibit a target cell. 2.) chemical messengers, synthesized from food that transmit instructions from the brain to the nervous system. The health of neurotransmitters is dependent on the quality of nutrients in food.

stress triggers: situations that bring on a stress response.

CHAPTER 10

ADVANCED SKIN DISORDERS: SKIN IN DISTRESS

CHAPTER OUTLINE

- THE INFLAMMATION CASCADE
- WOUND HEALING
- INJURIES FROM LASER AND OTHER TREATMENT THERAPIES
- SHORT-TERM SUN DAMAGE
- LONG-TERM PHOTOAGING
- SKIN CANCERS
- OTHER SUN-RELATED SKIN GROWTHS
- ACNE
- ROSACEA
- WHEN TO REFER FOR MEDICAL EVALUATION

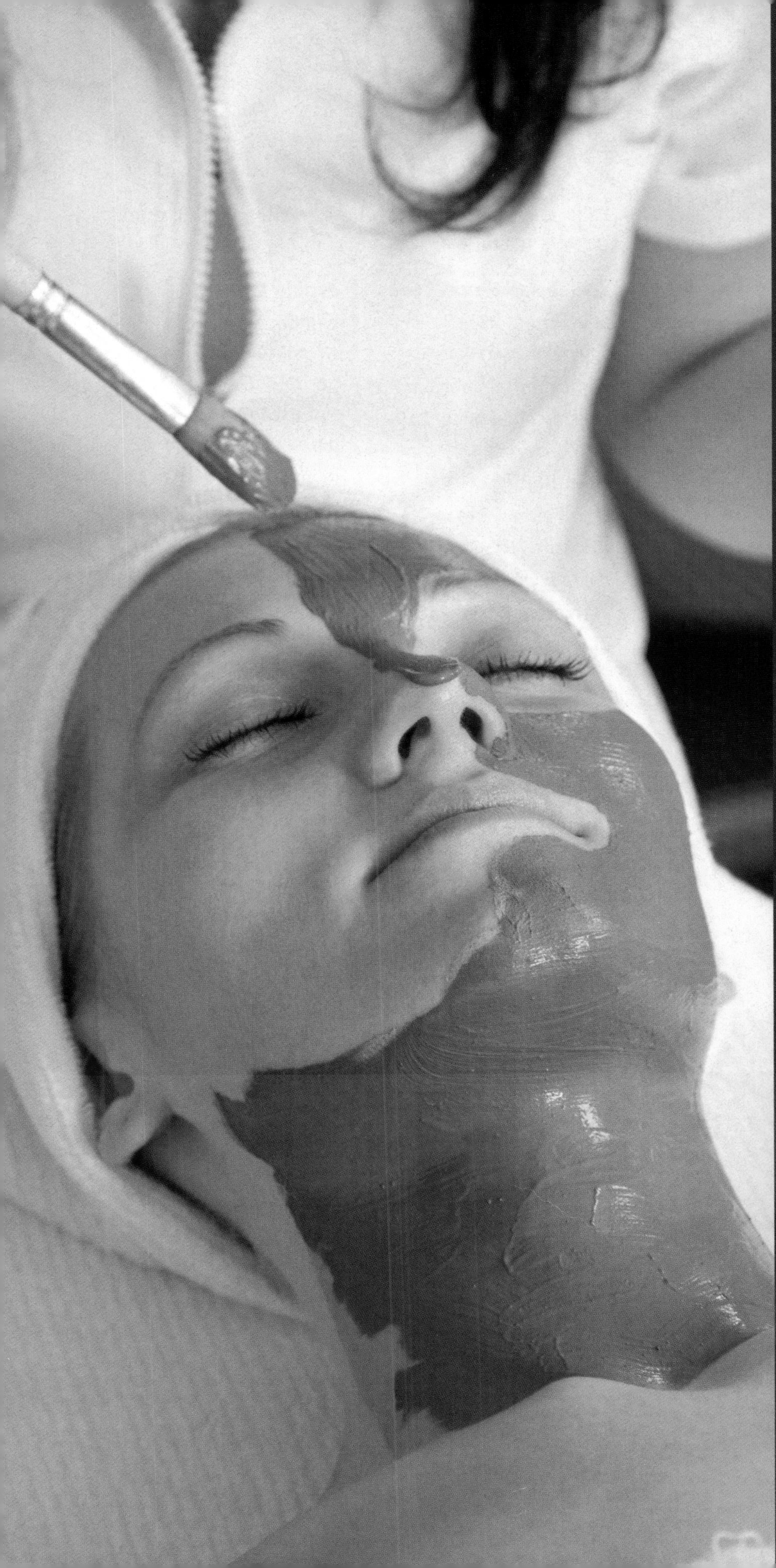

LEARNING OBJECTIVES

After completing this chapter, you should be able to:

- Understand the inflammation cascade.
- Understand wound healing.
- Identify injuries from laser and other treatment therapies.
- Recognize short-term sun damage.
- Identify long-term photo damage.
- Describe the factors that influence acne.
- Better understand rosacea.
- Recognize skin disorders that should be referred to a medical professional.

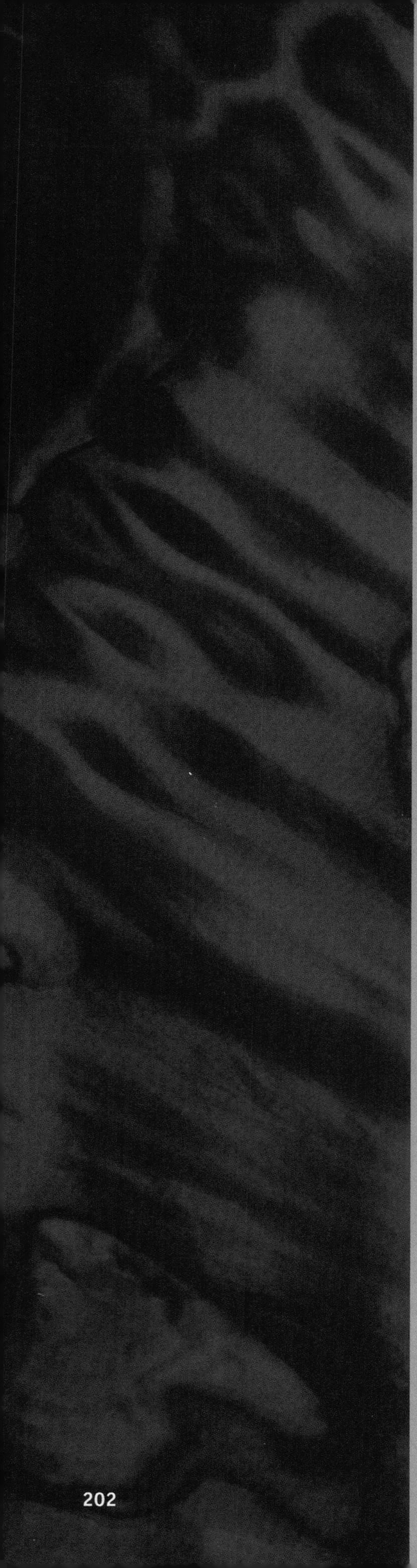

KEY TERMS

Page numbers indicate where in the chapter the term is used.

actinic keratosis 216
adult acne 227
chalazia 230
clinical inflammation 203
closed comedones 219
couperose 227
cross-linking 213
cryotherapy 214
cytokine 203
demodex folliculorum 228
dermatoheliosis 212
dihydrotestosterone (DHT) 222
dysplastic 216
erythematotelangiectatic rosacea 229
exudates 207
flare 228
flushing 227
granulomatous rosacea 231
helicobacter pylori 228
hemostasis 204
hordeolums 230
inflammatory mediators 203
keratosis pilaris 224
mucosa 206
ocular rosacea 230
open comedones 219
ostium 219
papulopustular rosacea 229
perifollicular inflammation 222
perioral dermatitis 227
phymatous rosacea 229
pilosebaceous 204
pityrosporum ovale 226
post-inflammatory hyperpigmentation 225
proliferative phase 204
propionibacterium acnes (P. acnes) 219
reepithelialization 204
remodeling 206
rhinophyma 229
seborrheic dermatitis 226
seborrheic keratoses 217
subclinical inflammation 203
superficial 204
telangiectases 227
telangiectasia 227
transient erythema 229
vascular 227
vascular growth factor (VGF) 228
vasodilation 228

Skin that is not healthy is distressed skin. This skin will commonly exhibit symptoms such as wounds, sun damage, or skin lesions as in acne and rosacea. As you move into more advanced treatments or work in a medical setting, you need a thorough knowledge of distressed skin, how the skin heals, and what can go wrong. This will better enable you to assist clients, plan for series treatment protocols, or refer clients to the best qualified people when necessary. For example, many clients will come to you for removal of what they think are blemishes but are in fact sun damage. The ability to identify what can and cannot be treated is critical. In addition, the more you know about acne and rosacea, the better you will be able to evaluate treatment products for effectiveness and appropriateness for an individual client.

THE INFLAMMATION CASCADE

The inflammation cascade is a series of chemical reactions that occurs when the skin is irritated (Figure 10-1). When a cell is irritated, it releases special chemicals called **inflammatory mediators** (chemicals released by irritated cells that alert the immune system to the irritation). The immune system then sends leukocytes, or white blood cells, to the site of irritation, and the leukocytes release another special chemical called **cytokine** (a chemical released by cells that signals other chemical immune responses). The cytokine signals cells to produce "self-destruct" enzymes, chemicals that break down substances in the skin. These enzymes break down collagen, elastin, and hyaluronic acid, which are responsible for the smoothness, firmness, and moisture content of the skin.

There are two levels of inflammation, clinical and subclinical. **Clinical inflammation** is visible upon inspection. **Subclinical inflammation** is not visible. This is

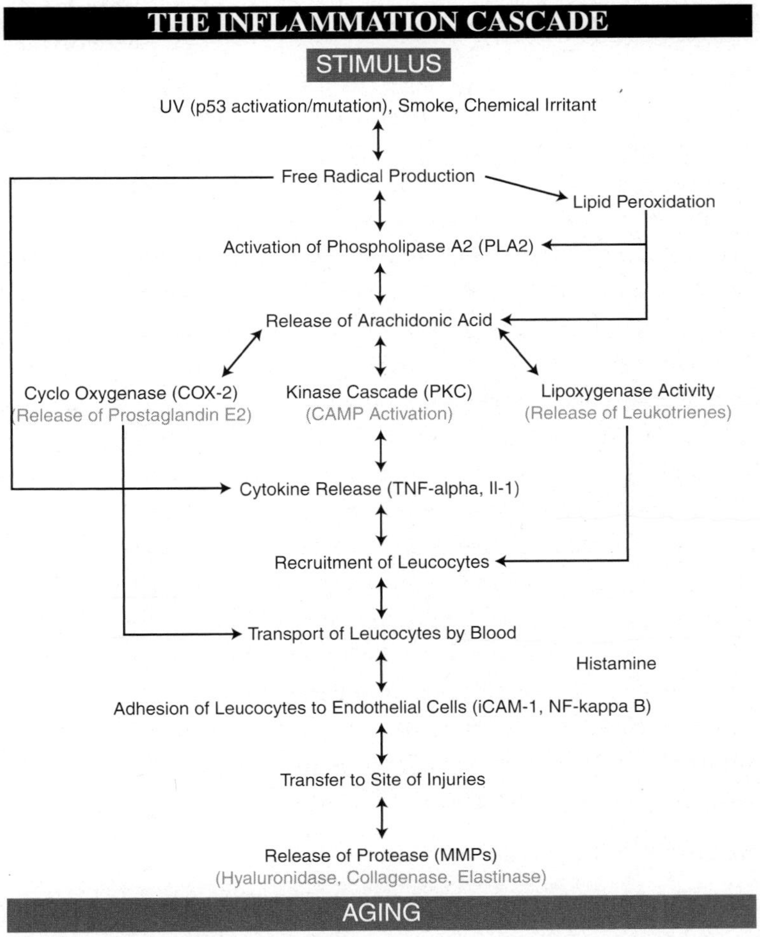

Figure 10–1 Inflammation cascade.

potentially more damaging, because you do not treat what you cannot see. Also, you may not know that a specific aggressive treatment is causing subclinical inflammation and it is time to stop the treatment. For example, a peel or microdermabrasion treatment produces some mild redness, but the redness should be allowed to heal completely before the treatment is repeated. You, the esthetician, will have to walk a fine line to determine when the skin needs to rest and repair rather than be insulted again. Therefore, it is extremely important to avoid chronically irritating the skin, whether from sun exposure or constant stripping from harsh chemicals or treatments.

FYI

Chronic skin irritation has a cumulative effect on skin aging and deterioration due to the irritation cascade of reactions.

WOUND HEALING

When the integrity of the skin is interrupted, a complex orchestration of cellular and physiological events is triggered depending on the depth and extent of the trauma. Whenever a client comes in with a compromised epidermal barrier, you know you are seeing a wound. Your first question to the client must be about the source of the wound; then you must visually determine the wound's depth. Wounds can be divided into two categories—**superficial** (surface only) and deeper—and into four stages. Stage 1 wounds are only to the epidermis, or superficial. You may see a lot of these. A mild sunburn is classified as an epidermal injury and a Stage 1 wound. A second-degree sunburn is an example of a Stage 2 wound. This may involve a blister where epidermolysis is occurring: the epidermis is lifting off the dermis. This is classified as a dermal injury and no esthetic services should be performed due to the heightened risk of infection. A Stage 3 wound, or third-degree burn, extends into the dermal tissue and is classified as a subcutaneous injury. The deepest injuries involve muscle and bone exposure and are termed Stage 4 wounds.

Superficial Injuries

Superficial injuries are those where trauma is just sustained to the epidermis, or those classified as Stage 1. **Reepithelialization** (in which epithelial skin cells

CAUTION!

As an esthetician, you cannot deal with any wound that extends into the dermal tissue. Refer clients with wounds beyond a Stage 1 to a physician.

cover a wound) is essential when the skin surface is violated by a scrape, superficial burn, or incision. Within 12 hours of the damage to the epidermis, epithelial cells from the wound margin and the **pilosebaceous** units (hair follicles) begin to migrate to repair the damage. It is essential to keep the wound moist as it heals, because dryness impairs efficient migration of the epithelium.

Deeper Wounds (Epidermis and Dermis)

Wounds that extend into the connective tissue of the dermis cause damage to the microvascular system and invoke a more complicated healing process. These are the Stage 2, Stage 3, or Stage 4 wounds. The upper papillary layer of the dermis can heal from injuries without scarring; however, when the lower reticular layer is damaged, scars may result. At this level of injury, the healing process is divided into three overlapping phases: inflammatory, proliferative, and maturation (Figures 10–2, 10–3, and 10–4).

Inflammatory Phase

The inflammatory phase is the period immediately after an injury. This is a period of vasoconstriction that lasts several minutes, which establishes **hemostasis** (control of bleeding), followed by a couple of days of vasodilation that allows a buildup of the necessary cells and protein to repair deeper wounds. During this phase, fibroblasts are stimulated to regulate the production of collagen (Figure 10–5).

Proliferative Phase

The **proliferative phase** usually begins about one week after the injury or incision (Figure 10–6). During this phase, there is an increase in the wound's vascularity to provide critical nutrients and oxygen to sustain the metabolism of the healing wound, particularly the deposit of collagen. Wound contracture begins at the tail end of the proliferative phase.

Approximating the wound margin with sutures, staples, butterfly stitches, or a superficial adhesive agent will minimize the granulation tissue and accelerate wound healing. This is known as *healing by primary intention*. The natural (unrepaired) process of wound

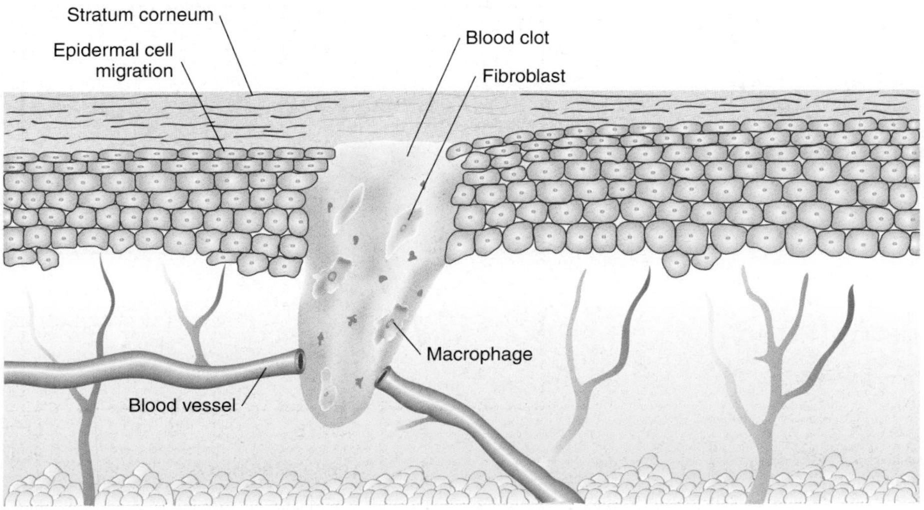

Figure 10–2 Wound healing phase 1.

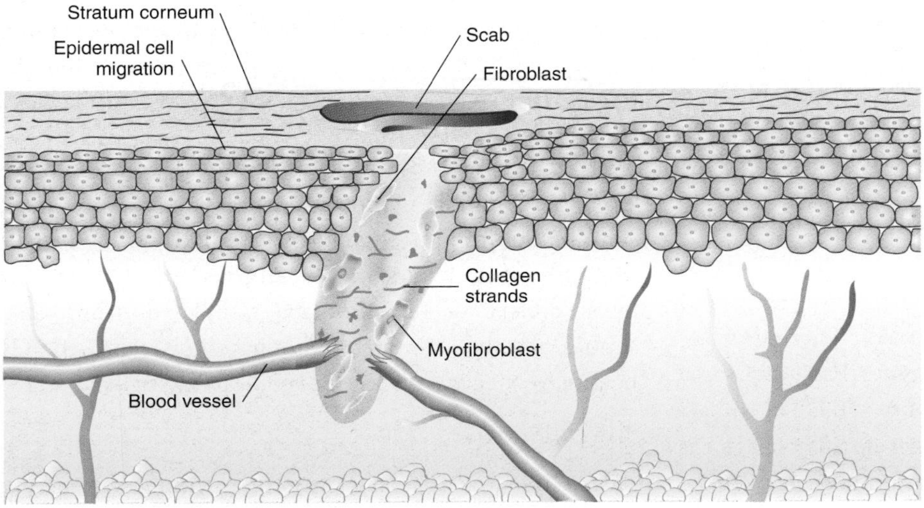

Figure 10–3 Wound healing phase 2.

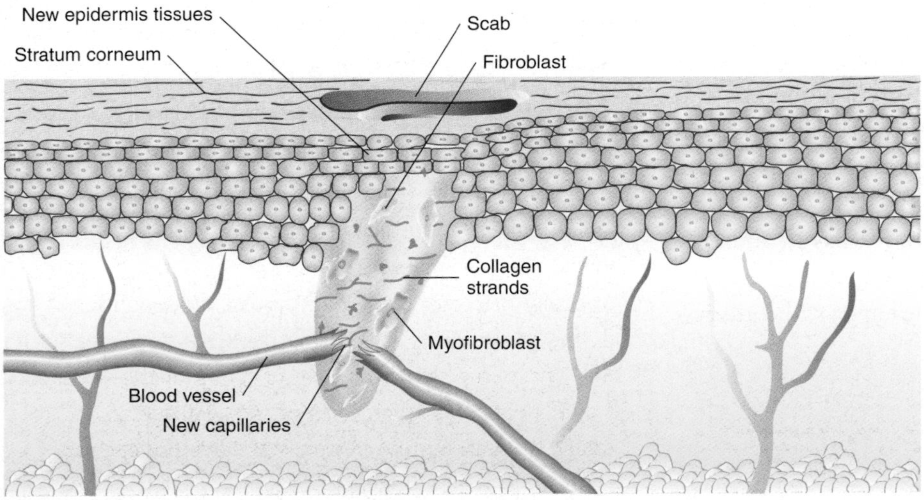

Figure 10–4 Wound healing phase 3.

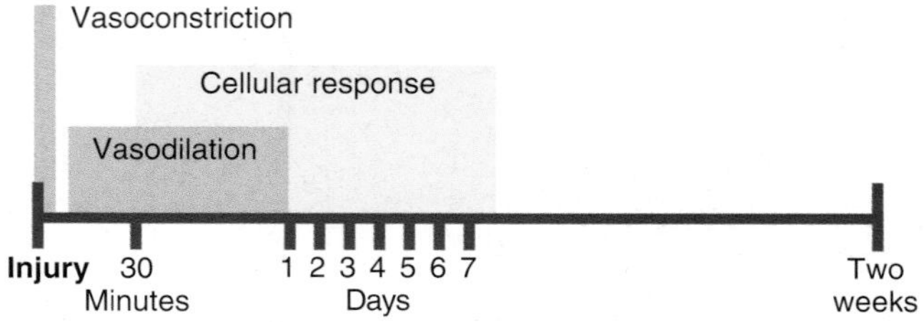

Figure 10–5 Inflammatory phase.

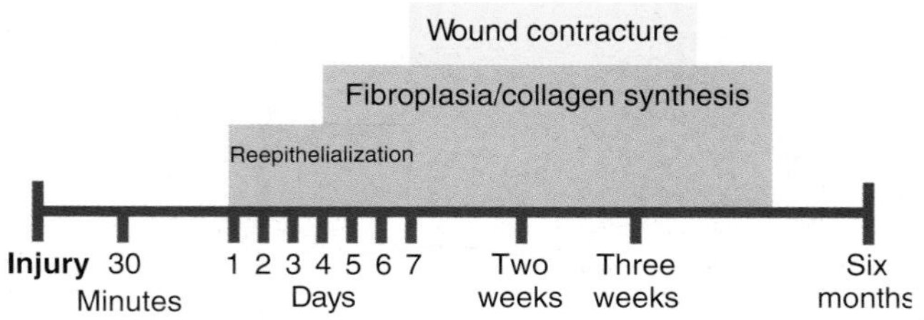

Figure 10–6 Proliferative phase.

healing is termed *healing by secondary intention*. In these wounds, wound contracture can account for up to a 40% decrease in wound size. In contrast, superficial injuries that only involve the epidermis will contract very little, if at all.

Maturation Phase (Remodeling)

Maturation, or **remodeling**, the final phase of wound healing, is characterized by an increase in strength without increase in collagen content (Figure 10–7). By three to six weeks, the maximum amount of collagen has been laid down in the wound; however, this collagen is then remodeled and aligned to maximum wound tensile strength. During this phase, special enzymes serve to ensure that the breakdown and production of collagen is balanced to keep a constant amount of collagen in the wound. This equilibrium serves to maximize mature configurations of the resulting collagen, which allows cross-linking and alignment in the wound along the axis of maximum tension, thereby increasing tensile strength. Cross-linking enhances the strength of the healed skin. This topic will be revisited later.

Within one month after the injury, the tensile strength of the wound will have increased to about 40% of the pre-injury tensile strength. This tensile strength will continue

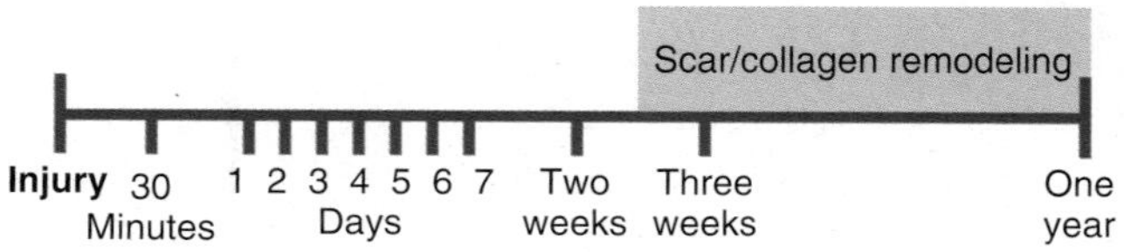

Figure 10–7 Maturation phase.

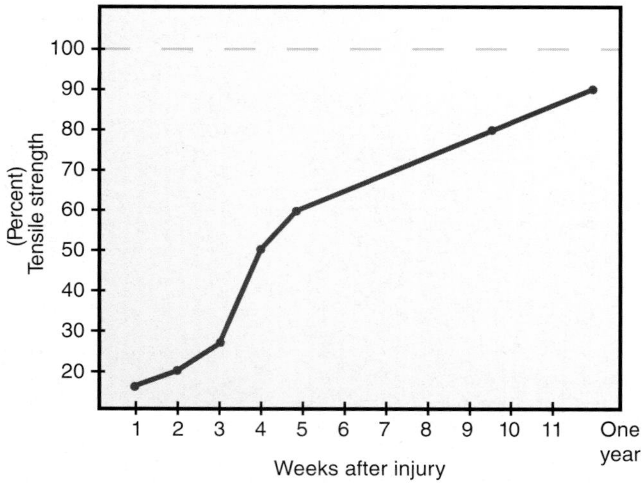

Figure 10–8 Wound tensile strength over time.

to increase for up to one year post-injury; however, the repaired wound will never be as strong as the pre-injured skin. It usually peaks at about 80% of its original strength (Figure 10–8).

Wound Repair Techniques

The most common method of repairing a deeper wound is suturing. Suturing, or stitching, is a method of wound repair using thin thread made of different materials. Stitches can be absorbable or nonabsorbable. Unlike nonabsorbable sutures, absorbable sutures do not need to be removed. It is helpful to be familiar with the methods physicians use.

Simple Suture

This is the most basic of the suture techniques, involving the approximation of the tissue margins with interrupted single loops of sutures (Figure 10–9). Superficial, simple, or running sutures are usually nonabsorbable, and sub-Q sutures (see below) and sutures used to close **mucosa** (moist tissue) are usually absorbable.

> **FYI**
>
> Depending on the radiation used, the amount administered, and other factors, the skin in the vicinity of the treated area may become red, sensitive, or easily irritated in the days, weeks, and months during and after radiation treatment, most commonly for cancer. The skin may swell or droop or the texture may change. Most symptoms of skin damage are temporary, although a person may have permanent changes in the skin tone or texture.

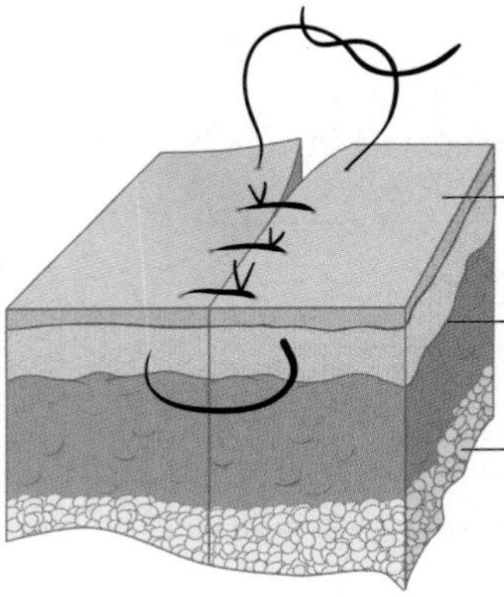

Figure 10–9 Simple interrupted sutures.

Buried Sutures

This is simply an inverted form of the simple suture technique that is placed beneath the skin or mucosa (i.e., the knot is placed at the deepest point of the loop). As the skin is closed, the "buried" suture is no longer visible. This technique is often referred to as subcuticular or sub-Q (Figure 10–10). Based on the injury, these sutures can be placed as interrupted or running (continuous).

Running Sutures

This technique uses one continuous suture in a series of running loops that is held with a knot at the beginning and end of the incision line. They can be superficial or buried (Figure 10–11).

Suture Removal

The appropriate time for suture removal varies with the area of the body injured and how well the wound is healing (Table 10–1).

Aftercare Impacts

Following a medical procedure, the client needs to keep the wound surface clean and moist. Watch for any signs of infection (Figure 10–12), and apply dressings to protect the wound from contaminants, reduce pain, and absorb **exudates,** or oozing, as the wound heals. Anytime the client is in the clinic the wound should be inspected.

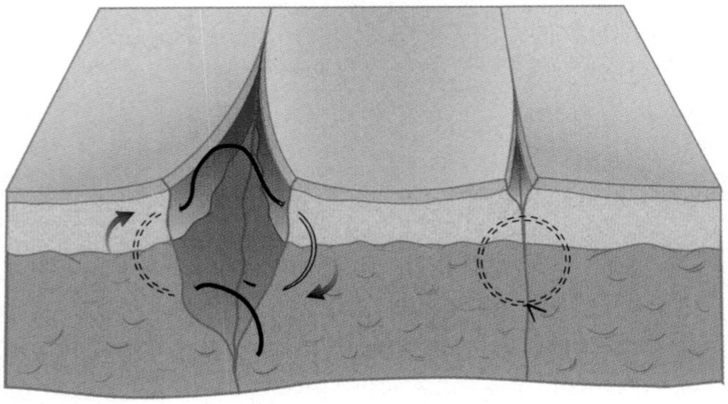

Figure 10–10 Buried suture.

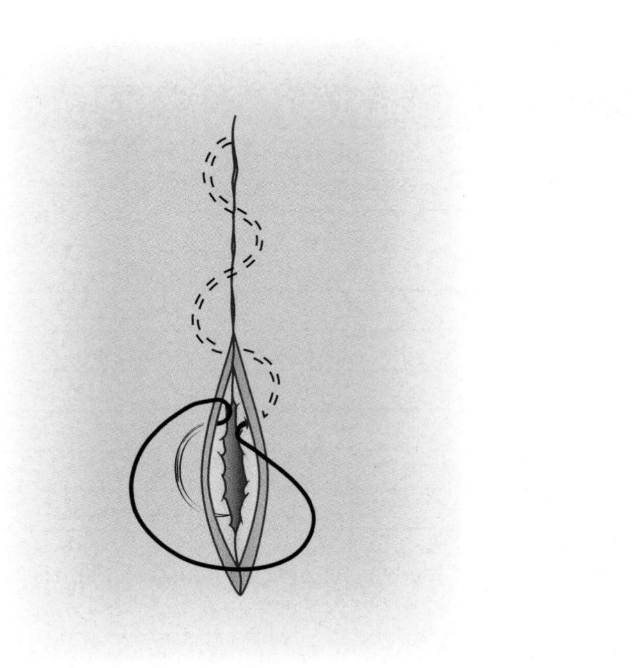

Figure 10–11 Running subcuticular sutures.

? Did You Know

Large wounds often require both buried, absorbable sutures as well as superficial, nonabsorbable ones.

A topical antibiotic ointment may assist in healing and keeping the wound surface moist to aid in the movement of migratory keratinocytes as they reepithelialize the wound. The client can apply the ointment lightly and cover it with semiporous, nonadherent gauze to absorb exudates, or he or she can apply it alone in a more generous amount. The client should remove and reapply the ointment according to the physician's instructions. This also gives the client an opportunity to cleanse the wound and check for signs of infection.

Bathing

During the initial phases of wound healing, the sebaceous gland's production of protective skin oils will decrease, resulting in decreased protection and increased water absorption by the healing tissue; however, there is minimal risk of contamination with "brief immersion" of wounds in soap and water after 24 hours.

Table 10–1 Recommended Suture Removal Based on Location

SUTURE LOCATION	SUTURE SIZE	RECOMMENDED REMOVAL
Scalp	3-0/4-0	7 to 12 days
Face	4-0 to 6-0	3 to 7 days
Ear	5-0/6-0	4 to 6 days
Neck	4-0/5-0	5 to 7 days
Chest		
Back	4-0/5-0	6 to 12 days
Abdomen		
Arms and legs	3-0 to 5-0	6 to 14 days
Oral cavity	*4-0*	
	(Absorbable)	*Absorbed*

Note: the higher the number of the suture material, the thinner it is.

Local Factors That Impair Wound Healing

Surgical Technique

- Rough handling of tissue may crush the wound edges and devitalize the tissue.
- Highly reactive suture material may increase inflammation and delay wound healing.
- Overly tight skin sutures may decrease blood flow through the capillaries in the dermis and cause tissue loss.

***Hematoma* Formation**

- Excessive bleeding can mechanically disrupt wound closure.
- Hematoma separates healing tissue from blood supply.
- Hematomas are an excellent culture medium for bacteria.

Wound Care

- Dryness of a wound will impair epithelial migration.
- Scabs inhibit healing and increase the distance epithelial cells must travel.

Foreign Bodies

- Foreign bodies prolong inflammation by attracting inflammatory cells.
- Necrotic tissue and pus contain proteolytic enzymes that damage cells and slow the healing process.
- Infection, which is defined as more than 10,000 organisms/gram of tissue, impairs healing by attracting inflammatory cells that compete for oxygen and nutrients, thereby damaging the cells/tissue.

Low Oxygen Delivery to the Tissue

- Decreases tissue growth
- Increases susceptibility to infection

Figure 10–12 Local factors that impair wound healing.

FYI

To understand brief immersion, think of washing hands versus doing dishes. Water immersion must be kept to a minimum.

Smoking and Healing

Nicotine decreases blood circulation in the skin and thus impairs blood flow to the tiny vessels that supply the dermis, causing delayed wound healing or complications, such as tissue loss and subsequent scarring. Therefore, smokers should not smoke for several weeks before and

Systemic Factors That Impair Wound Healing

Smoking

- Causes vasoconstriction, which decreases blood flow to wound
- Carbon monoxide preferentially binds hemoglobin, thereby reducing the delivery of oxygen to the wound

Circulatory Disease (atherosclerosis, congestive heart failure)

- Decreases delivery of oxygen, nutrients, and inflammatory mediators to the wound

Diabetes Mellitus

- Affects tiny blood vessels and thereby diminishes oxygen delivery to the tissues
- Insulin deficiency decreases white blood cell function
- Insulin deficiency impairs collagen synthesis
- Vitamin A supplements can decrease the effects of diabetes on wound healing

Diseases That Can Cause *Immunosuppression*

- Diabetes mellitus
- Liver failure
- Kidney failure
- Asplenism (no spleen)
- Alcoholism

Systemic Corticosteroids and Other Immunosuppressants

- Decreases the functioning of several cell types important in the healing
- Decreases epithelialization
- Decreases collagen production by fibroblasts
- Systemic vitamin A may reverse steroidal effect by promoting release of inflammatory mediators

Nutritional Deficiencies Such as Occur with Cancer or Alcoholism

- Protein deficiencies impair the proliferative phase of wound healing.
- Fatty acid deficiencies impair wound healing.
- Vitamin deficiencies (A, B, and C) impair wound healing.

Aging

- Fibroblastic activity decreases with age, reducing wound tensile strength.
- Increased proteolytic activity with aging results in greater tissue breakdown.
- Increased incidence of pulmonary and circulatory disease.

Figure 10–13 Systemic factors that impair wound healing.

after the medical procedure. Those who do not comply invariably have more trouble healing and end up with a less desirable result (Figure 10–13).

Sun Exposure and Wound Healing

Hyperpigmentation of a scar or wound can be avoided by staying out of the sun. Sunscreens are recommended once the skin has sealed, or about 7 to 10 days after initial treatment. Wide-rimmed hats and sunglasses are a must for patients who have had head, face, or neck surgery starting immediately after the surgery.

Nutritional Factors

It is important that a client consume an optimal diet and supplements prior to and following any invasive procedure. Deficiencies of vitamin A slow down the process of epithelization and the synthesis of collagen, and there is an increase of infection rates in clients who are low on these nutrients. If the client is lacking certain trace elements, including zinc, copper, iron, and manganese, the immune response and healing process will be affected. In addition, if the client has normal metabolic function and maintains adequate protein intake, the healing process is benefited.

Silicone Patches

Silicone patches have been tested extensively, and results show that when applied for at least 12 hours daily on both burns and incisions, they minimize scars and treat hypertrophic scaring. Results were visible in one to two months and remodeling continued for six months or more. The mechanism of how these silicone patches affect hypertrophic scars is not well understood but study continues. In the meantime these patches are being incorporated more and more to minimize scarring, especially in those individuals prone to it. The key to the success of these sheets seems to be in client education so that clients adhere to proper home use and wear the patches an adequate amount of time.

INJURIES FROM LASER AND OTHER TREATMENT THERAPIES

Most light therapy treatments do not result in injury to the client's skin beyond redness. The more aggressive the treatment is, however, the higher the level of skin trauma. Medical laser treatments such as CO_2 resurfacing are a controlled burn, and the client must follow strict home care to ensure a good result with no infection or scaring.

When properly done, esthetic therapies do not generate the intense heat associated with skin resurfacing. However, any light therapy treatment that heats the tissue may result in some localized redness for a couple of hours. Occasionally, a client will experience a mild burn, resulting in some crusting, which should be dealt with in the same way as any other burn appropriate for the severity of the wound (Figure 10–14). If the wound appears to be more than epidermal in nature, the client should be referred for medical attention to prevent scarring.

Pigmentation

Occasionally darker-skinned clients will respond to light therapies by hyperpigmenting. This is commonly treated with hydroquinone. There is also a risk of damage to melanocytes during the treatment, which can result in hypopigmentation (Figure 10–15).

Other Injuries from Light Therapy Treatments

Beyond a burn or hyperpigmentation, there is also the risk of a herpetic breakout if the area around the mouth is treated. To minimize this risk, advise the client to obtain and take an antiviral from his or her physician. Occasionally a client will respond to treatment with a mild to severe case of hives or stinging. There is also the risk of respiratory irritation from the inhalation of plume, the airborne result of light energy activity and the body. If the client experiences any of these side effects, refer the client to a physician for treatment.

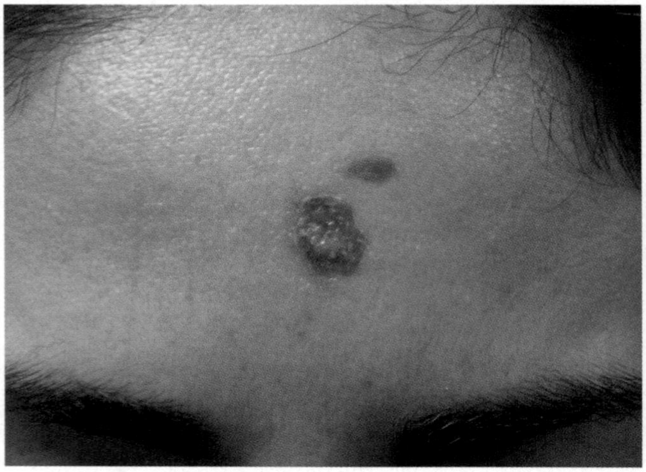

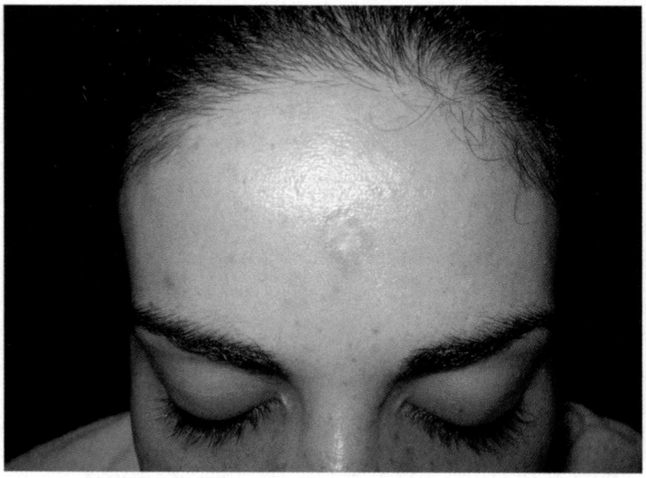

Figure 10–14 The result of epidermal separation and blistering.

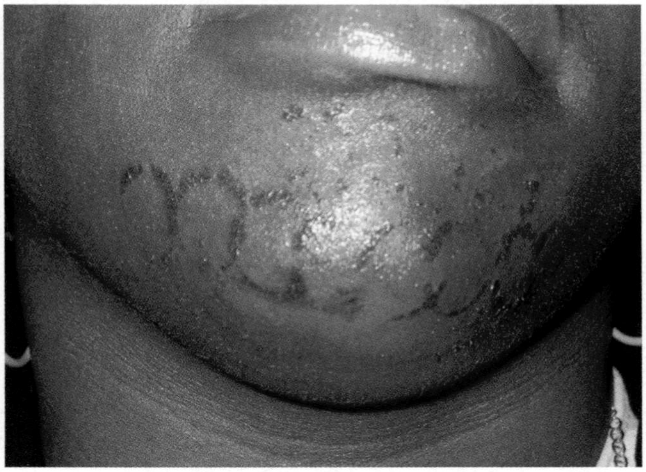

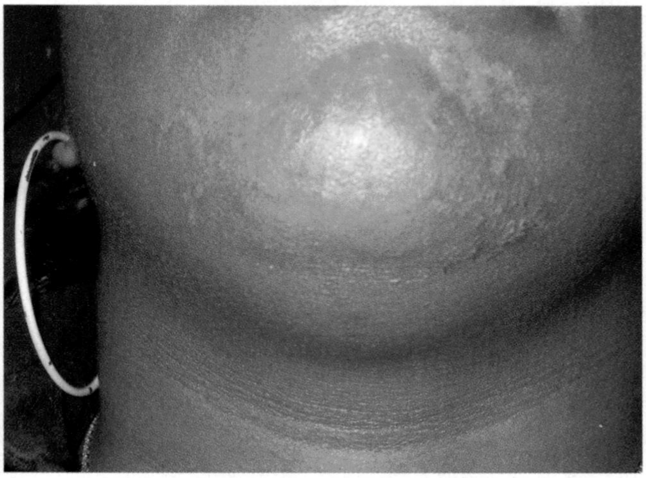

Figure 10–15 Hypopigmentation following laser hair removal.

SHORT-TERM SUN DAMAGE

Short-term sun damage is probably a misnomer. It refers to reddening of the skin as a result of too long an exposure—in short, a sunburn. Within a few days the redness will disappear and the skin may or may not take on a tan color as the result of melanocyte activity to protect the skin. But during these few days the skin is working overtime trying to repair itself as it undergoes the inflammation cascade.

As an esthetician, you already know that the sunburn has residual effects that may not show up until years later. Incidental exposure, regardless of duration, creates a cumulative effect that inevitably results in signs of accelerated aging. This being said, sunburns happen very frequently, especially during the summer months. They can be mild to severe. While the damage will be more evident on the lighter Fitzpatrick skin types, damage still does occur on darker skins. Not seeing redness on a Fitzpatrick V does not mean it may not be burned internally. With a burn the skin becomes very red, sore, and sensitive to the touch, caused by dilation of blood vessels and stimulation of nerve endings in the skin. The skin will eventually peel due to the extreme dryness associated with the sunburn. The skin literally bakes to a very dehydrated condition, just as cookies will burn and become dry if baked too long in the oven. Beyond the teen years when everyone seeks the golden tan, many people experience sunburns when they are out of their normal environment or are ignorant about sun protection. Whereas those from normally sunny areas are familiar with sun protection, those from cooler areas tend to overdo themselves in their exuberance to enjoy sunny warmth. Sunburns can also occur even on overcast days. People do not see the sun, so they assume they are "safe." Their skin temperature does not rise from solar heat so they do not realize until it is too late that UV rays certainly do penetrate clouds and can result in a nasty burn.

FOCUS ON: *Sunburn*

A sunburn is really a medical condition and therefore not the domain of the esthetician. Suggest cool packs, a cool bath with vinegar added to the water, applying plain yogurt to the area, or the use of over-the-counter anesthetic sprays, if the client is not allergic to them.

It is important that you are familiar with sun protection methods to help clients protect themselves from sunburn as well as from long- and short-term sun damage.

Other Short-Term Sun-Related Problems

Hyperpigmentation is both a long- and short-term cosmetic problem caused by the sun. It is dark splotching and is one of the first visible signs of skin aging. *Hyperpigmented* literally means "overpigmented."

Sun-induced skin discoloration begins in the late teens and early 20s and gets continually worse. Skin that has been repeatedly burned or has not healed from a sunburn before additional sun exposure is especially vulnerable. If you compare the skin of a 15-year-old to that of a 25-year-old, the biggest difference you will notice is in the skin pigmentation. The main noticeable difference between teenaged skin and skin in the early 20s is discoloration caused by deposits of melanin.

Almost completely caused by long-term sun exposure, chloasma, also known as liver spots, are directly related to cumulative sun exposure (Figure 10–16). These dark-brown patches, primarily on the face and hands, are areas of concentrated pigment. You may notice many clients do not exhibit hyperpigmentation on the body as much as they do on the face, décolleté, shoulders, arms, and hands. Although there are exceptions to this rule, these are areas that are chronically exposed to the sun for many years; hence, the pigmentation is much worse in these areas.

Hyperpigmentation may appear suddenly, especially on women, after years of sun exposure. It may first appear as subtle splotching that you may not notice when examining the skin under a magnifying lamp

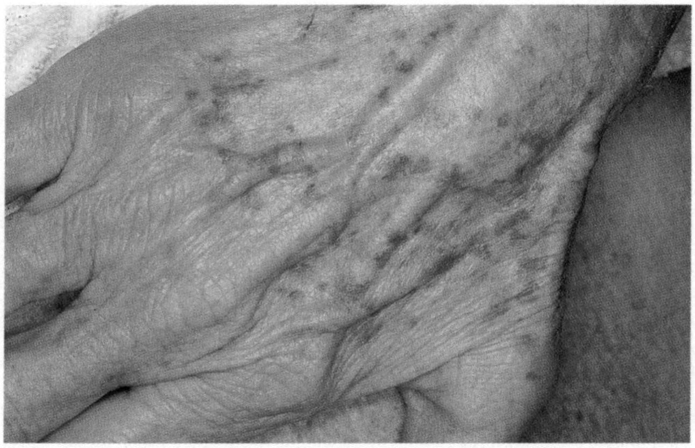

Figure 10–16 Chloasma is concentrated melanin caused by sun damage.

or, especially, a Wood's lamp. From this relatively mild splotching, darker, larger splotches may develop.

Tinea versicolor is what many refer to as sun spots or sun fungus. These white splotches, which usually appear on the chests and backs of avid sunbathers, are actually a fungal condition. The fungus interferes with the melanocytes' ability to make melanin, which causes the white splotches to appear when the body is tanned. Refer clients with this condition to a dermatologist for treatment (Figure 10–17).

The Real Damage from the Sun

Continual exposure to sun results in the formation of more and more damaging free radicals. Although not visible at the time or even for years, the routine damage to the cells eventually accumulates, resulting in wrinkles, hyperpigmentation, elastosis, and rough-textured skin.

Sun-exposed skin falls victim to the inflammation cascade, resulting in breakdown of collagen and elastin due to self-destruct enzymes manufactured through the immune system's defense against the sun exposure and damage to the cells of the skin. When enough damage occurs, it becomes visible in the skin's appearance.

What You Do Not Know about Short-Term Sun Exposure

We now know that sun exposure may actually suppress the immune functions of the skin. Exposure to sunlight "chases off" your protective macrophage "guard cells," the Langerhans, allowing substances and organisms to enter the skin, increasing the chance of infection. A good example of this immune suppression is the flare-up of herpes simplex that occurs in some individuals when they are exposed to the sun. Many cases of lupus, an autoimmune disease, are diagnosed after a sunburn, when the immune system has overreacted to the injury.

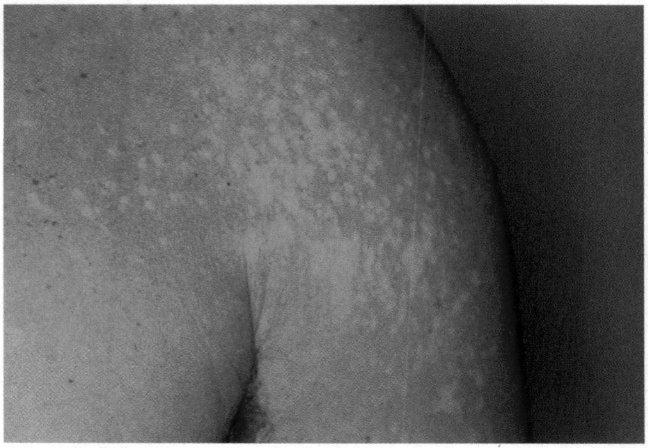

Figure 10–17 Tinea versicolor.

? Did You Know

Have you ever noticed how many people get colds after a vacation where they got too much sun? Without the Langerhans cells on guard duty, it is much easier to catch a cold.

It is so important to teach young children to use sunscreen daily. Humans receive about 80% of the sun's damage to the skin in childhood and adolescence. Sun freckles appearing on teenagers represent problem areas in the future. Most sun exposure is not from sunbathing but from day-to-day exposure. Think abut how many children play outdoors. Every time they go outside, they expose themselves to harmful UV rays. That's why every time they go outdoors they should be protected with a good sunscreen. Sunscreen is not just for summer; it is for use year-round.

LONG-TERM PHOTOAGING

Almost every skin symptom connected to aging is directly related to sun exposure. Some researchers have proposed that a "wrinkle" is not a "normal" skin condition. It is sun damage that would not exist without UV exposure. Even intrinsic aging symptoms, such as facial expression lines, are made worse because of sun damage. Hyperpigmentation, leathery texture, roughness, wrinkles, some forms of hypopigmentation, severe elastosis, chest and cleavage wrinkling, splotchiness, couperose and telangiectasias, flares of rosacea, neck texture problems, severe dehydration, and barrier function problems are all directly related to sun exposure.

For some clients sun exposure is a lifestyle, and the results of that lifestyle have generated the medical term **dermatoheliosis** to describe long-term damage to the

FYI

Wrinkles are not "normal." They are the result of cumulative sun damage. This means that with good sun protection and good skin care at an early age, they can be prevented.

skin caused by UV. Collagen and elastin fibrils in the dermis begin a process called **cross-linking,** collapsing due to cumulative effects of cell damage from repeated sun exposure, causing the support system for the skin to also collapse. Esthetically, this results in deep wrinkling of the skin, sagging, and elastosis.

Sun-damaged skin appears much more severely aged than skin that has aged solely from intrinsic factors. The wrinkling does not only appear in expression lines. Many lines develop in all areas and in all directions. Wrinkles may be both horizontal and vertical. Normal expression lines are much deeper in sun-damaged skin (Figure 10–18).

The abnormal structure of the dermis and epidermis give the skin a "leathery" appearance and feel. This type of skin is also severely discolored due to melanin deposits and hyperpigmentation. The skin of a person with sun damage is very rough to the touch, and the surface is actually uneven. This is caused by damage to the cells, which causes the corneum and other epidermal cells not to shed in a normal, even manner. This is due to the altering of the DNA from chronic sun exposure. The cells become "confused," divide unevenly, and no longer retain their normal shape. In a cross section of normal skin, the cells in the epidermis form layers that look like layers of brick in a brick wall. In sun-damaged skin, the same structure looks like a brick wall that is collapsing, made with uneven bricks that are poorly made. The epidermis of sun-damaged skin becomes progressively thinner, and the dermis slowly begins to atrophy or collapse and fall apart. This is how the sun eventually destroys the skin.

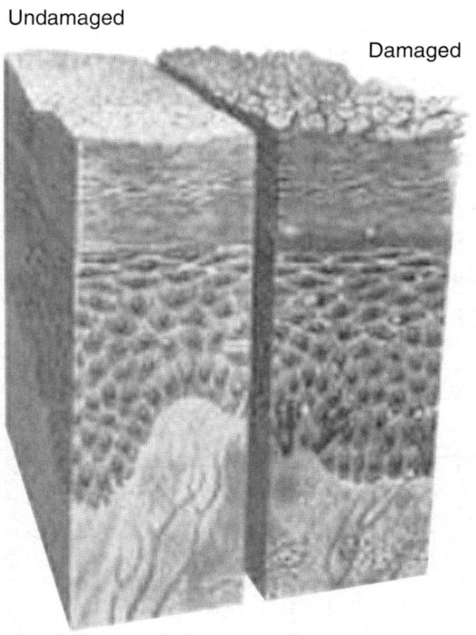

Figure 10–18 Cross section of healthy epidermis and a sun-damaged epidermis.

Clients with sun damage have multiple wrinkles, not just around the eyes and neck, but all over the face. They have many more pronounced wrinkles than other clients do. Their skin is literally a multitude of uneven colors, very freckled. The skin has a leathery look and feel. There may be patches of dryness, and clients may complain about how dry their skin is. The truth is that as the skin cells become disfigured, they also fail to produce sufficient amounts of intercellular cement, causing an impaired barrier function and making proper hydration of the skin practically impossible.

Sun-damaged skin may also have many telangiectasias or couperose areas. Sun damage also causes the collapse of some of the blood vessels and decreased blood flow. The small capillaries look like tributaries of a river. These vessels may be very fragile, and bruises may appear easily. You may notice how easily some of your older clients bruise. Although this may be due to many medical factors, sun-damaged skin bruises much more easily than normal, healthy nondamaged skin. You will also notice that these clients who bruise easily have very thin-looking, dry, hyperpigmented skin. This is because the skin is almost always severely sun damaged.

SKIN CANCERS

Skin cancer is caused by cells dividing unevenly and rapidly, while the genetic material in the cells' DNA is damaged by the sun. When first exposed to UV, the melanocyte responds by sending melanin to surrounding cells. The melanin situates itself between the cell nucleus and the source of the UV in an effort to protect it from "sun strikes" and damage. Think of it as putting on a sun hat when going outdoors. If the UV gets past the melanin and damages the cell, this can cause incomplete information or misinformation to be transmitted to the cell when it divides. It is a damaged cell. If the cell is re-damaged while it is still recuperating (as in the case of a sunburn), it can cause further cellular damage or even apoptosis—programmed cell death—to prevent the formation of a mutant cell and possibly the small tumors we know as skin cancer. There are three major kinds of skin cancer: basal cell, squamous cell, and melanoma.

CAUTION!

Estheticians' scope of practice does not include diagnosing skin cancer. However, you should know the signs of the major forms of skin cancer and be able to refer clients with suspicious-looking lesions and areas to a dermatologist.

Basal Cell Carcinomas

Basal cell carcinomas are the most common kind of skin cancers. They are almost always found on the sun-exposed areas, typically on the face, hands, legs, back, and chest. They look like small pearls. Sometimes they have a small blood vessel running through them. They are not usually perfectly round like a milium. On older hyperpigmented skin, they may be hard to differentiate from milia. You must look carefully to tell the difference (Figure 10–19).

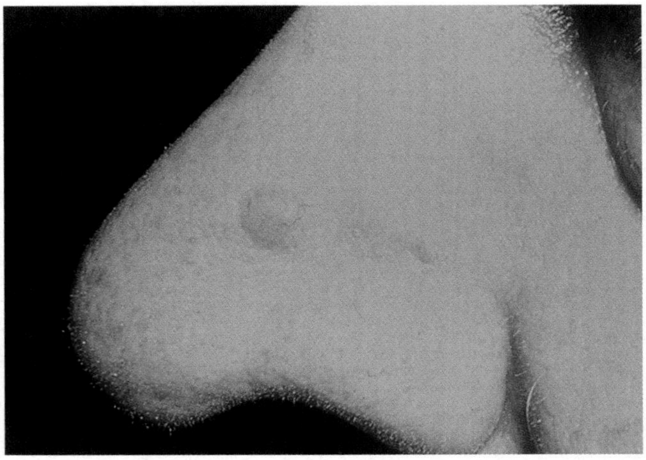

Figure 10–19 Basal cell carcinoma.

Basal cell carcinomas are very often curable and are treated either by surgical or laser excision or by **cryotherapy** (freezing). In fact, 95% of these cancers are cured and there is a 99% survival rate after five years. They rarely spread to the internal parts of the body, but they can grow, and if they are not treated, they can affect large areas of the skin.

Squamous Cell Carcinomas

Squamous cell carcinomas are the second most frequently diagnosed form of skin cancer. They may look like red or pink solid bumps on the skin. They may appear as open sores or ulcers that do not seem to heal. They may look crusty, or they may be a crusty area that bleeds easily (Figure 10–20). Many clients notice this when washing or cleansing the face. Again, these lesions appear on

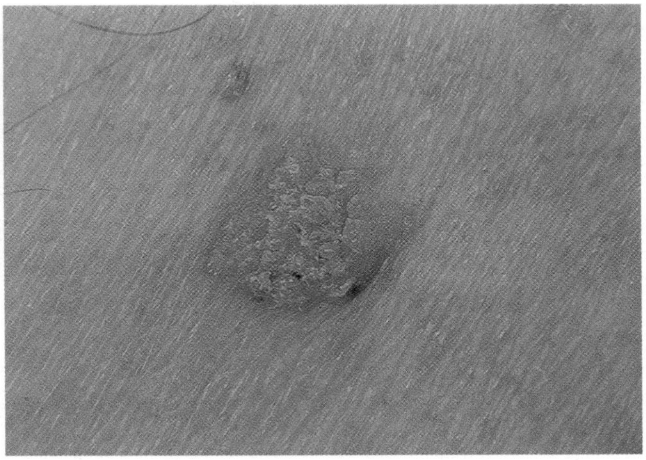

Figure 10–20 Squamous cell carcinoma.

chronically sun-exposed areas. Treatment is similar to treatment for basal cell carcinoma, but squamous cell carcinoma may sometimes spread to other areas of the body. In Mohs' surgery—a specialized surgical technique, named after its developer, Frederic Mohs, M.D.—the dermatologist trims more and more tissue from the cancer lesion, carefully checking each sample of tissue for cancerous cells using a microscope until all of the cancerous tissue is removed.

Melanomas

The least frequently seen form of skin cancer is also the most deadly. Melanoma is characterized by moles or mole-like lesions that are dark in color.

FOCUS ON: *The ABCDEs of Skin Cancer*

- A **stands for** asymmetric. **The melanoma lesion is usually growing to one side of the lesion and is uneven.**
- B **stands for** border. **The borders of melanomas are uneven and not smooth.**
- C **is for** color. **Melanomas are often dark brown and black and are usually splotchy and not of one color.**
- D **stands for** diameter. **Melanomas are usually at least the size of a pencil eraser or larger. Regular moles are usually smaller than this.**
- E **(a new addition) stands for** evolving **moles. Changes may include darkening or variations in color, moles that itch or hurt, and changes in the shape or growth of the mole.**

The Skin Cancer Foundation has coined an expression that is easy to remember when looking at suspicious lesions (Figure 10–21). They call this the ABCDEs of Melanoma (see the box on page 214).

Melanomas can be found on any area of the body but are most likely, again, to be found on areas that have had repeated sun exposure. They are most typically found on individuals with a history of sunburn and light-skinned individuals.

Skin Cancer Treatment

After a dermatologist treats skin cancer, he or she may suggest that the client not have skin care treatments until the lesion is healed completely. As a general rule, a client should not have a facial treatment if there are still sutures present in a treated lesion. Clients being treated with fluorouracil (sometimes sold under the brand name Efudex®) should not have facial treatments until the

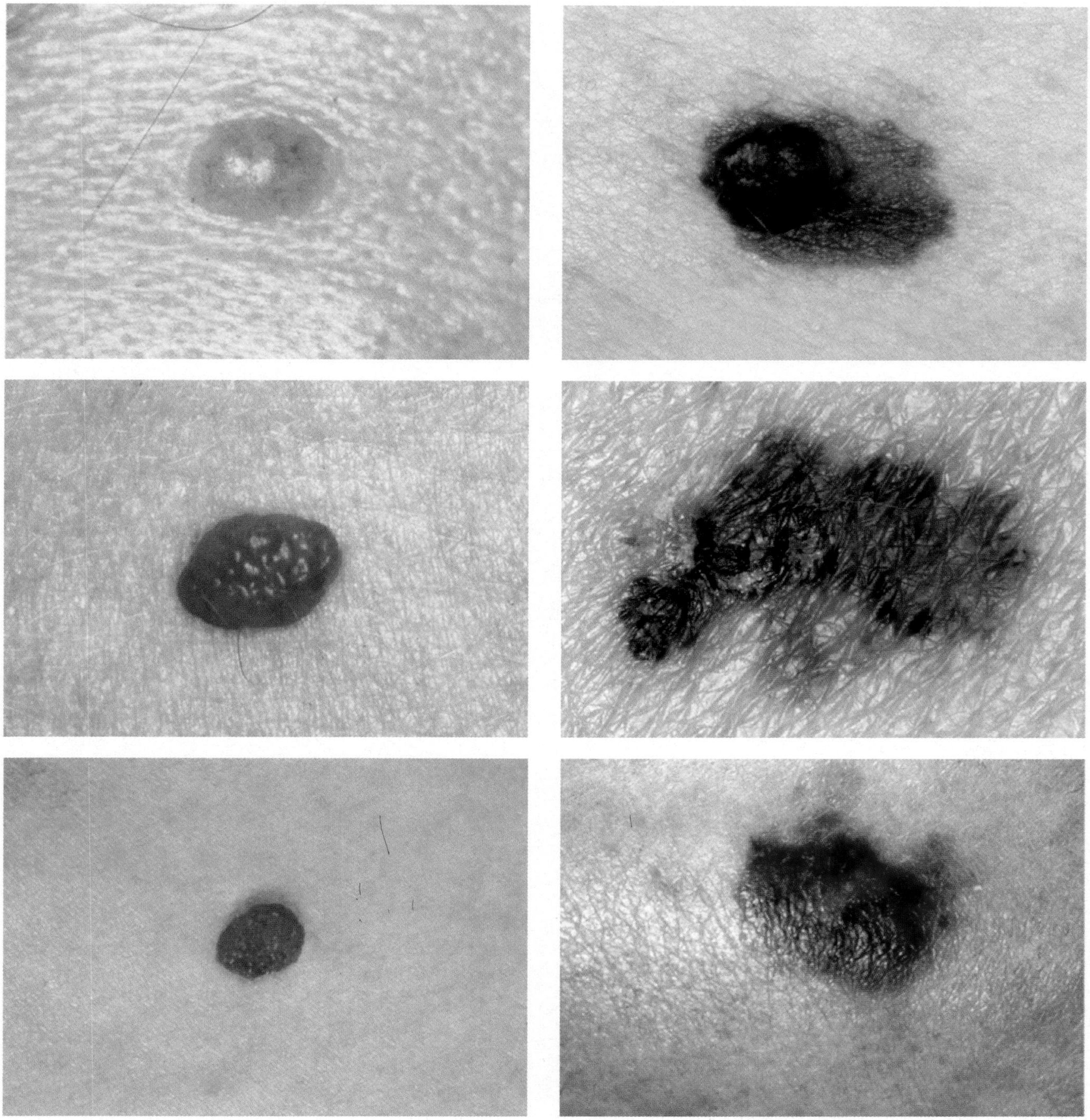

Figure 10–21 Suspicious lesions.

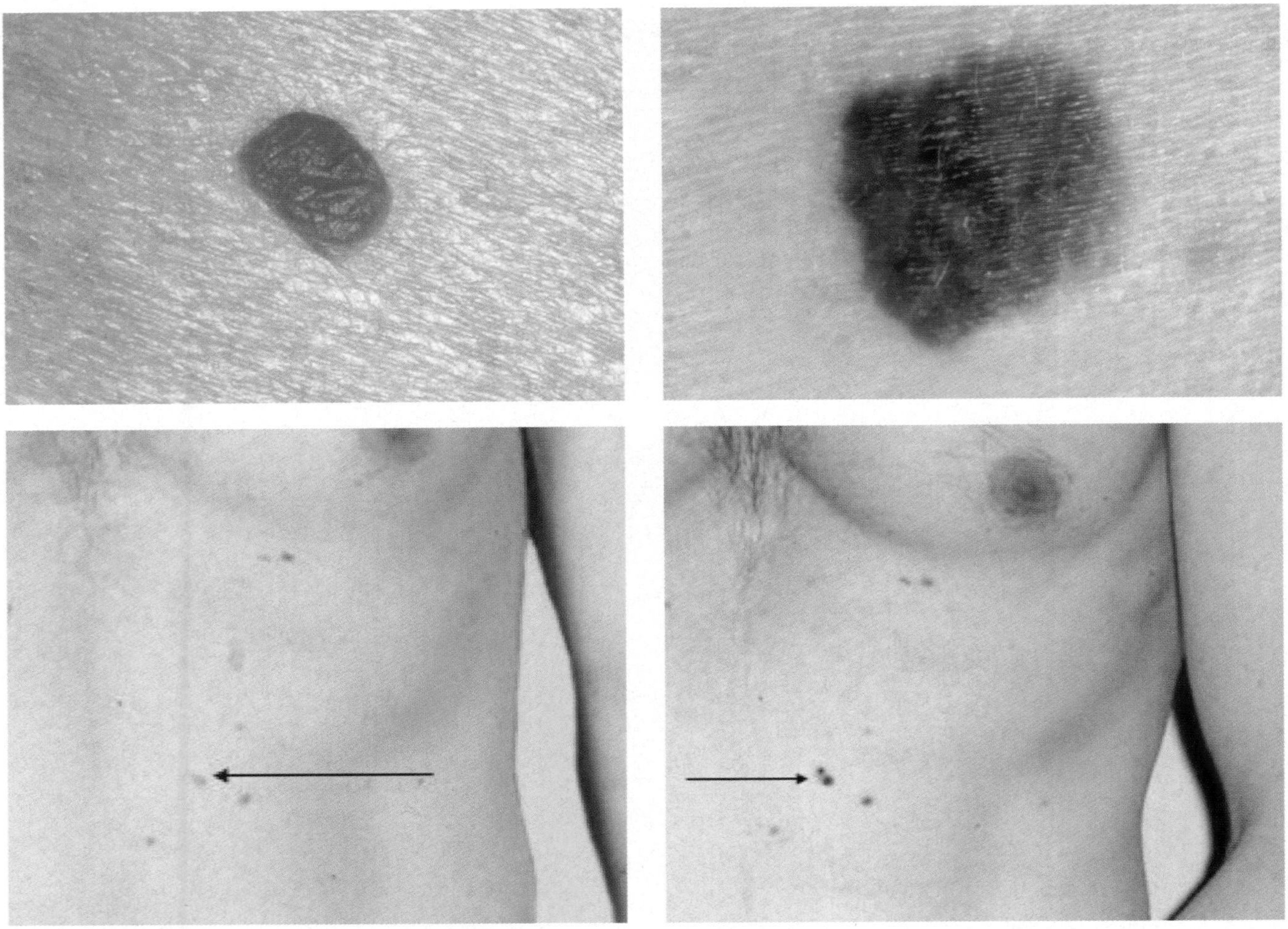

Figure 10–21 (*continued*).

therapy is completed, unless approved by the dermatologist, who may occasionally refer such a client for help with side effects. Make sure you have been properly trained by the doctor before treating these clients.

Other forms of growth treatment, such as electrosurgery or cryosurgery, generally do not cause any problem for treatment, except that facial treatment should not be performed until the lesion is healed or unless the doctor advises otherwise. Avoid these areas completely, and simply treat the rest of the untreated areas of the face. If you have any questions, contact the dermatologist, and remember—when in doubt, do not!

OTHER SUN-RELATED SKIN GROWTHS

Actinic Keratosis

Actinic keratosis are rough areas of sun-damaged skin, indicated by dysplastic cell growth. **Dysplastic** means abnormal growth. Actinic keratoses are frequently found on the faces of individuals who have had chronic sun exposure. They are also prevalent in light-skinned individuals. They are rough patches of skin and can be crusty, scaly, and rough to the touch. Sometimes they feel like small needles or splinters sticking out of the skin when they are touched with the fingers. They frequently occur in small groups or patches. Because they are dysplasic cells, they can become cancerous and are often referred to as pre-cancers (Figure 10–22).

FOCUS ON: *Moles*

Unusual-looking moles or moles that are changing should be checked by a dermatologist. If you or your client notices changes in a wart or mole, refer the client to a dermatologist for diagnosis and treatment.

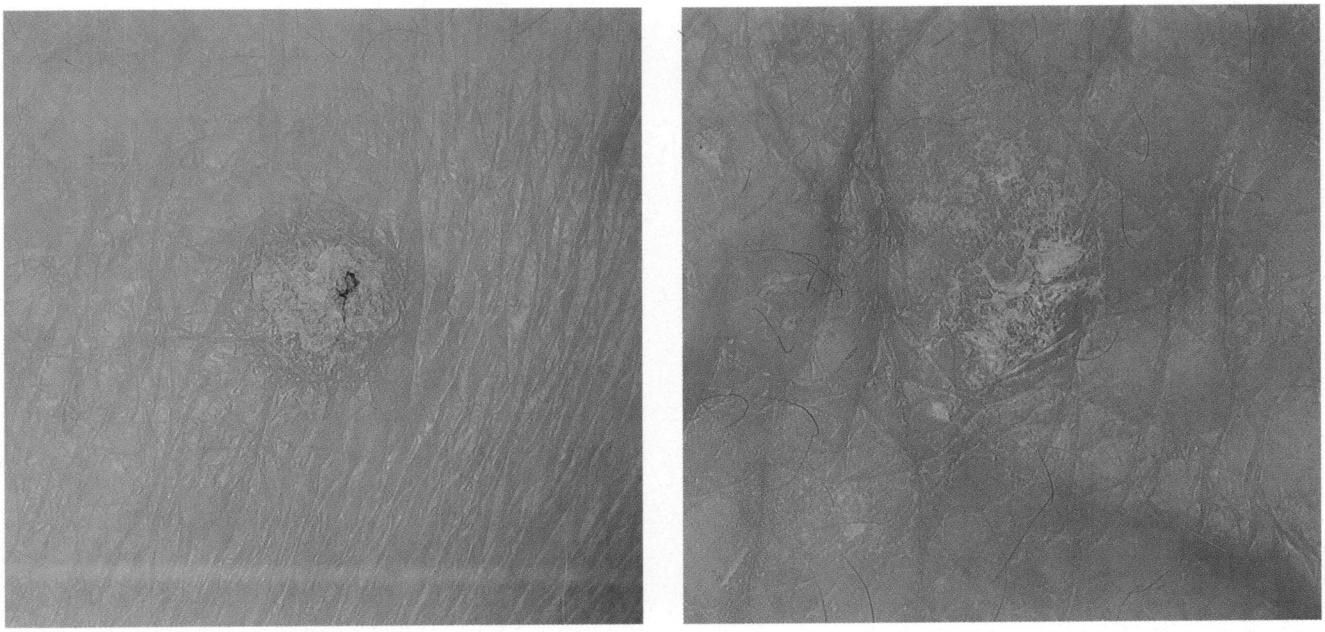

Figure 10–22 Actinic keratosis is frequently seen in sun-damaged clients.

Actinic keratoses may be treated surgically with cryotherapy (freezing with liquid nitrogen), or with chemical therapy with a chemical called florouracil (also commercially known as Efudex®). Unusual-looking moles or moles that are changing should be checked by a dermatologist. If you or the client notices changes in a wart or mole, refer the client to a dermatologist for diagnosis and treatment.

Sebaceous Hyperplasias

Sebaceous hyperplasias are small, donut-shaped lesions that often look like large, open comedones (also called *blackheads*) surrounded by a ridge of skin. Clients may come to you seeking the extraction of their "blackheads." Upon inspection, you will see it is not really a comedo but sun damage. *Sebaceous hyperplasia* actually means "overgrown oil glands." They are frequently seen on oily skins that have had repeated sun exposure, but they can appear on any skin, usually on someone 25 years old and older. You will frequently find them on the forehead and temples, although they may appear anywhere on the face. Sebaceous hyperplasias are beign lesions that rarely cause any problems, except esthetically. They are rarely removed surgically, because the scar from excision is usually worse than the appearance of the lesion. Sebaceous hyperplasia can be treated with electrodessication with an electric needle or sometimes cryosurgery. This helps flatten the lesion, but it may need to be retreated periodically, because the oil glands are deep within the skin and will continue growing. Estheticians frequently see sebaceous hyperplasias, and clients are often concerned about them.

Seborrheic Keratoses

Seborrheic keratoses are large, flat, crusty-looking, brown, black, yellowish, or gray lesions that are often found on the faces of older, sun-damaged clients. They are frequently found on the temples or cheekbones, although they can appear anywhere on the skin. They look almost like a scab, and clients will sometimes pick at them, which they obviously should not do. They are usually harmless growths but can occasionally turn into other more serious lesions, such as basal cell carcinomas. They are treated by a dermatologist, usually by curettage, in which a curette, a small, scoop-like instrument, is used to "scoop" the lesion off the face. Seborrheic keratoses are more of a cosmetic nuisance than anything else in most cases. Nevertheless, they should be referred to a dermatologist for treatment. Also, they may indicate other areas or other forms of sun damage that may require treatment.

Solar Freckles

Solar freckles, or lentigenes, are also known as *liver spots*. They are clumps of hyperpigmentation caused by sun exposure. They can appear on any area but frequently appear on the face and hands. These can be treated by an esthetician, and more severe cases can be treated by a dermatologist.

ACNE

Acne is a distressed skin condition that results in inflammatory and noninflammatory lesions. Commonly associated with teenage and adolescent skin, it actually affects many age groups at different stages of life. An esthetician sees acne and acne-related conditions every day. Although many forms of acne require the care of a dermatologist, many clients can benefit from esthetic treatments for problem skin.

The most common form of acne is called *acne vulgaris*. This is the type of acne often associated with teenagers. It usually begins at the onset of puberty, at which time teenagers begin producing larger amounts of sex hormones. (See Chapter 4 on hormones.) These hormones stimulate the sebaceous gland, which produces an overabundance of sebum.

Hereditary Factors in Acne

We inherit certain genes from our parents that determine how our bodies and our skin function and behave. These are known as *hereditary factors*. If either parent had acne or excessively oily skin, there is a good chance that the child will have a strong tendency to develop acne.

There are two major factors in acne development that are hereditary. As we learned in Chapter 3, the epidermal cells, particularly the corneum, are constantly shedding and being replaced by younger cells. Retention hyperkeratosis is a hereditary condition in which these cells are retained. The dead cells stick to the surface of the skin and begin lining the inside walls of the follicle ("cell buildup"). Much like wax tends to build up on the surface of furniture, the cells inside the follicle build up.

This process of buildup is complicated by the fact that the cells continue to push to the surface of the epidermis at a faster rate. *Hyper* means more than normal, so hyperkeratosis means the process of keratinization (turnover of cells) occurs at a rate much faster than normal.

Some researchers believe that retention hyperkeratosis is caused by an inability of the body to produce intercellular structures called *lamellar granules*. It is thought that these granules release an enzyme that causes dead cells to break away from the corneum in the normal manner. It has been determined that chronic acne patients do not have as many of these active structures present in their follicular cells.

The second major hereditary factor in the tendency to develop acne is oiliness. The amount of sebum produced by the skin is largely hereditary. People who have acne or excessively oily skin have inherited this tendency. The excessive sebum "bathes" and "waxes over" the cell buildup. The sebum becomes sticky and solidifies, much like the fat in chicken broth hardens and solidifies when it is refrigerated.

When enough cells and waxy sebum build up in the bottom of the follicle, they form a small impaction called a *microcomedo*. Microcomedones (plural) are a mixture of dead cell buildup, bacteria, fatty acids from the sebum, and other cellular debris. They are the beginning phase of any acne lesion. Microcomedones cannot be seen on the surface of the skin. They are deep in the follicles and can only be seen by microscopic examination of skin tissues (Figure 10–23).

Noninflammatory and Inflammatory Acne Lesions

As microcomedones continue to retain more and more dead cells and are coated by more and more sebum, they develop into larger, visible acne lesions. They may become either inflammatory or noninflammatory lesions. Inflammatory acne lesions are, like they sound, inflamed, meaning that they are red and swollen lesions.

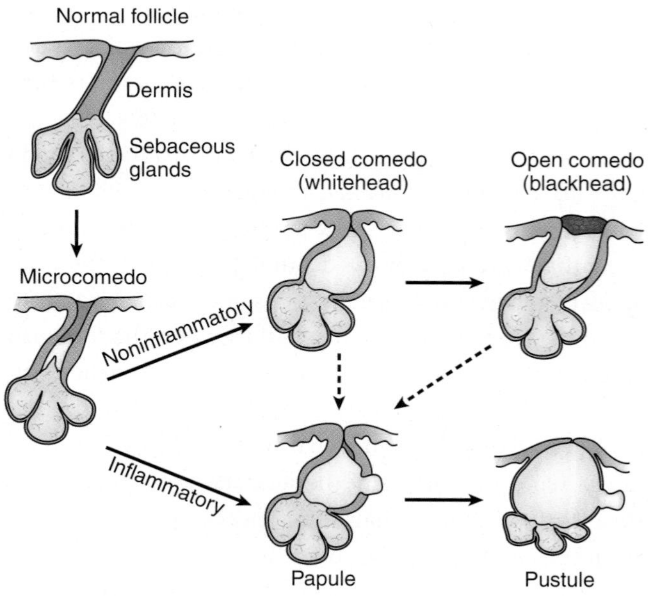

Figure 10–23 The progression of acne.

A typical acne pimple is an inflammatory lesion. Noninflammatory lesions are not red or inflamed. Examples of noninflammatory acne lesions are **open comedones** (blackheads) and **closed comedones** (whiteheads) (Figure 10–24).

Open comedones occur when the follicle is large enough to hold all of the debris retained by the follicle. The **ostium**, or opening, in these follicles is dilated by the mass of the impaction, allowing the comedo to push toward the surface opening.

Propionibacterium acnes (P. acnes) is the scientific name of the bacteria that causes acne vulgaris. These bacteria are anaerobic, which means they cannot survive in the presence of oxygen. These bacteria are constantly present in all follicles in small numbers. They are kept from reproducing in large numbers by the oxygen that is constantly aerating the open follicle. However, when the follicle is blocked from oxygen circulation, these bacteria multiply in great numbers, feeding off the sebum produced by overactive sebaceous glands (Figure 10–25). Open comedones do not encourage development of this bacterial growth because the follicle opening is large enough to expose the follicle to oxygen. The oxygen is also what causes the "blackhead" to form at the exposed part of the impaction. This darkening is caused by the exposure of the top of the comedo to the oxygen in the air outside the follicle. The sebum turns a brown color, similar to the way mayonnaise will turn yellow if left out on a picnic table for a period of time. The darkness is also caused by clumps of melanin (skin pigment) present in the dead cells in the comedo. This theory is easily demonstrated by observing an extracted open comedo. It is a solid cylindrical plug, topped by a dark area that gets lighter as the deeper parts of the impaction are extracted.

Open comedones, therefore, rarely develop into inflammatory lesions. Unfortunately, the same cannot be said for closed comedones. Closed comedones have very small pore openings, which prevents oxygen from

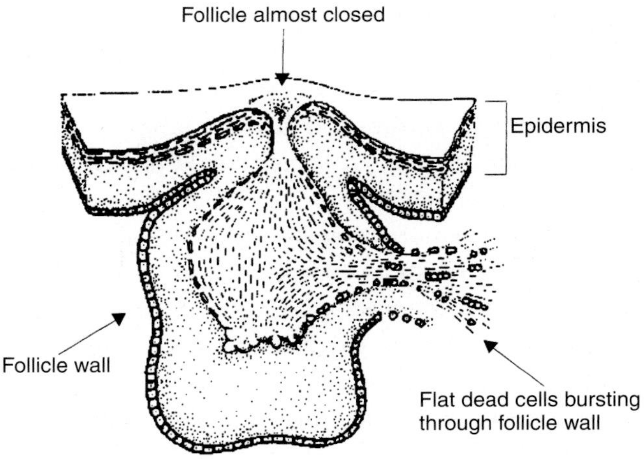

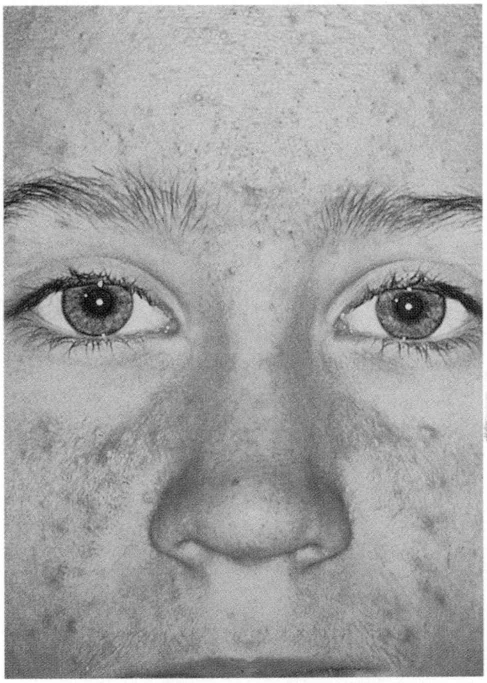

Figure 10–25 Development of acne in a young girl.

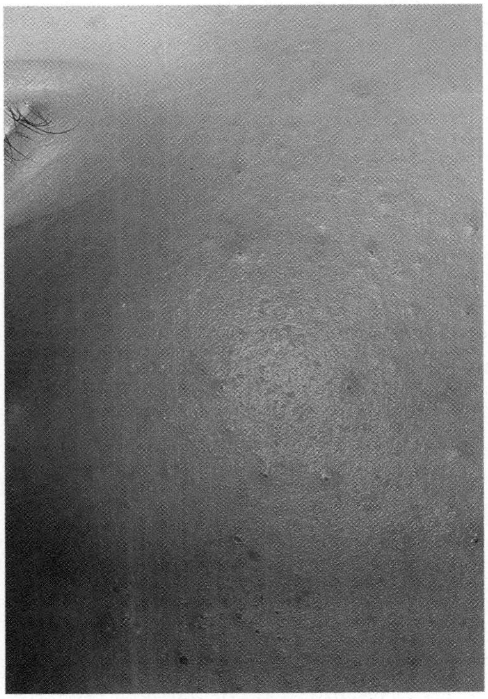

Figure 10–24 Open and closed comedones.

readily penetrating the follicle. The walls of the follicle stretch to hold the contents of the impaction, but the follicle opening does not. Because of this lack of oxygen, the lesions can easily become inflamed due to the increasing number of bacteria multiplying in the anaerobic environment.

Closed comedones are easily recognizable. They are frequently seen in adult women, often in the blush line of makeup users. They are small "underground" bumps and are not easily extracted. They are frequently associated with the use of comedogenic cosmetics.

When enough bacteria form inside the closed comedo and the impaction becomes large enough, a small tear occurs in the follicle wall, which stimulates the immune system to investigate, releasing white blood cells into the area. These white blood cells arrive via the blood vessels, causing the lesion to become red. This is an inflammatory lesion.

A papule is a red, sore bump without a "whitehead," the beginning of the "rescue" by the white blood cells. When enough white blood cells arrive, they may form a "clump" and rise to the surface, creating what is known as a *pustule* (Figure 10–26), the common name for this "clump" of white blood cells. For practical purposes, a papule is often described by the client as a large, red,

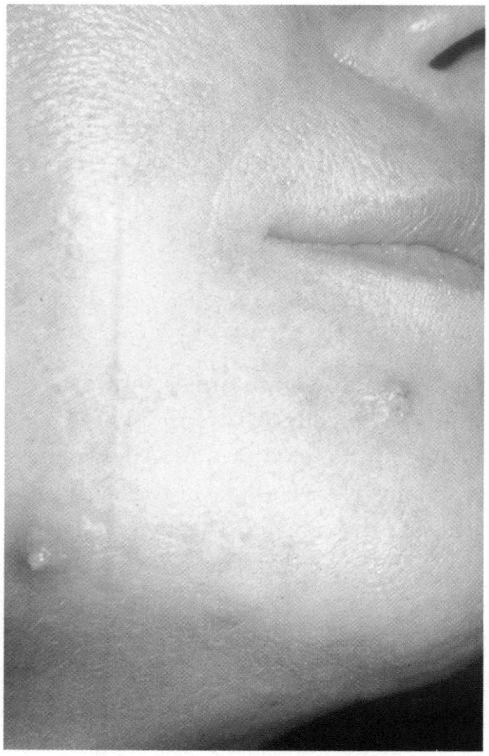

Figure 10–26 The pustule.

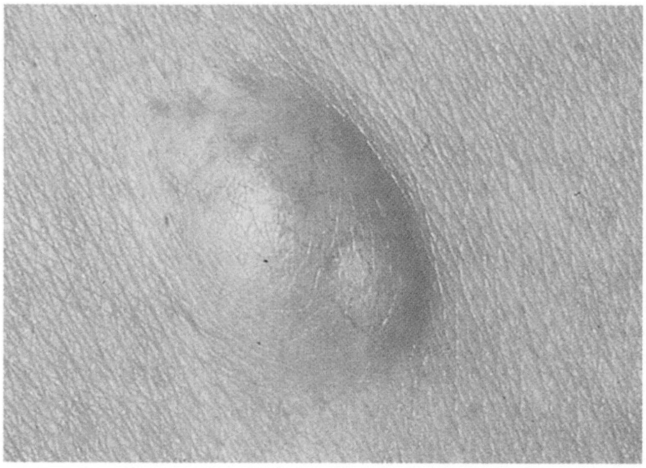

Figure 10–27 Cyst.

sore bump that never "comes to a head." Papules seem sometimes to "magically disappear." This is because the immune system has "won the battle" and disposed of the impaction through enzymes and absorption, and the body has disposed of the remains through normal blood excretion. Papules affect the nerve endings more than pustules because they are deeper in the skin. This explains the soreness. Pustules have "migrated" the impaction toward the skin surface, dilating the follicle opening and relieving the pressure on the nerve endings, resulting in less pain.

A nodule is similar to a papule, but it is deeper in the skin and feels very solid and sore. Cysts are deep infections caused by a deep, massive invasion of white blood cells (Figure 10-27). They are very pustular and very large. It is important to refer dermal cysts and nodules to a dermatologist for treatment.

The Grades of Acne

Acne is "graded" by dermatologists on a four-point scale (Figure 10–28):

GRADE 1 ACNE: Mostly open and closed comedones with an occasional pimple. Grade 1 acne is typical of a teenager just beginning puberty.

100

GRADE 2 ACNE: Very large number of closed comedones, with occasional pustules or papules.

GRADE 3 ACNE: Thought of by most people as "typical teenage acne." Very inflamed and red, it involves a large number of open and closed comedones and many papules and pustules as well.

GRADE 4 ACNE: Commonly referred to as cystic acne, with many deep cysts and scar formation (Refer the client to a physician.)

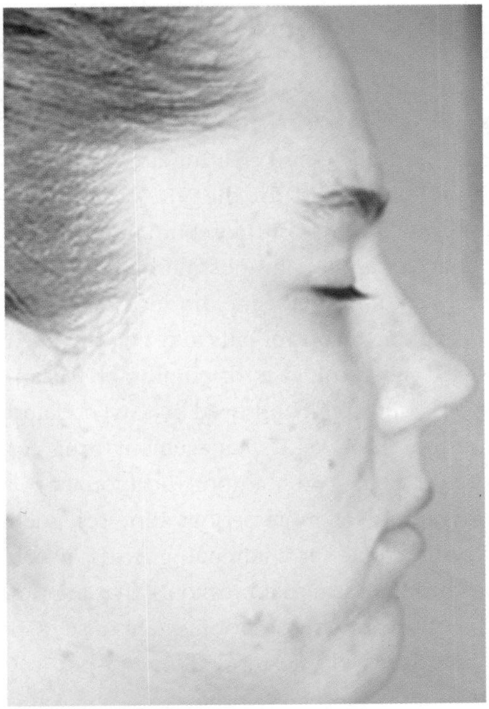

Grade 1

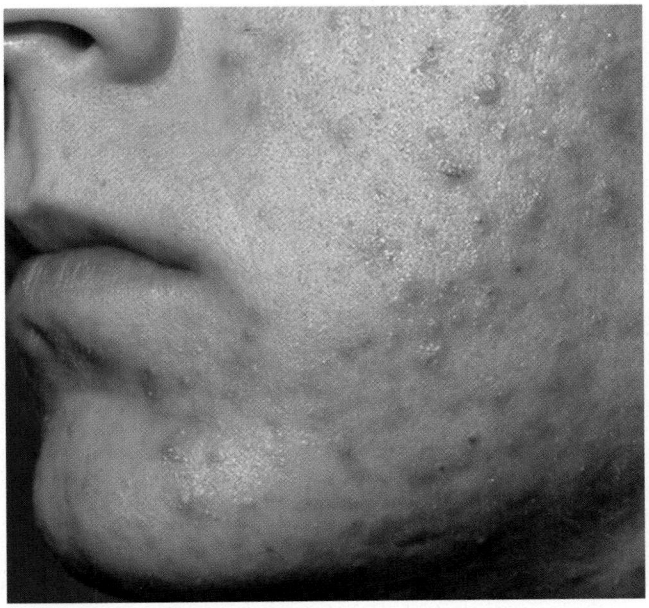

Grade 3

Grade 2

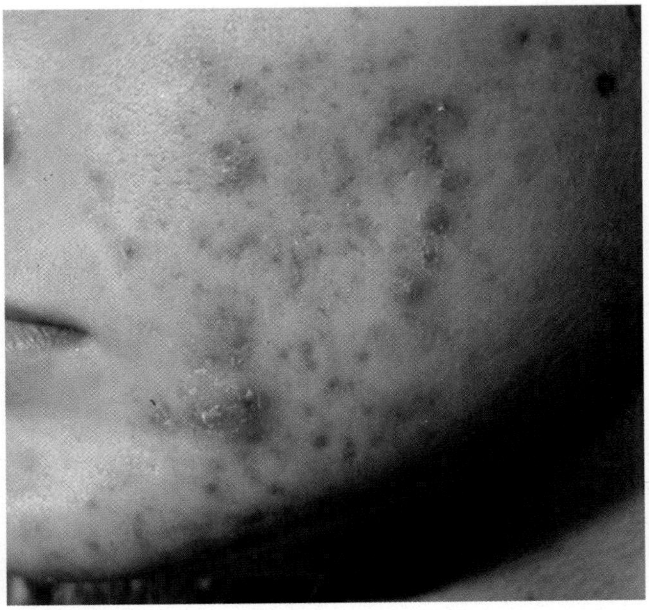

Grade 4

Figure 10–28 The grades of acne.

Why Scars Form

Scars form when the skin, in a desperate attempt to heal itself, produces lots of collagen to try to compensate for the lack of normal skin functioning. This type of scar is usually raised. Acne "pit" scarring occurs from actual destruction of the tissue during the inflammatory process. Cystic acne is almost always associated with scarring (Figure 10–29).

Hormones

As discussed in Chapter 4, males and females produce both male and female hormones, which are transported around the body via the circulatory system. Hormones, specifically male hormones, or androgens, are the mechanisms that cause stimulation of the sebaceous glands, which, in turn, produce more sebum. This sebum causes inflammation in the follicles, coating the

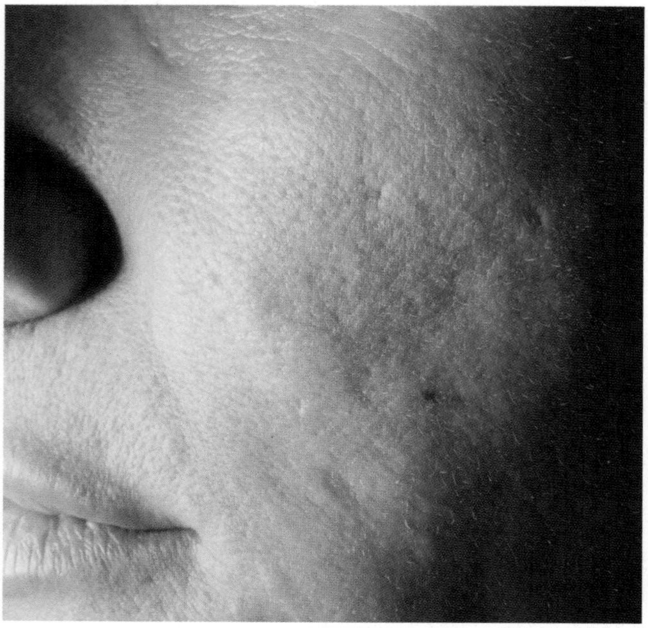

Figure 10–29 Cystic acne scarring.

cell buildup and providing a source of fatty acids, which is the food of *P. acnes* bacteria.

Testosterone, an androgen, converts to **dihydrotestosterone (DHT),** another form of male hormone, which "switches on" the oil gland. The oil gland is stimulated via receptor sites on the cells of the sebaceous glands, which are little "switches" that are "turned on" by hormonal stimulation.

Premenstrual, Hormonal, and Adult Acne

Premenstrual acne flares are often referred to as *adult acne*. Often, women who have never had problems with acne as a teenager suddenly develop a problem in their 20s or 30s. Although this can be related to comedogenic cosmetics, stress, and hereditary acne factors, hormones play a significant role in adult female acne.

Again, flares of the male hormone, or androgen, in the bloodstream cause this type of flare-up. Premenstrual flares are caused by a sudden predominance of androgen, which corresponds with the eventual loss of the egg during menses.

The elevation of testosterone in the bloodstream begins 8 to 10 days before a woman's period. This elevation is actually not an increase in androgen as much as a decrease in the female hormone estrogen. Nevertheless, there is suddenly a larger percentage of androgen in the bloodstream and therefore a sudden likely increase in stimulation of the sebaceous glands.

A sudden flow of sebum in the follicle causes **perifollicular inflammation,** inflammation around the inside of the follicle. This irritation causes swelling inside the follicle, decreasing the flow of oxygen to the lower part of the follicle and creating an "anaerobic pocket," an ideal environment for the *P. acnes* bacteria. The bacteria multiply, feeding off the sebum and causing a sudden flare of acne papules and pustules.

In chronic cases of hormonal acne, hormonal therapy using special kinds of birth control pills may be prescribed by a dermatologist, gynecologist, or family physician. Tricyclen® is a birth control pill approved by the Food and Drug Administration (FDA) as a management drug for hormonal acne. In extreme cases, chronic hormonal acne may also be a symptom of more serious illnesses, such as ovarian polycystic disease and adrenal growths. If you notice a client's chronic hormonal breakouts that are not responsive to topical treatment, do not hesitate to suggest that the client consult her physician.

Chin Acne

Many women suffer from premenstrual acne flares, predominantly in the lower part of the face, the chin, and the jawline (Figure 10–30). Many researchers believe that this is the area most responsive to male hormone sebaceous stimulation. It is also believed that many women have large sebaceous glands in these areas and relatively small

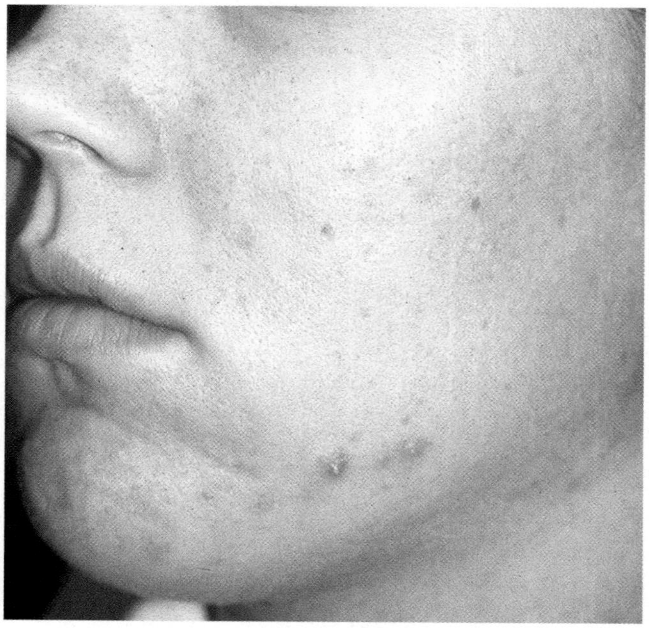

Figure 10–30 Acne on the chin and jawline can be related to hormone imbalances.

follicles. When a sudden sebaceous stimulation occurs, these follicles fill very quickly, causing inflammation due to the large amount of sebum. Women who suffer from chronic chin acne should see a dermatologist. There are hormone treatments available to help this problem.

Stress

Stress is what causes "pimples on prom night." Many acne sufferers, as well as dermatologists and estheticians, have noticed acne flare-ups in a patient under stress. A final exam at school, dating problems, financial problems, or difficulties at work seem to frequently trigger breakouts.

There is a fairly simple explanation for this relationship. Stress causes the brain to manufacture a hormone that, in turn, causes the adrenal gland to make more hormones, which causes an abundance of oil to be produced. The reaction is very similar to the premenstrual reaction.

> **Here's a Tip**
>
> Stress is one of the biggest contributors to acne flare-ups. Teach your client methods to alleviate stress and the skin care techniques to use under stress.

Birth Control Pills

Birth control pills can cause an androgenic flare-up that can contribute to acne. When starting birth control pills, a client might find her skin gets better or worse. The same may be true when discontinuing birth control pills. Women using birth control pills may find that their monthly premenstrual breakouts occur at different times in the cycle.

The reason is that birth control pills affect hormone levels and may affect different women in different ways. If a client seems to experience flares of acne when starting, stopping, or changing birth control pills, refer her to her doctor.

Pregnancy

Pregnancy may also produce unpredictable flare-ups or clearing of acne. The usual course is that acne gets worse during the first 3 months of pregnancy and then gets dramatically better. The acne may flare up again after childbirth or after breastfeeding is discontinued. Theoretically, this is due to obvious hormone changes, but stress levels may be partially responsible.

Menopause

During menopause, similar hormonal changes are very prominent and may cause flares. Because menopause is a time of more permanent hormonal change, some women will experience even more acne flares and other androgen-induced symptoms, such as facial hair growth. Hormone replacement therapies may help or aggravate breakouts. What helps one client may cause another to flare. Suggest they bring the problem to the attention of their prescribing physician as often they will not think of the HRT and the flares as related.

Inflammatory versus Comedonal Acne

Many women notice that premenstrual flares result in sore, inflamed papules. Hormonal acne is more inflammatory and less comedonal. In other words, it is the sudden irritation, rather than the traditional and slower buildup of cells in a comedo, that causes these papular lesions. The soreness is due to the swelling and relatively deep inflammation inside the follicle. This deep swelling is more likely to cause pressure on nerve endings, creating a painful lesion.

Inflammatory acne is not just caused by hormones. Acnegenic skin care products that cause overnight flares of pimples are a good example of inflammatory acne. Overtreated skin that has had too many peeling agents, or peeling agents applied too often, will show signs of dry irritation and often flares of inflammatory acne. Be observant of your clients' habits in these cases. Often they are overtreating their skin or may be using a new product that causes a flare.

Unfortunately, professional products are not immune from being acnegenic. Products labeled as "natural" are not assured to be nonacnegenic. Check to make sure that the products you use and sell have been properly tested to make sure they do not cause acnegenic or follicle irritancy reactions.

The Beginning of Teenage Acne

The beginning of teenage acne is characterized by minor breakouts in the nose area. Small blackheads and clogged follicles, small papules, and small milia are found. You may only see the beginning of visible pores in the nose and chin and sometimes the forehead. This is the beginning of adolescent pore structure, and usually, puberty and adolescence. Usually within six months more pimples will develop. Boys may notice small pimples in the lower cheeks. This may be caused by the beginning of beard hair growth. The hair is beginning to grow, but the follicle is not large enough to accommodate the hair.

This condition is known as **keratosis pilaris**, which essentially means there is a very small hair trying to force its way out of the follicle, resulting in irritation. This condition, which may affect girls or boys, is usually red or pink and has a "sandpaper" texture. It is often seen in the lower cheeks. If you look carefully at the area, you may notice very small whiteheads, which are responsible for the bumpy feel. Keratosis pilaris also frequently occurs on the upper arm and is more likely to affect adults in this area. Keratosis pilaris is best treated with alphahydroxy home care lotions and gels, and use of mild mechanical exfoliating cleansers helps bump off dead cells to allow the hair to come out (Figure 10–31).

Environmental Factors That Influence Acne

Heat and Humidity

There is no question that acne is more likely to flare up in the summer months when heat and humidity are high. Heat causes the skin to swell slightly, and humidity causes tremendous swelling of the outer epidermis. It is reasonable to assume that this could possibly exert enough pressure on the follicles to further complicate an already existing condition.

It has been observed over the years that people who live in tropical, warm climates with high humidity experience a fairly predictable seasonal pattern of flare-ups. Bring this to your clients' attention and encourage them to come to the salon more often for treatments during this type of weather.

Sun Exposure

Although sun exposure may have an immediate drying effect on acne lesions, sun-damaged skin is documented to cause more "cell buildup," which can add to or increase the chances of acne flare-ups.

Many patients with acne claim their acne improves with sun exposure. Tanning masks the redness, and as the buildup of tan cells occurs on the surface of the skin, acne may appear better. As soon as beach season is over, however, these same patients notice reoccurrence of their acne. What actually happens is that the tan fades and the cell buildup subsides, suddenly exposing a tremendous number of clogged follicles and closed comedones. The most unfortunate part of this situation is that these clients have a strong tendency to neglect treating their acne during beach season, making it more complicated when the tan fades. It is up to you, the esthetician, to educate the client before sun season to avoid this problem.

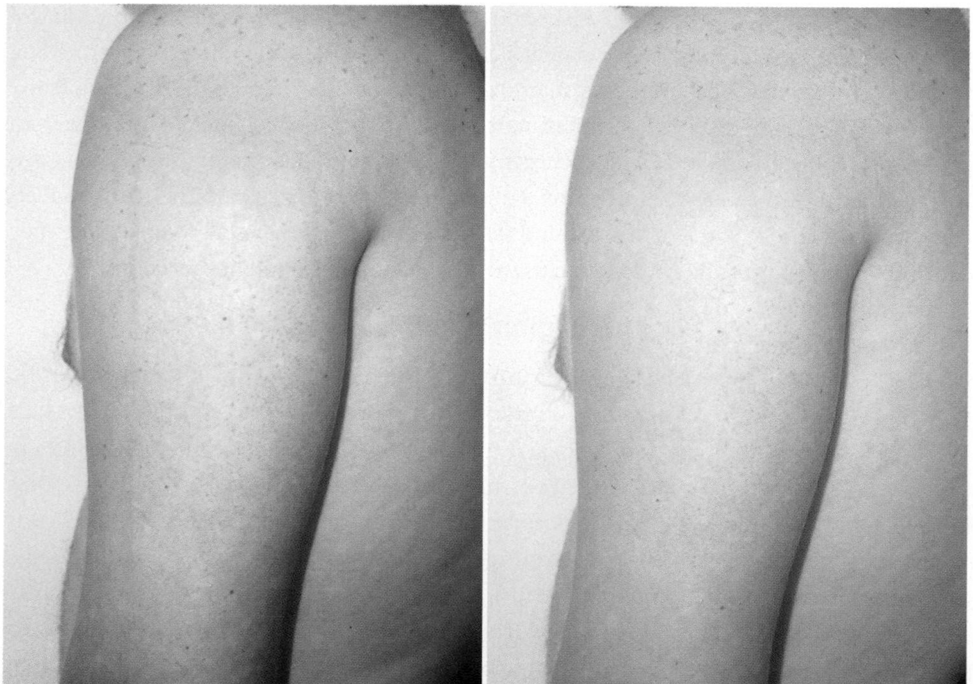

Figure 10–31 a) Keratosis pilaris and b) improvement using glycolic hydrator.

Here's a Tip

For those clients that think hiding their acne under the coloration of a tan is a good approach, suggest the use of a mineral powder makeup. It will camouflage the breakout and offer SPF protection at the same time.

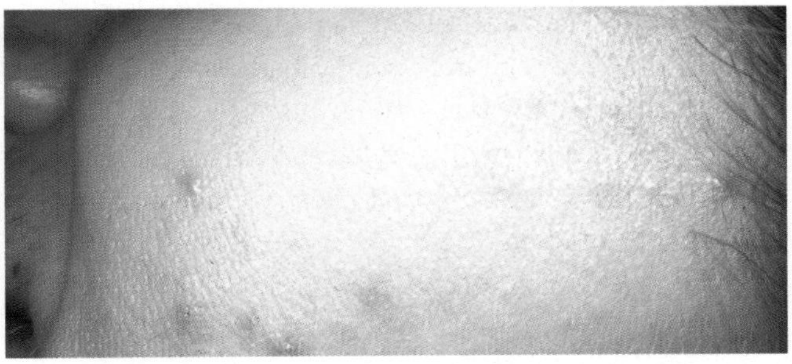

Figure 10–32 Acne excoriée.

Greasy Workplaces

Acne clients who work in environments where their skin is constantly exposed to large amounts of occlusive grease or airborne grease, such as in garages and fast-food restaurants, may notice a strong flare-up. It is best for these individuals to avoid working for prolonged periods of time under these conditions. Advise clients who must work in these types of jobs to cleanse their skin at regular intervals (about twice during an eight-hour period) with a mild cleanser that will remove the environmental oil without drying the skin too much.

Overcleaning

Clients are constantly under the impression that acne is directly caused by lack of cleansing. Although keeping skin as clean as possible is certainly important, acne is not caused by dirt. In fact, acne can be aggravated by too much cleaning. Repeated exposure to detergents in facial cleansers, for example, can aggravate acne if the client uses the cleansers too often. Estheticians often find that their clients are cleaning the face numerous times daily (eight to ten times). This causes enough irritation to precipitate not only an acne aggravation, but other sensitivities as well. Instruct these clients to cleanse two or three times a day only.

Self-Trauma Excoriations

Acne excoriée is a condition in which the client constantly picks at the skin. An excoriation is a scrape or scratch on the skin, in this case caused by the client. Most of the time, these clients are scratching or picking at small closed comedones and papules. Often the raised portion of the acne lesion is literally scraped off the face, usually with the fingernails.

An esthetician will notice acne excoriée during skin analysis because the acne lesions are flat, red, and sometimes raw, where the client has scraped off the entire epidermis to the point of bleeding. They often look like a freshly scraped knee or a brush burn (Figure 10–32). Sometimes there are scabs, which these clients have trouble leaving alone. Sometimes the esthetician will notice round, dark, hyperpigmented lesions. This is hyperpigmentation, either caused by trauma, known as **post-inflammatory hyperpigmentation**, or from exposure to sun after the client has picked the lesions raw.

Clients who have obvious excoriated acne lesions should be advised not to pick at the lesions. The lesions will never heal properly if the scabs are constantly being scratched off. Also, fingernails carry many germs that can cause other infections besides acne. Encourage "picker" clients to use a mask at home instead of picking, or tell them to call and move their treatment appointment to an earlier date. Suggest that they wear cotton gloves while reading or watching television. The touch of the glove material will signal them and make them aware when they are picking at their skin.

Clients sometimes absentmindedly pick at an occasional pimple. However, when clients constantly have several scraped areas on the face, this is a different situation. Some chronic pickers are often troubled mentally or suffer from a psychological disorder such as obsessive-compulsive disorder. Some may need referral to a psychologist or other mental health professional.

Nutrition and Diet

There are numerous falsehoods regarding the effects of food on acne. Chocolate, nuts, seafood, greasy "teenage" foods such as burgers and french fries, pizza, and candy have all been falsely accused of causing or worsening acne. Although some of these foods are not healthy in large quantities because they may be high in sugar, cholesterol, or triglycerides, they do not directly or indirectly cause acne. Many patients with acne and, unfortunately, some estheticians are still under the mistaken impression that these foods cause acne.

The food group that has consistently been implicated in aggravating acne conditions is iodides. Foods that are high in iodides include some types of shellfish, kelp, squid, asparagus, and iodized salt in salty foods. Iodine causes a follicular irritancy when ingested in large quantities. Consumed in reasonable quantities occasionally, these foods probably do not cause serious problems. It stands to reason, though, that excessive consumption of foods high in iodides can cause acne to flare up.

Milk and some milk products have been found to cause problems, primarily in females. The fat in milk does not appear to be associated with acne. Researchers have theorized that the hormones present in milk (from the cow) are the probable culprits for causing acne flares. If a client experiences chronic acne and does not seem to clear through topical treatment, ask if he or she consumes a lot of milk or milk products. Milk is a very important part of the diet, especially for calcium needs of the body and should not be discontinued unless the client associates a direct correlation between milk consumption and flares of acne.

Although foods are *not* the major cause of acne, many estheticians put too much emphasis on diet when treating problem skin, blaming foods when their treatments seem not to be working. Failure of the treatment plan is more likely to result from poor product choices or incomplete home-care programs. If you are truly concerned about a client's diet, refer the client to his or her doctor or to a registered dietician.

Dermatologists prescribe zinc supplements to some acne patients to reduce redness and inflammation. The usual dosage is 100 mg per day. It is best to check with a dermatologist before suggesting zinc supplements to your clients, because estheticians are not registered dieticians and therefore are not authorities on nutritional science. It is best to leave advice to the specialists in this area.

Acne and Cosmetics

So many factors cause or contribute to acne, but the esthetician has control over only a few. Heredity and hormones are not part of the practice of esthetics. Even though we may know a lot about these subjects, there is little the esthetician can do to control or affect these factors. Estheticians can temporarily reduce stress by administering soothing treatments, but the stress-reducing effects of these therapies are not long lasting when the client gets in an argument with the boss or forgets when a term paper is due.

Probably the best service you, the esthetician, can render to a patient with acne is helping the patient choose cosmetics and skin care products that are noncomedogenic. It is imperative that you fully understand comedogenicity for clients with acne or problem skin. The client may come in for treatment only once a month, but she exposes herself to cosmetics and skin care up to 60 times a month. Keep in mind that comedogenicity refers to the "risk" factor associated with an ingredient. With acne clients, estheticians work to reduce exposure risks by eliminating all possible comedogenic factors from the client's home-care and cosmetic regimen. Cosmetics, skin care, and topical drugs are the only things that are in constant, direct contact with the skin.

Acne-Related Conditions

Seborrheic dermatitis is a sometimes-chronic inflammation of the skin associated with oily skin and oily areas. Seborrheic dermatitis is characterized by dry-looking, flaky, crusty patches. Redness is often apparent under these flaky patches. Seborrheic dermatitis is most often seen in the T-zone of the face, eyebrows, hairline, inside the ears, along the sides of the nose, and the scalp (Figure 10–33). The exact cause of seborrheic dermatitis is unknown, but it is believed to be associated with a type of yeast called **pityrosporum ovale**.

Seborrheic dermatitis is often misdiagnosed by the client or an inexperienced esthetician as "dry skin";

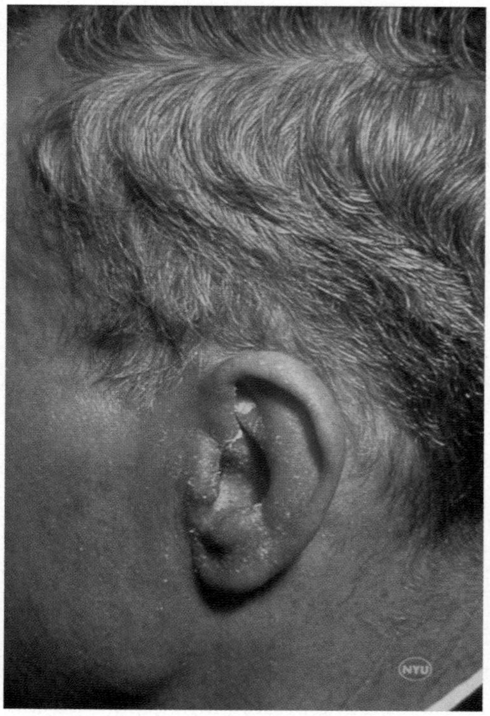

Figure 10–33 Seborrheic dermatitis.

it is actually an inflammation of the oil glands. Seborrheic dermatitis is best treated by a dermatologist, but you may be involved in choosing the correct skin care program. Sometimes a flare may be triggered after a client first uses a cream or product that is too rich or fatty-based. It is, again, important to avoid fatty, comedogenic products. Suggest a gentle but thorough rinseable cleanser toner and a very light, noncomedogenic moisturizing fluid. Overmoisturizing can be a contributing factor to flares of seborrheic dermatitis. Sunscreen is important for all skin types. Fragranced products, essential oils, or stimulating products and products with drying alcohols may aggravate or cause seborrheic dermatitis to flare.

Clients who suffer from seborrheic dermatitis are likely to experience flares as the seasons change. Lack of routine cleaning occasionally has been associated with the disorder. Dermatological treatment usually includes topical hydrocortisone, coal tar shampoos, salicylic acid, selenium sulfide, and zinc pyrithione. Anti-yeast topicals and oral medications are used in severe cases.

Perioral dermatitis, which is dermatitis around the mouth, is also considered an acne-related disorder, presenting as red papules and pustules in the mouth, nose, and chin area, usually small in size and in clusters of several lesions. Almost always found in women, perioral dermatitis often occurs during the childbearing years, ages 20 to 35 years (Figure 10–34). The condition is sometimes accompanied by scaliness and stinging dehydration. Moisturizers may complicate the condition. If a moisturizer is used, it should be water-based and noncomedogenic and used sparingly. Perioral dermatitis is, again, in the domain of the dermatologist. There is no known cause for perioral dermatitis. Because it is almost exclusively seen in females, it is thought to be somehow hormonally related.

Clients may report that their normal acne treatments are not working on this area of the face. This is not typical acne and needs medical referral. The usual course of treatment is oral antibiotics. Sometimes a physician will prescribe topical antibiotics or antibacterials, but topicals are not usually effective. It is not unusual to have recurrences, and they must be treated by the doctor.

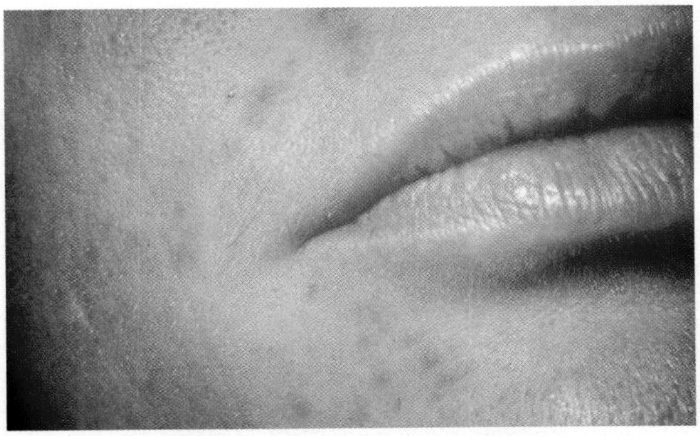

Figure 10–34 Typical pattern of perioral dermatitis on the chin. Perioral dermatitis can also appear on the cheeks or anywhere around the mouth.

ROSACEA

Rosacea, formerly known as *acne rosacea* and sometimes referred to as **adult acne,** is a disorder of the skin characterized by redness (erythema), **flushing** (sudden dilation of capillaries causing sudden diffuse redness, often accompanied with a feeling of heat, and turning red very easily), **telangiectases** (dilated or distended capillaries; Figure 10–35), and sometimes acne-like papules and pustules. A single distended capillary is known as a **telangiectasia**. Areas of telangiectases are also known by the European term **couperose.**

It is important to note that not all clients with telangiectases have rosacea, but almost all clients with rosacea have telangiectases. Telangiectases are also seen in clients with sun damage and injuries to the skin and can be more apparent in clients with high blood pressure.

Rosacea is a **vascular** disorder, meaning that it is related to blood vessels and circulation of the blood. Rosacea normally affects persons older than 30 years of age, but it can appear as early as age 20 or as late as age 70 or 80. The sudden rushing of the blood to the facial skin can stimulate sebaceous glands and irritate follicles, causing large red papules and pustules in the nose, cheeks, and chin areas. When patients with rosacea have

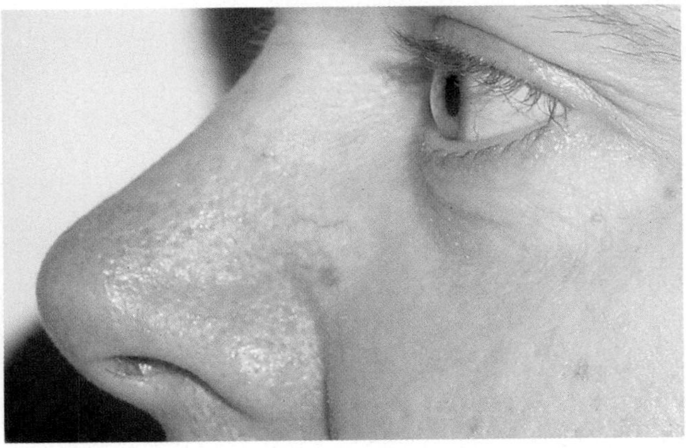

Figure 10–35 Nose telangiectasias.

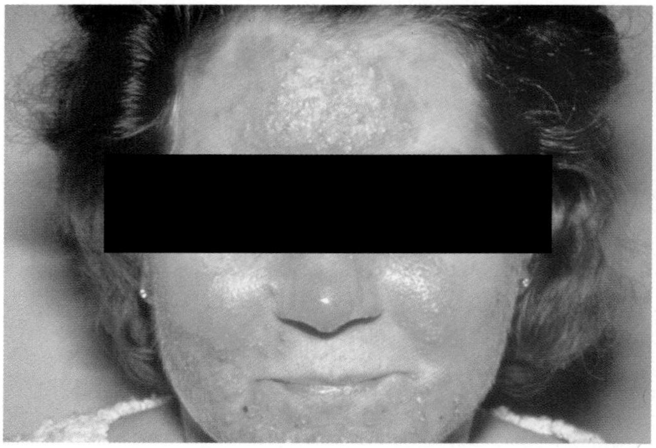

Figure 10–36 Flare of rosacea.

sudden redness or breakouts due to their condition, this is known as a rosacea **flare** (Figure 10–36). Rosacea is most prominent in light-skinned persons of Irish, Celtic, or western European origin.

The sudden flushing of blood to the face triggers the release of a biochemical within the skin called **vascular growth factor (VGF).** As its name implies, VGF triggers the growth or expansion of new blood vessels, specifically arterial capillaries in the skin. The addition of these new capillaries further increases the chances of flushing. Therefore, the disorder is self-perpetuating, or it continually progresses because of the formation of new blood vessels.

Rosacea may first appear as chronically red cheeks or a chronically red nose (Figure 10–37). Clients may notice flushing, which also produces a warming of the facial skin. Flushing can occur when the client becomes hot, drinks alcohol or wine (especially red wine), or eats spicy foods. Clients with rosacea are very likely to redden whenever they get physically hot, and some may notice flushing during or just after exercising. All these activities cause **vasodilation,** or increased blood flow due to dilated blood vessels, resulting in flushing or a rosacea flare.

Causes of Rosacea

No one is completely sure of the exact cause or causes of rosacea, but it appears to be hereditary and strongly related to how easily a person blushes. Theories for the cause of rosacea have included the presence of a mite called ***demodex folliculorum.*** It is thought that the microscopic mite feeds on the oil in the sebaceous gland and that heat makes these mites more active, resulting in itching. It has also been theorized that the presence of excessive yeast on the skin might be a factor. The topical drug used to treat rosacea is an anti-yeast medication, although the reason it works is thought to be because of anti-inflammatory action. An intestinal bacterium found in patients with ulcers, ***helicobacter pylori,*** is also thought to be involved. None of these theories has ever been confirmed to be a cause of rosacea because

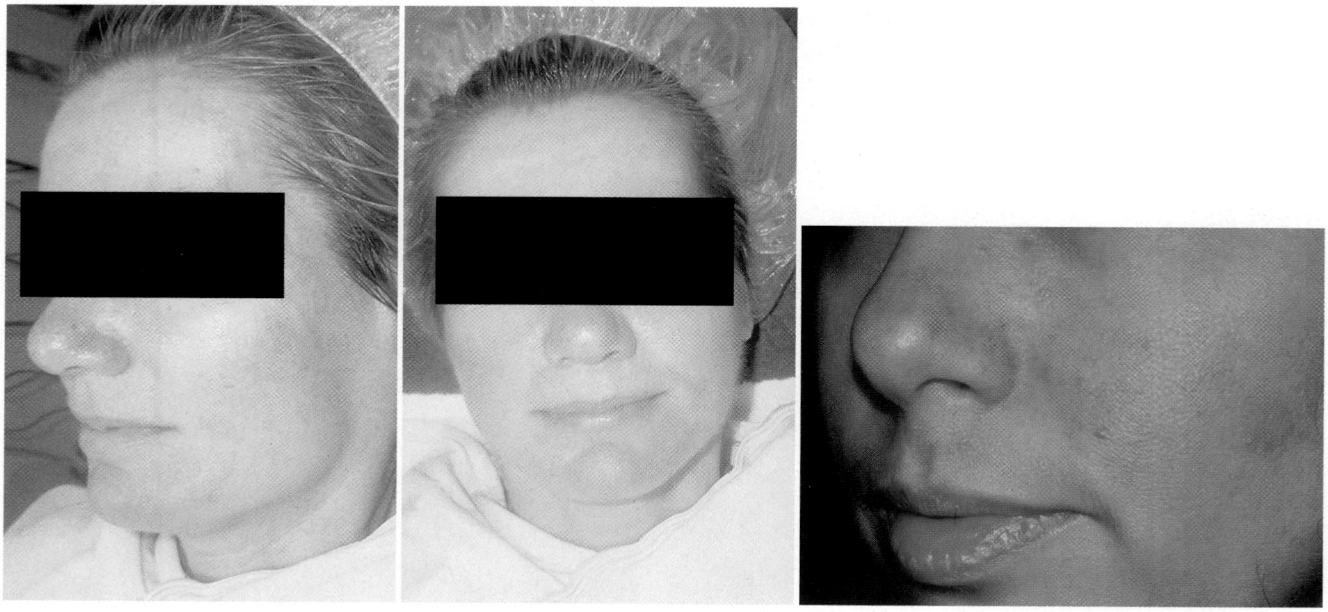

Figure 10–37 Beginning stages of rosacea.

the presence of mites, yeast, and bacteria vary among patients with rosacea. The search for real causes and a cure continues. As of the time of this writing, there is no confirmed cause or cure for rosacea. There are, however, many known ways to control and manage rosacea and to keep its symptoms under control for long periods through the use of medical treatment and lifestyle and skin care changes. When the flares of rosacea are under control for a long time, this is referred to as *rosacea remission*.

Subtypes of Rosacea

The National Rosacea Society is a nonprofit organization founded for research, education, and support of persons who have rosacea. The society estimates that as many as 14 million Americans have some form of rosacea. They conduct frequent surveys to determine factors that may trigger flares or flushing and assemble committees of dermatologists and other experts to conduct and interpret research about rosacea and its management. An expert committee of the society has divided rosacea into the following four subtypes:

Erythematotelangiectatic rosacea (subtype 1) is characterized by diffuse facial redness, patchy redness in the nose and cheeks, and a tendency to turn red extremely easily (Figure 10–38). Clients may or may not have distended capillaries (telangiectases). Persons with erythematotelangiectatic rosacea may have **transient erythema,** which means that the redness and symptoms can come and go. Facial swelling, skin roughness, dry-looking patches, tightness, and a grainy texture that feels much like fine sandpaper to the touch also may be seen. This grainy texture occurs primarily in the forehead and cheeks. The skin can sting and burn periodically.

Papulopustular rosacea (subtype 2) often resembles acne (Figure 10–39), but often there are no clogged pores or comedones present. These larger-than-normal pimples primarily occur on the nose and upper cheeks. There may be a lot of redness in the skin around the papules and pustules. There may be a dehydrated, crinkled appearance to the surface skin in these areas. Subjective symptoms of burning and stinging may also be present.

Phymatous rosacea (subtype 3) has a thickened appearance and results in an enlargement of the nose or other facial areas (Figure 10–40). An enlarged nose resulting from rosacea is known as **rhinophyma** (Figures 10–41 and 10–42). The famous comedian W. C. Fields suffered from rhinophyma, with his well-known red, bulbous nose. Many people thought that his big, red nose was caused by alcoholism, but it was actually phymatous rosacea. Alcohol use can cause flares and flushing, but it does not directly cause the thickening of tissues associated with rhinophyma (Figure 10–43). Phymatous rosacea can affect either women or men, but it is more prevalent in men. It is interesting to note that rosacea is more common in women, but phymatous rosacea is more common in men.

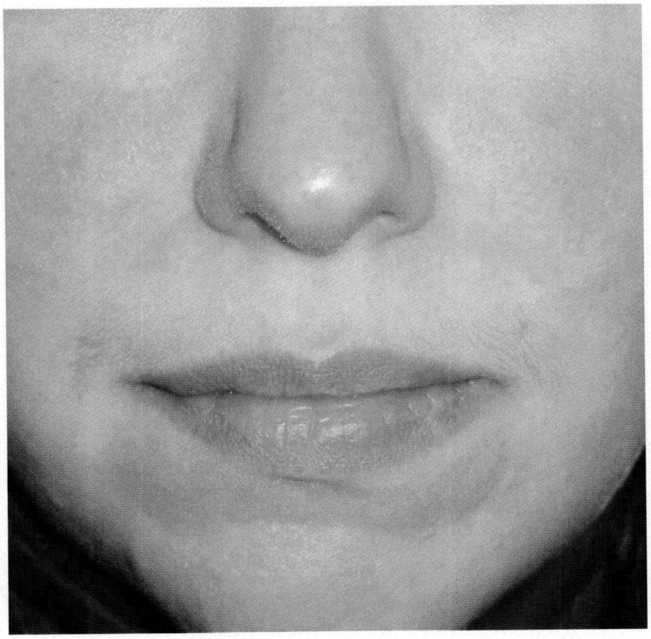

Figure 10–38 Rosacea subtype 1.

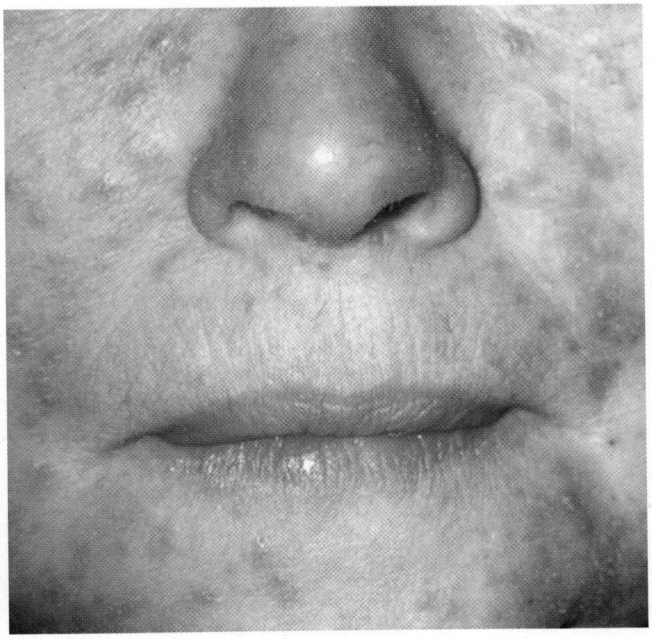

Figure 10–39 Rosacea subtype 2.

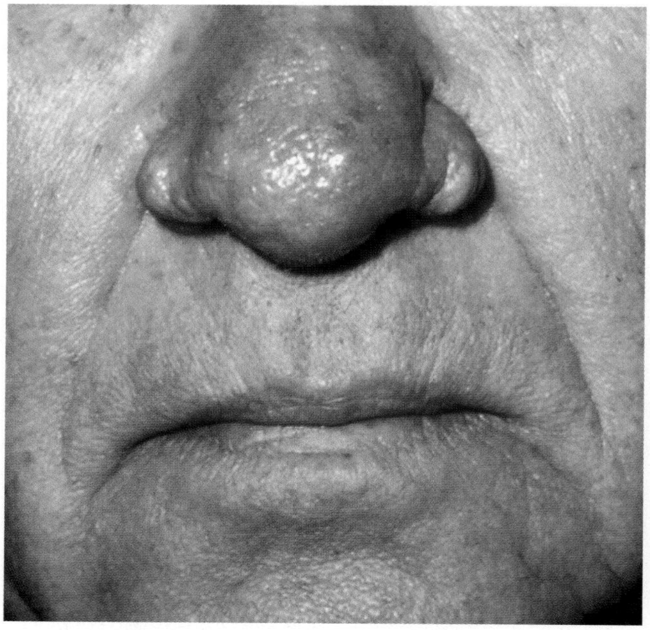

Figure 10–40 Rosacea subtype 3.

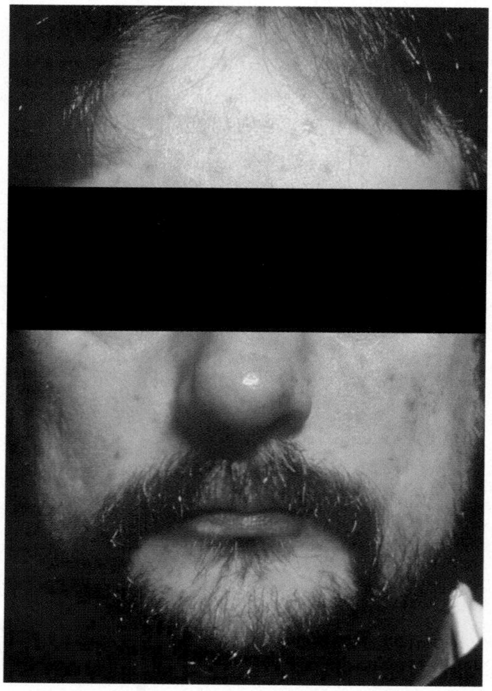

Figure 10–41 Red swollen nose can be the beginning of rhinophyma.

Ocular rosacea (subtype 4) occurs in the eye and eyelids, resulting in eye redness (bloodshot eyes), swollen eyelids, **chalazia** (small lumpy, cysts in the eyelids), **hordeolums** (better known as styes), eyelid skin telangiectases, stinging and burning, and other visual problems (Figure 10–44).

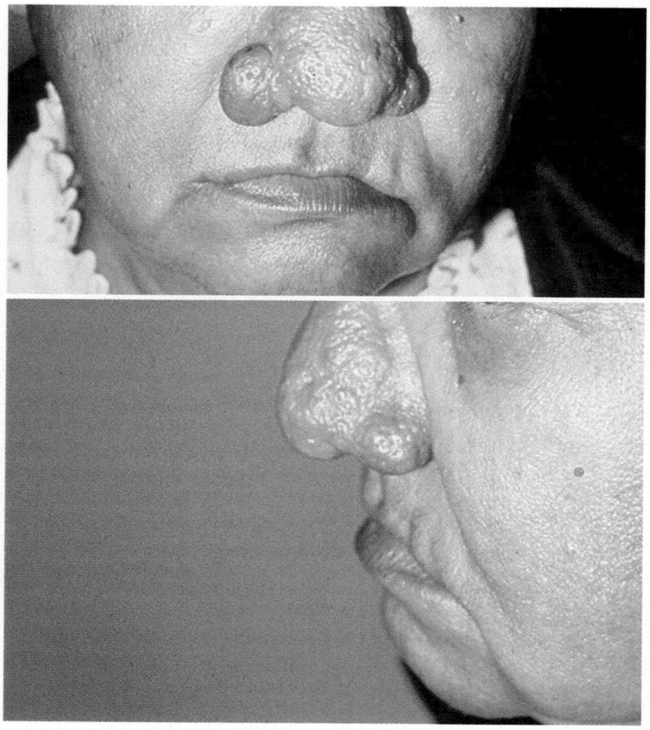

Figure 10–42 Rhinophyma.

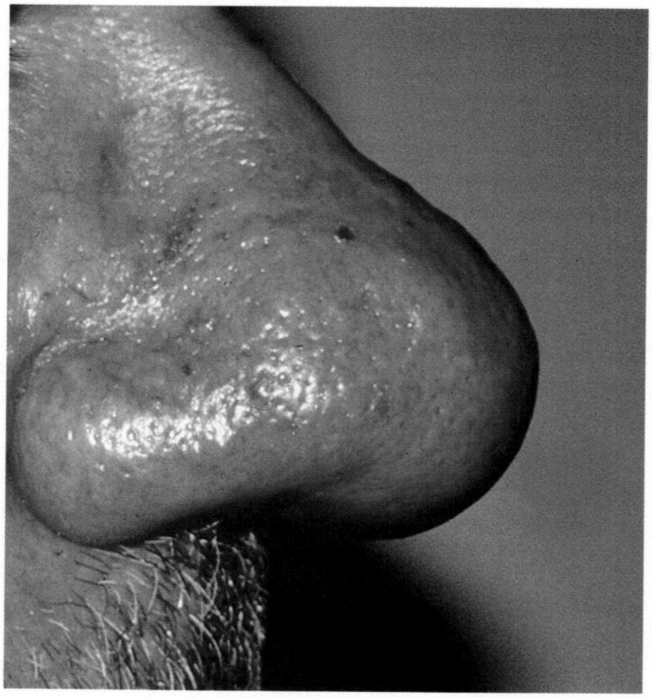

Figure 10–43 Dark and red distended capillaries, enlarged pores, and nose of rhinophyma patient.

It is possible for a client to have more than one subtype of rosacea. Subtypes 1 and 2 are frequently seen together. Some patients with rosacea have all four subtypes.

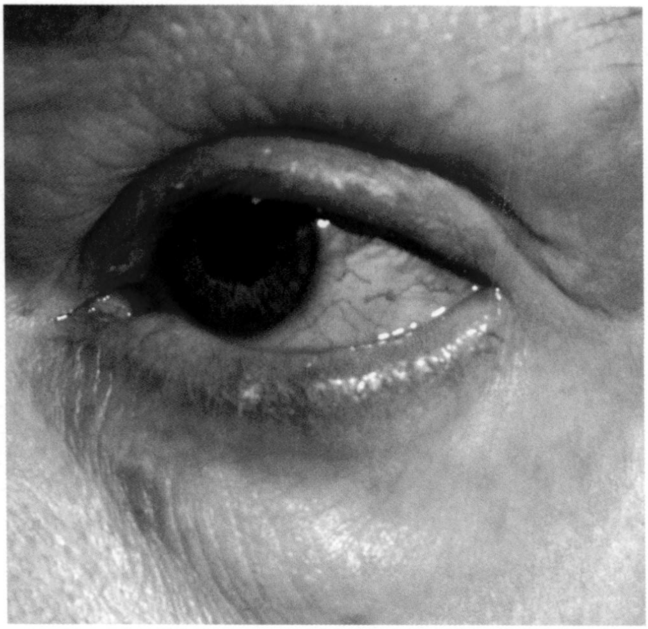

Figure 10–44 Subtype 4 ocular rosacea.

There is another factor that may affect any subtype of rosacea, known as **granulomatous rosacea**. This is not a subtype; it is more a factor that can affect the four basic subtypes. Granulomatous rosacea causes hard, nodular papules in the cheeks and around the mouth. They may be red, yellowish, or brown in color, and multiple papules will be identical in size and shape on an individual client.

Why Is There More Rosacea?

The most common question concerning rosacea is why estheticians are seeing more of it. Estheticians are not the only ones asking this question. According to the National Rosacea Society (NRS) in Barrington, Illinois, rosacea now affects an estimated 14 million Americans, ranking it among the top five most-diagnosed disorders by U.S. dermatologists. One reason for this increase could be, as a nation, people are getting older. The most common age group in which rosacea becomes noticeable is 30- to 55-year-olds, a time when most women, who outnumber men with rosacea two-to-one, enter menopause. However, other causes may also be suspect.

In the article "Drug and Cosmetic Ingredients That May Trigger Rosacea Episodes," Rebecca James Gadberry states that the drugs and cosmetic ingredients commonly used by members of this age group often appear on the lists. Flush-inducing drugs such as anti-inflammatory corticosteroids, blood pressure medications, cholesterol-lowering medications, and progesterone for relief of menopausal symptoms count among the most-prescribed drugs for baby boomers, while alpha hydroxy acids (AHAs), sunscreens, vitamin C, retinoids, mica, and other popular skin care and makeup ingredients are the most-used anti-aging cosmetics on the market today. Irritating procedures such as microdermabrasion and chemical peels, a tendency toward drier skin after age 30, and the likelihood of more stress as one gets older are all common tripwires for rosacea clients.

Activity

Visit the NRS or AAD Web sites and see what new information you can find on the causes or treatments of rosacea: www.rosacea.org or www.aad.org.

Anyone can get rosacea. While it may be the most common in pale-skinned individuals whose gene pool derives mainly from the British Isles or Scandinavia, people with darker skin, including Hispanics and African Americans, also experience rosacea, although the redness that typifies the disorder may be more difficult to detect. In these cases, rosacea may be misdiagnosed and treated as acne. Unfortunately, most acne drugs make rosacea worse, so the client may appear to be noncompliant or the condition may seem resistant to therapy. Switching a client to an ongoing rosacea treatment program should relieve the symptoms.

Medical Intervention

Even though rosacea is a vascular disorder, the traditional medical treatment for rosacea—a broad-spectrum oral antibiotic like tetracycline, minocycline, or doxycycline in combination with the topically applied antibacterial and antiprotozoal drug, metronidazole—has been shown to bring rosacea flares down within a few weeks for the majority of patients. To keep rosacea in check, metronidazole is continued on a long-term basis. For advanced cases of pustular rosacea, Accutane may be prescribed, while patients who experience severe and uncontrollable flushing may be put on beta-blocker propranolol or other blood-pressure medications, such as clonidine, lofexidine, or methyldopa, which are reported to reduce flushing by managing heat-regulating chemicals in the brain in the same way estrogen does.

These medical therapies are highly advised for rosacea patients displaying aggravated symptoms or frequent flare-ups. In a six-month study of rosacea patients using long-term therapies like metronidazole, 77% reported they remained in remission while 42% of those who did not maintain therapy experienced a relapse. That being said, those with milder symptoms often are more comfortable adopting drug-free methods that include lifestyle changes and cosmetic controls. In some cases, these drug-free methods may even help control aggravated symptoms. Of course, if rosacea worsens, a dermatologist should interve. Ideally, you and the dermatologist would work together to make sure your client gets the best care possible.

WHEN TO REFER FOR MEDICAL EVALUATION

Follow some simple guidelines for knowing when to refer a client for medical evaluation:

1. When there are undiagnosed rashes on the skin. Recall that estheticians cannot diagnose rosacea or any other disorder. This needs to be done by a physician.
2. When you see any blemish or growths on the skin that are changing, enlarging, oozing, or do not fit into one of the standard skin blemish classifications.
3. When a client has expectations that are beyond your scope of practice as an esthetician, such as the elimination of wrinkles or the removal of age spots.
4. Any time you see something unusual on the skin that you do not recognize or are unsure of. Many times you will be the first to look at a "spot" your client is concerned about. Even if you think you recognize it, you cannot diagnose it. If it is possibly a cancerous or precancerous lesion, a physician must be the person to determine that. Never alarm your client, but suggest he or she see a dermatologist.

If you follow these guidelines, your client and medical professionals will both have increased respect for you as you work for the client's best interests.

The more an esthetician knows about skin in distress, the healing process, and the skin disorders that can affect their client, the better they will be able to deal with the conditions that they see on the skin in the clinic. Recognizing and understanding the issues is the first step to finding a resolution for the client.

REVIEW QUESTIONS

1. Discuss the inflammation cascade.
2. Describe the phases of wound healing.
3. What are some possible wounds from treatments and how should they be handled?
4. What is short-term sun damage?
5. What can an esthetician do for short-term sun damage?
6. When should an esthetician not treat short-term sun damage?
7. What are the symptoms of long-term sun damage?
8. What happens to the skin histologically after long-term sun exposure?
9. Discuss esthetic problems caused by long-term sun damage.
10. What are the ABCDEs of melanoma?
11. Trace the development of the comedo.
12. Explain how hormones affect acne.
13. Name some environmental factors influencing acne development.
14. Discuss some acne-related conditions that should be referred to a dermatologist.

15. Why should an esthetician never tell a client she or he has rosacea?

16. Discuss the possible causes of rosacea.

17. When should an esthetician refer a client to a dermatologist or other medical practitioner?

CHAPTER GLOSSARY

actinic keratosis: pink, sometimes sealy, abnormal skin lesions that are regarded to be precancerous. These lesions develop as the result of sun damage and may present on the face, ears, neck, shoulders, arms, and most commonly on the hands.

adult acne: acne that develops in the 20s and above; often caused by hormone fluctuations, or external factors, such as comedogenic (pore-clogging) skin care products.

chalazia: small, lumpy cysts in the eyelids.

clinical inflammation: inflammation that can be seen with the naked eye or with the aid of a magnifying loop.

closed comedones: non-inflammatory follicle impactions that appear as small bumps just under the skin surface. Called closed comedones because the follicle opening is extremely small.

couperose: areas of small, red, enlarged capillaries of the face and other areas of the body.

cross-linking: a process in which collagen and elastin fibrils in the dermis collapse, causing the support system for the skin to collapse.

cryotherapy: the dermatological removal of lesions by freezing, usually with liquid nitrogen.

cytokine: (Gr. *Kytos*, "hollow vessel" + *Kinein*, "to move") molecule secreted by an activated or stimulated cell (for example, microphages) that causes chemical immune responses in certain other cells.

***demodex folliculorum*:** a skin mite that has been associated with rosacea.

dermatoheliosis: coined term describing damage to the skin caused by long-term sun exposure.

dihydrotestosterone (DHT): a form of male hormone that stimulates the sebaceous glands to produce sebum.

dysplastic: abnormal growth; often used to describe cancerous lesions.

erythematotelangiectatic rosacea: a subtype of rosacea that is characterized by diffuse, patchy redness, and a grainy texture.

exudates: fluid oozing from a healing wound.

flare: an episode in which pimples and redness occur in a person who has rosacea.

flushing: sudden facial redness caused by blood rushing to the skin.

granulomatous rosacea: any form of rosacea that includes hard, nodular papules.

***helicobacter pylori*:** a type of intestinal bacterium that has been associated with rosacea.

hemostasis: control of bleeding.

hordeolums: infected tear ducts: also called styes.

inflammatory mediators: chemicals released by inflamed cells that alert the immune system to the irritation.

keratosis pilaris: redness and bumpiness common on the cheeks or upper arms caused by blocked hair follicles. The patches of irritation are accompanied by a rough texture and small pinpoint white papules that look like very small milia.

mucosa: epithelial membranes that line internal orifices that lead to the outside of the body; mucous membranes secrete mucous which provides protection and lubrication for the internal surface. Examples are the inside of the nasal cavity or the inside of the intestine.

ocular rosacea: a subtype of rosacea that affects the eyes, resulting in eye redness, swollen eyelids, and other eye lesions.

open comedones: non-inflammatory acne lesions appearing as large, clogged follicles with solidified sebum and dead cell buildup. Often called blackheads.

ostium: the opening of a follicle on the skin surface.

papulopustular rosacea: subtype of rosacea that often resembles acne vulgaris, with large red pustules and papules.

perifollicular inflammation: inflammation of the follicle walls inside of the follicle.

perioral dermatitis: an acne-like condition around the mouth. These are mainly small clusters of papules, primarily seen in women of child-bearing age. Must be treated with internal antibiotics.

phymatous rosacea: a subtype of rosacea in which the nose has a thickened appearance and the individual sometimes has rhinophyma, which is a substantial enlargement of the nose.

pilosebaceous: the hair follicle.

pityrosporum ovale: a type of yeast sometimes associated with seborrheic dermatitis.

post-inflammatory hyperpigmentation: dark melanin splotches caused by trauma to the skin; can result from acne pimples and papules.

proliferative phase: the phase of wound healing in which there is increased vascularity to supply nutrients and oxygen to the wound.

propionibacterium acnes (P. acnes): the scientific names of the bacteria that causes acne vulgaris.

reepithelialization: the formation of new epidermis and dermis over an area of injury. The epithelial cells from the wound margin and the philosebaceous units migrate to repair damage.

remodeling: the maturation phase of a wound.

rhinophyma: enlarging of the nose, resulting from a severe form of acne rosacea.

seborrheic dermatitis: a skin disorder characterized by flaky, red, patchy skin primarily in the eyebrows, T-zone, and scalp, caused by inflammation of the sebaceous gland and resulting in patches of inflamed flakiness in oily areas of the skin; a common form of eczema.

seborrheic keratoses: crusty-looking, slightly raised lesions in mature, sun damaged skin. Often appear in the cheekbone area. They may be black, brown, gray or sometimes plesn-toned or sallow.

subclinical inflammation: biochemical inflammation that cannot be seen with the naked eye or a magnifying loop.

superficial: outermost parts of the skin.

telangiectases: capillaries that have been damaged and enlarged with distended blood vessels, commonly called *couperose skin*.

telangiectasia: a dilated or distended red capillary.

transient erythema: redness that comes and goes.

vascular: related to blood vessels.

vascular growth factor (VGF): Biochemical within the skin that triggers the growth of capillaries.

vasodilation: Vascular dilation of blood vessels; resulting in flushing.

CHAPTER 11

SKIN TYPING AND AGING ANALYSIS

CHAPTER OUTLINE

- FITZPATRICK SKIN TYPING
- THE GLOGAU SCALE
- RUBIN CLASSIFICATION
- KLIGMAN ROSACEA CLASSIFICATION
- ORIENTAL REFLEX ZONES OF THE FACE
- HORMONAL BALANCE FOR SKIN IDENTIFICATION
- SKIN CATEGORIES

LEARNING OBJECTIVES

After completing this chapter, you should be able to:

- **Discuss the various ways skin can be evaluated.**
- **Identify various Fitzpatrick skin types.**
- **Identify various Glogau classifications.**
- **Identify various Rubin classifications.**
- **Describe how estrogen-androgen balances define useful isotypes.**

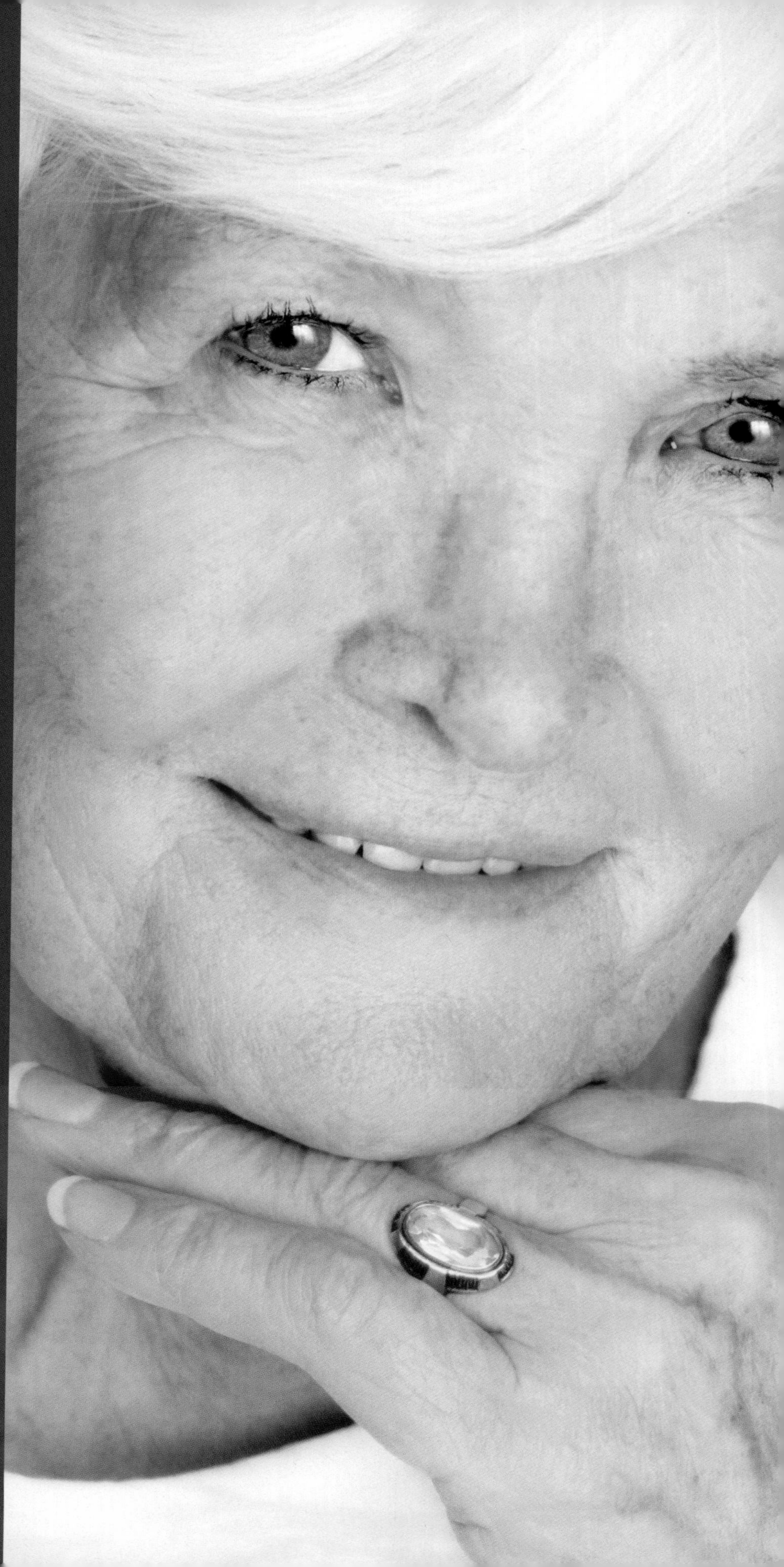

KEY TERMS

Page numbers indicate where in the chapter the term is used.

Fitzpatrick skin typing scale 237
Glogau scale 240
isotypes 245
Rubin scale 240

In a basic esthetics course you learn about the **Fitzpatrick skin typing scale** as a method of identifying various skin colorations. Here you will learn additional techniques for making a more accurate evaluation. Medical professionals have developed methods for classifying the stages of aging; these methods help them to determine the protocol needed for improving a patient's skin. A thorough understanding of these techniques can help you regardless of where you practice.

It is important to observe the skin thoroughly, using both a magnifying lamp and a Wood's lamp. The magnifying lamp allows you to determine a client's overall skin texture, tissue elasticity, and visible conditions. The Wood's lamp shows different skin conditions, including hyperpigmentation, hypopigmentation, oiliness, sun damage, or dehydration. You should record this information on the treatment form with other protocol or home-care notes. Continue observation throughout the treatment by noting how the skin responds to products, massage, and the overall facial.

There are three levels of information gathering that are important for making a proper skin analysis: determining the client's Fitzpatrick type, determining his or her skin type based on genetics, and observing any existing skin conditions. You can see these easily under a Wood's lamp and a magnification loop, sometimes referred to as a *mag lamp*. Once you record this information on a client assessment form, you have reference material that will be helpful in creating a treatment plan and home-care regimens.

FITZPATRICK SKIN TYPING

In its simplest form, the Fitzpatrick skin typing method measures the amount of pigment in the skin and its tolerance to the sun (Figure 11–1). Additionally, Fitzpatrick skin typing helps you predict the skin's response to treatments. Table 11–1 describes the characteristics of each of the six Fitzpatrick skin types. To classify a client's skin, you must first administer a thorough examination and ask a number of questions, which are shown in Tables 11–2, 11–3, and 11–4. Each table shows a numeric score that corresponds to each question. After you have supplied answers and have accorded each answer a score, you total the score for each of the three tables and write those in Table 11–5. Add those three numbers for the total Skin Type Score.

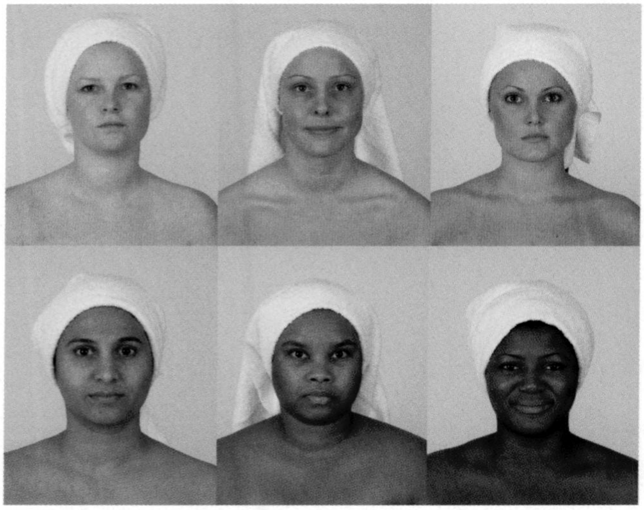

Figure 11–1 Fitzpatrick skin typing will help us predict the skin's response to treatments.

Activity

Answer the questions in Tables 11–2, 11–3, and 11–4 and determine your own Fitzpatrick skin type.

Then look at Table 11–6 to see where the score falls on the Fitzpatrick scale.

Keep in mind that fairer skin is more likely to display visible redness as a result of any trauma because capillaries show though its translucent layer. Darker skins, with their more active melanin, do not show redness as much. Their response to skin trauma is more apt to be hyperpigmentation, which may resolve readily or may take up to two years to dissipate. Use the Fitzpatrick scale to help determine which type of response a client's skin is most apt to have. Fitzpatrick types I–III are more prone to the red response, while Fitzpatrick types IV–VI are apt to hyperpigment.

This Fitzpatrick scale score gives you information on which to base a treatment decision. There have been some arguments made that skin treatments need to be designed based on ethnicity. It is probably more realistic to base skin treatments on the visible conditions with which the client is dealing, regardless of the client's ethnic background. For example, any Fitzpatrick skin type may suffer from dehydration, sensitivity, or acne flares. What skin coloration may indicate to us is the propensity of a given skin to react in a predictable manner to a given treatment. Fitzpatrick IV, V, and VI are more prone to hyperpigment. Fitzpatrick I and II are more apt to show redness from stimulating exfoliation treatments. It is prudent to do a thorough skin analysis and treatment

Table 11–1 Fitzpatrick Skin Typing Scale

SKIN TYPE	SKIN COLOR	HAIR AND EYE COLOR	REACTION TO SUN	COMMON ETHNIC CONSIDERATIONS
Type I	White	Blond hair and green eyes	Always burns, freckles	English, Scottish
Type II	White	Blond hair and green/blue eyes	Always burns, freckles, difficult to tan	Northern European
Type III	White	Blond/brown hair and blue/brown eyes	Tans after several burns, may freckle	German
Type IV	Brown	Brown hair and brown eyes	Tans more than average, rarely burns, rarely freckles	Mediterranean, southern European, Hispanic
Type V	Dark brown	Brown/black hair and brown eyes	Tans with ease, rarely burns, no freckles	Asian, Indian, some Africans
Type VI	Black	Black hair and brown/black eyes	Tans, never burns, deeply pigmented never freckles	Africans

Table 11–2 Fitzpatrick Identification Form Genetic Disposition Part I

	POINTS					
Question	**0**	**1**	**2**	**3**	**4**	**Score**
What color are your eyes?	Light blue, gray, green	Blue, gray, or green	Blue	Dark brown	Brownish black	
What is the natural color of your hair?	Sandy red	Blond	Chestnut/Dark blond	Dark brown	black	0
What color is your skin (unexposed areas)?	Reddish	Very pale	Pale with beige tint	Light brown	Dark brown	
Do you have freckles on unexposed areas?	Many	Several	Few	Incidental	None	
					Genetic Disposition Total	

Table 11–3 Reaction to Sun Exposure Part II

	POINTS					
Question	**0**	**1**	**2**	**3**	**4**	**Score**
What happens when you stay too long in the sun?	Painful redness, blistering, peeling	Blistering followed by peeling	Burns sometimes followed by peeling	Rare burns	Never had burns	4
To what degree do you turn brown?	Hardly or not at all	Light color tan	Reasonable tan	Tan very easy	Turn dark brown quickly	0
Do you turn brown with several hours of sun exposure?	Never	Seldom	Sometimes	Often	Always	0
How does your face react to the sun?	Very sensitive	Sensitive	Normal	Very resistant	Never had a problem	4
					Reaction to Sun Exposure Total	8

Table 11–4 Tanning Habits Part III

	POINTS					
Questions	**1**	**2**	**3**	**4**	**5**	**Score**
When did you last expose your body to sun (or artificial sunlamp/tanning cream)?	More than 3 months ago	2–3 months ago	12 months ago	Less than a month ago	Less than 2 weeks ago	
Did you expose the area to be treated to the sun?	Never	Hardly ever	Sometimes	Often	Always	
					Tanning Habits Total	

Table 11–5 Skin Type Scores

SKIN TYPE SCORES	
Total for Genetic Disposition	
Total for Reaction to Sun Exposure	
Total for Tanning Habits	
Total Skin Type Score	

Table 11–6 Fitzpatrick Skin Type

SKIN TYPE SCORE	FITZPATRICK SKIN TYPE
0–7	I
8–16	II
17–25	III
25–30	IV
Over 30	V–VI

of the existing conditions while keeping in mind any possible reactions based on ethnicity.

THE GLOGAU SCALE

The **Glogau scale** evaluates the level of photodamage to skin based on wrinkling. Dr. Richard Glogau, who developed this classification system a number of years ago, designed it to determine the level of peel a physician needed to use to address a visible condition. Glogau's system is specifically focused on the evaluation of photodamage present on the skin. It helps physicians standardize their approach in addressing problems and to communicate with each other about a client's issues. Because it is based on visual assessment, it is a quick tool for you to use to further evaluate a client (Table 11–7). You may do this before or after doing a Fitzpatrick evaluation.

One of the confusing aspects of the Glogau system is the incorporation of acne scarring and the use of makeup in addition to photodamage. As an esthetician you have most likely seen women who fall into all four categories and who all wore makeup differently than described in the chart. Also, a client may fit into Glogau Type IV but have no acne scarring. The key factors defining a Glogau category may be how wrinkles appear and the presence of photoaging. If you focus on the visible signs of aging as your determiner you will find this scale more useful.

RUBIN CLASSIFICATION

Dermatologist Mark G. Rubin created a slightly different method for determining the level of photodamage that eliminated the consideration of makeup and acne. The **Rubin scale** looks at the histologic depth of visible skin changes (Table 11–8). His method of evaluation is based on where in the skin the damage is present. If a client has only mild epidermal photoaging, you would select a different peel than if the damage extends into the dermis. Keep in mind that some clients may exhibit alterations from more than one category. They may have epidermal skin discoloration but fine lines that extend into the dermis. Esthetic superficial peels will help the skin discoloration but not dermal wrinkles. The Wood's lamp may help you determine this, and you can also use the DermLite® for close-up spot skin analysis (Figure 11–2). While the Wood's lamp

Table 11–7 Glogau Classifications of Photodamage

GLOGAU CLASSIFICATIONS OF PHOTODAMAGE	
Type I	**Type III**
No wrinkles while client is at rest or while moving Early photoaging Mild pigment changes No keratosis Minimal to no wrinkles Ages 20s–30s or younger Minimal acne scarring can be seen, if present No makeup or minimal makeup necessary	Wrinkles at rest; you see the wrinkles when the person is not moving Advanced photoaging Hyperpigmentation Telanglectasia Keratosis Wrinkles even when not moving Ages 40s–50s Makeup always worn Acne scarring, when present, shows through makeup
Type II	**Type IV**
Wrinkles only in motion, visible when the person is talking, laughing, frowning, and so on Early-to-moderate photoaging Lentigines, other pigment Changes showing Wrinkles forming Light keratosis Nasolabial lines beginning to form Ages 30s–40s Minimal makeup	Wrinkles as predominant characteristic; you see only wrinkles Severe photoaging Sallow-ashy skin color Prior skin cancers Wrinkles all over Makeup not worn, sets in cracks Severe acne scarring

Table 11–8 Rubin's Classifications of Photodamage

DESCRIPTION OF LEVEL	TREATMENT INDICATED
Level 1	
Alterations are in the epidermis only. These changes are primarily superficial pigment changes, roughness, lentigines, a dull or ashy appearance, and increased thickness.	This client will benefit from a superficial peeling such as glycolic acid and a steady home-care program combining AHA and/or BHAs, nourishers, antioxidants, and sunscreens.
Level 2	
Alterations are in the epidermis and papillary dermis. These conditions may include all of those seen in Level 1, as well as actinic keratosis, stronger pigmentation values, flat seborrheic keratosis, and an increase in wrinkles.	This client will benefit from medium-depth peels such as TCA (trichloracetic acid) and a more aggressive home-care program that includes retinoids and hydroquinone.
Level 3	
Changes are not only in the epidermis and papillary dermis but also in the reticular dermis. This is the most severe level of photodamage, and skin will be leathery and yellow in color and exhibit open comedones.	This client likely will benefit from laser resurfacing and possibly other cosmetic procedures, along with a progressive home-care program, depending upon the client's age and sensitivity to performance and active agents.

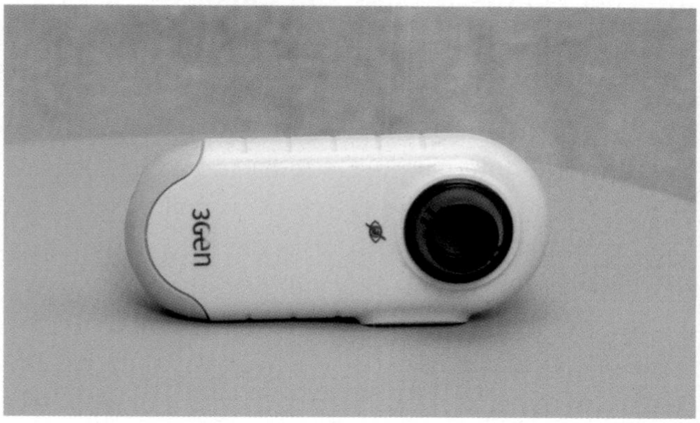

Figure 11–2 DermLite.

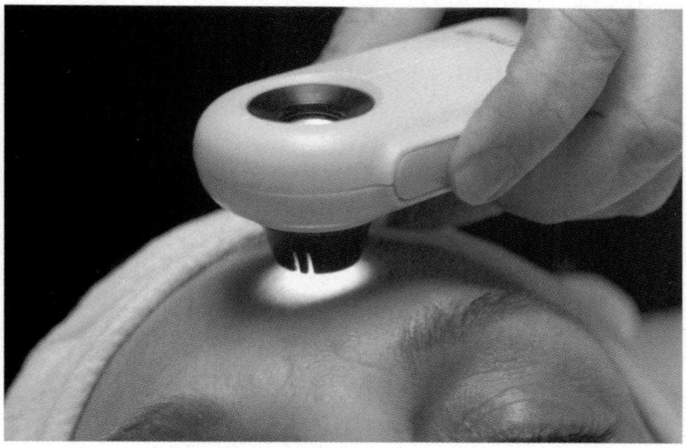

Figure 11–3 DermLite in use.

uses black light, the DermLite uses extreme magnification (Figure 11–3). Its 10x lens offers good superficial views as well as deeper views into the dermis. Dermatologists carry this little handheld device in order to do quick evaluations of skin imperfections that need a closer look. Permanent makeup artists use the DermLite to evaluate how much pigment they are getting into the skin.

In order to make the most comprehensive evaluation, use your Wood's lamp in a very dark room. The DermLite is not dark-dependent and may be a helpful alternative if your treatment room has windows. You may find other devices that offer high resolution analysis to be of assistance in obtaining the best possible results.

You may find the Rubin classification easier to use than the Glogau, but it is important to understand both. The Rubin classification can help you determine how close you will be able to come to achieving your client's goals. If a client has Level 1 damage, you can successfully assist him or her in your clinic. You may be able to offer a client with Level 2 damage some benefit, depending on his or her objectives, or you may advise that client to seek medical assistance. In either case, it is important to gain a clear understanding of the client's goals for results. She or he may be comfortable with a few wrinkles but may want to focus on improving the feel or texture of the skin. The client may not want the experience or the down time of medical intervention and would be happier with good home care and a series of esthetic exfoliation treatments.

If a client with Level 2 or Level 3 damage wants it reversed, you should work with a physician, because these cases involve deeper work, a higher risk of complications, and an alteration of the epidermis and the dermal tissue. It will take a combination of your esthetic skills, the services of a medical specialist, and the client's dedication to home care to achieve the best result. Your role will not only involve treatments but your ability to motivate the client and keep him or her focused on the importance of home care.

KLIGMAN ROSACEA CLASSIFICATION

Dermatologists Albert M. Kligman and Gerd Plewig have developed guidelines for classifying levels of rosacea. (For a full discussion of rosacea, see Chapter 10.) Being able to recognize and classify rosacea levels will help you communicate with medical professionals as well as select an appropriate treatment.

It is important to keep in mind that untended, rosacea can become progressively worse over time. It is more prevalent in women than in men, but it can be more aggressive and disfiguring in males. Stage I rosacea is the most common form seen in clinics; it responds well to appropriate esthetic treatments. For Stage II conditions, calm and soothe the skin, working to lower its surface temperature and using nonstimulating methods to reduce bacteria levels on the skin. In the case of severe rosacea—Stage III—refer the client to a physician for medical intervention.

Table 11–9 Kligman Rosacea Classification

KLIGMAN ROSACEA CLASSIFICATION
Stage I Erythema in the areas of the nasolabial folds, cheeks, and glabellum (forehead); skin seems to itch and burn in the presence of cosmetics.
Stage II Inflammation, pustules, and papules present, and pores seem larger; condition may spread over other parts of the face, including hairline and chin.
Stage III The most serious form of rosacea: large nodules present, orange-peel, and coarse appearance.

ORIENTAL REFLEX ZONES OF THE FACE

All energy medicines, of which Aryuveda and traditional Chinese medicine (TCM) are great examples, have a common fundamental philosophy, namely, the belief that the body is not, as we are taught in Western schools, made only of matter (solids and fluids) but also of energy. We are not talking about the constant energy released by the multitude of chemical activities taking place within the body. Vital energy, as it is called in Western countries, is a very subtle form of energy essential to all life-forms. It has a specific flow throughout the entire body. In China it is called *chi*; in Japan, *Ki*; and in India, as all yoga practitioners know, it is *prana*.

Those who use energy medicines, or vibrational medicines, have a view of the body that is holistic because of the interconnection of all parts and functions caused by energy flowing all over, from head to toes and back, from one side to the other and back, and from the inner parts to the outer parts. Nothing within the body is isolated from vital energy.

Internal Energetic Flow and Balance

In vibrational medicine, illness is a disruption, an imbalance, or a blockage of the natural energetic flow. Therefore, a health-oriented regimen aims to maintain or restore the internal energetic balance. The focus of such treatments is not the symptoms as much as the root cause of a problem. In both cases the field of attention is the energy flow, its quality and quantity through very specific pathways. In TCM these pathways are called the *meridians of acupuncture*, and in Ayurveda they are the *energetic centers* or *chakras*. Treatments might involve having a client ingest certain herbs and other natural ingredients with specific energetic properties, or they might involve treating the skin itself, where the energy flow can be accessed, on acupuncture points in particular.

Put "Energy" in Your Practice

The skin is connected to all other parts of the body by way of the energetic web that interconnects all organs and all tissues. As a result, it is a reflex-like organ, reflecting the internal condition of the body and providing useful indicators of the internal energetic and health condition. Esthetic conditions are signs pointing to energetic imbalance(s). Beauty and wellness treatments are highly desirable for restoring the vital energy flow and its balance to address the energetic root cause of problems. The question is how to do this in beauty salons or spas.

The energetic qualities of particular herbs, essential oils, and other natural products, including plants, clays, and trace elements—properly used and applied topically—can help put *chi* back in balance. Manual massages, baths, and the use of additional tools such as stimulation of selected acupuncture points and light therapy, in conjunction with the application of energetic products, will further correct the esthetic manifestations as well as address their inner cause(s). All of this is achievable by the use of a coherent method such as the Five Elements Theory of TCM.

The Body and the Five Elements of TCM

Following is a list of the five elements of TCM and their relevant components:

WOOD

The energies of liver (yin) and gallbladder (yang) and of overall vital energy circulation

FIRE

The energies of heart (yin) and small intestine (yang) and of red blood circulation

EARTH

The energies of spleen (yin) and stomach (yang) and of lymph circulation

METAL

The energies of lungs (yin) and large intestine (yang) and of venous circulation

WATER

The energies of kidney (yin) and bladder (yang) and of water movement

The Five Elements and Skin Conditions

Each one of the five elements, when out of balance, creates some undesirable conditions for skin and body shape that can be tell-tale signs that some energetic disturbances are at work within the body. The skin conditions are:

WOOD

Oily skin, blackheads, hyperpigmentation
Oily scalp and hair
Issues of vital-energy circulation

FIRE

Redness; irritated, sensitive, allergic skin; excessive heat and perspiration; couperose
Irritated, red, sensitive scalp
Issues of red blood circulation

EARTH

Blemishes, toxicity, acne, psoriasis, enlarged pores
Heavy-looking hair, pimples on scalp
Lymph circulation problems

METAL

Dry, dull, lifeless skin
Dry scalp and brittle hair
Issues of *red blood circulation*

WATER

Dehydration, lack of tone, wrinkles
Scalp lacking tone
Limp hair with no volume
Water retention

Skin from the Oriental Perspective

Practitioners of energy medicines believe that all esthetic conditions are the result of an internal energy imbalance. The condition of the skin, as well as the body shape, can also indicate when and where there is an energetic lack, or excess, from any of the five energies.

Because the skin is such an important indicator of health, then, it is to be valued as more than a covering that needs to be cleansed and moisturized. Energy medicines teach us that the skin is an organ with the gift of intelligent silent communication. It is most useful to pay attention and learn the language of the skin, not only to look better, but also to improve the overall state of wellness.

Increasingly, naturopaths and other medical professionals have come to share an enhanced view of the skin. Indeed, when the tissues in an embryo go through the process of specialization, the tissues that form the envelope of the body come from the same ones that specialize as the tissues of the nervous system and of the brain. Because of the way the skin reacts to what occurs both inside and outside the body, some naturopaths see the skin as a sort of external brain, capable of providing a large amount of psychosomatic information.

As a vital organ, then, the skin cannot be excessively stripped—mechanically or with acids—injected with chemicals, cut, stretched, or sewn without consequences. Likewise, what we eat, drink, and breathe and how we exercise our body, or not, has consequences on our health as much as on our skin. Skin care involves caring for the entire body. That is why it is a holistic proposition and a lifestyle decision.

Points of Acupuncture

Each of the ten organs of the body has its own energy pathway, following specific channels, or highways, called *meridians*. Acupuncture points are like the on and off ramps on those highways, allowing access to the energy in the meridians.

An acupuncture point is a small area where the natural resistance of the skin to an electrical stimulation is less than on the rest of the skin surface. As a result, a point can be located precisely with a simple electric device. However, a point detector cannot tell which point it is. It simply confirms the location of a point. Very sophisticated modern electronic devices are available to identify the nature and the flow of energy in a meridian at a given point.

While there are several hundred acupuncture points, spa technicians find that only a few on the face and the body are really useful. While an acupuncturist needs an exact location, a spa technician does not. The application of an energetic product, or light, therapy over a broad enough area will do.

Zones of the Face

All five elemental energies, as well as hormonal energy, are reflected on the face, making the face a mirror of our internal activity. Following is a list of the energies and the acupuncture points for each:

WOOD

Liver: in between the eyebrows

Gallbladder: temple areas

FIRE

Heart: upper lip and tip of nose and around nostrils

Small intestine: forehead

EARTH

Spleen: bridge of nose and sides above the nostrils

Stomach (extension of the spleen area): over the cheekbones, on both sides; also the frontal part of the neck, below the jaw and between the large intestine areas

METAL

Lungs: cheeks extended from the jawbone to the ears, on both sides

Large intestine (extension of lung area): down the side of the neck, on both sides

WATER

Kidney: lower part of the circle around the eyes

Bladder: upper part of the circle around the eyes, as well as the hairline, above the forehead

HORMONAL

Chin area: from below the lower lip, the width of the mouth, down to the jawbone

For face treatments, all points are conveniently located on the face itself.

Note that *any reflex zone* can express *any of the skin conditions* of the five elements. Therefore, when analyzing a client's face for an energy imbalance, consider the following:

The type of skin condition(s) according to the five elements

The location—reflex zone—where the condition exists

For example, excessively red and sensitive skin (which has not been caused by a sunburn or overexercising) is a sign of Fire energy imbalance (heart and small intestine energies), but if the Fire condition recurs chronically on the cheeks, which is the reflex zone of lungs (Metal), it is an indication of a Fire problem on a Metal zone. Both energies need to be rebalanced, each in its own way.

Treatments

It is not enough to define the nature of a problem; face reflexology should be used to provide an energetic solution. It should include work at the two levels of matter and energy. Certain tools are more adapted to one than the other. For example:

A clay mask is matter and it is used on the skin (matter). One of its primary functions is to draw out to the skin surface, be it water to hydrate or wastes to detoxify. More specific functions can be attributed to the clay with the addition of specific essential oils.

Essential oils can penetrate more deeply in the skin, working in the opposite direction of the action of the clay. But they also have energetic qualities that can make them useful when applied to reflex zones and on acupuncture points.

Light is a very energetic tool to work on the acupuncture points and chakras concerned, it can be used according to the colors of the five elements (green, Wood; red, Fire; yellow, Earth; blue, Metal; and violet, Water).

As a result of the diversity of tools, an advanced treatment uses a multi-tiered approach to work simultaneously at three different levels:

1. The level of matter (the pimples) with matter (topical products)
2. The level of matter (skin) with the energy of essential oils
3. The level of vital energy (points of meridians and chakras) with the energy of light

The result is that treatment can be highly personalized to specific conditions.

There is never a single version of any skin condition but five versions; for example, acne on the forehead is Fire energy. The treatment for acne varies and depends on what reflex zone it is on. That points to the energetic problem, and from that information you can select the right energetic tool. For example, acne (an Earth imbalance) on the forehead, namely the small intestine area (Fire), is a different version than acne on cheeks (lung area or Metal imbalance).

The same manifestation on different areas indicates different problems needing different solutions. Treating them all in a standard fashion without consideration for the reflex zone where the problem occurs is not as advanced an approach as looking at the reason for the problem as indicated by where it appears.

HORMONAL BALANCE FOR SKIN IDENTIFICATION

All women have both estrogen and androgen in their bodies, and the balance of these creates impacts on their bodies. As women age and lose estrogen, they take on some of the more androgen-related characteristics. The esthetics community has become increasingly interested in this balance. Dr. Peter Pugliese, MD has done extensive study on the variations of this balance and its impact on body shape, skin conditions, and the aging process. In his book *Advanced Professional Skin Care* Dr. Pugliese, writes of the relationship between increasing androgen levels and increasing hair volume and spread of hair growth patterns. In *Skin Care Beyond the Basics*, Mark Lees describes the relationship between estrogen and androgen balances and their impact on the client.

Recently, in an attempt to make the correlations simpler to understand, Dr. Pugliese shared an easy way to identify a client's potential problems and needs based on body typing. He described two main categories, which he called **isotypes:** estrogen-dominant women and androgen-dominant women. Each isotype is further broken down, for a total of four categories. This analysis technique has nothing to do with personal beauty or culture, as beautiful women of all ethnicities are found in all four of the categories. In addition, it is important to remember that all women lose estrogen and have a higher androgen balance as they age. It is common for a woman to move from one isotype to the next higher androgen type as she matures. This change may lead to increased unwanted hair growth as well as skin thinning and other signs of aging.

In the studies, bust size was also evaluated, but with the popularity of breast implants this is a less reliable factor. Also, the level of sun exposure a client receives during her life will exacerbate the aging factor for all of the skin types. Estrogen-androgen typing is a quick way for you to assist a new client and determine additional services she may be interested in receiving.

Estrogen Isotypes

Women who have more estrogen in their systems are generally smaller-boned with fine, delicate, or pointed features, such as nose and chin. Their brows tend to be sparse and their skin thin with refined, very small pores (Figure 11–4). They tend to carry their weight in hips and thighs with smaller more defined waists. Think of the classical hourglass body shape (Figure 11–5). These clients do not suffer much from breakout (especially once past adolescence), but due to their thin, fine skin, they show early signs of aging if not properly cared for. If they avoid sun exposure, they can stay quite youthful in appearance, but photoaging will exacerbate their natural predisposition. Due to their higher levels of estrogen, they are more prone to autoimmune disorders at a young age.

Estrogen-dominant clients can be further broken down into two categories: X and Y. The EX category has the most estrogen. The EY client will have a little less.

FOCUS ON: *Estrogen-Dominant Clients*

Clients who have estrogen-dominant skin types need lots of anti-aging skin therapies in the clinic and for home care.

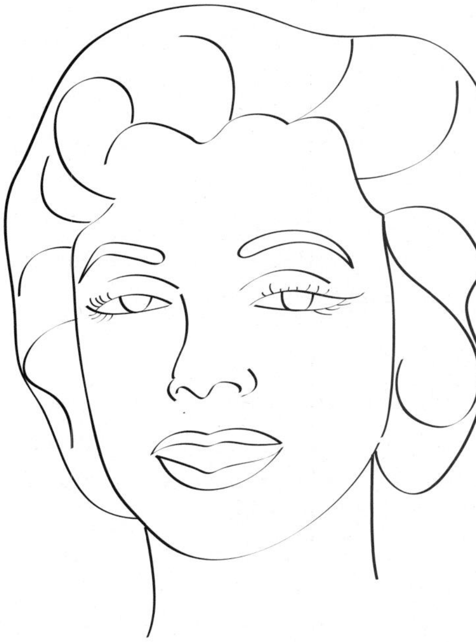

Figure 11–4 Estrogen isotype.

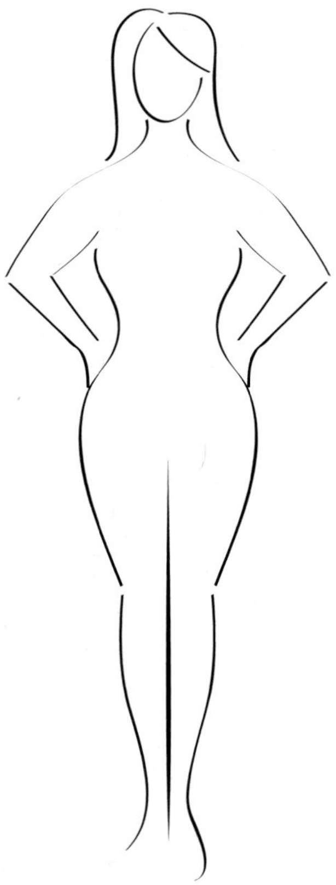

Figure 11–5 Estrogen hourglass body shape.

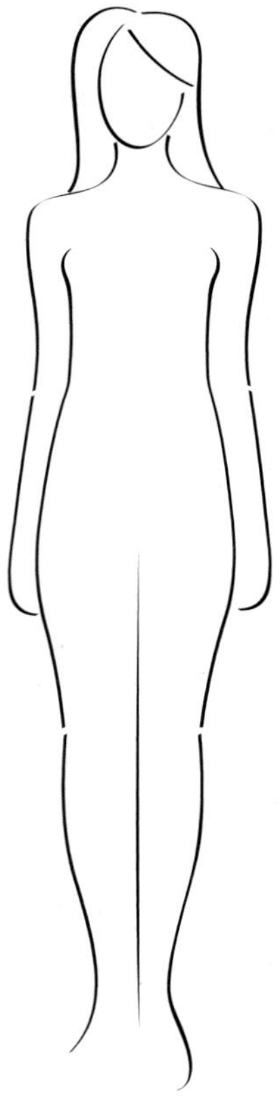

Figure 11–6 Androgen T-build body shape.

This can make the EY group a little more resistive to visible signs of aging, but they also have a little more androgen and may have more of a tendency for breakouts. EX clients seldom have terminal hair on the face, but an EY client will experience more terminal hair growth, especially as she moves toward menopause. The key difference in identifying an EX verses an EY will be in the nose and the chin. The EX will be narrower and pointier in these features than her EY counterpart. The EY's chin and nose are usually a little larger or rounder/broader. An EY's pores will be slightly more visible and she may have more T-zone oiliness when young. An EY will generally have more substance to her eyebrows than her EX counterpart.

Androgen Isotypes

Having more androgen in the body does not make a woman more masculine in appearance, but she will have narrower hips and broader shoulders than an estrogen-dominant woman (Figure 11–6). Generally women who are androgen-dominant are taller with larger, denser bone structure than their estrogen-dominant counterparts. The features are stronger and less pointed, although they may be angular. The jaw will be squarer with denser eyebrows that can grow closer to the center of the nose. The skin is thicker and oilier with larger pores (Figure 11–7). There is more facial hair and more terminal hairs as these women move toward menopause. Androgen-dominant women tend to have more body hair, making them prime clients for hair-removal services. Their higher levels of androgen can cause more breakout issues.

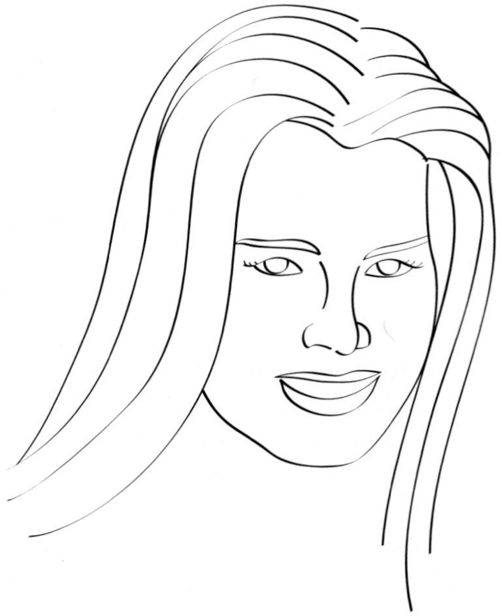

Figure 11–7 Androgen facial shape features.

FOCUS ON: *Androgen-dominant Clients*

Androgen-dominant clients need hair removal services and treatments and home care products to control problem skin issues.

Activity

Evaluate yourself and your classmates to determine the estrogen-androgen isotype of each and practice recognizing each isotype.

This isotype also has two main categories: AX and AY. The AX client is a step above an EY in terms of androgen levels, with thicker skin and a jaw that is more oval to square. An AX is straighter in the torso with a less defined waist and smaller in the hips and thighs proportionately. The AY client has the most androgen in her system. Many models who are tall and broad-shouldered and have small buttocks, are in the AY category. With the thicker skin, these clients tend to show the visible signs of aging more slowly.

SKIN CATEGORIES

During basic esthetics training, you learned to recognize different skin conditions. These conditions can be broken into easily recognizable categories that you can incorporate into your analysis of a client's skin. Moreover, if you see conditions that fall into multiple categories, you will be able to prioritize which condition needs treatment first. Following are five basic categories of skin conditions that can be dealt with on a hierarchal scale of priorities:

- Traumatized
- Sensitized or dehydrated
- Inflamed acne
- Non-inflamed acne
- Congestion
- Aging

We always must treat skin conditions in order of priority. The first issue we must deal with is redness or possible wounding. Next, skin sensitivities or inflammation can be addressed. Once these are under control we can deal with breakouts. First we deal with inflamed breakouts and once under control then the non-inflammed varieties. Once breakouts are under control we can deal with congestion. Lastly, once we have all of the other categories under control we can deal with the signs of aging. Of course not every skin will exhibit all of the catagories of conditions. In this case start with any inflamed type of issues before moving to non-inflamed ones.

All of the different methods or styles of skin evaluation and categorization are tools that can be used by estheticians to make treatments more successful. This is the ultimate goal.

REVIEW QUESTIONS

1. What does the Fitzpatrick scale measure?
2. Which Fitzpatrick type is the most prone to a sunburn?
3. Which Fitzpatrick type is the most resistant to sun trauma?
4. What are the four categories of the Glogau classification system?
5. How does the Rubin system differ from the Glogau?
6. Discuss the three levels of Kligman's Rosacea Classification system.
7. Which estrogen-androgen isotype is prone to early signs of aging?
8. Which isotypes are more prone to problem skin issues?

REVIEW QUESTIONS

9. What are the keys to differentiating between an EX and an EY isotype?
10. Discuss how treatments might differ for an estrogen-dominant client versus an androgen-dominant client.

CHAPTER GLOSSARY

Fitzpatrick skin typing scale: a scale used to measure the skin type's ability to tolerate sun exposure.

Glogau scale: a scale used to evaluate the level of sun damage based on wrinkling.

isotype: in biology, one of several biological types. A physical example or representation of that type.

Rubin scale: evaluates skin based on the depth of the photodamage into the skin.

CHAPTER OUTLINE

- CATEGORIES OF COSMETIC INGREDIENTS
- TYPES OF FUNCTIONAL INGREDIENTS
- PERFORMANCE INGREDIENTS
- INGREDIENTS FOR AGING SKIN
- READING INGREDIENT LABELS

CHAPTER 12

SKIN CARE PRODUCTS: INGREDIENTS AND CHEMISTRY

LEARNING OBJECTIVES

After completing this chapter, you should be able to:

- Describe the different types and categories of cosmetic and skin care ingredients.
- Define the difference between a drug and a cosmetic.
- Demonstrate how to interpret an ingredient label on a product.
- Discuss the difference between a functional and performance ingredient.
- Identify the functions of many functional and performance ingredients.
- Describe how products are made.
- Read and understand a product's ingredient label.

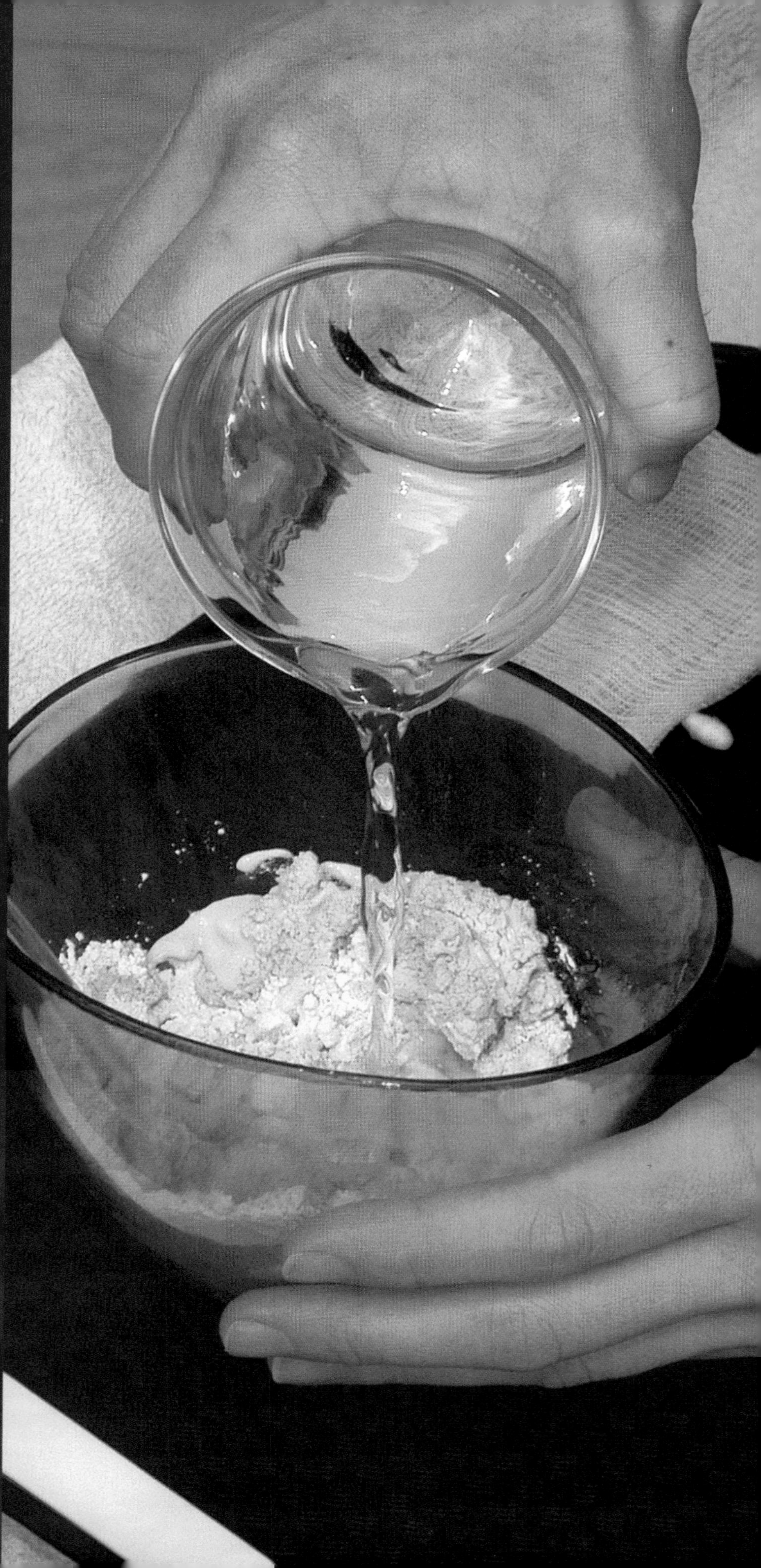

KEY TERMS

Page numbers indicate where in the chapter the term is used.

active ingredient 253
anecdotal 272
bioavailable 275
biologically inert 254
buffering 262
catechins 275
collagenase 274
crosslinking 275
defatting agents 264
deionization 253
distillation 254
drug 252
drug claim 253
elastase 274
ester 257
external phase 259
free radicals (reactive oxygen species) 274
gellant 263
globules 259
glucans 277
glycolic acid 271
homogenizers 260
hyaluronidase 274
hydroxy radical 274
inactive ingredients 253
internal phase 259
isopropyl alcohol 256
keratolytics 271
lactic acid 271
lipid peroxide 274
lipophilic 258
malic acid 271
micelle 260
micellized 260
microencapsulation 260
microsponge 261
natural moisturizing factors (NMFs) 267
non-acnegenic 255
non-comedogenic 255
parfum 264
physical emulsions 260
polyphenols 275
pressing agents 254
proanthocyanidins 275
proteases 274
protectants 254
proteolytic enzymes 271
rancid 262
SD alcohol ("specially denatured") 267
sodium PCA 268
subclinical 274
substantives 268
superfatted 265
superoxide dismutase 275
tartaric acid 271
viscosity 256

Estheticians work with both skin care products and color cosmetics. Cosmetic chemistry is the science of formulating and producing the products used in the esthetics profession and by consumers at home. Cosmetic chemistry includes the formulation of skin care products and color cosmetics, such as lipstick or eyeshadow. Cosmetic chemists often specialize in either skin care or color cosmetics. Using chemicals as well as ingredients obtained from plants and nature, the cosmetic chemist produces cleansers, moisturizers, foundation makeup, and dozens of other products. Cosmetic chemists must understand many scientific subjects, including:

- **Biology:** They need to know how products will be absorbed and how the skin and individual cells will react to ingredients and combinations of ingredients.

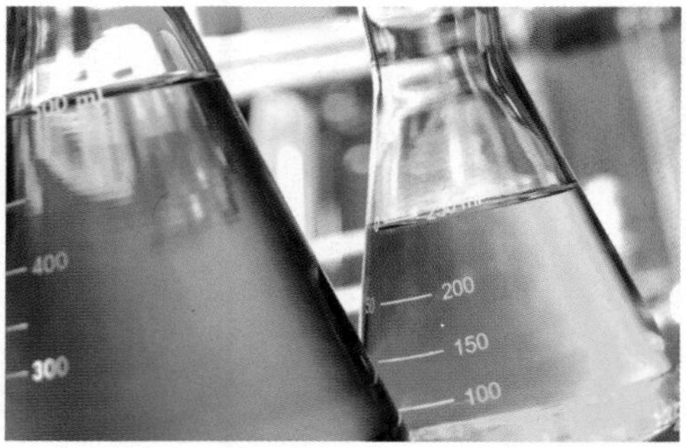

Figure 12–1 Chemistry lab.

- **Chemistry:** Chemists study how different chemicals interact and how ingredients are mixed to produce products (Figure 12–1).
- **Medicine:** Some products made by cosmetic chemists are actually drugs. For example, a topical acne medication may be formulated by a cosmetic chemist. The chemist must understand how the cells and body functions to properly formulate products.
- **Pharmacology:** This is the study of how drugs and chemicals affect the body's function. Cosmetic chemists are sometimes also pharmacists, and universities that offer training for cosmetic chemists often operate these programs through their college of pharmacy.
- **Cosmetology:** The cosmetic chemist must also be familiar with why a product is needed, how it will be used, and the appearance change achieved by the use of that product. Cosmetic chemists frequently work with estheticians to determine the need for a specific product and the practical application techniques and usage of the product. While the chemist is an expert at formulating and developing products, estheticians are experts at using the products.

CATEGORIES OF COSMETIC INGREDIENTS

Functional and Performance Ingredients

There are two basic categories of cosmetic ingredients: functional ingredients and performance ingredients. Functional ingredients are those that cause a product to spread across the skin, keep a product properly mixed, determine a product's texture and feel, regulate the pH of the product, or keep a product from spoiling or being contaminated with bacteria. Functional ingredients do not usually cause the appearance changes associated with the use of skin care products and cosmetics. Ingredients that cause actual physical changes to the appearance of the skin are called performance ingredients, performance agents, or active agents. (Sometimes people use the term *active ingredient* to describe a performance ingredient. This is not correct. *Active ingredient* is the term used to describe drug ingredients.) Some ingredients are both functional to the formulation and act as performance agents on the skin.

Drug versus Cosmetic

It is imperative to understand the legal difference between a drug and a cosmetic. The U.S. Food and Drug Administration (FDA) defines a **drug** as "articles (other than food) intended to affect the structure or any function of the body." The FDA defines cosmetics as "articles intended to be rubbed, poured, sprinkled, or otherwise applied to the human body or any part thereof for cleansing, beautifying, promoting physical attractiveness, or altering the appearance." As defined by the FDA, a drug causes physiological changes and is *intended* to cause this change. It is meant to affect the structure or function of the body.

An **active ingredient** in a drug is the specific chemical or chemicals that cause the change when the drug is used. Active ingredients affect the biochemical activity of the body, which may also include the skin. An active ingredient in a drug is similar to a performance ingredient in a cosmetic. It causes the changes desired by its use.

Inactive ingredients in a drug product do not specifically cause a physiological change but are necessary for the drug to work. For example, if penicillin capsules are used to treat a bacterial infection, the penicillin itself is the active ingredient; the gelatin in the capsule is an inactive ingredient. Inactive ingredients in a drug are similar to the functional ingredients in a skin care product or cosmetic. They do not cause the change but are necessary for the change to take place.

To imply that a skin care product causes changes in the structure or function of the skin is to make a **drug claim.** *Making such a claim is a violation of federal law.* On the other hand, in television or print advertising you may hear specific terminology such as "this product makes the skin *appear* younger." The key word here is *appear*. The skin that experiences this product will *not be* younger—it will only *look* younger. This is clearly a cosmetic claim.

"Cosmeceutical" Ingredients

In 1938 the U.S. Congress passed the Food, Drug, and Cosmetic Act, which lists the drug and cosmetic definitions above. Obviously, much more is known today about the skin, the aging process, and the structure and function of the skin. It is now known that although the epidermis is technically dead, it is biochemically active, and there are many biochemical reactions that take place in the epidermis. It is also known that there are many topical ingredients that affect the appearance of the skin and the biochemical reactions that occur within the skin. It is often the changes that occur in these biochemical reactions that produce the appearance changes we see when we use certain skin care products. Although this is known to be true, no one can tout these physiological reactions because that would constitute making a drug claim for a cosmetic product. One can only talk about the appearance effects caused by the product.

Many scientists, including cosmetic chemists, pharmacists, and physicians, believe that there should be a third product category defined by the Food, Drug, and Cosmetic Act. Cosmeceuticals are products that are not drugs intended to treat diseases, but they do benefit the skin in a positive way, helping to maintain or restore normal skin behavior and enhancing or preserving the skin's health. Although not officially recognized by the FDA, the term *cosmeceuticals* refers to products or ingredients that promote skin health and also make the skin look better. Until there is a change in the law, however, estheticians must keep in mind the current legal definitions when describing products. To that end, this chapter offers detailed information on how different performance ingredients affect the behavior of the skin and therefore affect the skin's appearance.

TYPES OF FUNCTIONAL INGREDIENTS

Vehicles

The largest part of any skin care or cosmetic product is a functional ingredient that acts as the spreading agent or vehicle. Without vehicles, estheticians could not deliver the performance ingredients to the skin.

Water

Water is the most common vehicle ingredient, and it is almost always listed first on the ingredient label of most products. The FDA requires that all companies must list the ingredients of cosmetics on a label or product package, and they must list the ingredients in descending order of concentration. This means that the ingredient that makes up the largest part of the product must be listed first, the second largest part second, and so on. When water is listed first, it means that there is more water in the product than any other ingredient. The thinner the product, the more water is in the formula.

Water must be purified before being used in skin care and cosmetic products. There are several different ways of refining water:

- **Deionization** neutralizes ions that can cross-react with other ingredients, which can make a product unstable. Using deionized water is particularly important in the emulsifying process, which keeps a product well mixed and uniform.

- **Distillation** removes mineral and trace elements from water. These minerals and elements can possible interfere with product stability.
- **Sterilization** kills all bacteria, viruses, and spores that might be in water. This process is used primarily in the manufacture of drugs.

Water can be both a functional and performance ingredient. It serves as a functional ingredient when it is a spreading agent or solvent for other ingredients. Water is also very important as a performance ingredient because it is literally what hydrates the skin. When mixed with moisturizing ingredients and applied to the skin, water helps soften the skin, hydrating dead surface cells and plumping the surface, which makes wrinkles look much better. Because bacteria grows in water, a preservative is required to prevent this growth.

Emollients

Emollients are ingredients that coat the skin. Oils are a good example of emollients. Emollients can serve as a vehicle or spreading agent, helping to deliver performance ingredients. They are also used to help other ingredients like powders and color foundations adhere to the skin's surface, and they are most often responsible for the softness and silky feel of skin care and cosmetic products.

Emollients can also be performance ingredients as they lubricate the skin, creating a surface barrier that helps the skin retain water, blocking evaporation, and keeping the skin from dehydrating. Ingredients that keep water from evaporating from the skin are performance ingredients called **protectants,** which can also keep substances from penetrating the skin. A good example is baby oil, which is simply mineral oil with fragrance. Baby oil keeps urine from irritating the delicate skin of an infant and also keeps the baby's skin from dehydrating. Emollients help to smooth cracks in the skin surface caused by dehydration, making skin look smoother and feel softer. Following are some emollients commonly used in skin care products.

PETROLATUM Petrolatum, commonly known as *petroleum jelly,* is a well-known protectant. It can serve as a vehicle or performance agent. Like mineral oil or other oils, petrolatum can help prevent dehydration, provide protection and lubrication for severely dry skin, and work as a barrier to keep substances from penetrating the skin. Petrolatum is commonly used in drugs as both a vehicle and protectant, and many dermatologists regard it as the best protective agent known. As a vehicle it is often used to carry antibiotics for skin infections and topical steroids to treat dermatological conditions, such as eczema and psoriasis. One advantage of using petroleum is that almost no one is allergic to it, so it is often used in topical drug formulations. A disadvantage of petroleum is that it feels greasy and cannot be used in large concentrations in skin care or cosmetic products without the product also feeling greasy. It is often used as a vehicle in camouflage makeup to cover scars and birthmarks because foundation products made with petrolatum are very easy to apply, suspend enough pigment to give excellent coverage, and are waterproof.

SILICONES Silicones are a group of chemicals and derivatives frequently used in many modern skin care, cosmetic, and hair products. The silicones are one of the most state-of-the-art chemical groups used in skin care and makeup products today. They are lightweight, have a very silky feel, and help make products feel soft and appealing. Like many emollient ingredients, silicones and their derivatives can serve as either functional or performance ingredients. They are excellent spreading agents for sunscreens, creams, fluids, and serums and are also frequently used in makeup foundations.

Silicones offer a number of advantages. First, many silicone derivatives are polymers forming a web-like molecular structure. They lie across the skin like a window screen, allowing air to touch the skin while helping to prevent water from escaping from the skin surface. Therefore, they are also performance ingredients. As functional ingredients, silicones are often used to help sunscreen actives spread evenly across the skin. Another advantage of silicones is that they make the skin soft but not greasy, like other emollients can. Silicones can also be used as **pressing agents,** helping blushes and powders stay in cake form, and they can help powder cosmetics adhere or stick to the skin. In addition, silicones are **biologically inert**—a trait they share with petrolatum and mineral oil—so they will not cross-react with natural skin-functioning reactions. This means they are extremely unlikely to cause inflammation, irritation, or allergic reactions, making them excellent ingredients for sensitive-skin products. These state-of-the-art substances have replaced heavier and occlusive oils used in older formulations. Following are some silicones frequently used in skin care products:

- Cyclomethicone
- Dimethicone

- Dimethiconol
- Phenyl trimethicone
- Cyclopentasiloxane

Here's a Tip

When reading a cosmetic product label, you will find silicone-based ingredients usually shown with the letters *con, sil,* or *cone* somewhere in the ingredient name. Also, these vehicle ingredients are usually near the top of the ingredient list, because they are often used in higher concentrations than other ingredients.

EMOLLIENTS AND COMEDOGENICITY Comedogenicity is the tendency of topical agents, primarily emollients, to cause the development of comedones. A product or ingredient that causes comedones to develop is called comedogenic. In clog-prone and acne-prone skin, cell buildup, known as retention hyperkeratosis, occurs on the follicle walls. Dead cells build up and are coated by the sebum overproduced by this same skin type. Acne bacteria feed off fatty acids, which the bacteria break down from the sebum. When applied to the skin surface, some oils and oil-derivative emollients, particularly natural oils, further coat these follicle walls, worsening acne conditions. For people who do not experience acne issues, the incorporation of these ingredients is not a problem.

Silicones and their derivatives are **non-comedogenic,** which means that they do not cause comedones or clogged pores to form. They are also **non-acnegenic,** meaning that they will not irritate the inside of follicles and cause flares of acne. Unfortunately, silicones, as well as mineral oil and petrolatum, have been incorrectly blamed for causing problems because they are not "natural," having been derived from other sources in the laboratory. The truth is that many natural substances, including plant oils, are much more likely to cause allergies and irritation and to be comedogenic and acnegenic.

NATURAL EMOLLIENTS Most natural oils are emollients (Figure 12–2). Again, they are used as both vehicle functional ingredients and moisture-guarding performance ingredients. Some oils are used by themselves in skin care, particularly in massage treatments and aromatherapy treatments. Commonly used plant oils include:

- Coconut oil
- Grapeseed oil
- Palm oil
- Sweet almond oil
- Soybean oil
- Rice bran oil
- Castor oil
- Sunflower oil
- Safflower oil
- Jojoba oil

Many plants from which these oils are derived can provide waxes, which are basically hardened forms of natural oils. Following are some commonly used waxes that are derived from plants:

- Carnauba wax (frequently used in lipstick, from the carnauba palm)
- Candelilla wax
- Soy wax
- Jojoba wax

Other waxes come from animal sources:

- Beeswax
- Lanolin (from wool processing)

Some come from petroleum sources:

- Paraffin wax
- Microcrystalline wax

Other waxes are synthetic:

- Polymer wax
- Polyethylene wax

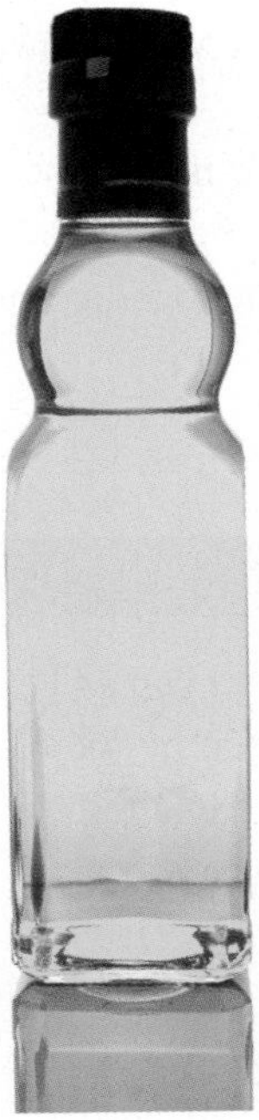

Figure 12–2 Natural oil.

FATTY ACIDS Fatty acids are fatty ingredients derived from plant or animal sources. Many people think of an acid as being corrosive or capable of inflicting burns. A fatty acid is a noncorrosive triglyceride that has been broken down in the process of removing glycerin from fat. Fatty acids are used as emollients, both as functional spreading agents or texture softeners for creams and lotions, as well as performance ingredient hydration protectants and skin smoothers.

Fatty acids are used in many moisturizers, shaving creams, lipsticks, foundations, and cleansers and as pressing agents in cake powder blushes and powders. Although there is a trend to derive fatty acids strictly from plant oils, many can also be derived from animal fat. Following are common fatty acids used in skin care and cosmetic formulations. All of these acids are derived from natural sources.

- **Stearic acid:** Derived from animal fat or plant oil; frequently used in creams, including shaving cream; also used in making soap and candles
- **Caprylic acid:** Derived from coconut oil, palm oil, or animal fat
- **Oleic acid:** Derived from animal fats and olive and grapeseed oils
- **Myristic acid:** Derived from coconut or palm seed oil, nutmeg butter, animal fat, and other vegetable fats
- **Palmitic acid:** Derived from palm oil or palm kernel oil, but occurs naturally in many dairy products
- **Lauric acid:** The main fatty acid in coconut and palm oil; used in manufacture of the well-known surfactant sodium lauryl sulfate

Note that although fatty acids have many good uses in the manufacturing of skin care and cosmetic products, in large concentrations many are comedogenic and can irritate acne-prone skin.

Here's a Tip

When reading a cosmetic product label, you will usually find fatty acid ingredients listed by their actual names, unless they are chemically altered. If they are chemically altered, the name of the related ingredient will still contain a few letters of their fatty acid name. For example, lauryl alcohol and ammonium lauryl sulfate are derivatives of lauric acid.

FATTY ALCOHOLS When most people think of alcohol, they think of isopropyl alcohol, which is poured on cuts as an antiseptic. They may also think of alcoholic beverages. These forms of alcohol have negative connotations and may explain why people have a fear of alcohol in skin care and cosmetic products. The word *alcohol* is actually a reference to a particular type of chemical structure in which a hydrogen atom and an oxygen atom have attached themselves to the end of a chain of carbon atoms.

Many people also think of alcohol as being a drying cosmetic chemical. This may be true of isopropanol, also known as **isopropyl alcohol**, which is sometimes used in products for very oily skin. Another common stripping alcohol is SD (specially denatured) alcohol. The truth is that most alcohols used in skin care and cosmetic formulations are actually more like waxy or oily emollients, although less sticky or heavy than fatty acids. They are certainly not drying. They are fatty acids, like the ones discussed previously, that have been exposed to hydrogen. Fatty alcohols can be used as emollient vehicles or skin smoothers and sometimes enhance the texture of lotions and creams. Fatty alcohols are also frequently used to improve the thickness and liquidity, or **viscosity**, of lotions and creams. Some common fatty alcohols include:

- **Cetyl alcohol:** Derived from petroleum products, coconut and palm oils; used as an emollient, an emulsifier for keeping creams mixed, and a cream thickener
- **Lauryl alcohol:** Also known as *dodecanol*; used as an emollient and emulsifier
- **Stearyl alcohol:** Can be derived from animal or plant sources; used as an emollient, emulsifier, thickener, or foam booster for foaming cleansers
- **Cetearyl alcohol:** A mixture of cetyl and stearyl alcohol used as a foam booster, stabilizer, and thickener, or to give a silky feel to products
- **Oleyl alcohol:** Multi-use functional ingredient used as an emollient, thickener, and emulsifier; used in superfatted soaps and has an oilier feel than other fatty alcohols

Here's a Tip

When reading a cosmetic product label, you will find that a fatty alcohol ingredient has its fatty acid component in the first part of the name, followed by the word *alcohol*.

FATTY ESTERS An **ester** is formed when an organic (carbon chain) acid, such as a fatty acid, chemically combines with an alcohol. Fatty esters are used as emollients in skin care and cosmetic products. Fatty esters are lighter weight than many other emollient ingredients. They can be used as either functional emollients or emulsifiers or as performance ingredient protectants, and they can also be used to reinforce barrier function (discussed later in this chapter).

Fatty acids vary greatly in molecular weight and size, which can affect how each ester is used in formulation. Like fatty acids and alcohols, fatty esters are often comedogenic and must be carefully selected and used in low concentrations when formulating products for oily or acne-prone skin types.

Frequently used fatty esters in skin care and cosmetic formulations include:

- **Isopropyl myristate:** Isopropanol reacts with fatty acid myristic acid to form this ester. Isopropyl myristate is comedogenic and should be avoided for oily skin.
- **Isopropyl palmitate:** Isopropanol reacts with fatty acid palmitic acid to form this ester. Isopropyl palmitate is comedogenic and should be avoided for oily skin.
- **Ethylhexyl palmitate:** Used as an emollient
- **Ethylhexyl stearate:** Used as an emollient
- **Isopropyl isostearate:** Lighter weight emollient
- **Glyceryl stearate:** Used as an emollient and emulsifier
- **Propylene glycol dicaprate/dicaprylate:** Non-comedogenic emollient ester
- **Cetyl palmitate:** Used as a lighter weight emollient

Surfactants

One of the largest categories of cosmetic chemicals, surfactants are chemicals in cosmetics that lower surface tension on the skin to allow cosmetic vehicles to slip across or onto the skin. a surfactant differs, though, from an emollient vehicle. Surfactant ingredients are used in personal care as well as household products like laundry detergents, industrial chemicals, and even agriculture. Personal-care applications of surfactants include detergents and soaps.

> ***Here's a Tip***
>
> When reading a cosmetic product label, you will find that fatty ester ingredients usually have the letters *-ate* at the end of the last word in the ingredient name. The first part of the last word reflects the ester's fatty acid component relation. For example, *stearate* is an ester of stearic acid.

DETERGENTS Detergents are surfactants that are used for cleansing. They break up oils, fats, and other debris and cause the debris to separate from the skin. When detergents are applied to the skin and are mixed with water, they begin to bubble. This bubbling is a good example of how surfactants and detergents reduce surface tension and allow water to spread more easily across the skin. Bubbling is the air that has come between the surfactant and the surface of the skin. The surfactant removes surface oils from the skin, as well as makeup, dirt, pollutants, and other agents that have come in contact with or adhered to the skin during the day.

Another good example of reduction of surface tension by a surfactant is in your kitchen. You cooked hamburgers for dinner and you left the pan with the hamburger grease on the stove while you ate dinner. During that time, the grease, which is fats and fatty acids, has solidified in the pan. After dinner, you add hot water to the pan, which liquefies the fat. It is the temperature, not the water, that liquefies the fat. If you leave the water in the pan, the grease will remain liquid for the most part, but we know that hot water alone will not remove beef grease from a pan. So you pour in some dishwashing liquid. If you look closely while you are pouring in the dishwashing liquid, you will notice that the fat has a tendency to "run" from the dishwashing liquid. This "running" is actually the surfactant or detergent improving the water's ability to remove the grease from the pan's surface. The grease will break up much faster with the detergent added to the pan.

During the process of cleaning the pan, you accidentally rub grease from the hamburgers on your hand. When you remove your hand from the sink, you discover that your hand is greasy. Dipping your hand into the dishwater seems to loosen the grease from your hand. This is because the surfactant (detergent) works on skin in the same way that it works on the dishes or pan (Figure 12–3).

Of course, the surfactant used in dishwashing is much too strong a detergent to use routinely on your skin. Similar detergent agents may be used in dishwashing liquids, but the concentration of detergent in the formula is far greater than that used in a facial cleanser. Facial cleansers also may vary in strength and concentration.

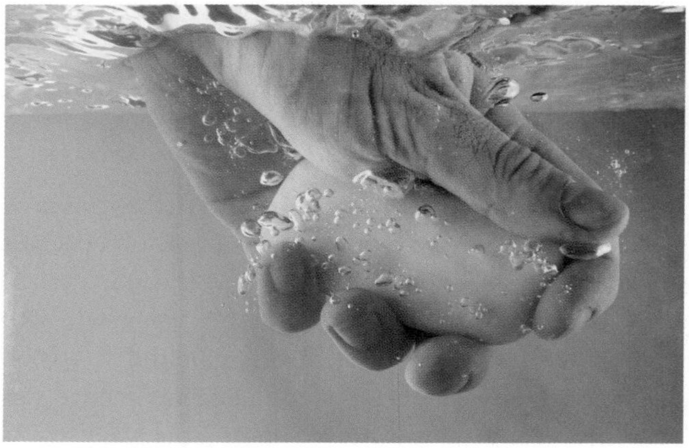

Figure 12–3 Soap in use.

The four major types of surfactants vary with the pH of the water being used in the formulation. The four basic types of surfactants are as follows:

1. **Anionic surfactants,** which have a negative ionic charge. Anionic surfactants are strong cleansers and are frequently used in household products.
2. **Cationic surfactants** have a positive ionic charge. They are frequently used in cosmetics and hair shampoos.
3. **Amphoteric surfactants** may have either a positive or negative ionic charge. They will adapt to the pH of the water used in the solution. Because they are so adaptable to both acid and alkaline water, they are frequently used in facial lotions and creams. The neutrality of the surfactant is important to the mildness of the cosmetic product.
4. **Nonionic surfactants** are used in heavier creams such as hand creams.

Following are some surfactant ingredients that are frequently used in cosmetic cleansers. All of these surfactants help remove oils, dirt, and other debris from the skin's surface. How much they remove depends on the amount of surfactant in the individual cleanser.

- Sodium laureth sulfate
- Sodium lauryl sulfate
- Disodium lauryl sulfosuccinate
- Ammonium lauryl sulfate
- Cocoamphocarboxyglycinate
- Cocamidopropyl betaine
- Alpha-olefin sulfonate
- Decyl polyglucoside

For sensitive and drier skin types, cosmetic manufacturers often add a fatty acid, oil, or wax to cut the contact of the surfactant with the skin. The fatty substance prevents too much of the surfactant from coming in contact with the skin. Too much detergent can be irritating or dehydrating to sensitive, dry, or thin skin.

Cleansers can also vary in strength depending on the concentration of surfactant that is in the formula. A cleanser for oilier skin generally contains more, or a higher concentration of, surfactant than a cleanser for dry skin. Most cleansers are carefully prepared so that they prevent irritation on most skin types. Surfactants are also added to creams to improve the cream's slip (how well the product flows across the skin) and adhesive qualities. Some surfactants may irritate skin when used in creams.

Surface active agents (which reduce surface tension of water for the spreading of cosmetic products), detergents (cleansing and foaming agents), and emulsifiers (which keep water and oils in emulsion state) are all surfactants. If they are all surfactants, why do these three surfactants do different things? The difference among the three functions has to do with their molecular structures. The size of a particular molecule determines the different properties that the particular surfactant will have in a cosmetic solution. Surfactants are polymer molecules. This means that there is a chain of carbon atoms that are connected to one another. Surfactant polymer molecules have two ends. One end is attracted to water, and this is called the hydrophilic ("water loving") end; the other end is repelled by water and is attracted instead to fatty substances, so it is called the **lipophilic** ("fat loving") end. The size of the lipophilic end of the polymer determines which kind of surfactant group the molecule will be.

- Shorter-chain carbon polymers—chains with 8 or 10 carbon atoms—have a shorter lipophilic end and are surface active agents used in creams to improve slip and spreadability.
- Medium-length-chain molecules with a medium-sized lipophilic end are the detergents used in cleansers that help foam and remove surface debris.
- Long-chain polymers, which have a large lipophilic end, are emulsifiers.

This makes sense, because these molecules must have a strong attraction to fat. Remember, these molecules are the ones that "surround" or form the "shell" around the oil droplets and spread themselves throughout the water solution. The other end of the emulsifier (the hydrophilic end) is attracted to the water in the solution, so the molecule produces a "tug-of-war" between the oil and the water. The emulsifier is attracted to the oil and is more or less wrapped around the oil, but the other end is attracted to the water in which it is floating. This constant "pulling" keeps the oil or fat evenly suspended in the water solution or, in the case of a water-in-oil suspension, the water is evenly suspended in the oil or fat solution. The oil droplets in an oil-in-water emulsion are referred to as **globules.** They are the dispersed part of the emulsion and are referred to as the **internal phase.** The water in an oil-in-water emulsion is called the **external phase.**

A suspension is a liquid solution in which the internal and external phases do not stay mixed for any period of time. Suspensions always separate, like salad dressing, and must be shaken before use. In esthetics, there are suspension foundations (generally designed for very oily skin), suspension drying agents for acne, and other suspension products.

We have only talked here about lotions. Many types of cosmetic emulsions are not lotions and contain components other than water and oils. Makeup, for example, is a solid such as talc that is emulsified in a liquid. The external phase of a makeup base is usually water, possibly mixed with propylene glycol or another solvent. Aerosol hair spray is an example of a liquid that is emulsified within a gas. Mousse is an example of a gas that is emulsified within an external phase liquid.

PHYSICAL EMULSIONS The barrier function of the epidermis is extremely important to maintain hydration and protect the skin from irritating substances penetrating the skin surface. As you know from previous chapters, the barrier function resembles a brick wall. The "bricks" are the epidermal cells, and the "mortar" comprises lipids that have been secreted during the keratinization process. The complex of lipids between the cells prevents epidermal dehydration as the lipids "seal" the moisture in the skin and helps to repel potential inflammatory agents that might penetrate the skin surface.

EMULSIONS AND EMULSIFIERS Oils or fats are often mixed with water in an emulsion to form a fluid, lotion, or cream. If you have ever mixed oil and water in a bottle, or mixed vinegar and oil in salad dressing, you know that water and oil repel each other. They do not mix and stay mixed. Emulsions are stabilized and uniform mixtures of water and oil. An emulsifier is an ingredient that keeps water and oil mixtures uniformly mixed. Emulsifiers work by forming a sort of "shell" around oil droplets, allowing them to remain mixed in a solution with water. Like detergents, they reduce the surface tension of the components of the mixture. In fact, some detergents can also be emulsifiers.

Some of these mixtures may be fluids, lotions, or heavier creams. In general, the more water in the formula, the more liquid the product will be. Emulsions that are mostly water are called oil-in-water (o/w) emulsions. Most lotions available today are oil-in-water emulsions. They are lighter weight and have light textures, do not feel greasy, and are easy to remove. "Water-based" generally means that the emulsion or lotion is an oil-in-water emulsion. It does not necessarily mean that the emulsion is oil-free. The main reason cosmetic companies refer to a product as being water-based is to appeal to the consumer. Consumers who have oily or problem skin and consumers who do not like greasy products look for products that are watery textured because they are lighter weight and non-greasy. Most oil-in-water products are packaged in bottles or tubes.

Emulsions that are mostly oil are called water-in-oil (w/o) emulsions. Water-in-oil emulsions tend to be thicker and heavier, because they are mostly oil. Old-fashioned cold cream is a good example. Thicker, heavier mixtures also tend to have more emulsifier ingredient in the product. Most water-in-oil products are packaged in jars. They are too heavy and thick to be poured out of a bottle.

Have you ever found an old bottle of lotion in your cabinet? Did it look "watery"? Over time, generally a year or more, emulsifiers can stop working in an emulsion. When this happens, the lotion begins to separate back into its water and oil phases. It is said to "fall out of emulsion." Another way to determine a particular product's emulsion type is to check the ingredient label. The FDA requires that cosmetics list their ingredients in descending order. If oil is listed before water, it is a water-in-oil emulsion. If water is listed first, then it is oil-in-water.

Emulsifiers help to provide stability and texture to lotions and creams. They make the cream feel even and smooth. If they were not used in moisturizers, the lotion would feel wet and oily when applied. Following are some frequently used emulsifiers:

- Amphoteric 9
- Ceteth-20
- Beeswax
- Polyethylene glycol (PEG)
- Polysorbate
- Carbomer

- Carbopol
- Stearamide

Emulsifiers can sometimes cause problems for thin, sensitive, or dry skin types. What happens in these cases is that the emulsifiers actually start breaking down the natural intercellular lipids that form the barrier function of the skin. Although this is not a problem for all types of skin, it can cause sensitivity for already thin, sensitive skin with impaired barrier function.

There is a relatively new technology that uses high-speed mixers, called **homogenizers,** to emulsify products. Most of these products are creams and lotions for sensitive skin. These products use special blends of emollients and nonsurfactant emulsifying agents, which are mixed at high speeds under pressure. This process produces a suspended effect without using traditional surfactant emulsifiers, eliminating further disturbance of the barrier function. These types of products are **physical emulsions** and are known as excellent moisturizers for sensitive skin.

Solvents

Solvents are the liquid part of a solution. A solute is the material mixed into the solvent. Solvents are used in cosmetic formulations either as vehicles for the product or as vehicles for other ingredients. a solution is a solvent plus a solute.

Plant extracts used in skin care products have to be extracted from the actual plant, and a solvent, propylene glycol, is normally used for the extraction. If you see "arnica (arnica montana) extract" on a cosmetic label, it often means that the arnica extract is present in a solution of propylene glycol or another solvent. Both the extract and the solvent must be listed on the cosmetic product label. However, both ingredients still must be listed in the exact order of predominance in the final formulation. Alcohols of various types are also often used as solvents for plant extracts.

High-Tech Vehicles

As we learn more about the skin's anatomy and physiology, the intercellular cement, and penetration of the skin, we learn more about formulating products that are more easily accepted by the skin and that penetrate the skin's surface better. We know, for example, that the intercellular cement is made of various lipids. Making products and using vehicles that are compatible with the intercellular lipids can increase a product's permeability and efficacy. Lipid-based products are good examples. Of course, not every product should easily penetrate the skin. Many ingredients would irritate the skin if they penetrated more deeply, and there are many that are too large in molecular size to penetrate, regardless of what type of vehicle is used.

The concept and technique of how performance ingredients or active ingredients are spread across the skin or set up to adhere to the skin or absorb into the skin's surface is known as the product's delivery system. The delivery system is often more than just a common vehicle-spreading agent; it is often the combination of the primary vehicle ingredient, polymers added to adhere ingredients to the skin in a uniform fashion, or lipids to help penetrate important ingredients through the intercellular lipids.

Micelles

A **micelle** is a protective sphere that is created by emulsifiers surrounding an internal phase ingredient. When you add emulsifier to a solution of water and oil, the emulsifier surrounds the internal phase of the solution. As the emulsifier lines up around the oil, for example, there are small spaces between emulsifier molecules.

In a micelle, the emulsifier completely surrounds the oil, creating a sort of bubble. The bubble encloses the oil, or whatever internal phase ingredient is being emulsified. a cosmetic that has micelles present in it is said to be **micellized.** Micelle technology is important in helping to protect antioxidant ingredients, vitamins, and other performance ingredients that could easily deteriorate chemically if they were not protected.

Liposomes And Microencapsulation

Microencapsulation is the process of using barrier and intercellular-compatible materials like lipids to form special micro-shells to protect and better penetrate certain ingredients. Many ingredients that are unstable or highly reactive can be protected from becoming unstable and can be delivered in a more effective way through microencapsulation. A good example is tocopherol, or vitamin E. Vitamin E, if unprotected, will serve as an antioxidant for the product, keeping the product itself from oxidizing. But if tocopherol is microencapsulated, it will serve as an antioxidant for the skin's protection, instead of the product's protection. A good example of microencapsulation is the liposome.

Liposomes are hollow spheres made of lipid materials, often phosphololipids. Think of a liposome as a spherical bubble envelope made of lipids that are compatible with the lipids making up the intercellular cement. The liposome may be loaded, which means that the liposome may contain a performance ingredient. What is put into a liposome depends on many factors, including the size of the liposome, the size of the ingredient to be carried by the liposome, the shape of the liposome, the ionization of any components, and the purpose of the product. Liposomes may be used to transport moisturizers, vitamins, antioxidants, peptides, or drugs. (Drugs, of course, are not used in cosmetic formulations.) Many ingredients are simply too big to put inside a liposome. Empty liposomes, or unloaded liposomes, are sometimes used in cosmetics to improve the penetration of a cream or moisturizer.

The lipid "mortar" that makes up the barrier function is similar to the lipid material that comprises a liposome, and those lipids can be used to enhance the structure of the barrier function. The lipid barrier accepts lipids similar to its own lipid composition. Therefore, liposomes are allowed to pass through the barrier function, carrying a performance ingredient deeper into the epidermis. Eventually, the liposome begins to dissolve, releasing the ingredient into the intercellular cement to carry out whatever function it is meant to complete. The theories behind liposome functions are still being confirmed. Although chemists have a good idea of how liposomes work, more is being learned all the time about their value in cosmetics.

Other Innovative Vehicles

Other vehicles similar to liposomes have recently been launched. One type is a **"microsponge"** that releases an active ingredient once inside the skin. Microsponges have been used for both skin care ingredients and drug ingredients.

> **Here's a Tip**
>
> When reading a cosmetic product label, you will find that liposomes are never listed as liposomes on the ingredient label. The fact that the product contains liposomes is usually pointed out on the label description or the name of the product. Ingredients that indicate liposomes include soya lecithin, lecithin, phospholipids, or ceramides.

Nanoparticle technology or nanotechnology is the science behind making micronized absorbable delivery systems. Some of these are targeted particular tissue to deliver an ingredient to where it is the most bioavailable or available for the skin (the biology) to use.

Delivery innovations may be used and developed for drugs before they are developed for cosmetics. As we learn more about the functions of the epidermis and the ways chemicals react with the surface of the skin, we will learn more about transport mechanisms for various cosmetic as well as pharmaceutical ingredients.

Antimicrobials and Preservatives

Because of the many fats and natural materials used in skin care and cosmetic formulations, products are more susceptible to invasion by microorganisms than are other types of chemical formulations. Preservatives are chemical agents that inhibit the growth of microorganisms in creams or cosmetic products.

The three main types of microorganisms present in cosmetic formulations are bacteria, fungi, and yeast. Cross-contamination is the process of spreading bacteria or other germs by touching the skin or a surface and then touching the product. This happens when the user applies the cream to the skin and then dips the hand that has touched the skin back into the jar of cream. When the fingers touch the cream, bacteria and other microorganisms come in contact with the product in the jar. Cosmetics must contain preservatives that kill these contaminating bacteria as well as bacteria that are present in small amounts in the raw ingredients used to make the cosmetic. Preservatives are usually one of the first ingredients used in the cosmetic production process, because, if the preservative is already in the mixing tank, bacteria introduced into the formula will be killed as ingredients are added.

Preservatives work by either directly poisoning or releasing other chemicals that poison the microorganisms. Because these substances are poisonous, a user may experience allergies and irritation. Chemists must be careful to use enough preservative to kill microorganisms in the product without adding so much preservative that a user's allergies will be more likely to flare.

A trend in skin care products is the use of botanical (plant) ingredients and other natural materials. Natural materials are more likely to break down than synthetic materials and are more likely to be contaminated with microorganisms such as fungi, frequently present on plants. Therefore, the use of natural materials actually increases the need for more preservatives.

The most commonly used preservatives are methylparaben, propylparaben, phenoxyethanol, and imidazolidinyl urea. Other paraben groups such as ethyl and butyl paraben are also used. These are generally included at less than 1% of the product. Following are other, more frequently used preservatives:

- Ethylparaben
- Butylparaben
- DMDM hydantoin
- Methylchloroisothiazolinone
- Methylchlorothiazolinone
- Methylisothiazolinone
- Quaternium-15
- Diazolidinyl urea

Preservatives are used in very small quantities so they do not cause unnecessary irritation.

Other Types of Preservatives

Microorganisms are not the only threat to cosmetics; chemical reactions can take place that can alter or even ruin skin care products. Oxidation is a chemical reaction in which oxygen is exposed to certain ingredients, which results in a breakdown of the ingredient. It is also the process by which free radicals form. Fats and fatty substances are particularly vulnerable to oxidation. Have you ever been to a picnic and noticed that the potato salad was a yellowish color on the top but when you spooned some onto your plate, noticed that the potato salad below the surface was lighter? This is oxidation. One of the main ingredients in potato salad is mayonnaise, which is mainly oil. The oil in the mayonnaise oxidizes very quickly, causing the yellow color on the top of the potato salad.

The exact same reaction takes place in the fats, fatty acids, and esters in cosmetic products. Oxygen constantly comes in contact with the product during the manufacturing process. After the user opens the product, it is exposed to more oxygen. Every time the user opens and shuts the container, the product is exposed to oxygen. To prevent these reactions, chemists add preservatives such as antioxidants, chelating agents, and buffering agents to cosmetics.

> **Here's a Tip**
>
> Remember, federal law says that ingredients must be listed in descending order of their proportion of the product. Because preservatives are present in products in small quantities, they are almost always the very last ingredients to be listed on a label.

ANTIOXIDANTS Antioxidants are used as both functional as well as performance ingredients. They not only prevent oxidation of product components; they also keep creams and other products from developing color and odor changes caused by oxidation. a bad odor may develop in creams that do not contain enough antioxidant. An oxidized cosmetic product that has discoloration and/or odor due to oxidation is said to be **rancid.** Following are common antioxidants:

- Butylated hydroxyanisole (BHA)
- Butylated hydroxytoluene (BHT)
- Tocopherol (Vitamin E)
- Benzoic acid

CHELATING AGENTS A chelating agent is a chemical that is added to cosmetics to improve the efficiency of the preservative. Chelating agents work by breaking down the cell walls of bacteria and other microorganisms so that the preservative is more easily absorbed by the microorganism. Common chelating ingredients are disodium EDTA, trisodium EDTA, and tetrasodium EDTA. EDTA stands for the chemical name *ethylenediaminetetraacetic acid.* These ingredients appear further down on an ingredient list because they are not used in large quantities.

BUFFERING AGENTS **Buffering** refers to adjusting the pH of a product to make it more acceptable to the skin. Sometimes the pH of a product may be too high or too low. These pH levels may irritate the skin if they are not adjusted. To remedy this problem, a chemist will add a small amount of an acidic or basic chemical to bring the pH up or lower it appropriately. Citric acid is commonly used to lower the pH of a product. Tartaric acid is another acidic agent used in small quantities to bring pH down to an acceptable acid level.

Some products have the opposite problem and turn out to be too acidic for the skin. Ammonium carbonate, calcium carbonate, potassium, sodium, or ammonium hydroxide is sometimes added to a product to raise the pH. These buffering agents are added in very small quantities and will be seen lower on the ingredient label.

Gellants and Thickening Agents

A **gellant** is an agent that is added to a product to give it a gel-like consistency. It improves the appearance of the product and gives it more body, making it stiffer and less runny. Thickening agents make the product spread more easily, easier to handle, and more acceptable to the eye. Many thickening agents can also be used as emulsifiers. Following are examples of thickening and gellant agents:

- **Methyl cellulose:** Derived from plants and chemically altered, this ingredient is both a thickener and an emulsifier.
- **Xanthan gum:** A natural sugar complex but often produced through biotechnology, xanthan gum is a thickener used in foods and cosmetics and also has industrial uses.
- **Beeswax:** This is a natural chemical comprising largely fatty esters and alcohol and used as an emulsifier and thickener.
- **Carbomer:** This synthetic polymer, which is often used in gel formulations, can stabilize emulsions or can be a thickener.

Coloring Agents

Colors are added to products for one reason only: to make them more appealing to consumers. Of course, color agents are used extensively in makeup, appearing on ingredient labels under a variety of names. Color agents are used extensively in the formation of foundations, mascara, eye shadows, eye pencils, lip pencils, powders, blush, lipstick, and contour and camouflage products. The one exception to colors being used in cosmetics only for appeal would be a moisturizing bronzer, designed to moisturize or protect and still give a slight hint of color to the skin's surface.

The FDA regulates two types of colors, certified and noncertified. Certified colors are pigments, or lakes, in blue, green, orange, red, and yellow. They are listed on ingredient labels by color name followed by the number assigned to that color agent by the FDA and the metal associated with the chemical structure. One example is *D & C* (Drug and Cosmetic) *Red No. 4 Aluminum Lake*. On food packages, you might see a color ingredient listed as, for example, *F, D, & C* (Food, Drug and Cosmetic) *Yellow*. Some colors are approved for use in drugs, cosmetics, and foods (Figure 12–4), but, in general, you will rarely see *F, D, & C* listed on a cosmetic ingredient label.

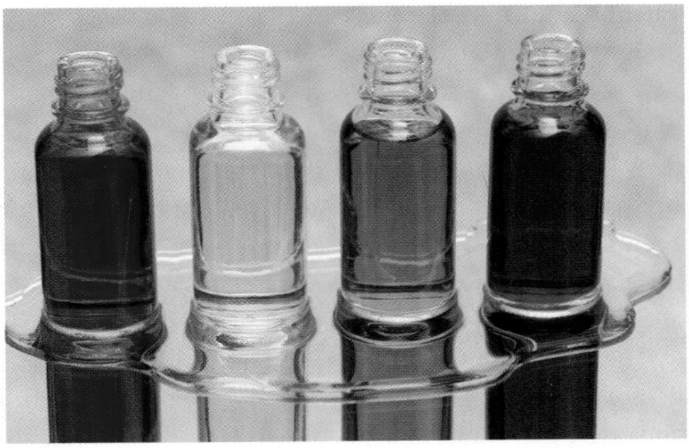

Figure 12–4 Colors.

Noncertified colors are a second list that the FDA uses that are not metal salts. Most noncertified colors are natural plant or animal extracts, mineral pigments, and sometimes synthetic colors. Although these colors are regulated by the FDA, they do not have a specific certification number. They include a variety of common cosmetic color agents, such as:

- Iron oxide
- Zinc oxide
- Carmine
- Beta-carotene
- Chlorophyllin-copper complex
- Annatto
- Ferric ferrocyanide
- Mica
- Ultramarine colors
- Henna

Iron oxide is actually rust, but it is used extensively in the development of foundations and frequently gives makeup its color. There are various shades of iron oxide, and, of course, the shade can vary with the amount used in a particular solution.

When the FDA first began regulating colors, there were about 116 certified colors. Over the years the agency determined that many of these colors were not safe for continual use, and therefore the list has dwindled to about 35 certified color agents. Some individuals are allergic to certain color agents. Therefore, you must pay attention to a client who tells you she is allergic to a particular color and check ingredient labels of products you wish to use on her or sell her.

Certified colors require the processing lab to submit test results to the FDA to be certified. Non-certified colors are generally accepted as "safe" so do not require testing. All colorants used in cosmetics must come from one of these two lists.

The FDA does not permit the use of certified colors in any cosmetics intended for use around the eyes.

Chemists must use noncertified colors in eyeshadow, eyeliner, and other cosmetics intended for the eye area. At any rate, many cosmetic companies now totally eliminate color from their skin care products, because the public is becoming more aware that these chemicals are not necessary in skin care formulations. Also, because color agents can occasionally cause allergic reactions, eliminating coloring agents cuts down on the likelihood of an allergic reaction to the product.

There are countries other than the United States that do not have strong laws governing the use of color agents and therefore may produce cosmetics with color agents that are not permitted in the United States. The European Union and Japan have regulations regarding color, but even those regulations may differ significantly from those of the United States. If you use imported cosmetics, check to see if the maker has complied with FDA rules concerning color.

Fragrances

Consumers often buy a product because they like the smell, which is an important factor in the cosmetic chemistry, especially in bath products. Fragrances are ingredients added to products to give them a pleasant odor. Fragrance can be derived from animal or plant sources or can be synthetically produced.

Essential oils are plant-derived extracts that can be used for their fragrance but also may have aromatherapy characteristics. There are more than 400 essential oils. Plant oils are by far the most popular type of fragrances.

Sometimes products do not smell good because of particular ingredients, and fragrance is added, not to enhance the product but to cover up a bad smell. These fragrance ingredients are known as masking fragrances.

Here's a Tip

When a product contains fragrance, the ingredient is listed as **parfum** on the product label. Many products contain plant extracts that have an odor but are not listed as parfum; rather, they are listed by their Latin and common names, such as camellia oleifera (green tea) extract or vitis vinifera (grape) seed extract. Ingredients such as lavender extract may be used in a skin care product for soothing properties, yet the extract also imparts a powerful fragrance.

Fragrance-free Products

Many skin care products are now marketed as being fragrance-free. Because many consumers have sensitive skin or are allergic to fragrance, fragrance-free products are popular with these clients. Fragrance-free products should not have much odor but may still smell like their other ingredients. Sunscreens often have a very distinctive smell, even if they contain no fragrance ingredients.

PERFORMANCE INGREDIENTS

As discussed earlier, ingredients within a skin care product or cosmetic that actually cause changes to the appearance of the skin are known as *performance ingredients* or *active agents*. They are intended to affect the *appearance* of the skin. *Active ingredients* are chemicals or substances within a drug that are intended to cause *physiological changes*, meaning they are intended to affect a structure or biochemical function of the body, including the skin. Performance ingredients are, by far, the most important ingredients in cosmetic chemistry. In this section, we will discuss many different performance ingredients used in cleansers, moisturizers, and treatment products for various skin types and conditions, as well as active ingredients used in over-the-counter (OTC) drugs like sunscreens and acne products. Every skin care product or cosmetic has at least one performance ingredient. Performance ingredients may also be functional ingredients, or vehicles. For example, an emollient that helps to spread a moisturizing cream can also serve as a barrier to keep moisture from leaving the stratum corneum. In that case the emollient is both a functional and a performance ingredient.

Cleansing Agents

Performance ingredients in cleansers may be of two types: detergents or emulsion cleansing agents. Detergents cause cleansers to foam. a performance ingredient detergent is present in any foaming cleanser, rinseable cleanser, or shampoo. Detergents work by loosening sebum and debris from the skin surface. They are essentially **defatting agents**, which means the surfactant separates fats and lipids, along with dirt, makeup, and debris, from the surface of the skin.

Following are commonly used detergent ingredients used in cleansers:

- Sodium lauryl sulfate
- Sodium laureth sulfate
- Ammonium lauryl sulfate

- Disodium lauryl sulfosuccinate
- Decyl polyglucoside
- Lauramphocarboxylglycinate
- Cocamidopropyl betaine

Individual detergents can be stronger than others. A cleanser's strength is also related to the concentration of detergent ingredients in the cleanser and how long the cleanser is left on the skin. Other ingredients that may be in the formulation may also enhance or reduce the cleansing action of the detergent ingredient.

Foaming Cleansers

Foaming cleansers are popular because they are easily rinsed away and because they are quick and easy to use. Many consumers report their skin feels cleaner when they use a foaming cleansing product. This is common with former soap-and-water users.

Foaming cleansers vary in strength and in the levels of oiliness they target (Figure 12–5). The main differences in these cleansers are the amount and type of detergent ingredient used and the amounts of buffering oils and fats that may be included in the formulation to lessen skin contact, as well as other ingredients such as exfoliants or granules that enhance dead cell removal during cleansing or soothing ingredients that may be included to help soothe sensitive skin types.

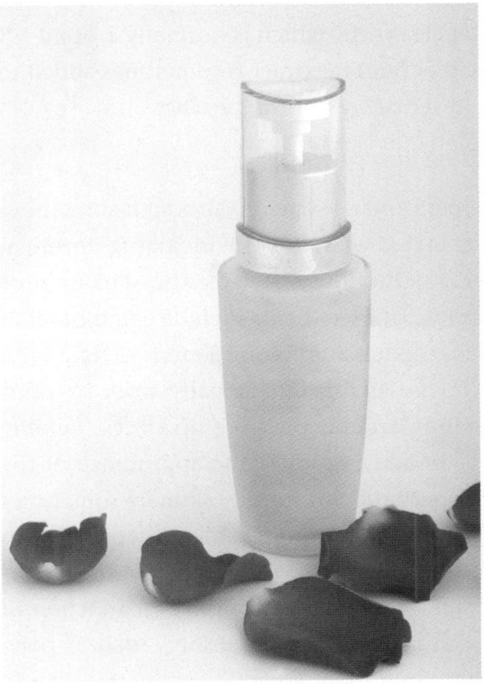

Figure 12–5 Lotion cleanser.

Soap

Like foaming cleansers, soap also defats the skin's surface. There are two basic disadvantages to soaps, which are usually made of salts of fatty acids. First, many soaps have a high pH, which can irritate and dry the skin, impair the barrier function by removing too much sebum, and begin removing intercellular lipids from the corneum. Both fatty acid salts in soap and detergents in foaming cleansers can strip too much sebum if the soap or detergent is too strong for a certain skin type, such as dry or sensitive skin. When this happens, the skin can become dry, flaky, tight, and irritated. The cleanser can "eat" into the lipids within the intercellular cement, "the mortar," damaging the barrier function and making the skin susceptible to dehydration and irritation. Continued use of the soap or cleanser may further damage the barrier function and further dry and irritate the skin.

Second, because of their fatty content, many soaps leave a residue or film on the skin that is created by insoluble salts, which are formed when the soap is used. Because of this overdrying factor, fats and oils are often added to cleansers and soaps to prevent too much of the irritating cleansing agent from coming in contact with the skin for too long. Think of these fats and oils as "buffer zones" set up to keep the product from stripping too much oil from fragile, dry, or sensitive skin. Cleansers that have added fat to buffer contact with skin are called **superfatted** soaps or cleansers. Of course, the fats that are added to these products can also leave a film on the skin. This can be a problem for oily skin types because the fats may cause comedone development. In dry skin, the fats may actually help retain moisture. Fats used in true bar-type soaps include the following:

- Sodium tallowate
- Sodium oleate
- Sodium cocoate
- Sodium stearate

Emulsion Cleansers

Emulsion cleansers are what most estheticians think of as cleansing milks. They are primarily used for removing makeup and are often recommended for sensitive skin because of their gentleness. Most do not have detergents, but detergents can be used in these products to help them foam slightly, to make them easy to rinse and easier to remove, or to keep them emulsified.

> **Here's a Tip**
>
> Notice that the names of fatty additives in soap almost always start with the word *sodium* and end in a fatty ester (suffix-*ate*) of one of many fatty acids listed earlier in this chapter: stearic, myristic, oleic, and so on. Sometimes potassium is used instead of sodium.

A lot of ingredients used in makeup are not water-soluble. In other words, the product is not easily removed with water. It takes some sort of oil or fat to work as a solvent to loosen non-water-soluble makeup products from the skin. Cleansing milks are liquids made mostly of water, with oil or fat mixed in the emulsion; therefore, they are oil-in-water emulsions. The oil or fat is the active agent used to create a slippery surface to facilitate the removal of makeup or other debris from the skin's surface. The advantage to these cleansing milks is that they remove makeup products effectively, and they are less drying and irritating to the skin. The disadvantage is that they generally leave a residue on the skin. This residue is usually an emollient, the same one often used as the active cleansing agent.

The emollient film left on the skin can be good or bad. For drier skins that do not make enough oil, the film can actually help condition the surface. It can be a problem, though, for oily skins or acne-prone skins, because it leaves a residue of fat to further clog the problem skin. It is important to make sure the emollient left on oily facial skin is non-comedogenic or that the emollient is thoroughly removed by following makeup removal with a toner or a foaming detergent cleanser and toner. In fact, emulsion cleansers should always be followed with a toner.

Another type of emulsion cleanser is cold cream, which is often made primarily of mineral oil, making it a water-in-oil emulsion. It is certainly a more oily emulsion cleanser, although very effective for removing heavy makeup, including theatre makeup. It often leaves a significant amount of oil on the skin after use. Clients often complain about a greasy feeling after using a cold cream cleanser, so these cleansers are slowly losing popularity.

Performance Agents in Toners

The main function of toners is to lower the pH of the skin after cleansing. Toners also help remove any excess cleanser or residue left on the skin after cleansing.

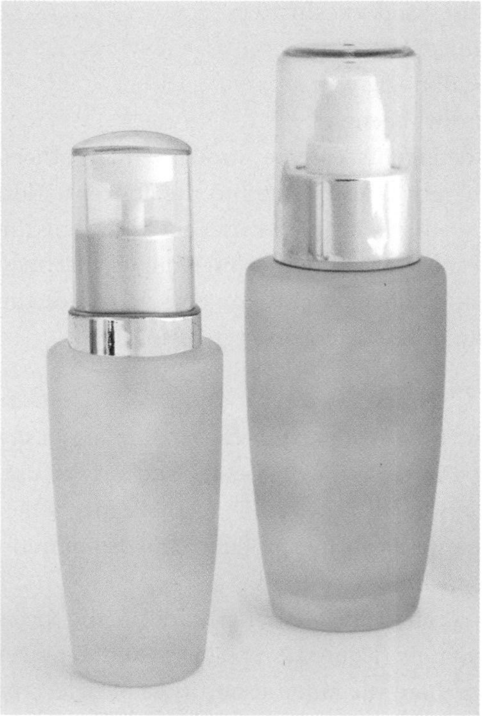

Figure 12–6 Toners.

Performance agents in toners vary greatly, depending on the skin type (Figure 12–6).

pH Adjusters

Most toners have a low pH, usually around 4.0 to 5.5. This low pH helps to restore the normal pH of the skin's acid mantle after cleansing, which is normally around 5.5 to 6.2. Citric acid or lemon extract is sometimes added to toners to help lower the pH of the product.

Toners for Oily Skin

Astringents are performance agents (although sometimes they are active ingredients if used in a drug formulation) that have a tightening effect on the skin or pore appearance. Astringent ingredients include witch hazel or hamamelis extract, potassium alum, lemon extract, and other citrus extracts. Astringents actually work by causing a slight swelling around the pore openings, helping to tighten the skin and minimize the appearance of the pore opening. Toner products for oily skin are sometimes referred to as astringents, although to call a product an astringent is technically a drug claim.

Removal of surface sebum is an important function of toners for oily skin. Sometimes, emulsifiers such as polysorbate are used in toners for oily and combination skin to help disperse sebum on the skin surface. Salicylic or glycolic acid may be included in an oily or problem skin toner to help exfoliate the skin. Soothing agents such as chamomile extract may also be included for their soothing properties.

Alcohol is often used as a performance agent for oily skin. **Isopropyl** and **SD alcohols** are drying alcohols, unlike cetyl alcohol, which is a fatty alcohol used in creams. SD alcohol is **"specially denatured" ethyl alcohol,** also known as ethanol. The term *denaturing* means the alcohol is not suitable for drinking. Bittering agents are added to the ethanol to make it taste terrible and ensure safety, so that infants who might try to ingest the product will leave it alone after only a small taste. SD alcohol is listed on the ingredient label followed by a number. This number indicates the technique used to denature the alcohol.

SD alcohol and isopropyl alcohol are strong cleansing agents or defatting agents that help remove excess quantities of sebum from oily skin or oily areas. In larger quantities, they are antiseptics, helping to kill surface microorganisms. This, of course, is a drug claim. Isopropyl alcohol is an even stronger drying alcohol. The drying effect of these alcohols on the skin can also have an astringent effect on the oily skin and pore appearance.

> **FYI**
>
> Alcohol has an undeserved terrible reputation in the cosmetics industry. Many companies tout that their products are "alcohol-free," because of the drying effect of certain alcohols on the skin. Although large amounts of SD or isopropyl alcohol can be irritating or overdrying to dry or sensitive skin, these substances are useful in helping to control oiliness in very oily and some acne-prone skin. Do not reject a product simply because it has some SD or isopropyl alcohol. Make your decision based on the skin type you are treating.

Toners for Dry Skin

Toners for dry skin, which have an acidic pH, often contain performance ingredients, such as azulene, chamomile, or bisabolol, which might be added for their soothing effect on dry, sensitive skin. In addition, toners for dry skin may contain humectants, ingredients that attract water and help restore moisture to dehydrated skin after cleansing. Toner humectants include butylene glycol, propylene glycol, and sorbitol. These ingredients are also known for softening the skin. (Humectants are discussed further in the next section of this chapter.)

Performance Ingredients for Dehydrated Skin

Dehydrated skin suffers from a lack of water after water leaves the skin surface and evaporates into the atmosphere. Cold weather, dry climates, and low humidity can cause dehydration, because the skin is exposed to air that is lower in water contact than the skin. Exposure to the sun dehydrates skin and damages the skin's barrier function. Harsh cleansers or the overuse of detergent cleansers can remove lipids within the barrier function and allow water to escape. Aging skin is often sun-damaged, and because the cell renewal process slows with age, the replenishment of the barrier function also slows. This sets up a perfect anatomical condition for the skin to become dehydrated. Impaired barrier function can result not only in flaking and esthetic problems but also in increased skin sensitivity.

Humectants

Humectants are water-binding agents that have a strong attraction to water. Many chemically bind water to them, holding water molecules. Natural humectants, lipids, or hydrating agents found within the intercellular cement are known as **natural moisturizing factors** or **NMFs.** The NMFs in the skin help to preserve water or hydration within the epidermis, keeping the barrier function intact and keeping the skin soft and supple. Impaired barrier function can mean a lack of NMFs from missing lipids or other components and can cause dehydration, which is sometimes severe. It can also cause the skin's surface to have a wrinkly, unfirm appearance.

NMFs include sodium PCA, sphingolipids, and glycosphingolipids (also known as *ceramides*), phospholipids, fatty acids, glycerol, squalane, and cholesterol. These intercellular components are produced during the cell renewal process as cells migrate from the basal layer to the stratum corneum. During the aging process, cell renewal slows down and, therefore, skin produces fewer NMFs. This reduces the ability of the skin to hold hydration, making it dry, tight, flaky, and dull. In recent years, scientists have been able to isolate and prepare special ingredients that help to "repair" or "patch" the moisture barrier. These ingredients can now be used in products for dry, dehydrated, aging, and sun-damaged skin.

Lipid replacement is accomplished by applying a group of lipid ingredients to the skin. These include ceramides or sphingolipids, phospholipids, cholesterol, and fatty acids. These lipid ingredients can actually be derived from plant or animal sources, although most are derived from plant materials such as soy sterols or soy lecithin. Linoleic acid can be derived from numerous plant sources, including evening primrose oil, sunflower oil, or borage oil. These lipid components occur naturally in the intercellular material at a ratio of 4:1:1:1. In other words, it is four parts ceramides to one part of each of the other components. This complex of performance lipid ingredients literally patches the impaired barrier. Its function is to hold water within the intercellular matrix. However, lipids alone are not as effective without the use of humectants or hydrophilic ingredients. These ingredients work like "water magnets," attracting water while the lipids hold the water within the intercellular spaces between the cells. This combination of lipid complexes with hydrators is excellent for restoring essential moisture to dry, dehydrated, and sensitive skin.

Sodium PCA is an excellent hydrator and a natural moisturizing factor. It has a strong ability to attract water and is readily accepted by the skin. Sodium PCA is used frequently in night creams, day creams, sunscreens, and other hydrating products. It can be used without lipids to hydrate oilier or combination skin. It is lightweight on the skin and does not cause clogged pores.

Glycerin, a strong water binder, is a humectant that has been used for many years. It is, in fact, so strong that it should not be used by itself. Glycerin can actually make the skin drier over a period of time because it does not just pull water from cosmetics and the atmosphere when applied to the skin. In large amounts, it can pull water from the lower levels of the epidermis, causing transepidermal water loss (TEWL), which results in drier skin. Used in a moderate amount in a good hydrating cream, it is an excellent hydrating agent.

Propylene glycol is another widely used humectant. It penetrates the skin fairly easily, making it a good hydrating agent. However, because propylene glycol can increase permeability of the skin, it can cause problems for sensitive or dry skin with impaired barrier function. Butylene glycol is now being used more frequently in products for dehydrated or sensitive skin. It has less potential for sensitive skin irritation than its chemical cousin, propylene glycol. Sorbitol is another excellent hydrating agent that is frequently used in hydrating lotions.

Alpha hydroxy acids (AHAs) are surface exfoliants and hydrators. One of these, lactic acid, is actually used in prescription-strength moisturizers. Glycolic acid is also a hydrating agent. Alpha hydroxy acids are excellent for dehydrated skin because they stimulate epidermal cell renewal, which stimulates natural production of skin lipids and natural repair of the barrier function.

Other Humectants

Other water binders work very differently than the standard hydrophylic agents. Following is a list of a few and their purposes. All of these ingredients are known as **substantives,** which are ingredients that attach themselves well to the surface of the skin, spreading out across the skin to protect and hydrate the surface.

A molecule of hyaluronic acid, also known as sodium hyaluronate, is quite large and cannot penetrate the skin to any degree. It can, however, hold up to 400 times its own weight in water, and because of its excellent water-binding properties, it is a frequently used hydrating performance ingredient. Hyaluronic acid is expensive, and creams and lotions containing hyaluronic acid may be more expensive than others.

Mucopolysaccharides are carbohydrate–lipid complexes that are also good water binders. Considered a "mother-molecule" to hyaluronic acid, it is capable of holding large amounts of water and is an excellent hydrator. Again, it is too large to penetrate the skin.

Collagen and elastin are large, long-chain molecular proteins that lie on top of the skin and bind water, also helping to prevent water loss. Collagen and elastin have been used in creams for many years. They are too big to ever penetrate the skin, but they do a good job hydrating. Because they lie on top of the skin, they also help to "fill in" small lines and wrinkles, making skin look smoother.

Some of the more recent discoveries in humectants include algae and seaweed extracts. These are quite remarkable hydrators. They are substantive, forming a surface gel. Some forms of algae are now being used as hydrating base materials for sensitive skin products without using traditional emulsifiers that can decrease the barrier function in sensitive skin with loss of lipid barrier.

Ingredients for Treating Dry Skin

Skin that is dry and dehydrated suffers from a lack of barrier protection that allows the skin to become dehydrated. We have already discussed impaired barrier function and how the NMFs and intercellular lipids can be replaced. There is a second barrier naturally produced by the skin's sebaceous glands. The lipids in sebum are different than the lipids in the epidermal barrier function. Sebum provides a natural moisture guard on the surface of the skin and is the first line of defense against dehydration. Alipidic skin is skin that does not produce enough sebum. Alipidic skin can be recognized during analysis by the absence of visible pore structure or extremely small pores. Without the protective layer of natural sebum, the skin can become dehydrated and is likely to have impaired barrier function between the epidermal cells as well. When treating dry, dehydrated skin, it is important to use humectants to bind water, lipids to help repair the barrier function, and surface moisture guarding ingredients such as occlusives and emollients.

OCCLUSIVES An occlusive is a large, heavy molecule that sits on top of the skin and prevents moisture loss. Occlusives are exactly what they sound like, forming a barrier on top of the skin to shield it from transepidermal moisture loss from the inside out, much like the barrier function, except on top instead of within the skin.

A good example of an occlusive is the emollient petrolatum, or petroleum jelly. As discussed earlier, petrolatum is both a vehicle and a protectant. It can be used by itself or incorporated into a cream or lotion. The amount of occlusion created by petrolatum depends on the amount used in the cream formulation. The advantages of using petrolatum in formulations are many. It is extremely hypoallergenic, rarely causing a problem with allergies or irritations. Hence, it is often used in formulas, both drug and cosmetic, for sensitive or irritated skin. Petrolatum provides an excellent occlusive barrier both to keep water in the skin and to keep allergens, antigens, and foreign bodies out of the skin. Petrolatum is also very inexpensive.

There are some disadvantages to using petrolatum. First, it is extremely sticky, slippery, and greasy. Most clients do not like this greasy feeling. It is also hard to accomplish any task when your hands are too slippery to handle anything. It is extremely greasy on the face, creating esthetic problems as well. Second, it is disadvantageous to use petrolatum for oily and problem skin. Although petrolatum is not comedogenic in its pure state, it is very greasy and heavy. Many estheticians do not like petrolatum because it is not "natural." This is simply not true. Petrolatum comes from minerals in the Earth. What could be more natural? In short, petrolatum is a useful product, but it should not be used in all cases of dehydration.

Emollients

Emollients are somewhat like occlusives in that they mostly lie on the surface of the skin and prevent water loss. Emollients help to smooth the surface of wrinkled skin, filling in the cracks of dry and dehydrated skin (Figure 12–7). They are much lighter weight than occlusives. Emollients are often used not only for dehydrated or water-dry skin but also for oil-dry or alipidic skin. They have a second use as spreading agents, which was discussed in the section on functional ingredients.

Emollients help to supplement skin that suffers from a lack of sebum and lipid production. They serve as a substitute, helping to keep the surface lubricated and protected. There are several categories of emollients. Fatty acids, already discussed in the section on functional ingredients, are emollients. Fatty alcohols and fatty esters are also emollients. Other new types of ingredients that are, again, actually a synthetic version of intercellular cement lipids include cholesterol, ceramides, lecithin (also a humectant), squalane, and glycosphingolipids.

Mineral oil is another emollient. Like petrolatum, it is a petroleum derivative. It has many of the same advantages and disadvantages as petrolatum. It is hypoallergenic and a good emollient, helping to soothe irritated, dry, scaly skin, but it also can have a greasy feeling, particularly in its pure state. However, when formulated properly into a cream, this is not the case, and it can be an excellent active agent emollient for dry, dehydrated skin. This is especially true when mixed with good humectant active agents.

Silicones are often used instead of traditional fatty-type emollients. Silicones include cyclopentasiloxane, cyclomethicone, dimethicone, and phenyl trimethicone, often used in combination. Referred to as "breathable barriers,"

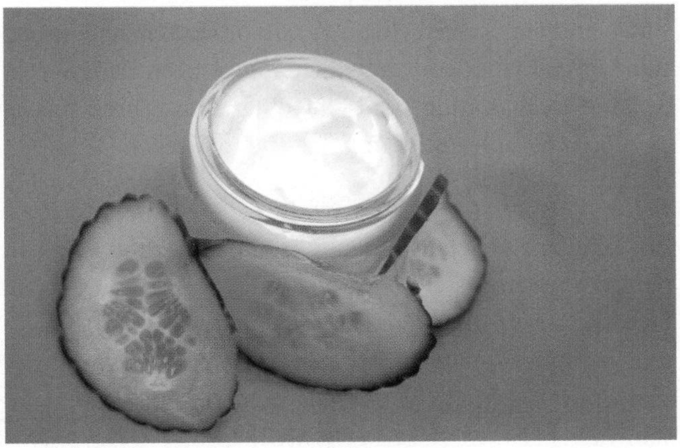

Figure 12–7 Emollient cream.

these lightweight and unique ingredients help block water to prevent it from escaping from the surface of the skin, while keeping the skin feeling light and comfortable. Another advantage is that silicones are biologically inert, which means they are chemicals that are unlikely to cause reactions with the skin, making them ideal for sensitive skin formulations also. The silicones are noncomedogenic and do not irritate the pores; thus, they are ideal for oily and acne-prone skin types. They can be used in creams, lotions, cleansing milks, and foundations and are often used in concentrated lipid serums for dry and sensitive skin with impaired barrier function.

NATURAL OILS AS EMOLLIENTS There are many natural oils that also can function as emollients. These include sunflower, safflower, jojoba, soybean, grapeseed, and others. In most cases, these, as well as other emollients, are blended with proper levels of humectant into a cream or lotion.

Moisturizing Products

Most products designed for dry skin contain a combination of humectants and emollients to help boost moisture levels and improve the skin's ability to hold the moisture. Dry skin products often contain lipid replacement ingredients to improve barrier function within the epidermis. Normally these products are water-based, or oil-in-water emulsions, although some may be water-in-oil emulsions (creams) designed for more severely alipidic skin.

These moisturizing products vary greatly in the amount of emollients and humectants they contain. The more oil-dry (alipidic) the skin is, the more emollient should be used. Treatments with larger amounts of humectants and fewer emollients are designed for oilier and combination skin. Hydration fluids that are designed for younger or oilier skin types may contain just enough emollients to serve as a vehicle to spread the product on the skin. Because some emollients often clog oily skin or worsen acne-prone skin, special emollient ingredients have been designed to be used in hydrating fluids for oilier skin. These special emollient complexes do not clog the follicles.

Exfoliants

An exfoliant is a performance ingredient that helps to remove dead cells from the skin surface (Figure 12–8). Exfoliants help improve the appearance of the skin by removing dead cells, making the surface look smoother and more refined, and they actually stimulate the skin to replace these old cells with fresher cells. This is particularly helpful for mature and sun-damaged skin.

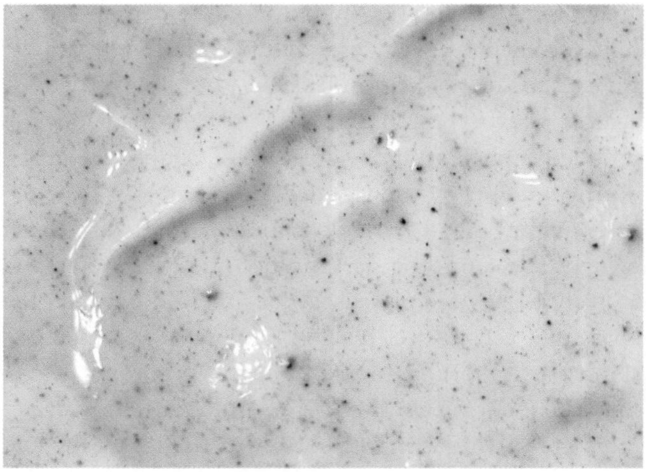

Figure 12–8 Exfoliating cream.

When the cell cycle is stimulated, the cell renewal process speeds up, increasing skin moisture, skin smoothness, and intercellular lipid production, improving barrier function.

There are two major types of exfoliants: mechanical exfoliants and chemical exfoliants. These can be combined into a product that has both types of exfoliation in it.

MECHANICAL EXFOLIANTS Mechanical exfoliants are usually granular particles that bump or scratch the skin surface to remove cells. Polyethylene, ground shells or nuts, salt crystals, and hydrogenated jojoba oil beads are examples of these types of particles. Sometimes these ingredients are mixed into cleansers to increase their ease of rinsing. Applied with the fingertips and gently massaged, these agents bump off excess dead cells on the skin's surface.

The main crystal ingredient used in microdermabrasion treatments as a mechanical exfoliant, aluminum oxide, is also often used as a mechanical exfoliant in manual microdermabrasion scrubs. Scrubs are frequently designed for use in the shower or in exfoliating body salon treatments.

CHEMICAL EXFOLIANTS Chemical exfoliants include alpha hydroxy acids, such as glycolic and lactic acids, and a beta hydroxy acid, salicylic acid. They help improve the appearance of wrinkles, fine lines, rough textures, and clogged pores, and they improve cell renewal and the lipid content in the barrier function. They also encourage the shedding of discolored cells, helping with hyperpigmentation. On oily skin they loosen clogged pores and remove dead cell buildup within the follicles. They are best used when applied to the skin in a gel, serum, or cream and worn under a moisturizer or sunscreen. Gels are usually used for oily skin types; serums for combination skin; and creams for dry, mature, or sensitive skin types. These acids work by dissolving surface intercellular lipids in the top of the corneum, loosening the cells so they can shed. Sometimes these acids are added to cleansers or scrubs, but they work best when left on the skin.

Benzoyl peroxide, salicylic acid, sulfur, and resorcinol are stronger exfoliants and are used in OTC acne products. They help to shed cells from both the surface of the skin as well as inside the follicle, helping to break loose dead cell buildup that is clogging pores, kill acne bacteria, and prevent new comedones from forming.

Enzymes such as papain (derived from papaya), bromelain (derived from pineapple), and pancreatin (a pancreatic enzyme derived from beef or pork processing) work by dissolving keratin protein in dead cells. They are **keratolytics** known as **proteolytic enzymes.** *Proteolytic* literally means "protein dissolving." Enzymes are often used in professional salon skin care treatments. Enzymes can be used in "vegetal" peels or gommages, roll-off surface exfoliation treatments, or they can also be in powder form and mixed with water to activate them.

ALPHA HYDROXY ACIDS (AHAS) In the history of cosmetics, no ingredient or family of ingredients has had the impact or efficacy of alpha hydroxy acids. Alpha hydroxy acids (AHAs) are a family of naturally occurring mild acids. Most AHAs are present in fruits and vegetables, but some actually occur in human cells. Most AHAs used in cosmetics have been purified in a laboratory or are the side product of other industrial chemical processes, such as the making of film.

AHAs have a large number of applications in skin care and can help many conditions, including oily and acne-prone skin, sun damage, dryness, and hyperpigmentation. There are several AHAs used in skin care treatment. These include **lactic acid, tartaric acid, malic acid,** and by far the best-known AHA, **glycolic acid.** Salicylic acid and citric acid are also often included when discussing hydroxy acids, but they are actually beta hydroxy acids (BHAs).

130

The chemical difference between alpha hydroxy and beta hydroxy acids is the location of the hydroxy group on the carbon chain of the acid. *Alpha* indicates that the group is on the first carbon atom, whereas *beta* means that the group is on the second carbon atom. Glycolic acid is the smallest, molecularly, of all the alpha hydroxy acids. It has been widely researched, and, because of its size, penetrates between cells more readily than the other AHAs.

AHAs work by loosening the bond between dead corneum cells, dissolving part of the surface intercellular cement that holds dead epidermal cells together. This makes it easy to remove dead cells from the skin surface, which has a positive effect on many conditions:

- Removal of dead cell buildup smoothes the surface of dry, sun-damaged, or aging skin, improving roughness and making wrinkles appear much less deep. Results on aging skin can become apparent in a very short period of time.
- By removing dead surface cells, cell renewal is stimulated, bringing younger, fresher cells to the surface more quickly and increasing the production of intercellular lipids, improving barrier function and, therefore, improving hydration of the skin. Well-hydrated skin is smoother and firmer looking and is generally healthier, helping all activities of the skin proceed.
- Removing dead cell buildup from the inside of follicles helps loosen clogged pores, comedones, and other impactions on oily skin or an oily area. Continued use helps keep dead cells from accumulating on the follicle wall, which prevents impactions that can lead to inflammatory acne lesions. This property of AHAs and BHAs make them good ingredients to use for acne-prone and oily skins.
- Removal of dead cells can mean the removal of hyperpigmented cells, which helps to lighten discolored or splotchy skin. Used in combination with a melanin suppressant, such as hydroquinone, AHAs help remove stained cells, whereas hydroquinone helps suppress the activity of the melanocytes. a broad-spectrum sunscreen with an SPF of 15 or higher should always be used with AHA products, especially if the client has hyperpigmentation.
- AHAs can also be used on body skin, removing dead, dry cells and helping to improve retention of moisture. This has some affect on conditions such as dry, winter skin and helps dermatologists treat medical conditions such as eczema and icthyosis. Alpha hydroxy acids are also helpful in removing calluses on feet, elbows, and hands.
- New information indicates that routine use of alpha hydroxy acids improves both barrier functions of the epidermis, and long-term studies indicate the improvement of collagen content in the dermis.

Alpha hydroxy and beta hydroxy acids can be used in many products, including cleansers and toners, but are most effective when used in leave-on products such as treatment gels, serums, or moisturizing creams.

STRENGTHS AND EFFECTIVENESS OF AHAs The strengths of alpha hydroxy acids vary extensively. Products have been formulated with as little as 2% or 3% being AHAs to as high as 20% in higher-strength treatment preparations, which are generally available only through dermatologists and plastic surgeons. There has been a great deal of controversy over the irritation potential of higher-strength products. The esthetics industry generally accepts that products contain 8% to 10% AHA in order to show results in helping the various conditions previously discussed, although even 5% can show gradual improvements in skin conditions.

pH is also a very important factor in AHA efficacy. The lower the pH, the higher the strength of the acid and the more cells will be removed from the skin. However, the lower the pH, the more potentially irritating the acid will be to the skin. AHA leave-on products of 8% or higher sting slightly when applied, indicating some irritancy, even though this is probably very small at this concentration.

The Cosmetic Ingredient Review (CIR) is a special panel of scientists and dermatologists who investigate cosmetic ingredient safety for the Cosmetic, Toiletries, and Fragrance Association, the largest cosmetic manufacturers association. The CIR shares its findings with the industry as well as with the Food and Drug Administration (FDA). The CIR conducted an extensive investigation of the safety of alpha hydroxy acids and many derivatives of AHA. The CIR determined that home-use products were generally safe, as long as they contained no more than 10% AHA and had a pH of no less than 3.5.

> ***FYI***
>
> Remember, the lower the pH, the stronger the acid.

Vehicles and Other Ingredients with AHAs

The cosmetic spreading agent or vehicle for AHAs can vary greatly. AHAs can be incorporated into leave-on gels (used frequently on oily, acne-prone, and combination skin types) and lotions or creams (which are more suitable for dry skin and body skin). Other ingredients may also be combined with AHAs in different formulations. Hydrating ingredients or emollients may be included for dry skin, hydroquinone may be included for hyperpigmented skin, and salicylic acid may be included for acne-prone skin.

Plant Extracts

There are literally hundreds of plant extracts used as performance ingredients in skin care products. One-third of all prescription drugs are made from plants. Plant extracts are generally liquids that are pressed, boiled, or chemically extracted from different plants. They can be extracted from plant leaves, flowers, bark, peel, or roots.

Most plant extracts are used for their **anecdotal** properties, meaning that the ingredient is reputed to have certain benefits for improving the appearance of the skin, but the benefits have not been substantiated, or proved, by accepted scientific means. Many plant extract ingredients are studied individually for their effects on the skin and are studied on cells in a laboratory, but that does not necessarily mean that those ingredients will work on a live person or in a particular product, unless the finished product has also been studied. Research is ongoing on some plant extracts to substantiate their effectiveness and understand which chemicals within the particular extract cause the appearance changes and other effects on the skin.

Plant extracts are simply natural complexes of various chemicals. Many estheticians like plant extracts because they believe they are "natural." Nevertheless, they *are* chemicals. a single plant extract might comprise literally hundreds of chemicals. Some plant extracts are used solely for their fragrance properties.

Plant extracts are normally used in relatively small quantities in skin care products. Usually they are listed as

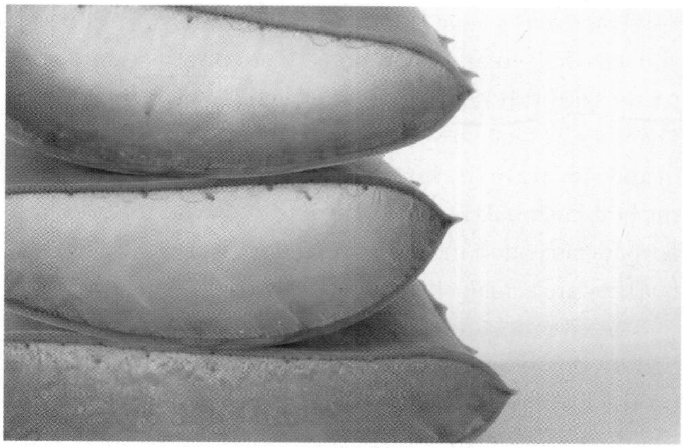

Figure 12–9 Aloe plant ready for extraction.

CAUTION!

AHAs should not be used on the following clients:

- Those who are using or have recently used Accutane®
- Those who have recently had laser resurfacing, chemical exfoliation, dermabrasion, or any other exfoliating procedure
- Those who have recently had a professional microdermabrasion treatment
- Those who have recently been waxed in the area of treatment
- Those who are using tretinoin (Retin-A®, Renova®), tazarotene (Tazorac®), adapalene (Differin®), or other exfoliating prescription drugs
- Those who are known to be allergic to AHA or BHA
- Those who are sunburned or have visibly irritated skin
- Those who have cuts; abrasions, including open acne lesions that have been scratched; or blisters
- Those who are using other topical medications, unless approved by a physician
- Those who are planning to deliberately expose their skin to the sun or sun beds
- Those who have not had a thorough consultation and may be using products that are contraindicated
- Those who are pregnant or nursing; AHA safety has not been determined for pregnant or nursing women

In addition, AHAs should be used carefully with other exfoliating agents such as salicylic acid, benzoyl peroxide, sulfur, resorcinol, or products with large amounts of alcohol. Combining exfoliating agents can increase irritation. Using AHA products on skin that has recently had a microdermabrasion treatment may also increase irritation. Overall, it is not advisable to combine mechanical and chemical exfoliation procedures. Be careful when using any stimulating product with AHAs, because this may increase irritation.

It is a good idea to supervise a client's entire home-care program when using AHA products. This way you can determine exactly what he or she is using with the AHA product for best results and the least irritation. Last, but certainly not least, the client *must* use a daily sunscreen with an SPF of at least 15 while using AHA products!

extracts, but if they are in a solution of water or alcohol, which most of them are, they may be listed near the top of the ingredient label. This simply means that water is the main ingredient in the extracts and that the extracts were prepared before the formula was actually combined.

Following are some commonly used plant extracts and their properties:

- **Aloe vera extract:** Used for soothing, reducing redness, and improving hydration (Figure 12–9)
- **Centella asiatica:** Also known as *gotu kola;* used for skin firming
- **Grapeseed extract:** Used for antioxidant, soothing, and anti-redness properties
- **Green tea:** Used for antioxidant and soothing properties
- **Hamamelis (witch hazel):** Used for astringent effects and soothing effects
- **Horse chestnut extract:** Used for reducing diffuse skin redness
- **Licorice extract:** Used for soothing properties and also for skin lightening properties
- **Matricaria extract:** A specialized type of chamomile, know for soothing properties
- **Seaweed/algae extracts:** Primarily used for moisturization and hydration, but different types of seaweed have different properties; some can be used for exfoliation, some for soothing skin, and so on.

When extracts are listed on an ingredient label, they must be listed by their Latin name, and their common name must be listed in parentheses, such as citrus medica limonum (lemon) peel extract.

INGREDIENTS FOR AGING SKIN

So much of aging, sensitive skin, redness, and inflammation are related to chemical changes that occur every day from sun exposure and other inflammatory factors. Before looking at the chemical treatment and prevention of the reactions that affect the appearance of the skin, you must understand the reactions themselves.

Free Radicals and Their Effect on the Skin

Many scientists believe that **free radicals,** or **reactive oxygen species,** which are different types of free radicals, are responsible not only for aging of the skin, but of the body. Free radicals are essentially unstable oxygen atoms that rob electrons from the surface of skin cell membranes, creating another form of free radical called *lipid peroxide* and starting a domino effect of chemical reactions that lead to skin damage and even damage to DNA. Free radicals are caused by forms of inflammation such as sun exposure, smoking, pollution, and certain types of chemical exposure. The inflammation cascade is a series of biochemical reactions that lead to the production of self-destruct enzymes in the skin called **proteases.**

FYI

Free radicals are wild molecules or atoms, usually of oxygen or an oxygen-based compound, that are created by inflammation such as sun exposure, smoking, pollution, and certain types of chemical exposure. Free radicals wreak havoc in the skin and eventually lead to the effects of aging.

Collagenase, elastase, and **hyaluronidase** are three of these self-destruct enzymes. As you might guess by their names, they cause destruction of collagen, elastin, and hyaluronic acid. Collagen and elastin are fibers responsible for elasticity, firmness, and smoothness of the skin, and hyaluronic acid in the lower dermis makes up the ground substance that gives the skin further cushion and support. Constant, cumulative free-radical damage eventually results in the skin damage we think of as aging skin.

Oxygen exists in the environment as O_2, or two oxygen atoms with a covalent bond, sharing electrons. This is a stable form of oxygen. Sun exposure causes this molecule to split, creating one stable and one unstable oxygen atom, which has lost electrons to the stable atom. This unstable oxygen atom is a free radical, and is also known as superoxide.

Because of the loss of electrons, the free radicals are desperately trying to regain enough electrons to regain stability. They will actually steal electrons from other atoms. One of the best sources of electrons is the membrane of the cell. Superoxide radicals often steal electrons from the lipids in the membrane of the cell. When these electrons are stolen, more free radicals are formed, because now the atoms in the cell membrane are missing electrons. The free radicals formed when the membrane is damaged are called **lipid peroxides.**

So, one free radical can form another. The damage to the membrane of the cell can affect the ability of the cell to function properly. The cell membrane is responsible for nutrient, water, and oxygen absorption as well as disposal of cellular waste. The cell membrane also contains the receptor sites that allow the cell to communicate chemically with other cells.

Remember that life and biological functions are really nothing more than chemical reactions. One chemical reaction is often necessary for another to take place, forming a chain of reactions leading to a biological function. Also, remember that all chemical reactions involve the exchange of electrons. This is how molecules react and interact to form new substances. If a chemical lacks electrons, it cannot perform in normal chemical reactions required by the cell. It can perform in abnormal chemical reactions.

Iron is one of the most reactive elements and loses electrons or oxidizes very readily. Surely you have noticed how easily iron rusts. Rust is a reaction of iron and oxygen that forms iron oxide, which is rust. Peroxides can react with iron, which is abundantly present in the hemoglobin in blood, to form **hydroxy radicals,** the most dangerous free radical. Hydroxy radicals (abbreviated as -OH) can react with many different molecules, including the DNA in the cell nucleus, causing permanent damage to the cell and causing damage to the DNA in future cells produced from cell division. This is what really causes skin aging.

This causes many problems for the skin and results in what is now recognized as **subclinical** inflammation, or inflammation that is not easily seen. However, this does not mean that they are not happening. Instead, they are happening but not showing visible redness and symptoms.

Inflammation and Free Radicals

When a skin cell is inflamed—creating free radicals—it releases special chemicals that signal the immune system within the blood that it has been damaged. Blood rushes to the site in a large enough response to create redness, or what we think of as inflammation. (This may not be as visible in subclinical inflammation.) The white blood cells release chemicals that signal skin cells to make "self-destruct" enzymes—primarily elastase, collagenase, and hyaluronidase—that destroy elastin, collagen, and hyaluronic acid.

Any skin inflammation causes free-radical activity. The inflammation can damage the skin, and chronic inflammation will result in more severe skin damage, creating symptoms we think of as "aging." It is, therefore, important to prevent and treat the skin for inflammation and to do all we can to stop inflammation from occurring. This makes sense from a sun-damage perspective, because one of the most prevalent immediate signs of sun exposure is redness, or erythema, a primary sign of inflammation.

Long-Term versus Short-Term Damage

Free radicals can damage collagen over time. Collagen fibers normally slide over one another to give the skin flexibility. Free radicals attack the proteins in the collagen in a process known as **crosslinking.** This process binds the fibers together, making them inflexible and resulting in the appearance of "old" skin. This takes years to accumulate, but some crosslinking occurs with any unprotected sun exposure. If this process suddenly occurred at age 20, more people would be aware of sun protection earlier. Unfortunately, because younger people believe that sun damage will never happen to them, they take few or no precautions, and years of non-protection result in all the symptoms of photoaging—wrinkles, elastosis, pigmentation disorders, roughness, leathery texture, dilated capillaries, and skin cancers.

Antioxidants

Antioxidants are free-radical scavengers. Some neutralize free radicals before they attack cell membranes, beginning the inflammation cascade. Others squelch other forms of free radicals. Antioxidants work by supplying electrons to radical oxygen atoms, which need electrons to be stable. This prevents the need for the free radical to attack the cell membrane, avoiding the start of the inflammation cascade.

The routine use of topical antioxidants can help improve the visible signs of aging and help prevent the inflammation process that leads to cell and skin damage. Because there are numerous types of free radicals that form during the inflammation cascade, it is now theorized that different types of antioxidants should be combined to squelch the different types of free radicals at all levels of the inflammation cascade. When different types of antioxidants are combined in a formulation, the formulation is said to be a broad-spectrum antioxidant.

Antioxidants are, by nature, unstable substances. Because they are so reactive, they must be stabilized to remain effective in a skin care product. Antioxidants have been used for many years to keep products fresh by neutralizing free radicals within the product. This helped prevent rancidity, but the ingredient worked in the product, not on the skin. Only in the past few years have antioxidants been stabilized so they could be used as performance ingredients.

The invention of liposomes and other forms of microencapsulation helped provide a way to keep these reactive substances stable until they could be used. Besides acting as protective "shells" to keep antioxidants **bioavailable,** or able to be used as a performance ingredient in the skin, the lipid-based microencapsulation also improved penetration of the antioxidants.

Some of the best-known antioxidants are vitamin C and vitamin E. These have been known as health supplements for many years, but we are now able to better understand how they work. Vitamins C and E work together to neutralize free radicals and then to replenish themselves to work again. One form of vitamin C, magnesium ascorbyl phosphate, is a melanin suppressant and is helpful in treating hyperpigmentation. Beta carotene, a form of vitamin A, is another well-known antioxidant. **Superoxide dismutase** and minerals like zinc and copper also help prevent reactions from starting. Above all, though, sunscreen protection alone is a good first step in preventing the original creation of free radicals.

Other more contemporary antioxidants are grapeseed extract and maritime pine extract (also known as its trade name Pycnogenol®). These are called **proanthocyanidins** and are very powerful antioxidants. They are important because they help to neutralize the most dangerous free radical, the hydroxyl radical. Grapeseed extract has been documented to have significant anti-redness properties.

Another powerful antioxidant that has received much acclaim is Japanese green tea extract (Figure 12–10). Green tea contains components called **catechins** and **polyphenols** that are very strong antioxidants. Common antioxidant ingredients include the following:

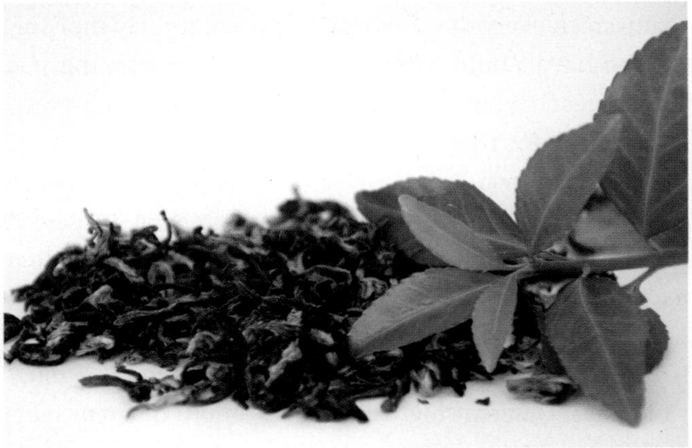

Figure 12–10 Green tea leaves.

- **Superoxide dismutase:** An enzyme that helps prevent the start of the cascade
- **Tocopherol:** Vitamin E; helps prevent lipid oxidation and also helps replenish vitamin C
- **Tocopherol acetate:** A more stable form of stabilized vitamin E
- **Ascorbic acid:** Vitamin C acid
- **Magnesium ascorbyl phosphate:** Vitamin C ester; known to help prevent lipid oxidation and also has a suppressive effect on hyperpigmentation
- **Grapeseed extract:** Contains very strong antioxidants known as proanthocyanidins; used in soothing, anti-redness and anti-wrinkle formulations; often used in liposomal form
- **Green and white tea extracts:** Contain strong antioxidants called *polyphenols*, well known as both a topical and internal antioxidant; have been used as soothing, anti-redness, and anti-wrinkle ingredients
- **Stearyl glycyrrhetinate:** A strong anti-inflammatory antioxidant derived from licorice
- **Malachite extract:** Derived from the mineral
- **Silymarin:** Derived from milk thistle
- **Elagic acid:** Derived from pomegranate
- **Hypericin:** Derived from St. John's wort
- **Lipoic acid**
- **Coenzyme Q-10:** Also known as *ubiquinone*; a very strong, naturally occurring fat-soluble antioxidant that exists in almost every cell in the human body but in great quantities in the liver, heart, and lungs; thought to be helpful in topical forms for aging skin
- **Idebenone:** a newly discovered powerful topical antioxidant, related to coenzyme Q10

Sunscreen Ingredients

Many free radicals are caused by sun exposure. One of the best ways to prevent free radical damage is to use a sunscreen every day. It is now common for day moisturizers to have a built-in sunscreen. This is something you should teach your clients: Help them find a sunscreen that is right for their skin and lifestyle.

There are two basic types of sunscreen ingredients: absorbing sunscreen ingredients and physical sunscreen ingredients. Absorbing sunscreen ingredients are often referred to as *chemical sunscreens*. This is a misleading term since all sunscreen ingredients are chemicals. Absorbing sunscreens work by absorbing and chemically neutralizing ultraviolet rays. Different ingredients may absorb different parts of the ultraviolet spectrum, and therefore several ingredients may be used in one sunscreen product. Some common absorbing sunscreen ingredients include:

- **Octinoxate:** Probably the most-used absorbing ingredient; formerly known as *octyl methoxycinnimate*, it absorbs UVB light
- **Octisalate:** Also known as *octyl salicylate*; a UVB absorber, but absorbs a different area of UVB rays than octinoxate; they are often combined in a sunscreen product
- **Oxybenzone:** Formerly called *benzophenone*; absorbs some of the UVB and some of the UVA ranges of ultraviolet light
- **Avobenzone:** Also called Parsol 1789, absorbs all UVA rays
- **Ecamsule:** Also known as Mexoryl®; a recently approved UVA absorber that is considered a very stable and complete UVA absorber

Physical sunscreen ingredients work by scattering or reflecting the sun's rays. There are only two physical sunscreens approved for use in sunscreens in the United States, and these screen both UVA and UVB rays:

- Zinc oxide
- Titanium dioxide

Titanium dioxide and zinc oxide work by physically reflecting the sun. Both ingredients are opaque and must go through a micronization process to avoid being seen laying on the skin surface as a white mask. You may have noticed that surfers often wear a white substance on their noses. This is a zinc oxide paste and is a very effective sunscreen.

Peptides and Collagen Stimulants

Peptides are a recent discovery for treatment of wrinkles and lack of elasticity. They are chains of amino acids that can cause various responses when applied to aging skin. Palmitoyl pentapeptide-3 is the most commonly used peptide for aging skin. Also known as Matrixyl®, palmitoyl pentapeptide-3 has been demonstrated to significantly increase collagen synthesis, improving the appearance of wrinkles and sagging of aging skin. Palmitoyl pentapeptide-3 is basically a sequential piece of a collagen molecule. It is theorized to work by "tricking" the skin into "believing" that too much collagen has been broken down, curbing the production of collagenase, the enzyme that destroys collagen, and stimulating fibroblasts, the cells that produce collagen. The results are remarkable, and the performance ingredient does not cause the irritation that can be caused by other anti-aging ingredients such as retinol.

Acetyl-hexapeptide-3 is another peptide ingredient and is used in "wrinkle-relaxing" creams. This ingredient is reported to prevent certain reactions in the skin that create skin folding as a result of facial expressions, softening pronounced wrinkles and expression lines.

Hydrocotyl (*Centella asiatica*) and coneflower (*Echinacea purpurea*) extracts are a patented complex of botanical ingredients that has been demonstrated to stimulate collagen production. Often, peptides are combined with this complex in products to improve collagen content, soften wrinkles, and improve skin firmness.

Other, newer peptides are being developed that help with eye puffiness, wrinkling, and increasing skin elasticity. These include palmitoyl oligopeptide, dipeptide-2, and palmitoyl tetrapeptide-3. Peptide technology is an area that is very promising, and new ingredients will surely be developed that have other appearance effects on the skin.

More Performance Ingredients for Aging Skin

Glucans, also known as beta glucans, are a saccharide compound found in the cell wall of yeast but can also be found in oats, barley, and other sources. Beta glucans are stimulants to the immune system, signal tissue repair, and are thought to also stimulate collagen synthesis. They also have antioxidant properties. They are frequently used in products for aging skin.

Also derived from yeast is the tissue respiratory factor (TRF). This ingredient increases the ability of cells to utilize oxygen and has skin care applications, primarily in products for aging skin. It is also used as a soothing and calming agent and is famous for its use in a well-known product for treating hemorrhoids.

Glycoproteins are molecules that combine proteins and carbohydrates. In the body, some hormones, antibodies, connective tissue, and surface membranes all are made of or are related to glycoproteins. Like glucans and TRF, glycoproteins help improve skin cells' ability to utilize oxygen, help with immune function, and enhance membrane quality.

Combining Anti-Aging Ingredients

All of these anti-aging ingredients definitely help the appearance of sun-damaged and aging skin. However, the best results are achieved by combining products and performance agents. Choosing just one ingredient modality will not provide the benefit that you will see when you combine all of the types of ingredients discussed here. Use of a good sunscreen in a lipid-based hydrating vehicle, antioxidant/peptide collagen-stimulating serums, and AHA gels or creams provide a program approach to helping the appearance of aging or sun-damaged skin.

READING INGREDIENT LABELS

The FDA requires that makers of all skin care and cosmetic products available for retail sale provide a list of all of a product's ingredients. This list must appear on the outermost packaging of the product. Companies are not required to list percentages of concentration, and professional back bar products used during services by cosmetology professionals are exempt from the label requirement. Drug products such as sunscreens and acne medications are required to have drug labels. The active drug ingredient(s) are listed separately, and the inactive ingredients (so-called by the FDA in drug products) are listed separately. The ingredients used in these product must be listed in descending order. In other words, the ingredient that makes up the largest concentration of the product must be listed first, the second-largest ingredient concentration listed second, and so on.

You will notice that water is listed first on almost all products. This is because most products are primarily made of water, and these are known as water-based products. The vehicle and spreading agent ingredients are usually the first few ingredients listed, again, because they make up the majority of the product. After the spreading

Ingredients: Water (Aqua), Butylene Glycol, Caprylic/Capric Triglyceride, Stearic Acid, Propylene Glycol Dicaprylate/Dicaprate, Ethylhexyl Palmitate, Glyceryl Stearate, PEG-100 Stearate, Aloe Barbadensis Leaf Juice, Dimethicone, Glycerin, Glycoproteins, Glycosphingolipids, Phospholipids, Cholesterol, Sodium Hyaluronate, Sodium PCA, Retinyl Palmitate, Ascorbic Acid, Tocopherol, Ceteth-20, Carbomer, Disodium EDTA, Cetyl Alcohol, Triethanolamine, Propylene Glycol, Diazolidinyl Urea, Methylparaben, Propylparaben.

Figure 12–11 Ingredient label for a moisturizer.

agent ingredients, the next ingredients listed are usually the emulsifying and thickening ingredients. The last ingredients listed are most often the performance ingredients, which are often not needed in large concentrations to produce the desired appearance effects. Other ingredients toward the end of the list are fragrance components, preservatives, and color agents. Figure 12–11 shows an ingredient label for a moisturizer.

Water is listed first, so it makes up the biggest part of the product. Butylene glycol is a strong humectant and is listed second. Caprylic/capric triglyceride, stearic acid, propylene glycol dicaprylate/dicaprate, ethylhexyl palmitate, glyceryl stearate are all emollient ingredients, probably serving as both functional spreading agents and performance moisture-guarding agents. Note that the emollients are a mixture of fatty acid and a variety of esters. PEG-100 stearate, ceteth-20, triethanolamine, cetyl alcohol, and carbomer are all emulsifier and thickeners used at different levels in this product. Dimethicone, a silicone, is used as a moisture guard. Glycosphingolipids, phospholipids, and cholesterol are all performance lipids to support the barrier function. Sodium hyaluronate and sodium PCA are both hydrating ingredients (humectants). Retinyl palmitate, ascorbic acid, and tocopherol are antioxidant vitamins a (palmitate is vitamin a ester), C (ascorbic acid), and E (tocopherol). They may be included as antioxidants or may be part of the product preservative system. Disodium EDTA is a chelating agent, and diazolidinyl urea, methylparaben, and propylparaben are all preservatives placed in the product as a system. Because of where it is listed, propylene glycol is most likely a solvent for the preservative system.

As you move through your career as an esthetician, you will become more knowledgeable about ingredients and their functions. In this era of cosmeceuticals, consumers are educated about what ingredients to look for, making it necessary for you to be knowledgeable about all skin care and cosmetic ingredients.

REVIEW QUESTIONS

1. What are the two basic categories of cosmetic ingredients? Discuss the difference between the two different categories.
2. According to the FDA, what are the differences between a drug and a cosmetic?
3. Why should estheticians not use the term *active ingredient* to discuss ingredients that are in a product that is not a drug?
4. What makes up the largest part of any cosmetic product?
5. Describe two possible functions of an emollient ingredient. Name some frequently used emollients.
6. What are some advantages to using silicone-based ingredients? Name several silicone ingredients.
7. What does *biologically inert* mean?
8. What does *comedogenic* mean?
9. How are fatty acids used in cosmetics? Where do fatty acids come from? List several examples and their sources.
10. Discuss the term *alcohol*. Are all alcohols drying?
11. How do detergents work?
12. Name the four types of surfactants and how each is used.
13. What do emulsifiers do in a cosmetic formulation?
14. What is a liposome? What are some advantages of using liposomes in skin care products?

15. Why are preservatives so important in products?
16. What are humectants? What skin type can benefit from a humectant?
17. What are NMFs and why are they important?
18. Moisturizers are a mixture of what two performance ingredients? How would moisturizers for oily and dry skin differ?
19. What are the two basic types of skin exfoliants? Discuss their differences and list some examples.
20. Discuss six reasons why alpha hydroxy acids are important performance ingredients.
21. What role does pH and concentration play in alpha hydroxy acid products?
22. What is a free radical? How do free radicals affect the skin?
23. What is the inflammation cascade?
24. Why are antioxidants important for the skin? List several antioxidant ingredients.
25. What is a broad-spectrum antioxidant?
26. What are the two types of sunscreen ingredients? How does each work? List examples of each.

CHAPTER GLOSSARY

active ingredient: ingredient in a drug that causes a change to the structure or function of the body.

anecdotal: based on observation and theory, rather than scientific experimentation.

bioavailable: describes a substance's ability to be used as a performance ingredient by the skin.

biologically inert: describes ingredients that will not cross-react with chemicals that occur naturally in the body.

buffering: refers to adjusting the pH of a product to make it more acceptable to the skin.

catechins: a crystalline flavinoid compound with antioxidant properties.

collagenase: self-destruct enzyme that destroys collagen.

crosslinking: a process in which collagen and elastin fibrils in the dermis collapse, causing the support system for the skin to collapse.

defatting agents: agents that remove fats and lipids, along with dirt, makeup and debris, from the surface of the skin.

deionization: a process that neutralizes ions in water to be used in the manufacture of skin care and cosmetics.

distillation: 1. process that removes mineral and trace elements from the water 2. process used to extract essential oils from a plant using hot water, hot water and steam, or steam alone.

drug: according to the FDA: "articles (other than food) intended to affect the structure or function of the body."

drug claim: to make a claim that a product affects the structure or function of the body.

elastase: self–destruct skin enzyme that destroys elastin.

ester: a compound structure that is formed through the reaction of an acid with an alcohol.

external phase: the component of an emulsion that is of the largest concentration.

free radicals (reactive oxygen species): a major contributor to aging, free radicals are unstable molecules that have broken away from weak molecules. In an attempt to stabilize themselves, they steal electrons from stable molecules, creating more and more unstable molecules. The result is tissue damage, accelerated aging, and vulnerability to disease.

CHAPTER GLOSSARY

gellant: an agent that is added to a product to give it a gel-like consistency.

globules: oil droplets in an oil-in-water emulsion.

glucans: a saccharide compound found in the cell wall of yeast but can also be found in oats, barley, and other sources. Beta glucans stimulate the immune system, signal tissue repair, and are thought to also stimulate collagen synthesis. They also have anti-oxidant properties. Also known as *beta glucans.*

glycolic acid: an alpha hydroxy acid used in skin treatments.

homogenizers: high-speed mixers used to emulsify products.

hyaluronidase: A self–destruct skin enzyme that destroys hyaluronic acid.

hydroxy radical: the most dangerous free radicals, which can react with many DNA in the cell nucleus, causing permanent damage to the cell and to the DNA in future cells produced from cell division.

inactive ingredients: ingredients within a drug that do not specifically cause a physiological change but are necessary for the drug to work.

internal phase: component of an emulsion that is of the least concentration.

isopropyl alcohol: a fairly strong on drying alcohol used as a cleansing and drying agent to remove excess oil.

keratolytics: also called proteolytic, means "protein dissolving." These agents work by dissolving keratin protein within dead surface cells, helping to remove these cells and making the skin look cleaner and smoother.

lactic acid: an AHA occuring naturally in milk. It is both an exfoliant and a hydrophilic.

lipid peroxide: free radicals formed when the cell membrane is damaged by other free radicals.

lipophilic: having an affinity or attraction to fat and oils.

malic acid: an AHA derived from apples.

micelle: a protective sphere that is created by emulsifiers surrounding an internal phase ingredient.

micellized: refers to ingredients encapsulated in a micelle.

microencapsulation: the process of using barrier and intercellular-compatible materials like lipids to form special micro-shells to protect and better penetrate certain ingredients.

microsponge: A variety of microencapsulation that releases a performance ingredient once inside the skin.

natural moisturizing factors (NMFs): natural humectants, lipids, or hydrating agents found within intercellular cement.

non-acnegenic: refers to ingredients or products that will not irritate the inside of follicles and cause flares of acne.

non-comedogenic: describes ingredients or products that do not cause comedones or clogged pores to form.

parfum: scent, fragrance.

physical emulsions: products emulsified using special blends of emoillients and non surfactant emulsifying agents that are mixed at high speeds.

polyphenols: antioxidant phytochemicals.

pressing agents: ingredients that help powders stay in cake form and also help powder cosmetics adhere or stick to the skin.

proanthocyanidins: very strong family of antioxidants found in grapeseed extract and maritme pine extract (pycnogenol).

proteases: enzymes that digest proteins; includes proteinases and peptidases.

protectants: ingredients that keep substances from penetrating the skin.

proteolytic enzymes: protein dissolving enzymes.

rancid: describes an oxidized cosmetic product that has discoloration and/or odor.

SD alcohols: are specially denatured to make them not drinkable. Also known as ethanol.

sodium PCA: a humectant that helps to bind water in the epidermis.

subclinical: describes a situation in which normal clinical symptoms are not visible.

substantives: ingredients that attach themselves to the surface of the skin to protect and hydrate the surface.

superfatted: describes soaps or cleaners that have fat added to buffer their contact with the skin.

superoxide dismutase: an enzyme that helps squelch reactions early in the cascade of reactions.

tartaric acid: an AHA occuring naturally in grapes and passion fruit.

viscosity: the thickness and liquidity of a solution.

CHAPTER 13

BOTANICALS AND AROMATHERAPY

CHAPTER OUTLINE

- WHAT ARE BOTANICAL INGREDIENTS?
- PLANT COMPOUNDS AND EXTRACTS
- METHODS OF BOTANICAL EXTRACTION
- ELEVEN BOTANICALS FOR SKIN CARE
- AROMATHERAPY AND ESSENTIAL OILS
- WHAT ESSENTIAL OILS CAN DO
- ESSENTIAL OIL CHEMISTRY
- CONTRAINDICATIONS
- THIRTEEN ESSENTIAL OILS
- APPLICATION OF ESSENTIAL OILS
- RECIPES FOR SKIN AND SPA
- THE AROMATHERAPY AND BOTANICAL PRACTICE
- HOLISTIC CONSULTATION
- LEGAL CONSIDERATIONS

LEARNING OBJECTIVES

After completing this chapter, you should be able to:

- Define herbal ingredients and extracts.
- Discuss benefits and uses of botanicals in skin care.
- Understand plant compounds.
- Discuss the methods of botanical extraction.
- Know 11 botanicals for skin care.
- Discuss aromatherapy and essential oils.
- Understand the sense of smell and olfactory response.
- Discuss essential oils and their chemistry.
- Know contraindications to essential oils.
- Name 13 essential oils.
- Discuss how essential oils are blended.
- Prepare recipes for skin and spa.
- Discuss issues surrounding an aromatherapy practice.
- Understand a holistic consultation.
- Discuss legal considerations of using essential oils and botanicals.

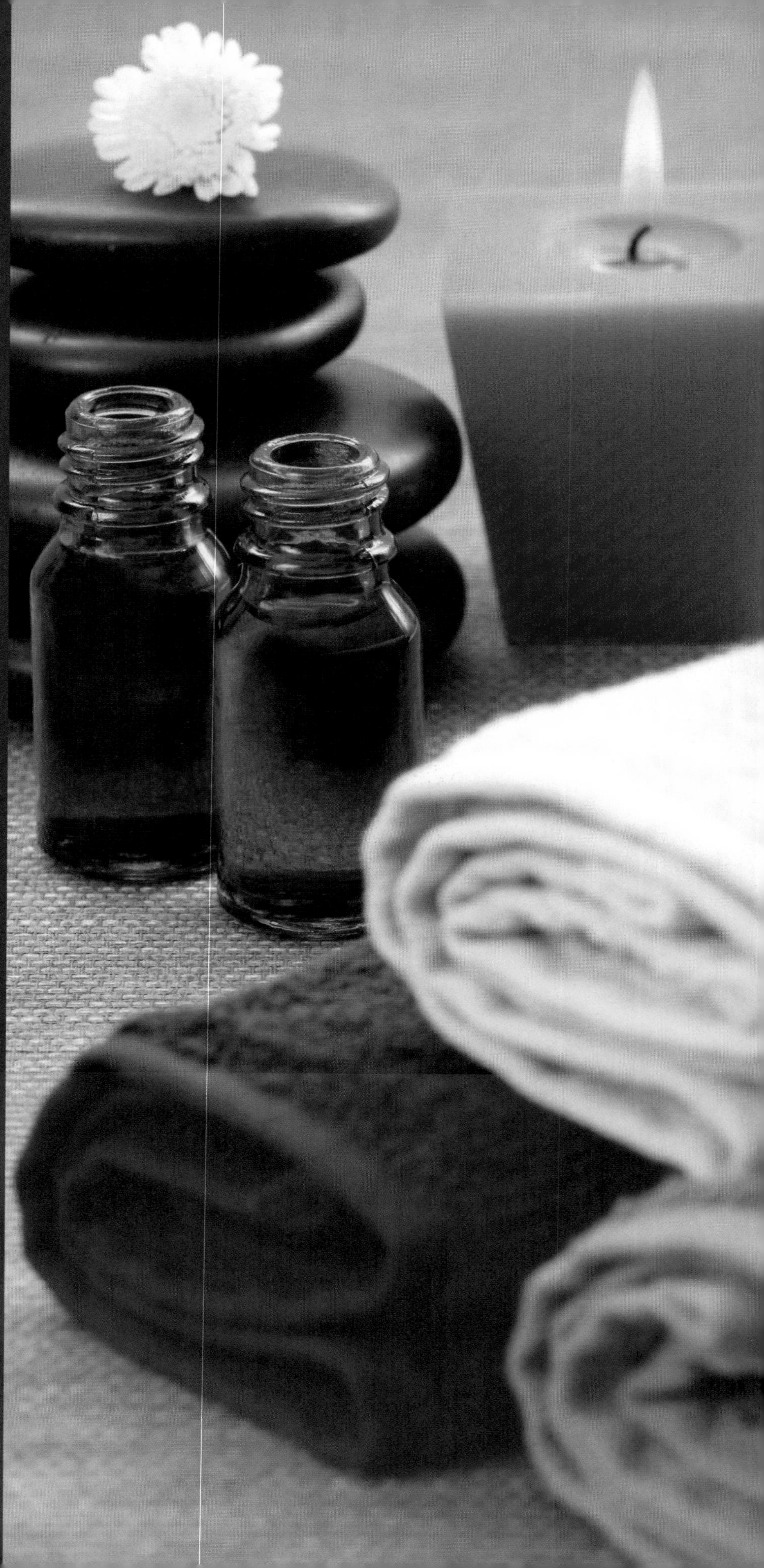

KEY TERMS

Page numbers indicate where in the chapter the term is used.

absolutes 290
adulteration 294
allantoin 284
alpha d-tocopherol 284
aqueous extract 285
autonomic motor systems (autonomic nervous system) 291
dilution amount 300
distillation 290
dl-tocopherol 284
emulsifier 301
endocrine system 291
expeller pressed 285
fixed oil 285
genuine and authentic 294
herbal infusion 285
holistic health 302
homeostasis 290
hydrosol 290
hypothalamus 291
isolates 284
limbic system 291
nonvolatile 285
olfaction 290
phytotherapy 283
rectified 295
refined 284
supercritical carbon dioxide (CO_2) 285
synergy 292
tincture 284
whole extract 284

Throughout history, plants have provided humans with food, shelter, clothing, medicine, energy, and skin care. The study of plants for therapy is sometimes called **phytotherapy**. Today there is increased awareness of how botanicals and their extracts work to create health and well-being of the body and skin. Botanical fixed oils, essential oils, herbal extracts, and other plant-based therapies are utilized in cosmetic preparations and treatments to enhance the vitality and healing of the skin. This chapter discusses plants, their properties, and their uses in skin care. This knowledge will assist you in fine-tuning your personalized botanical formulas for more precise treatment results and will give you a better understanding of products containing botanical ingredients (Figure 13–1).

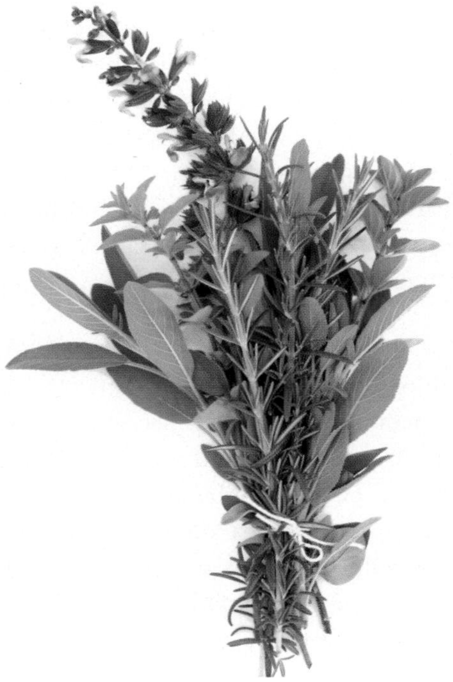

Figure 13–1 Herbal bouquet.

WHAT ARE BOTANICAL INGREDIENTS?

The term *botanical* means relating to plants or plant life. In the world of esthetics and spa therapy, botanicals are often categorized under the umbrella term *natural ingredients*. The term *natural* has become vague and meaningless due to product marketing and random overuse. It is important to have a clear knowledge of plant-based, or botanical, ingredients, where they come from, and their properties and use in skin care.

Plant-derived medicines have been utilized throughout history. It is well known that plants contain compounds that have therapeutic benefits to human health. Plants offer the following benefits to the skin:

- Anti-inflammatory
- Antimicrobial
- Antioxidant
- Antiseptic
- Astringent
- Cellular protection and rejuvenation
- Moisturizer
- Decongestant
- Regulator
- Strengthener (tonifies)
- Wound healing

As you can see, the benefits of botanicals in skin care are extensive and wide-ranging. Plant-derived ingredients are utilized topically in skin lotions, creams, wraps, masks, compresses, sprays, and a variety of other application preparations.

PLANT COMPOUNDS AND EXTRACTS

Plants produce a variety of compounds to assist in their structure, survival, and protection against parasites, herbivores, wounds, and environmental stresses. In essence, they are a plant's immune system and serve to keep it alive. When used in skin care products, these compounds share their therapeutic benefit with humans.

Botanical ingredients are seldom used in their whole state, such as a dried herb. Plants "give up" their compounds through a variety of extraction procedures usually defined by the name given to the extract. When selecting extracts, it is vital to determine that the extraction method does not alter the plant's composition or damage the therapeutic value. It takes a great amount of study to thoroughly understand plant extractions.

A **whole extract** is one that has not been changed from its natural state, or **refined.** Refining is the process of removing colors, odors, or other naturally occurring compounds from the plant's extract. There may be a loss of therapeutic activity or potential irritation when extracts are altered from their natural state.

Some useful therapeutic components are individually separated from a plant or extract. These are called **isolates** or isolated compounds. An example of an isolate is **alpha d-tocopherol,** the popular form of vitamin E that is isolated from soy and other botanicals. Some isolates are created synthetically. For instance, the synthetic forms of vitamin E are **dl-tocopherol** and tocopherol acetate. Isolates are individual compounds recognized for specific therapeutic activity, such as the antioxidant properties of tocopherol and the anti-inflammatory compound **allantoin,** isolated from the herb comfrey.

METHODS OF BOTANICAL EXTRACTION

Several methods are used to extract active properties from plants. Each method results in an extract that directly relates to the process used. Some compounds are water-soluble so are best extracted using water. Vegetable oils and alcohol are best for extracting fat-soluble compounds. Following is a discussion of some of the more common methods.

Tinctures

When alcohol or glycerin is used to extract the compounds from a plant, the result is called a **tincture.** This is the most common method of plant extraction and is often used in medicinal herbology. Plant material is placed into the alcohol. After a specified amount of time, the plant material is removed. The compounds that are soluble in alcohol will remain in the alcohol and the resulting tincture. This would be the same if glycerin were used. Tinctures come in varied strengths.

Dried Herbs

Plants can be dried for use in medicines and skin care. There is no extraction method used. Because the plant material is left in its most whole and natural state, there are limits to the use of dried herbs in skin care. Dried herbs do not dissolve in skin preparations so must be used in procedures that will be left on for a lengthy period of time and then removed from the skin, such as masks and wraps. Benefits depend on the specific herb used.

Infusions

The most historically common extraction method of plant material is the infusion. When the plant material is soaked in hot water—though sometimes cold water is used—for a given period of time, the result is an **herbal infusion.** The best example of this method is tea. Infusions can also be extracted using vegetable oil, juices, vinegar, and glycerin. Infusions are a great addition to skin care and are adaptable in almost any preparation.

Activity

Make an infusion by placing sprigs of fresh, organically grown chamomile in distilled water and soaking to make a strong tea. Strain and use for soothing eye pads. Since there are no preservatives, this product can be kept for only a few days and must be refrigerated.

FYI

A term you might see on product labels is **aqueous extract,** which is an infusion. It is common to see an aqueous extract as first on an ingredient list, such as "aqueous extract of rose, chamomile, lavender, comfrey, horsetail and clover." This does not necessarily mean the formula contains high amounts of the herbs mentioned; extracts are not well regulated and may contain few to no plant compounds. One of the challenges in working with botanical ingredients is to recognize the quality of the extracts and the language used on labels. Question manufacturers of botanical products to be sure they are working with extracts that offer the greatest potential therapeutic benefits.

Expeller Pressed Oils

A fatty oil derived from vegetables and fruits that does not evaporate, or is **nonvolatile,** is called a fixed oil. **Fixed oils,** such as olive oil, grapeseed oil, and jojoba oil, are of the purist quality and therapeutic strength when they are **expeller pressed.** This involves using a mechanical press to extract the oil from the seeds, nuts, or plant material, (Figure 13–2). This extraction method is preferred for fixed oils over using other methods involving caustic chemicals or solvents. Expeller pressed oils are the only fixed oils that should be used in organic or natural skin care that is considered to be "clean."

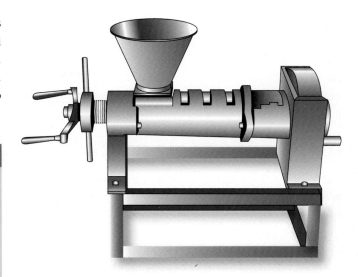

Figure 13–2 Mechanical press used for expeller pressed oils.

Expeller pressed fixed oils contain a fatty acid content that nourishes and protects the skin. Often these oils are refined, bleached, and deodorized (RBD oils). Oils left in their whole state (non-RBD oils) offer increased therapeutic benefit. There are beneficial properties to color and scent. This is evident in foods, like carrots, that offer powerful antioxidant protection, which is attributed to the compounds that give them their deep red, yellow, and green colors. Scent compounds also contain worthy properties, as we will find later in this chapter.

Supercritical Carbon Dioxide

The most recently developed method of extraction involves placing plant material in a high-pressure container with **supercritical carbon dioxide (CO_2).** The CO_2 is in a state midway between being a liquid and a gas. This process is popular in the fragrance industry as it is gentler than essential oil distillation and it extracts heavier therapeutic and fragrant compounds that do not easily evaporate in the distillation process. The resulting fragrance is truer to the plant from which it is extracted. Supercritical extractions are highly concentrated and used in small amounts in a formula.

Solvent Extraction

Methods that utilize synthetic or petroleum-based solvents are solvent extracts. Solvents are used to extract fatty acid components from plants. Propylene glycol and hexane are commonly used solvent extracts. It is important to know if your extracts were processed using solvents. Solvent extracts have a potential for contamination and also destruction of the vital composition of the plant extracts. Solvent extracts are generally not acceptable when a manufacturer is making a purity claim, though there are no regulations or standards that require a manufacturer to provide information regarding solvent or expeller pressed fixed oil content on their label.

ELEVEN BOTANICALS FOR SKIN CARE

There are a multitude of botanical extracts currently being used in skin care, offering endless possibilities for uses. Following is a list of eleven botanicals, their botanical names, and the properties that make them an asset in any skin care program. These botanicals were selected for their common use in cosmetics and their diversity of properties, uses, and extraction methods.

FYI

What Is Organic?

The term organic, when used to define a botanical ingredient, refers to the growing practice and was created to regulate foods claiming to be grown under well-defined, "organic," conditions. The conditions relate to pesticide use, fertilizer and other factors that are selected for their ecological harmony and positive environmental impact. Only organics that are properly certified, such as USDA NOP (National Organic Program) certified organic, are guaranteed organically grown. The main reason for purchasing or using organic foods, ingredients, and personal care is because they are an environmentally safer, "greener," choice. Organic farming avoids soil erosion and the pesticides and fertilizers that cause environmental harm and pollution.

Aloe Vera (Figure 13–3)
BOTANICAL NAME: *Aloe barbadensis*
EXTRACTED PARTS: Whole leaves
CHEMICAL STRUCTURE: Mucopolysaccharides, enzymes, amino acids
PROPERTIES: Anti-inflammatory, regenerative, moisturizing, soothing, healing
USES: Burns, irritation, general skin care and conditioning
QUALITY AND PREPARATION: Available as a whole juice or powder; it has a pale yellow color, bitter taste, and distinctive "aloe" odor; best when bought without any color or other additives, except the preservative sodium benzoate or sodium citrate

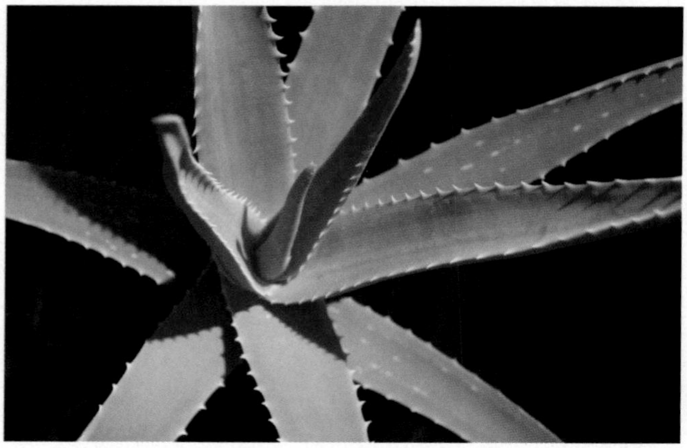

Figure 13–3 Aloe plant.

Arnica (Figure 13–4)
BOTANICAL NAME: *Arnica montana*
EXTRACTED PARTS: Flowers
CHEMICAL STRUCTURE: Alkaloids, flavonoids, tannins, essential oils
PROPERTY: Anti-inflammatory
USES: Arthritis, bruises, inflammation, pain
QUALITY AND PREPARATION: Available as a dried herb, infusion, and tincture

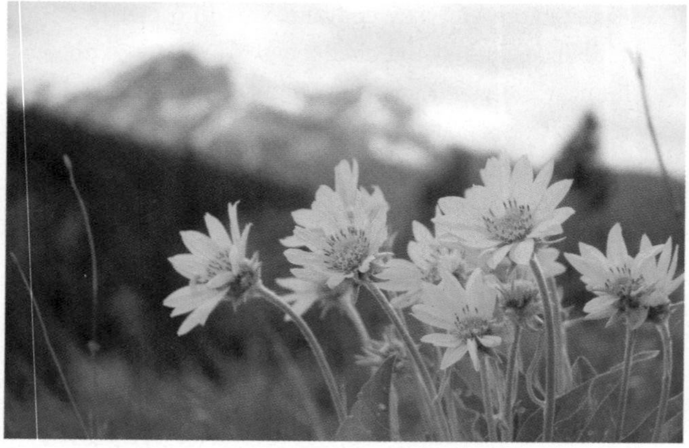

Figure 13–4 Arnica flower.

Bamboo (Figure 13–5)
BOTANICAL NAME: *Bambusa vulgaris*
EXTRACTED PARTS: Stalk, leaves
CHEMICAL STRUCTURE: Silica
PROPERTY: Assists in organization of connective tissue
USES: Skin strength and conditioning
QUALITY AND PREPARATION: Available as a powdered extract and tincture

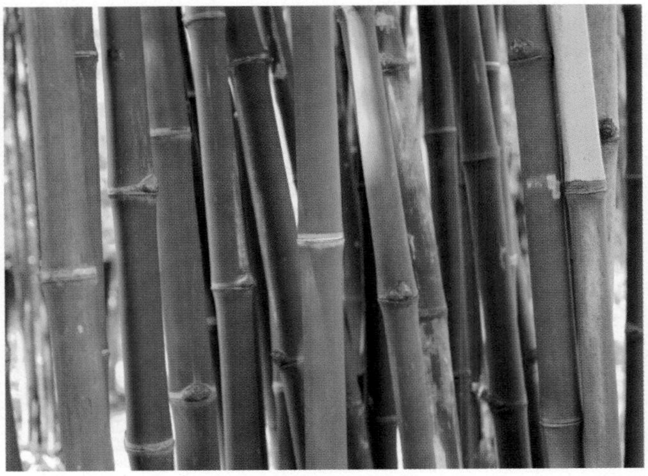

Figure 13–5 Bamboo.

Cocoa (Butter and Powder) (Figure 13–6)

BOTANICAL NAME: *Theobroma cacao*

EXTRACTED PARTS: Seeds

CHEMICAL STRUCTURE: Butter—oleic, stearic, and palmitic fatty acids; Powder—theobromine, proteins, fats, volatile oils, amines, alkaloids, caffeine

PROPERTIES: Anti-inflammatory, antioxidant, emollient, regenerative

USES: General skin care and conditioning, regenerative, moisturizing

QUALITY AND PREPARATION: The butter is light brown with a definite chocolate butter fragrance; the powder is unmistakably rich dark chocolate.

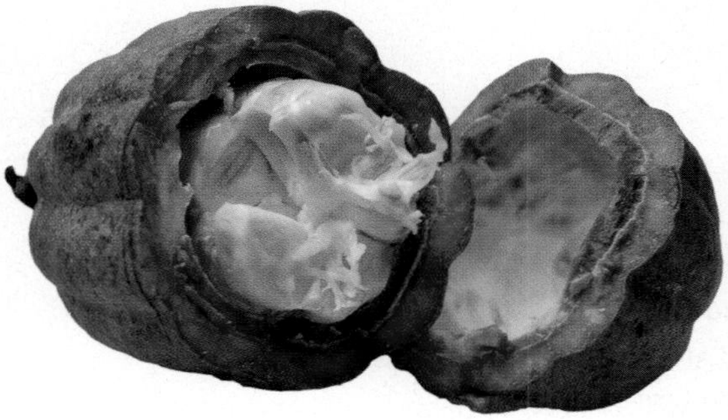

Figure 13–6 Cacao seed.

Comfrey (Figure 13–7)

BOTANICAL NAME: *Symphytum officinale*

EXTRACTED PARTS: Roots

CHEMICAL STRUCTURE: Mucilage, allantoin, alkaloids

PROPERTY: Stimulates cell proliferation

USES: Wound healing, general skin care and conditioning

QUALITY AND PREPARATION: Available as dried herb, infusion, tincture

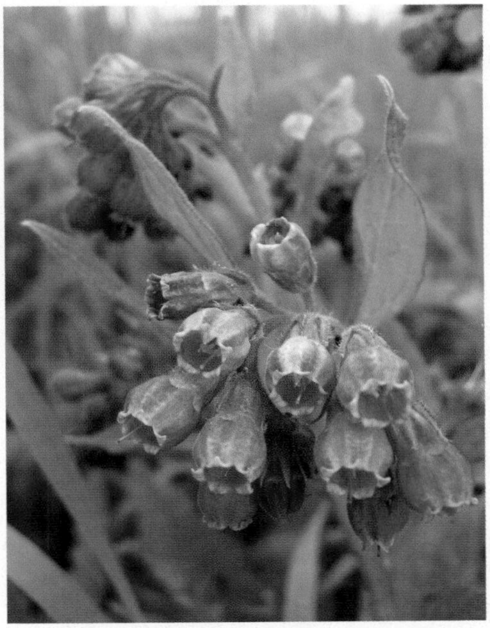

Figure 13–7 Comfrey.

Cranberry Seed Oil (Figure 13–8)

BOTANICAL NAME: *Vaccinium macrocarpon*

EXTRACTED PARTS: Seeds

CHEMICAL STRUCTURE: 1-to-1 ratio of omega-6 to omega-3 fatty acids, lauric acid, tocopherols (vitamin E)

PROPERTIES: Anti-inflammatory, antioxidant, emollient, UV protection

USES: General skin care and conditioning, barrier protection, moisturizing

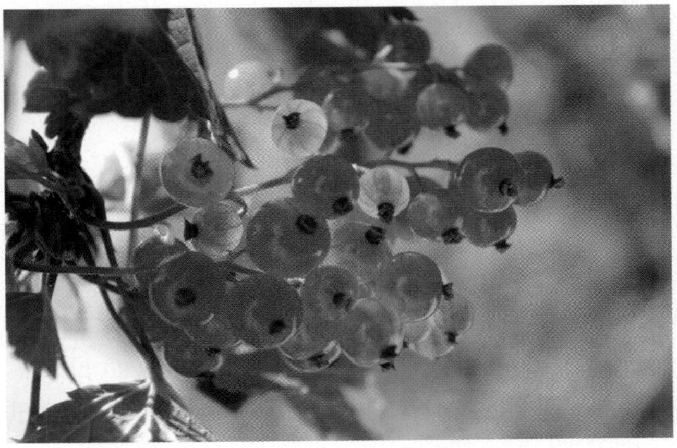

Figure 13–8 Cranberries.

QUALITY AND PREPARATION: Available both refined and—though harder to find—as an unrefined oil; the unrefined has a deeper brownish red color and fruity fatty acid odor. An organic cranberry seed oil is very difficult to find.

Green Tea (Figure 13–9)
BOTANICAL NAME: *Camellia sinensis*
EXTRACTED PARTS: Leaves
CHEMICAL STRUCTURE: Polyphenols, tannins, alkaloids, volatile oils
PROPERTIES: Anti-inflammatory, antioxidant, astringent, decongestant, circulatory stimulant
USES: Acneic skin, strengthening, protective, general skin care and conditioning
QUALITY AND PREPARATION: Available as dried herb, infusion, tincture. Green tea can be prepared as a tea and added to any skin treatment.

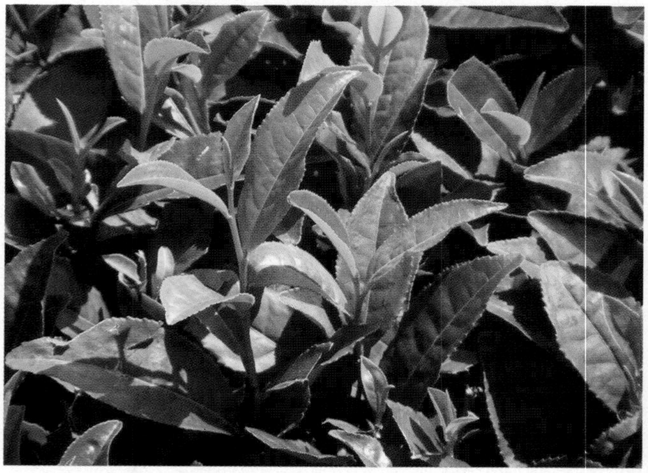

Figure 13–9 Green tea.

Kelp (Figure 13–10)
BOTANICAL NAME: *Laminaria digitata; Laminaria ochroleuca*
EXTRACTED PARTS: Leaves
CHEMICAL STRUCTURE: Mucilage, minerals
PROPERTIES: Wound healing, detoxifying
USES: Wounds, skin congestion, general skin care and conditioning
QUALITY AND PREPARATION: Available as dried powder and tincture. There are a variety of sea plants used in skin care offering a wide variety of beneficial properties. Sea botanicals tend to give off a typically pungent seaweed odor.

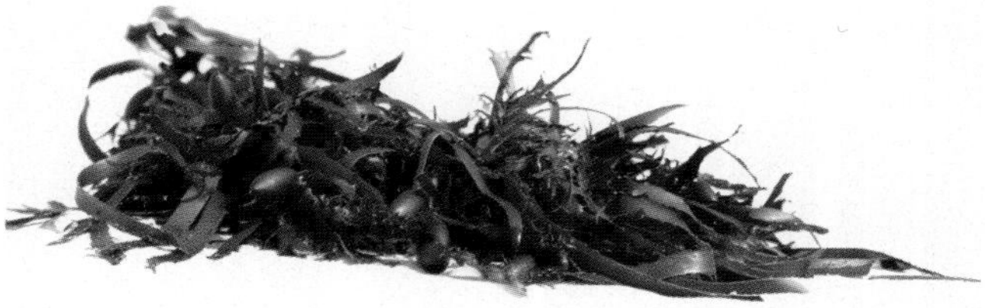

Figure 13–10 Kelp.

Marigold (Calendula) (Figure 13–11)
BOTANICAL NAME: *Calendula officinalis*
EXTRACTED PARTS: Flowers
CHEMICAL STRUCTURE: Carotenoids, flavonoids, polyphenols, volatile oils
PROPERTIES: Anti-inflammatory, astringent, antifungal, regenerative
USES: Inflammation, cell regeneration, wounds, general skin care and conditioning
QUALITY AND PREPARATION: Available as dried herb, tincture, infusion, and supercritical CO_2 extract (contains higher amounts of carotenoids); CO_2 extract is a deep golden yellow color.

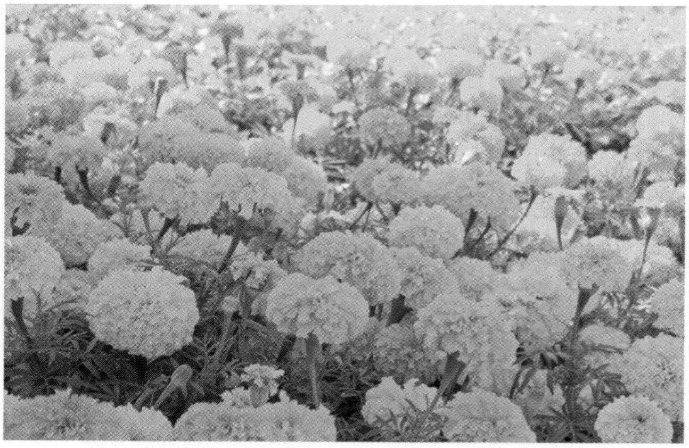

Figure 13–11 Marigold.

Sea Buckthorn Supercritical CO_2 Extract (Figure 13–12)
BOTANICAL NAME: *Hippophae rhamnoides*
EXTRACTED PARTS: Berry seeds and pulp
CHEMICAL STRUCTURE: Carotenoids, omega-6 and omega-3 fatty acids, and a unique omega-7 fatty acid, volatile oils
PROPERTIES: Anti-inflammatory, antioxidant, antimicrobial, emollient, immune modulator, regenerative
USES: Inflammation, cell regeneration, skin strengthening, soothing, moisturizing, general skin care and conditioning

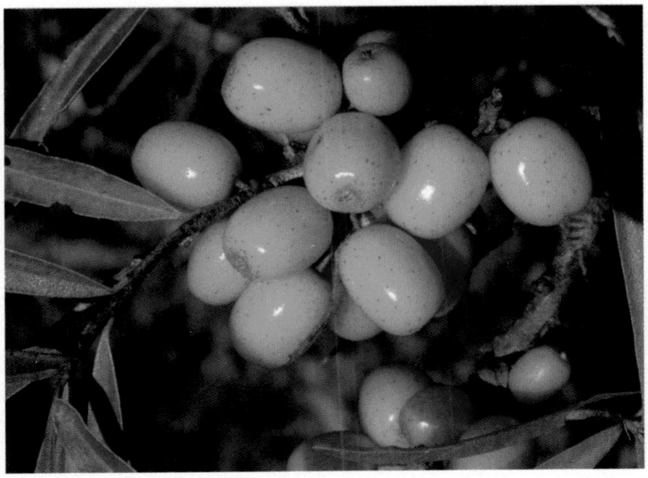

Figure 13–12 Sea buckthorn.

QUALITY AND PREPARATION: Available as an oil infusion and supercritical CO_2 extract, which is a deep reddish brown and adds color to any formula that contains it

Shea Butter (African Karite Butter) (Figure 13–13)
BOTANICAL NAME: *Butyrospermum parkii*
EXTRACTED PARTS: Nuts
CHEMICAL STRUCTURE: Triglycerides, fatty acids, polycyclic triterpene, cinnamic acid
PROPERTIES: Anti-inflammatory, emollient, regenerative, UV protection
USES: Inflammation, wounds, irritation, rash, moisturizing, general skin care and conditioning

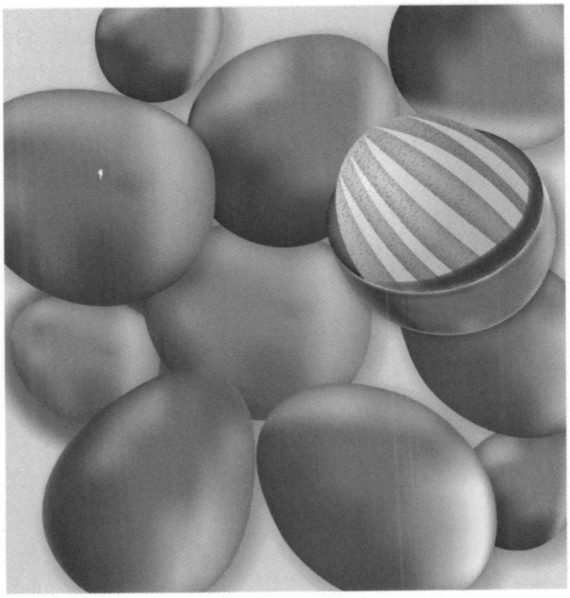

Figure 13–13 Shea nut.

QUALITY AND PREPARATION: Available as an expeller pressed butter. It can be produced refined or unrefined. Select a shea butter that is unrefined and has been prepared and stored properly and has not lost its integrity. The unrefined has a slight musty fat odor, a brownish color, and a smooth to somewhat chrystalized texture.

FYI

There are many resources available on botanicals. One of the best botanical Web sites is Dr. Duke's Phytochemical and Ethnobotanical Databases (www.ars-grin.gov), which allows you to search for a vast number of facts about a chosen plant. For example, you can begin by searching for "plants with a specific activity." This brings you to a page that asks you to select criteria. Selecting "All" widens your options. Type in which activity you are looking for, such as anti-inflammatory. The next page is a list of botanicals with names of anti-inflammatory compounds and how many of these compounds the plant contains. Click on a plant name, and you will see a list of its anti-inflammatory compounds and the part of the plant from which each comes. This is helpful if, for instance, you are curious about an extracted seed oil you have and the list tells you that the anti-inflammatory compounds are in the leaf. You will then know that the oil is not anti-inflammatory. This easy-to-use Web site offers great insights into herbs, oils, and other skin care ingredients.

AROMATHERAPY AND ESSENTIAL OILS

Aromatherapy, or the therapeutic use of essential oils, is a valuable tool for the care and treatment of the skin. Introducing essential oils into an esthetic practice increases the ability to work holistically, addressing a client's physical and emotional aspects that affect skin conditions and imbalances. To use essential oils effectively, you must be able to identify essential oils and differentiate them from fragrance oils. A solid foundation in basic essential oil chemistry and the therapeutic properties will help you develop the means to blend and formulate effective aromatherapy treatments.

Combining this with an awareness of how human behavior is significantly impacted by scent gives you the expertise to offer treatment for a vast array of skin conditions.

What Is Aromatherapy?

Aromatherapy is the art, skill, and science of using essential oils for the health and well-being of the body, mind, and spirit. The earliest known use, or suspected use, of fragrant materials goes back to 7000 B.C. However, it was not until the sixteenth century that distilled essential oils, as we know them today, were used, though they were relegated mainly to royalty, alchemists, and perfumers.

The practice we now know as aromatherapy was introduced by René-Maurice Gattefossé in the early twentieth century. Gattefossé was a French perfume chemist whose interest in the medicinal properties of essential oils was triggered by a laboratory accident. He burned his hand and, after treating it with lavender essential oils, was amazed by how quickly it healed. In 1928 he coined the word *aromatherapy* when writing a paper describing his research in essential oil chemistry. The practice of aromatherapy blossomed in the 1970s and continues to be one of the world's most effective healing modalities.

Essential Oils

Essential oils are volatile fatty acid substances extracted from plants, flowers, seeds, woods, and fruit by means of dry steam, water/steam, or water distillation. The composition of carbon-based chemical structures provides the essential oils with diverse therapeutic activity. Essential oils are extracted from plants using the **distillation** process. Distillation is a method using water, water and steam, or just steam to extract the essence from a plant (Figure 13–14). The essence evaporates in the water vapors and is carried through a cooling condensing tube to become liquid again. This then flows into another container. The essential oil floats to the top of the water and is separated. The water that results from this procedure is called a **hydrosol,** which is also used in aromatherapy and skin care.

There are other methods of extracting the essence from plant material. These are called **absolutes**. Absolutes use a solvent extraction method. Some plants cannot be distilled and are solvent-extracted, such as jasmine and tuberose. Some oils, such as orange blossom and rose, are produced through distillation and solvent extraction. Absolutes can vary in quality; they can be contaminated just as vegetable oils are in solvent extraction.

Essential Oils and the Sense of Smell

The effect of **olfaction,** the sense of smell, on human behavior, the nervous system, and emotions is commonly unrecognized and underestimated (Figure 13–15). Due to the interaction with the hypothalamus, scent has a profound effect on thirst, hunger, sexuality, and functions of **homeostasis,** the process of feedback and regulation that keeps the body in a state of equilibrium within its environment. Early humans relied on smell for survival. It warned of danger, was used to track food, and was a key sense in mating and reproduction. Humans today still use the sense of smell for these very things, though, in our visually dominant world, we do not recognize how profoundly we are affected and controlled by olfaction. Throughout the rest of your day, pay attention to all of the odors you detect. Be aware of the way they make you feel or if they trigger any changes in your body. Do you notice that your body tenses or relaxes when certain scents appear? Are you reminded of a distant memory? Are you attracted or put off by a person who enters your "smell space"? Most responses are subtle and may be difficult to associate with a scent.

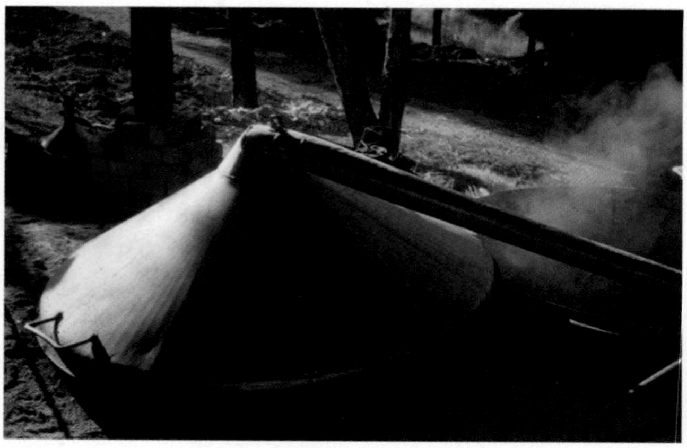

Figure 13–14 Distillation process.

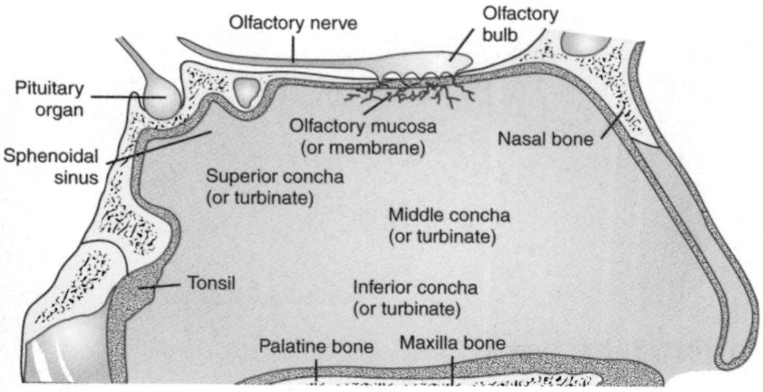

Figure 13–15 Olfactory nerve.

The sense of smell begins in the epitheleum, at the top of the nasal passage. Odor molecules attach to nerve endings, sending a signal through the olfactory bulb and to the limbic system and olfactory cortex, where scents are detected and processed. The **limbic system** is an important series of brain structures activated by odor, behavior, and arousal. This activation influences the **endocrine system,** the release of hormones, the **autonomic motor systems,** the control of the heart, respiration, and digestion. Olfaction greatly influences the **hypothalamus,** which regulates important metabolic functions, hormone release, and autonomic function.

Essential oils are accepted as having interaction within the limbic system, especially the hypothalamus. When a person inhales the oils, this interaction triggers specific functions, depending on the oil, and helps bring balance to mind and body.

> ***FYI***
>
> When working with essential oils, it is important to understand the relationship between scent and memory. Every memory has a scent association. This becomes obvious when the scent of a baking pie or flowers triggers a childhood memory. Essential oils also trigger memory, though rarely do they evoke vivid memory. Citrus oils tend to conjure up positive feelings due to their common use in goodies consumed during childhood. Often it is not the memory that is triggered but the emotion associated with this memory. For instance, think of a child who has a fearful experience when visiting a funeral parlor that is filled with the fragrance of roses. This leaves a deep emotional impact, and as an adult, when this person smells roses, he or she may experience a subtle, or even strong, anxiety or other stressful emotional response. This is the opposite reaction expected from the smell of rose. If you introduce this person to rose essential oil, it may cause him or her to feel uncomfortable, or in a worse case, cause a rash related to the stress of the emotion. Memory/emotion reactions seldom cause a rash or even a noticeable emotional response; often, emotional associations with essential oils produce more subtle reactions to the fragrances.
>
> Keep in mind that the scent/emotion association is related to all scent. Pay attention to your own feelings when you enter a fragrance zone, such as a dentist's or doctor's office.

WHAT ESSENTIAL OILS CAN DO

Following is a list of the wide-ranging properties that you can expect from essential oils. You may not think that all of these properties are related to an esthetic practice, especially one that is non-medical. When working holistically, though, you will find that you can use all of the properties of essential oils within the topical applications of your esthetic practice.

Antiseptic and Antimicrobial Properties

Essential oils are well documented for their action on microbes such as bacteria, viruses, and fungi. For example, the broad antiseptic action of tea tree oil is well known, making it one the most widely used medicinal essential oils. The most comprehensive study of essential oils and their effects on microorganisms was undertaken by Dr. Paul Belaiche, who published a three-volume work listing essential oils and their effectiveness against specific microorganisms.

Essential oils are used to prevent colds, flu, and bacterial infections of all kinds. When used in general skin care, the antimicrobial action of essential oils is present even if that is not the intent behind the use. For example, if you are using aromatherapy to detoxify an acneic skin condition, the oil's antimicrobial properties are present as well, eliminating a possible bacterial infection. In another example, say you are using essential oils to soothe a rash. If the rash is caused by a virus or fungus, the essential oils may eliminate the cause even though this was not your intention.

Anti-Inflammatory Properties

Inflammation is a major cause of many imbalances and diseases of the body. It is also a chief cause of the signs of aging. Reducing inflammation should be paramount to any skin care regimen. Essential oils, especially German chamomile and helichrysum, are superb anti-inflammatory and pain management tools.

Sedative and Stress Relief Properties

The skin and body are deeply affected by the ravages of stress, anxiety, and tension. Stress relief is likely the most popular use of aromatherapy products. This reputation is well deserved and well documented in numerous studies. When used in skin care preparations, the sedative and calming properties form a holistic treatment, because they address both the physical condition and the emotional and stress-related conditions that may be a direct reason of imbalance.

Antispasmodic Properties

Essential oils have the ability to reduce spasms, a therapeutic property helpful in relieving menstrual cramps, muscle spasms, and digestive cramping. Many antispasmodic essential oils also have sedative properties, relieving the stress that may be the cause of the spasms.

Expectorant and Mucolytic Properties

A common remedy for congestion due to the common cold is eucalyptus oil. The expectorant properties contained in this, as well as other oils like tea tree and ravensare, help to expel mucous from the lungs. The mucolytic properties of *Eucalyptus dives* and *Inula graveolens* assist in the breakdown of hardened mucous.

Cell Regenerative and Wound Healing Properties

The cell regenerative, or cytophylactic, properties of essential oils is highly praised and valued in skin care. Essential oils have been used to heal wounds and burns, reduce scarring and stretch marks, and repair damage due to aging and dermatitis. Oils such as rose, lavender, helichrysum, and cistus can be used in everyday treatment of the skin, resulting in vital and youthful-looking skin.

ESSENTIAL OIL CHEMISTRY

The properties attributed to essential oils are directly related to their chemical compositions. Essential oils can be constructed of up to several hundred compounds. The more complex the chemical structure of an oil, the more diverse and interesting that oil may be. As is common in essential oil study, the opposite is also true. Even the simplest of essential oils will surprise, delight, and astound with its therapeutic outcome.

Though the chemistry of the essential oils is recognized as defining the action, in reality, the activity of an essential oil is beyond clear-cut identification of its chemistry. The overall **synergy,** or how the parts act as a cooperative whole, along with the interaction within the complexities of the human body, will determine the final outcome in any aromatherapy treatment. The chemistry allows you to anticipate an oil's healing potential.

The chemical compounds in essential oils are grouped into families. Each family of chemical structures has common and known properties. If you know which group forms the majority, or most influential aspect, of an essential oil, you can identify its main properties through the association with that family and know what precautions to take in its use. Table 13–1 lists the chemical families.

Table 13–1 Essential Oil Chemical Families

CHEMICAL FAMILY	ESSENTIAL OILS WITH INFLUENTIAL AMOUNTS	PROPERTIES	CAUTIONS	EXAMPLES OF INDIVIDUAL COMPONENTS WITHIN THE FAMILY
Monoterpene Hydrocarbons These compounds are the most abundant in essential oils.	Needle tree oils, such as cypress, pine, and spruce Citrus oils such as grapefruit, lemon, and orange Frankincense	Diuretic, antiviral, stimulant, tonic	Potential skin irritant due to peroxidation of poorly produced and stored oil. Kidney irritant at continued high daily doses.	Alpha-pinene limonene
Sesquiterpene Hydrocarbons	German chamomile *Helichrysum italicum*	Anti-allergic, anti-inflammatory, cooling		Chamazulene beta-caryophyllene
Monoterpene Alcohols The most beneficial and safest of the aromatic molecules	Lavender MQV (*Melaleuca quinquenervia viridiflora*) Palmarosa Peppermint Rosemary Tea tree Ylang ylang	Antiseptic, immune stimulant, bactericide, and energizing (except linalool, a sedative monoterpene alcohol in lavender and other oils)		Linalool borneol menthol terpinen-4-ol

Table 13–1 *continued*

Sesquiterpene Alcohols	Sandalwood Cedarwood Ginger Patchouli	Properties vary according to the individual sesquiterpene alcohol. Overall, they are similar to the monoterpene alcohols.		Cedrol santalol (-)alpha-bisabolol
Aldehydes	Lemon verbena Melissa Lemongrass Citronella *Eucalyptus citriodora*	Antiseptic, anti-inflammatory, antiviral, hypotensor, sedative	Use caution on skin. May cause mild irritation, especially when used undiluted.	Citral citronellal
Esters	Lavender Bergamot Cape chamomile Clary sage Geranium Roman chamomile	Anti-anxiety, anti-inflammatory, antifungal, antispasmodic, balances central nervous system, calms		Geranyl acetate linalyl acetate methyl ester
Ketones	*Eucalyptus dives* Helichrysum Mugwort Rosemary verbenone Thuja	Promotes tissue and cell formation, mucolytic	Neurotoxic, abortive. Avoid most ketone containing oils during pregnancy and with people prone to seizures, especially mugwort, thuja, and pennyroyal. Euc dives, helichrysum and rosemary verbenone are safe as used in skin care.	Itallidone thujone verbenone
Lactones	*Inula graveolens*	Strong mucolytic	Use with caution	Alpha-lactone
Oxide	Eucalyptus oils (especially globulus and radiata) Tea tree Ravensare MQV	Antiviral, expectorant		1,8 cineole rose oxide
Phenols	Oregano Thyme thymol Savory	Antifungal, antiparasitic, strong antibacterial, heart tonic, immune stimulant	Skin irritant	Carvacrol thymol
Phenylpropanes	Cinnamon Clove	Similar to phenols, analgesic (clove)	Skin irritant Liver toxin at high dosages	Cinnamic aldehyde euganol
Ether (Phenylpropane Derivatives)	Anise seed Basil Fennel Nutmeg Tarragon	Antispasmodic, balancing, digestive (fennel, anise), mental stimulant (basil)	Toxic to the nervous system at very high dosages.	Anethol methyl chavicol myristicin

CONTRAINDICATIONS

Responsible Use of Oils

There is a great deal of confusion surrounding the potential hazards of essential oil use. A large amount of information stating the cautions of allergic reaction, irritation, and toxicity are unfounded or based on faulty research. Common sense is the best guide when dealing with aromatic oils. If essential oils are used irresponsibly, as with anything, there can be minor injuries and irritation. Avoid risk by using essential oils as recommended in this chapter and in other aromatherapy and essential oil literature. When the essential oils are used sensibly there is little risk of damage to the human body.

Despite the overall safety of using essential oils, there are cautions. Some clients may have negative or allergic reactions to an oil. Remember, for example, the effect scent has on memory and emotion. The reactions cannot be foreseen, even in a consultation, because they are specific to the individual. Placing a small amount of diluted oil behind the client's ear or on the skin of the inner elbow offers you one way of avoiding, though not completely, allergic responses.

Table 13–1 outlines the cautions concerning the chemical components. This is a useful guide to avoid any dangers. Most of the common essential oils you will use do not carry contraindications unless they are misused. The most cautious use by the aromatherapist is to use essential oils diluted in low concentrations in a vegetable oil or cream base.

Quality of Essential Oils

One of the main problems in using essential oils is low-quality fragrance oils or essential oils that contain synthetics and other compounds. Many oils said to be pure and/or organic essential oils are not and may cause irritation or allergic reaction. Essential oils may also react on the skin when they are poorly combined in cosmetic formulations.

When selecting essential oils, it is important to choose oils with the composition required for therapeutic purpose. Due to commercialization and the demand for cheaper product by the flavor and fragrance industry, finding quality essential oils can be challenging. This is an area of aromatherapy expertise that takes quite a while to master.

A good indication of the quality of an essential oil is price. For example, it is unrealistic to expect a quality French lavender to sell for $10 an ounce. Lavender would likely cost $25 to $50 an ounce.

Just to be safe, though, it is best to assume that many oils in skin care and mass-marketed aromatherapy products are adulterated or completely synthetic, because essential oils, especially expensive or hard-to-produce oils, are often adulterated. **Adulteration** is the process of adding natural or synthetic compounds, or cheaper but similar oils, to "stretch" an amount of oil. Lavender, for instance, is often adulterated. The main constituents in lavender are linalool and linalyl acetate. These compounds are generally used to extend lavender. Lavandin, a real but less-complex essential oil similar to lavender, is also a common lavender adulterant.

Although adulterated oils may contain natural compounds, they do not behave in the same way as essential oils that have not been adulterated. In many cases it is the adulteration that causes sensitivity and allergic reactions that people experience from essential oil use. A client may state he or she does not like the smell of lavender or some other oil. It could well be that the client has never smelled a real, unadulterated lavender essential oil.

Genuine and Authentic Oils

Many suppliers claim to have the best essential oils. Unfortunately, it can be difficult to recognize inferior quality oils, even for an expert. Experience will be your best guide, but even that is not always enough. There is a defined grade of essential oils for aromatherapy purposes called **genuine and authentic**. Many essential oil sellers do not use this definition. When buying oils, you may still use this to qualify your oils by asking if the seller's oils fit the definition of "genuine and authentic."

Several years ago French insurance companies instituted a policy of reimbursing patients for treatments using essential oils. The oils carried by the pharmacies could only be the regulated genuine and authentic oils, which are pure, natural, and complete (Table 13–2), not redistilled; and they are processed under conditions assuring maximum authenticity, meaning that the plant from which they are extracted is defined by its botanical name and the end product is known to contain only the oil from this plant. Genuine and authentic oils are produced using water or water/steam distillation; they are not dry-steam distilled.

Table 13–2 Pure-Natural-Complete

PURE-NATURAL-COMPLETE
Pure indicates there are no other essential oils or vegetable oils in the product.
Natural means there are no synthetic ingredients added to the essential oil.
Complete indicates the oil has not been decolorized or deterpenized.
Some essential oils are redistilled, or **rectified,** in a process that removes color and unwanted compounds from the oil. Tea tree and eucalyptus are commonly rectified. A pure, natural, and complete oil may or may not be redistilled. When the oil is also defined as genuine and authentic, it cannot be redistilled.

THIRTEEN ESSENTIAL OILS

There are hundreds of essential oils from which to choose. The best starting point is to select a handful of essential oils that offer complete and diverse healing potential. This would include oils from a variety of common botanical families, a collection that represents all of the chemical families, and a variety of fragrance choices. Following is a list of oils that fulfills the important criteria for a complete essential oil kit. All of the listed oils can be used in general skin care.

Cedarwood (*Cedrus atlantica*) (Figure 13–16)
BOTANICAL FAMILY: Coniferae
MAIN COMPONENTS: Cedrol (a sesquiterpene alcohol), atlantone-7 (a mild ketone)
HEALING PROPERTIES: Grounding, relaxing, antiseptic, fungicidal, tonic (glandular, respiratory)

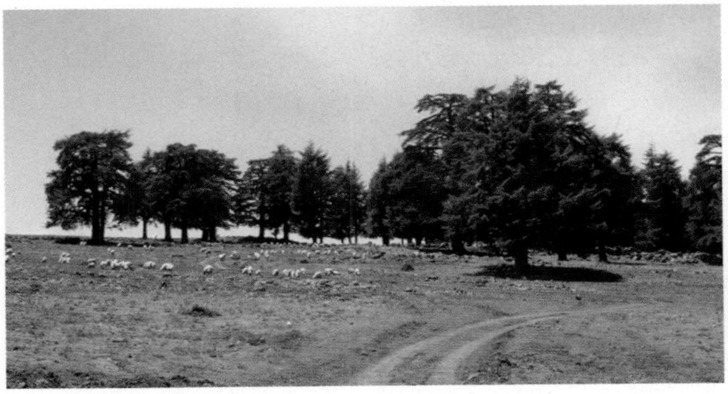

Figure 13–16 Cedarwood.

Cape Chamomile (*Eriocephalus punctulatus*) (Figure 13–17)
BOTANICAL FAMILY: Compositeae
MAIN COMPONENTS: Esters, sesquiterpene (chamazulene)
HEALING PROPERTIES: Anti-inflammatory, antispasmodic, skin balancing, soothing

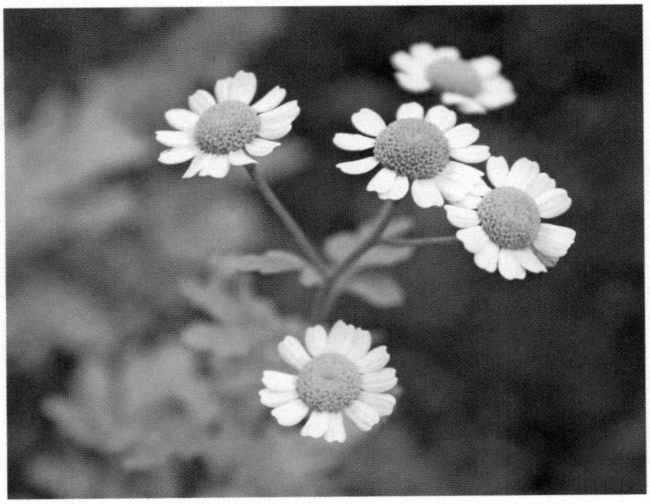

Figure 13–17 Chamomile.

Eucalyptus (*Eucalyptus radiata*) (Figure 13–18)
BOTANICAL FAMILY: Myrtaceae
MAIN COMPONENTS: Monoterpene alcohols, cineole (oxide), aldehydes
HEALING PROPERTIES: Expectorant, antiviral, antiseptic

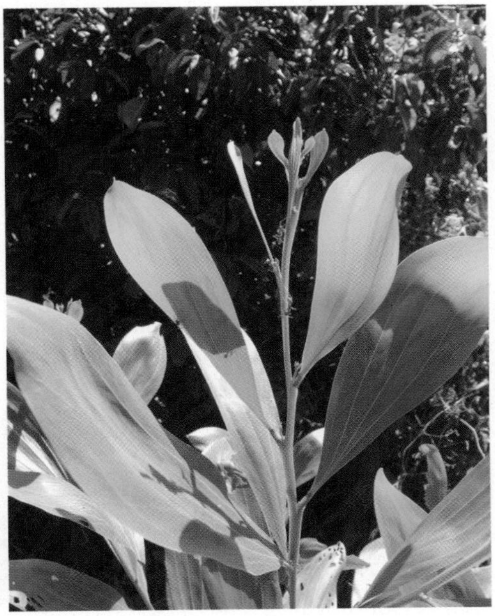

Figure 13–18 Eucalyptus.

Geranium (*Pelargonium asperum*) (Figure 13–19)
BOTANICAL FAMILY: Geraniaceae

MAIN COMPONENTS: Monoterpene alcohols, esters

HEALING PROPERTIES: Adaptogen (adapts to needs of the body), antiseptic, cell regenerative, fungicidal, tonic, and immune strengthening

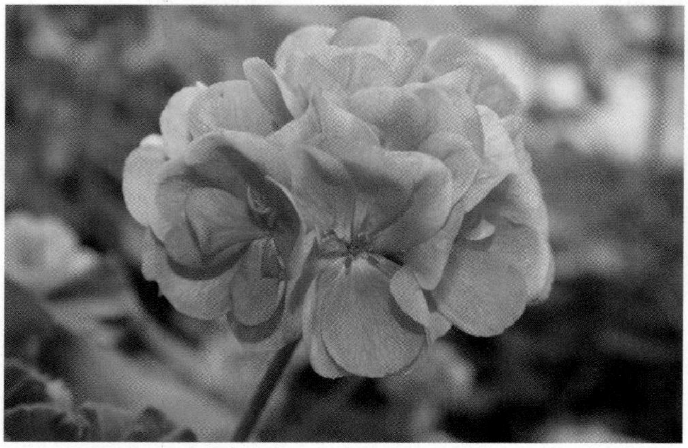

Figure 13–19 Geranium.

Grapefruit (*Citrus paradisi*) (Figure 13–20)

BOTANICAL FAMILY: Rutaceae

MAIN COMPONENTS: Monoterpene hydrocarbons (limonene)

HEALING PROPERTIES: Diuretic, drainer, detoxifier, lymphatic stimulant

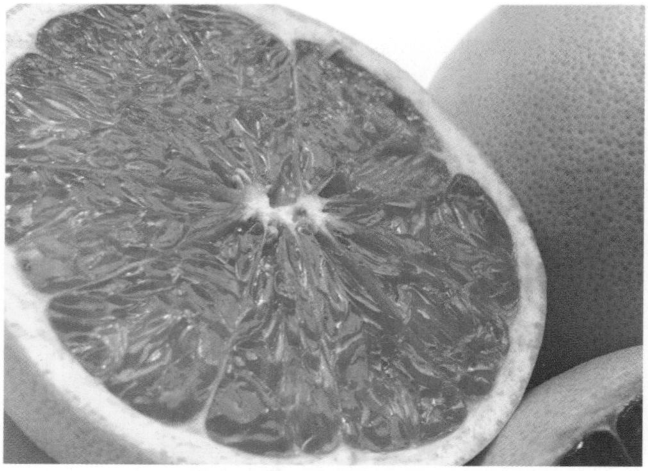

Figure 13–20 Grapefruit.

Helichrysum (*Helichrysum italicum*); Common name: Everlasting (Figure 13–21)

BOTANICAL FAMILY: Compositeae

MAIN COMPONENTS: Diketones, esters, sesquiterpenes

HEALING PROPERTIES: Anti-inflammatory, wound healing, cell regeneration

CONTRAINDICATIONS: Safe overall, but use some caution due to ketone content.

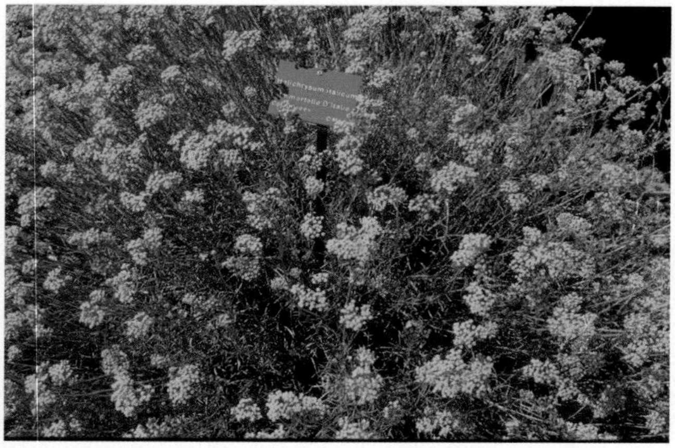

Figure 13–21 Helichrysum.

Lavender (*Lavandula angustifolia*) (Figure 13–22)

BOTANICAL FAMILY: Labiatae

MAIN COMPONENTS: Linalool (a terpene alcohol), linalyl acetate (an ester); a quality French oil contains the antispasmodic trace compound coumarin

HEALING PROPERTIES: Balancing to the CNS, antispasmodic, wound healing, sedative

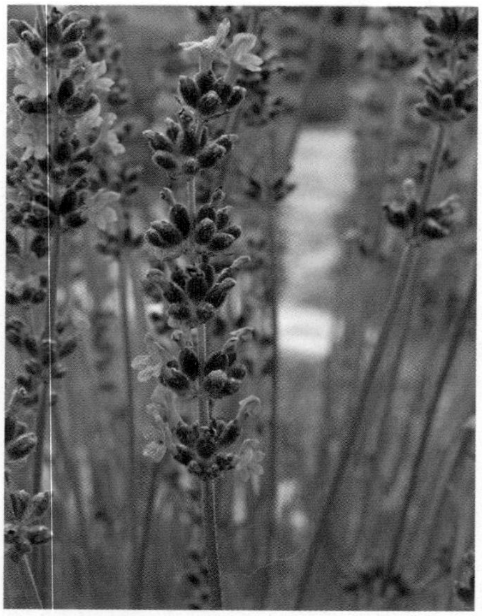

Figure 13–22 Lavender.

Neroli (*Citrus aurantium*) from orange tree blossoms (Figure 13–23)

BOTANICAL FAMILY: Rutaceae

MAIN COMPONENTS: Monoterpene alcohols, esters, aldehydes

HEALING PROPERTIES: Anti-inflammatory, antiseptic, calming, stress, tension and anxiety relief, soothing to skin

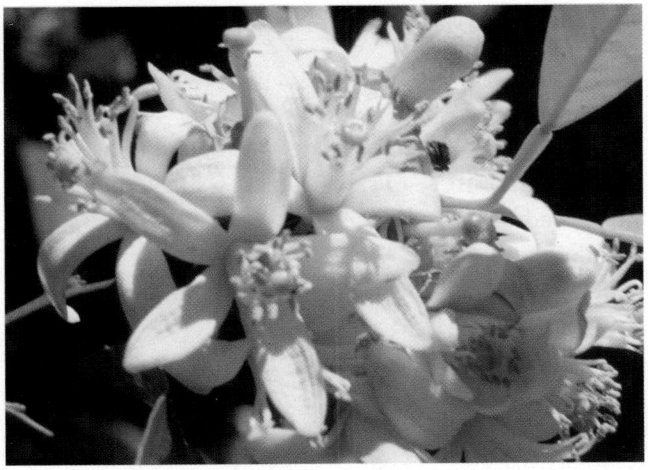

Figure 13–23 Neroli.

Niaouli (MQV) (*Melaleuca quinquenervia viridiflora*) (Figure 13–24)

Oil from Madagascar is referred to as MQV and is the preferred oil.

BOTANICAL FAMILY: Myrtaceae

MAIN COMPONENTS: Monoterpene hydrocarbons, terpene alcohols, sesquiterpene alcohols, oxide

HEALING PROPERTIES: Expectorant, strengthening, overall health and healing

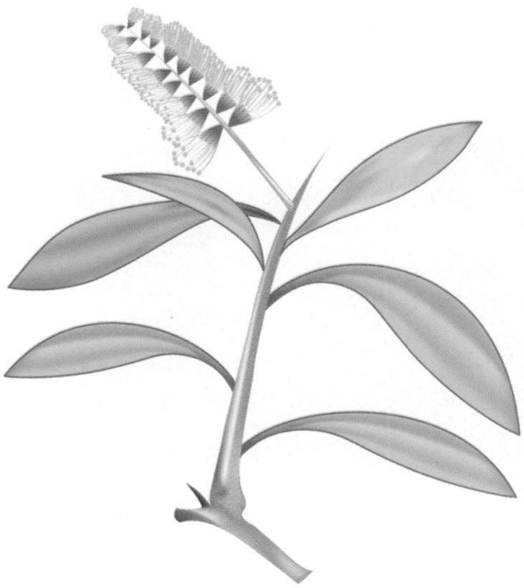

Figure 13–24 Niaouli.

Palmarosa (*Cymbopogon martini*) (Figure 13–25)

BOTANICAL FAMILY: Graminae

MAIN COMPONENTS: Monoterpene alcohols (geraniol)

HEALING PROPERTIES: Antiseptic (especially for infectious skin conditions), cell regenerative, viral and bacterial illness of throat and lungs

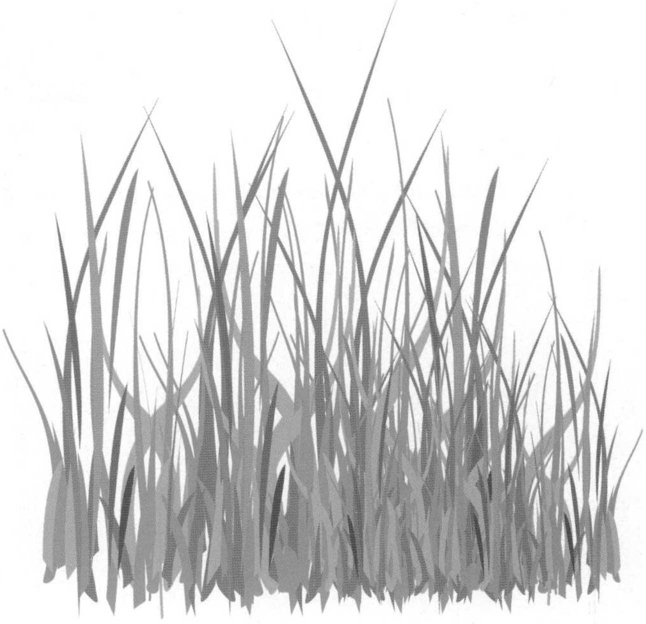

Figure 13–25 Palmarosa.

Rosemary verbenone type (*Rosmarinus officinalis* chemotype verbenone) (Figure 13–26)

BOTANICAL FAMILY: Labiatae

MAIN COMPONENTS: Ketones (verbenone), cineole, monoterpene alcohol

HEALING PROPERTIES: Mucolytic, cell regenerating, promotes digestion

CONTRAINDICATIONS: Contains ketones; young children and pregnant women should use with caution though normal dilutions of 1% or less are generally recognized as safe.

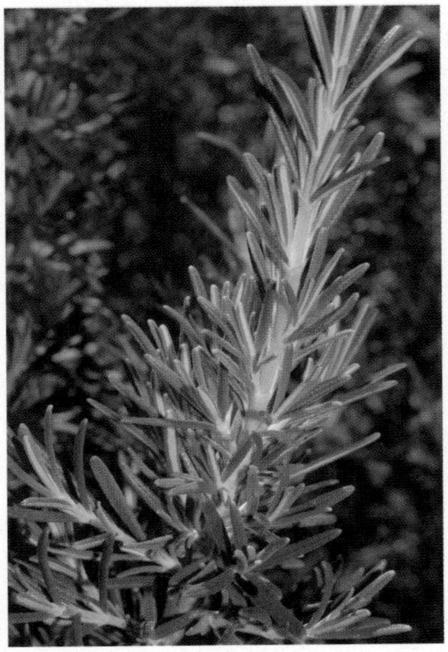

Figure 13–26 Rosemary.

Australian Sandalwood (*Santalum spicatum*) (Figure 13–27)

BOTANICAL FAMILY: Santalaceae

MAIN COMPONENTS: alpha and beta santalol, farnesol, alpha-bisabolol

HEALING PROPERTIES: Anti-inflammatory, antibacterial, antifungal, sedative, analgesic

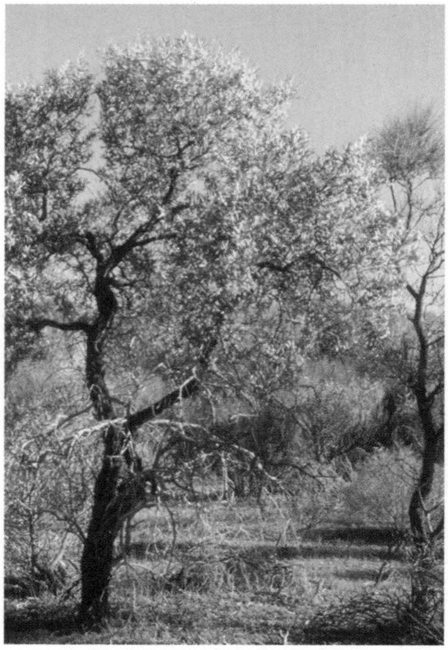

Figure 13–27 Sandalwood.

Ylang Ylang (*Cananga odorata*) (Figure 13–28)

BOTANICAL FAMILY: Anonaceae

MAIN COMPONENTS: Sesquiterpenes, esters

HEALING PROPERTIES: Euphoric, relaxing, heart palpitations

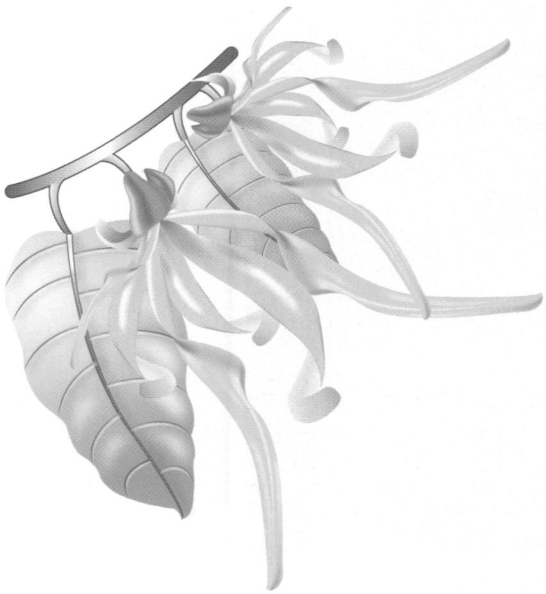

Figure 13–28 Ylang ylang.

APPLICATION OF ESSENTIAL OILS

The diversity of aromatherapy applications is one of its special qualities. The treatment may be complete with just one essential oil or by using a formulation incorporating a blend of three or more oils. The single oil or blend may be administered in a variety of methods, including:

- Massage
- Skin, hair, and body cosmetic formulations
- Inhalation
- Perfumes
- Baths
- Showers
- Body wraps
- Poultices
- Direct, undiluted application to the skin
- Suppositories (medical application)
- Capsules (internal medical application)

Each of these application methods includes a number of formulation techniques and choices. The flexibility of application methods allows for precision and range in aromatherapy treatment (Figure 13–29). Methods may be selected according to written aromatherapy protocol or according to the judgment and mood of the practitioner. There are no rules for using essential oils. Allow experience to be your guide.

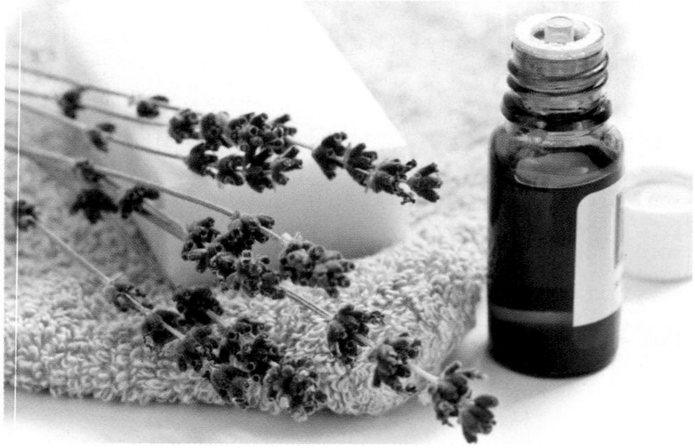

Figure 13–29 Bottle of essential oil.

Essential Oil Blends

Blending essential oils can be a simple process or, with proficiency, may become an artistic and scientific undertaking. Incorporating knowledge of essential oil chemistry and clinical research studies assist in precision therapeutic formulations. The art of aromatherapy blending relies on intuitiveness, spontaneity, and inspiration. The end fragrance is an important aspect in blending the oils and a skill that you will develop over time.

Essential Oil Synergy

A synergy occurs when two or more essential oils are combined, producing a sum, or result, greater than the individual parts. The unique character of each essential oil is a consequence of the combined synergistic activity of its chemical structure. In aromatherapy, *synergy* describes the resulting activity of a blend of oils.

Carrier Oils

Carrier oils are the fixed oils, such as olive, coconut, and rosehip seed, used for diluting essential oils. Carrier oils have healing benefits derived from their fatty acid compounds and their vitamin and nutrient content. Table 13–3 shows carrier oil suggestions based on the nourishing benefits to the skin. For best results an aromatherapy practitioner will use carrier oils that are unrefined, organic, and expeller pressed.

Dilution Amounts and Measurements

What is a safe and effective dosage amount in an aromatherapy application? Like other features of aromatherapy, seasoned aromatherapists hold differing opinions. It is agreed that essential oils deliver therapeutic efficacy at low dosages, though what this means, along with the term *high dosage,* is never thoroughly identified. Table 13–4 shows guidelines for dosage amounts, in terms of percentages of essential oils used topically, depending on the therapeutic intent and conditions of treatment.

Calculation for a Basic Essential Oil Blend

Essential oils are measured in drops. The percentage used in most massage and skin care blends is 2.5%. This means that your formula consists of 2.5% essential oils and 97.5% of carrier oil or base ingredients. There is a simple formula that is used to calculate how many drops are used to create a 2.5% blend of essential oils. Start with the size, in milliliters, of the container you are using to make your blend (1 ounce is approximately 30 milliliters). Divide this number by 2. This is the total number of essential oil drops that will be used to create a 2.5% dilution in a 30-milliliter bottle or jar.

Use this formula to calculate other percentage dosages (Table 13–5). Do your calculation for a 2.5% blend, double your answer, and you will have a 5% dilution amount; double this number and the formula gives you the number of drops for a 10% dilution of essential oils. For a lower percentage of essential oil in a blend, divide the original 2.5% dilution in half and you have the lower aromatherapy dilution of 1.25%.

Table 13–3 Carrier Oils; Skin Properties; Composition and Use

FIXED OIL	SKIN BENEFITS	COMPOSITION	PERCENTAGE USED IN AROMATHERAPY
Coconut oil (*Cocos nucifera*)	Antioxidant, conditioning, emollient	Saturated, monounsaturated, and polyunsaturated fatty acids, vitamin E	Can be used 100%; best when combined with other oils like sunflower and jojoba
Jojoba oil (*Simmondsia chinensis*)	Conditioning, emollient, UV protection	Polyunsaturated liquid wax (waxy esters)	Best for perfume blending 100% because it does not oxidize (go rancid); blends well with other oils
Kukui nut oil (*Aleurites moluccana*)	Antioxidant, conditioning, emollient, healing	Omega-3, -6, and -9 fatty acids, vitamins A and E	Use 15%–25% in a blend of oils.
Olive oil (*Olea europaea*)	Excellent all-around skin care, emollient, healing and nourishing	Complex fatty acid composition, vitamins, volatile compounds	Use 100% or in a blend.
Raspberry seed oil (*Rubus idaeus*)	Anti-inflammatory, antioxidant, nourishing, protective	High amounts of Omega-3 and -6, vitamin E	Use 5%–15% in a blend of oils.
Rosehip seed oil (*Rosa rubiginosa*)	Cell regenerative, wound and scar reduction	Omega-3 and -6, polyphenols, vitamin C	Use 5%–20% in a blend of oils.
Sunflower seed oil (*Helianthus annuus*)	Conditioning, emollient, and protective	High oleic fatty acids, vitamin E	Can be used 100% or blended

Table 13–4 Topical Use Blending Percentages

TOPICAL USE BLENDING PERCENTAGES	
Essential oils are combined as a percentage of the total formula when added to a cream, oil, or perfume blend. The percentages shown below tell you how much essential oil is in an entire product, or the **dilution amount** of that essential oil.	
0.5%–1% Blend	This is best for children, those with weak immunity or weak constitution, and people who are overly sensitive. For use in "subtle" or energetic aromatherapy.
1.5%–2.5%	This is the most basic dilution amount. The most common massage and skin dilutions are between 2%–2.5% of essential oils.
2.5%–5%	This amount is used to increase physical therapeutic activity or fragrance balance and may be used when treatment focus is on larger parts of the body, such as legs and buttocks, and for conditions like cellulite reduction.
5%–10%	This concentration of essential oils is used for specific areas, such as the abdomen, lower back, or larger muscle area, when a deeper concentration and detoxification of oils is desired.
10%–50%	Higher percentages of essential oils are used for physical conditions that require "medicinal-like" therapeutic activity, such as arthritis and joint pain, lower back pain, and parasitic infections. Skin care seldom, if ever, requires this higher concentration. Practice caution when blending any phenols (thyme thymol type, oregano), cinnamon, clove, wintergreen, and some aldehydes (lemongrass, eucalyptus citriodora) at this percentage.
APPROXIMATE CONVERSION OF ESSENTIAL OIL DROP TO WEIGHT AND VOLUME	
Approximately 20 drops equals 1 gram.	
Approximately 20 drops equals 1 milliliter.	

Table 13–5 Formula to Create a 2.5% Blend of Essential Oils

FORMULA TO CREATE A 2.5% BLEND OF ESSENTIAL OILS
Calculation for 2.5% blend: no. of milliliters ÷ 2 = total no. of drops of essential oil
To create a 2.5% blend using this formula, follow these steps:
1. Select the essential oils you will be using; you would commonly use 3 to 10 essential oils in each blend.
2. Calculate the total amount of drops using the dilution formula, such as 30 ml ÷ 2 = 15 drops. This is the total number of drops of essential oil you would use in a 30-ml container for a 2.5% dilution of essential oils.
3. Drop the essential oils into the 30-ml container, one at a time.
A formula using four essential oils in a 30-ml container might look like this:
5 drops cape chamomile
3 drops cedarwood
4 drops lavender
3 drops palmarosa
15 drops total/2.5% dilution
The remaining 97.5% of this blend would consist of carrier oils, or this blend of oils may be added to an unscented base formula such as a cream or shampoo base.

RECIPES FOR SKIN AND SPA

Formulating your own skin care preparations is much more involved than just tossing a few ingredients in a bowl and turning on the blender. There are many formulation protocols that require separate training and education (Figure 13–30; Table 13–6). A cream is a formula that combines water and oil, two ingredients that do not bond. An **emulsifier** is used to bond water and oil ingredients. When you see the oil floating at the top of a cream jar, it means that the oil ingredients have separated from the water. This happens when the cream is not well formulated or it has been exposed to extreme temperatures. Two emulsifiers used in cosmetics are vegetable emulsifying wax, a synthetic to semi-natural emulsifier, and lecithin, a derivative of soy. There are some petroleum based synthetic emulsifiers that most organic cosmetic manufacturers and aromatherapists do not recommend in combination with essential oils.

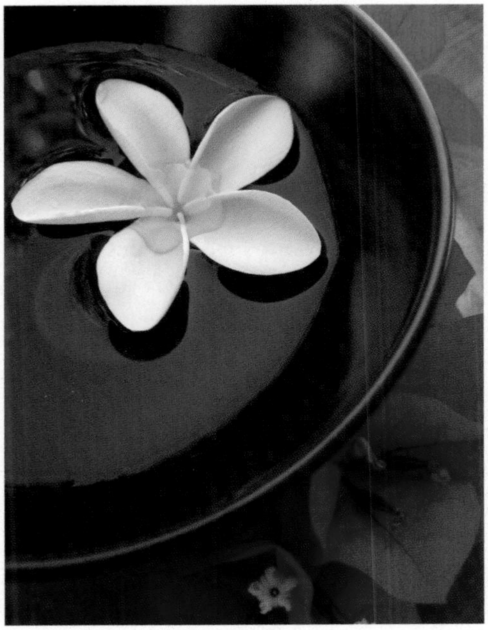

Figure 13–30 Aromatherapy treatment bowl.

THE AROMATHERAPY AND BOTANICAL PRACTICE

This chapter offers enough information for you to begin using essential oils. If you are hesitant to begin without further instruction, use pre-prepared essential oil products. Most beginning aromatherapists purchase a set of oils and use them at home. This will acquaint you with the oils and give you personal experience.

Table 13–6 Essential Oil and Fixed Oil Recipes

ESSENTIAL OIL AND FIXED OIL RECIPES
Blending fixed oils with essential oils does not require emulsifiers or special equipment. Here are some recipe ideas for specified skin conditions. Each blend will be formulated as a 2.5% blend of essential oils in a 1-ounce (30-ml) container. The fixed oils and other ingredients will be calculated in milliliter (ml) amounts with the percentage of the formula written in parentheses. The essential oil formula may be added to an unscented botanical cream or lotion base.
Mature Skin Conditioner
3 drops cedarwood
4 drops geranium
2 drops helichrysum
4 drops rosemary verbenone
2 drops rose
In a base of:
21.2 ml (70.5%) olive oil
3 ml (10%) cranberry seed oil
.06 ml (2%) sea buckthorn CO_2
4.5 ml (15%) rosehip seed oil
Acne Skin Treatment
This formula is applied in a small amount (about the size of a pea) on moistened skin, spread thoroughly over the affected areas.
4 drops cape chamomile
3 drops cedarwood
4 drops grapefruit
2 drops lavender
2 drops tea tree oil
In a base of:
24 ml (80%) unrefined grapeseed oil
4.5 ml (15%) raspberry seed oil
.75% (2.5%) rosemary verbenone type CO_2
Scar Treatment
7 drops helichrysum
8 drops rosemary verbenone type
24.75 ml (82.5%) olive oil
4.5 ml (15%) rosehip seed oil
For Cellulite/Detoxifying
This essential oil blend may also be added to 1 ounce unscented wrap or body mask formula instead of the carrier base formula (Figure 13–31). It is calculated as a 5% essential oil blend in a 30-milliliter container.
5 drops cedarwood

Table 13–6 *continued*

4 drops cypress
8 drops eucalyptus globulus
8 drops grapefruit
5 drops MQV
In a base of:
13.5 ml (45%) olive oil
13.5 ml (45%) jojoba oil
1.5 ml (5%) kelp alcohol extract

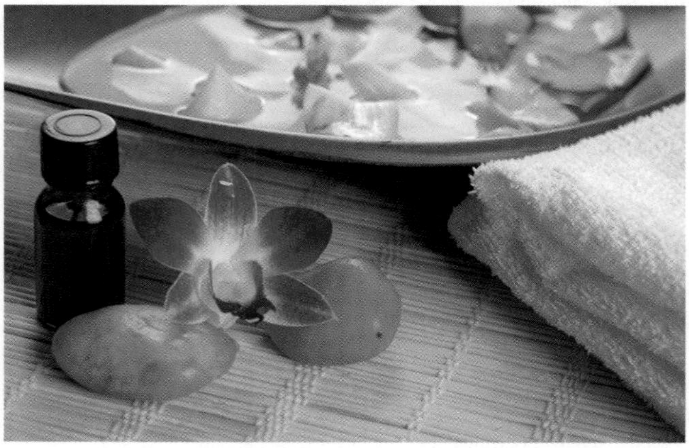

Figure 13-31 Aromatherapy essentials.

There are many books on aromatherapy offering an abundance of recipes, and these can be beneficial learning tools. You will find that some oils in the recipes will be oils you do not have. You can replace these with oils you do have by matching as closely as possible the main chemical components, therapeutic activities, and fragrances. Keep in mind that it takes knowledge, training, and practice to gain skill working with and mixing essential oils.

When incorporating aromatherapy into professional esthetic and spa treatments, you will often come across the issue of pricing the new service. Pricing depends on overhead cost, cost of materials, and your time. When adding essential oils to an existing unscented base formula or treatment, you may find that a per-drop charge is sufficient, charging more for expensive oils like rose, neroli, helichrysum, and jasmine. If you provide a special holistic aromatherapy consultation, you will want to be compensated at your hourly wage.

HOLISTIC CONSULTATION

The skin is affected by the internal functions of the body as well as external influence. You can increase the overall health of a client by utilizing a **holistic health** model, the practice of addressing all of the influences—including physical, emotional, spiritual (or philosophical) and environmental—that may affect health. Essential oils have naturally holistic properties. Cape chamomile will soothe irritated skin and, holistically, calm the nerves and tension that directly cause the skin irritation. As you learn more about essential oils and develop a holistic practice, you will find that many skin conditions that are difficult to treat in a one-dimensional, symptom-focused practice are alleviated through a proper holistic consultation and aromatherapy application. A holistic consultation, one that reviews all of the possible causes affecting the skin—emotional balance, lifestyle issues, and physical conditions—will guide appropriate, safe, and highly effective aromatherapy treatments. In holistic consultation, it is never necessary to prescribe, diagnose, or in any way step out of the confines of your professional practice and licensing.

LEGAL CONSIDERATIONS

In the United States there are no specific rules, laws, or regulations regarding the use of essential oils and botanicals. You are governed by your state licensing laws, health laws, and business liability. The best rule to follow is this: Do not make medical diagnoses or prescribe treatments outside of your professional practice and licensing. In addition, make no claims regarding efficacy or physiological changes for any material; those are regulated by the FDA.

As already expressed, essential oils and botanicals allow for holistic healing within your esthetic practice. The essential oils do what they do without any claims as to their efficacy. Your only concern, as with any products used, is to apply them in an educated and responsible fashion. As an esthetician, all you need to focus on is the soothing aromas, calming sensations, and clarity and youthfulness of the skin after an aromatherapy treatment. Any positive health results will happen without mention.

REVIEW QUESTIONS

1. In what ways do botanical ingredients benefit the skin?
2. What is the difference between a tincture and an infusion?
3. What are expeller pressed oils?
4. Name five botanical extracts with anti-inflammatory properties.
5. What is aromatherapy and who is responsible for its name?
6. What are essential oils, and how are they separated from plant material?
7. List five essential oil properties, and with each one, match at least one of the chemical families that contain the property.
8. What are the contraindications of using essential oils with a high ketone content?
9. Which compounds are most irritating when used topically on the skin and which oils contain these compounds?
10. What percentage of essential oil is used in massage and skin care preparation and what is the formula for calculating how many drops are used in a 30-milliliter container?
11. What are the legal considerations for use of essential oils and botanicals in an esthetic practice?

CHAPTER GLOSSARY

absolutes: an extraction method using a solvent (hexane) to extract the essence from the plant material.

adulteration: the process of adding natural or synthetic compounds, or cheaper but similar oils, to "stretch" or alter the fragrance of an essential oil.

allantoin: an anti-inflammatory compound isolated from the herb comfrey; used in creams, hand lotion, hair lotion, after shave, and other skin-soothing cosmetics for its ability to heal wounds and skin ulcers and to stimulate the growth of healty tissue.

alpha d-tocopherol: an antioxidant nutrient and popular form of vitamin E used in skin care and health supplements, generally isolated from soy or wheat.

aqueous extract: an herbal water infusion.

autonomic motor systems (autonomic nervous system): the system that controls involuntary functions of the circulatory, respiratory, endocrine, and digestive systems and controls the actions of involuntary muscles, such as the heart.

dilution amount: the amount, usually defined as a percentage, that essential oils are diluted in a formula when added to a cream, oil or perfume blend.

distillation: 1. process that removes mineral and trace elements from the watu 2. process used to extract essential oils from a plant using hot water, hot water and steam, or steam alone.

dl-tocopherol: synthetic form of vitamin E.

emulsifier: a substance used in creams, lotions and other skin and hair care products that allows oil and water to mix without separating.

endocrine system: the bodily system of specialized glands that affects the growth, development,

CHAPTER GLOSSARY

sexual activities, and health of the entire body.

expeller pressed: a mechanical process used to "press" the oil from seeds, nuts, or plant material.

fixed oil: a nonvolatile fatty oil derived from vegetables and fruits.

genuine and authentic: a definition and standard developed several years ago by French insurance companies to label the essential oils suitable for patient reimbursement.

herbal infusion: the result of using hot water, and sometimes cold, to release the compounds from plant material. For example, tea is an herbal infusion.

holistic health: the philosophy or practice that sees the body as a whole. The practice takes into consideration the effects of the emotions, lifestyle, and the environment on health.

homeostasis: the process of feedback and regulation that keeps the body in a state of equilibrium within its environment.

hydrosol: the water portion, or by-product, of essential oil distillation; used for aromatherapy purposes.

hypothalamus: regulator of important metabolic functions, hormone release, and autonomic function.

isolates: compounds that are isolated from a plant extract and have an active therapeutic property.

limbic system: an important series of brain structures activated by odor, behavior, and arousal.

nonvolatile: does not evaporate easily.

olfaction: the sense of smell.

phytotherapy: the use of plant extracts for therapeutic benefits.

rectified: the result of redistilling essential oils to remove color and unwanted compounds from the oil.

refined: name given to a plant extract, usually referring to a fixed oil, that has gone through the refinement process of removing colors, odors, or other naturally occurring compounds, such as a refined grapeseed oil.

supercritical carbon dioxide (CO_2): a modern method of extraction in which the plant material is placed in a high-pressure container with CO_2 that is in a state midway between being a liquid and a gas.

synergy: two or more agents working as a cooperative whole, producing a result that is greater than the total effect of the individual parts.

tincture: herbal extract using alcohol or glycerin to extract the compounds from the plant material.

whole extract: extracts from plant material that have not been changed or altered from their extracted form.

CHAPTER OUTLINE

- CLEANSERS
- TONERS
- DAY CREAMS AND TREATMENTS
- NIGHT CREAMS AND TREATMENTS
- AMPOULES AND SERUMS
- SPECIALTY CREAMS AND TREATMENTS
- HOW PRODUCTS ARE DEVELOPED
- ADDITIONAL ACNE CARE CONSIDERATIONS
- ADDITIONAL ROSACEA PRODUCT SELECTION TIPS

CHAPTER 14

INGREDIENTS AND PRODUCTS FOR SKIN ISSUES

LEARNING OBJECTIVES

After completing this chapter, you should be able to:

- **Examine a product and determine by its ingredients the type of client for whom it is suitable.**
- **Select specialty treatment products for skin issues based on ingredients.**
- **Understand the process of developing a product.**

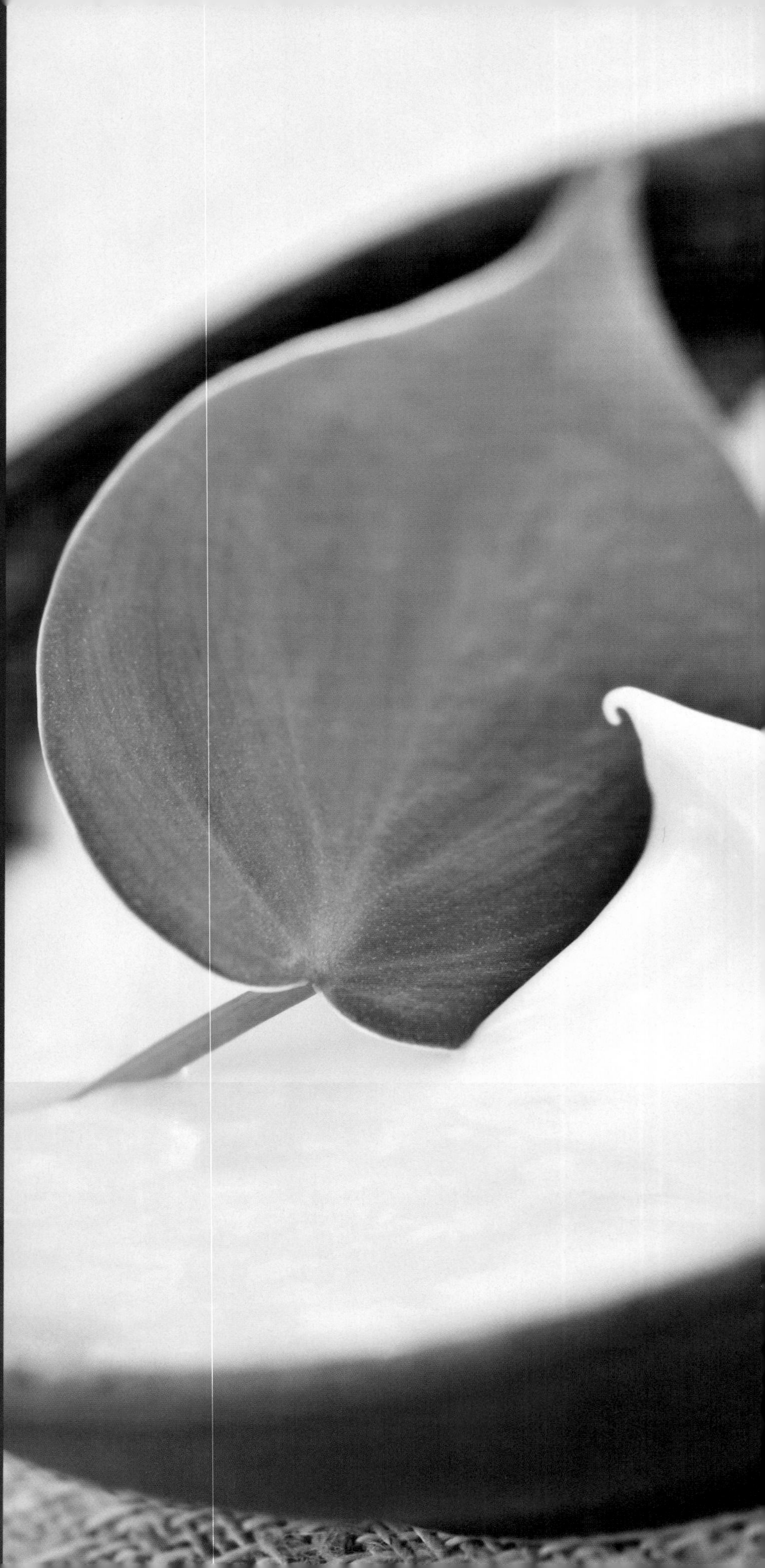

In Chapters 7 and 12 you learned about ingredients used in manufacturing cosmetics and their potential impact. Now you will learn about the practical application of various formulas of cleansers, toners, creams, and other products available for different skin types and problems and the chemical makeup of those products. It is easy to become overwhelmed by the variety of skin care products on the market. There are literally hundreds of different products available for you to use in the treatment room and recommend that your clients use at home (Figure 14–1). It is important to carry a variety of products to sell to clients for home use. There are many good esthetic product manufacturers, and the most successful skin care salons carry lines made by at least two or three of them (Figure 14–2). There is no one line that is the answer to every problem you will see. What your client is doing to his or her skin at home—twice a day, or 60 times a month!—is actually more important than your in-room treatments.

Although this chapter provides only an overview of available products, it does present the factors involved in choosing products for various skin problems and clients' needs. Keep in mind that the formulations included are only an example of what you may expect to find on the market. Examine available products to compare components. Most likely they will fall within the ingredient categories discussed here. The most important factor in prescribing the right home care for your clients is your education and knowledge of skin analysis. The more experience and expertise you gain in doing skin analysis the better. It is the biggest key to success in esthetics.

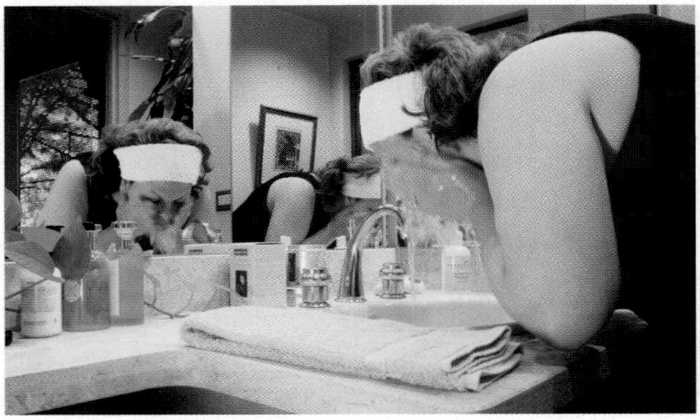

Figure 14–1 Client doing home care.

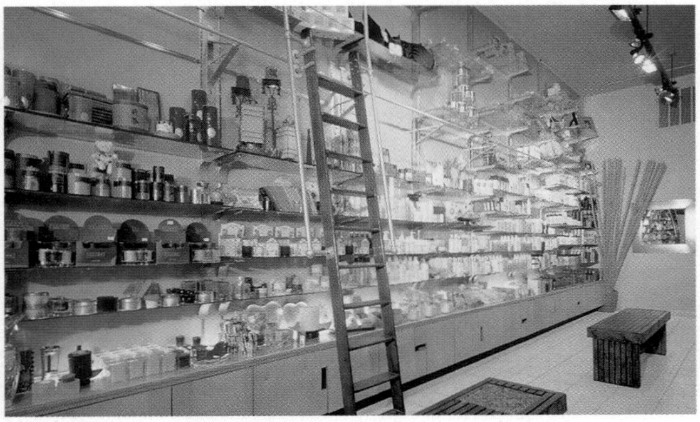

Figure 14–2 Well-organized retail area.

FOCUS ON: *At-Home Skin Care*

The success of any skin care program relies on the client using the products you recommend for at-home use.

CLEANSERS

There are various types of cleansers available on the market today, including milk-type cleansers and cleansing lotions, rinsable foaming cleansers, and specialty cleansers for acne- and clog-prone skin (Figure 14–3). In particular, rinsable cleansers vary in strength and texture. Rinsable cleansers are for clients who are used to washing their faces with bar soap. They like the foaming action, and do not feel "clean" without a sudsing action.

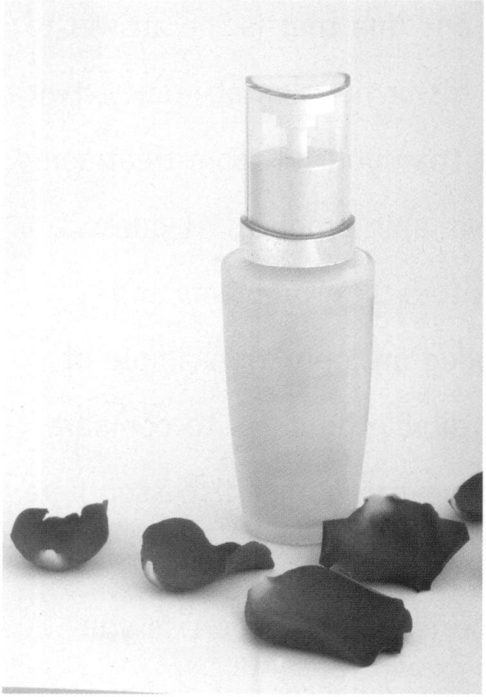

Figure 14–3 Lotion.

FOCUS ON: *Problem Solving for Clients*

Your clients come to you with issues looking for answers. Giving product recommendations is providing them with answers. If their products at home were working for them, would they be in your clinic looking for answers? It is not that their home product is good or bad, it is that the product is not doing the job.

Product Profile: Rinsable Cleanser for Oily and Combination Skin

Client and Skin Type: Clients with oily and combination skin are especially fond of rinsable cleansers because they need some solvent action to help cut excess amounts of oil. However, you should not recommend a cleanser that will overdry them or strip the acid mantle.

Product Characteristics: The product consistency feels almost like soap. When the client adds water, the product begins to foam moderately. It rinses completely, leaving the skin feeling fresh and clean but not too tight. This feeling is a good sign that the product has the correct blend of cleansing agent and emollient. It removes excess oil without damaging the barrier function causing dehydration.

Chemical Action and Design: Chemically, this product uses disodium lauryl sulfosuccinate as a detergent-surfactant (Figure 14–4A). It also contains smaller amounts of avocado oil and cetyl alcohol, emollient ingredients added to cut the detergent action on the skin's surface so that it will not strip the acid mantle. This cleanser is also fragrance-free, which is helpful for sensitive skin. This cleanser is good for adult oily and combination skin or for clients who are used to heavier moisturizers but really need to switch to a lighter program for oily or combination skin.

INGREDIENTS: Deionized Water, Disodium Lauryl Sulfosuccinate, Cetyl Alcohol, Ceteth-20, Propylene Glycol, Avocado Oil, Methylparaben, DMDM Hydantoin.

A

Figure 14–4A Ingredient label.

Product Profile: Rinsable Cleanser for Dry and Combination Skin

Client and Skin Type: This cleanser is designed for clients who have dry skin but still want the action of a foaming cleanser. You can recommend this one to a mature client with dry skin who prefers soap over a milk cleanser.

Product Characteristics: This cleanser foams very slightly and rinses well, leaving the skin feeling very soft. It is not aggressive enough for oily-combination skin, but it is excellent for more alipidic skin.

Chemical Action and Design: If you look at the ingredient label of this product, you will notice that its surfactant agent, sodium lauryl sulfate, is listed about halfway down the list of ingredients (Figure 14–4B). This means that the product is not nearly as strong a cleanser

INGREDIENTS: Deionized Water, Mineral Oil, Cetyl Alcohol,Sodium Lauryl Sulfate, Cetearyl Alcohol, Ceteth-20, Imidazolidinyl Urea, Methyl Paraben.

B

Figure 14–4B Ingredient label.

as the first cleanser listed on the label. The ingredients listed after water are different types of emollients, fatty alcohols, and esters. This cleanser is superfatted and contains lots of emollients because it is designed for dry skin. The large amounts of emollients keep the detergents from stripping too much lipid from the skin's surface.

Product Profile: Rinsable Cleanser for Very Oily Skin

Client and Skin Type: This stronger rinsable cleanser is designed for clients who have very oily skin. Their skin is covered with enlarged pores, and they almost never have any dryness or dehydration but experience extreme oiliness by early in the day.

Product Characteristics: The product has almost the consistency of shampoo. It foams quite strongly and rinses thoroughly, leaving the skin feeling very clean. It is much too strong for any skin type except extremely oily skin.

Chemical Action and Design: The active detergent in this rinsable cleanser is an anionic surfactant called ammonium laureth sulfate. This cleanser contains some glycolic acid, which, in a cleanser, is helpful in loosening surface cells. Glycolic and other alpha hydroxy acids (AHAs) can be used in cleansers but, of course, are rinsed off and do not have the same long-term conditioning effects as acids that are used in leave-on products. This cleanser is mixed with gelling agents, which give it the shampoo-like consistency. The surfactant concentration in a cleanser such as this is somewhat higher than other rinsable detergent cleansers designed for less oily skins. There are no emollients in this product, and therefore the product has no buffer against stripping oil from the skin's surface, but this is appropriate for a cleanser that is designed for very oily skin.

Product Profile: Rinsable Medicated Cleanser for Acne

Client and Skin Type: Medicated cleansers are made for mild to moderate acne, excessively oily, and chronic acne-prone skin, including teenage acne. This type of skin is not sensitive and is fairly thick because of the accumulation of corneocytes on the surface of the skin. This client may have an active acne condition or may tend to develop moderate acne frequently.

Product Characteristics: This cleanser is very similar to the one designed for chronically oily skin, except that it contains an antimicrobial agent to kill bacteria. Medicated cleansers such as this are usually registered as over-the-counter drugs. It is a strong foaming cleanser that may also exfoliate, depending on the ingredients.

Chemical Action and Design: Benzoyl peroxide serves as the antimicrobial in a product like this, or it may include another antimicrobial such as salicylic acid, sulfur. Benzoyl peroxide and salicylic acid are also keratolytic agents, which serve to lightly peel away dead corneocytes from the skin's surface as well as flush the follicular canal. Some products may also contain a mechanical exfoliant such as polyethylene granules. These small, bead-like granules are used for their grit and ability to literally "bump off" dead cell buildup.

Here's a Tip

When your client tells you about a product he or she is using at home, focus on attributes that the client likes while thinking of another product best suited to the client's skin issues.

Product Profile: Milk Cleanser for Oily and Combination Skin

Client and Skin Type: This cleanser is an emulsion to be used for makeup removal on oily and combination skin. Clients with acne rarely use a milk cleanser other than as a makeup remover, followed by a rinsable surfactant cleanser for extra cleansing action, but cleansing milk is a good choice for a mature person with oily or combination skin who has a tendency toward oiliness and minor but persistent breakout problems. This type of client may find twice-daily cleansings with detergents too dehydrating, because mature skin tends to dehydrate more easily than younger skin does. This client can use a rinsable cleanser in the morning and then a more gentle milk for nightly makeup removal.

Product Characteristics: A water-based fluid, this milk is slightly slippery to the touch and leaves the skin feeling fairly clean when removed. The product should be applied and removed with a room-temperature damp sponge cloth or cleansing sponge. Use a very soft cloth to apply and remove any cleansing milk, because it does not contain much detergent, and it does not rinse as easily as detergent cleansers. However, it will rinse well when used with a sponge or sponge cloth. This product removes makeup easily but should not be used on the eyes, because it is designed for oily and combination skin and is not chemically appropriate for the eye area.

Chemical Action and Design: The emollients used in this cleanser are tridecyl stearate, neopentylglycol dicaprate/dicaprylate, and tridecyl trimellitate, which are a complex of emollients designed to be a non-comedogenic oil replacement. They do not clog the skin and are easily removed. The emollients mix with the dirt, makeup, and oils and work to dissolve foreign materials so they may be removed from the skin's surface. This product has a pH of about 7.0, typical of a cleanser designed for oily and combination skin. The slightly higher pH makes the cleanser a more aggressive solvent. The cleansing process should be followed by a lower pH toner to lower the pH and remove any film left from the emollient.

Product Profile: Cleansing Milk for Combination Skin

Client and Skin Type: This thicker cleansing emulsion is made for clients who wear heavier makeup and therefore need a more oily cleanser to dissolve the thicker, oilier makeup. It is often prescribed for mature clients with combination skin and is considerably heavier than many other cleansing milks. Actors and other performers use it to remove heavy stage makeup.

Product Characteristics: Because of this cleanser's thickness, it must be used with a sponge or a soft cloth. Otherwise, it would leave a residue on the skin. Its emollients dissolve makeup very readily, making it an excellent product for heavy makeup wearers. This product should be followed by a toner designed for combination skin, and the toner needs to be strong enough to remove any residue left by this cleanser.

Chemical Action and Design: Petrolatum and mineral oil are the secrets of the slipperiness of this cleanser. There is enough emulsifier in this product to make it relatively thick. The petrolatum makes the product physically heavy, and the addition of the mineral oil makes it an excellent makeup dissolver. Plant extracts have been added to this product for soothing.

Product Profile: Cleansing Milk for Sensitive Skin

Client and Skin Type: This lightweight milk cleanser is designed for sensitive skin. It is designed for the client with thin, fragile skin that reddens easily. It is not specifically designed for oily skin; its emollient content is meant more for dry, irritated skin.

Product Characteristics: This is a lightweight cleansing milk designed to be used with a soft cloth or sponge. It does not leave much residue when rinsed and has very little fragrance. Many are designed to be water rinsable since these clients may be sensitive to toners or fresheners. It will remove liquid makeup well.

Chemical Action and Design: This water-based cleanser combines a relatively large amount of water with a mixture of emollients to dissolve makeup. It does not contain a traditional emulsifier. It is a physical emulsion, blended by homogenization. As discussed in earlier chapters, traditional emulsifiers can impair barrier function when used on sensitive skin, increasing reactivity. Using cleansers that are physically emulsified will not further damage an already thin barrier. This cleanser contains calming agents such as azulene, bisabolol, and chamomile extract, which are included for their soothing properties. Because of the potential for allergies, the only fragrance added might come from the plant extract used.

Product Profile: Cleansing Milk for Dry Skin

Client and Skin Type: Dry, mature skin will benefit from the use of this fairly lightweight milk for dry skin.

Product Characteristics: This is another product that should be applied and removed with a damp, soft cloth. This cleanser is slightly richer to the touch than other milk cleansers. It may leave a residue if not carefully removed and should be used with a toner designed for dry skin. Some products of this type are designed to leave a beneficial protective barrier on the skin that does not need to be removed.

Chemical Action and Design: The ultra-rich emollient oils in this cleanser are added to help condition the surface of the skin while cleansing, helping to avoid overstripping of the natural oils. This product contains no oil solvents. Some skin care companies add expensive conditioners to the cleansing product. These conditioning ingredients are normally used in creams, lotions, and fluids intended for day or night treatments. In other words, they stay on the face for long periods of time.

Many cosmetic scientists believe that it is useless to include expensive conditioning ingredients in cleansers, because they simply do not stay on the face long enough to do any good. Soothing agents and agents that are meant to strengthen or weaken the action of the cleanser are the only agents that should be added.

TONERS

Toners, clarifying lotions, fresheners, and astringents are all basically the same type of product. Products that are labeled "astringents" are considered to be over-the-counter (OTC) drugs. Toners vary in strength, drying ability, and alcohol content (Figure 14–5). They are made for three specific reasons:

1. They remove excess cleanser and residue from liquid cleansers.
2. They have a relatively low pH, helping to adjust the pH of the acid mantle after cleansing so it is not overstripped.
3. They provide a temporary tightening effect to both the skin and the individual follicle openings, helping to temporarily shrink the appearance of pore size.

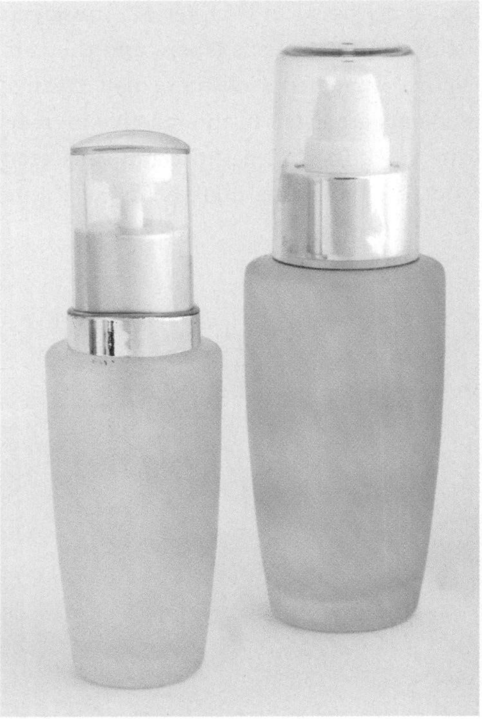

Figure 14–5 Toner.

Product Profile: Toner for Oily and Combination Skin

Client and Skin Type: This toner is designed for oily and combination skin. It is good for the client who develops clogs easily but still needs a hydrating moisturizer. Adult oily-combination skin benefits from this toner.

Product Characteristics: This toner is a clear, water-based liquid. It should be applied with a pre-dampened cotton pad, sponge, or soft cloth after using a rinsable cleanser or cleansing milk, or it can be atomized onto the skin with a fine-mist sprayer. Sprayers have become popular in nonalcoholic toners because they are so convenient. Sprayers cannot be used in toners containing alcohol because of possible accidental contact with the eyes or their potential of triggering a coughing response in some people. This toner may have a citrus fragrance such as lemon for its astringent characteristics. After use, the skin should feel clean and toned but not dry, and pores seem more refined. It is a good product for men, who can use it as an aftershave, because it is not femininely fragranced and has enough astringent action. This constricts the follicles, helping to keep the hair pointed in an outward direction so it does not become ingrown hair by growing into the side of follicle walls.

Chemical Action and Design: The pH of this toner is low due to the inclusion of lemon extract and citric acid. (The combination has an astringent action.) It is blended into a liquid with mostly water, but it also contains a glycerin derivative, which is a humectant that helps to restore water to dehydrated skin.

Product Profile: Toner for Extremely Oily Skin

Client and Skin Type: This toner is made for skin that becomes very oily after only a short period of time and has large pores that clog easily. This client's skin is never dehydrated because it is so oily.

Product Characteristics: This toner is a water-based liquid that is used after cleansing milk or rinsable cleanser. It should be applied on a pre-dampened cotton pad or damp sponge. With a strong astringent action, it leaves the skin feeling very clean and tight. Application to dry skin would be too drying.

Chemical Action and Design: This oily skin astringent contains plant extracts for oily skin as well as sulfur, a keratolytic peeling agent, and potassium alum, a strong astringent agent. They are in a base vehicle of water and propylene glycol, a hydrating agent.

Product Profile: Astringent for Acne-Prone Skin

Client and Skin Type: This very strong astringent is made for inflamed acne and extremely oily skin. It is a good product for teenage acne, grades II and III.

Product Characteristics: This astringent has a strong medicinal (alcohol) odor. Applied with a damp cotton ball after cleansing, it is very stripping, removes lots of sebum, and is very drying to the skin. It may burn or tingle slightly, especially if applied to open acne lesions. Some extremely oily skin needs this much oil removal.

Chemical Action and Design: This product is actually an OTC drug with isopropyl alcohol and water as the main ingredients. Isopropyl alcohol is often the active ingredient for its astringent properties and also for its oil-stripping action. Witch hazel distillate provides astringent properties and temporary pore "tightening." Camphor may be included as a soothing agent.

> **Activity**
>
> Compare all of the toners in your facility and determine the skin types for which they are appropriate according to their ingredients. Does this match the name of the product and the type of skin targeted by the marketing material? Why or why not?

Product Profile: Toner for Normal Skin

Client and Skin Type: This toner is a medium-strength tonic designed for normal and sensitive skin. It is for adult skin that basically needs moderate hydrating and has no particular problems.

Product Characteristics: This toner has a very mild astringent action. It is applied with cool, wet, cotton pads after cleansing. It does not pull on the skin and has a moist feeling and slight soothing effect when applied.

Chemical Action and Design: An example of a very simple formula made with water, rosewater, propylene glycol (as a humectant), cucumber extract for soothing, and allantoin, this product contains a smaller amount of witch hazel extract than toners for oily skin.

Product Profile: Toner for Extra-Dry Skin

Client and Skin Type: This toner has moisturizing properties and helps gently remove traces of cleanser from dry, sensitive skin. This dry skin can become so dehydrated that the face becomes tight even after a very gentle cleanser. Applied with a cool, damp cotton pad, this toner is designed for dry skin that becomes tender after cleansing.

Product Characteristics: This is a very moist toner, almost soft to the touch. It has practically no astringent action. It is designed to moisturize the skin with humectants that provide a buffer so that the skin will not become stripped if the toner is used after cleansing.

Chemical Action and Design: A large amount of butylene glycol provides humectant effects for the skin in this water-based, fluid, unusually moisturizing toner. Glycerin also has hydrating action on the surface of the dry skin. Extracts of chamomile, mallow, and cornflower are included for their softening and soothing properties.

DAY CREAMS AND TREATMENTS

Day creams are made for various skin types. Treatments for everything from acne to extremely dry and aging skin are available. These products vary greatly in texture and thickness, depending on the amount of fats or emollients that are added (Figure 14–6).

Many day creams now include sunscreen ingredients, offering an important health benefit to clients. It is becoming commonplace to find broad-spectrum UVA–UVB protection in day treatment products, making them OTC drugs. As discussed in Chapter 12, sunscreen ingredients are shown on drug facts labels, and they are shown as the active ingredients of these day creams, while other ingredients are listed in the inactive ingredients section of the label. (It is illegal to claim sunscreen protection and not list the active ingredients in a drug

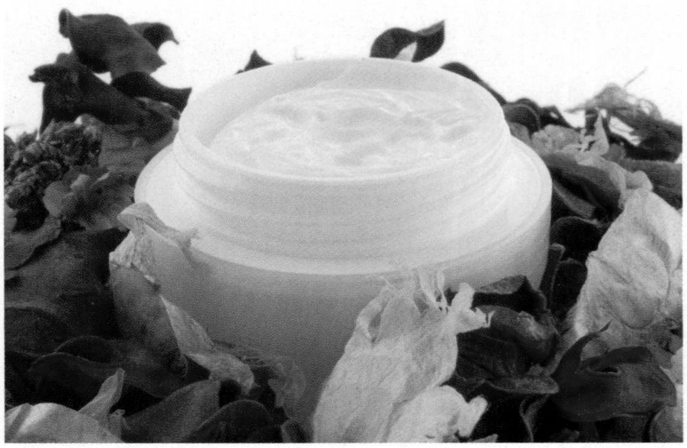

Figure 14–6 Cream.

facts label.) UVB ratings are listed using the now-familiar numbering system, such as SPF 30. UVA ratings will soon appear on sunscreen products and will guide consumers as to the level of protection offered by a product. This will incorporate the use of a one-, two-, or three-star system indicating low, medium, or high protection.

Day creams almost always contain either an occlusive agent or a protective ingredient that helps hold moisture in the surface layers of the skin. They may also contain various hydrating ingredients, emollients, or other performance ingredients, depending on the skin type for which they are included.

Some companies market day creams that are basically moisturizers with hydrating and protective inclusive ingredients but no sunscreen ingredients. Use of these day creams necessitates an application of sunscreen over the moisturizer. Again, most companies now have sunscreen built into their day creams, which include hydrating and protective ingredients. This is much more convenient for the client, who only has to apply one product.

Product Profile: Day Sunscreen Protection Fluid for Oily and Combination Skin

Client and Skin Type: Clients who have oily skin appreciate this type of product because it does not feel oily or greasy and is non-comedogenic. It is a good choice for 20- to 50-year-old clients who develop impacted pores easily and for people who need hydrating but become oily easily. These latter clients generally have trouble with makeup not staying on and becoming oily during the day. The lack of many emollients in this cream benefits the client who prefers a light-textured day product. It also serves well as a daytime moisturizer-protectant for oily skins during winter months.

Product Characteristics: This is not a thick product and feels very light and non-greasy. It absorbs quickly, helping to hydrate the skin and protect against daytime water loss, and it contains SPF-15 sunscreen to shield against daily sun exposure. While a higher SPF may be desirable, it gives the product a heavier feeling. The heavier-feeling products are very unpopular in hot, humid climates. Applied with the fingertips in the morning before makeup or alone, this product may hydrate, protect, condition, contain two sunscreens, and be non-comedogenic, which means it does not clog pores.

Chemical Action and Design: This fluid is water-based with small amounts of non-comedogenic emollients added. These emollients include tridecyl stearate, tridecyl trimellitate, neopentylglycol dicaprate/dicaprylate, and glyceryl stearate. The active humectants that help to bind water in this fluid include glycerin and sodium PCA. Other conditioning agents include allantoin, cornflower extract, tocopherol, and retinyl palmitate. Octinoxate (formerly called *methoxycinnimate*) and titanium dioxide are selected as sunscreen ingredients, and dimethicone is used as a water-loss shielding agent because of its lightweight characteristics.

Activity

Using the products in your facility, design a homecare regimen for yourself. Then try it for a fellow student. Last, design a regimen for a hypothetical client with specific skin conditions.

Product Profile: Day Cream for Dry and Dehydrated Skin

Client and Skin Type: Designed for oil-dry (alipidic), dehydrated, or mature skin, this cream will help the client who becomes dry very easily due to lack of oil production. It is for clients who have a slight amount of oiliness through the T-zone, but the large part of the outer perimeter of the face is dry and dehydrated.

Product Characteristics: This is definitely cream and normally contains a substantial amount of emollient. It also contains a broad-spectrum sunscreen and a protective agent. The product is not extremely greasy or heavy, so it may be worn by clients who prefer a lighter-weight day cream. Its color may come from botanical additives. It should be applied under makeup or alone.

Chemical Action and Design: This cream contains propylene glycol and aloe as hydrating agents. It contains dimethicone as a shielding protective agent, a broad-spectrum sunscreen combining UVA-UVB sunscreen active oxybenzone (formerly called *benzophenone*), and UVB actives octinoxate (formerly called *methoxycinnimate*) and octisalate (formerly called *octyl salicylate*). These active ingredients are mixed into a water-based blend of emollients, commonly including ingredients like sphingolipids, cholesterol, cetyl palmitate, and beeswax. Azulene provides soothing benefits.

Product Profile: Sunscreen Day Lotion for Sensitive Skin

Client and Skin Type: The client with sensitive, dehydrated, redness-prone skin will appreciate this product. It helps reduce the appearance of redness and provides sunscreen protection.

Product Characteristics: It can be applied under makeup or alone.

Chemical Action and Design: This lotion contains soothing performance ingredients such as aloe barbadensis gel, matricaria extract, green tea extract, and licorice extract. Its sunscreen active ingredients are octinoxate and zinc oxide, with glycerin as a hydrator. Protective emollients may include sunflower oil and caprylic/capric triglycerides. It does not contain fragrance or color agents, which is important for sensitive skin; it has been dermatologist-tested for irritancy potential; and it has been determined to be non-comedogenic.

NIGHT CREAMS AND TREATMENTS

Night treatment creams are normally intensive treatment products designed to help hydrate and condition skin during the night, a time when normal tissue repair is taking place all over the body, including the skin. Night treatments are often heavier in consistency and texture than day products. They normally contain more emollient than day creams and are not made for use under makeup. It is important that the skin be thoroughly cleansed before a night treatment is applied, and the cream should be applied all over the skin, according to manufacturer's instructions.

Product Profile: Night Treatment Fluid for Oily-Combination Dehydrated Skin

Client and Skin Type: Laboratory-tested and found to be non-comedogenic, this fluid is made to provide hydration to adult oily skin that is also dehydrated. It can be used on oily and combination skin. These clients are normally adults who need to use a hydrating agent but develop impacted pores and break out easily. It is also ideal for the client who prefers a lighter-weight night treatment.

Product Characteristics: Due to its low emollient content, this fluid is very light in texture and feel. It does not feel oily because it comprises mostly humectants, which attract water to the skin, rather than oils and fats that will clog this type of skin. This should be applied in moderate amounts to the entire skin before bedtime.

Chemical Action and Design: This fluid contains sodium PCA, a natural moisturizing factor (NMF), and glycerin as hydrating agents. It also includes allantoin, retinyl palmirate, and tocopherol in its formula for their conditioning properties. This fluid should be without comedogenic ingredients (see Chapter 10) to avoid clogging the oily and combination skin for which it is intended. The emollients added include tridecyl stearate, tridecyl trimellitate, and neopentylglycol dicaprate/dicaprylate. This fluid adds hydration to the skin without adding excess emollients that cause buildup of cells, which cause clogs to form.

Product Profile: Night Treatment for Oily, Clogged Adult Skin

Client and Skin Type: This product is for clients who have a tendency to break out but find that most drying agents overdry. Adult acne can benefit because the product can incorporate both a peeling agent and a hydrating agent as well as a protectant. It is also ideal for an adult client with oily skin who is used to using heavy moisturizers that are clogging the skin. It feels like a moisturizer but is actually a very light peeling agent.

Product Characteristics: This lightweight product can have an unusual texture somewhere between a gel and a cream. It is very light and dries quickly when applied. It can have a matte dry feeling when used. Applied in the evening after cleansing and toning, it takes the place of moisturizer and can be used under makeup or alone.

Chemical Action and Design: Salicylic acid, a beta hydroxy acid, is used in a very small quantity in this product to promote some exfoliation. This product contains glycerin and propylene glycol as humectants, and dimethicone provides protection against excess water loss.

Product Profile: Night Hydrating Cream for Combination Mature Skin

Client and Skin Type: Designed for maturing oily and combination skins that need hydration but do not need extra oils, this lightweight cream is good for more mature clients who still have a tendency to break out. It provides hydration without oiliness but can also be used as a night treatment for younger, extra-dehydrated skin types. The cream is laboratory-tested to be non-comedogenic.

Product Characteristics: The cream is extremely lightweight and is absorbed by the skin easily. It should be applied to clean skin before bedtime, and after use, the skin feels smooth and "plumped up." It contains no color or fragrance, which is helpful for sensitive and allergy-prone skin.

Chemical Action and Design: A mixture of lipids, including fatty acids, sphingolipids, phospholipids, and cholesterol, help to reinforce the barrier function of the mature combination skin. Hydrating agents include sodium hyaluronate, glycerin, and butylene glycol. Protective emollients that help prevent dehydration include caprylic/capric triglycerides and dimethicone.

Product Profile: Night Moisturizing Lotion for Dehydrated Combination Dry Skin

Client and Skin Type: This lotion is formulated to help skin that is both oil- and water-dry. This type of skin—found mostly on mature women—has a very narrow T-zone with little oil production or visible pore structure.

Product Characteristics: This treatment is a lotion packaged in a bottle. It is slightly oily to the touch, leaving a slight film on the surface of the skin. This characteristic is helpful for drier skin types. It should be applied before bedtime.

Chemical Action and Design: The lotion contains a mixture of oils, emollients, and humectants, providing both hydration and oils for the oil-dry skin. It contains the humectants urea, propylene glycol, and butylene glycol and is mixed with sesame oil, peanut oil, and various emollient esters and fats. Because it contains a large amount of hydrator and oils, it also contains sodium lauryl sulfate, used as an emulsifier to keep the oils in the water-based emulsion (Figure 14–7).

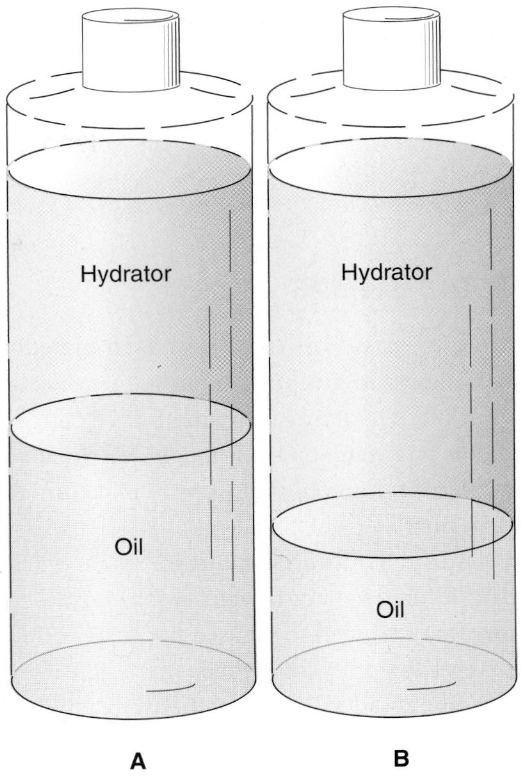

Figure 14–7 Differing levels of oil and water balance in products.

Product Profile: Night Cream for Dry, Dehydrated Skin

Client and Skin Type: Alipidic, dehydrated, mature skin is the target for this heavier cream. This type of client is very dry for most of the year and needs a richer cream.

Product Characteristics: This cream is rich in texture and leaves an emollient residue on the skin when applied on the skin and left on all night.

Chemical Action and Design: This cream is a mixture of humectants and emollients containing large amounts of the latter. The chief humectant is sorbitol, with emollients caprylic/capric triglycerides, jojoba oil, and squalane, which help to prevent moisture loss. It is non-fragranced and has been tested to be non-comedogenic, although it is intended for skin that does not tend to develop comedones.

Product Profile: Firming Night Cream for Mature Skin with Lack of Elasticity

mature.

Client and Skin Type: This is for clients with combination to dry, dehydrated, sun-damaged skin that needs more elasticity.

Product Characteristics: This cream has a fluffy, light texture and absorbs easily. It has no color or fragrance, helpful for sensitive skin. The product has been tested for irritancy potential and comedogenicity.

Chemical Action and Design: This high-tech cream is a mixture of humectants and emollients with a complex of botanical performance ingredients, such as hydrocotyl and coneflower extracts, that are helpful in firming the appearance of skin with poor elasticity. The chief humectants in this cream are sodium hyaluronate, glycerin, and butylene glycol, with protective cyclomethicone, a silicone derivative, which helps to prevent moisture loss.

Activity

Choose three specialty products for your clinic. What types of conditions do they address? What are the key ingredients you looked for?

AMPOULES AND SERUMS

Ampoules are sealed glass vials of concentrated ingredients. They are designed to give ultra-intensive treatment to the skin. They often contain larger amounts of performance ingredients in a water base, although occasionally they are in an oil base. Ampoules must be applied under a night cream or fluid.

Frequently found in European skin care lines, ampoules are available for a wide variety of skin types and problems. They are often designed to be used in a series once a month or several times a year. Others are designed to be used nightly. The disadvantages are that they are less environmentally friendly and are often very expensive. Clients who are extremely conscientious about home care will often take time to use ampoules and will not mind paying extra for them.

In the past decade, serums have replaced ampoules, at least in many American lines. Like ampoules, serums contain concentrated ingredients, often in liposomes or other advanced delivery systems, but they are easier to use. Many serums are designed to be used daily and sometimes twice a day. Serums are usually in pump or tincture bottles. Many contain antioxidants, peptides, lipids, or other intensive ingredients. Like ampoules, they are applied under a day or night cream or fluid. Be alert for oil-based serums in eyedropper-topped bottles. The oils in the serum can compromise the soft dropper top during the course of use and possibly cause product contamination.

Product Profile: Firming Serum for Mature Skin with Lack of Elasticity

Client and Skin Type: This product is an example of one for dehydrated, sun-damaged skin of any type that needs more elasticity.

Product Characteristics: This water-based serum has a liquid-gel consistency. Because it contains no fats or oils, it can be used on any skin type. It has no color or fragrances, which are helpful features for sensitive skin. The product has been tested for irritancy potential and comedogenicity.

Chemical Action and Design: This advanced serum combines palmitoyl pentapeptide-3, a peptide known for firming skin and improving the appearance of mature, sun damaged, and wrinkled skin. The base of the serum contains hyaluronic acid, boosting water levels; the peptides improve elasticity. Additionally, this serum contains four different liposomed antioxidants and a botanical complex of coneflower and hydrocotyl extracts, known for their firming effects.

Product Profile: Lipid Serum for Wrinkles and Dry Skin

Client and Skin Type: This exemplifies a product for dry, dehydrated, mature skin and wrinkled areas.

Product Characteristics: It has a slippery feel, but when applied to the skin it seems to absorb quickly, leaving a velvety feel. Applying this serum to wrinkled areas shows almost immediate smoothing effects. The serum does not contain color or fragrances, which are helpful features for sensitive skin. The product has been tested for irritancy potential and comedogenicity.

Chemical Action and Design: This serum is anhydrous, which means it contains no water. This means no preservatives are needed. The vehicle of this serum is a complex of three silicone derivatives: cyclomethicone, dimethicone, and phenyl trimethicone. A specific lipid complex has been added to mimic the natural proportions of lipids identical to the lipid complex in the normal barrier function.

SPECIALTY CREAMS AND TREATMENTS

Treatment creams are available for special problems or special areas, and these should be used in conjunction with other day and night treatments. These include performance-oriented products like alpha hydroxy acid formulations, antioxidant serums, melanin suppressant OTC formulations, and acne treatment products. The following profiles are just examples of formulations. The individual product your manufacturer may offer may be similar but different. The key is the ingredient action.

Product Profile: Alpha Hydroxy Treatment for Dry, Sun-Damaged Skin

Client and Skin Type: This product is designed for dry, dehydrated, mature skin that is wrinkled or sun-damaged.

Product Characteristics: This is an emollient, thicker cream that contains multiple AHAs. It should be applied after cleansing and toning and before sunscreen—which should be used daily with this product—or night hydration cream.

Chemical Action and Design: Alpha hydroxy acids and beta hydroxy acids (BHAs) work to exfoliate dead cells and smooth surface wrinkles and lines. Long-term use helps with barrier function and moisture retention. Emollients include hydrogenated polyisobutene, cetyl alcohol, dimethicone, and polyacrylamide, an appropriate combination for a drier skin type. Green tea extract is present in a fairly large concentration to soothe potential irritation. Even with a large emollient base, this product has tested non-comedogenic and has been dermatologist-tested for irritancy. The pH of this product is 3.5, in compliance with the Cosmetic Ingredient Review (CIR) recommendations discussed in Chapter 12.

Product Profile: Alpha Hydroxy Treatment Gel for Oily-Combination, Clogged Skin

Client and Skin Type: This product is designed for any skin with impacted pores and oily or oily-combination skin. It is appropriate for patients with acne and acne-prone skin.

Product Characteristics: A liquid gel, this alpha hydroxy and beta hydroxy blend should be used on oily-combination skin once or twice a day to help improve impacted pores and impacted areas. Sunscreen should be used daily with this product.

Chemical Action and Design: A 10% mixture of alpha hydroxy acids—glycolic, lactic, tartaric, and malic—with beta hydroxy acids—salicylic and citric—help to exfoliate the surface as well as the follicle, removing dead cell buildup and loosening pore accumulations. The gel base contains SD alcohol 40, aloe vera gel, and hydroxycellulose, which gives the product its gel-like feel. The pH of this product is 3.5 in compliance with CIR recommendations.

Product Profile: Lightening Treatment Gel for Hyperpigmented Skin

Client and Skin Type: This treatment gel is intended for clients who have splotchy hyperpigmentation, melasma, or chloasma on the face or hands.

Product Characteristics: A liquid gel in a dark bottle, this product should be applied every day for best results. Clients using this product must always wear a sunscreen, because the symptoms being treated are caused by sun exposure. This product oxidizes very quickly, easily turning brown, indicating decreased effectiveness.

Chemical Action and Design: An OTC drug, the active ingredient in this product is 2% hydroquinone, which suppresses the melanocytes' production of melanin in the basal layer of the epidermis. The gel also contains 10% glycolic acid, which helps remove stained surface cells, as well as magnesium ascorbyl phosphate, a vitamin C derivative antioxidant known for its melanin suppressive activity. Hydroquinone is a frequent allergen, so the product should be patch-tested before use on larger areas.

Product Profile: Benzoyl Peroxide Gel for Acne-Prone Skin

Client and Skin Type: This product is designed for acne prone skin, grades I and II. Both adults and teenagers can use this product.

Product Characteristics: A 5% benzoyl peroxide lotion is used at night only on active acne papules and pustules. A light application to all areas should be followed by dabbing a small amount on any raised lesions. Do not use in the eye area.

Chemical Action and Design: This is an OTC drug. A 5% concentration of benzoyl peroxide is the active ingredient, which helps flush and exfoliate debris from the follicle. The oxygen released from the benzoyl peroxide kills anaerobic *Propionibacterium acnes* bacteria. The lightweight, glycerin-based lotion is a simple emulsion that serves as a spreading agent for the benzoyl peroxide. Benzoyl peroxide acts as bleach to fabric and hair. It can be irritating if overused, and some clients are allergic to it.

Eye Creams

Eye creams are specially designed to be used twice daily on the skin around the eyes. This area of the skin is usually more oil-dry and more sensitive than other areas. Therefore, creams designed for these areas are generally higher in emollients and lower in humectants. Because the skin around the eyes is very thin, if it is "plumped up" with hydrating agents, the eyelid looks puffy. More emollient is added to these creams to help supplement the lack of oil production associated with the eye area. Some of the newest on the market look like an eye cream but are actually more of a serum formula designed to either firm the eye area or deal with under-eye circles or other specialty issues. Because this area is very sensitive, eye creams must be carefully designed not to irritate. Nevertheless, they often do cause irritation and allergic reactions.

Neck Creams

Neck creams are also made with more emollients and fewer humectants. The neck area has thinner skin that dries easily. Neck creams should be massaged into the skin twice daily. They are available in a variety of formulations, including those with peptides to firm and support this delicate tissue.

Masks

Masks are designed to treat a variety of skin problems, from oil-dryness to acne. They are formulated with less water than creams, lotions, and fluids and are considerably heavier than any of these products.

Masks for oily skin generally contain bentonite and kaolin; these clays are helpful in absorbing excess oil and drying the skin. They cause the drying of masks designed for cleansing oilier and combination skin types. These masks may contain other conditioning ingredients. For example, a mask for acne-prone skin might contain sulfur, salicylic acid, or benzoyl peroxide. For oily and combination skin it might contain camphor for soothing and antiseptic action or cornstarch for soothing action.

Dry-skin masks often do not dry tightly and contain large amounts of emollients. To give substance to the mask, the chemist may use titanium dioxide or may use a gelling agent or thickener to give the mask a thicker texture. These dry skin masks may contain a variety of plant extracts, conditioning agents, emollients, and humectants. They work by adding water and emollients to surface layers, temporarily filling in or plumpings up small lines and wrinkles. They can have a lasting effect on the skin, particularly if preceded by the use of a good humectant or other active agent. The effects may last up to several days.

Exfoliants

Mechanical exfoliants usually come in the form of scrubs. They are usually water-based products with a humectant, mixed with some sort of abrasive agent such as almond meal or polyethylene granules or hydrogenated jojoba oil beads (Figure 14–8). They are applied after cleansing and massaged over the skin. The granules literally "bump off" dead cells from the skin's surface. The humectant keeps the product from overdrying the skin. For best results, exfoliants should be used several times a week and followed with a toner and a night or day cream. New treatments are constantly being developed.

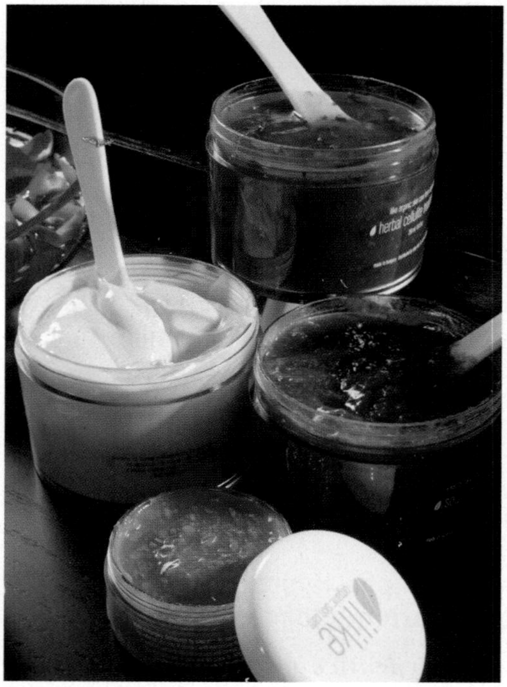

Figure 14–8 Scrub.

Chemical exfoliants are applied and absorb into the skin. In home care, they are left on and not removed. Once they are applied and have completely dried, moisturizing protection can be placed over them. Common ingredients include AHAs and vitamin A. These are generally recommended to be only used at night. Some are used on a daily basis, others less frequently depending on the individual formulation and the risk of irritation.

HOW PRODUCTS ARE DEVELOPED

Improvements in both active agents and vehicle and delivery transport systems for active ingredients constantly help to improve the quality of cosmetics and their positive effect on the appearance of the skin. There are many steps in developing new skin care and cosmetic products. Following are the steps involved in developing a new skin care product. As you will see, there is a lot involved in developing a new product. The more claims and more specific the skin condition, the more complicated the development.

Step 1: The Idea

The first step is, of course, recognizing the need for a new product. It must be determined that a product is needed and will sell. What is the appearance change that is desired? What type and condition of skin will benefit from this product?

As an example, these steps follow the development of a new cleanser for combination skin. The product must be strong enough to remove some oil from the oily areas of the skin but not so strong that it will strip areas of the facial skin that are more alipidic and prone to dehydration.

Step 2: Product Characteristics and Client Type

What characteristics should this product have? Will it be a foaming or non-foaming cleanser? Will it be a gel or lotion? How easily will it rinse? Will it have fragrance? How sensitive is the skin it is to cleanse?

What about the lifestyle of the client that will likely buy this product? The client type is best determined from day-to-day client interaction. What age is the client that is most likely to buy this product? Are those clients asking for a particular type of product? Have they asked for a particular characteristic?

Through this client-identification process, it is determined that this product will be targeted at a 30- to 40-year-old female client who is likely to have combination skin. This typical client has a family, and ease of use is important because she does not have a lot of free time. The best product for this client will be an easy-to-rinse, lightly foaming cleansing lotion.

Step 3: Choosing Ingredients and Budgeting

The next step is to choose the individual ingredients for the product. The person in charge of the product's development talks to the chemist, making sure the chemist understands the product idea, the product characteristics, and the client type.

Budgeting is an important part of product development. How much will this product cost, in terms of materials? What will packaging look like? A cheap container will not necessarily support a higher price for the product. Attractive packaging is important, but it is more important to be practical. Is the packaging type acceptable with the specific chemicals being used in the products? Sometimes packaging materials can cross-react with the chemicals in the product. The use of exotic or expensive ingredients may be prohibited to keep the cost and price of the product reasonable. How will that translate into the price for the final product?

If this product will foam, it needs a detergent foaming cleansing agent. There are many from which to choose. The example product will contain a classic detergent, ammonium lauryl sulfate. It is not the strongest detergent, and the chemist can vary the strength of the cleanser by deciding how much detergent to use in the formula. The more detergent, the more aggressive the cleanser will be. Ammonium lauryl sulfate might not be the best choice for ultrasensitive or delicate skin, but that is not the target client or skin type. With the chemist, the person in charge of the product's development decides what type of preservative, emulsifier, thickener, and fragrance to use with this product, based on the type and condition of the skin and the client's lifestyle.

Step 4: The Prototype and Use Testing

A *prototype* product is a product sample that has been developed by the chemist and is ready for actual people to test. The person in charge of the product's development gathers their opinions about the use of the product. Does the product smell nice? Does it rinse well? How does the skin feel after its use? Does it cleanse enough, or does the skin feel stripped? How did the skin feel after use of other products? Did the packaging work well during use?

Of course, it is important to obtain unbiased, honest opinions. If the majority of test participants like all of the characteristics of the product, it is an acceptable product. If most of the participants dislike a characteristic of the product, the characteristic needs to be changed and the product re-tested until all participants like it. This phase of development can take a substantial amount of time.

Step 5: Independent Testing

To make specific claims about the product, such as a claim that a product does not irritate skin, a company must have the product tests in an outside lab. This is called *claims substantiation testing*. The company must send that lab enough cleanser for testing on, say, 200 people. This testing can take a few months to perform, depending on the type of testing, the product, the claims, and other factors.

Step 6: Production

Once the budget and packaging are final and the tests have come back with acceptable results, it is time for production. This involves finalizing artwork for silkscreening on the product's bottle and making sure that all the labeling complies with FDA regulations. The next decision concerns the size of the batch to be made and how many bottles will be produced. The finished product must be tested using microbiology to make sure the product is not contaminated and that the preservative system is working properly. The company must know how long the preservative system will work for this product and what the shelf life will be. Clients and salons do not want to deal with products that have passed their "use by" date.

Step 7: Marketing

A marketing department starts working as soon as a company comes up with the initial idea for the product. They have to get the word out that the product is great and tell people why they need to use it. Marketing is involved in every step of the development, including the packaging. Without proper marketing, no one will know what the product does, and it will not sell well.

ADDITIONAL ACNE CARE CONSIDERATIONS

Keep in mind that estheticians can only treat the symptoms of acne, not cure it. What the client does at home is the biggest contributor to the success of any treatment.

Many clients with acne have very oily or oily-combination skin. Daily use of a good rinsable foaming-type cleanser with gel-based 10% alpha hydroxy acid and the elimination of comedogenic (clog-pore causing) products help to prevent comedones from forming and cut down on acne flares.

Care for Young Teens

For young teens, recommend a gentle, non-medicated, foaming cleanser, a toner for oily/combination skin, and a mild gel of alpha hydroxy or salicylic acid or 2.5% benzoyl peroxide. Used regularly, these products will help prepubescent teens through this period. Teenagers usually do not need a moisturizer except in cold weather. Regular use of non-comedogenic, daily-use, broad-spectrum sunscreen is also advised.

Young teenagers may not be disciplined when it comes to a regular facial care routine. Gently explain to them the need for consistent care. At this age, they usually will take advice from you before they will from their mothers.

Care for Adults

Teenagers are not the only age group that suffers from lack of skin hygiene. Even though acne is not caused by dirt, many adults neglect their skin. Sleeping in makeup is not only unhygienic; someone who did not remove makeup did not apply a night treatment. Explain to the client that she may come to the salon for treatment twice a month, but she is responsible for the other 60 times a month that the skin is cleansed and conditioned! Help her find simple routines that she enjoys doing. Teach her to clean her face as soon as she gets home for the evening. This is also a good time to floss her teeth, right after dinner. When she gets sleepy later in the evening, she can walk past the bathroom guilt-free!

ADDITIONAL ROSACEA PRODUCT SELECTION TIPS

A key factor in successful rosacea treatment is avoiding the triggers that cause a flare-up. There are a wide range of cosmetic ingredients, drugs, foods, salon procedures, and lifestyle events that can trigger a rosacea episode. The maddening thing about triggers, sometimes called *tripwires*, is that they are not the same for everyone, so it is difficult to create a one-size-fits-all solution when guiding a rosacea client around potential landmines that can set off a red, inflamed flare-up. "Drug and Cosmetic Ingredients That May Trigger Rosacea Episodes" lists oral, inhaled, and topical drugs and cosmetic ingredients that can trigger rosacea flares or worsen an existing episode.

It is easiest to teach a client how to decide if an event or substance causes flushing, redness, or vasodilation. Other responses that can signal a potential tripwire are stinging, itching, burning, and warming.

Here's where it gets confusing. The mere presence of a known irritant factor does not guarantee that someone will experience a reaction. There are many reasons for this. The most basic is that individuals are unique in their responses. One client may react consistently to an ingredient that has no effect in others. An individual's reactions also can vary from one exposure to the next. Climate change, stress level, food intake, and medications may cross-react to create a response once, but without the other conditions present, the client may not react at other times. Reactions can also be triggered when a higher percentage of the chemical is present, while no reaction occurs at lower percentages. Delivery vehicles that slow the penetration of otherwise irritating ingredients also can prevent a rosacea episode.

Here's a Tip

Have your client keep a journal of things that seem to trigger his or her rosacea. This may be much more accurate and productive than overwhelming the client with a list of things that may not bother him or her.

Advise rosacea clients to avoid skin care products or procedures known to set-off flares. Potential product tripwires include soap; extra-strength cleansers, usually with sodium lauryl or laureth sulfate; alcohol-based astringents; abrasive scrubs; chemical exfoliants such as AHAs, BHAs, and enzymes; dehydrating clay-based masks; cologne; perfume; aftershave; and hairsprays. Products featuring herbal ingredients extracted into ethanol or propylene glycol also have been known to trigger rosacea in some people, as have products with fragrance, essential oils, and formaldehyde-releasing preservatives; the most common are diazolidinyl urea, imidazolidinyl urea, quaternium-15, DMDM hydantoin and 2-bromo-2-nitropropane-1,3-diol.

While this seems like a lot to avoid, the reality is that most people usually find just a few factors that trigger their response lurking in the world of skin care and medications. In a survey of 1,066 rosacea patients conducted by the National Rosacea Society (NRS) in 2002, 41% of respondents identified skin care products that were tripwires and 27% identified cosmetics, while only 15% cited medication. On the high end of sure-to-trigger events, 51% identified hot baths such as a sauna or whirlpool, with 81% reporting sun exposure as the number one culprit behind their rosacea. The good news comes from another survey of 1,273 rosacea patients by the NRS in 2000. Of the 91% of rosacea patients who modified their skin care routine to help control the disorder, more than 91% reported the change helped improve their condition while 61% said simply wearing sunscreen reduced flare-ups.

One thing is certain: Since rosacea is a chronic disorder that frequently lasts a lifetime, rosacea clients will need to remain vigilant and stand by these changes permanently.

Sunscreen Ingredients

Many sunscreen ingredients are irritating to sensitive skin or cause heat and flushing when they chemically alter ultraviolet light into warming energy. For rosacea clients, these actions can develop redness that evolves into pustules and papules, giving the appearance of acne when it is actually rosacea. To keep skin under control, help your client find a product that works for them. While many rosacea clients do better with the physical sunblocks like titanium and zinc oxide, these ingredients may feel heavy and "hot" on a client in a hot, humid climate. While we would like clients to use an SPF of 30, if their skin will only tolerate a 15, then this is what they should use. Better that they use a lower level than none at all. Also recommend hats, dark glasses, and protective clothing.

Persons with rosacea should look for sunscreens that contain zinc oxide or titanium dioxide. These ingredients reflect, rather than absorb, energy from UV rays, allowing the skin to stay cooler. Zinc oxide and titanium dioxide may be mixed with a UVB-absorbing sunscreen ingredient such as octinoxate. Mixing an absorbing sunscreen ingredient with a reflecting physical sunscreen ingredient produces a lighter-weight, more user-friendly product.

Reducing Redness

Prolonged redness can come from a number of causes, but most researchers believe it is linked to inflammation that develops either before or after blood vessels expand and do not contract quickly. Antibiotics are thought to help calm this inflammation, but they need to be used judiciously and are not recommended for long periods of time. The same is true for the OTC drug hydrocortisone. Hydrocortisone can also worsen some cases of rosacea, so it is usually avoided as a treatment.

Some cosmetic ingredients are showing great promise as potent soothing agents; these are the cosmetic version of anti-inflammatories, which are drugs. Chemically standardized extracts of grapeseed, pomegranate, borage, kava kava, green tea or white tea, zinc oxide, allantoin, alpha lipoic acid, mangiferin from mango, bisabolol from matricaria, resveratrol from red grapes, glycyrrhizinates from licorice and quercetin from citrus, grapes, and tea are among the most promising cosmetic ingredients being used to calm rosacea.

Sea whip (*Pseudopterogorgia elisabethae*), a member of the gorgonian coral is a naturally occurring enzyme in the body that leads to the pain and swelling seen with rosacea. Pseudopterosin, sea whip's active compound, is currently under review as a new drug for the treatment of arthritis, burns, psoriasis, and contact dermatitis.

Since the superoxide free radical is usually at the heart of the inflammation response, antioxidants specifically

? Did You Know

The most common triggers for rosacea clients are the following:

81% sun exposure
60% stress
53% heat

targeted to the superoxides also should be of help. These include superoxide dismutase, glutathione, zinc, and copper. A new antioxidant derived from the green stone malachite appears to be the most effective superoxide-specific antioxidant found to date.

Lifestyle Modifications

The lifestyle modifications that will help control rosacea vary from client to client, just as the irritant factors vary from person to person and can vary in impact at different times for the same person. The most common tripwire is sun exposure. Avoiding known triggers is considered one of the most reliable methods to curbing rosacea episodes. Ninety-six percent of those who had identified personal irritant response agents reported that avoiding those triggers reduced their flare-ups. For further suggestions, recommend that clients with rosacea read the NRS's booklet "Coping with Rosacea."

REVIEW QUESTIONS

1. What are the differences between rinsable cleansers and emulsion cleansers?
2. What is one important ingredient for a rinsable cleansers that is used for acne?
3. Products that are titled "astringents" are considered to be what?
4. Describe a good day cream for oily or combination skin.
5. What is the biggest health benefit that can be contained in a day cream?
6. What is the difference between a day treatment and a night treatment?
7. What is the difference between a serum and an ampoule?
8. What are some things you might look for in a specialty serum/ampoule?
9. What will result if using an eye cream that contains excessive hydrating agents?
10. What are the steps in developing a new product?

CHAPTER OUTLINE

- CLIENTS AND THEIR MEDICATIONS
- THE FDA AND DRUGS
- PRESCRIPTION DRUGS
- OVER-THE-COUNTER (OTC) DRUGS
- DRUG CATEGORIES

CHAPTER 15

PHARMACOLOGY FOR ESTHETICIANS

LEARNING OBJECTIVES

After completing this chapter, you should be able to:

- **Recognize medications used by clients.**
- **Discuss the FDA and drug approval process.**
- **Name drug categories.**
- **Understand different conditions and the drugs used to treat them.**
- **Discuss common skin side effects of these medications.**
- **Understand the effects of these medications on the skin.**

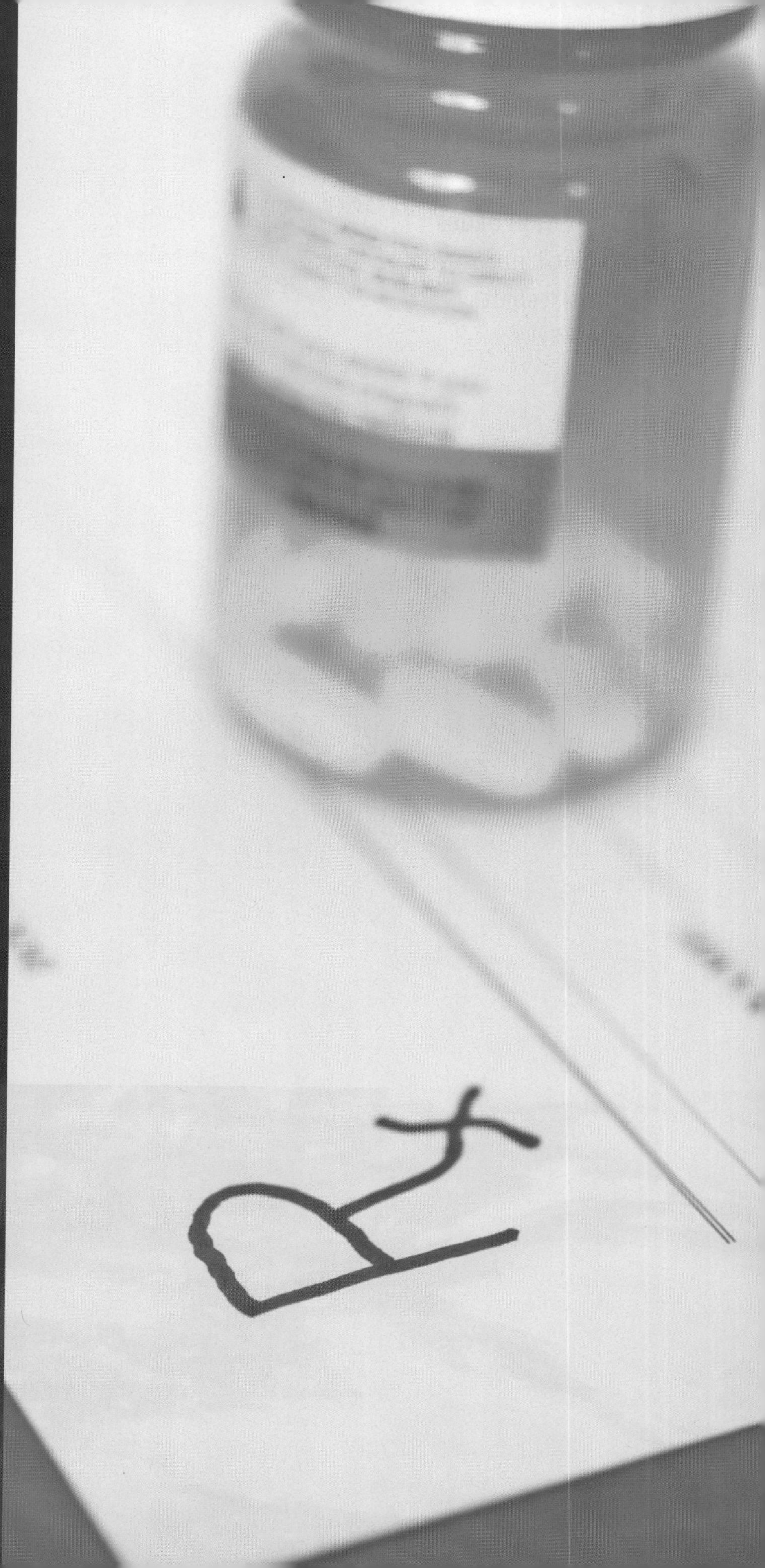

KEY TERMS

Page numbers indicate where in the chapter the term is used.

5-HT3 antagonists 334
acute coronary syndrome (ACS) 331
anaphylaxis 333
angina 332
antacid 335
antianginals 332
antianxiety drugs 328
antiasthmatics 333
anticholinergics 334
anticonvulsants 336
antidepressants 328
antiemetics 334
antigen 333
antihistamines 333
antipsychotic 337
antiretrovirals 339
antispasmodics 334
antithrombotics 331
antiulcer drugs 334
arrhythmia 332
barbiturates 336
benzodiazepines 336
bronchodilators 333
central serous retinopathy 341
Cushing syndrome 341
depression 335
dowager hump 340
epilepsy 336
erythema multiforme 332
generalized anxiety disorder (GAD) 336
glucose 337
hallucinations 337
hantavirus 339
histamine 333
hyperpigmentation 326
hypertension 331
hypertrichosis 335
hypopigmentation 326
immunocompromised 340
immunologic response 333
insulin 337
lymphocytes 337
lysosomes 337
metabolic alkalosis 341
monoamine oxidase inhibitors (MAOIs) 336
myocardial ischemia 331
norepinephrine 336
obsessive-compulsive disorder (OCD) 336
opportunistic mycoses 340
osteoarthritis 340
over-the-counter (OTC) 327
parenteral 332
pathogenic fungi 340
pathogens 337
peptic ulcer 333
phlebitis 331
phobias 336
photosensitivity 332
physical dependence 336
post-traumatic stress disorder (PTSD) 336
proton pump inhibitors (PPIs) 334
psychological dependence 336
psychoses 337
select serotonin reuptake inhibitors (SSRIs) 336
serotonin 336
subcutaneous mycoses 340
sublingual 332
superficial mycoses 340
systemic mycoses 340
toxic epidermal necrolysis (TEN) 340
tricyclics (TCAs) 336
unicellular 338

Your job as an esthetician does not include medication management or disease management; that is a physician's territory. However, sometimes what you see on the surface of the skin is a result of the drugs a client is taking. You need to know and understand how those drugs work in order to understand the effects on the skin. Will a treatment make any side effects worse for that client? Will his or her healing be impaired? Will the products you recommend for home care inflame the skin or leave it open to infection? The use of certain drugs may be contraindicated for a specific treatment or may trigger **hyperpigmentation** (too much pigment in the skin) or **hypopigmentation** (absence of pigment in the skin). These are questions to ask yourself when you see drugs listed on a client intake sheet. This chapter is a quick reference on common medical conditions, the drugs used to treat them, and potential impacts. The chapter includes a description of each category of drugs, followed by discussion of common drugs in that category, side effects, and skin side effects.

CLIENTS AND THEIR MEDICATIONS

When you first meet a client, it is important to get a complete picture of that client's past and current health, including detailed information about the client's allergies, current and past illnesses, pregnancy status, daily medications, and past surgeries, along with information on lifestyle, such as whether he or she smokes or not. This means that your initial questionnaire must ask these questions, along with queries about why the client is seeking a particular service. Encourage the client to be as accurate and complete as possible when filling out the form.

Once the client provides a complete list of the medications—both prescription and over-the-counter—that he or she is taking, take a moment and cross-reference the medication skin effects with the skin complaints for which the client is coming to see you. If you suspect that his or her complaints are a result of the medications, discuss that with the client. Suggest that the client consult his or her physician to discuss the possibility of finding a medication that does not affect the skin so adversely. Meanwhile, be aware of any treatment contraindications of the client's medications and things to watch for on the client's skin. While the tables included in this chapter list common drugs, you should also have a current drug reference guide on hand. This is especially important because of the constant influx of new drugs and new brand names.

Regardless of whether it is the first time or one hundredth time you are seeing a client, make sure you inquire and document about any medications they might be taking, including OTC medications, vitamins or homeopathic remedies, and dosage changes in prescription medications. Take a moment to investigate any skin consequences which might be associated with these items. This can be done in a Nurse's or Physician's Drug Reference or online from a reputable source. This ought to be done with consistency.

THE FDA AND DRUGS

As part of the U.S. Department of Health and Human Services, the Food and Drug Administration (FDA) is tasked with making sure that drugs that reach the marketplace are safe for consumption. This is done by holding trials of drugs in development, regulating labeling, and monitoring drugs that are already on the market. The FDA requires this process for both prescription and nonprescription medications but does not regulate cosmetics or herbal products.

The FDA as we now know it came into being in 1938, following the death of dozens of people who ingested an elixir that was heavily fortified with a poisonous agent. Public outcry led to the passage of the Federal Food, Drug, and Cosmetic Act. This law resulted in the formation of the FDA, which created a new drug application (NDA) and required that clinical studies be performed on potential drugs before they can be introduced into the marketplace. New drugs must undergo a four-phase clinical trial process prior to release, involving thousands of people and often taking years to complete.

Those who oppose the FDA argue that they prevent lifesaving medications from becoming available and often act in favor of political motives versus scientific ones, driving up overall health-care costs. Those who support the FDA argue that its policies and procedures save many more lives than the drugs it does not approve might.

The procedures for gaining FDA approval are complex but can be summed up by saying that provided that a new drug is safe for consumption, and it works as well as or better than similar products on the market, it will be approved by the FDA, which issues a patent to the manufacturer of each approved drug. Those products approved before June 8, 1995, had a 17-year patent, while those approved after that date received a 20-year patent. During this period, only the originating manufacturer can produce the drug. This gives that manufacturer authority to establish prices, and drive the demand. Following the expiration of the patent, other pharmaceutical companies can start making generic versions of the same product.

PRESCRIPTION DRUGS

Once approved by the FDA, these drugs are available for physicians to prescribe to their patients. A prescription drug requires a physician's "order," or prescription, which includes the name, strength, and quantity of the medication and appropriate directions for use (Figure 15–1), as well as physcian supervision while the patient takes the drug. If the medication is safe to use without a physician's supervision, it is classified as a non-prescription or **over-the-counter (OTC)** product and can be purchased at the local drug store or supermarket.

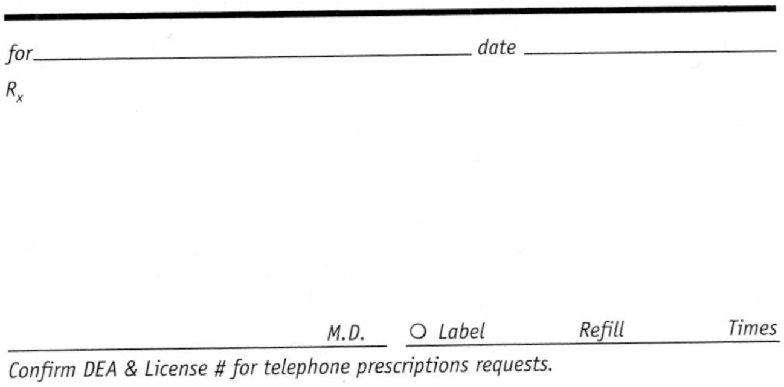
for ______ date ______
R_x
M.D. ○ Label Refill Times
Confirm DEA & License # for telephone prescriptions requests.

Figure 15–1 Blank prescription form.

Definition of a Prescription

A prescription is a physician's order for and recommended administration of a particular drug. Originally, ancient prescriptions comprised a detailed list of ingredients, which, when combined, formed a complex preparation. These recipes were often written in codes to protect the secrets of their purposes. Today, a universal language and process is used to write prescriptions. The process has a common format: patient information, the symbol Rx (which comes from a Latin word meaning "recipe"); the Signatura, which is the Latin name for the body of the prescription, or instructions to patient; and finally, the signature of the prescribing physician. In the modern United States, prescription-writing privileges for controlled substances are regulated by the Drug Enforcement Agency (DEA). This process is granted only to specific individuals in the medical, veterinary, and dental professions. Those who are given this privilege are physicians, dentists, physician's assistants, and nurse practitioners. In some states optometrists have limited authority to write prescriptions for eyeglasses. In all states prescriptions include the DEA number (for controlled substances) and, in some states, a prescriber's license number. Forgery of prescriptions is illegal and taken very seriously.

Common Prescription Drugs

You should be aware of the common prescription drug categories, such as oral medications for diabetes, heart disease, depression, and bacterial and viral infections, that might be on a client's chart (Table 15–1).

Table 15–1 Common Oral Prescription Drugs

CATEGORY OF DRUG	COMMON DRUG NAMES	COMMON REASONS FOR PRESCRIPTION
Antidepressants	Prozac, Zoloft	Depression
Antivirals	Zovirax, Valtrex	Prevent or treat herpes simplex (cold sores)
Antibiotics	Tetracycline	Acne or infections
Antifungals	Lamisil	Fungal infections
Diuretics	Hydrochlorothiazide	Hypertension
Hormones	Estrogen	Menopause symptoms
Hypoglycemic agents	Actos, Glucophage	Diabetes
Birth control medications	Many varieties	Prevent pregnancy

Table 15–2 Common Topical Prescription Drugs

CATEGORY OF DRUG	COMMON DRUG NAMES	COMMON REASONS FOR PRESCRIPTION
Anti-aging drugs	Renova	Lines and wrinkles
Antibiotics	Cleocin T	Acne
Antivirals	Denavir, Zovax	Cold sores
Anti-inflammatory drugs	Aclovate	Irritation from peel or treatment

Other prescription products are administered topically and clients use them for anti-aging, antibiotic, antiviral, and anti-inflammatory purposes (Table 15–2).

OVER-THE-COUNTER (OTC) DRUGS

Over-the-counter (OTC) medications are those that treat common conditions but do not require a prescription from a physician. These products are still regulated by the FDA but are proven safe enough for public consumption without the oversight required by a prescription. The safety of over-the counter products rests in the labeling. As part of its ongoing mission to protect the health of Americans with regard to drugs, the FDA requires that the labels of all OTC medications list required information in a particular order so that it is easy to see what is in the product and directions for its use. Common OTC drugs that you might find on an intake form of a potential client include anti-aging products, pain medications, and anti-diarrhea medications (Table 15–3).

DRUG CATEGORIES

Drug categories define groups of drugs. Each category is basically an umbrella for a group of drugs that target a particular condition or disease and provide the same or similar effect. According to the FDA, there are more than 35 drug categories. Among those categories examined here are analgesics, **antianxiety drugs**, antiarrhythmics, antibiotics, anticonvulsants, **antidepressants**, antifungals, antihistamines, antihypertensives, anti-inflammatories, antipsychotics, brochodilators, coritosteroids, diuretics, hormones, hypoglycemics, and muscle relaxants (Table 15–4). Multiple drugs have been developed in each category because different drugs work best for different people, and because some people may be allergic to a drug in a category but tolerate another drug in the same category.

> **REGULATORY AGENCY ALERT**
>
> It is important to remember that you have no authority to recommend medications or dosages to clients. Always refer a client to his or her physician if they have questions about medications.

Drugs Used to Treat Hormonal Imbalances and Birth Control

The endocrine system is a network of glands that secrete or excrete chemical substances or messengers, called *hormones,* into the blood (Table 15–5). These glands are sometimes part of a larger organ, such as the adrenal gland, which is situated on top of the kidney. The endocrine glands include the pituitary gland, parathyroid glands, adrenal glands, pineal gland, thymus glands, and the pancreas. Also included are the gonads, more commonly called the ovaries and testes. The hypothalamus is a major contributor to the endocrine system, even though it is typically recognized as a part of the nervous system.

The endocrine system secretes two types of naturally occurring hormones: amino-acid based or steroid. Prostaglandins, hormone-like substances, are a separate, often synthetic, category. Hormones regulate growth and development, sexual development, the body's ability to fight stress, the balance of nutrients,

Table 15–3 Common Over-the-Counter Drugs

CATEGORY OF DRUG	COMMON USE	COMMON PRODUCTS
Anti-aging medications	Accelerate epidermal turnover	Glycolic acid
Pain medications	Reduce minor pain	Ibuprophen
Anti-diarrhea medications	Treat minor diarrhea	Imodium AD

Table 15–4 Drug Categories

DRUG CATEGORY	EXPECTED RESULT	DRUG EXAMPLE
Analgesics (narcotic and non-narcotic)	Drugs to relieve pain	Narcotic: morphine Non-narcotic: aspirin
Antacids	Relieve indigestion	TUMS
Antianxiety drugs	Relieve anxiety	Xanax
Antiarrhythmics	Control heartbeat	Tikosyn, Ethmozine
Antibiotics	Treat infections	Ceclor
Anticoagulants	Prevent blood clotting	Coumadin
Anticonvulsants	Prevent seizures	Tegretol, Dilantin
Antidepressants	Mood-lifting	Wellbutrin
Antidiarrheals	Relief of diarrhea	Lomotil
Antiemetics	Treat nausea and vomiting	Zofran
Antifungals	Treat fungal infections	Lamasil
Antihistamines	Block histamine response	Benadryl
Antihypertensive	Lower blood pressure	Zestril
Anti-inflammatory drugs	Reduce inflammation	Motrin, Naprosyn
Antipsychotics	Treat psychotic disorders	Thorazine
Antipyretics	Reduce fever	Acetaminophen
Beta blockers	Reduce the oxygen needs of heart by reducing heart rate	Lopressor
Bronchodilators	Open the bronchial tubes	Proventil
Corticosteroids	Anti-inflammatories for arthritis or asthma	Medrol
Cough suppressants	Reduces cough	HOLD Lozenges
Cytotoxics	Kill cancer cells	Tamoxifen
Decongestants	Reduce membrane swelling	Sudafed
Diuretics	Increase urine	Lasix
Expectorants	Promote coughing	Mucinex
Hormones	Hormone replacement	Estrogen, progesterone
Hypoglycemics	Reduce blood glucose	Glucophage
Immunosuppressives	Treat autoimmune diseases	Azathioprine
Laxatives	Increase bowel movements	Metamucil
Muscle relaxants	Relieve muscle spasms	Flexeril
Sleep drugs	Sedatives	Ambien
Thrombolytics	Dissolve clots	Heparin
Vitamins	Promote good health	Vitamins C, A

water, and electrolytes, cellular metabolism, and energy. A malfunction in one part of the endocrine system often causes another part to malfunction. Assuming that the body does not malfunction, the endocrine system will function properly into old age. However, when the body malfunctions, it needs a synthetic version of the hormone to keep functioning normally. Hormones are used to treat a variety of conditions, but in the esthetic arena, clients will most often be using hormones for birth control or for hormone replacement therapy (HRT) during menopause.

Drugs used to prevent pregnancy are called *contraceptive hormones*, or more commonly, birth control pills (BCP). Birth control medications comprise the hormones estrogen

Table 15–5 Hormones

DRUG CATEGORY	EXAMPLE	COMMON SKIN EFFECTS
Hormones	Calcitonin, Danazol, Desmopressin, Epoetin, estrogens, Estropipate, Fludrocortisone, Glucagon, insulins, Leuprolide, Levothyroxine, Liothyronine, Liotrix, Megestrol, Nafarelin, Nandrolone decanoate, progestins, Teriparatide, vasopressin	rashes, acne, hirsutism, oily skin, itching, flushing, hyperpigmentation, hives
Birth control medications	estradiol acetate, estradiol cypionate, estradiol cypionate, estradiol valerate, estradiol topical emulsion, estradiol transdermal system, estradiol vaginal tablet, estradiol vaginal ring, ethinyl estradiol/desogestrel, ethinyl estradiol/drospirenone, ethinyl estradiol/ethynodiol, ethinyl estradiol/etonogestrel, ethinyl estradiol/levonorgestrel, ethinyl estradiol/norelgestromin, ethinyl estradiol/norethindrone, ethinyl estradiol/norgestimate, ethinyl estradiol/norgestrel, levonorgestrel, levonorgestrel/ethinyl estrodiol, medroxyprogesterone, mestranol/norethindrone, norethindrone, norethindrone/ethinyl acetate, norgestimate/ethinyl estradiol, Norgestrel	acne, hirsutism, oily skin, rashes, itching, flushing, hyperpigmentation, hives

and progesterone. Some birth control medications block ovulation, while others hinder sperm transport, and others manipulate the fallopian tubes or the endometrium. Birth control is delivered in a variety of ways, including by pills, intravenously, topical patches, and slow release systems (such as rings and skin implants). Ideally, the medication controls the menstrual cycle with minimal side effects. The most effective medication varies from one individual to the next. Patients work with their physician to find out which form and dose is best for them, often changing their prescription a few times.

The types of birth control are named by the doses of progestin and estrogen in each of the active pills. The four dosages are referred to as *monophasic, biphasic, triphasic*, and *progesterone-only pills (POP)*. Monophasic pills have a constant dose of both estrogen and progestin in each of the hormonally active pills throughout the entire cycle (21 days of active pills). Several brands may be available in differing strengths of estrogen or progesterone, from which the physician chooses according to a woman's individual needs. Biphasic pills typically contain two different progesterone doses. The progesterone dose is increased about halfway through the cycle. Triphasic pills gradually increase the dose of estrogen during the cycle. (Some pills also increase the progesterone dose.) There are three different increasing pill doses in each cycle. Progesterone-only pills (POPs), also known as mini-pills, are not used widely in the United States. Fewer than 1% of oral-contraceptive users take these as their only method of birth control. These include women who are breastfeeding and women who cannot take estrogen.

Among the most important to know about BCP is the decreased efficacy with certain antibiotics, such as penicillin or tetracycline. Since tetracycline is often used in the treatment of acne, a client should be educated about the possible interference with BCP. It should also be mentioned that BCP can be used for the management of acne. The most common BCP used for this purpose is Ortho Tri-Cyclen. You can suggest a client discuss this option with a qualified physician. The client should seek out a patient physician who is empathetic to the problems of acne.

The most common skin complaints associated with hormones are mild and easily treatable. Skin discolorations, like those associated with rashes or hyperpigmentation, and mild allergic reactions like hives or itching are often mild and will often go away.

Drugs Used to Treat Blood Conditions

The blood is one of the body's most interesting body fluids. It can be affected by several serious conditions, which can be addressed by drugs in several categories (Table 15–6).

The cells that make up the blood include erythrocytes, leukocytes (five types), and platelets. Platelets are blood cells that are involved in the clotting process. If an injury to the body occurs, platelets and other blood factors

Table 15–6 Drugs That Affect the Blood

DRUG CATEGORY	EXAMPLE	COMMON SKIN EFFECTS
Lipid-lowering agents	Choletyramine, colesevlam, colestipol, atorvastatin, fluvastatin, lovastatin, pravastatin, rosuvastatin simvastatin	Irritation, rashes
Antithrombolytics	Argatroban, bivalirudin, desirudin, lepirudin, anistreplase, streptokinase, tenecteplase	Ecchymoses, flushing, hives
Anticoagulants	Heparin and warfarin	Alopecia, rashes, hives, dermal necrosis
Antiplatelets	Dalteparin, enoxaparin, fondaparinux, tinzaparin, eptifibatide, tirofiban	Ecchymoses, itching, rash, hives, bruising

clump together, causing a clot to form. This process stops the bleeding. However, in some cases unwanted clots can occur. Antiplatelet drugs keep platelets from becoming sticky and creating unwanted clots in the arteries or veins, including the vessels of the heart. These drugs are used to treat individuals that are at risk of stroke or myocardial infarction. Antiplatelet drugs can also be used after certain types of surgery, such as cardiac surgery, to prevent clots from forming. In low dosages aspirin is an antiplatelet drug.

Anticoagulants are used to prevent the formation of clots. These medications are especially useful in the treatment of deep vein thrombosis, pulmonary embolisms, and some heart problems. Anticoagulants will not dissolve clots that have already developed but will help to prevent a clot from getting larger. This is why drugs are used in combination to achieve the best result for the patient.

Antithrombotics work by prohibiting clotting factors from traveling and are used to treat a variety of problems, including clots in the legs, secondary to blood infections, such as **phlebitis,** and some heart problems.

Another group of drugs used to treat blood conditions are those that address cholesterol, or lipids, in the bloodstream. There are three types of cholesterol found in the body: HDL, LDL, and VLDL. Too much LDL cholesterol clogs the arteries. Cholesterol is especially attracted to the coronary arteries or those arteries that supply blood to the heart. High cholesterol increases the chances of heart disease and may contribute to heart attacks. Therefore, a lot of attention has been given to the research and development of drugs that lower lipids.

Because of the skin's proximity to the vascular system, effects on the skin can be wide ranging from flushing to skin necrosis (skin death). While some of these side effects are unappealing and unflattering, they are certainly better than the alternative. If you are unable to treat the side effects, as in the case of tissue necrosis, be sure to refer your client to see his or her doctor, as such a condition can be of great detriment to your client and is outside your own scope of practice.

Drugs Used to Treat Heart Conditions

As steady and reliable as the heart is, it is prone to wear and tear, which can manifest itself in a variety of problems. Heart problems include rhythm disruptions (arrhthymias), **hypertension** (more commonly referred to as high blood pressure), and the deadliest of all, **acute coronary syndrome,** which is an umbrella term used to describe those problems associated with blood flow to the heart. There are a number of categories of drugs to treat the conditions of the heart (Table 15–7).

Like other muscles, the heart needs blood flow directed specifically to it. When that blood flow is blocked or compromised in any way, acute coronary syndrome or **myocardial ischemia** (lack of blood flow to the heart) occurs. Acute coronary syndrome accounts for one-third of all deaths among Americans, making it the nation's leading killer.

Strokes are a cardiovascular disease that involve the arteries in the brain rather than the heart. According to the National Stroke Association, strokes are the third largest killer and the number one disabler of Americans. After age 55, the rate of strokes doubles with each 10 years of age. Risk factors include ethnic considerations (African Americans have a greater incidence), age, smoking, and high blood pressure. While men are more commonly affected than women, it is still important for women to be aware of the symptoms of stroke and act immediately as well.

Table 15–7 Common Drugs Used to Treat Heart Conditions

DRUG CATEGORY	EXAMPLE	COMMON SKIN EFFECTS
Beta blockers	Atenolol, carteolol, labetalol, metoprolol, nadolol, propranolol	Dermatitis, **erythema multiforme**, flushing, increased sweating, itching, rashes
Calcium channel blockers	Diltiazem, felodipine, isradipine, nicardipine, verapamil	Dermatitis, erythema multiforme, flushing, increased sweating, hives
Nitrates	Isosorbide mononitrate, isosorbide dinitrate, nitroglycerin	Skin rash, yellowing of the skin, contact dermatitis, flushing of face and neck, bluish-colored lips, fingernails, or palms of hands
Antiarrhythmics	Disopyramide, moricizine, procainamide, quinidine, fosphenytoin, mexiletine, tocainide, acebutolol, diltiazem, atropine	Itching, skin rash, yellowing of the skin, dermatitis, erythema multiforme, flushing, increased sweating, **photosensitivity**, pruritus/urticaria
Antihypertensives	Clonidine, eplerenone, benazepril, captopril, lisinopril, moexipril, ramipril, guanfacine methyldopa, doxazosin, candesartan	Flushing, rash, itching, hives, sweating

Another cardiovascular event is **angina**, the medical term for chest pain. A condition that should be taken very seriously, angina is a symptom of myocardial ischemia and is often mistaken for a heart attack. While not as deadly, it could be considered a symptom of heart disease. It may feel like pressure or a squeezing pain in the chest. The pain cans also occur in the shoulders, arms, neck, jaw, or back, or it may feel like indigestion.

There are three different types of angina: stable angina, unstable angina, and variant angina. Stable angina is rhythmic in nature, overexerting the heart at a fairly predictable schedule. Usually this discomfort ceases after rest and/or medication. People who suffer from stable angina are at increased risk for heart attacks. Unstable angina is a much more risky condition. Those who suffer from this subtype experience pain at unpredictable times. It can occur either while the body is at work or at rest. People who have unstable angina are at immediate risk for a major cardiac event. The effects of variant angina usually occur when the body is at rest. Medication will often resolve it. This condition is fairly rare, and like stable angina, those who experience this subtype are at increased risk for a cardiac event.

Antianginals are those drugs used to treat angina. These medications are typically nitrates, but beta blockers and calcium channel blockers can also be used for angina. The usual method of administering nitrates is **sublingually** (placed under the tongue), a sublingual spray, transdermal patches, orally, or **parenterally** (by injection). (Medications that are only administered parenterally have not been included in the table.)

Drugs in several categories are used to treat heart-related issues. The drugs in each category work in a different way. Nitrates work by dilating the coronary arteries (vasodilation). Beta blockers work by decreasing the heart rate, thereby decreasing the need for oxygen in the myocardium. Calcium channel blockers dilate the arteries in the heart, allowing greater blood flow to the heart muscle.

Disturbances in normal heart rhythm, also known as **arrhythmia**, are common in older adults. In fact, an estimated four million Americans are live with arrhythmia. Arrhythmia can occur in a healthy heart and may be of minimal consequence. It also may indicate a serious problem and lead to heart disease, stroke, or sudden cardiac death.

Researchers continue to develop new medications that can control arrhythmia. Most common are beta blockers, or beta adrenergic blocking agents. These medications target the adrenaline response of nerve impulses, so that the heart does not need to work as hard.

Table 15–7 lists some of the more common skin effects associated with heart medications. Like medications used to treat blood disorders, a heart patient will need to either deal with the side effects or switch drugs, as the heart condition is more severe than its side effects. Some of the more mild effects, such as itching, can be relieved with OTC products designed to do as much. But in the case of these, and all other medications, you should not suggest this to your client, as to prevent a medication conflict. As an esthetician, your role is to be an advocate to your client. If you suspect that his or her complaint may be the result of a medication they might be taking, refer them to seek the permission of their physician prior to treating the side effects.

Drugs Used to Treat Lung Disorders

Antihistamines, antiasthmatics, and bronchodilators are prescribed by physicians to treat a variety of respiratory conditions (Table 15–8). The most common of these conditions are allergies and asthma, and as many as one in three Americans suffer from one or both. Since the conditions are so common, so are the medications used to treat them.

As many as 45 million Americans suffer from allergies. Hay fever, asthma, and eczema are the most common symptoms of an allergic reaction. Allergy symptoms surface when the body's immune system responds to a trigger substance as though it were a dangerous invader. This invading substance is called an **antigen** or allergen. The **immunologic response** is accomplished by sending defenders called *antibodies* to the entry site (most often the nose or skin). The release of chemical mediators, most often **histamine,** into the bloodstream cause the symptoms that we call *allergic reactions*. Symptoms caused by allergic reactions are itching eyes, sneezing, nasal congestion and drainage, and sometimes headache. Some people experience scratchy sore throats, hoarseness, and coughs. Other less-common symptoms include balance disturbances, swelling in face or throat tissues, skin irritations, respiratory problems, and asthma. Anaphylactic reactions are much more serious and may include difficulty breathing, rash, and a slowed pulse. **Anaphylaxis** requires immediate medical attention from a qualified medical professional.

Antihistamines are drugs that block the release of histamine, thereby reducing allergy symptoms. Most antihistamines produce drowsiness as a side effect. Newer non-sedating antihistamines, many available only by prescription, do not produce this adverse effect. The first few doses may cause sleepiness; subsequent doses are usually less troublesome. Most antihistamines are available in lower over-the-counter (OTC) dosages, which are sufficient for mild allergy sufferers. Those who experience regular allergies should ask a physician for a daily allergy medication that is available by prescription.

Antiasthmatics treat asthma symptoms from a multitude of attack modes. They are further classified according to short-term and long-term symptom management. Long-term asthma relief targets the causes and triggers of asthma attacks, whereas short-term asthma relief is meant to target relief of the symptoms of asthma attacks once they occur.

Bronchodilators are drugs that relieve airway constriction caused by a number of conditions, including asthma. Because they relieve symptoms quickly, they are often referred to as short-term relief. The drugs may be administered by inhalation, orally, or by injections. Most of these medications are delivered via inhalation. It is commonly thought that inhaled medicines are strong and a person will become dependent on inhalers. This is false. In fact, inhaled medications work fast and are quite safe because they are available in much lower doses and have fewer side effects.

As you may have noticed, the consequences of most lung medications are similar. As a general rule, most different medications which are used to treat the same condition will do so. Often these side effects are temporary or will wane with time. As an advocate for your client's skin, you will need to gauge your client's patience for the side effects. Be empathetic and proactive, without making promises.

Drugs Used to Treat Gastrointestinal Disorders

Conditions associated with disruptions in the normal functioning of the gastrointestinal tract and urinary functions include everything from frequent heartburn to urinary incontinence to **peptic ulcers.** Most of the conditions are rather benign, but they are often painful and inconvenient. Because the conditions are so common, the medications that are used to treat them are equally

Table 15–8 Common Drugs Used to Treat Lung Disorders

DRUG CATEGORY	EXAMPLE	COMMON SKIN EFFECTS
Antihistamines	Azatadine, clemastine, bromopheniramine, diphenhydramine, fexofenadine, loratadine, epinephrine	Erythema, photosensitivity, excessivse sweating, rash, and hives
Antiasthmatics	Cromolyn, nedocromil, zafirlukast, albuterol, formoterol, levalbuterol, salmeterol, montelukast	Rash, erythema, flushing, hives, photosensitivity
Bronchodilators	Formoterol, levalbuterol, terbutiline, theophylline	Rash, erythema, flushing, hives, photosensitivity

Table 15–9 Common Drugs Used to Treat Gastrointestinal Disorders

DRUG CATEGORY	EXAMPLE	COMMON SKIN EFFECTS
Anticholinergics	Atropine, darifenacin, dicyclomine, hyoscyamine, oxybutynin, solifenacin, tolteradine	Urticaria, flushing and decreased sweating
Antidiarrheals	Bismuth subsalicylate, difenoxin/atropine, diphenoxylate, kaolin/pectin, loperamide	Flushing
Antiemetics	Dolasetron, ondansetron, granisetron	Pruritis
Antiulcer drugs	Aluminum hydroxide, magnesium hydroxide/aluminum hydroxide, esomeprazole, lansoprazole, omeprazole, rabeprazole, cimetidine, famotidine, nizatidine, randitine, sodium bicarbonate, calcium acetate, magnesium hydroxide	Pruritis, flushing, sweating, photosensitivity and rash

common. Therefore many of the medications listed in Table 15–9 will appear often on client intake paperwork.

The **anticholinergics**, also called **antispasmodics**, are drugs used to treat cramps (spasms) of the stomach, intestines, and bladder. Such cramping results in upset stomach, nausea, vomiting, and a variety of bladder conditions. Anticholinergics are also used in certain surgical and emergency procedures. In surgery, some are given by injection before anesthesia to help relax the patient and to decrease secretions, such as saliva. During anesthesia and surgery, they are often used to help keep the heartbeat normal and to prevent a side effect of anesthesia, nausea. Anticholinergics can also be used to treat painful menstruation and runny nose and to prevent urination during sleep. As you can see, drugs in this category have a variety of uses.

Antidiarrheals are drugs used to prevent of relieve the symptoms of diarrhea. They operate according to one of two separate mechanisms: They either thicken the stool or regulate intestinal spasms. The remedies that operate by thickening stool usually contain clay or other substances, which absorb bacteria or toxins that cause diarrhea. Stool thickeners are safe because they do not enter the blood. However, long-term usage can be problematic since the flora needed for normal functioning is absorbed as well.

The other mode of antidiarrheals regulates or reduces intestinal spasms that result in diarrhea. Loperamide (the active ingredient in products such as Imodium A-D and Pepto Diarrhea Control) is an example of this type of remedy. Some products contain both thickening and antispasmodic ingredients.

Two other gastrointestinal conditions, nausea and vomiting, occur for many reasons. The most common causes are motion sickness or self-limited illnesses that last a few hours to a few days. However, nausea can also be caused by more serious conditions that may require the care of a physician. For most, nausea is a temporary, and bothersome, condition that is easily treated with many over-the-counter and many prescription drugs. **Antiemetics** are drugs that are effective against vomiting and nausea. They are typically used to treat motion sickness and the side effects of other medications. Often, they are prescribed to prevent chemotherapy-related nausea in cancer patients. There are several different types of antiemetics, which are classified according to their mode of operation.

The **5-HT3 antagonists** are selective serotonin inhibitors, which inhibit the binding of serotonin to 5-HT3 receptors, resulting in a reduction in the symptoms of nausea and vomiting. 5-HT3 antagonists are most often prescribed for cancer patients undergoing chemotherapy; however, they are also prescribed for people prone to prolonged nausea or motion sickness, such as people who suffer from motion sickness and are flying a long distance.

Anyone who suffers from peptic ulcers knows that they are painful and persistent and can have a great effect on the quality of life for those who suffer from them. A peptic ulcer is a hole in the gut lining of the stomach, duodenum, or esophagus. An ulcer occurs when the lining of these organs is corroded by the acidic digestive juices that are secreted by the stomach cells. A peptic ulcer of the stomach is called a *gastric ulcer;* of the duodenum, a *duodenal ulcer;* and of the esophagus, an *esophageal ulcer.* Left untreated, ulcers can have serious consequences that may require surgery to repair.

Medications used to relieve the symptoms of ulcers are called **antiulcer drugs.** This is a drug category that is further subcategorized according to mode of operation. Antiulcers include antacids, H2 histamine inhibitors, and **proton pump inhibitors (PPIs).** Some are prescription, while others are available in over-the-counter (OTC) dosages. Aside from the antiulcer drugs whose purpose is specific, many minerals which our bodies require normally can be used to treat the symptoms of peptic ulcers.

Antacids are taken by mouth to relieve heartburn, sour stomach, or acid indigestion. They work by neutralizing excess stomach acid. Some antacid combinations also contain simethicone, which may relieve the symptoms of excess gas. Antacids alone or in combination with simethicone may also be used to treat the symptoms of stomach or duodenal ulcers. These medicines are generally available without a prescription.

Another drug category used to treat acid is H2 blockers. Studies have shown that the protein histamine stimulates gastric acid secretion, which is responsible for ulcer irritation. Histamine antagonists are drugs designed to restrict histamine on gastric cells, reducing acid output. While H2 blockers are effective in reducing the symptoms of ulcers, they do not cure the underlying conditions. Therefore, ulcers frequently return when H2 blockers are stopped.

As with some other medications, the side effects of those used to treat gastrointestinal disorders are relatively mild. The temptation to try to relieve these irritable side effects will be great. All but very few will require a consult with a physician. The exception: photosensitivity. Tell your client to stay out of the sun. This helps accomplish your skin care goals with minimal interference!

Drugs Used to Treat Mental Disorders

At any given point, roughly 10% of the population of the United States suffers from a mental illness. However, many go undiagnosed and untreated because many people do not realize that the feelings that they have are symptomatic of a condition, let alone a condition that can be treated with medications. A mental illness is a condition that produces disturbances in an individual's thoughts, emotions, or behavior. Scientists believe that these conditions are due to an imbalance of chemicals in the brain. Most pharmacologic remedies target these chemicals in order to achieve stabilization of the afflicted individual's mood or behavior.

The term *mental illness* encompasses a wide variety of treatable conditions, which have an equally wide range of symptoms. On one end of the spectrum, mild **depression** leaves an individual feeling sad and lethargic, while psychotic disorders, such as multiple personality disorder, can render an individual incapable of performing even the most perfunctory task. These disorders all have one thing in common: They interfere with a person's ability to live a normal life. People with severe mental illnesses cannot hold a job, relate to other individuals, or cope with ordinary events. Different medications are used to treat various mental conditions, and there is some overlap (Table 15–10).

Table 15–10 Common Drugs Used to Treat Mental Disorders

DRUG CATEGORY	EXAMPLE	COMMON SKIN EFFECTS
Antianxiety drugs	Alprazolam, chlordiazepoxide, diazepam, lorazepam, midazolam, oxazpam	Rashes
Anticonvulsants	Buspirone, doxepin, hydroxyzine pamoate, hydroxyzine hydrochloride, paroxetine hydrochloride, venlafaxine, phenobarbital, phenytoin, divalproex sodium, valproate sodium, valproic acid	Rashes, **hypertrichosis**, exfoliative dermatitis, pruritis, ecchymoses, photosensitivity, rashes, flushing
Antidepressants	Citalopram, duloxetine hydrochloride, escitalopram, fluoxetine, paroxetine, sertraline, mirtazapine, nortriptyline, phenelzine, trazodone, bupropion	Ecchymoses, pruritis, photosensitivity, rashes, itching, hives, alopecias
Antipsychotics	Clozapine, olanzapine, haloperidol, quetiapine, risperidone, ziprasidone	Rash, hives and sweating, dry skin, sun sensitivity, ecchymoses, pruritis
Central nervous system stimulants	Amphetamine mixtures, dextroamphetamine, methylphenidate	Unusual bruising, hives, rash and itching
Sedatives	Chloral hydrate, droperidol, eszopiclone, ramelteon, zaleplon, zolpidem	Rashes, photosensitivity, sweating

Currently, there are about 50 different approved medications that treat mental conditions. Some of their side effects can make them difficult to take, but it comes down to weighing the benefits of the medication versus the side effects. If a patient experiences undesirable side effects, they often consult with the prescribing physician and switch to a medication that might not have the undesired side effects.

Collectively, anxiety disorders are the most common mental illnesses in the United States. More than 20 million individuals have one of the several diseases that make up this disease category. Everyone experiences normal levels of anxiety in their lives. But anxiety in its most extreme cases can render an individual paranoid, alone, and often housebound. Fortunately, drugs are available to ease the fear and paranoia while improving quality of life as well. Under the general category of anxiety disorders, there are five specific disorders, which all have their own unique characteristics and symptoms: panic disorder, **obsessive-compulsive disorder (OCD)**, **post-traumatic stress disorder (PTSD)**, **phobias**, and **generalized anxiety disorder (GAD)**. There are several different types of drugs used to treat anxiety disorders. One of these are **benzodiazepines.** Benzodiazepines are a type of central nervous system (CNS) depressant, meaning that they slow down the nervous system. Most benzodiazepines are used to relieve anxiety but only in the most extreme cases. When used regularly, they usually are not effective for more than a few weeks.

Another class of drugs used to treat conditions of the brain are anticonvulsants. **Anticonvulsants** are a category of drug used to reduce the frequency and severity of seizures resulting from a variety of conditions. The most common of these conditions is **epilepsy**, a neurological condition with an unknown etiology. It might be the result of genetics, serious illness, or a head injury. Other situations, such as chemical withdrawal, prolonged sleep deprivation, or low blood sugar can also result in patient seizures. There are several types of anticonvulsant medications that depress the central nervous system in a variety of ways, including **barbiturates**, benzodiazepines (see above), hyantoins, and valproates.

One of the most common mental disorders is depression. Collectively, the medications that are used to treat depression are called antidepressants. Antidepressants were first developed in the 1950s and have been used regularly since then. The exact mechanisms under which they operate are not entirely clear; however, it is known that they affect neurotransmitters in the brain, particularly dopamine, **serotonin**, and **norephinephrine**. There are three major categories of antidepressants: tricyclics (TCAs), select serotonin reuptake inhibitors (SSRIs), and monoamine oxidase inhibitors (MAOIs).

Tricyclics were the first antidepressants to become available. They are powerful drugs that beef up the brain's supply of norepinephrine and serotonin. The down side is that the side effects can often be severe and are not tolerated by some patients. Also, the failure rate is around 30%, a statistic that is common to all antidepressants.

Select serotonin reuptake inhibitors (SSRIs) are best for individuals who are in the early stages of less-severe depression. These drugs are newer and accompanied by less severe side effects. While they are generally better tolerated, their success rate is not any greater than TCAs, about 60% to 70%. Another down side to these drugs is their price: They are expensive. The good news is that since the patents for many of these drugs will expire in coming years, the costs should go down.

Monoamine oxidase inhibitors (MAOIs), like TCAs, affect the levels of norepinephrine and serotonin in the brain, but they also affect dopamine levels, which can result in other neurological conditions. An enzyme in the brain called *monoamine oxidase* destroys neurotransmitters before they have an opportunity to convey their messages to the receptors. MAOIs inhibit this enzyme, allowing a buildup of neurotransmitters.

While antidepressants have proven to be effective and have helped millions of people, finding the right one is a complicated process. Whether it is the failure of a particular drug to achieve positive outcomes, or the inability to tolerate the drug, many patients have to switch medications several times before finding one that works and can be tolerated.

Psychotic disorders are among the most dangerous, not only for the individual, but for those around him or her as well. The distortion of thought processes and reality can be

FYI

Benzodiazepines may be habit-forming (causing **psychological dependence** or **physical dependence**), so care must be taken in the use of these medications.

so extreme that an affected individual loses sight of right and wrong, as well as what is and is not real. The good news, however, is that psychotic disorders are only temporary by definition. The major symptom of these disorders is **psychoses,** or delusions and hallucinations. Delusions are false beliefs that significantly hinder a person's ability to function—for example, believing that people are trying to hurt you when there is no evidence or believing that you are somebody else. **Hallucinations** are false perceptions. They can be visual (seeing things that are not there), auditory (hearing), olfactory (smelling), tactile (feeling sensations on skin that are not really there, such as the feeling of crawling bugs), or taste. The cause of one of these disorders is typically an extremely stressful event or trauma.

Psychotic disorders are usually treated with talk therapies and the family of medicines known as *thioxanthenes,* also called **antipsychotics.** Whereas central nervous system depressants slow down the functions of the CNS in people suffering from anxiety disorders.

Sleep disorders are common in the stressful times in which we live. Sleep disorders include trouble getting to sleep, trouble staying asleep, and ineffective sleep. For the millions of people who suffer from a sleep condition, medications, particularly sedatives and hypnotics, are the only resort. Most clients using the medications listed on Table 15–10 will likely be using them for sleep disorders. Conversely, those who suffer from conditions like narcolepsy or certain types of depression will sleep too much or without warning. For these individuals, central nervous system stimulants increase the activity for people suffering from conditions such as narcolepsy.

FYI

Many medications used to treat mental disorders have troubling side effects and are often habit-forming.

Drugs Used to Treat Diabetes

Diabetes is a common and potentially catastrophic condition that affects more than 20 million American adults and children. It is a condition in which blood sugar, or blood **glucose,** is too high. Glucose is a vital carbohydrate that is used by animals to supply energy to the body. While a certain amount of glucose in the blood is healthy and essential, too much can be toxic. For diabetics, a daily balancing act of calculating and responding to glucose levels is a way of life.

A main source of glucose is foods; however the liver and muscles also produce a small amount. A hormone produced in the pancreas, **insulin,** helps the cellular intake of glucose for energy. Diabetics either fail to produce insulin or their cells do not respond to it. While an overabundance of glucose in the blood is the end result of diabetes, ineffectual or nonexistent insulin supplies are the root cause. For this reason, diabetics need to fortify insulin supplies externally. This may be done via diet, tablets, or shots. While the exact etiology of the condition has yet to be discovered, researchers believe that genetics and environmental factors, such as obesity, contribute greatly.

There are two major types of diabetes, Type 1, or insulin-dependent, and Type 2, or non-insulin-dependent. One other type, gestational diabetes, occurs in pregnant women who have high blood glucose levels. About 4% of woman who become pregnant will develop gestational diabetes. The cause is unknown but it is speculated that the hormones that are secreted by the placenta may block the insulin in the mother, causing blood glucose levels to rise. Typically, gestational diabetes disappears after delivery, but the chances of reoccurrence are greater with future pregnancies.

You need to be especially aware of Type 1 diabetics, as they do not heal well and are at a high risk of infection. In 2006, two diabetics who received minor cuts during a pedicure developed infections that resulted in their deaths. This condition cannot be taken lightly.

Drugs Used to Treat Bacterial Infections

Bacteria are single-celled organisms that can be innocuous or have far-reaching consequences for their hosts. The human body has evolved to include three major lines of defense to protect from **pathogens.** The primary immune responses, the first line of defense, include **lysosomes** found in tears and saliva, enzymes in the stomach, and the acid mantel of the skin. These mechanisms seek to destroy or block pathogens to prevent their invasion and growth in or on the body. The next line of defense is the body's nonspecific immune responses. Immune responses use inflammation to isolate and flush out pathogens. The final line of defense uses **lymphocytes** (T-cells) to destroy specific pathogens and create specific immunity (B-cells). While the human body's innate immune responses are complex and effective, many bacteria are equally cunning. Their ability to evolve quickly keeps the body's mechanism hard at work.

As is often the case, an infection can outwit an immune response and do its damage.

Until the discovery of penicillin in the 1940s, many common bacteria had devastating or dire consequences for those who contracted an infection. People lost limbs and lives due to infections which are now easily remedied. In the Western world, thanks to the explosion of antibiotics in the pharmaceutical industry. However, overuse of antibiotics has caused ever-adaptable bacteria to evolve antibiotic-resistant strains, creating a demand for newer and more powerful antibiotics.

MRSA, or methicillin resistant *Staphylococcus aureus*, was first discovered in the 1960s just after methicillin was introduced. There are five strains of MRSA. Those persons who carry MRSA pick it up the same way as other bacteria—through physical contact, especially if the organism is on the skin. The 1990s saw a sharp rise in the number of patients infected with MRSA. It is typically found in younger people, individuals who have been in a hospital, and also those with suppressed immune systems. It is much more likely to be the cause of a skin or soft-tissue infection. There has been concern over the past decade that MRSA is becoming antibiotic-resistant, but new drugs have been developed to address this concern, including linezolid, quinupristin-dalfopristin, daptomycin, and others.

Antibiotics work to kill bacteria. Since bacteria are responsible for disease and a list of unpleasant symptoms, the goal is to kill the bacteria and eliminate the disease. When immune systems fail to take care of this matter, antibiotics are required. There are two main groups of bacteria: gram-positive and gram-negative. Gram staining, the process used to decipher the type, is the first step to identifying the particular bacteria affecting an individual. It takes much less time than a culture and can indicate the best means of applying an appropriate treatment.

In reality, an antibiotic is a selective poison. It has been chosen so that it will kill the desired bacteria but not the cells in the body. Each type of antibiotic affects different bacteria in different ways (Table 15–11). For example, an antibiotic might inhibit a bacterium's ability to turn glucose into energy or its ability to construct its cell wall. When this happens, the bacterium dies instead of reproducing.

> **Here's a Tip**
>
> Most skin infections can be attributed to three pathogens: *Staphylococcus, Streptococcus,* and *Pseudomonas.*

Drugs Used to Treat Viral Infections

Viruses are microscopic, **unicellular** entities that straddle the fence between living and non-living. They come in a variety of shapes and sizes and exist everywhere there are cells to infect. They are in the air, in soil, and in water. They exist for one purpose and one purpose only: to reproduce. There are thousands of different viruses. Some infect plants, some infect animals, and some even infect bacteria.

Viruses are basically a microscopic bundle of genetic material (either DNA or RNA) housed within an envelope. They float around in an inert state, waiting to attach to a suitable host cell that they then infect and commandeer. Once they have infected a host cell, they use the operations of the cell to reproduce. However, viruses are rather picky about what types of cells they infect. Viruses that infect plants are capable of infecting animals, and vice versa.

Table 15–11 Common Antibiotics

DRUG CATEGORY	EXAMPLE	COMMON SKIN EFFECTS
Antibiotics	Amikacin, kanamycin, neomycin, streptomycin, tobramycin, ertapenem, meropenem, cefadroxil monohydrate, cefazolin, cephalexin, cefotetan, cefuroxime, loracarbef, cefoperazone, ceftriaxone, piperacillin, ticarcillin, ciprofloxacin, levofloxacin, moxfloxacin, norfloxacin, ofloxacin, azithromycin clarithromycin, erythromycin, amoxicillin, ampicillin, cloxacillin, dicloxacillin, oxacillin, nafcillin, penicillin, doxycycline, minocycline, tetracycline, clindamycin, metronidazole, vancomycin	Rashes, itching, burning, photosensitivity, rashes and hives with topical use, mild dryness, skin irritation, transient redness, epidermal necrolysis, erythema multiforme

Table 15–12 Common Drugs Used to Treat Viruses

DRUG CATEGORY	EXAMPLE	COMMON SKIN EFFECTS
Antivirals	Acyclovir, amantadine hydrochloride, cidofovir, docosanol, entecavir, famciclovir, ganciclovir, lamivudine, oseltamivir, penciclovir, ribavrin, valacyclovir, valganciclovir hydrochloride, vidarabine, zanamivir, delavirdine mesylate, efavirenz, nevirapine, abacavir, didanosine, emtriciabine, stavudine, zalcitabine, zidovudine	Acne, hives, rashes, sweating, Stevens Johnson syndrome, hair loss, dry, itchy skin, photosensitivity, erythema multiforme, hives, ecchymoses, nail pigmentation, lipodystrophy

However, viruses that infect one species can easily move to a closely related species. Furthermore, viruses behave differently in different species. For example, the **hantavirus** infects rodents with no apparent detriment. Once it infects humans, however, the results are often fatal.

The body has means to protect itself from viruses. One such means is the skin itself. The skin acts as a barrier to hold in what is needed and keep out what is not needed. However, being the opportunistic entities that they are, viruses are adept at finding alternative entries to the body. Once a virus has found a way to enter the body, the body uses its internal mechanisms to fight. The immune system responds and white blood cells begin to fight. If the virus does not survive this battle, the white blood cell responds by remembering the virus, and the means to defeat it, rendering an individual immune to further infection. Vaccination is another means of combating viruses. By introducing a small, easily combated dose of the virus into the body, the body develops immunity before a full-blown attack.

In humans, viruses have a wide variety of physical expressions. Since viruses usually infect only one type of cell, different viruses have different expressions. For instance, the virus that causes the common cold only infects respiratory cells, and the virus that causes AIDS only affects immune system cells.

The viruses that cause more common skin diseases are the herpes simplex virus and the human papilloma virus. Together, these viruses are responsible for cold sores (HSV-1), genital herpes (HSV-2), and warts (HPV). Viruses that are responsible for respiratory distress include the common cold, influenza, and sinusitis. A few viruses infect the nervous system, but they are rare. They include encephalitis and West Nile Virus.

Treating viruses poses a unique challenge. Unlike bacterial infections, in which antibiotics can target the infecting agent, viruses are more difficult to treat since they are in a constant state of genetic flux. Drugs that are used to treat viruses are called antivirals (Table 15–12). Since viruses reside in commandeered cells and replicate by means of those cells, antiviral drugs target the DNA of infected cells to hinder replication. As a consequence, antiviral drugs are much more expensive to develop. Furthermore, viruses can develop a resistance to antiviral drugs, requiring a constant influx of new antiviral drugs.

The Human Immunodeficiency Virus (HIV) disables specific immune cell functioning. It attacks the cells that provide immunity for the body—typically the T cells and the CD2+ cells—causing a gradual deterioration of immune defenses. Eventually the body's immunity becomes seriously compromised, and at that point a disease called AIDs, or Acquired Immunodeficiency Syndrome, takes hold. HIV and AIDS are treated with **antiretrovirals,** which have been developed specifically to fight the virus.

Antiretrovirals are specific in their treatment. There are four categories of antiretrovials: nonnucleoside reverse transcriptase inhibitors, nucleoside reverse transcriptase inhibitors, protease inhibitors, and fusion inhibitors. Each drug functions differently but helps to treat HIV and AIDS. Both non-nucleoside reverse transcriptase inhibitors and nucleoside reverse transcriptase inhibitors work by prohibiting the HIV enzyme from converting HIV RNA to HIV DNA. Protease inhibitors work in a completely different way by interfering with the protease enzyme that HIV uses to produce infectious viral particles. Finally, fusion inhibitors work to interfere with the virus's ability to fuse cellular membrane. This action blocks the entry to the cells host. Knowing these different drug functions, it is easy to see why a patient might be on a "cocktail" of several drugs to manage their disease.

Drugs Used to Treat Fungal Infections

Fungal infections usually occur in darker moister areas of the body, often where skin surfaces join together—for example, where the toes meet the trunk of the feet. Fungi are a species of parasite that feeds from hosts and reproduce both sexually and asexually. **Pathogenic fungi,** or fungi that cause or are a result of disease, also known as *mycoses,* are classified according to the depth to which they invade the skin. The most common, **superficial mycoses,** are localized to the exterior layers of the dermis in the skin and its appendages. The fungi live and produce in the area of infection. This includes *Tineas* and ringworm. **Subcutaneous mycoses** are rare and occur mostly in tropical regions. They usually result from the introduction of vegetative matter to an open wound. Like superficial mycoses, the infection is limited to the dermis. They tend to have a slow onset and are chronic. Equally rare, **systemic mycoses** affect the internal organs. **Opportunistic mycoses** usually occur in **immunocompromised** patient, such as someone who is undergoing chemotherapy or who has just undergone surgery. These infections can be localized or they can spread throughout the body. They can sometimes be fatal.

The human body contains natural flora, which are harmless and often vital, to overall bodily health. However, there are some fungi that can cause a fungal infection of the skin. These fungi can spread easily from one person to the next. The associated infections are generally not considered to be serious conditions and are typically easily remedied. However, rare systemic mycoses can be more problematic. The symptoms and appearances of a fungal skin infection depend on the type of fungus causing it and the part of the body affected. Usually, fungal infections will present with a rash. Different types of fungal infections are named for the part of the body in which they present (Table 15–13).

Drugs Used to Treat Skeletal Conditions

Bones and cartilage that are healthy work together, providing a smooth system of operation for the joints. Healthy cartilage is slippery and allows the bones to glide and function unnoticeably, without pain. But over the course of a lifetime, the bones and the associated cartilage undergo wear and tear. For some the use is greater—for example, runners who pound their feet against the pavement, jarring their knees. In this example, the cartilage is worn down over a period of time and the bones do not glide as they once did. This in turn causes the pain associated with **osteoarthritis** and degenerative joint arthritis. As time goes on, the joint may collect debris, such as chips of bone or cartilage and the movement may become limited. Other factors that may contribute to osteoarthritis include obesity and joint injuries. The good news is that osteoarthritis is a localized condition.

Rheumatoid arthritis, on the other hand, is considered an autoimmune disease and can affect not only the joints but internal organs as well. The term *autoimmune disease* refers to a varied group of serious, chronic illnesses that involve almost every human organ system. In all of these diseases, the underlying problem is similar—the body's immune system becomes misdirected, attacking the very organs it was designed to protect. Rheumatoid arthritis is one of those diseases, chronic but typically with times of disease flare and remission. During a flare, the joints, as well as the tissues around the joints, will be inflamed and sore. If the disease has progressed to a systemic state, the involved organs will also be inflamed. During this time, the patient will be lethargic and the joints and muscles will be painful and ache. The patient may also be inactive due to the pain. Remissions can occur without reason and last weeks or even years. During times of remission, the patient will feel good, typically without pain.

Another bone disease is osteoporosis. Osteoporosis occurs in both men and women, but it is more common in postmenopausal women when significant bone absorption is likely to occur. Bones that were once strong become porous and brittle. In the spine, the vertebrae begin to compress and the torso becomes shorter. The appearance of a **dowager hump** or outward curvature of the upper spine

Table 15–13 Common Drugs Used to Treat Fungal Infections

DRUG CATEGORY	EXAMPLE	COMMON SKIN EFFECTS
Systemic antifungals	Amphotericin B, fluconazole, itraconazole, terbinafine, voriconazole	Flushing, exfoliative skin disorders, Stevens Johnson syndrome, rash, itching, **toxic epidermal necrolysis,** and photosensitivity
Topical antifungals	Butenafine, butoconazole, ciclopirox, clotrimazole, econazole, haloprogin, ketoconazole, miconazole, nystatin, oxiconazole, sulconazole, tolnaftate	Burning, itching, local sensitivity, redness, stinging, local irritation, sensitization, rash or itching, hives, toxic epidermal necrolysis

Table 15–14 Risk Factors for Osteoporosis

INFLUENCES FOR OSTEOPOROSIS	HOW OSTEOPOROSIS DEVELOPS
Gender	Postmenopausal women are at the greatest risk.
Age	Bones get thinner with age. As aging progresses, osteoporosis is more likely.
Body Size	Slight-sized women are at greater risk.
Ethnicity	Caucasians and Asians are at greater risk.
Family history	Individuals with parents who developed osteoporosis may be more likely to develop the disease themselves.
Sex hormones	Absence of periods or low estrogen influences the development of osteoporosis.
Anorexia	Malnourished individuals are at greater risk.
Calcium and vitamin D intake	Poor bone growth related to less calcium and vitamin D
Medication use	Corticosteroids and anticonvulsants inhibit bone density.
Exercise	Lack of exercise causes the bones to be less dense.
Cigarette smoking	Increases bone loss
Alcohol	Increases bone loss

Table 15–15 Common Drugs Used to Treat Skeletal Conditions

DRUG CATEGORY	EXAMPLE	COMMON SKIN EFFECTS
Osteoporosis drugs	Alendronate, Etidronate, Pamidronate risedronate, Tiludronate, Zoledronic acid, Raloxifene	Itching, swelling, skin rash, sweating, flushing, photosensitivity, erythema multiforme
Rheumatoid arthritis drugs	Anakinra, Etanercept, Hydroxychloroquine, Infliximab, Leflunomide, Methotrexate, Cyclosporine, Sulfasalazine	Tashes, exfoliative dermatitis, photosensitivity, yellow discoloration of the skin, hirsutism, acne, hives and skin ulcers, alopecia, painful plaque erosions, photosensitivity

becomes more pronounced with time. Certain women are more at risk than others, including Caucasian and Asian women of slight build (Tables 15–14 and 15–15).

Corticosteroids

Cortisones were first introduced in 1949 for the treatment of rheumatoid arthritis. These drugs worked so well they were deemed "miracles" by the patients using them. Since that time the use of corticosteroids has broadened to include the treatment of other autoimmune diseases, such as lupus. Corticosteroids are now also used to treat asthma, adrenal insufficiency, hepatitis, ulcer bowel disease, and athletic injuries. Topical conditions can also be treated with cortisone; the skin and eyes typically respond well to cortisone (Table 15–16).

When produced naturally, corticosteroids attend to the body's stress, immune responses, inflammation, carbohydrate metabolism, protein catabolism, and blood electrolyte levels. Unfortunately, the use of corticosteroids also comes with a price—side effects. The most common side effect is **Cushing syndrome**, or moon face. Other side effects include high blood pressure, low potassium in the blood, high sodium levels in the blood, and a condition called **metabolic alkalosis.** Recent studies show that a condition called **central serous retinopathy** or CSR can occur with the use of topical cortisone, nasal sprays containing cortisone, and eye drops containing cortisone.

Drugs Used to Treat Pain

The description of pain is divided into two categories, chronic and acute. Chronic pain is that experienced every day, such as with arthritis, while acute pain is associated with injury or surgery. Whether the pain is chronic or acute, relief is important.

Table 15–16 Corticosteroids

DRUG CATEGORY	EXAMPLE	COMMON SKIN EFFECTS
Corticosteroids	Beclomethasone, budesonide, flunisolide, fluticasone, triamcinolone, beclomethasone, budesonide, fluticasone, mometasone, loteprednol, prednisolone, rimexolone, hydrocortisone, cortisone, prednisolone, prednisone, dexamethasone, alclometasone, clocortolone, desoximetasone, diflorasone, flucinonide	Acne, delayed wound healing, ecchymoses, fragile skin integrity, hirsutism, petechiae, allergic contact dermatitis, skin shrinking, burning, dryness, swelling, folliculitis, hypersensitivity, hypertrichoses, loss of pigmentation, irritation, maceration, **miliaria,** perioral dermatitis, secondary infections, stretch marks

Table 15–17 Common Drugs Used to Treat Pain

DRUG CATEGORY	EXAMPLE	COMMON SKIN EFFECTS
Narcotic analgesics	Buprenorphine, butorphanol, codeine, fentanyl citrate, fentanyl transdermal system, hydrocodone, hydromorphone, meperidine hydrochloride, methadone, morphine, nalbuphine, oxycodone, oxymorphone, propoxyphene	Pruritus, rash, flushing, urticaria, exfoliative dermatitis
Non-steroidal anti-inflammatory agents (NSAIDs)	Celecoxib, diclofenac, diflunisal, etodolac, fenoprofen, flurbiprofen, ibuprofen, indomethacin, ketoprofen, ketorolac, meloxicam, nabumetone, naproxen, oxaprozin, piroxicam, sulindac, tolmetin	Stevens Johnson syndrome and exfoliative dermatitis, ecchymoses, skin rash, and itching
Non-narcotic analgesics	Acetaminophen, butalbital compounds, capsaicin, choline and magnesium, salicylates, salsalate	Dermatitis, rash, exfoliative dermatitis, Stevens Johnson syndrome, toxic epidermal necrolysis
Muscle relaxants	Baclofen, carisoprodol, chlorzoxazone, cyclobenzaprine, dantrolene, diazepam, metaxalone, methocarbamol, orphenadrine	Flushing, pruritis, rash, urticaria, sweating

Often the relief is associated with a medication that manages and improves the pain (Table 15–17). Pain medications can reduce inflammation and help control pain when taken properly. They cannot stop the effects of aging and wear and tear on the body and they do not remedy the underlying cause, but they do make certain conditions more manageable.

Pain medications are associated with a certain amount of risk. A lot of pain medications are addictive and often abused. Great concern and restraint must be executed when taking pain medications.

If you have clients using pain medications, watch for rashes, which are usually associated with allergic reactions to those medications. If you suspect that a client is experiencing an allergic reaction, refer him or her to a physician. These reactions can sometimes be severe and are outside your scope.

On certain occasions, clients will complain of skin conditions that are not previously linked to medications. For instance, pruritis and erythema are common skin effects from many medications. If the client finds the condition unbearable, refer him or her to the prescribing physician to consider a substitute medication.

Obviously, the conditions, medications, and side effects are all equally varied. As mentioned, some of these conditions will be ones which you see regularly. Itching, pigmentary irregularities, and dermatitis clients will come into your office on a daily basis. It might be a challenge, at first, connecting the condition to the medication. In fact, oftentimes, it will require you to do some detective work—prying the names of medications from your clients lip.

Once you begin to suspect a medication side effect, it is vital that you do not rush into treating it. Doing so could cause a drug interaction, exacerbate the problem, or cause irreparable damage to your client and your career. Think ahead, and always advise your client to consult with his or her physician prior to trying to resolve the side effects.

REVIEW QUESTIONS

1. Why should you be aware of a client's medical conditions and his or her medications?
2. Describe the role of the FDA regarding drugs.
3. Discuss how a drug becomes approved.
4. What is the difference between a prescription drug and an over-the-counter drug?
5. What does *Signatura* mean on a prescription?
6. Are there any skin side effects to blood pressure medications? What are they?
7. Discuss common heart conditions and any skin impacts of drugs used to treat those conditions.
8. What are gastrointestinal drug types? What common skin issues are associated with them?
9. Discuss anxiety and sleep disorder drugs and the skin impacts of them.
10. What are antibiotic drugs and what are the skin impacts?
11. List the factors that create vulnerability for osteoporosis.
12. What are pain-relieving drugs and what, if any, are the skin impacts?
13. Did you discover a common group of skin impacts caused by many drugs? What are they?
14. What should the esthetician do if they see possible side effects of drugs on their client's skin?

CHAPTER GLOSSARY

5-HT3 antagonists: antienemic which is a selective serotonin inhibitor, which inhibits the binding of serotonin to 5-HT3 receptors.

acute coronary syndrome (ACS): general term used for any condition which causes chest pain resulting from limited blood flow to the heart.

anaphylaxis: serious hypersensitive allergic reaction characterized by respiratory distress, hypotension, edema, rash, and tachycardia. Immediate medical attention is necessary.

angina: chest pain resulting from the heart experiencing a lack of oxygen.

antacid: any agent that neutralizes stomach acid.

antianginals: class of drugs used to prevent the onset of an anginal attack.

antianxiety drugs: any drug that prevents or limits the severity of the symptoms of an anxiety disorder.

antiasthmatics: any drug that prevents or limits the severity of the symptoms of an asthma attack.

anticholinergics: class of drugs used to limit spasms and cramping, particularly of the digestive and urinary tracts.

anticonvulsants: class of drugs used to prevent or limit the of severity of spastic activity resulting from certain neurological conditions.

antidepressants: class of drugs used to prevent or limit the severity of the symptoms of depression.

antiemetics: class of drugs used to prevent or limit the severity of the symptoms of nausea and vomiting.

antigen: 1. a modified type of serum globulin synthesized by lymphoid tissue in response to antigenic stimulus. 2. any material that elicits an immune response.

antihistamines: class of drugs used to block the action of histamine.

CHAPTER GLOSSARY

antipsychotic: class of drugs used to prevent or limit the severity of the symptoms of psychosis.

antiretrovirals: class of drug used to treat retroviruses, viruses that use the infected individual's DNA to replicate.

antispasmodics: *see* anticonvulsants.

antithrombotics: class of drugs used to prevent platelet coagulation.

antiulcer drugs: class of drugs used to prevent or limit the severity of the symptoms of peptic ulcers.

arrhythmia: heart condition characterized by irregular heartbeats. Arrhythmias can be harmless or potentially serious.

barbiturates: addictive central nervous system depressants.

benzodiazepines: group of drugs with a sedative effect; predominantly used to treat anxiety and sleep disorders.

bronchodilators: group of drugs which are used to reverse acute bronchial constriction.

central serous retinopathy: occular condition characterized by fluid leaking from the macula resulting in blurred vision.

Cushing syndrome: condition of the endocrine system characterized by a multitude of disorders.

depression: condition characterized by low mood, loss of interest, loss of energy, weight changes, changes in appetite, changes in sleep patterns, fatigue, inability to concentrate, feelings of low self-worth, and possible thoughts of suicide.

dowager hump: a bump that forms along the spine due to slow bone loss over time.

epilepsy: neurologic condition characterized by sudden seizures.

erythema multiforme: macular eruptions in a patchy formation on the extremities.

generalized anxiety disorder (GAD): condition characterized by unspecific or unwarranted anxiety.

glucose: simple blood sugar which is an important source of energy.

hallucinations: abnormal visions associated with certain psychoses.

hantavirus: virus transmitted to humans through mice feces with potentially fatal consequences.

histamine: amino acid vital to human immunologic response.

hyperpigmentation: skin condition characterized by overproduction of melanin resulting in patches of colored skin.

hypertension: high blood pressure.

hypertrichosis: excessive hair growth where hair does not normally grow.

hypopigmentation: skin condition characterized by under production of melanin resulting in patches of non-colored skin.

immunocompromised: refers to limited or reduced functioning of the immune system.

immunologic response: a bodily defense reaction that recognizes an invading substance and produces antibodies specific against that antigen.

insulin: essential hormone needed for the normal metabolic breakdown of glucose in the body.

lymphocytes: (L. *lymphia,* "water, goodness of water" + G. *kytos,* "hollow vessel") 1. a type of white blood cell; a component of the immune system produced by stem cells in the bone marrow. 2. type of white blood cell which is important to the immune system for its ability to digest foreign invaders.

lysosomes: 1. cytoplasmic, membrane-bounded organelle that contains digestive and hydrolytic enzymes, which are typically most active at the acid pH found in the lamen of lysosomes. 2. cell organelle that digests foreign matter considered potentially threatening to the body.

metabolic alkalosis: increased alkalines in the body resulting from decreases acids.

monoamine oxidase inhibitors (MAOIs): class of drugs used to treat depression; however, the exact mode of their action is not quite understood.

myocardial ischemia: temporary restriction in normal blood flow to the heart and cardiac muscles.

norepinephrine: neurotransmitter responsible for heartrate and the fight or flight reaction. Overproduction or underproduction are associated with several psychological conditions including depression.

obsessive-compulsive disorder (OCD): anxiety disorder characterized by perpetual and excessive thoughts and activities that interfere with the normal functioning of the affected individual.

opportunistic mycoses: fungi that use breaks in the skin or abnormal immunity to infect the body.

osteoarthritis: joint condition characterized by inflammation of weight-bearing joints.

over-the-counter (OTC): any drug that has FDA approval to be sold or consumed without a doctor's order.

parenteral: piercing of mucous membranes or the skin barrier through such events as needlesticks, human bites, and abrasions; any drug delivery route other than through the mouth.

pathogenic fungi: any fungus that results in disease.

pathogens: a microorganism or substance capable of producing disease.

peptic ulcer: wearing down of stomach and esophagus tissue resulting in frequent stomach pain, especially after eating.

phlebitis: inflammation of the wall of a vein.

phobias: anxiety conditions characterized by unwarranted fear such that it interferes with the normal fuctioning of the affected individual.

photosensitivity: responsive to sunlight.

physical dependence: chemical dependence in which the body thinks it needs a particular substance to continue to function.

post-traumatic stress disorder (PTSD): anxiety condition resulting from stress brought on by a traumatic event.

proton pump inhibitors (PPIs): type of antacid that works to reduce the production of acid.

psychological dependence: type of chemical dependence characterized by the affected individual thinking he or she needs a substance in order to function.

psychoses: any psychological condition that affects an individuals ability to live their lives in a normal and healthy manner.

select serotonin reuptake inhibitors (SSRIs): type of antidepressant that allows for more productive use of the neurotransmitter serotonin.

serotonin: neurotransmitter which is associated with many psychoses, especially depression.

subcutaneous mycoses: fungal infections occurring below the skin.

sublingual: below the tongue.

superficial mycoses: skin condition that results from the introduction of vegetative matter to an open wound; infection is limited to the dermis.

systemic mycoses: fungi that affect the internal organs.

toxic epidermal necrolysis (TEN): tissue death on the epidermis.

tricyclics (TCAs): a strong peel used to diminish sun damage and wrinkles; the most commonly prescribed type of antidepressant used to treat milder cases of depression or anxiety.

unicellular: single-celled organism.

PART 4

ESTHETICS

Chapter 16 Advanced Facial Techniques

Chapter 17 Advanced Skin Care Massage

Chapter 18 Advanced Facial Devices

Chapter 19 Hair Removal

Chapter 20 Advanced Makeup

CHAPTER OUTLINE

- TREATMENT VARIATIONS
- ROSACEA AND SENSITIVE SKIN TREATMENTS
- CLINIC EXFOLIATION TREATMENTS
- MASK THERAPIES

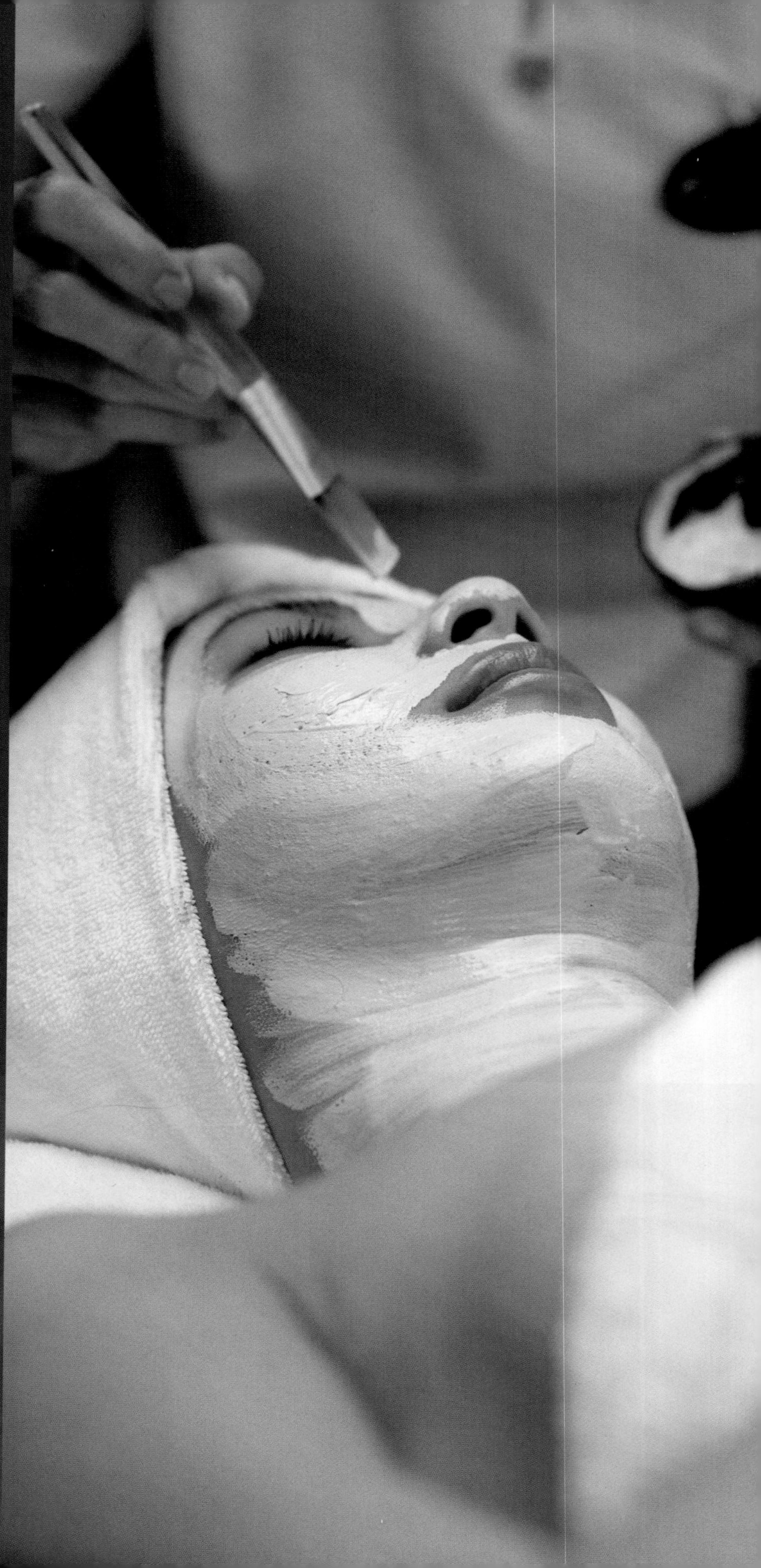

CHAPTER 16

ADVANCED FACIAL TECHNIQUES

LEARNING OBJECTIVES

After completing this chapter, you should be able to:

- Understand and employ variations in skin treatments.
- Develop and employ protocols for specific skin conditions.
- Treat sensitive skin and its issues.
- Perform manual microdermabrasion.
- Select and use superficial peels that are appropriate for a client.
- Select and employ different mask technologies.

KEY TERMS

Page numbers indicate where in the chapter the term is used.

rubifactants 383

In your work as an esthetician, you need to be equally comfortable using techniques that involve equipment and those that do not. Every treatment has its own strengths and weaknesses, indications, and contraindications. The more you know about each, the more choices you can offer a client. For example, there are any number of variations in facials, including the arrangement of the steps, the types of exfoliants used, masks, and temperature. Other variations involve the use of different devices during treatments. Layering technologies use both cosmetic chemistry as well as one or more equipment techniques in the same treatment. Understanding the options and how to safely incorporate them gives you a wide-ranging repertoire of treatments and the ability to customize treatments to a client's needs.

TREATMENT VARIATIONS

While a basic facial has a standard pattern, variations can enhance your treatment results. Consider the basic treatment steps as building blocks (Figure 16–1). If you give several children the same pile of blocks, each will build something different based on his or her own vision for the result. Estheticians can do the same thing. Keep in mind that you must perform a thorough consultation and analysis of the skin prior to a treatment so that you find the best way to assemble "the building blocks" needed to treat a client's skin.

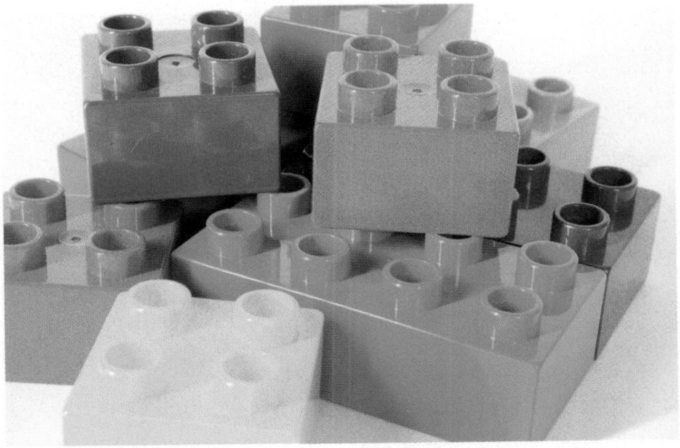

Figure 16–1 Building blocks of treatment.

The Building Blocks of Treatment

BLOCK 1—BASIC CLEANSE: All treatments start with removal of a client's makeup and then a complete facial cleansing. During this time, you continue to analyze and evaluate the client's skin.

BLOCK 2—TONERS/FRESHENERS: You can incorporate these blocks as needed throughout the treatment. The type of product will vary depending on whether your goal is to strip, pH balance, hydrate, or soothe the skin.

BLOCK 3—WATER: This step contributes to hydration of the skin and can be either stimulating or soothing. You can administer it using a steamer, compresses, spray device, or wet towels.

BLOCK 4—EXFOLIATION: You may use scrubs, enzymes, acids, or equipment to remove layers of dead stratum corneum. You may determine that more than one is necessary to achieve your treatment goal. Steam may be used to soften the skin and to keep an exfoliating agent, such as an enzyme, active.

BLOCK 5—MASSAGE: Massage duration and placement will vary with treatment goals. If you do massage before extraction, it stimulates the circulatory system and gets the body working with you. You may do massage after extraction, but you will have to take more care—using calming rather than stimulating movements—because the skin will already be stimulated.

BLOCK 6—EXTRACTION: While not a component in all treatments, extraction must be performed carefully and only when the skin is properly prepared for it. Generally extraction should be done after the skin is warmed and hydrated using steam or hot towels, stimulated, and exfoliated.

BLOCK 7—MASK: Depending on your goal for the client's skin, you can use masks that include enzymes, creams, gels, clays, and a host of other diverse technologies.

BLOCK 8—PENETRATION OF AMPOULES OR TREATMENT SERUMS: Use these as needed, depending on that client's skin and the goal for the treatment. While you might apply some nourishing serums at the end of a treatment, you can use a skin-calming or soothing serum multiple times if dealing with sensitive skin. You may also incorporate steam or sonophoresis equipment to soften and hydrate the skin.

BLOCK 9—PROTECTION (MOISTURIZATION AND SPF): Consider this finishing step as the smallest block, perfectly placed to top off the building project.

Using these building blocks or steps, you can create treatment guidelines based on your goals. Following are suggestions to help you create your own protocols.

Activity

Use these treatment ideas and the products you have available to you to create your own protocols for differing skin conditions.

For Dehydrated Skin

In very dehydrated skin the stratum corneum is more resistive to the penetration of products. Think of how little water a dry sponge will pick up as opposed to a moist one or how water runs off parched earth as opposed to how moist soil accepts it. One answer is to employ massage early in a treatment with hydrating serums under the massage vehicle; this can start to soften this skin and provide for a better exfoliation process. A second massage, this time using effleurage following exfoliation, enables better penetration of desired ampoules. Follow this by masking and finishing with protective creams or SPF products. Depending on the products and manufacturers' guidelines, you can decide on the number of uses of the toning building block. If you wish to incorporate equipment, a hydrating ultrasonic procedure or iontophoresis might be good choices.

FOCUS ON: *Dehydrated Skin Treatment*

- **Cleanse.**
- **Tone/freshen.**
- **Use hydrating ampoule.**
- **Massage, to help ampoule penetrate.**
- **Tone/freshen.**
- **Exfoliate.**
- **Tone/freshen.**
- **Use penetrating serums or ampoules.**
- **Massage.**
- **Use hydrating mask.**
- **Freshen.**
- **Apply protection.**

For Clogged Resistive Skin

Clogged resistive skin has a very different set of issues and re-arranging the blocks can allow you to better dilate follicles to facilitate extraction. First, administer a brief massage to stimulate circulation and activate the body's own self-cleansing mechanism, followed by exfoliation and then a warm stimulating mask to further dilate the impacted openings. Masking is followed with extraction and brief penetration of appropriate serums, finishing with a soothing mask and protection. This type of skin may require multiple treatments, and you may choose multiple modalities. Once you are familiar with the client's skin, you may perform microdermabrasion, ultrasonic treatments, galvanic desincrustation, or peels.

While the traditional approach of cleansing, exfoliating, extraction, and applying a clay mask will work for this skin type, the protocol shown below will also facilitate extraction and minimize residual redness.

FOCUS ON: *Clogged Resistive Skin*

- **Cleanse with massage to stimulate blood circulation.**
- **Apply stripping toner (so that exfoliant will better penetrate).**
- **Exfoliate.**
- **Use stimulating mask (to facilitate extraction).**
- **Extract.**
- **Apply antiseptic toner.**
- **Use penetrating ampoules or serums.**
- **Apply a calming mask.**
- **Apply protection.**

For Sensitive Skin

Sensitive skin requires a gentle approach. The first objective is to reduce redness, irritation, or skin reactivity that may have been triggered by dehydration or very reactive nerve endings. (As you recall from *Fundamentals*, skin sensitivities may result from internal or external factors.) Eliminate extraction at least until the you are comfortable with the response of the client's skin. Massage should be effleurage only. While you may incorporate exfoliation, it should be a product compatible with this skin type. Often a gentle enzyme exfoliant is the best choice. Do not use physical scrubs or abrasive mechanical devices. Following exfoliation, apply soothing serums to the skin, followed by masking. This is a skin that responds better to a gel, cream, or collagen sheet mask. Since ultrasonic treatments are non-irritating and hydrating, this device generally promotes a good skin response from the sensitive skin client. For the complete protocol, see Procedure 16–2.

FOCUS ON: *Sensitive Skin*

- **Cleanse with gentle effleurage.**
- **Apply gentle toner/freshener.**
- **Use soothing serum (to help skin tolerate exfoliation).**
- **Apply enzyme exfoliant.**
- **Use soothing toner.**
- **Use penetrating soothing serums or ampoules.**
- **Apply calming mask.**
- **Apply protection.**

FYI

These are just three examples of protocols you can create based on skin conditions. Use this format to create additional protocols for specific skin conditions.

Treatment Arc and Theory

When you go to the gym and work with a fitness trainer, he or she has you follow a pattern for a safe and effective routine. First they will have you warm up, then do the workout, and then finish with a cool down. The trainer will always have you follow this pattern to prevent injury, but variety is necessary for effective cross-training, so in the workout the trainer will vary the routine to ensure that you exercise all muscles and not just a few.

Here's a Tip

Like cross-training the body, cross-training the skin works wonders.

These fitness activities can be seen as forming an arc: starting with the warm up, rising to the workout, and finishing with the cool down (Figure 16–2). You can apply this same arc structure to activities in the treatment room. The initial cleanse warms and prepares the client's skin, and the massage, exfoliation, extraction and penetration steps stimulate the circulatory system. When you reach the finishing mask, the client should be in cool-down mode. This slows down the circulatory system and ensures that he or she doesn't leave the clinic with a pink or red face. If you wish to use a clay mask to complete the treatment, applying a cool wet towel on top of it prevents the mask from drying. The benefits of the clay are maintained but the removal process is now in sync with the cool-down pattern rather than a stimulating one. If you have a client that you feel must have a drying clay mask, soak the mask with a tepid towel or cotton compresses to soften it and facilitate removal. Avoid rubbing.

You can add diversity to a treatment by timing components and not following the same protocol every time. As the client's skin improves, you can change the focus of the treatment from sensitive skin to dealing with congestion, signs of aging, and so on. You can use an enzyme in one treatment and use ultrasonic, microdermabrasion, or an AHA in another. Just as when you do a variety of exercises for the body, you can keep the client's skin more responsive and achieve better results when you incorporate diversity into treatments. It is cross-training for the face.

Here's a Tip

Educate your clients that you can be their facial fitness trainer. It will help clients understand their specialized treatment programs.

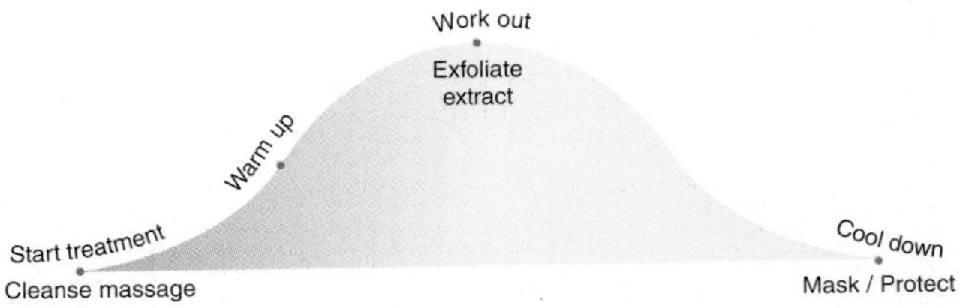

Figure 16–2 Treatment arc.

Thermotherapy and Pressure Therapy

Both of these therapies employ the activation or calming of the body's natural self-cleansing mechanism—the circulatory system. Temperature is an effective way to enhance treatment results. Hot steam, stones, or hot, wet towels stimulate the circulatory system. Likewise, cool steam, Lucas spray, cool stones, or cool towels are vasoconstrictive. Wrapping the face in hot, wet towels is not a new technology, but it is a valuable one (Figure 16–3). Not only is there a heat effect, but the towels add a layer of occlusion to better penetrate the product underneath. The base towel should feel hot to the client but not uncomfortable. To keep that towel warm, add a second one on top of it. This towel can be as hot as you can handle. To prevent irriation, do not allow this towel to touch the client's skin directly. The weight of these towels adds the benefit of pressure therapy. This is the same philosophy as placing a warm stone on a muscle, triggering slow relaxation.

The temperature of cold wet towels can be divided into three categories: cool, cold, and refrigerator cold. The cool range would be just below tepid. This will feel cool to the skin but not shocking. For a stronger skin response, use a towel soaked in very cold water. Some therapists like to keep a supply of wet towels in a plastic bag in the refrigerator. This level of cold causes the strongest skin response. Warn the client that the towel will feel very cold, but if the skin is red or irritated, it will quickly adjust and feel very soothed. The towel will also reduce redness and irritation.

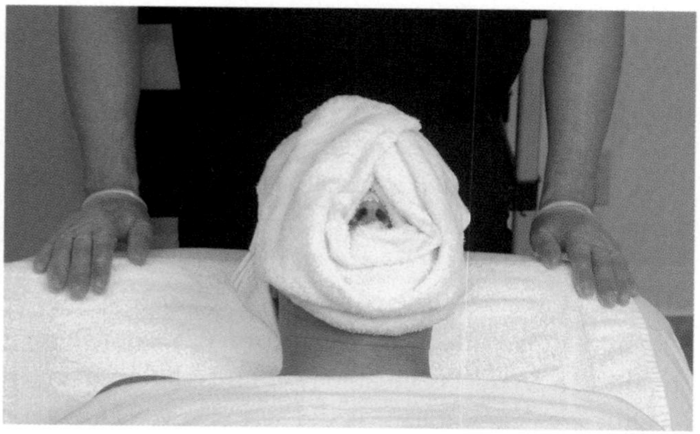

Figure 16–3 Face wrapped in double hot towels.

CAUTION!

Always alert the client before applying a hot or cold towel and make sure the temperature is acceptable to them.

PROCEDURE 16–1 THERMOTHERAPY FOR CLOGGED PORES

This procedure is designed to prepare and soften the impactions for extraction. Thermotherapy facilitates this process and calms the skin following the procedure.

IMPLEMENTS AND MATERIALS

- Cleanser to remove makeup
- Stimulating massage vehicle
- Antiseptic toner
- Typical facial lounge, client draping, and linen setup
- Gloves
- Disposable compresses, cloths, or sponges for removing product
- Water and bowl
- Steamer (optional)

Preparation

1. Set up the facial lounge with linens.
2. Prepare towels and cotton and gather supplies.
3. Decant and set up products.

Procedure

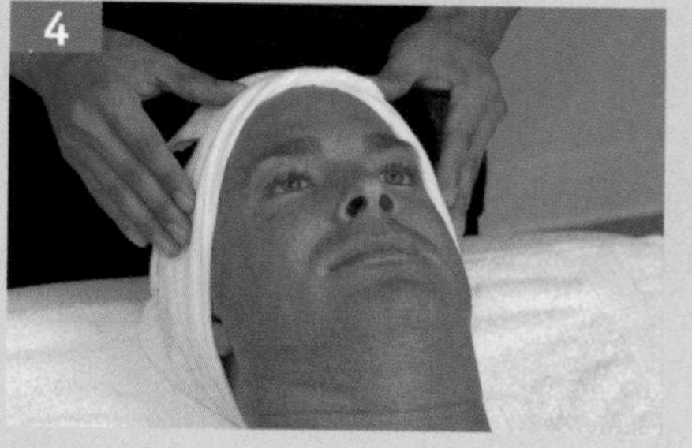

Prepare client.

4. Prepare the client for treatment.

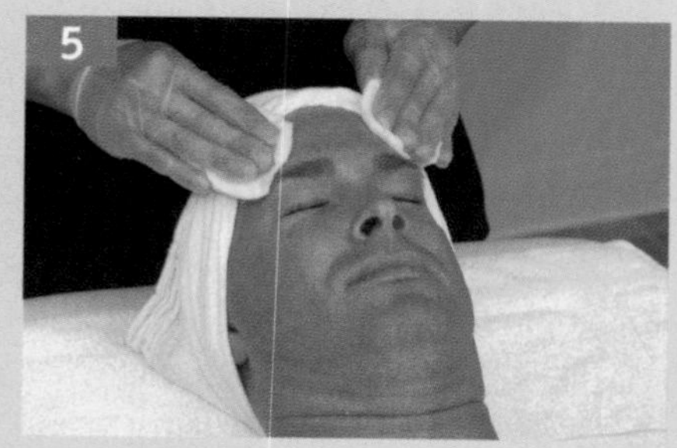

Moisten the skin.

5. Cleanse. Moisten the skin using warm cotton compresses or sponges.

- Treatment brush
- Enzyme exfoliant
- Cotton swabs or comedo extractor
- Serum to facilitate extraction
- Serum to soothe or calm the skin
- Hydrating serum
- Cool globes, high-frequency or sonophoresis
- Hot wet towels
- Cool wet towels
- Sun protection

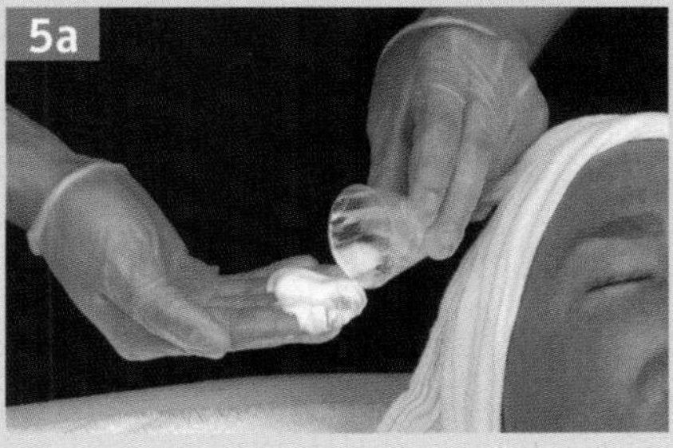

Apply a cleanser.

a. Apply a cleanser suitable to remove makeup with your gloved hands (optional).

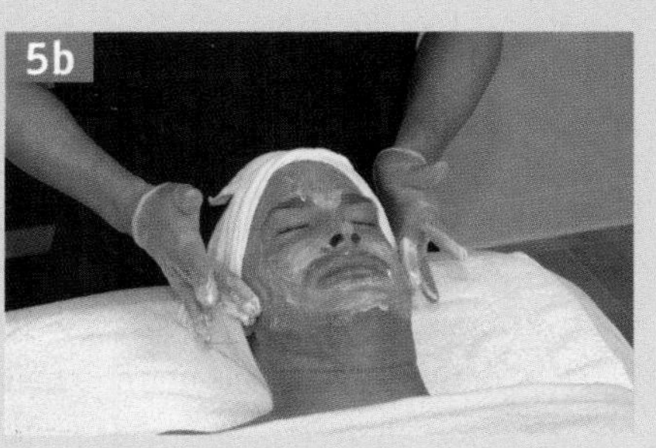

Massage the cleanser.

b. Massage the cleanser to loosen makeup.

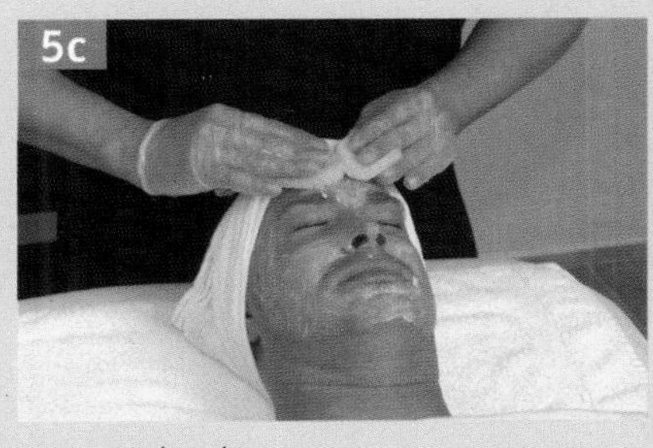

Remove the cleanser.

c. Remove the cleanser using warm cloth, sponges, or compresses.

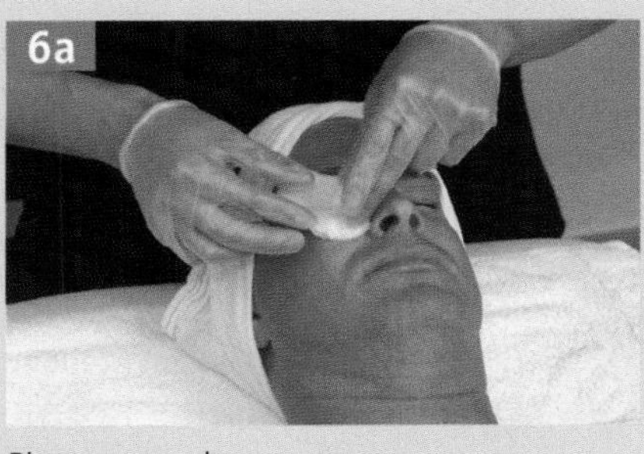

Place eye pads on eyes.

6 Analysis and consultation

a. Place moistened eye pads on eyes.

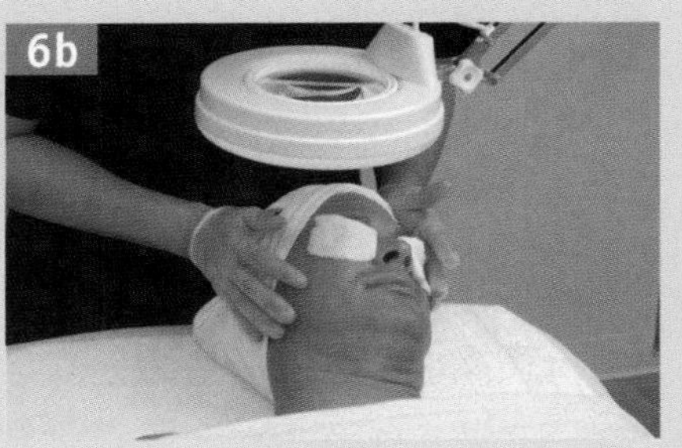

Examine skin.

b. Examine the client's skin under magnifying lamp. Observe for the level of sensitivity and skin response to cleansing. Confirm that the selected products will be appropriate.

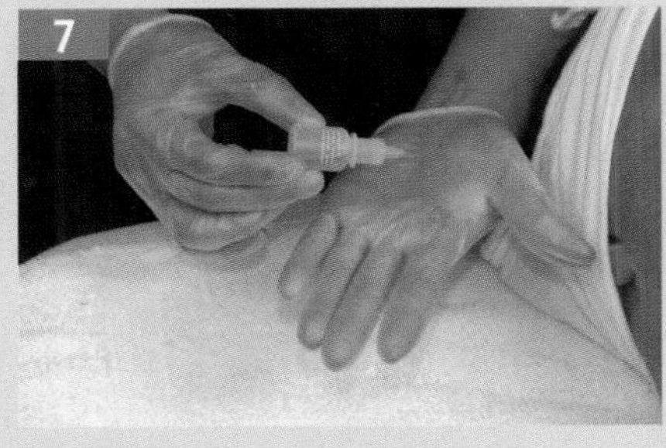

Apply a serum.

7 Apply a serum designed to loosen impactions. If you use warm steam, stand at a distance of 18 to 20 inches from the client's face.

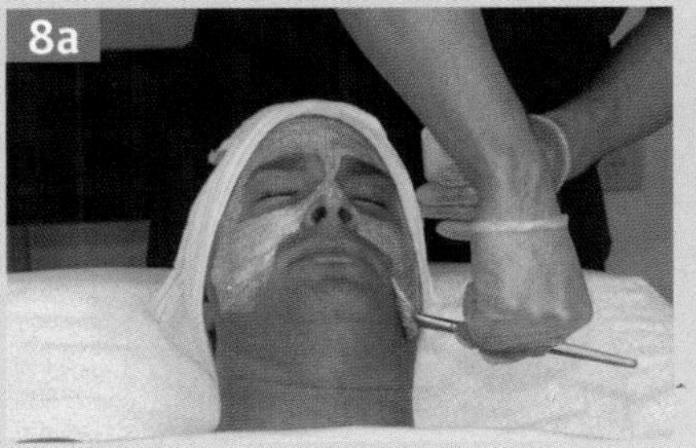

Use an enzyme exfoliant.

8 Exfoliation

a. Use an enzyme exfoliant following manufacturer's guidelines.

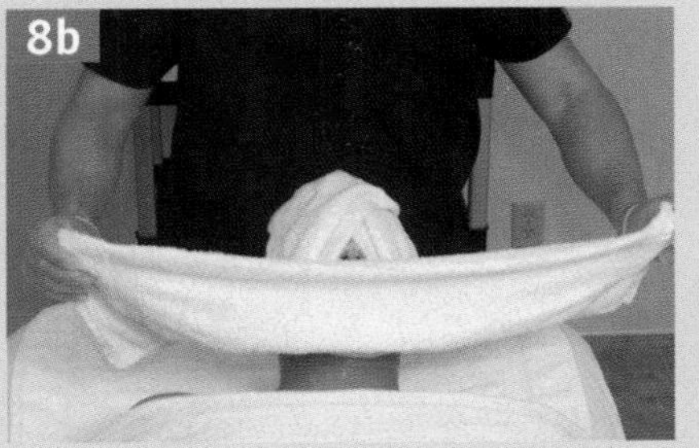

Wrap the face in a classical barber warp.

b. Wrap the face in two hot towels in a classical barber wrap. The first towel should

continues on next page

PROCEDURE 16-1, CONT. THERMOTHERAPY FOR CLOGGED PORES

be hot but comfortable. Place the second towel on top of the first. It should be as hot as you can handle.

c. Leave the towel on the skin approximately 8 to 10 minutes. If the towel cools too quickly, use steam to keep it warm or replace the top towel with a fresh one.

8e

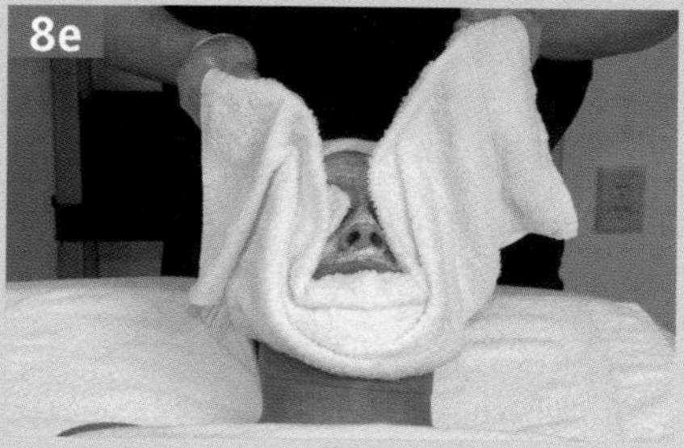

Remove enzyme.

d. Remove top towel.

e. Use the lower towel to remove enzyme from the skin.

9b

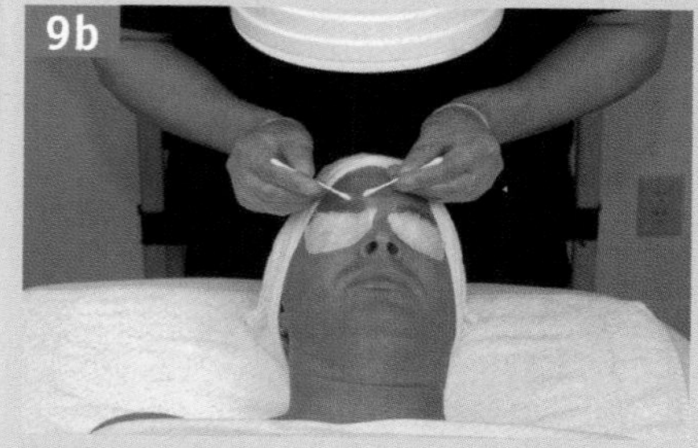

Perform extraction.

9 Extraction. Before starting, refresh gloves if necessary.

a. Apply a pre-extraction serum if desired. Follow manufacturer's guidelines.

b. Use cotton swab technique or comedone extractor to perform extraction.

9b-1

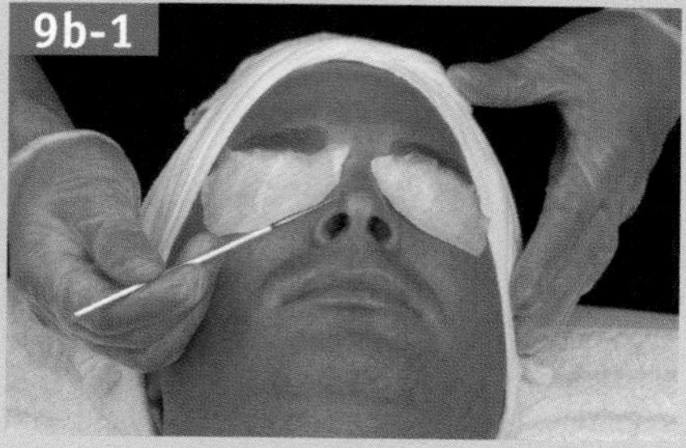

Continue to perform extractions.

c. If skin begins to welt, redden severely, or swell, stop extraction immediately.

d. Limit the extraction to 5 to 10 minutes only, particularly during the first visit.

10

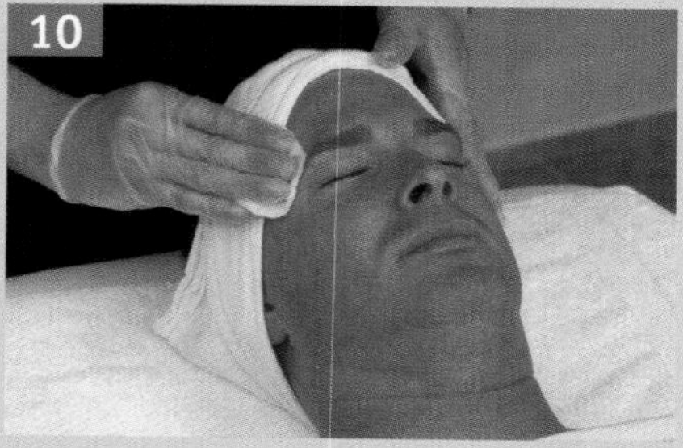

Wipe skin with toner.

10 Wipe the skin with an antiseptic toner.

11a

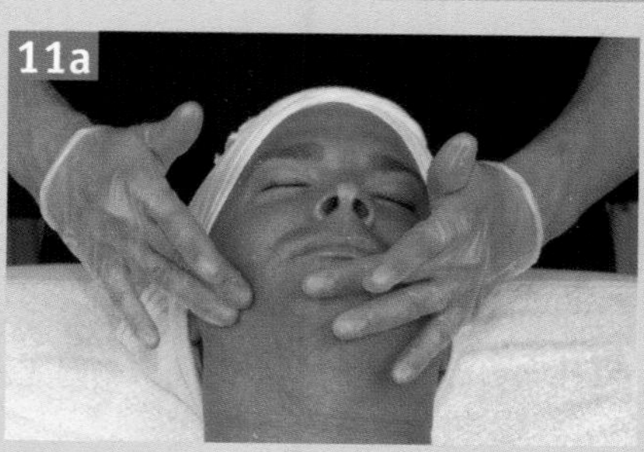

Apply serum.

11 Calm.

a. Apply soothing serum.

11b

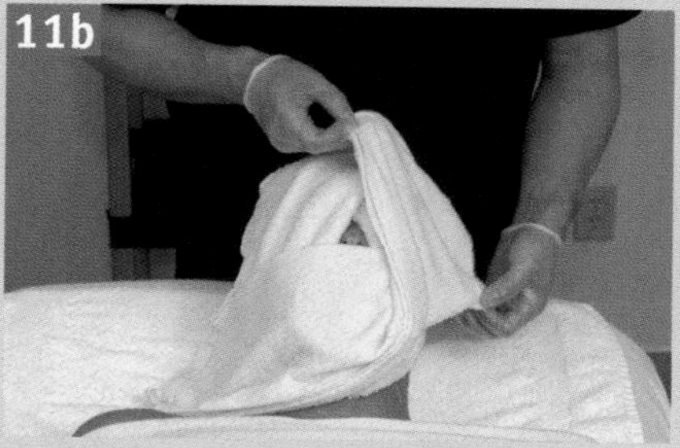

Apply cold wet towels.

b. Apply cold wet towels wrapping the face in classical barber wrap. As an alternative, you can use cold globes, slowly stroking across the entire face, one area at a time.

11d

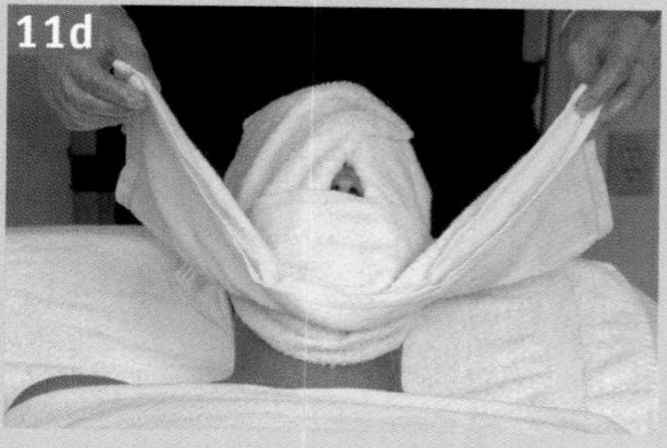

Remove towels.

c. Allow the skin to calm about 10 minutes.

d. Remove towels.

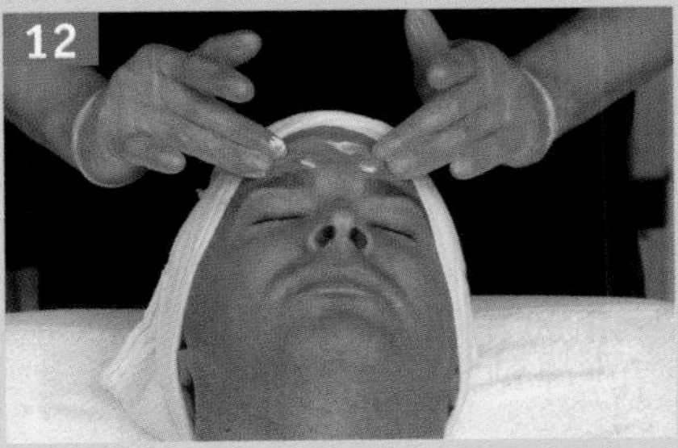

Apply sunscreen.

12 Apply a hydrating fluid and sunscreen.

Post-procedure

13 Advise the client to treat any extracted area carefully, avoiding touching it to minimize contamination with bacteria.

14 Remind the client to avoid the sun.

15 Determine if the client is using appropriate home-care products for his or her skin.

Clean-up and Disinfection

16 Follow clean-up and disinfection procedures in accordance with state guidelines.

17 Reset and prepare the room for the next client.

ROSACEA AND SENSITIVE SKIN TREATMENTS

Not all clients who have sensitive skin will have rosacea, but all clients who have rosacea will have sensitive skin.

Treatment Concepts for Sensitive Skin

There are several basic concepts that are widely accepted when treating sensitive skin:

1. Be very careful to protect the barrier function of the skin. Use products that support the barrier function, and avoid any product or procedure that might strip or impair it, including strong foaming soaps and cleansers.
2. Avoid materials, products, or procedures that are known to irritate and sensitize skin (see Chapter 10). This includes fragrances, certain preservatives, many "natural" ingredients, stimulating products, or products that can injure the barrier function, such as strong soaps, surfactants, solvents, and emulsifiers. Avoid any ingredient to which the client has had a previous allergic or irritant reaction.
3. Use products that have been shown through independent testing to have low irritancy potential. This means that the product has been determined to be unlikely to cause irritation or allergy. It does *not* mean that the product is appropriate for every client. Remember, somewhere in the world, there is someone allergic to any given ingredient.
4. Incorporate products with ingredients that have been shown to decrease sensitivity. These include chamomile extract, cornflower extract, licorice extract, bisabolol, matricaria extract, and azulene. Also, look for ingredients that protect or enhance the barrier function, such as lipid complexes.

Treatment Contraindications for Treating Sensitive Skin

It is advisable to avoid the following procedures when treating clients with sensitive or redness-prone skin:

1. Avoid heat exposure, including close or prolonged exposure to steam. A cool steamer may be helpful in providing the hydration of steam without the heat.
2. Avoid paraffin, electric heat masks, or exothermic mineral-type heating masks.
3. Avoid extremely cold compresses.
4. Use non-fragranced products. Fragrances are the number one cause of cosmetic skin allergies and may also be irritants.
5. Microdermabrasion, brushing machines, enzyme treatments, gommages (roll-off treatment products), and granular scrubs may be too aggressive.
6. Use of low pH exfoliation chemicals, such as low pH alpha hydroxy (AHA or glycolic) acid or enzymes. AHA exfoliants with pHs of 3.5 or greater (check the MSDS sheet or manufacturer labeling) are usually acceptable as long has the client's skin is not already inflamed. When in doubt, do not use it! Avoid exfoliating sensitive skin too often.

7. Avoid waxing on sensitive skin.
8. Avoid prolonged or vigorous massage, such as petrissage or any deep or rapid manipulation, which may be too stimulating and increase redness. Effleurage, shiatsu, gentle tapotement, and manual or machine lymph drainage (if you are trained on this technique) are usually acceptable for use on sensitive skin.
9. Avoid overdrying masks or leaving clay masks on too long. Drying clay masks are often not appropriate for sensitive skin.
10. Many essential oils or aromatherapy products may be too stimulating for sensitive skin.
11. Extraction must be gentle and limited to a brief period to avoid redness. As you become better acquainted with an individual client's skin, you can adapt procedures.
12. Avoid heavily mentholated or alcohol-based treatment products.
13. Avoid using isopropyl or SD alcohol-containing products on sensitive skin.

PROCEDURE 16–2 TREATMENT FOR SENSITIVE SKIN

IMPLEMENTS AND MATERIALS

- Typical facial lounge, client draping, and linen setup
- Gloves
- Cotton compresses (Sponges and other cleansing implements are often too rough-textured for sensitive skin.)
- Water and bowl
- Gentle cleanser
- Non-fragranced hydrating fluid for sensitive skin
- Steamer (optional)
- Treatment brush
- Exfoliant (optional; must be mild)
- Cotton swabs for extraction, if necessary
- Gentle alcohol-free freshener
- Serum for sensitive skin
- Cool globes, high-frequency or sonophoresis
- Non-setting mask for sensitive skin (gel, wet collagen blanket, dry collagen sheet, etc.)
- Sun protection

Preparation

1 Set up the facial lounge with linens.

2 Prepare towels and cotton and gather supplies.

3 Decant or set up products.

3
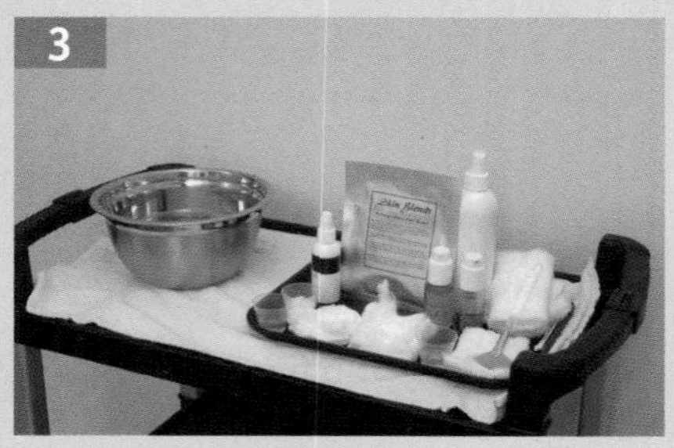

Set up products.

Procedure

4
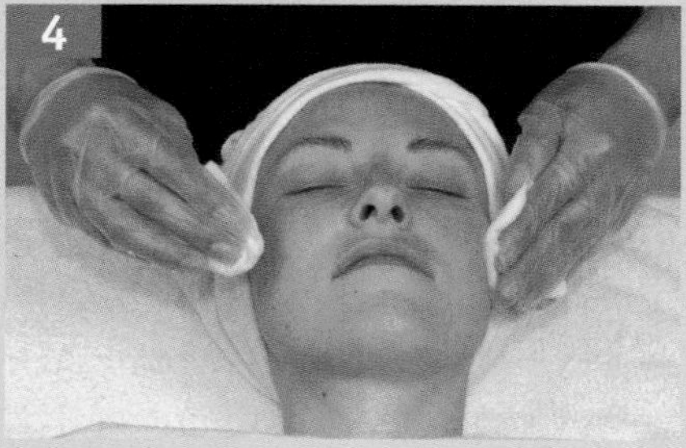

Dampen the skin.

4a
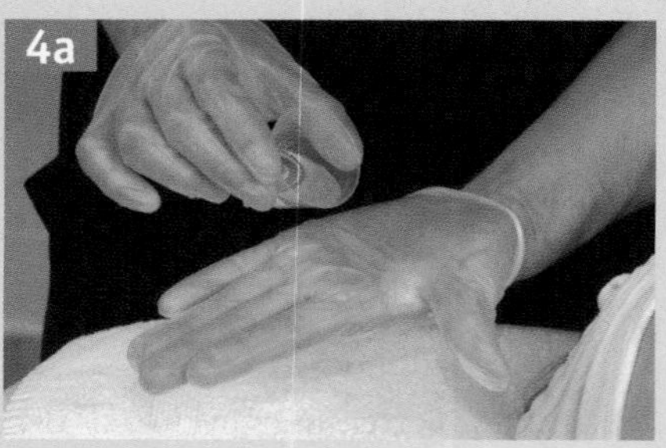

Apply cleanser.

4 Cleanse. Dampen the skin using cool (not cold), wet cotton compresses.

a. Apply a gentle, non-fragranced cleanser with your gloved hands.

4b
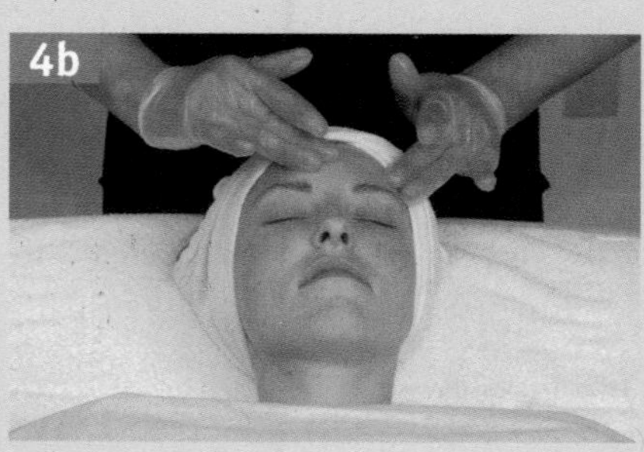

Massage the cleanser.

4c
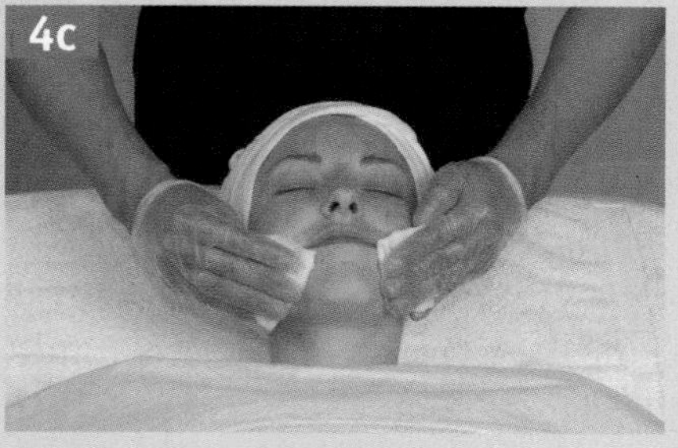

Remove the cleanser.

b. Gently massage the cleanser using light effleurage.

c. Remove the cleanser using cool, wet cotton pads.

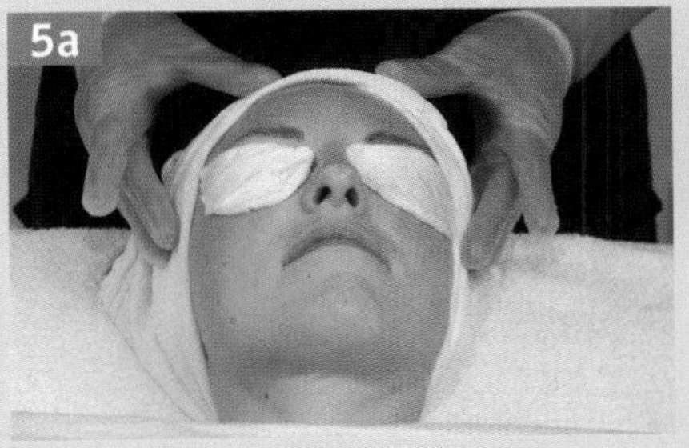

Place eye pads on eyes.

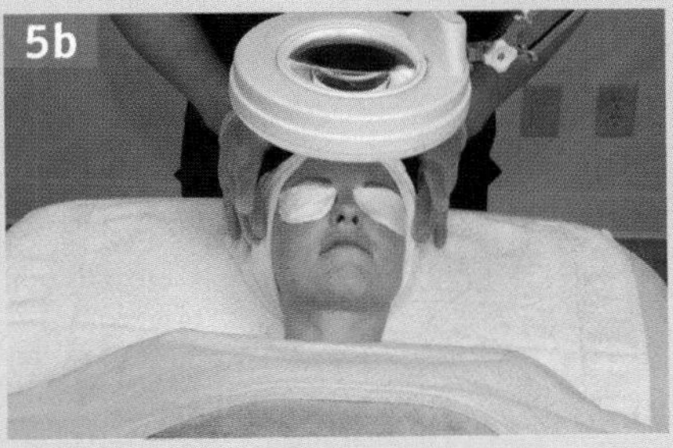

Examine skin.

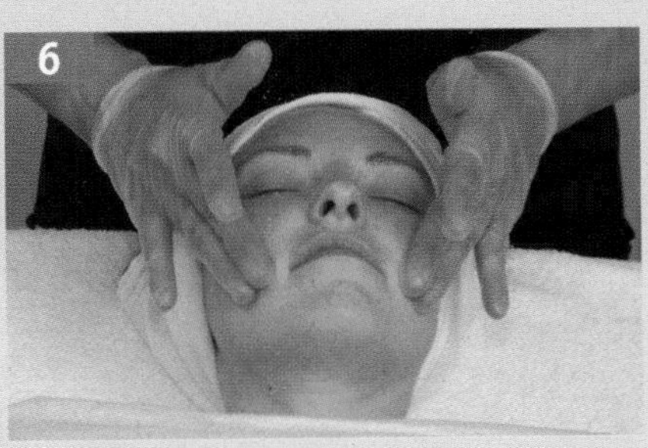

Apply hydrating fluid.

5 Analysis and consultation

a. Place moistened eye pads on eyes.

b. Examine skin under magnifying loop. Observe for level of sensitivity and skin response to cleansing. Confirm that selected products will be appropriate.

6 Apply a lightweight, non-fragranced hydrating fluid designed for sensitive skin to the face.

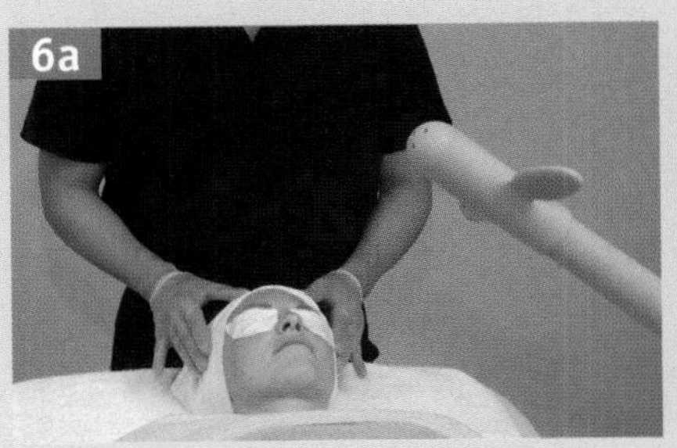

Steam should be used 18 to 20 inches from the face.

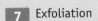

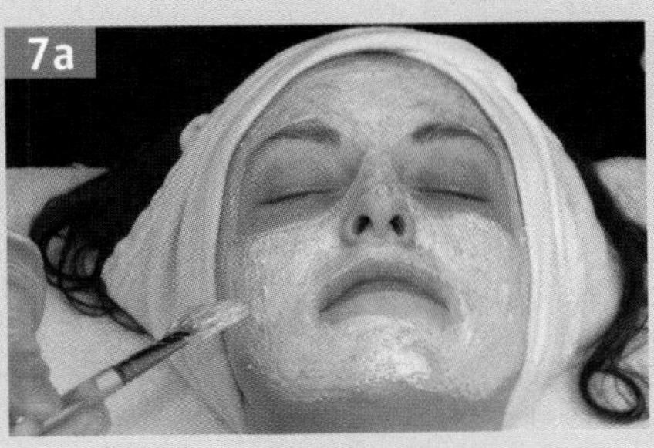

Use a gentle enzyme exfoliant.

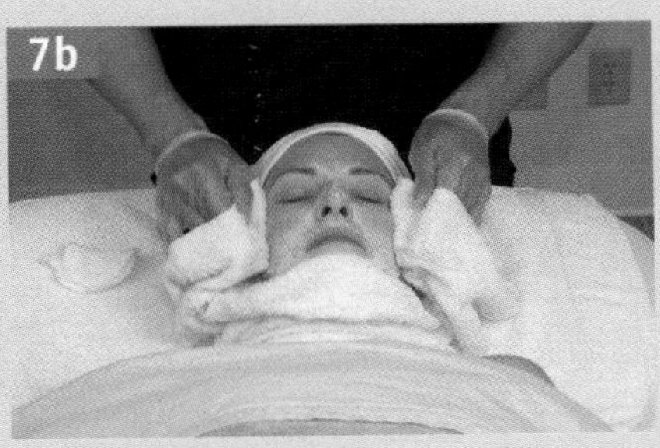

Remove the exfoliant.

a. If you use warm steam, stand at a distance of 18 to 20 inches from the face and use for only a few minutes.

b. Cool steam, if available, is preferable.

7 Exfoliation

a. Use a gentle enzyme exfoliant following manufacturer's guidelines. (Please note that exfoliation is not appropriate for most sensitive skin types.)

b. Remove the exfoliant with lukewarm towels, disposable sponges, or gauze. Follow manufacturer's guidelines.

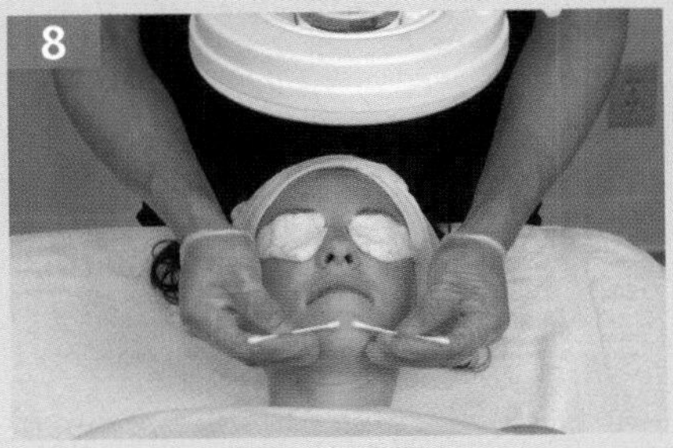

Perform gentle extractions.

8 You can perform gentle extraction using the cotton swab technique. Avoid using comedone extractors on sensitive skin.

a. If skin begins to welt, redden severely, or swell, stop extraction immediately.

b. Extraction should be limited to 3 to 4 minutes only, particularly during the first visit.

continues on next page

PROCEDURE 16-2, CONT. TREATMENT FOR SENSITIVE SKIN

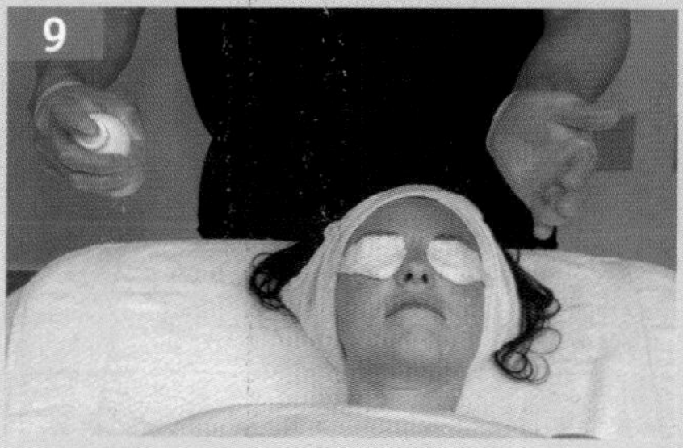

Spray skin with toner.

9 Spray the skin with a mild, non-fragranced, non-alcohol toner designed for sensitive skin.

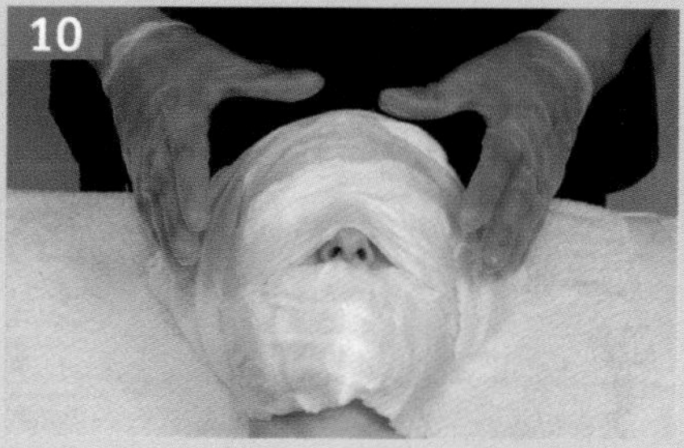

Calm the skin.

10 Calm. If the skin is still very red after extraction, apply cool, wet compresses for about 5 minutes. Do *not* apply any product.

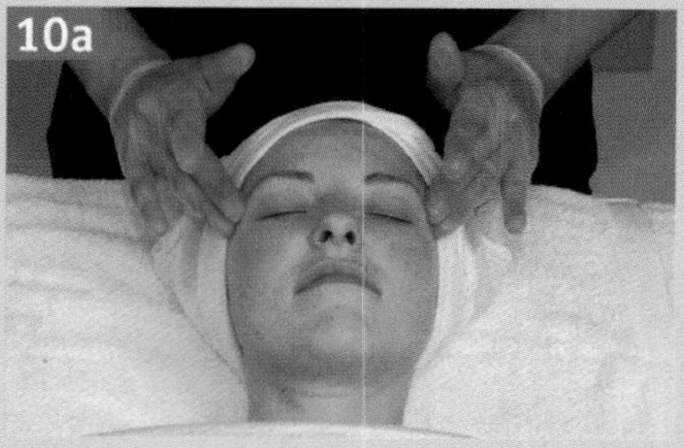

Apply hydrating fluid or serum.

a. After the skin has cooled down, apply a non-fragranced hydrating fluid or serum designed for sensitive skin.

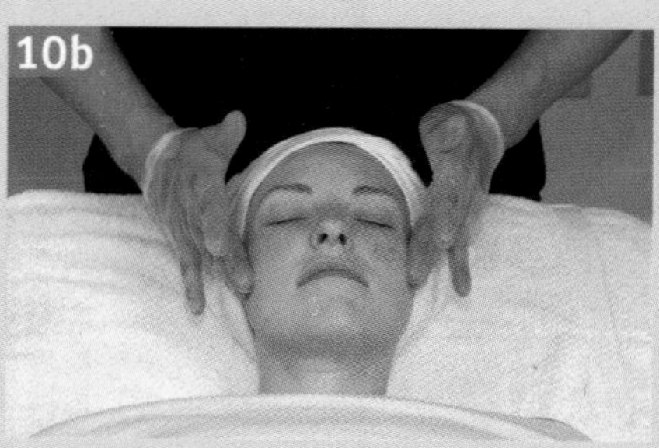

Gently massage the face.

b. With gentle movements such as effleurage, massage the face for a short period of time, using the fluid as the treatment product for massage. If redness increases, discontinue the massage immediately and remove the product with cool, wet cotton compresses.

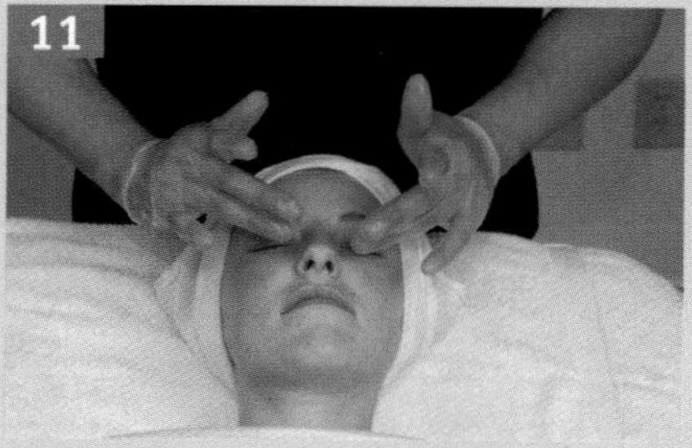

Apply hydrating fluid/serum.

11 Treat. Apply hydrating fluid/serum designed for sensitive skin (if the skin is not still inflamed).

a. Unfold a 4×4 piece of gauze and place across the client's face. Move cool globes over the gauze to help the hydrating fluid penetrate. Do *not* apply the globes without the gauze buffering the contact.

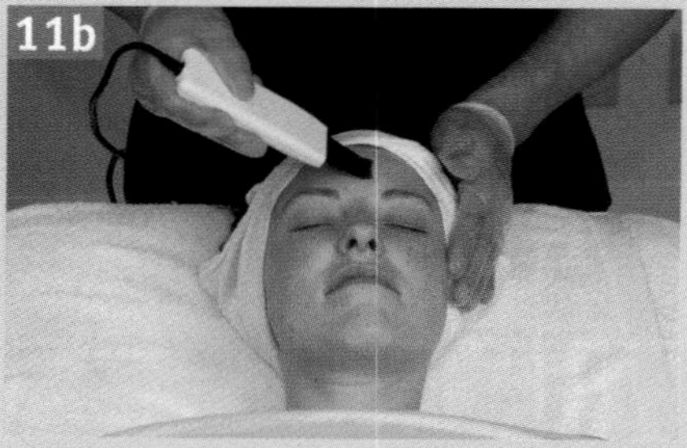

Sonophoresis may be used in place of a mask.

Treatment should be cool but not cold.

OR

b. As an alternative, perform sonophoresis at low settings. This may be used in place of a mask step. Be sure to follow manufacturer's guidelines.

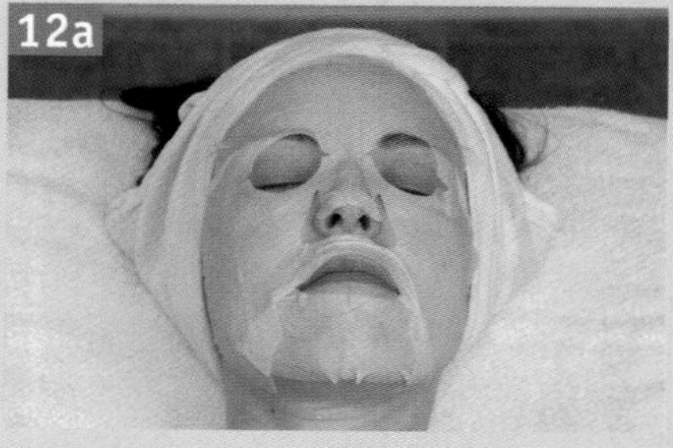

Wet collagen mask in place.

12 Mask

a. Apply a non-setting, non-drying, non-fragranced gel mask designed specifically for sensitive skin. It should contain soothing agents such as matricaria, chamomile, or licorice extract. If using wet or dry collagen, follow manufacturer's directions.

b. Allow the mask to sit on the face for 10–20 minutes. Check frequently with the client to

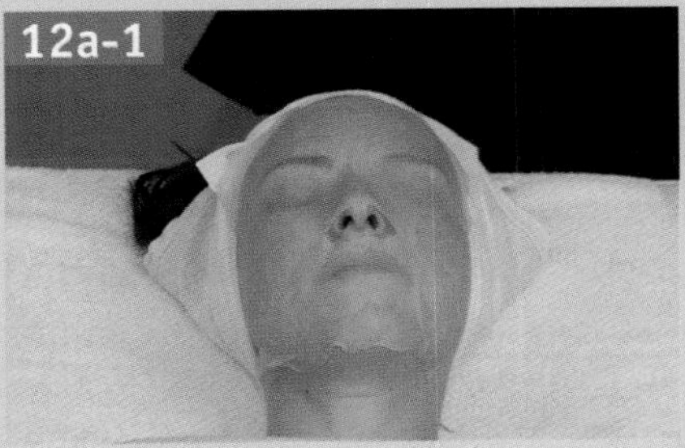

Dry collagen mask in place.

make sure the treatment is not stinging or burning.

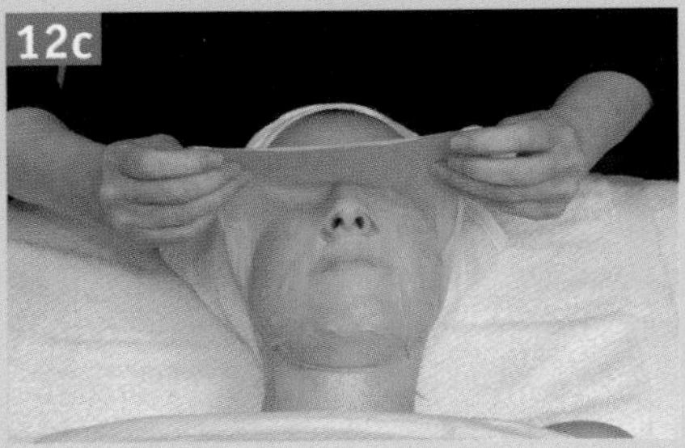

Remove the mask.

c. Remove the mask with cool, wet cotton pads. Collagen blankets can simply be lifted off.

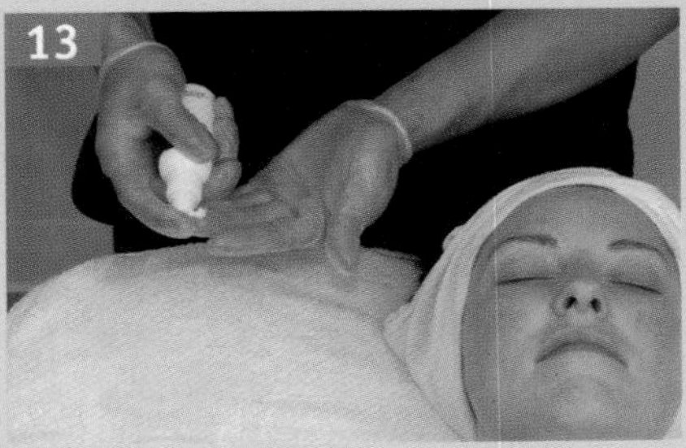

Apply a moisturizer and sunscreen.

13 Apply a gentle, non-fragranced hydrating fluid and sunscreen.

Post-procedure

14 It is best to avoid applying makeup immediately after a treatment on sensitive skin. Suggest that the client wait at least 2 hours before makeup application to minimize skin reaction.

15 Remind the client to avoid the sun.

16 Determine if the client is using home-care products that are appropriate for sensitive skin.

Clean-up and Disinfection

17 Follow clean-up and disinfection procedures in accordance with state guidelines.

18 Disinfect and prepare the room for the next client.

Client Reactions in the Treatment Room

Occasionally, a client will experience a reaction in the treatment room. Most reactions are irritant reactions and are mild. This is different from what a true allergy produces. A client may complain of a particular product stinging or burning. Some products such as alpha hydroxy acids are supposed to cause a mild tingling sensation. Most of the time these minor sensations quickly dissipate.

Red, rashy, and swollen skin, however, is not normal. Severe burning and stinging are not normal. If a client experiences extreme burning, redness, or swelling, remove whatever is on the face immediately with cool cotton pads. Apply cool, wet compresses or spray atomized water on the skin to soothe it. Many times simply removing the irritant greatly reduces the inflammation. If a client has a reaction, it is best to end the treatment. Applying further products, even if you are trying to help, may only aggravate the reaction. Use only cool water or compresses. Wait several days until the reaction has completely subsided before trying a different plan. As always, refer clients with severe reactions to a dermatologist.

Rules for the Retinoid Client

Retinoid users are among those with sensitive or sensitized skin. Here are some guidelines for dealing with this skin type.

1. Tretinoin and tazarotene and other prescribed retinoids are prescription drugs. The client must follow the advice of the dermatologist regarding usage.
2. Clients using retinoids may find that they are more sensitive to cosmetic and skin care products and procedures. Guide the client to choose soothing hydrating products and ingredients that can co-exist with retinoids.
3. Facial treatments may need to be adapted for the patient using a retinoid. This includes discontinuing the use of any exfoliation treatment; using gentle,

fragrance-free hydrators; and avoiding heat and any alcoholic or stimulating skin care products.

4. Redness and peeling are normal transitional side effects, particularly when a client is first using a prescription retinoid. These side effects can be minimized with the use of good hydrators and by being careful with the amount and frequency of application of the retinoid. Some patients find it helpful to "phase in" retinoids, using the retinoid every second or third night and slowly switching to every night.
5. Clients using retinoids should avoid sun completely. Deliberate sun exposure is contraindicated and counter productive.
6. Avoid using scented and fragranced products, alcohol-based lotions, stripping products, abrasive scrubs, microdermabrasion, alpha hydroxy or beta hydroxy acid products, benzoyl peroxide, sulfur-resorcinol, and other exfoliating agents on clients who are using retinoids.
7. *Do not wax clients who are using retinoids!* After the transitional side effects have passed, electrolysis is usually acceptable.

CLINIC EXFOLIATION TREATMENTS

Clinic exfoliation treatments use either chemical or physical exfoliation methods. They may include the use of scrubs, manual microdermabrasion, equipment exfoliation, enzymes, AHA or BHA products. Chemical exfoliation is sometimes appropriate when mechanical exfoliation is not appropriate. While the client may use the term *peel* to describe these services, they are actually forms of superficial exfoliation.

Manual Microdermabrasion

Manual microdermabrasion is a technique that is rather like a classic scrub on steroids. It is used both by estheticians and medi-spa staff. Studies have documented that the use of microdermabrasion as the exfoliating step in a treatment can improve the appearance of the skin and has a side benefit of enhancing collagen production, possibly caused by the vertical massage and the suction activity. More recently, anecdotal studies have noted that a manual method of this microdermabrasion can produce similar benefits. However, individual results depend on the skill of the technician performing the service. Just as machine pressure may vary with each stroke, so do hand strokes vary in pressure and intensity.

There are a variety of products available for manual microdermabrasion. These vary from loose crystals to creams or gels with a crystal incorporated. With loose crystals, you must take care as the crystals tend to creep into the hairline and orifices, such as the mouth and ears. This is a similar problem with the machine devices that use crystals. Because of the issue of crystals ending up in the ears and mouth, some manufacturers have developed special bases as carriers for aluminum oxide, salts, or pumice crystals. Crystals are more angular than the components of traditional scrubs, allowing for more intensive exfoliation of the stratum corneum. The carrier base facilitates removal and enhances the gommage-style technique used to do the treatment.

The esthetician administering a manual microdermabrasion treatment controls the result with the amount of pressure applied in the strokes and the number of repeated strokes in any area. For best results, you want to make strokes as alike as possible in terms of pressure. Treat more sensitive skins with lighter pressure and more resistive skins with deeper pressure. Stretch a section of skin very taunt between the fingers of one hand and use firm rolling strokes with the other hand (Figure 16–4).

Just as when using machine microdermabrasion, you divide the client's face into areas, and then you systematically work your way around the face. Generally, you make about 10 strokes in each area of the skin (Figure 16–5). If no redness results, you may perform an

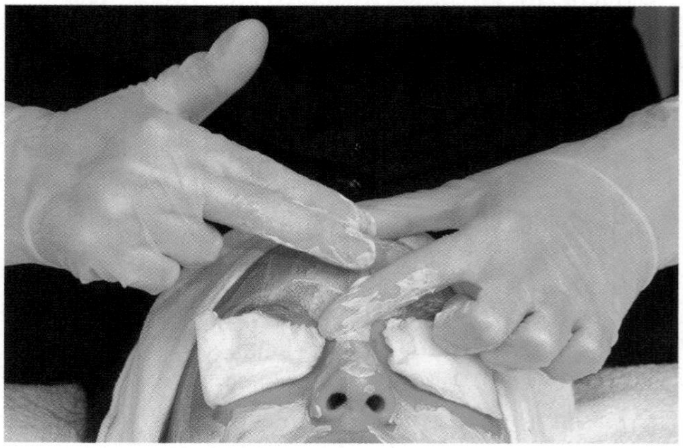

Figure 16–4 Manual microdermabrasion in process, showing the stretch and stroke.

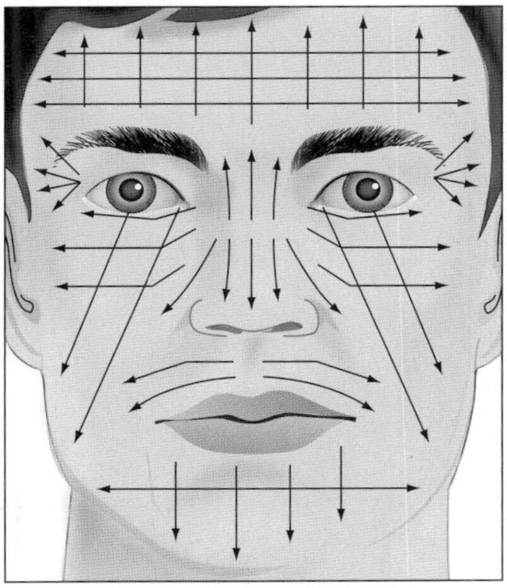

Figure 16–5 Showing direction of strokes in each area of the face.

additional 10 strokes. Make the strokes deep and firm, and roll the fingers from first to little finger in a scooping action. When you have treated the entire face, remove the product and resume the facial treatment.

CAUTION!

Always wear gloves when performing this or any other exfoliation technique.

PROCEDURE 16–3 MANUAL MICRODERMABRASION

Manual microdermabrasion is an exfoliating scrub treatment and may be a useful alternative for clients in salons or spas where machine devices are not allowed or where equipment is not available. It may be employed as the scrub/exfoliation step in a facial treatment.

IMPLEMENTS AND MATERIALS

- Facial lounge, client draping, and linen setup
- Disposable sponges, cotton compresses, or facial cloths
- Water and bowl
- Gloves
- Cotton rounds
- Cotton gauze squares (optional)
- Cleanser to remove makeup
- Cleansing massage product
- Microdermabrasion scrub
- Toner (appropriate for client skin)
- Serum(s)
- Moisturizer and sunscreen

Preparation

1 Set up the facial lounge with linens.

2 Prepare towels and cotton and gather supplies.

3 Decant or set up products.

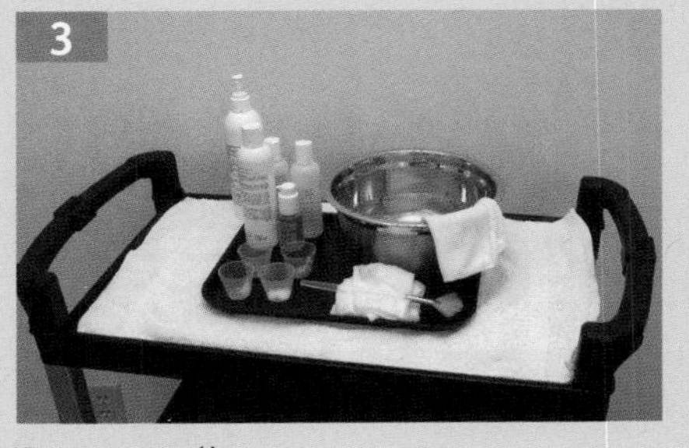

Set up supplies.

Procedure

4 Wash and disinfect your hands.

5 Cleanse. Remove all makeup and prepare for skin evaluation.

a. Remove eye makeup and lipstick with cleansing agent and cotton rounds.

b. Remove face makeup with cleansing lotion. Rinse with wet sponges or warm moist towels.

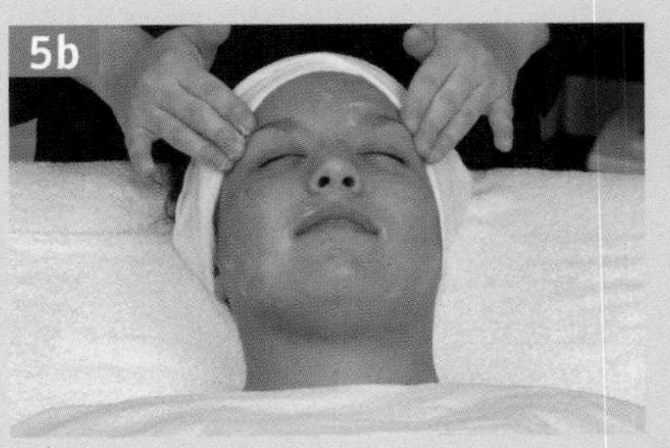

Remove makeup.

continues on next page

PROCEDURE 16–3, CONT. MANUAL MICRODERMABRASION

5c
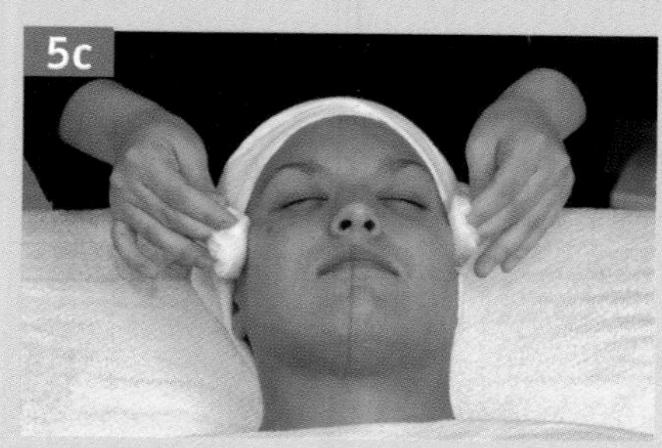
Wipe face with toner.

c. Wipe face with cotton pads soaked in toner.

6a
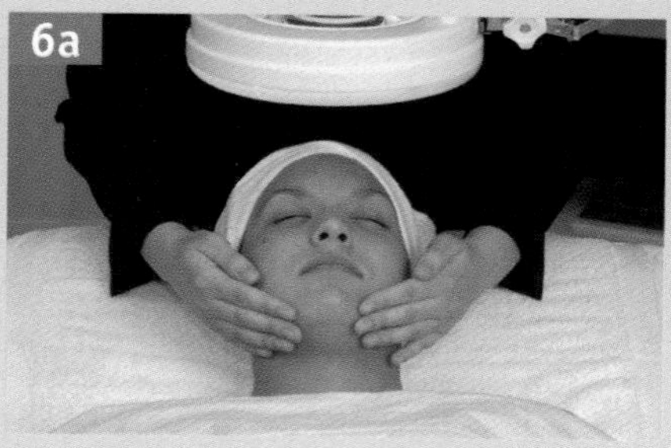
Perform skin analysis.

6 Analysis and consultation

a. Reevaluate the client's skin to assure this is an appropriate treatment for his or her skin at this time.

b. Discuss possible results with the client and confirm the appropriateness of the treatment before continuing. Make home care suggestions and discuss a treatment series, if appropriate.

7
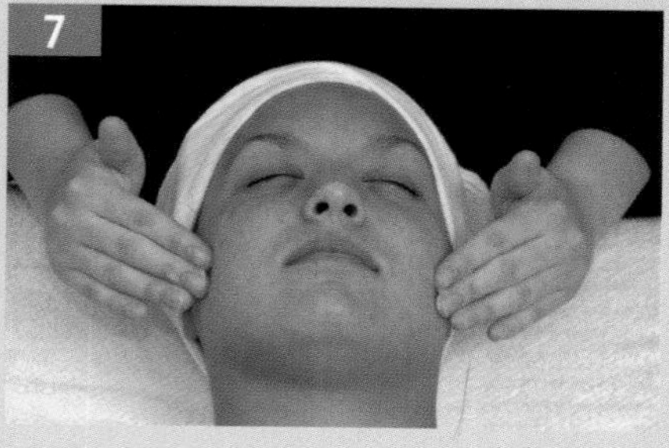
Massage.

7 Massage. Perform massage as usual for your treatment.

8a
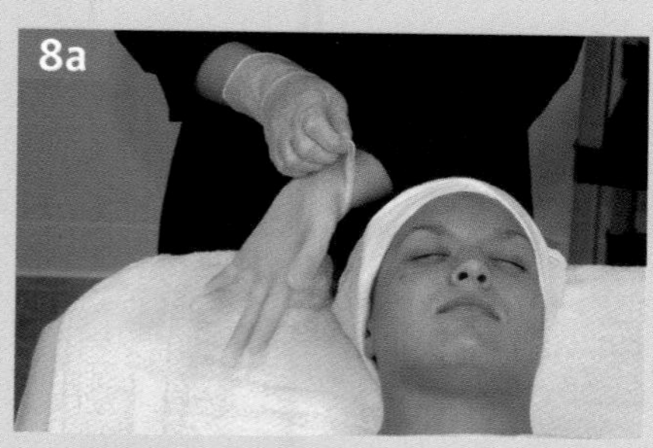
Apply eye protection.

8 Manual microdermabrasion

a. Put on gloves and then apply eye protection on the client.

8b
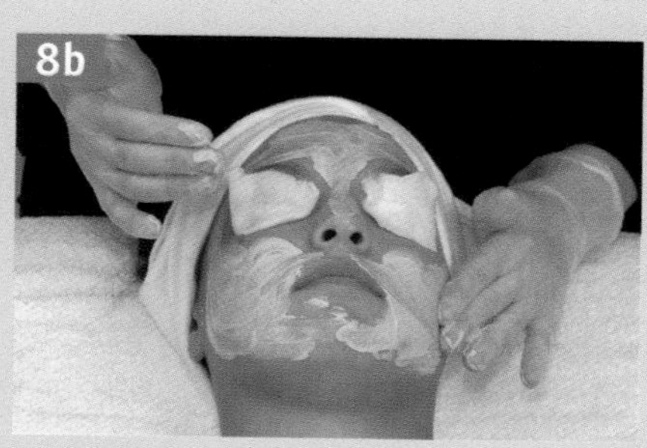
Apply microdermabrasion product.

b. Apply the microdermabrasion product to the skin following manufacturer's guidelines.

8c
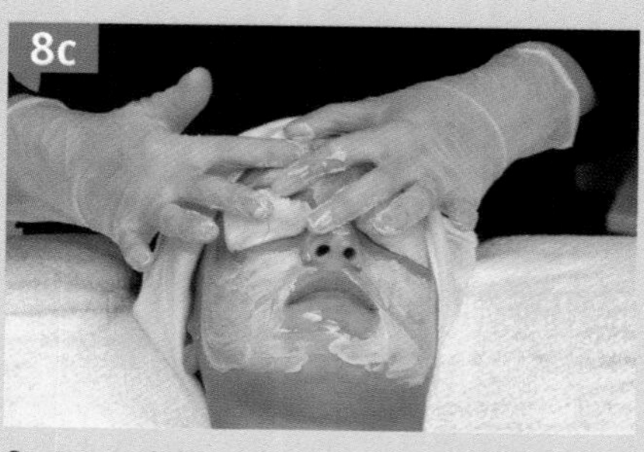
Start on right side of the forehead.

c. Starting with right side of the forehead, firmly stretch the skin between the thumb and fingers of one hand; then using the fingers of the other hand, perform firm vertical strokes on the taut skin in a rolling action. After 10 strokes, evaluate the skin for any sign of redness or irritation. If none exist, perform 10 more strokes, this time in a horizontal direction.

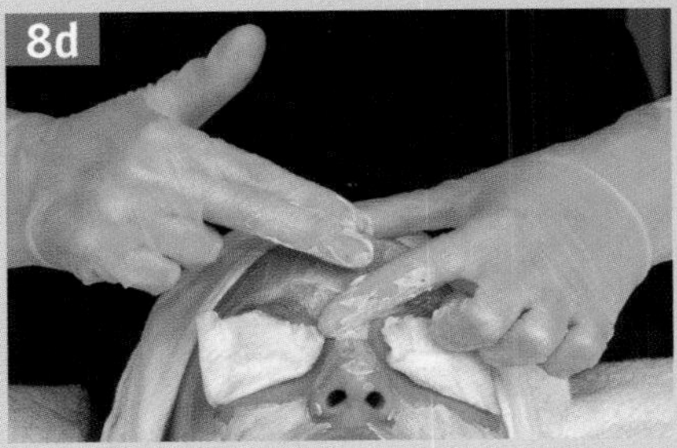

Move to the center of the forehead.

d. Move to the center of the forehead and repeat.

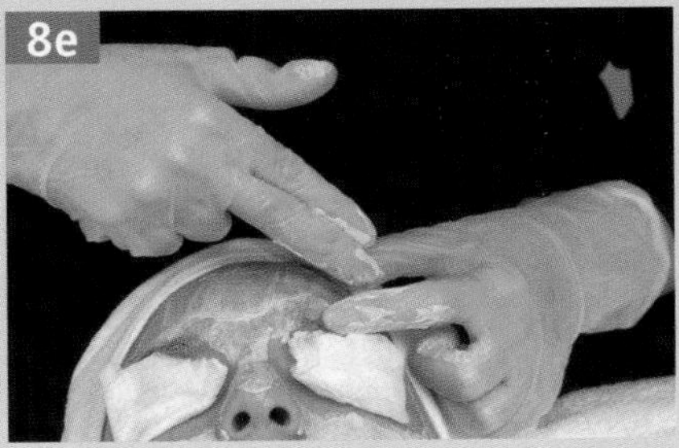

Move to the left side of the forehead.

e. Move to the left side of the forehead and repeat.

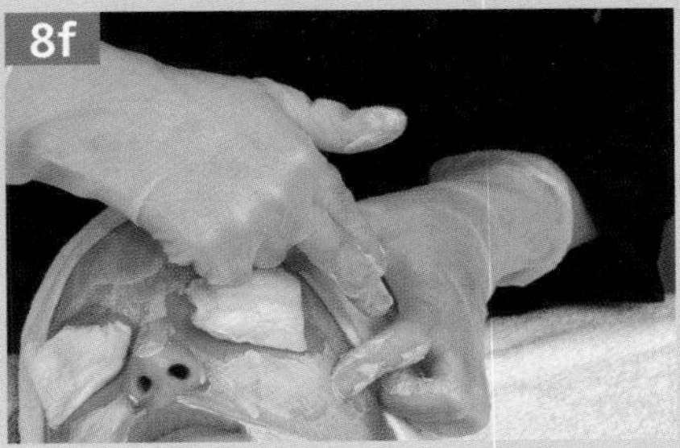

Move to left temple.

f. Move to left temple and repeat.

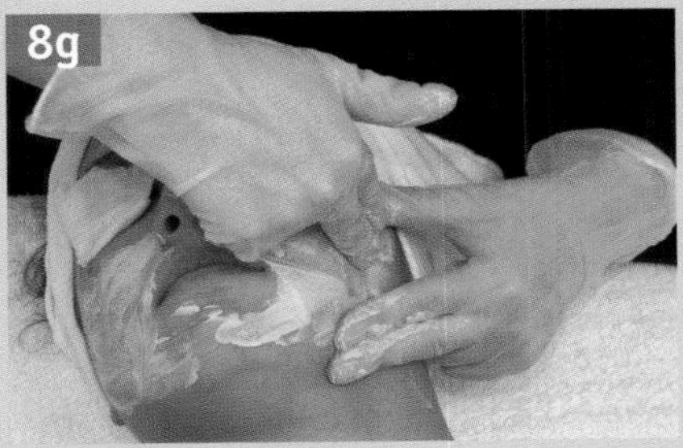

Move to left cheek.

g. Move to left cheek and repeat. (Depending on the size and shape of the face, you may need to break this area into more than one segment).

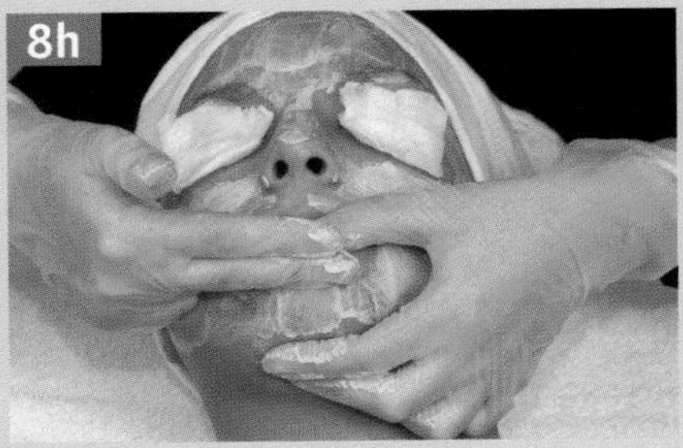

Move to the chin.

h. Move to the chin and repeat.

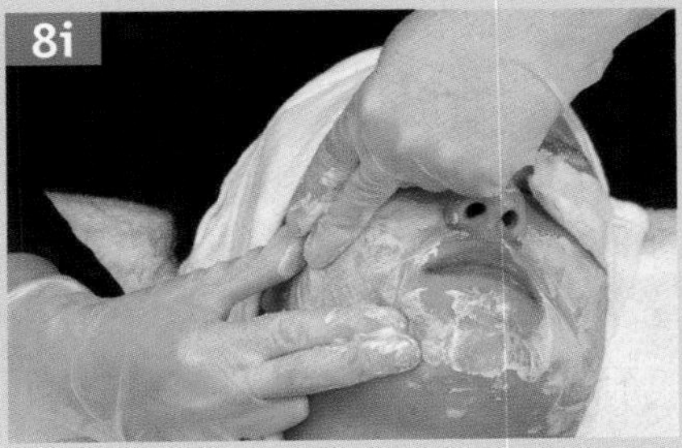

Move to the right cheek.

i. Move to the right cheek and repeat.

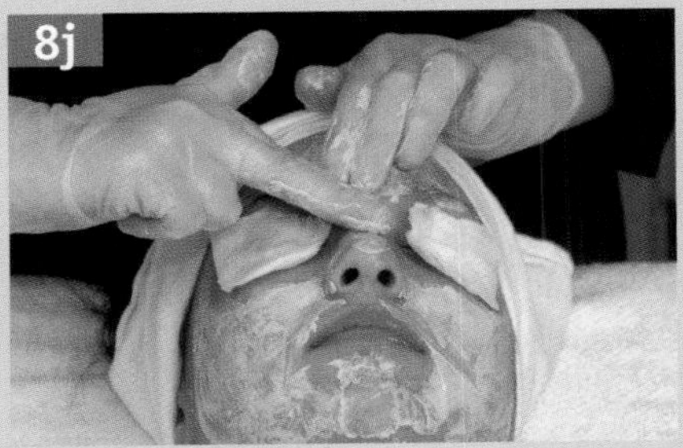

Move to the nose.

j. Move to the nose and repeat.

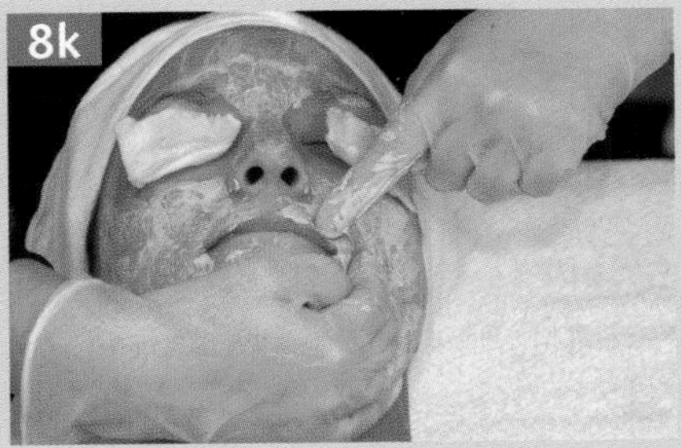

Repeat procedure on upper lip area.

k. Repeat procedure on each half above the upper lip, stroking outward from the centerline.

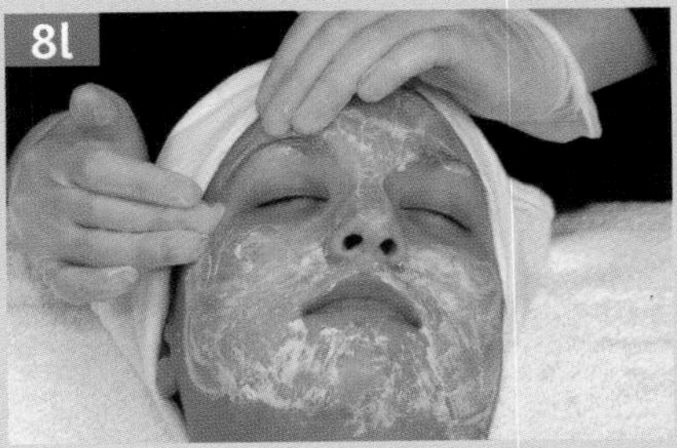

Stroke along the lower obicularis occuli.

l. Using *gentle* pressure, stroke along the lower obicularis occuli, following the orbital bone and classical massage stroke pattern.

continues on next page

PROCEDURE 16–3, CONT. MANUAL MICRODERMABRASION

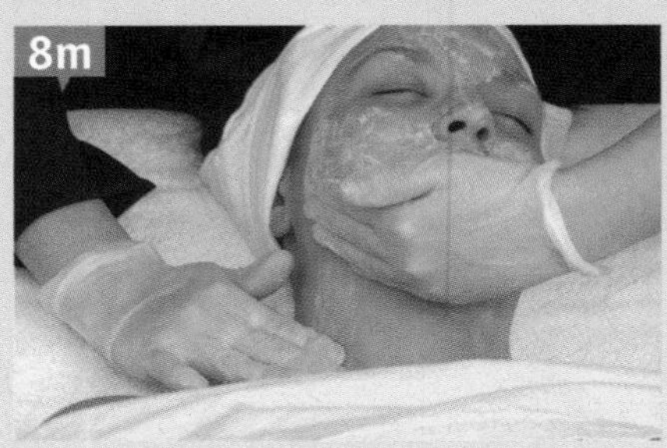

Move to the left side of the neck.

m. Move to the left side of the neck and repeat stroke patterns in two segments (adjust to fit the client).

n. Move to the right side of the neck and repeat in two segments (adjust to fit the client).

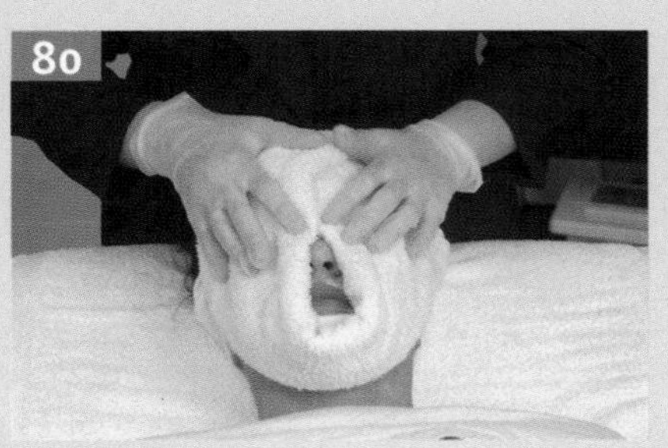

Remove product.

o. Use warm moist towels (or cotton gauze) to remove all product from the skin.

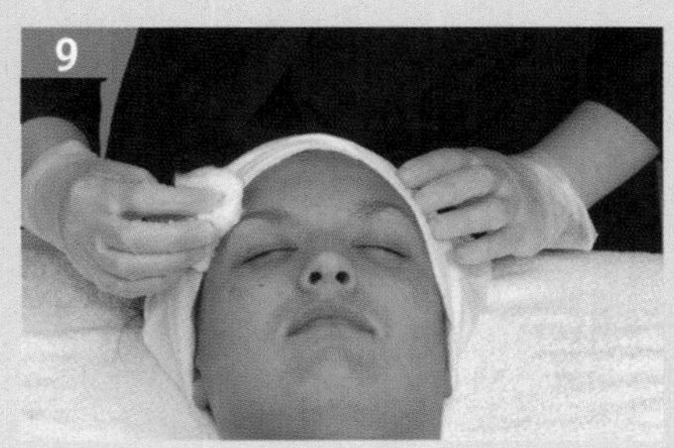

Wipe skin with toner.

9 Tone. Apply toner appropriate for the client's skin with wet cotton rounds. Wipe the skin with cotton rounds.

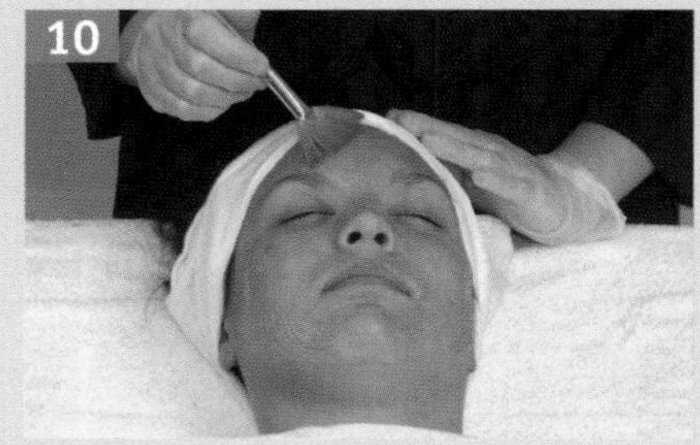

Use appropriate mask.

10 Treat and mask as appropriate for client's skin to conclude the treatment. Apply serum(s) appropriate for client's skin.

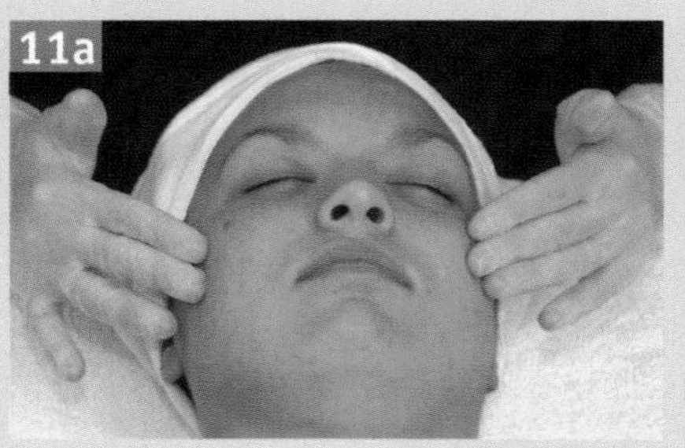

Apply serum.

11 Protect

a. Apply additional serum if desired.

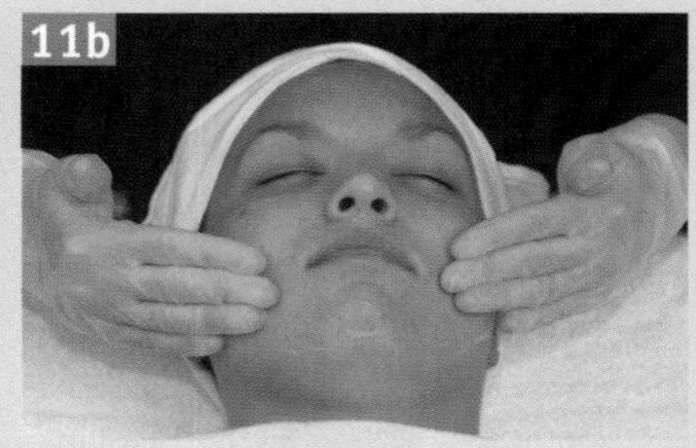

Apply sun protection.

b. Apply sun protection.

Post-procedure

12 Remind the client to stay out of the sun and to wear appropriate protection.

13 Assure that the client has appropriate products for home care.

14 If this is part of a series, schedule the next appointment.

Clean-up and Disinfection

15 Follow clean-up and disinfection procedures in accordance with state guidelines.

16 Reset and prepare the room for the next client.

Enzymes

Enzymes are proteolytic and protein-dissolving. They work to destroy the keratin in dead cells on the surface of the skin. These treatments are often referred to as *enzyme peeling, enzyme masks,* or *enzyme treatments*. In Europe, enzyme therapy is known as a lysing or lysis.

Papain, an enzyme often included in exfoliation, is derived from the papaya fruit. This ingredient is also used as a meat tenderizer for its ability to soften tissue and dissolve protein. Bromelain from pineapples and pancreatin and trypsine derived from meat by-products are also used. Papain cannot be blended with any activator that has AHA in it, as this neutralizes the enzyme. However, bromelain and AHA can be co-mingled.

Pancreatin and trypsine enhance exfoliation activity. When mixed with a liquid activator trypsine has less odor than does pancreatin. Some manufacturers add fruits to improve the smell and enhance activity through the chemical components of the incorporated extract.

There are two basic types of proteolytic enzyme peeling used in facial treatments. One is a cream that is applied to the skin after cleansing and steaming. This cream contains paraffin, which dries and forms a hardened crust. The cream sets up in about 10 minutes and then is massaged or "rolled" off the skin. Treatments of this type are often called *vegetal* or *vegetable* peelings. This treatment is actually a combination of chemical and mechanical peeling. The "rolling" or gommage action provides friction that physically removes dead cells. The flakes coming off the skin are not dead cells but dried paraffin. The actual dead cells that are removed are not visible without a microscope.

The second, and probably more popular, type of enzyme treatment uses a powdered form of enzyme. Mixed with warm water or an activator immediately before application, this treatment generally is kept soft during application by using warm steam or placing a hot towel over the treatment and not allowing it to dry. It is easily removed because it is soft and moist. This type of enzyme treatment generally produces a more even peeling of the cell buildup and helps to dilate the follicle openings slightly, which makes extraction much easier. While water will work, an activator may significantly enhance exfoliation because it also contains exfoliants, such as more of the enzyme or AHAs.

FOCUS ON: *Enzyme Peelings*

Enzyme peelings are often available in varying strengths and suitable for the following conditions:

1. **Oily, clogged skin with open and closed comedones and minor acne breakouts**
2. **Dry or dehydrated skin with cell buildup, flaking, and a tight dry surface**
3. **Dull, lifeless-looking skin. This skin condition actually has a tremendous buildup of dead cells that produces a slight gray color on the surface of the skin.**
4. **Skin with multiple milia**
5. **Clients who desire a smoother appearance to their skin or a more even surface for makeup application**

Enzyme treatments are generally gentle enough to repeat even on an every-two-week schedule, although most clients have them with regular monthly facial treatments. Most clients notice an immediate softening of the skin after the very first application of the enzyme. Because enzyme treatment slightly dilates the pore openings, which helps with extraction, clients notice that extraction is more comfortable and only gentle pressure is needed. Follow the manufacturer's directions for mixing, application, and removal of any enzyme treatment.

Acids

While physical exfoliants work to slough off dead cells sitting on the surface, alpha hydroxy acids work by loosening the "glue" of lipids that hold the cells together, helping to continually shed this sheath of cells. This removal of dead cells is also beneficial to acne-prone skin, helping to loosen both surface cell buildup and impacted dead cells inside the follicle, which can lead to comedones and, possibly, acne.

Alpha hydroxy acid (AHA) and beta hydroxy acid (BHA) treatments are probably the most effective tools that you have to treat photoaging skin (Figure 16–6). They are an integral part of any program The terms *alpha hydroxy acid* and *glycolic acid* are often used interchangeably. However, technically, glycolic acid is an alpha hydroxy acid, and treatments may involve both alpha hydroxy and beta hydroxy acids.

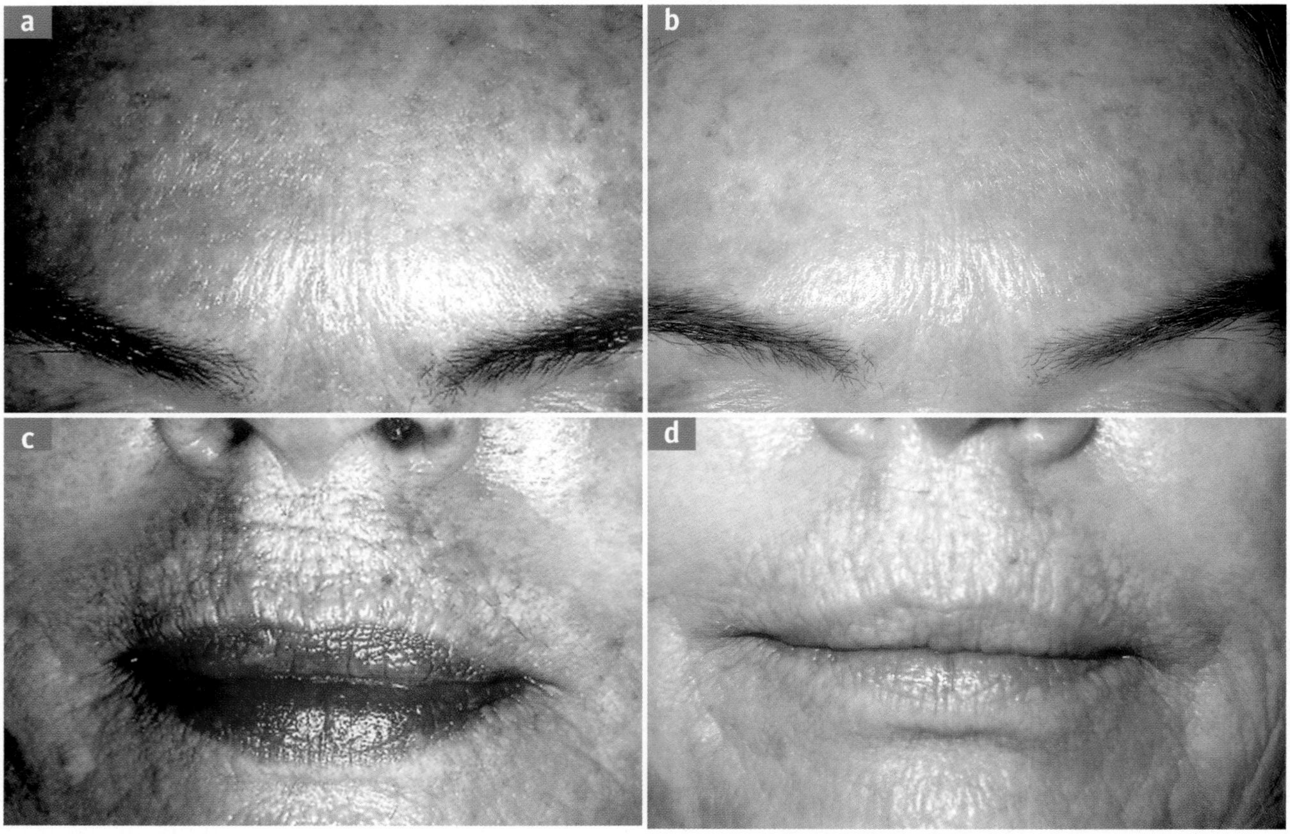

Figure 16–6 Treating photoaged skin with AHA.

Although very different from retinoids, AHA and BHA agents also help to "reorganize" the epidermis. There is only a small molecular difference between AHAs and BHAs, but that difference affects the way they function. AHAs are water-loving and work through the hydrophilic aspect of the epidermis. BHAs are oil-loving and work through the lipophilic aspect of the epidermis and sebaceous follicle. The most commonly used BHA is salicylic acid, which is less apt to trigger an inflammatory response in acne clients than AHAs. Because they are oil-loving, BHAs are metabolized differently than AHAs. You would remove any excess during treatment, but you should advise a client to drink water as it is metabolized through the body. Salicylic acid has been used by estheticians for more than 50 years with great results. Commonly esthetic strengths are less than 20% and designed not to work on living tissue.

Long-term use of acids helps to replenish intercellular lipids that decrease with age and sun damage. As discussed in previous chapters, intercellular lipids make up the barrier function and are responsible for epidermal hydration and the appearance of the skin. The mild trauma triggered by the application of these acids causes a "skin healing" response, which in turn triggers increased cellular renewal and increased production of epidermal and dermal cells, often resulting in a more youthful appearance.

Besides typical aging and wrinkles, alpha hydroxy acids can help improve hand and foot calluses, dry and dehydrated skin, and dry body skin. Low levels of salicylic acid (BHA) in cleansers are commonly used to help control acne.

Alpha Hydroxy Acid Exfoliations

Glycolic or lactic acids are available in a variety of strengths for salon use. The typical concentration of these acids used in salon treatment is between 15% and 30%. Higher strengths are used only by dermatologists due to the risk of skin damage. These applications will be discussed in a later chapter.

Before administering alpha hydroxy acid exfoliation, make sure the client has been using an 8% to 10% concentration gel, lotion, or cream at home for at least two weeks. Home use of the AHA before AHA exfoliation should be mandatory because it helps to acclimate the

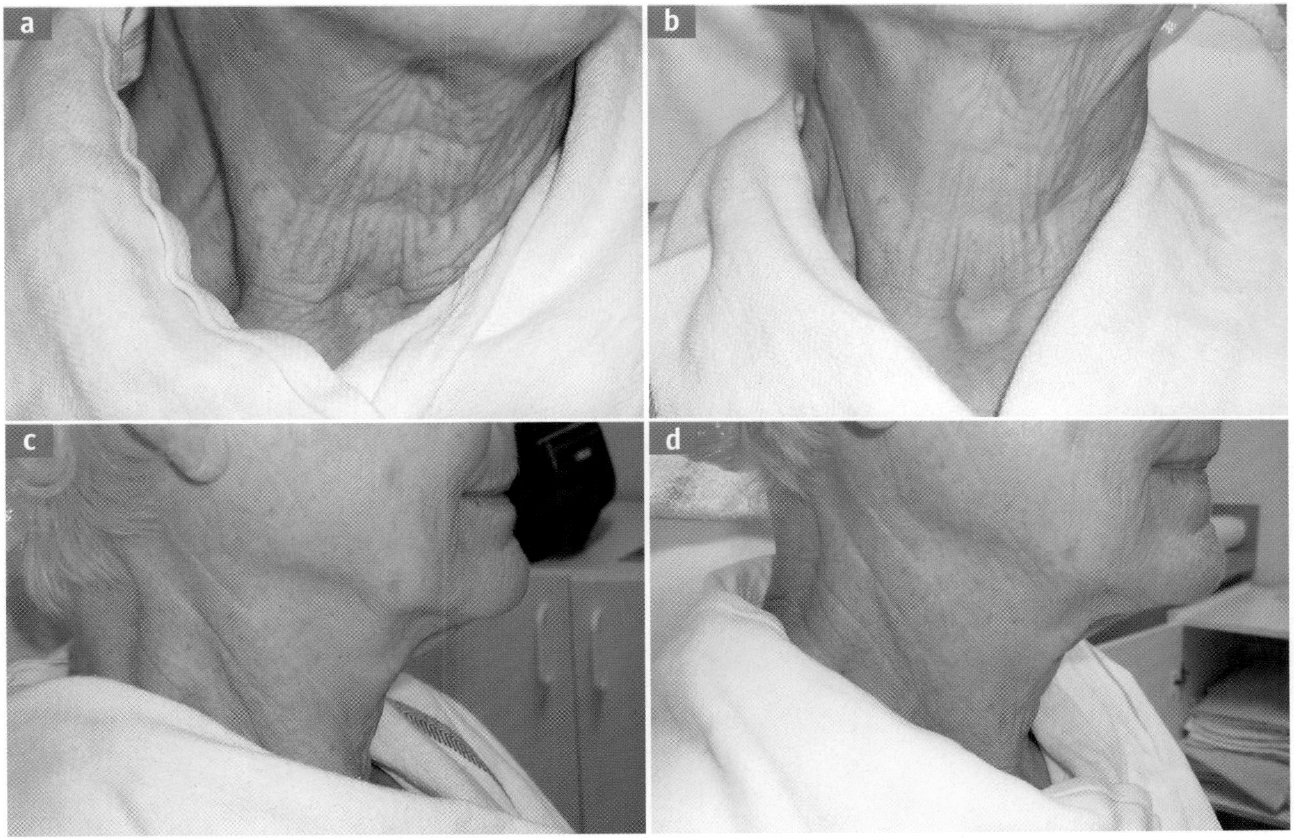

Figure 16–7 Client being treated for loss of elasticity.

skin for higher strength salon products. Failure to use AHA at home as described may result in increased discomfort during the procedure and increased chances of redness and irritation after the exfoliation treatment.

The standard treatment consists of an application of 30%, pH 3.0 gel or solution (Figure 16–7). This is administered twice a week for three weeks, or following manufacturer guidelines, for a client beginning AHA treatments. Maintenance treatments are usually twice a month but vary with client needs, budgets, and sensitivity levels.

Mild glycolic or lactic acids or blends of the two used in AHA treatment may be influenced by the cleansing procedure that takes place before extraction. The cleansing procedure determines how much surface oil is removed before applying the AHA peeling treatment. A typical protocol for an AHA treatment follows; however, before implementing this or any protocol, read and follow the manufacturer's instructions for the particular product you are using.

CAUTION!

Do *not* experiment with higher percentages of AHA products. Higher levels carry with them heightened risk of skin trauma or damage for the client. Hyperpigmentation, a wound, or scarring can all occur.

? Did You Know

The Cosmetic Ingredient Review of the Cosmetics, Toiletries, and Fragrance Association has issued a recommendation that licensed estheticians use alpha hydroxy acid salon exfoliation products that do not exceed 30% in concentration and have a pH of 3.0 or above. Higher concentrations or lower pH can cause irritation.

CAUTION!

It is very important to follow manufacturer's instructions, which may vary from brand to brand or product to product from the same manufacturer.

PROCEDURE 16–4 ALPHA HYDROXY TREATMENT (AHA)

IMPLEMENTS AND MATERIALS

- Typical facial lounge, client draping, and linen setup
- Makeup removing cleanser
- Pre-peel cleanser
- Toner
- Cotton rounds
- Disposable sponges, cotton compresses, or facial cloths
- Cotton swabs
- Petrolatum
- Bowl and warm water
- Peel solution
- Soothing serum
- Moisturizer and sun protection
- Gloves
- Small decanting containers

Preparation

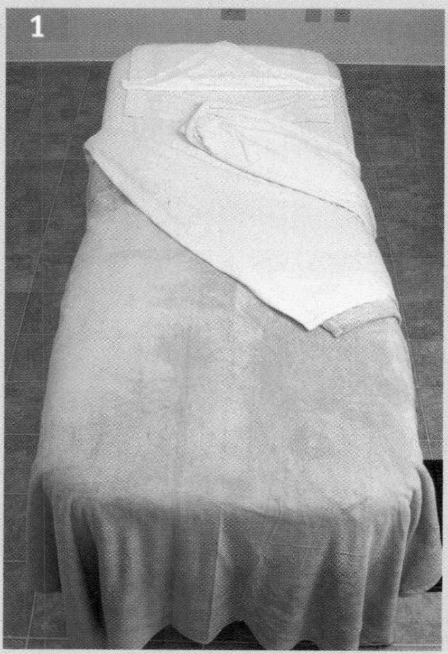

Prepare treatmemt bed.

1 Set up the facial lounge with linens.

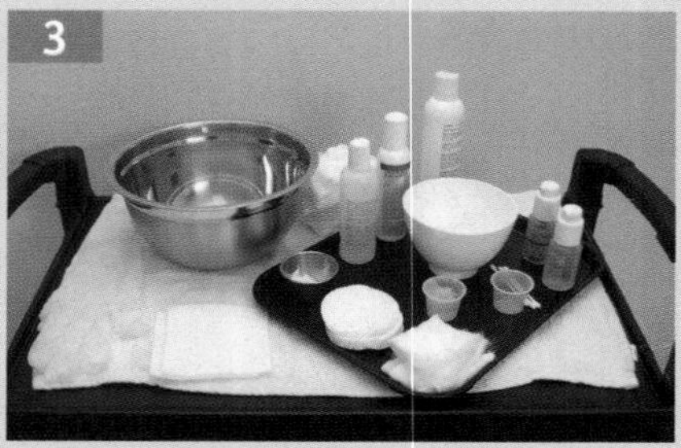

Set up supplies.

2 Prepare towels and cotton and gather supplies.

3 Decant or set up products.

Procedure

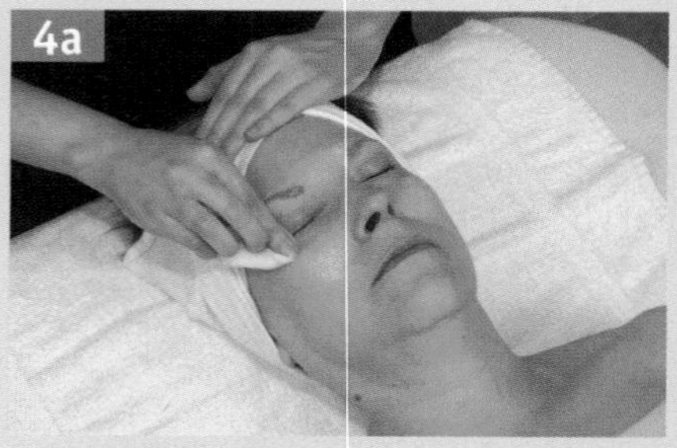

Remove eye makeup.

4 Cleanse the skin with makeup-removing cleanser.

a. Remove eye makeup.

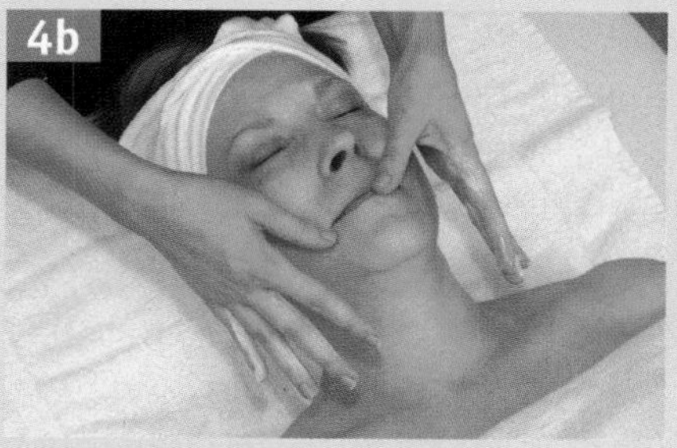

Remove lipstick.

b. Remove lipstick.

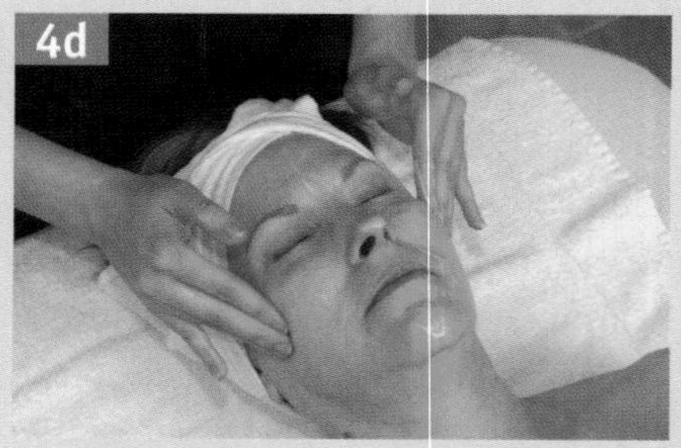

Remove facial makeup.

c. Remove makeup.

d. Re-inspect the skin to assure procedure is appropriate for client.

5 Perform a second cleansing using the manufacturer's recommended stripping cleanser.

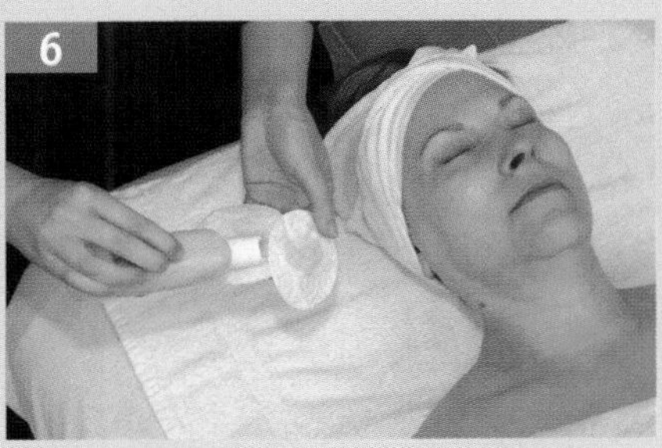

Use toner.

6 Tone the skin with moist cotton rounds and an appropriate stripping toner per manufacturer recommendations.

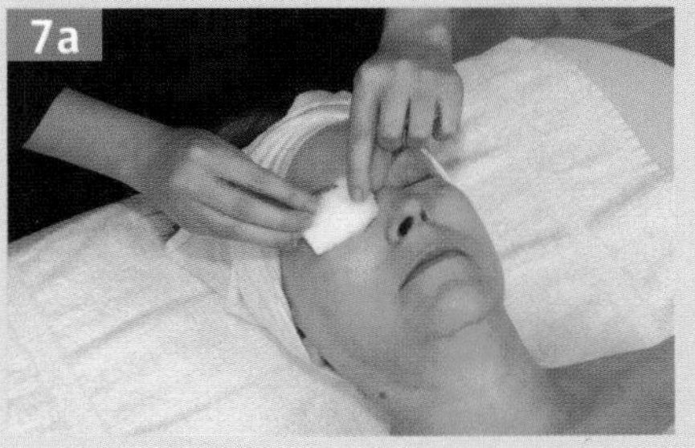

Apply eye protection.

7 Protection

a. Apply cotton compresses to the eyes to protect them.

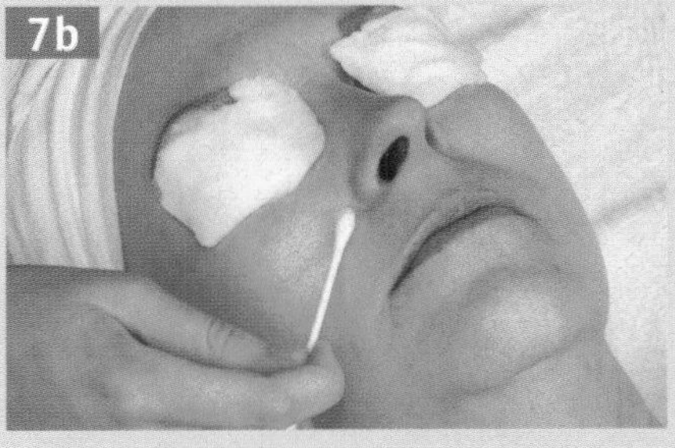

Apply petrolatum in nasal curve.

b. Apply small amount of petrolatum in the nasal curve and nasal labial fold, if recommended by manufacturer.

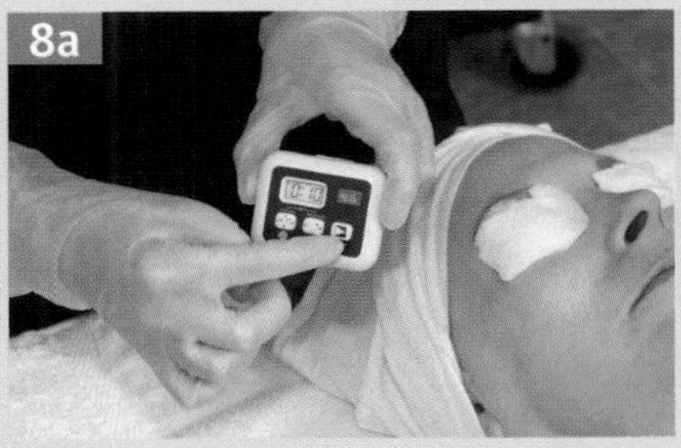

Put on gloves and set timer.

8 Acid treatment

a. Put on gloves. Set a timer for 10 minutes or the length of time recommended by the manufacturer.

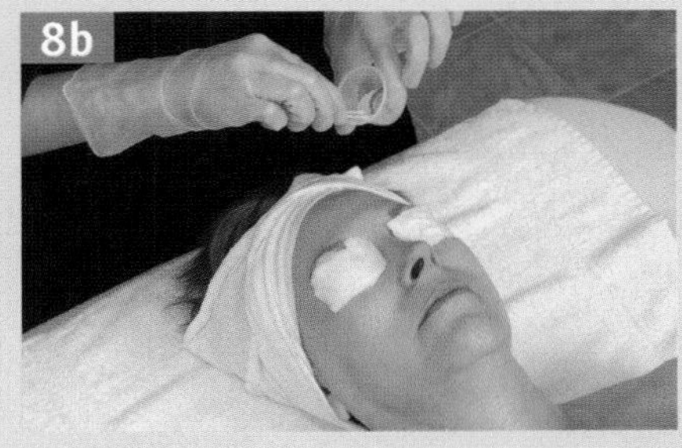

Apply acid with cotton swabs.

b. Apply the acid by holding two cotton swabs together and dipping them in acid solution or gel.

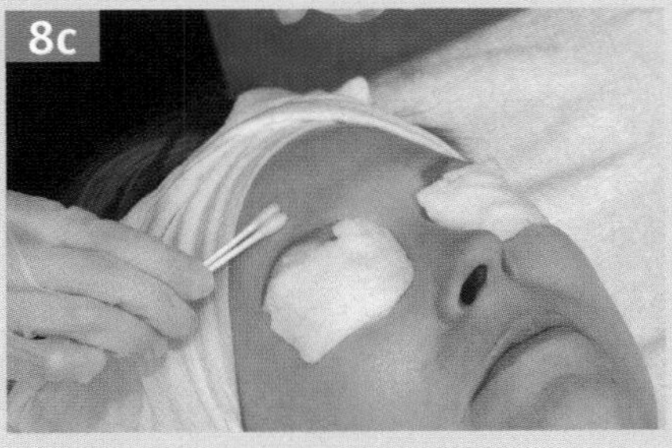

Use small, circular motions.

c. Begin with the forehead, and apply the product using small, circular motions with the cotton swabs. The product is clear so it may be difficult to see where you have been. Avoid going back over areas or leaving puddles of product on the skin.

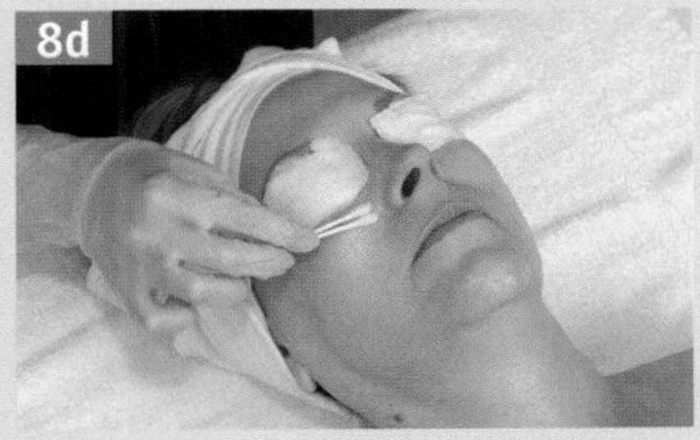

Follow a precise pattern to ensure even application.

d. Proceed to other areas in a precise clockwise pattern. It is important to be precise to ensure an even application of the acid. Work carefully.

e. Allow AHA to stay on the skin for the manufacturer-recommended amount of time.

continues on next page

PROCEDURE 16–4, CONT. ALPHA HYDROXY TREATMENT (AHA)

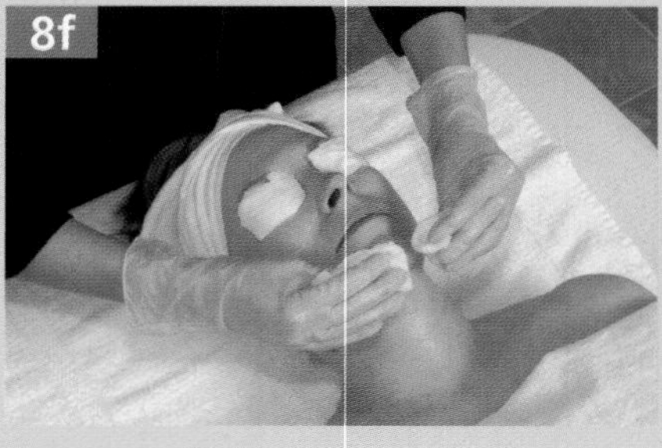

Remove product.

f. Remove the AHA from the face with cool, wet pads.

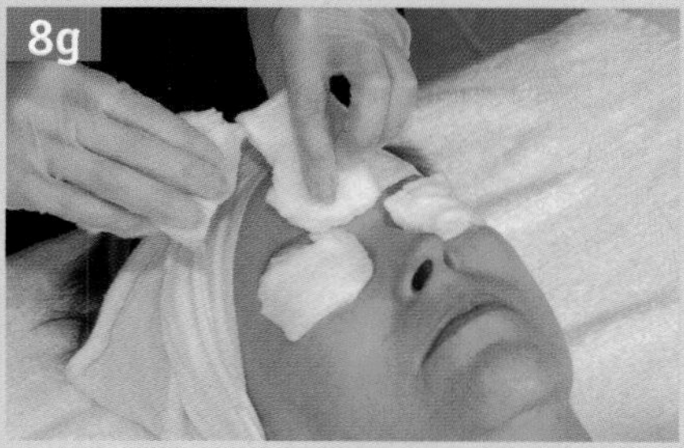

Rinse well.

g. Rinse the face well with the wet pads.

h. Optional: You may follow this with a cool spray of plain water in an atomizer and another clean-up with wet gauze.

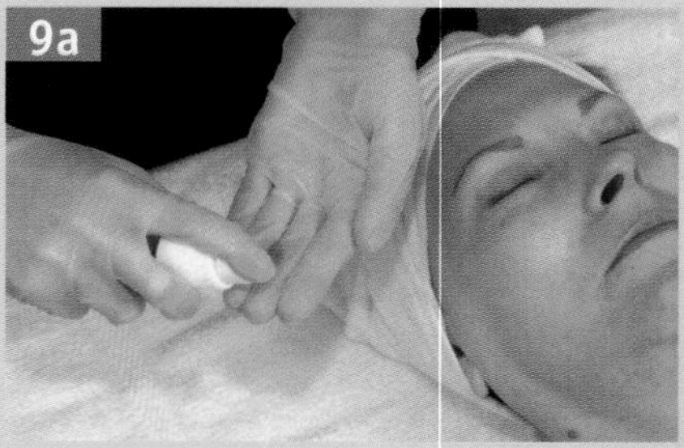

Apply serum.

9 Protect

a. Apply soothing, hydrating serum if desired.

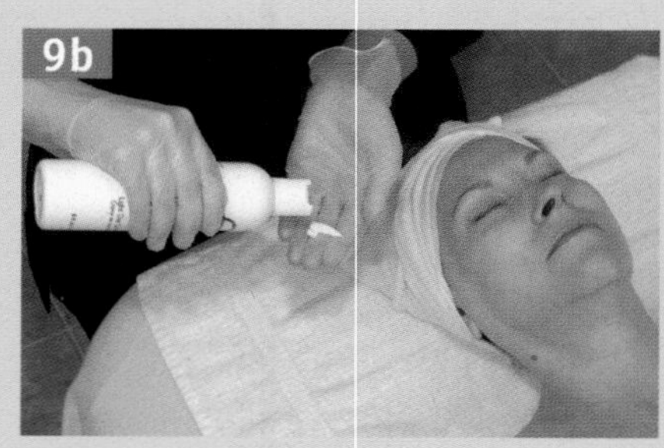

Apply sunscreen moisturizer.

b. Apply sunscreen moisturizer.

Post-procedure

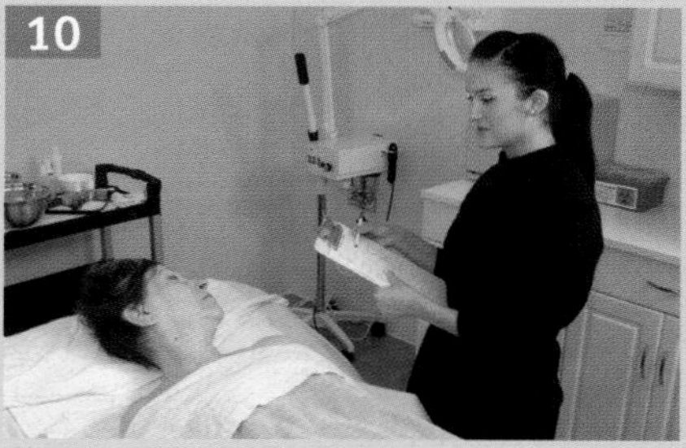

Remind client of post-procedure care.

10 Remind the client to stay out of the sun.

11 Advise the client not to use exfoliants (scrubs or chemical) for at least 48 hours following treatments.

12 Assure client has appropriate home care.

Clean-up and Disinfection

13 Follow clean-up and disinfection procedures in accordance with OSHA or state guidelines.

14 Reset and prepare the room for the next client.

The strength of the cleansing products influences the amount of surface oils and corneum cells removed before application of the solution. During the first treatment, cleanse with a mild cleansing lotion. If the first treatment does not produce any redness or irritation, you can precede the second treatment with a slightly stronger cleanser. For the third visit—again assuming there is no irritation—you may add a mild toner to complete the cleansing. Strengthen the fourth treatment by using a slightly stronger cleanser with a slightly stronger toner. Do not use extremely strong cleansers and toners or those with an alcohol base.

BHA treatments are nearly identical to procedures for AHAs, employing the same setup and supplies. The variation between the treatments occurs in step 5 of the protocol. When applying a BHA product, you may use a Wood's lamp to determine that you have applied the product evenly. The Wood's lamp will illuminate the product.

You can include the face, neck, and chest in a single treatment but do not treat the back on that same day. There is a risk of salicylic poisoning if too large an area of the body is treated at one time. Most importantly, do not use salicylic treatments on clients who are pregnant.

You should reassess the condition of the skin after the first few applications to determine a further treatment course. Results are not particularly dramatic after one treatment, so do not attempt to assess results until after six treatments. It takes several applications of 30% alpha hydroxy acid, over several weeks, to produce appreciable results in many cases (Figure 16–8). It takes time for new, healthier skin to develop.

Precautions for AHA Exfoliations

1. Make sure the client is pretreating his or her skin with lower-strength alpha hydroxy acid at home for at least two weeks before you administer a 30% AHA treatment. Failure to do this may cause skin irritation.
2. Do not use the alpha hydroxy acid treatment if the client is currently using prescription keratolytic drugs, including tazarotene (Tazorac®), tretinoin (Retin-A or Renova®), adapalene (Differin®), azelaic acid (Azelex®), or any other prescription peeling agents. The client should discontinue use of any of these drugs for several weeks before a salon alpha hydroxy exfoliation treatment.
3. Do not use glycolic or alpha hydroxy acid on patients who have taken Accutane® within the past 12 months.
4. Do not administer AHA treatments to a client who is under a dermatologist's care for any skin disorders without first obtaining written approval from the dermatologist.
5. Be careful to use eye pads on the client, and avoid getting the alpha hydroxy acid close to the eyes.
6. Do not use the peeling agent on a male client immediately after he has shaved. It is best to wait several hours after shaving before applying an acid treatment.
7. After waxing, wait at least 24 hours before performing an AHA treatment.
8. Check with the client before each successive treatment to make sure he or she has not experienced any irritation from the previous treatment. If irritation developed after the previous treatment, do not add pre-cleansing steps. Avoid any area that is peeling, red, or irritated, or wait a few days before resuming treatment.
9. Do not administer AHA treatments to any skin that is already irritated. This includes rosacea flares, seborrheic dermatitis, eczema, wind-burned or sunburned skin, or skin that is irritated from a previous treatment of any type.
10. Apply a broad-spectrum sunscreen of SPF-15 or higher that is appropriate for the skin type after any exfoliation treatment. The client should use that sunscreen daily at home.
11. If the client has a history of herpes simplex outbreaks (cold sores), refer him or her to a doctor for preventative medication before administering any chemical exfoliation treatments. Remember: When in doubt, don't!
12. Check manufacturer's instructions for information regarding combining AHA treatment with other types of salon skin care treatments.

AHA treatment can be administered indefinitely on a weekly, biweekly, or monthly basis, depending on the client, the skin type and the manufacturer's guidelines (Figure 16–9). Supporting this treatment with soothing products, ingredients, or techniques will enhance results.

AHA Treatment for Acne

Because AHA is an exfoliating treatment, using it on acne uncovers closed comedones and loosens open comedones while exfoliating the dead-cell layer on the surface, which can be fairly heavy on oily, problem skin.

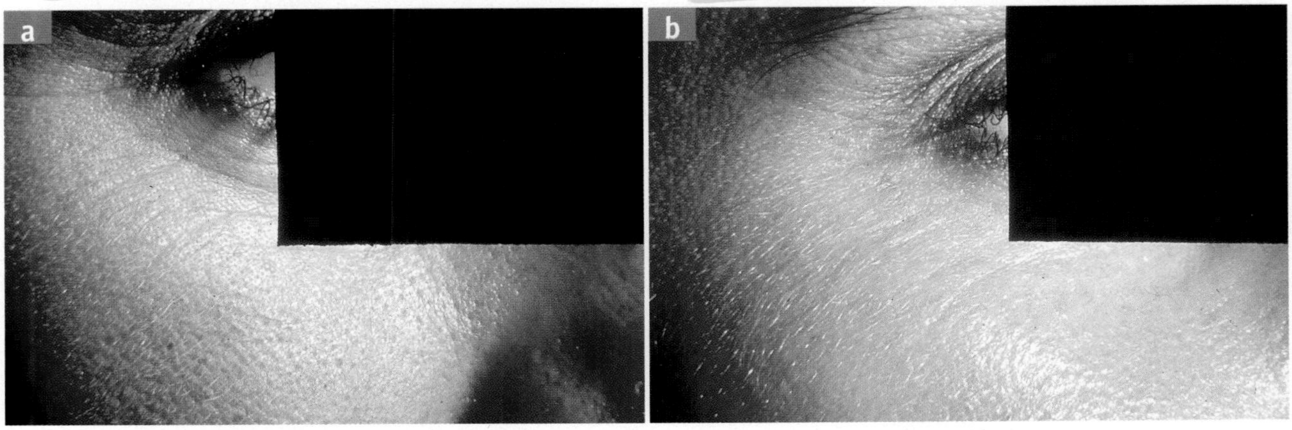

Figure 16–8 Gylcolic acid used for treating facial wrinkles.

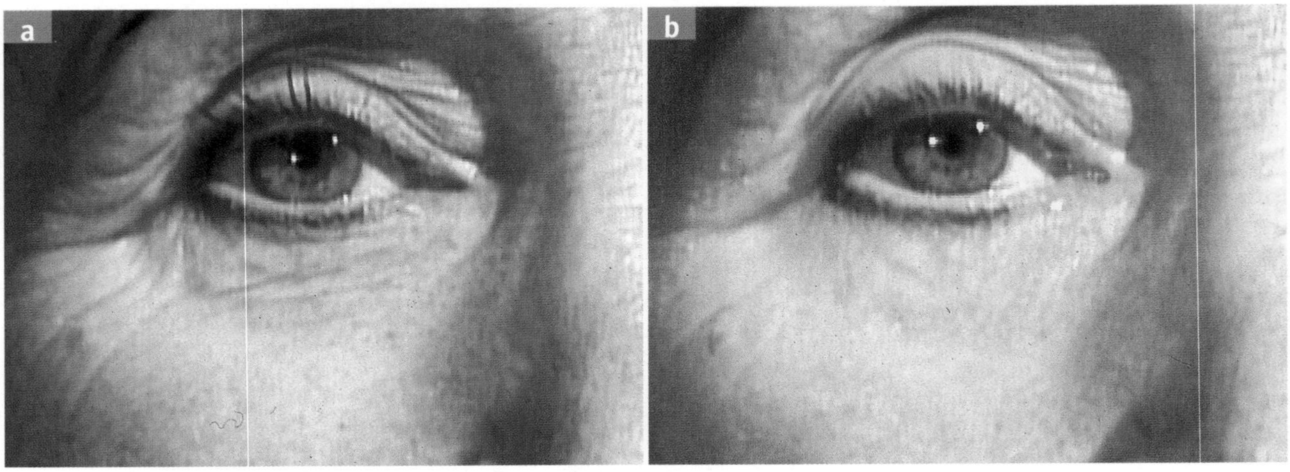

Figure 16–9 Routine home AHA and skin treatments to reduce signs of aging.

Before this treatment, explain to the client the possibility that the skin may seem to get worse before it gets better (Figure 16–10). Continued treatment, along with alternating extraction treatments on different days, will help loosen the acne impactions (Figure 16–11).

AHA Treatment for Hyperpigmented Skin

You can administer AHA treatments to a client's hyperpigmented skin, removing already stained corneum cells while suppressing melanin production in the melanocytes (Figures 16–12 and 16–13). Several weeks before such a treatment, the client should use home care products that include a melanin suppressant such as hydroquinone, kojic acid, magnesium ascorbyl phosphate, arbutin, asafetida extract, or a combination of these agents. There are premixed solutions available that include combinations of melanin suppressants with alpha hydroxy acids. Needless to say, hyperpigmented clients should wear a daily broad-spectrum sunscreen of SPF-15 or 30 and should avoid sun exposure completely.

Deeper Exfoliation (Superficial Peels)

The deepest type of chemical exfoliation performed by estheticians are called *superficial peels*. Unlike deep and

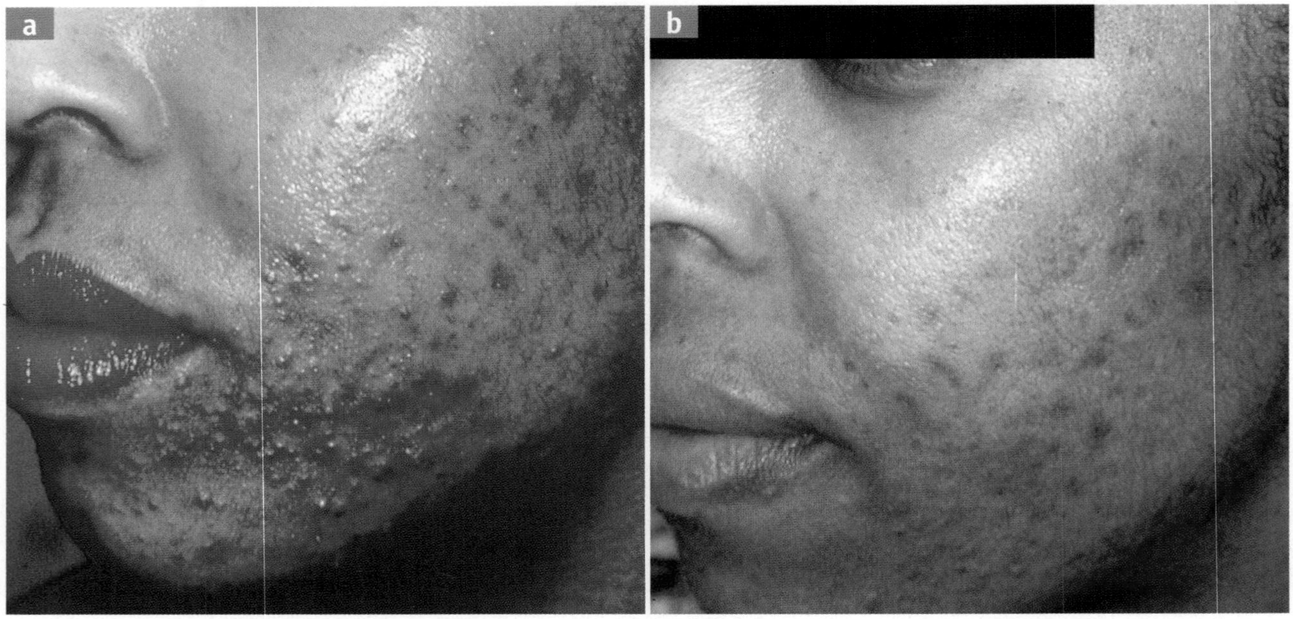

Figure 16–10 Glycolic acid before and after for acne.

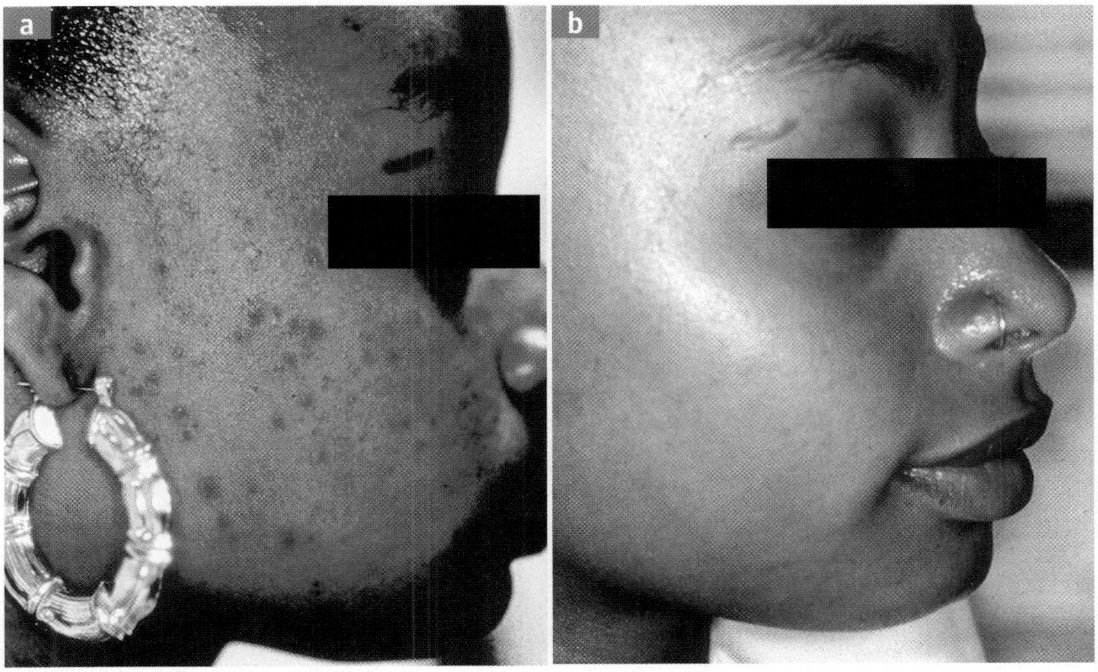

Figure 16–11 Before and after treatment results.

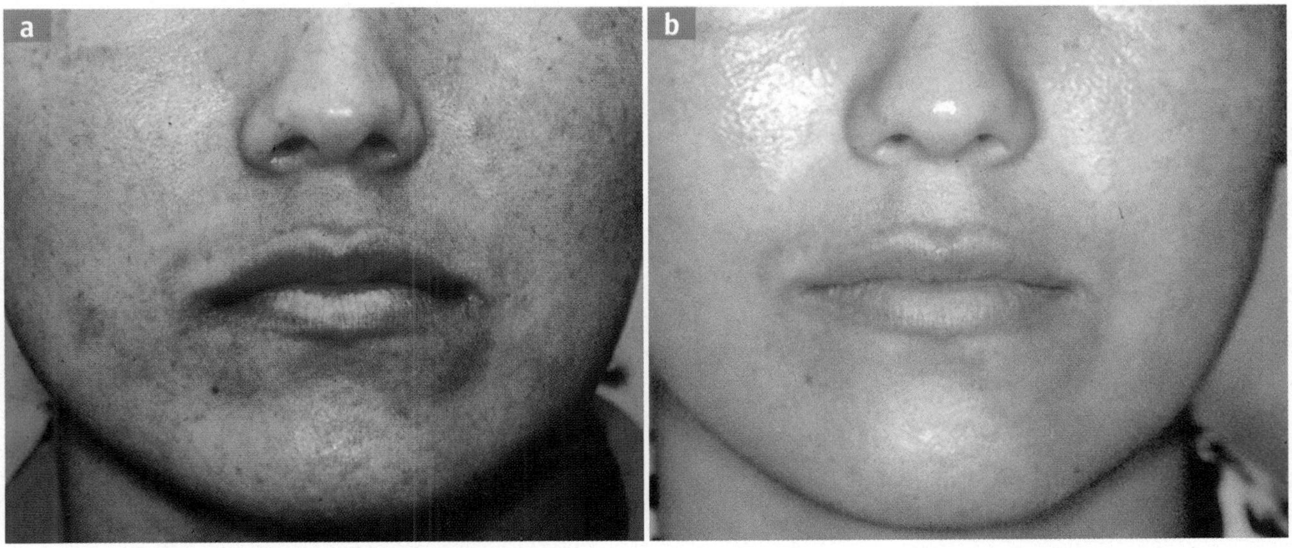

Figure 16–12 Successful treatment of hyperpigmentation.

medium medical peelings, superficial peels only remove cells from the epidermis. While the consumer thinks of all exfoliation as a peel, this is a misnomer. Estheticians exfoliate, physicians peel.

These chemical exfoliations are helpful for treating small, superficial wrinkles, dark spots, and other forms of hyperpigmentation, melasma, and acne-prone skin. They are designed to even the surface skin pigment, smooth the appearance of the skin, and dry the surface of acne and problem skin. Like AHA, deep exfoliation may also increase the amount of surface acne lesions, because it loosens impactions and causes them to move toward the surface. In other words, it may cause acne to get worse before it gets better.

The most frequently used type of chemical for a superficial peel is known as Jessner's solution, which is a

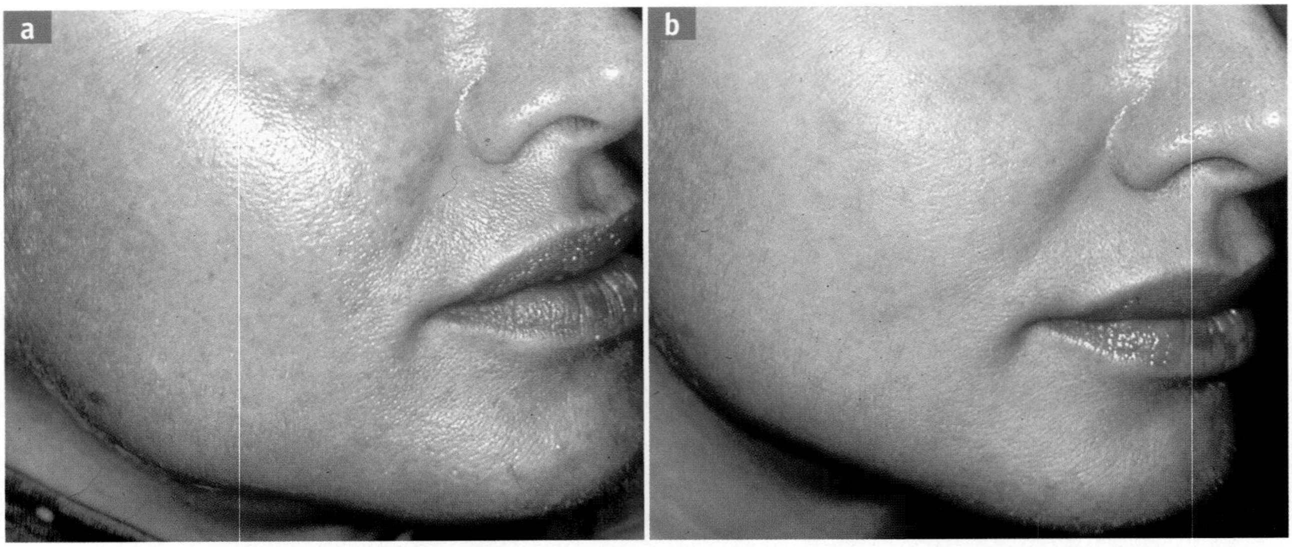

Figure 16–13 Treating hyperpigmentation.

REGULATORY AGENCY ALERT

Some states prohibit the use of all forms of phenol by estheticians. Know your state laws before you buy products.

mixture of salicylic acid, resorcinol, lactic acid, and ethanol. Some of these formulas also contain a small amount of phenol, usually 2%, and sometimes sulfur. Although Jessner's solution is a liquid, some cream forms produce similar effects on the skin.

Candidates for Clinic Deep Exfoliation

Clients who have sun-damaged skin, hyperpigmented skin, or other forms of melasma are the best candidates for superficial peeling. Technically, most adult clients can benefit from these peelings, because most adults do have some form of fine wrinkling or hyperpigmentation.

Most estheticians attempt to treat these cosmetic conditions with more conservative treatments before resorting to deeper exfoliation. AHA acid, hydroquinone solutions, or a combination can be very effective for many forms of hyperpigmentation. Low-strength AHA peelings are another alternative.

Make sure that your client has started on home care before you administer deeper exfoliation. This pretreatment ensures that the client's skin is in better shape before you use the chemicals. Many estheticians insist that a client have facial treatments for a period of time before they administer a chemical exfoliation. This allows an esthetician to learn about a client, the client's skin, and the client's needs before using exfoliation products.

Many clients call a clinic asking about chemical peels. Ask a client to make an appointment for a consultation before you issue an opinion about his or her skin. Many clients have cosmetic problems that can be treated by other, simpler methods than chemical exfoliation. In addition, some clients do not use proper home care. Good home care plus salon care—including lighter exfoliation, such as with enzymes or AHA—are the basis for a healthy program for the client's skin for a lifetime.

Deeper chemical exfoliation is probably the most drastic and dramatic treatment administered by an esthetician, so a client should never view it as a "magic bullet" for skin problems. There are some disadvantages to this technique. These include discomfort, temporary discolorations, a small risk of allergic reaction, a bad appearance to the skin during the actual procedure, and a possibility of hyperpigmentation.

These few paragraphs are not meant to discourage the use of deeper exfoliation products. They are meant to clarify that clients do not always fully understand the process or for what conditions it is intended.

Clients Who Should Avoid Superficial Peels

Clients who are not familiar with good skin care and do not use a regular skin care program will generally not have as good or as long-lasting results with superficial peeling as clients who have regular salon treatments and are consistent with home care. Following is a list of other clients who should not have chemical peeling:

1. Clients who are pregnant or are lactating
2. Clients who have a history of heart problems
3. Clients who have a history of medical problems, such as eczema, lupus, seborrhea, rosacea, psoriasis, bacterial skin infections, mental disorders, extremely sensitive or hyperallergic skin, and other systemic problems that could contribute to poor healing. These clients should have written permission from a physician. If during an interview about the client's health history, you have questions about his or her eligibility for the treatment, refer the client to a medical doctor.
4. Clients who have a history of fever blisters or herpes simplex, which can be stimulated by chemical exfoliation; refer these clients to a physician for pretreatment.
5. Clients who have used Accutane within the last year
6. Clients using retinoic acid (Retin-A); these clients should discontinue use of this medication about three months before the superficial peeling.
7. Clients who have extremely thin skin with telangectasias or couperose veins

The Pre-exfoliation Consultation

Consultation with a candidate for exfoliation should take place at least a week before the scheduled peeling. Explain to the client what normally happens during the procedure, step-by-step. Make sure he or she understands the discomfort and how he or she will look during the procedure. Show the client pictures of what a normal peel looks like. Take pictures of the client's skin before and after the procedure. This will allow you to show him or her the improvement in the skin's appearance. Explain that the client should not have any sun exposure for eight weeks after peeling and must use a broad-spectrum sunscreen at all times. Clients who are being treated for hyperpigmentation should be especially careful about sun exposure.

Have the client sign a release saying that he or she has been fully informed about the possible disadvantages of peeling and the actual procedure that takes place. It is very important to be honest. Chemical exfoliation at this level is uncomfortable, and during the procedure the skin looks terrible. A nervous client or one who becomes hysterical easily should not have deep chemical exfoliation. You will save yourself a world of trouble by getting to know your client well before performing these services.

FOCUS ON: *Superficial Exfoliation*

Superficial exfoliation will not do the following:

Remove deep wrinkles.
Reduce deep acne scarring.
Repair severe sun damage to any appreciable degree.
Cause a lifting effect on the skin.

Superficial exfoliation will do the following:

Improve the skin's texture.
Even the coloring.
Help lighten hyperpigmentation.
Improve fine lines and rough textures.

Deep Exfoliation Guidelines

Several different procedures are used for deep exfoliation, which vary according to the manufacturer. Following are two examples of typical procedures for liquid and cream deep exfoliations. These are meant to serve only as examples. *Although these procedures sound fairly simple, you must be thoroughly trained and experienced to perform them correctly.* You must have hands-on training to perform this type of deep chemical exfoliation. Do not think you are qualified simply from reading this chapter or a manufacturer's handbook. You should observe several procedures and have hands-on supervision doing a treatment before attempting to perform this procedure on your own. You must also work within the legal guidelines for your state and license.

LIQUID EXFOLIATION One liquid used for exfoliation is normally Jessner's solution; another is a 20% solution of salicylic acid (a BHA). Both are applied to the face with cotton swabs. Remember to follow directions furnished by the manufacturer before any treatment.

CAUTION!

Always follow the manufacturer's direction for the preparation that you are using.

REGULATORY AGENCY ALERT

Percentages of acids used for this process vary from manufacturer to manufacturer. Follow state guidelines as to whether it is within your scope of practice to use them.

PROCEDURE 16–5 JESSNER'S SOLUTION OR 20% BHA TREATMENT

IMPLEMENTS AND MATERIALS

- Typical facial lounge, client draping, and linen setup
- Client eye protection
- Gloves
- Disposable sponges, cotton or gauze
- 4×4 cotton gauze squares
- Solution applicator swabs
- Water and bowl
- Cotton rounds
- Peel solution
- Pre-peel solution (if recommended by manufacturer)
- Makeup-removing cleanser
- Pre-peel cleanser
- Toner
- Neutralizer (if needed due to a reaction)
- Post-peel serum, lotion, or balm as recommended by manufacturer
- Sun protection, SPF 30

Preparation

1. Set up the facial lounge with linens.
2. Prepare towels and cotton and gather supplies.
3. Decant or set up products. Set up supplies.

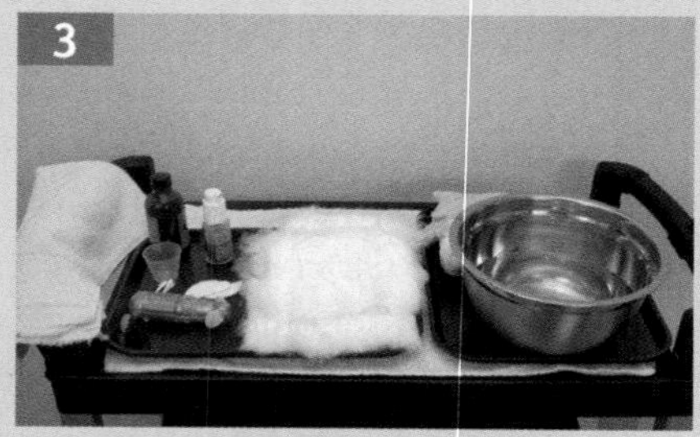
3
Set up supplies.

Procedure

4. Complete all the pre-exfoliation consultation procedure forms and discuss procedure with client.
5. Drape client and secure hair away from the face.
6. Remove the client's makeup thoroughly with cleanser.
   a. Remove eye makeup.
   b. Remove lipstick.
7. Put on gloves.
8. Perform a second cleansing, if recommended by manufacturer.

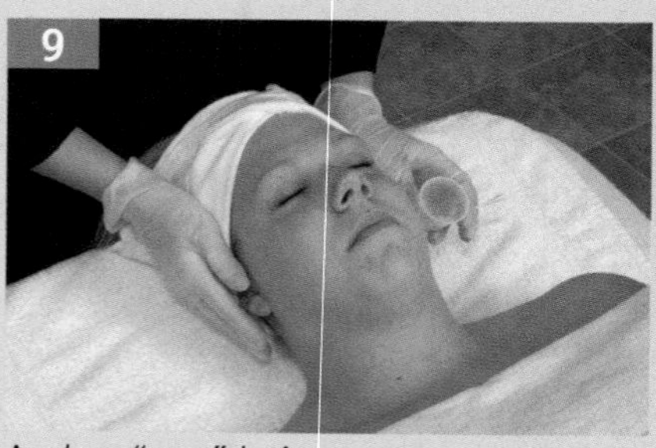
9
Apply a "prep" lotion.

9. Apply a "prep" lotion, if furnished or recommended by the manufacturer. This solution is usually acetone, which removes excess oils and surface dead cells. (Avoid the upper lip due to inhalation of fumes.)

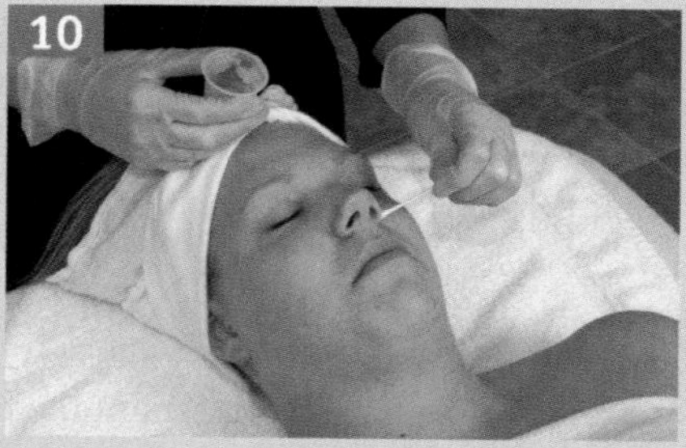
10
Apply occlusive barrrier.

10. Follow manufacturer's directions for application of occlusive barrier to corners of the mouth and nose and around the eyes.

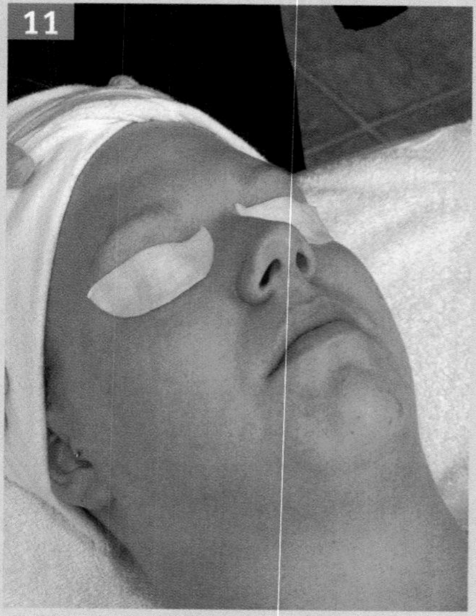
11
Place eye protection on client.

11. Place eye protection on client.

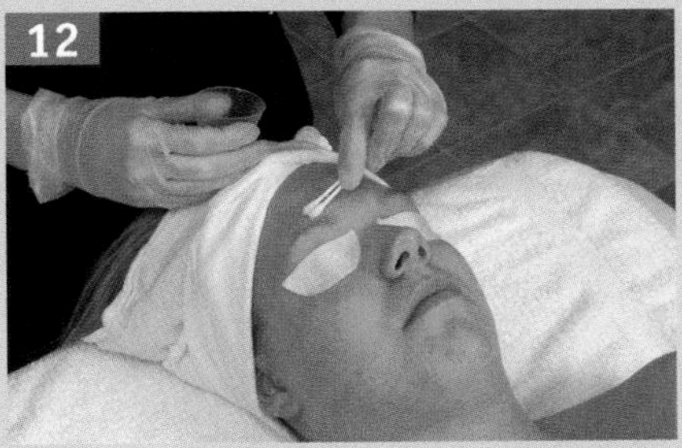

Apply liquid solution.

12 Apply the liquid solution on the face using two cotton swabs held closely together or a 4 × 4 gauze.

a. Begin with the forehead and apply the solution in small, gentle, circular motions. Do not apply pressure with the swabs.

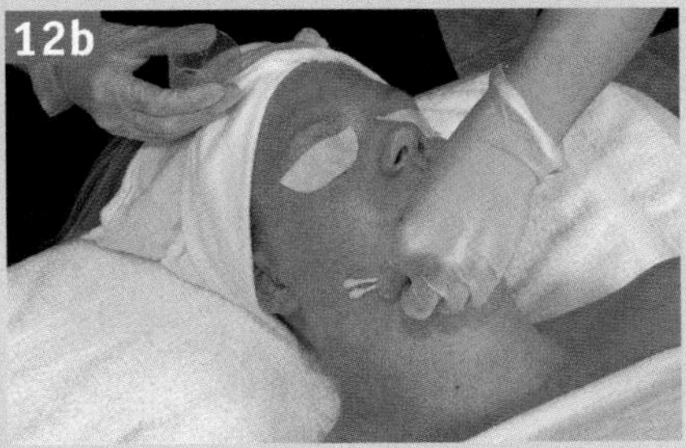

Feather solution below the jawline.

b. Proceed down the cheek and around the face. It is very important that the application be as even as possible. Feather solution below the jawline.

c. Be sure to apply the solution to the cheeks, chin, upper lip and nose area.

d. Do *not* apply the solution to the lips, ears, or upper lids. Below the eye may be treated, but stay at least 1/8 inch away from the lower lid edge outside of the area where the occlusive barrier product was placed. Follow the manufacturer's recommendations. Assure eye protection remains in place.

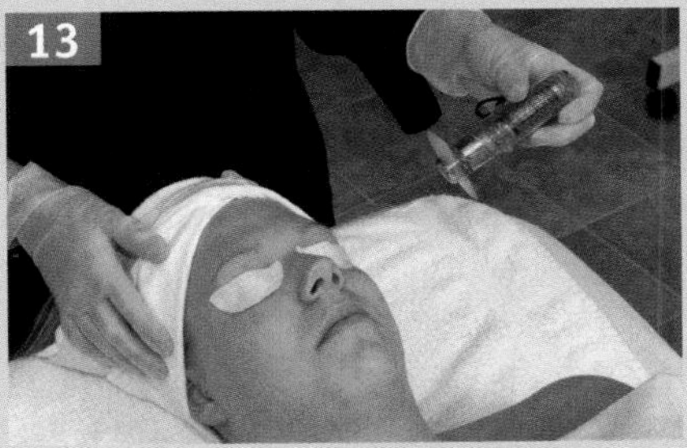

A small fan can alleviate burning sensation.

13 Place a small fan so that it blows gently on the client's face. (Do not turn the fan to high speed, because this may blow the liquid. Some companies do not recommend using a fan at all for this reason or because it accelerates the drying process too much. Some fans are small enough for clients to hold in their hands.) The fan also helps cool the strong burning sensation that he or she will feel when you start the application. The intensity of the burning sensation varies with the client. As an alternative to the fan, do a scalp massage and talk to the client so he or she does not concentrate on the burning sensation. After about 15 minutes, this sensation will stop, and the skin will feel numb and slightly tingly.

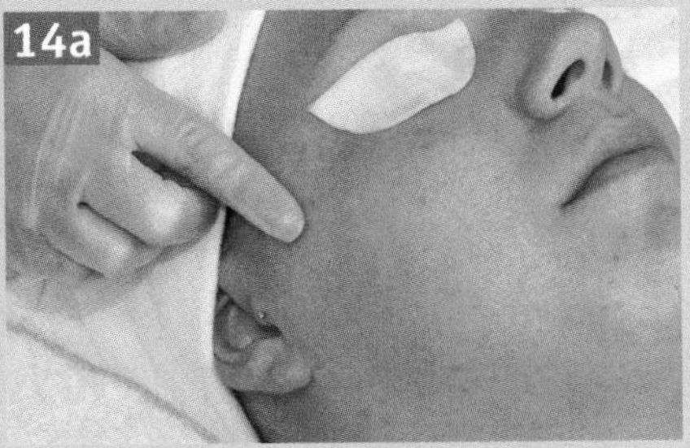

Frosting occurs when the peel is complete.

14 Allow this coat to "dry" for 2 minutes.

a. Look for any white areas forming on the face. This is known as *frosting*, which occurs when the peel is complete. Some clients will frost after one coat and some after two or three coats of solution.

b. If frosting does not occur after the first coat, repeat the application procedure and wait for another 4 minutes. Occasionally, some areas of the face will frost and others will not. If this happens, reapply the solution to the unfrosted areas only.

c. Apply the solution at 4-minute intervals until frosting occurs. Most clients require only one to three coats; do not apply more than three coats.

continues on next page

PROCEDURE 16–5, CONT. JESSNER'S SOLUTION OR 20% BHA TREATMENT

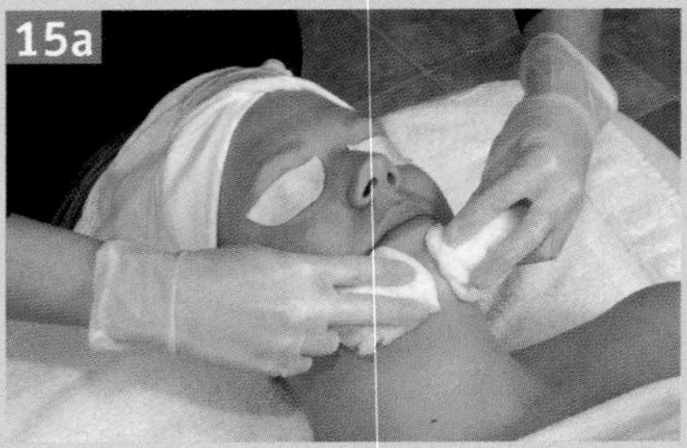

Cold compresses for 3 to 5 minutes will minimize redness.

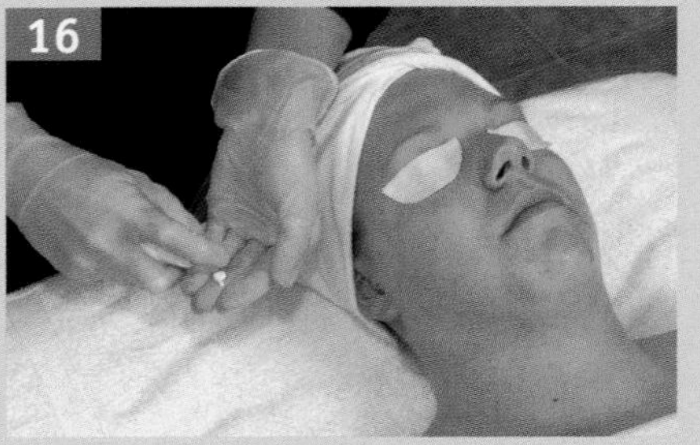

Apply post-peel product.

15 Following the manufacturer's directions, rinse frost and residue from the skin using neutralizer as recommended.

a. For a BHA, remove the frost and residue with 4×4s. If the skin is flushed, cold compresses for 3 to 5 minutes will minimize redness.

b. For Jessner's treatments, the frost and residue remain on the skin. This will subside in approximately 2 hours.

16 Apply post-peel product and sun protection per manufacturer's directions.

Post-procedure

17 The client's skin may be sensitive or look flushed after the treatment and for 1 to 2 days.

18 Only gentle products should be used at home during the healing process. Assure that the client has appropriate home care, including non-AHA cleanser, non-AHA toner, non-AHA moisturizer, and post-treatment balm that he or she can apply to alleviate any tight feeling of the skin.

19 Give the client written home-care guidelines following the manufacturer's guidelines.

20 Remind the client of the following:

a. Do not pick at flaking skin as this may cause scarring.

b. Do not apply makeup for 7 days.

c. Avoid the sun and exercise and wear appropriate sun protection.

21 Schedule a follow-up visit 7 to 10 days later.

Clean-up and Disinfection

22 Follow clean-up and disinfection procedures in accordance with state and OSHA guidelines.

23 Reset and prepare the room for the next client.

THE CREAM EXFOLIANTS The preparation procedure is the same as for the liquid peel. No prep solution is used with the cream peel and the basic steps include the following:

1. With gloved hands apply the cream peel to the forehead, cheeks, nose, chin, and neck and finish with a very light application to the lower lids using a cotton swab. Apply evenly. The face will begin to burn and sting. Again, this sensation can be lessened by the use of a fan, and the feeling usually subsides after 15 to 20 minutes.
2. You do not have to watch for frosting with this treatment. It will happen automatically. There is no need for a second application until the next day. This thick treatment stays on the face for 1½ hours. After this time, gently remove the cream with a tongue depressor and then cleanse well with cool, wet, cotton compresses.
3. After removing the treatment, apply the thick moisturizing cream furnished in the peeling kit. The client will continue to apply this emollient cream to the face at home. The skin should be well lubricated with the emollient at all times.
4. On the second day, repeat the procedure in the salon. The client continues to keep the skin moist with the emollient cream.

After the Treatment

Immediately after a chemical exfoliation treatment, the skin will often look slightly red and flushed. There is often little change on the first day. On the second day of either peel, the skin will become tan-looking, sometimes splotchy.

On the third day the skin will becomes very dark and often splotchy and will feel very tight and dry. Peeling will begin around the mouth and chin first, then the cheeks, then the eyes. The neck and forehead are the last to peel. The skin will usually show flakiness or mild peeling from the third through the sixth or seventh day. Occasionally, the peeling will continue for several more days. Warn the client not to pull on the loose skin. This can cause infection and possible hyperpigmentation. It is best for the client to visit the clinic daily for a quick check, and you can gently peel off areas that are ready. Clients should not wash the face at all during the peeling procedure. They may use moisturizer, depending on the manufacturer's instructions, and cool water but no cleanser. Clients should avoid granular scrubs and other keratolyic preparations for at least the first two weeks after peeling. These include glycolic acid, benzoyl peroxide, sulfur, resorcinol, Retin-A, salicylic acid, lactic acid, or any other peeling or exfoliating agent. Clients should protect their skin with a daily sunscreen for at least eight weeks after peeling, and they must avoid direct sun exposure.

Reactions to Chemical Exfoliation

Rarely, a client will have an allergic reaction to a chemical exfoliation. The symptoms may include severe itching, swelling, severe redness, and stinging. Refer this client to a dermatologist who is familiar with your services, particularly your exfoliation procedures. Normally, a doctor will prescribe a steroid cream, which willl quickly alleviate the problem.

Dark skin types have a tendency to hyperpigment after chemical exfoliation. Many estheticians will not administer chemical exfoliaiton to Fitzpatrick skin levels V and VI. If the client pulls off skin that is not ready, splotchy hyperpigmentation can occur. Normally this fades within a few weeks, as long as the skin is protected with a sunscreen. Sometimes, if the hyperpigmentation does not decrease within two or three weeks after exfoliation, you may need to treat the skin with a mild bleaching cream.

Your proficiency in chemical exfoliation will increase as you perform more and more procedures. This is why it so important that you thoroughly train with someone accomplished in the practice of deep exfoliation and observe the actual peeling that takes place during the six or seven days after the procedure is performed (Figure 16–14). With this training you can become proficient at deeper chemical exfoliation.

Stronger Exfoliating Treatments

Some companies sell low-percentage TCA to estheticians. However, most experienced professionals agree that TCA belongs in the hands of dermatologists and plastic surgeons only. TCA is too unpredictable and is beyond the scope of esthetic exfoliation. See Chapter 26 for more information on medical peels.

MASK THERAPIES

Masks are a defining component of nearly all facial treatments. They can be implemented at different points during a facial to assist in treating skin conditions or to stimulate or calm the skin. Estheticians may use a single mask to conclude a therapy or multiple masks to accomplish different objectives.

Mask Theory

Masks are products applied to the skin in an occlusive manner; they trigger a skin response based partially on the duration of time they are in contact with the skin. As the skin's visible conditions change, or treatment goals change, so then does the chosen mask. A key part of the response they achieve is a result of the activation or calming of the body's own self-cleansing mechanism, the circulatory system. This impact occurs with all masks regardless of their base. Any time a coating is applied to the skin, the circulatory system enhances blood flow to the area to try and remove the substance. Consider how wearing a plastic glove makes the hand grow moist. The body responds to the occlusive nature of the glove and tries to remove it. The benefits include increased nutrient flow to the area, hydration, and a purging of waste materials. Masks may also have thermal factors that cause a warming or cooling sensation on the skin.

Employing a variety of masks can enhance treatment results and keep both you and the client focused on the facial's benefits (Table 16–1). As you rotate through customized treatments for cross-training the skin, mask diversity can enhance the process.

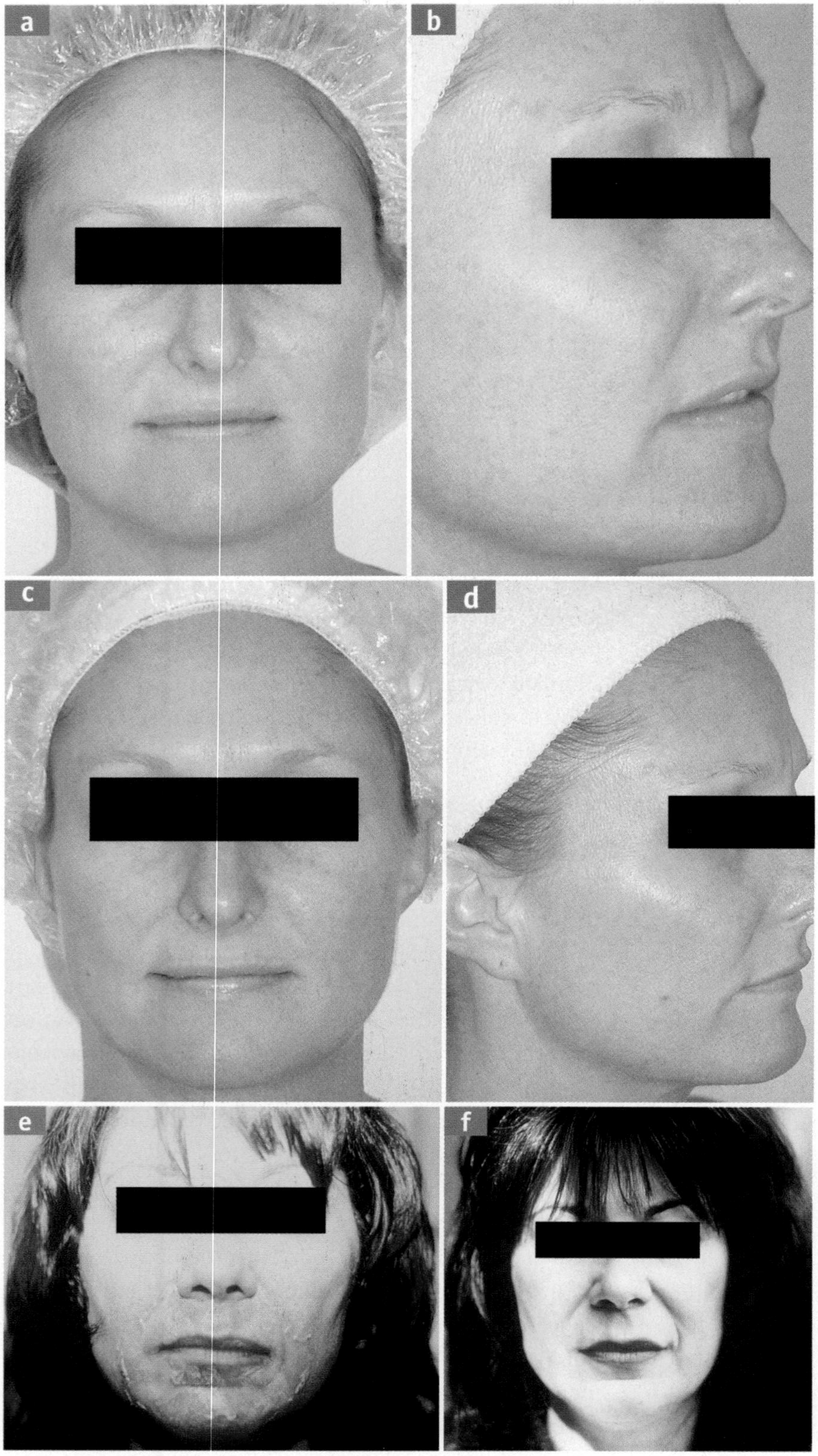

Figure 16–14 Changes in skin post peel.

Basic Masks

While clay, cream, and gel masks are standard components of every treatment room, you need to be alert to your ingredients to determine if they are soothing or stimulating in nature. Keep in mind that stimulating and soothing are two key impacts you can effect on the body's

Table 16–1 Mask Functions on Skin Conditions

MASK FUNCTIONS ON SKIN CONDITIONS	
Suffocation	Triggering increased circulation to the area
Hydration	Adding moisture
Purification	Purging, drawing, absorption of impurities
Calming	Soothing
Nourishing	Rejuvenating
Exfoliating (as in enzyme mask)	Smoothing to the skin

circulatory system: speeding it up or calming it down. This cannot be assumed by the base. The bases themselves are neutral but manufacturers incorporate additional ingredients in order to enhance or achieve specific results. Stimulating or purifying masks may include ingredients such as mint, camphor, clove, or other **rubifactants** that enhance blood flow to the skin. Soothing, calming, healing masks may include ingredients like aloe vera, grapeseed extract, green tea, sea whip, amino acids, panthenol, allantoin, plantain, chamomile, or comfrey. Nourishing regenerating masks may incorporate vitamins, caviar, avocado, amino acids, peptides, antioxidants, collagen, elastin, and hylaruonic acid. Hydrating masks include hydrators such as NMF (Natural Moisturizing Factor), collagen, elastin, ceramides, or hylauronic acid. It will take more than one mask to meet the diverse needs of your clients.

Zone Therapy

For enhanced results in clients with a mixture of skin conditions, you can apply these masks in a zone treatment pattern (Figure 16–15). If the forehead or T-zone is more oily/problematic, apply a clay mask in this area. If the cheeks are more dehydrated, then a gel mask would be appropriate. Specialty eye masks can be applied to treat delicate orbital tissue and perhaps a cream mask on the throat to fight signs of aging. Apply each mask with a mask brush, and then allow the masks to remain on the skin about 10 minutes before removing, unless the manufacturer's directions say to do otherwise. To intensify the activity of the mask, apply a cool to cold wet towel over it.

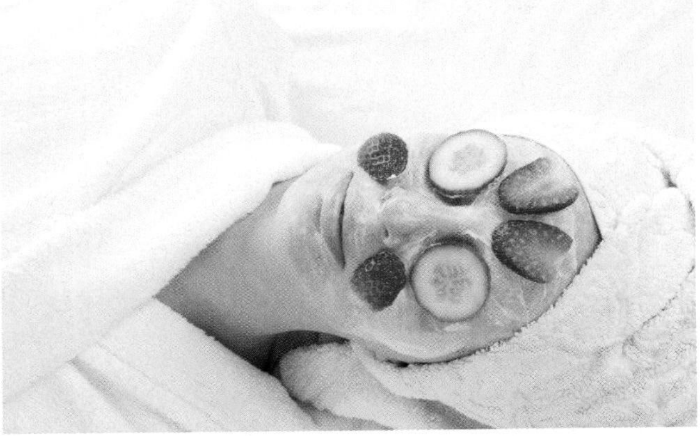

Figure 16–15 Zone therapy mask.

Collagen Sheet Masks

Collagen masks are made of collagen fibers (Figure 16–16). Other ingredients may include ceramic powder, gelatin, sorbitol, and carboxymethycellulose. Collagen masks are available in wet and dry formulas. These masks are beneficial for hydration, rejuvenation, soothing, and calming of the skin. They can be applied over an ampoule or serum for enhanced penetration. Collagen patch masks enhanced with algae and organic mud patches, vitamin C, and AHA designed for problem-area spot treatments are all available. Other specialty ingredients commonly incorporated into the collagen or the serum in which it is packed are aloe vera, allantoin, panthenol, L-ascorbic acid, fruit acids, DNA, ginko biloba, vitamins, and other botanical extracts.

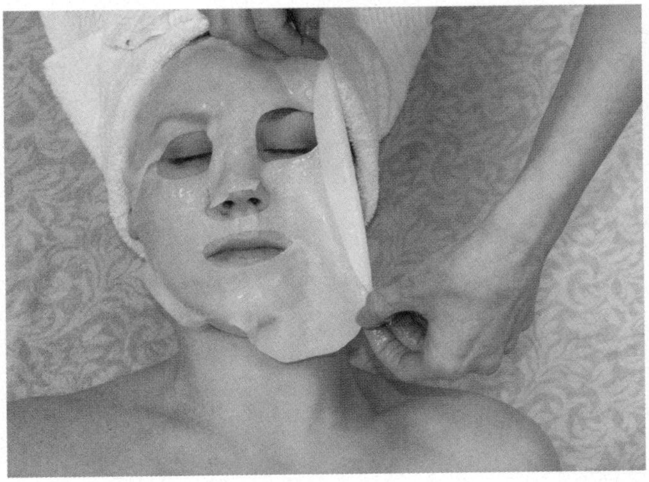

Figure 16–16 Wet collagen sheet applied to the skin.

The wet or pre-moistened mask comes in a foil pouch. When you cut open the package, you can slide out the mask and carefully lay it on the client's face (Figure 16–17). This form generally has precut openings for the eyes, nose, and mouth. If the client has a small face, you can pleat the fabric to fit and allow it to set 10 to 20 minutes. When you remove the mask, you can work the remaining hydrating fluids into the skin or rinse them off before applying finishing creams.

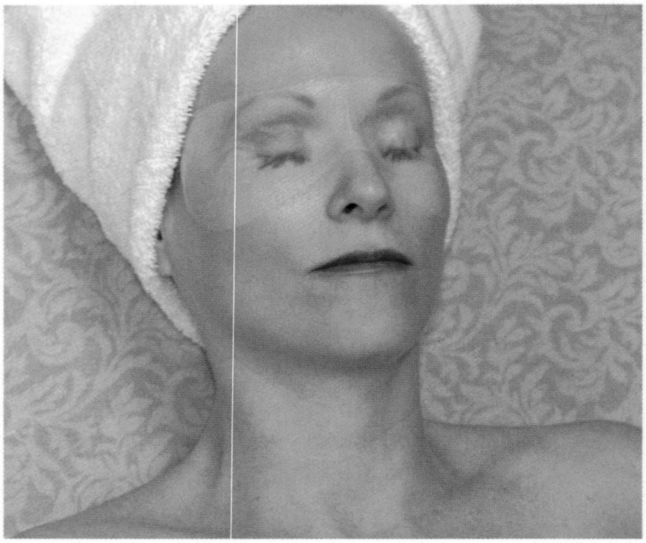

Figure 16–17 Wet collagen eye pads.

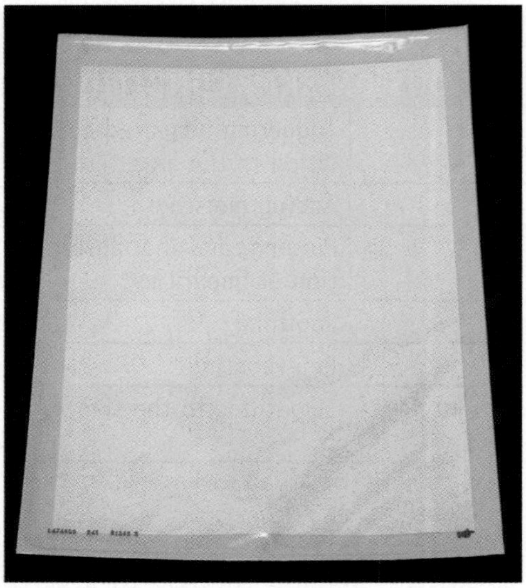

Figure 16–18 Dry collagen mask in package.

Dry collagen sheets come in plastic covers and may or may not have precut facial openings (Figure 16–18). Before hydrating this mask, premeasure and make slits for the eyes, nose, and mouth as needed, because it is nearly impossible to do so once the mask is wet (Figure 16–19). You can hydrate with water or a pre-formulated liquid and a spray unit, very wet cloths, or disposable sponges; then allow the mask to set 10 to 20 minutes as directed. The dry sheets also can be used for the décoletté or cut for spot treatments such as eye patches. Any cutting should be done prior to hydration and the unused portion returned to the plastic sheet to protect it from moisture.

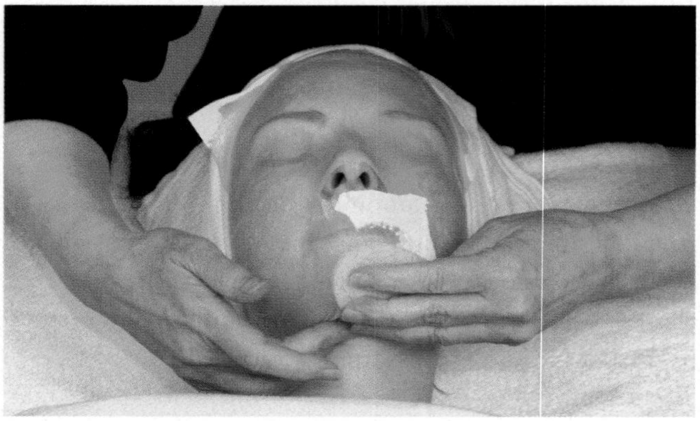

Figure 16–19 Dry collagen mask on face.

Powder Masks

Most powder masks come in a powder form that is mixed with water and then applied. They are commonly divided into hard- and soft-setting varieties. Attributes for skin improvement include sculpturing, tightening, hydrating, rejuvenating, oxygenating, and stimulating. The hard-setting form is sometimes termed either a *plaster* or *thermal modelage* mask due to the heat response that occurs as the mask cures. To facilitate application and removal of the thermal mask, apply treatment serums and a cream. Then place a gauze mask on the client's face before applying the mask product thickly with a tongue depressor.

PROCEDURE 16–6 APPLICATION AND REMOVAL OF POWDER MASK

This mask procedure may be incorporated into any appropriate facial treatment.

IMPLEMENTS AND MATERIALS

- Typical treatment lounge, client draping, and linen setup
- Disposable sponges, 4×4 gauze squares, or facial cloths
- Water and bowl
- Soft rubber mask bowl
- Wood or plastic tongue depressor (for mask blending and application)
- Cotton rounds
- Facial gauze sheet
- Cleanser
- Toner
- Powder mask
- Premeasured water for mask
- Balm
- Serums appropriate for skin
- Rich moisturizer
- Sunscreen

Preparation

Perform general treatment room setup:

1 Prepare treatment table, linens, and towels.

2 Assemble and set up products.

3 Pre-cleanse the client's skin and remove makeup.

4 Perform any desired exfoliation and massage steps.

5 Remove massage product and rinse well.

6 Make sure the client's hairline is well protected.

Procedure

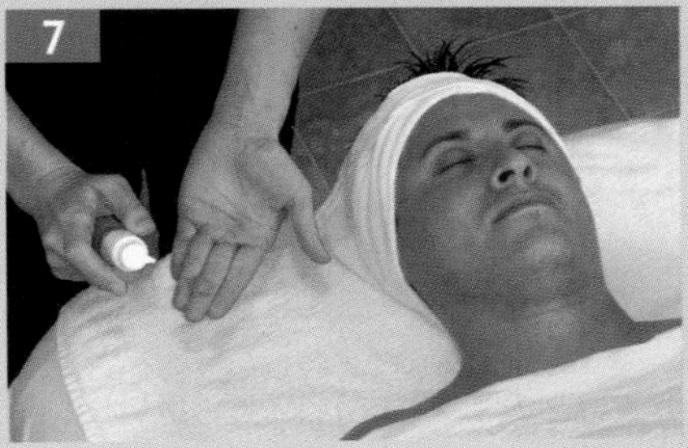

Apply serum.

7 Apply appropriate serums for the skin.

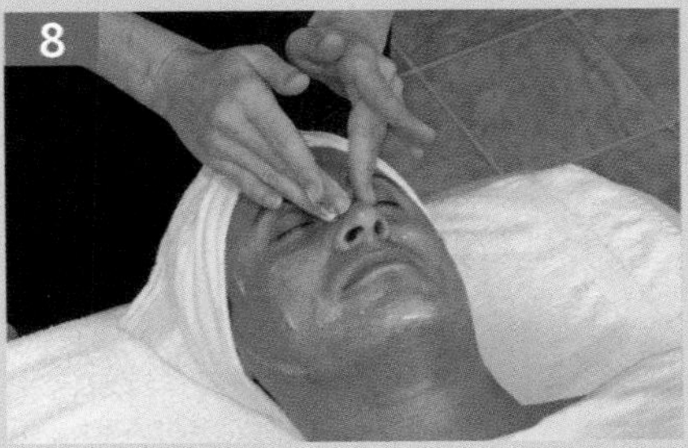

Apply moisturizer to skin.

8 Apply a layer of moisturizer to skin.

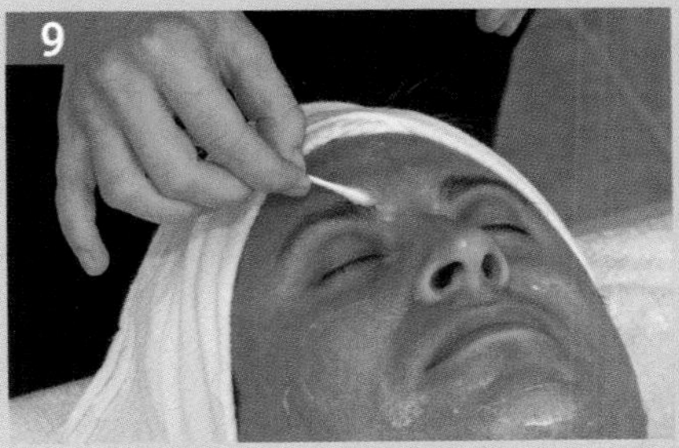

Apply balm to eyebrow hair and to lips.

9 Apply balm to eyebrow hair and lips.

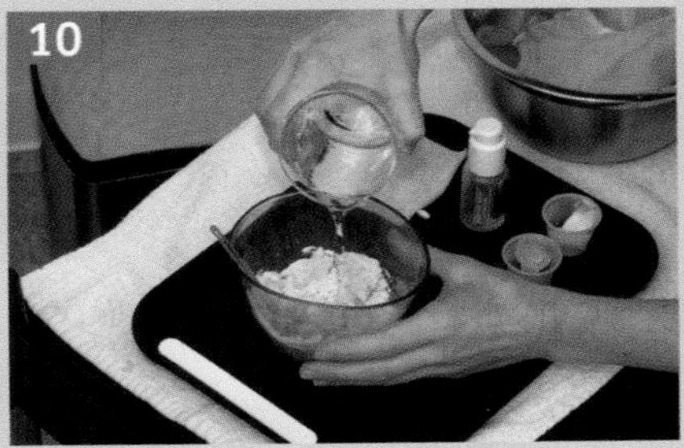

Blend mask and water.

10 Following the manufacturer's directions, blend the mask and water in a rubber bowl using a tongue depressor. Stir quickly but carefully to prevent powder spillage. The mask will thicken and start to set up, so do *not* premix this product.

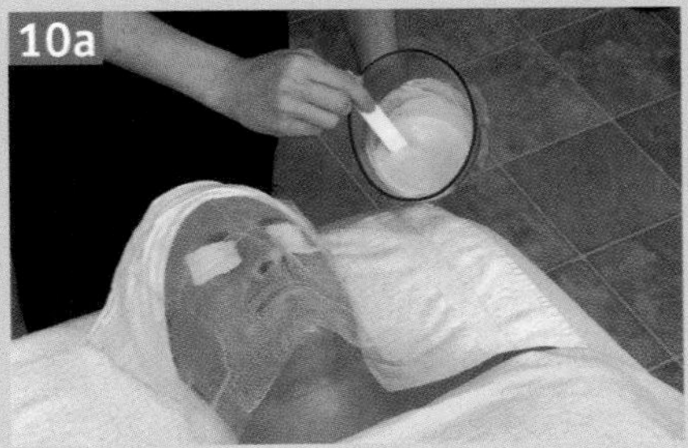

Stir quickly as mask thickens.

continues on next page

PROCEDURE 16-6, CONT. APPLICATION AND REMOVAL OF POWDER MASK

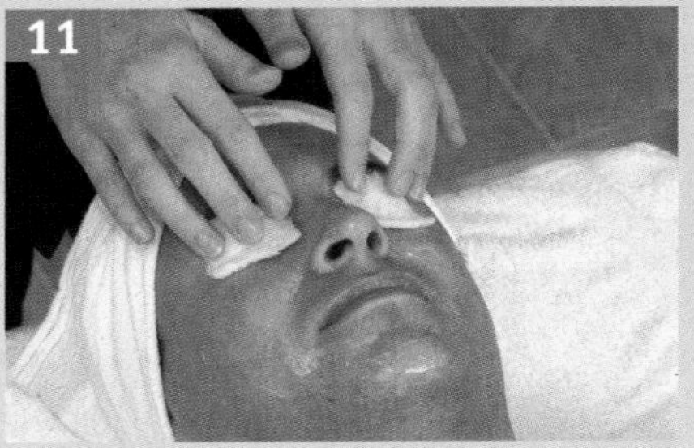

Protect eye area.

11 Apply damp cotton rounds to protect the eye area.

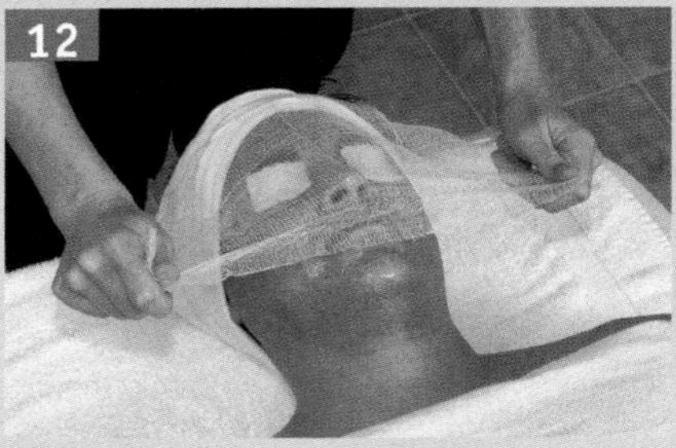

Use gauze to facilitate removal.

12 Apply a single-layer gauze sheet over the client's face to facilitate removal.

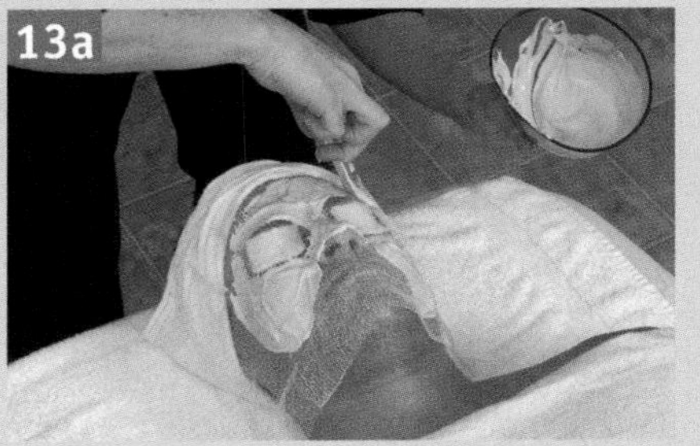

Spread the mask thick; clear to the edges.

13 Apply the mixture to the mask with the tongue depressor as you would frost a cake.

a. Keep mask thick to edges to avoid crumbling during removal.

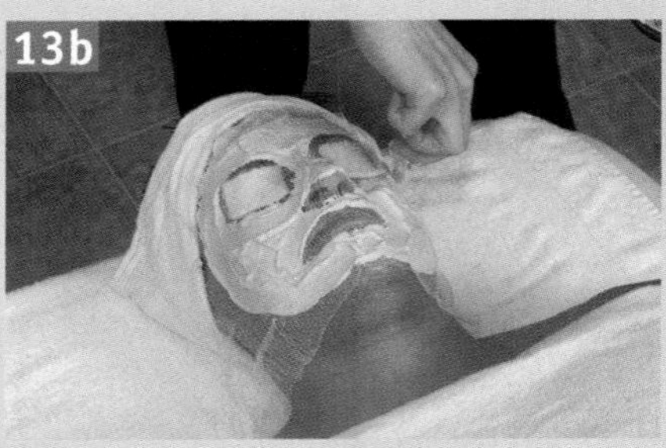

Stop application at the edge of the mandible.

b. Stop application at the edge of the mandible and do not extend down the neck.

14 Allow the mask to set according to manufacturer's guidelines.

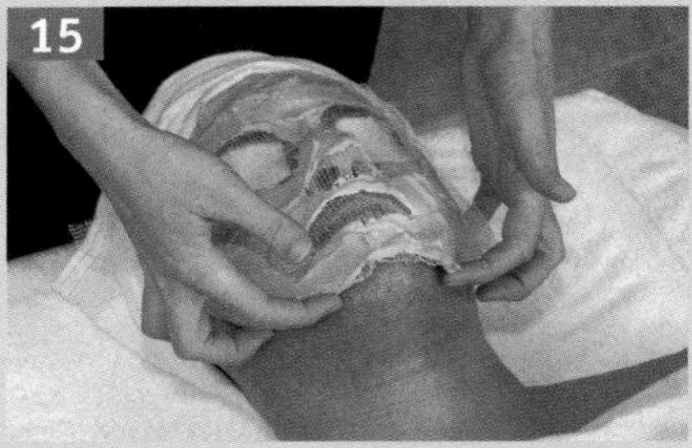

Remove mask.

15 Remove the mask by placing your fingers along the hairline perimeter of mask just above jaw level.

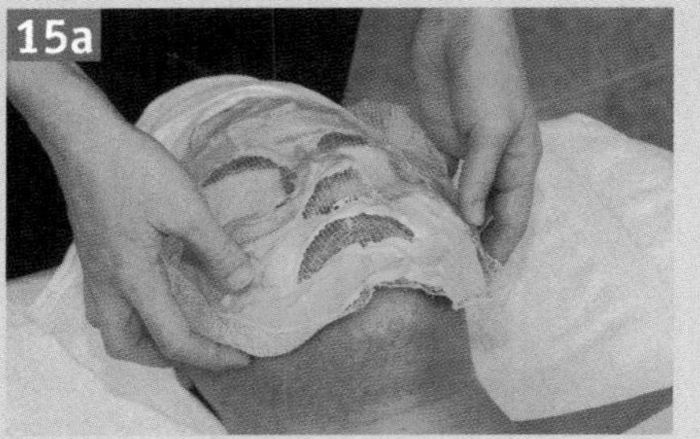

Rock mask to loosen.

a. Rock the mask just slightly to loosen. Lift from the neck toward the forehead.

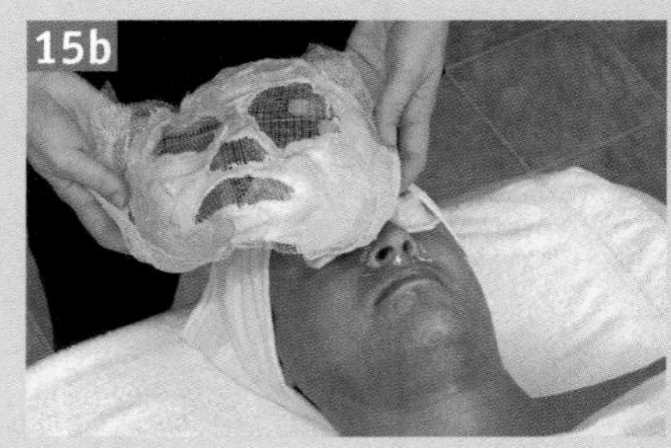

The mask can be removed in a single piece.

b. Properly applied, the mask can be removed in a single piece.

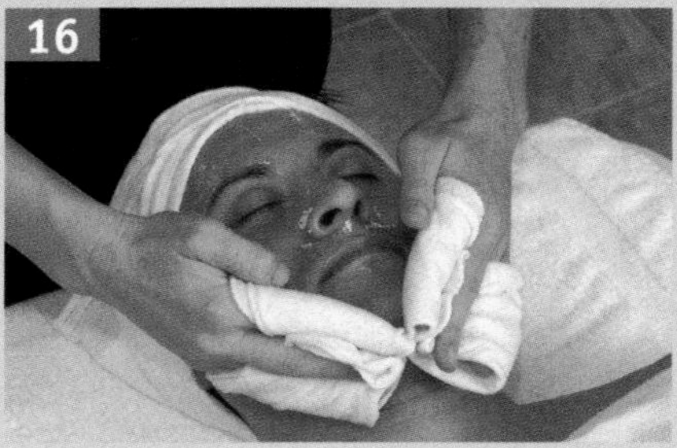

Rinse the skin.

16 Rinse the skin.

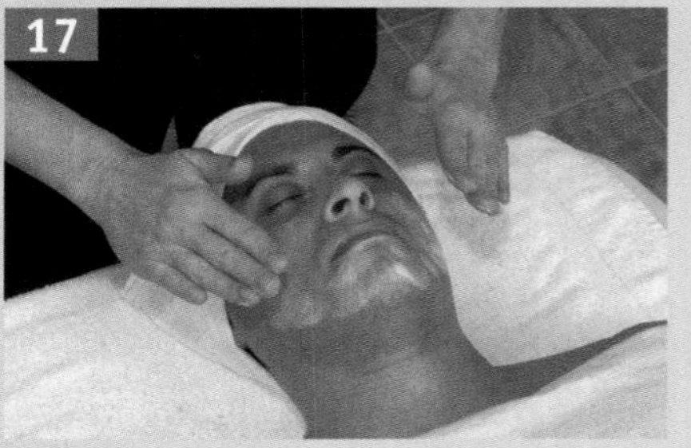

Apply sun protection.

17 Apply sun protection.

Post-procedure

Assure that the client has appropriate home care.

Clean-up and Disinfection

18 Perform clean-up and disinfection according to OSHA or your state's regulations.

19 Always dispose of all hard-setting mask remnants in the trash, never in a sink; it will clog it.

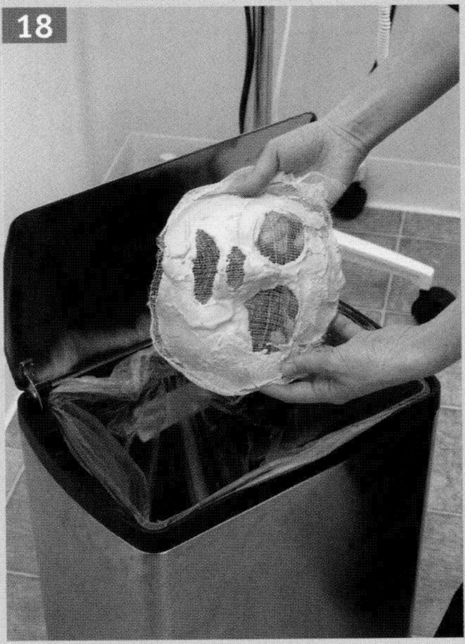

Clean up and disinfect.

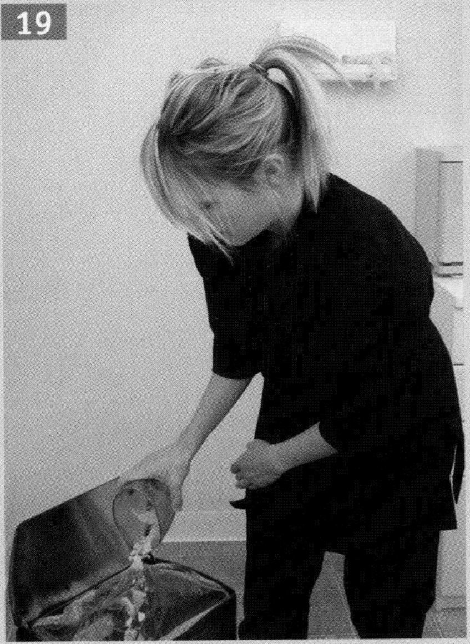

Dispose of mask remnants in the trash.

Here's a Tip

If there is any residual mask in the rubber bowl, allow it to dry. Once dry, flex the bowl and the mask will break loose cleanly. Wipe out the bowl with a dry paper towel and place the residue in trash. Now the bowl is ready to be cleansed and sanitized.

Soft-setting masks such as alginates, latex, and liquid rubber are applied in the same manner as the hard-setting variety, only less thickly (Figure 16–20). They are applied over a serum/ampoule, a cream or basic mask, and often a layer of gauze. They set to a point at which fingerprints will not show in the mask, but they stay soft and pliable. Some of these masks cool as they set up on the skin, triggering a soothing, vasoconstrictive response. These masks often include common ingredients such as pearl powder, silica, algin, rubber latex, diatomaceous earth, proteins, talc, calcium sulfate, and calcium carbonate. Specialty ingredients sometimes include seaweed, algae, aloe vera, spirulina, allantoin, or centella. Always dispose of soft-setting mask remnants in the trash and never in a sink; the residue will clog the sink.

CAUTION!

Avoid using masks on clients who suffer from claustrophobia.

Here's a Tip

For best control in removing the soft mask, start at the forehead and roll it on top of itself as if you were rolling up pastry.

Rubber-type Masks

These masks are sold in a somewhat pliable block. Treatment portions are cut off the block and the remainder stored in air-tight plastic. The product is melted and applied over gauze (Figure 16–21). The mask takes on a rubbery consistency as it cools but remains pliable. Depending on the formula, the mask triggers a warming or cooling effect on the skin. The warming variation is designed for pre-extraction. It provides a softening of sebum and follicular material as it promotes oxygenation by activating the body's self-cleansing mechanism. The cooling variation of this mask soothes, reduces redness, and enhances

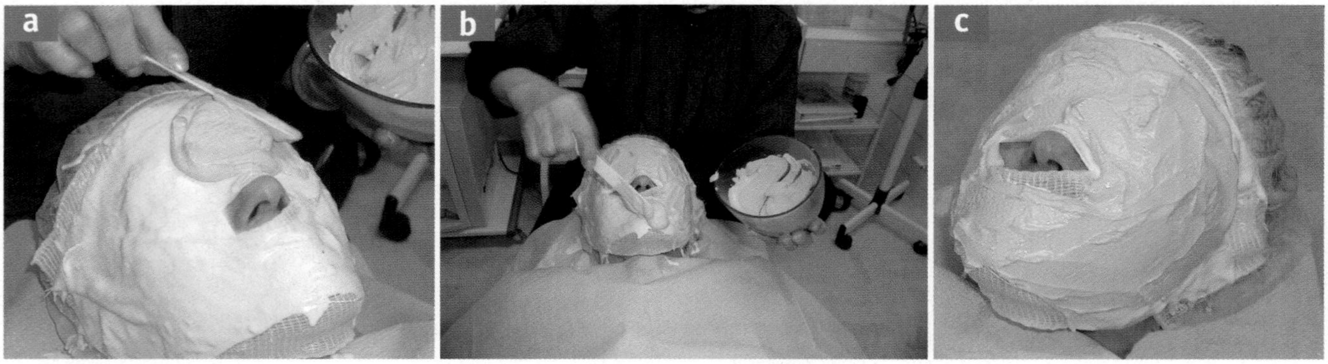

Figure 16–20 Applying and removing soft latex mask.

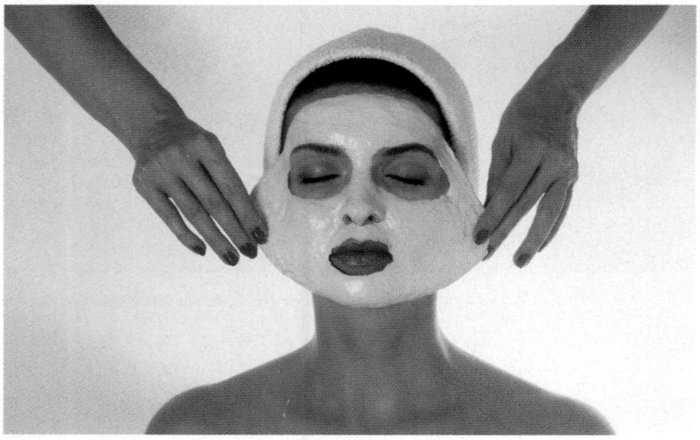

Figure 16–21 Rubber-type mask on client.

absorption of performance ingredients applied underneath the mask. Common ingredients found in these masks are paraffin, plastics, and rubber gel.

Specialty Layered Masks

Specialty layered masks use multiple layers of product and mask to achieve intensive hydration and rejuvenation. They may be sold in a kit or created from within an esthetician's existing treatment line. Often these kits include the same components discussed for other masks. Generally a layered mask therapy incorporates a serum layer, rich cream layer, and two layers of mask which may be powder base or a variety of other combinations to create an equivalent result. One mask may be of the soft-setting variety with a hard plaster mask on top. Common ingredients vary greatly depending on the intent of the mask and manufacturer's goals. Consult product manuals for specific guidelines and information on compatibility of masks to be layered.

These treatments may take a little longer to accomplish and require extra steps for preparation and application. When applying two mask layers, it is important to allow the first soft mask layer to set up before attempting to apply the plaster. The use of gauze over the moisturizer and under the masks will facilitate removal. Extra treatment time may be necessary for this mask procedure to achieve optimal setting results. The skin responds with deep hydration and excellent absorption of product. It is particularly nice for maturing or sun-damaged skin.

Here's a Tip

- The use of intensives (ampoules or serums) on the skin under the mask allows for enhanced penetration of these agents.
- The use of a hot, wet towel over an enzyme mask or other pre-extraction mask will cause increased activity of the body's self-cleansing mechanism.
- Applying a cool to cold wet towel over an appropriate finishing mask will reduce skin temperature, redness, and irritation.
- The weight of wet towels on the epidermis intensifies the body's circulatory response, resulting in skin being either pinker or more blanched.

The ability to customize treatments and blend modalities to achieve the best result for the client's skin is a skill all estheticians need for success. Establishing a treatment plan that cross-trains the skin and works with it while nurturing new cellular development enhances results even more. Combining customized treatments, a diverse treatment plan and appropriate home care that can help the client achieve their goals is an exciting part of an esthetician's career.

REVIEW QUESTIONS

1. Discuss the building blocks of a facial.
2. Discuss treatment arc theory.
3. Discuss treatment enhancers.
4. What is thermotherapy and how does it apply to facials?
5. What are some basic and advanced mask therapies?
6. Discuss some advanced masks and their benefits.
7. What is exfoliation therapy?
8. Discuss the different forms of exfoliation therapy.
9. What are the Cosmetic Ingredient Review Committee's guidelines for chemical exfoliation?
10. What are the contraindications for esthetic exfoliation?
11. Discuss some of the different exfoliation used in the clinic.
12. What is manual microdermabrasion?
13. Discuss the technique of manual microdermabrasion and client selection.
14. What are some of the possible complications or side effects of exfoliation techniques?
15. What are the guidelines for sensitive or rosacea skin treatments?

CHAPTER GLOSSARY

rubifacant: an agent that causes the skin to redden.

CHAPTER 17

ADVANCED SKIN CARE MASSAGE

CHAPTER OUTLINE

- ADVANCED FACIAL MOVEMENTS
- SELECTING AND INCORPORATING ADVANCED MOVEMENTS
- ADVANCED NECK AND DÉCOLLETÉ MOVEMENTS
- ADVANCED BACK MOVEMENTS
- SHIATSU MASSAGE FOR THE FACE
- REFLEXOLOGY FOR THE FACE
- EAR REFLEXOLOGY
- STONE MASSAGE FOR ESTHETICIANS
- LYMPHATIC MASSAGE FOR THE FACE AND NECK
- MACHINE-AIDED LYMPHATIC MASSAGE TREATMENTS

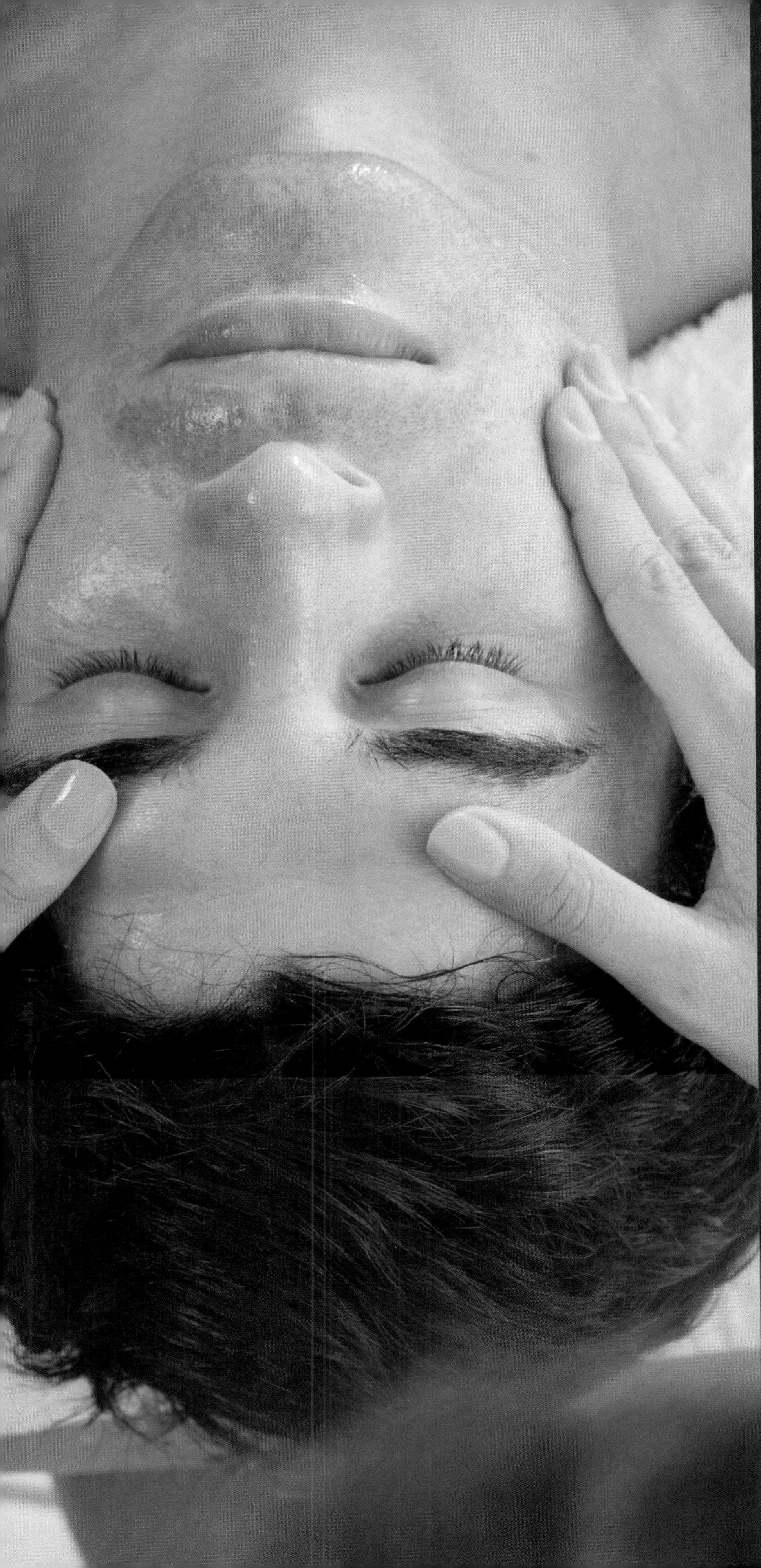

LEARNING OBJECTIVES

After completing this chapter, you should be able to:

- Incorporate advanced facial massage movements into current massage.
- Include advanced neck and décolleté movements in current massage.
- Add back application movements into your back treatments.
- Select movements that meet the needs of your client.
- Perform Shiatsu face massage.
- Provide a reflexology ear massage.
- Incorporate stones into facial massage.
- Perform manual lymph drainage of the face.
- Perform machine-aided lymph drainage of the face.

KEY TERMS

Page numbers indicate where in the chapter the term is used.

acupuncture 402
basalt 410
conduction 410
igneous 410
metamorphosed 410
reflexology 407
sedimentary 410
Shiatsu massage 402

Growing in knowledge and expertise is an important part of an esthetician's profession. For many clients, there is no step in the facial that is more important than the massage. This is a fast-paced and busy world where stress is commonplace. When a client has a facial, he or she wants to relax and be pampered. For just a little while, he or she needs to let go of problems and the stress of life and just unwind. Providing a great massage keeps clients coming back again and again. Being able to offer different massages and to include specialty treatments such as Shiatsu, lymph drainage, and stone therapy sessions helps attract a broader range of clients and delights your current client base. For those who want to focus on medi-spa work, lymph drainage techniques are an important skill to master because they reduce swelling and accelerate healing with no pressure to the skin.

FOCUS ON: *Massage Contraindications*

- **Inflamed skin conditions**
- **Burns (sunburn, chemical burns)**
- **Open wounds or rashes**
- **Sensitive skin**
- **High blood pressure**
- **Cancer**
- **Contagious disease**
- **Recent facial injections (within last 2 weeks)**
- **Recent surgery in area (within last 2 months)**
- **Autoimmune disorders**
  If in doubt about suitability get clearance from client's physician.

ADVANCED FACIAL MOVEMENTS

Whether you have practiced esthetics for many years or are new to esthetics, learning new massage movements is like adding spices to a recipe. Both you and your clients will enjoy these specialty techniques. You can select any of the face, back, and neck movements based on the client's skin and your personal preferences.

A good massage is like a dance choreographed between you and your client. Fluidity, continuity, and suitability for the client are key components. To build your skills, practice these movements and start blending them into the massage you have already learned. Vary the massage slightly from time to time so clients do not find your work predictable. A client may comment that he or she especially enjoys a specific movement, which you can note and include in every treatment that client receives.

FYI

Adding new massage movements does not mean you have to learn a new massage. You master the new movements and incorporate them at logical points in your current massage where they flow smoothly and rhythmically.

SELECTING AND INCORPORATING ADVANCED MOVEMENTS

Advanced facial massage movements can be incorporated into your existing massage easily and effectively. You may choose a single movement or several movements to add into your basic massage procedures.

To add movement to your existing procedure, simply place it so that the flow of your massage is even,

> **Here's a Tip**
>
> The addition of movements to your basic massage procedure will lengthen the time of your massage. To stay on schedule in the treatment room, practice and plan accordingly.

smooth, and connected. Whichever movement you choose to add should feel connected to the massage pattern. A client can tell when something does not flow, even if he or she has not had a massage before. Before adding any new techniques, it is important to know the client's skin care history, health history, likes, dislikes, and any massage contraindications. This allows you to provide a safe, effective, relaxing, and enjoyable skin care experience. Following is a list of advanced movements, along with a detailed description and illustration of each.

Eye Express

Using the ring finger, start at the temple and perform tiny circles, moving under the eye toward the inner corner of eye (Figure 17–1).

Around We Go

Beginning at the center of the forehead, perform friction circles from center to temples (Figure 17–2). When you reach the temples, lightly glide to just above the eyebrows and repeat the circular motion to the center of the forehead and then up to the hairline. Glide across hairline to temples and perform larger circles at the temples. End by circling the eyes and gliding up the forehead to the hairline and off or on to the starting position for the next movement.

Center Point

Placing the middle finger and index finger in the center between the eyebrows, perform friction circles down onto the tip of the nose and back to center between the brows

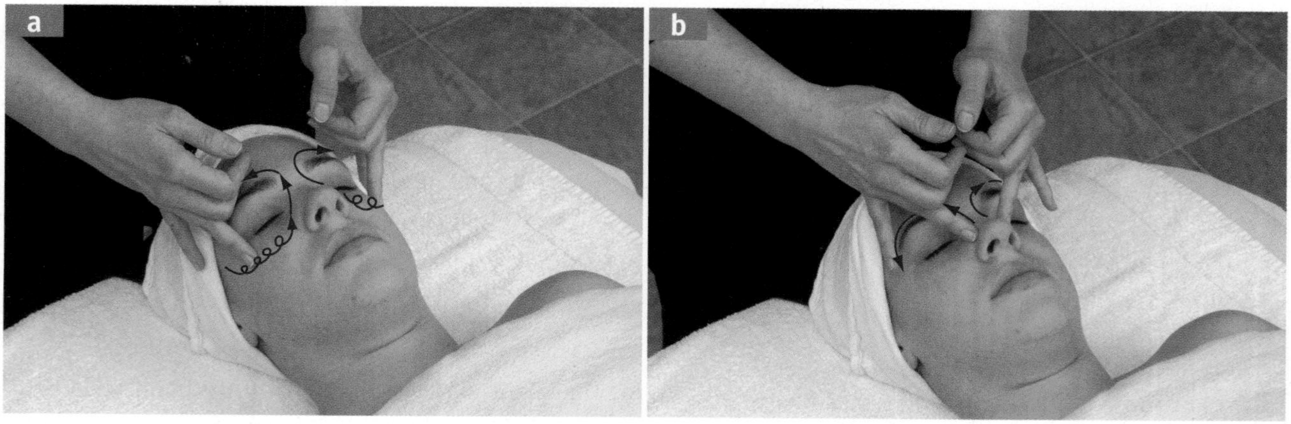

Figure 17–1 Eye Express.

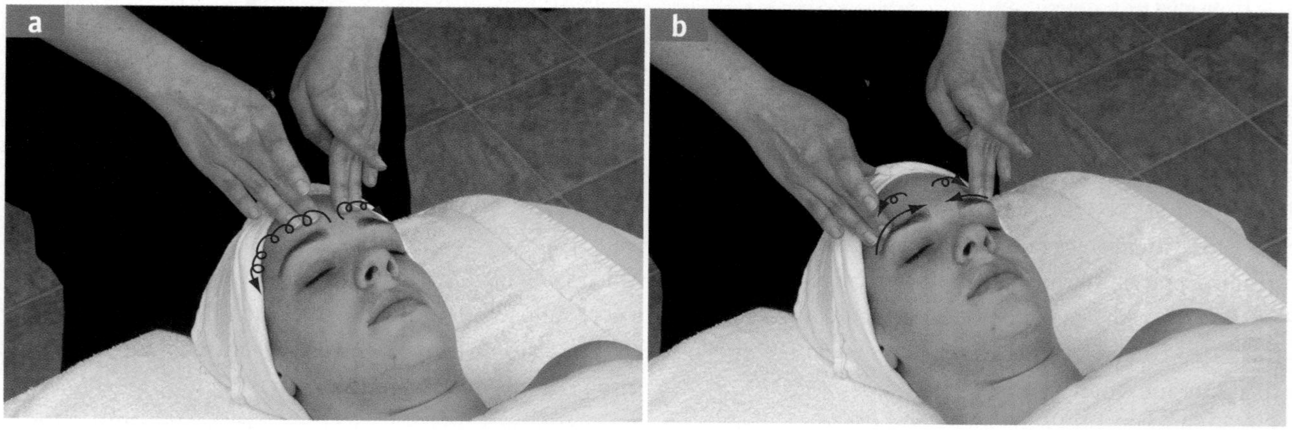

Figure 17–2 Around We Go.

(Figure 17–3). Drag fingers up the forehead to the hairline, and then glide to the next starting position.

Sinus Relief

Using four fingers on the bottom of the maxilla next to the nostrils, lightly and slowly slide the fingers up under the eyes and then down next to the nostrils. Apply firm pressure with finger pads, knuckles to tips, and hold for 10 seconds before releasing (Figure 17–4). Hook fingers under the maxilla and apply light pressure and release. Glide fingers around the bone toward the ears and over the temples, across the brows and down the sides of the nose, ending at the nostrils.

Paddlewheel

Use the palm and surface of the fingers of both hands to create a rolling motion, moving rapidly from the clavicle to the chin (Figure 17–5). Begin under the left ear and move across to the right ear. Movement should be in rapid succession, creating a paddlewheel motion.

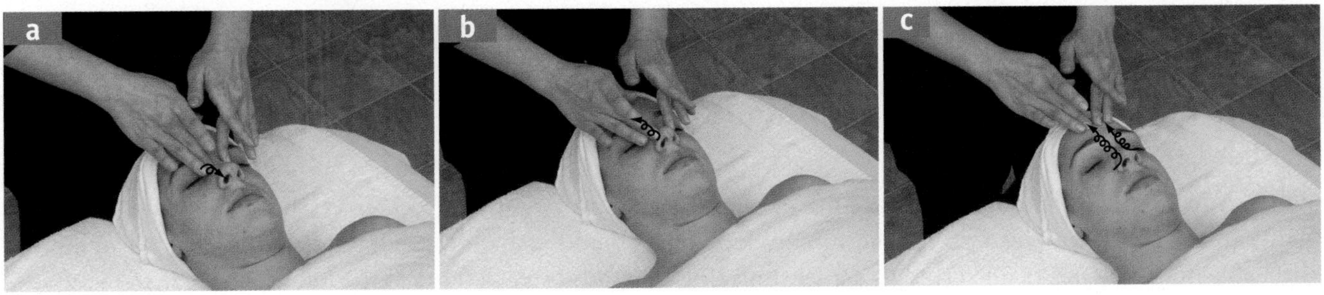

Figure 17–3 Center Point.

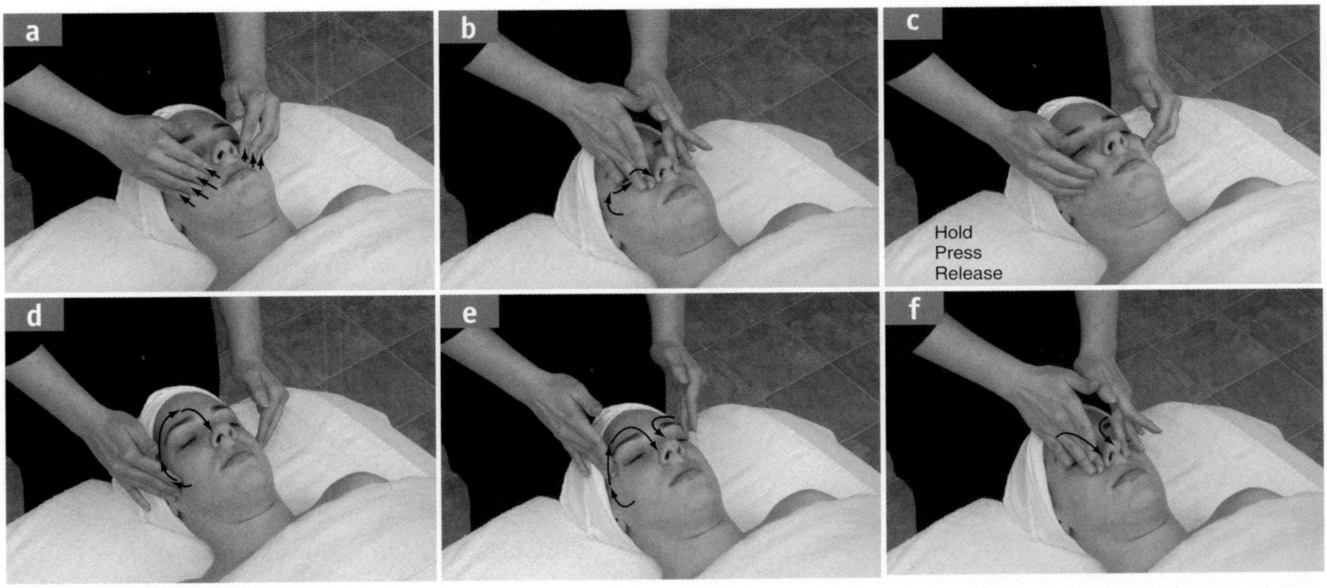

Figure 17–4 Sinus Relief.

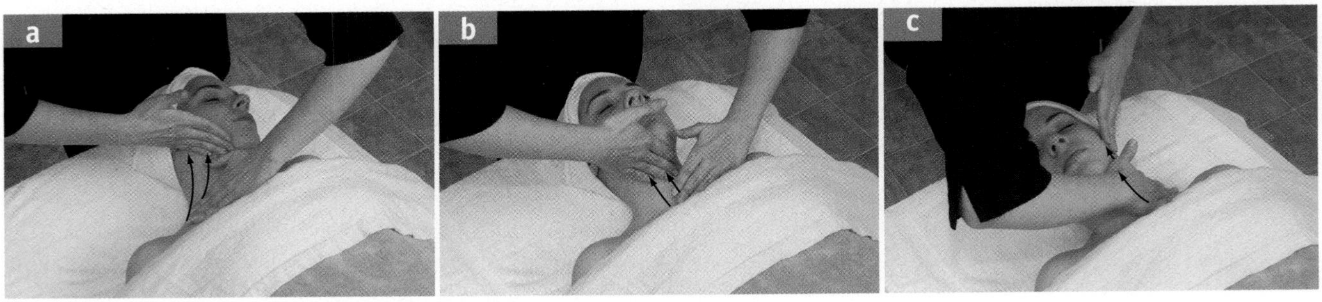

Figure 17–5 Paddlewheel.

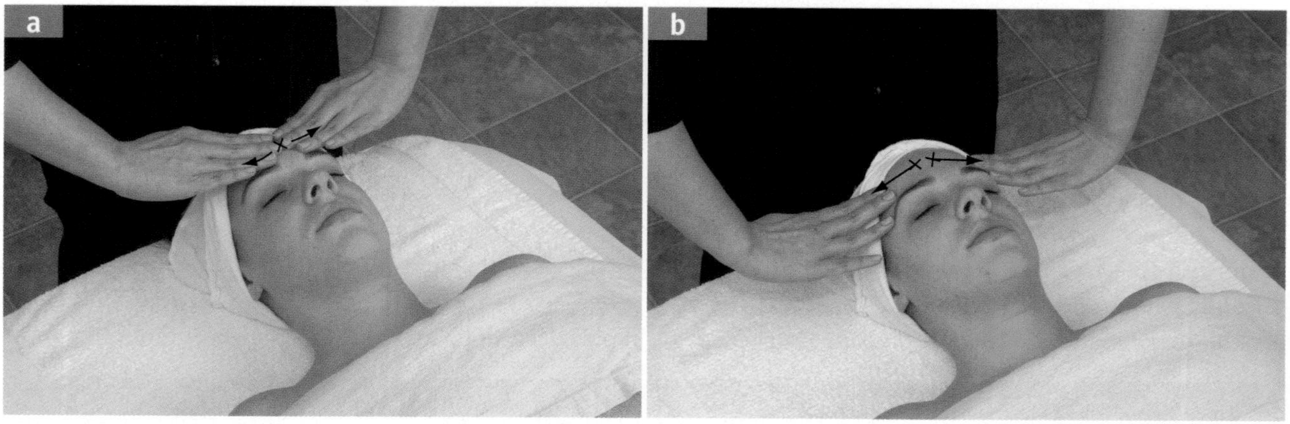

Figure 17–6 Feather Off.

Feather Off

With hands on the forehead, fingers meeting in middle, gently glide to the temples and off the forehead, as if with a feather (Figure 17–6). (This is a nice finishing movement.)

Forehead Press

Place your right hand flat on the forehead. Then place your left hand over the top of the right and press down on the forehead (Figure 17–7). Release. Repeat three to six times.

Gallop 1-2-1

Begin at the mandible bone at the center of the chin. Apply a light lifting and tapping motion, using two taps with the right hand followed by one tap with the left hand. Move from the center to the left side of the face, back across to the right side of the face, and end at the center of chin (Figure 17–8).

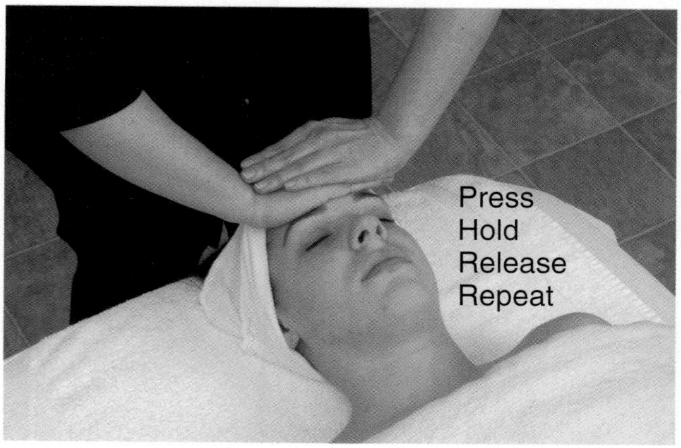

Figure 17–7 Forehead Press.

Full-Face Sweep

Starting with the center of the chin, glide the hands around the outer perimeter of the face, passing your hands by each other at the forehead. Circle the face three to six times (Figure 17–9).

ADVANCED NECK AND DÉCOLLETÉ MOVEMENTS

Neck, décolleté, and shoulder movements are an important addition to any massage service. The neck and shoulders are one of the principal storage areas for tension in the body. Working these areas will help to release the build up of tension and further relax and energize the client.

Rolling Along

Make your hands into fists. Then start on the back on the outside point of each shoulder and work in clockwise circles until your hands meet at the neck. Rotate up the neck to the occipital. With hands still in fists, work back down the neck and across the shoulders (Figure 17–10). Repeat the full movement six to eight times.

Feels Good

At the outside back of the shoulders, with your palms open and fingers spread slightly apart, slide across the back of the shoulders, dragging the tips of your fingers

> Check with your client to see if they have any neck or shoulder conditions or concerns that would not allow you to massage these areas.

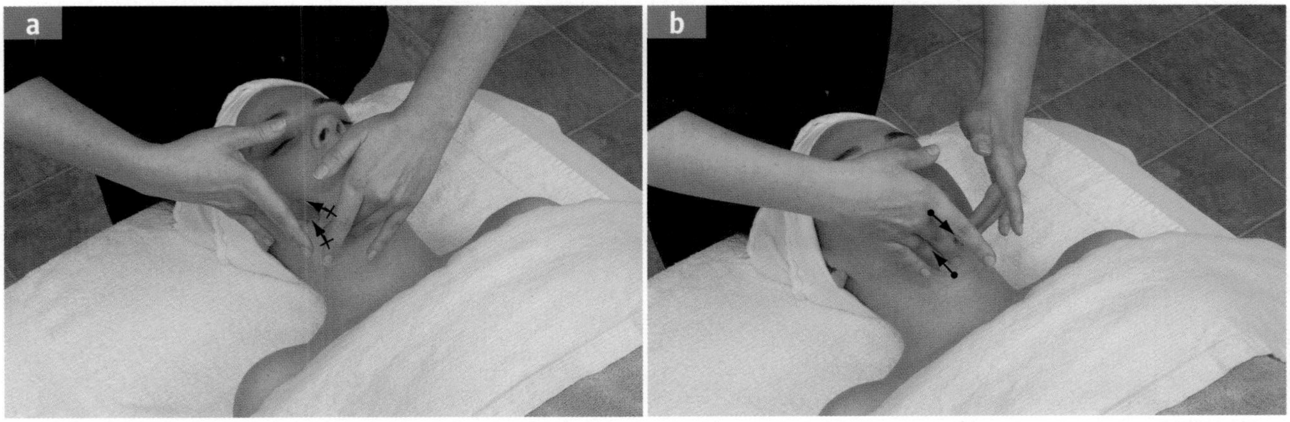

Figure 17–8 Gallop 1-2-1.

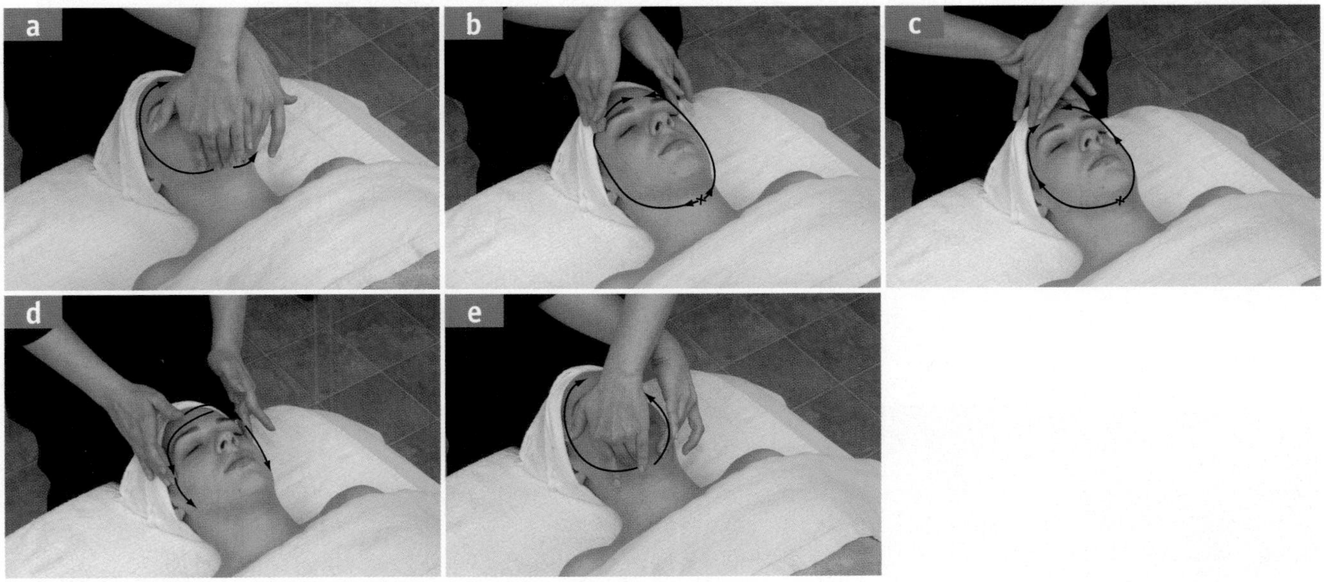

Figure 17–9 Full-face Sweep.

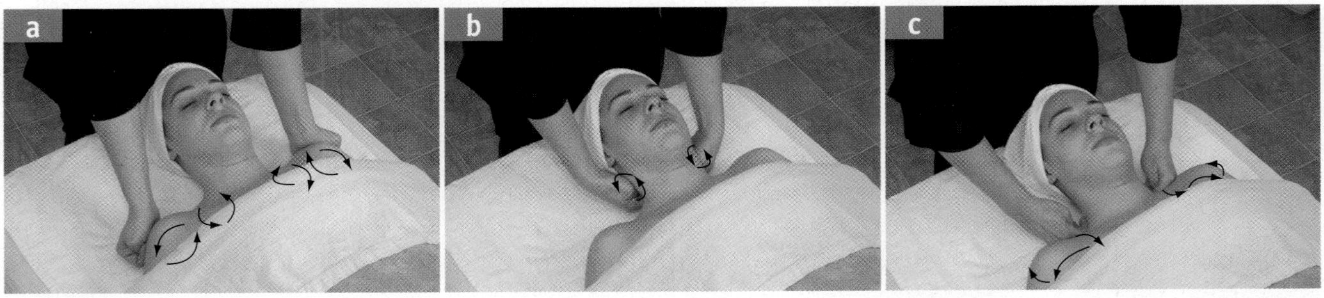

Figure 17–10 Rolling Along.

across the shoulders and up the back of the neck to the occipital ridge (Figure 17–11). Apply light pressure with fingertips to the hollow just under the occipital ridge. Then release and glide your hands down and back to the outside of shoulders. Repeat this movement six to eight times.

Décolleté Sweep

Starting with your left hand, sweep from the right shoulder across the décolleté and over the left shoulder, around the back of the shoulder, continuing to sweep across the back and up the neck (Figure 17–12). As your left hand moves across the back of the shoulder,

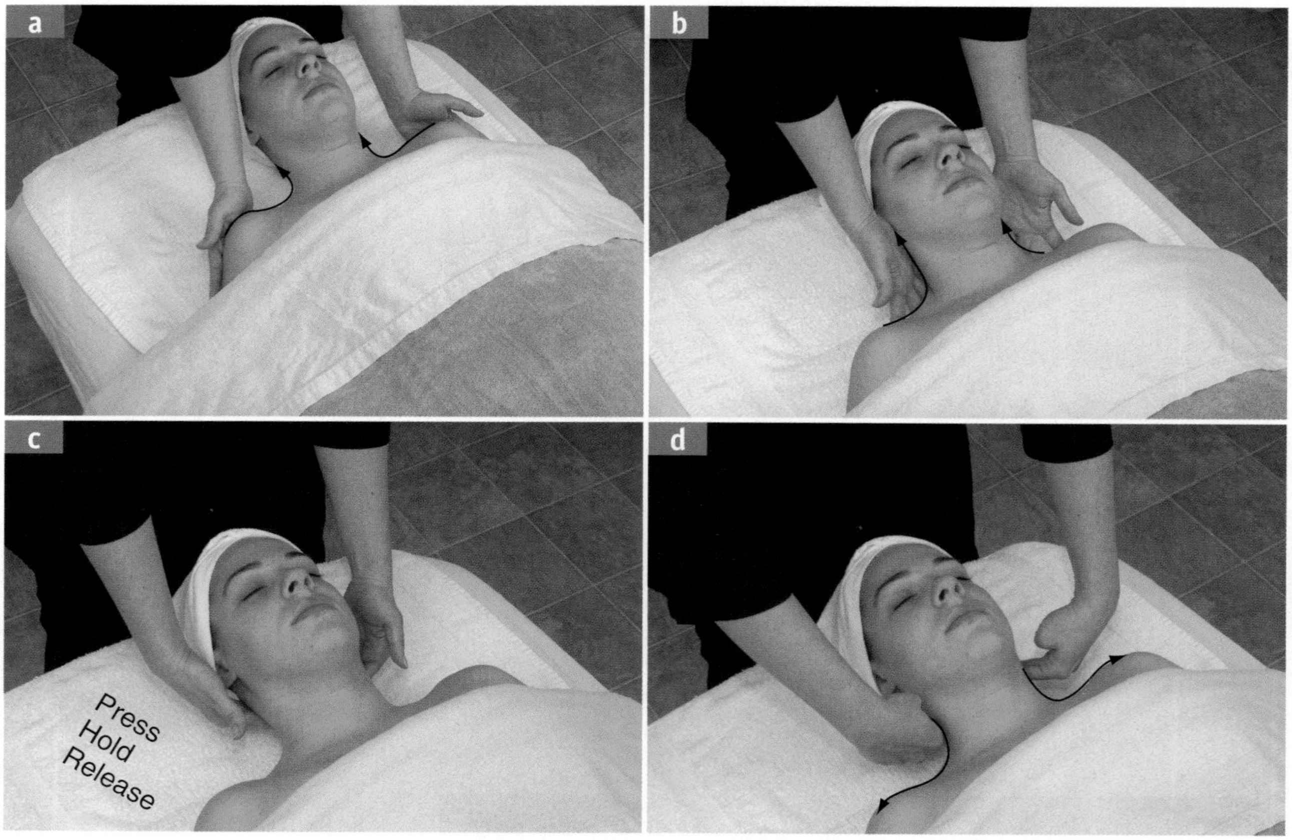

Figure 17–11 Feels Good.

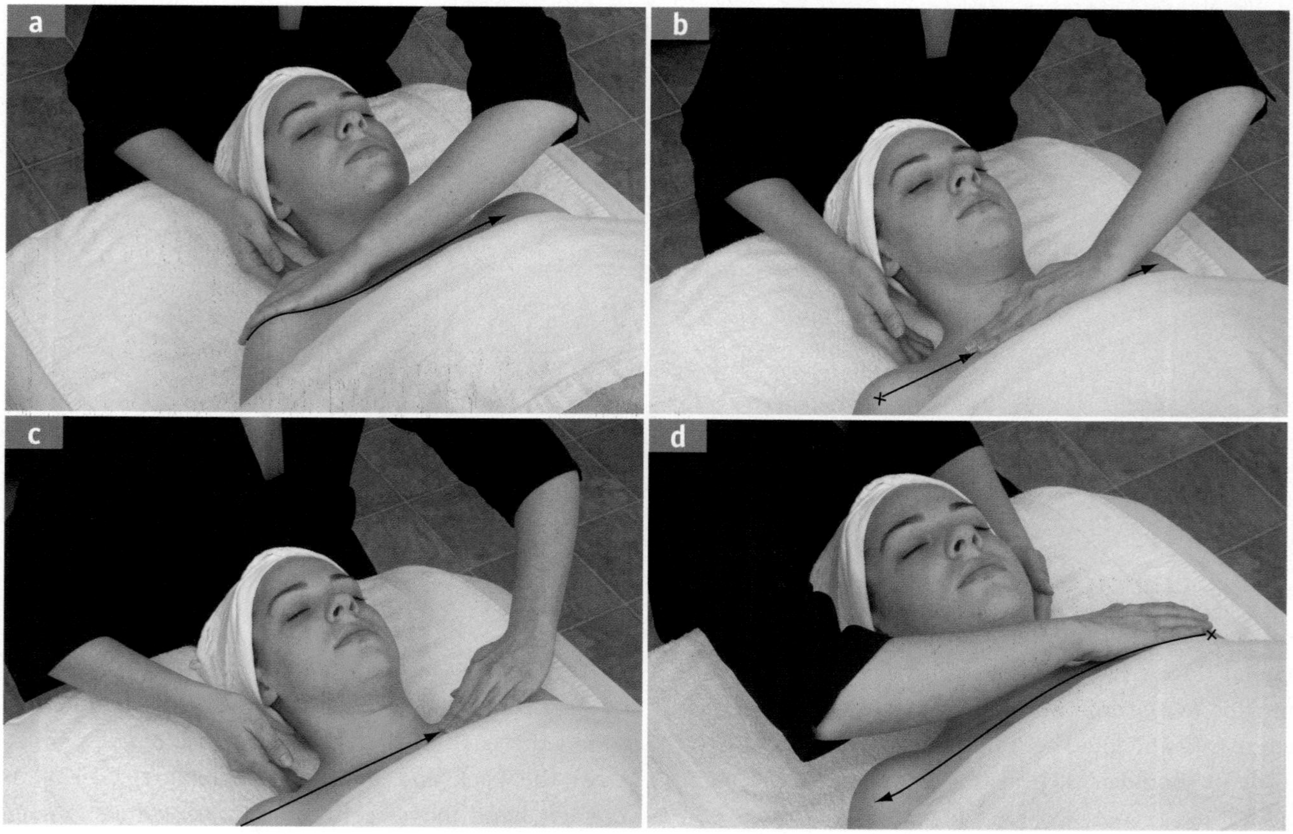

Figure 17–12 Décolleté Sweep.

your right hand begins the same movement, working in the other direction.

Ski Up

With the client's head turned towards the right shoulder, stroke hand over hand, from below the left ear down the neck and off the shoulder. Turn the client's head and repeat on right side of neck. (Figure 17–13).

Neck-Shoulder-Arm

Place right hand under client's neck gently holding client's head in hand. Place left hand below client's ear and glide down the side of neck, down the front of the arm to the elbow. Glide over the elbow and then up the back of the arm, continuing up the neck to the right-hand. Roll the left hand out occipital (Figure 17–14).

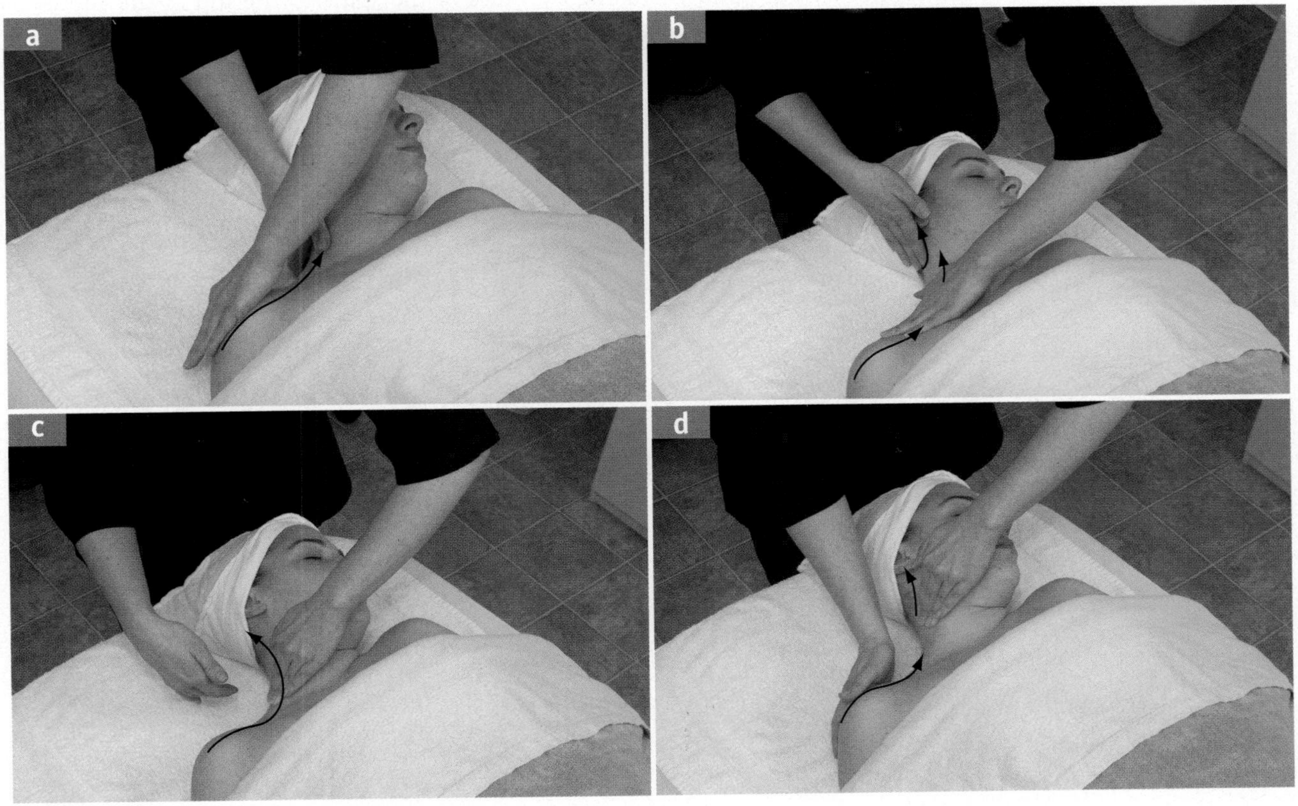

Figure 17–13 Ski Up.

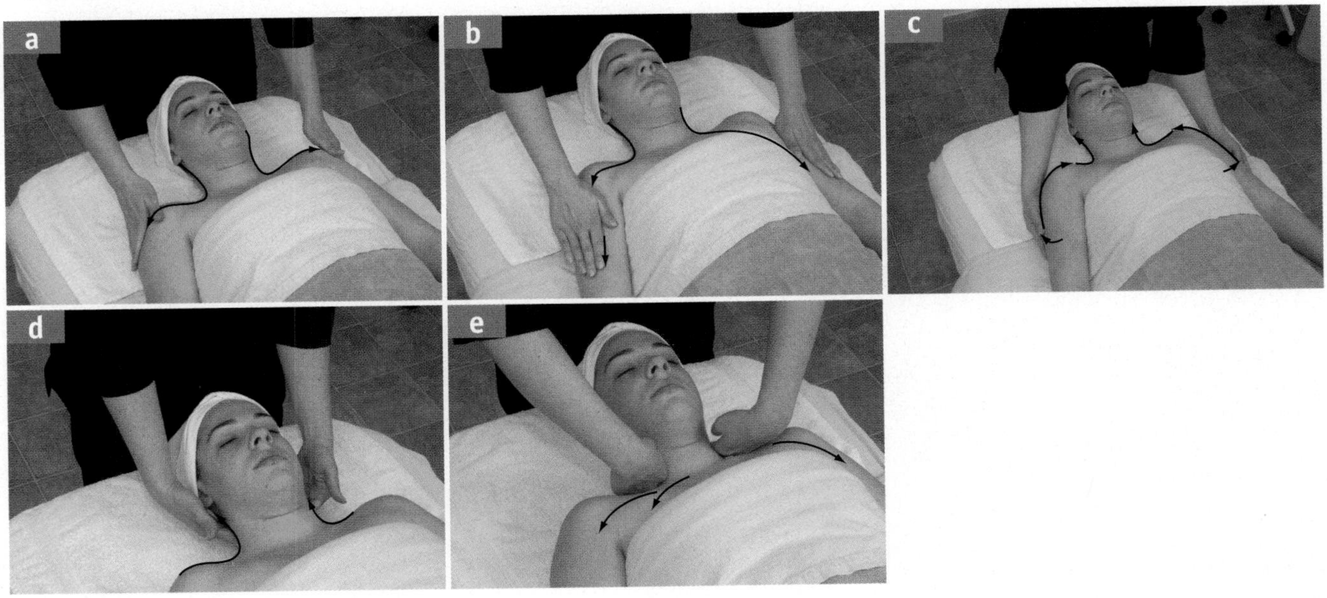

Figure 17–14 Neck-Shoulder-Arm.

Twirl over and out onto the neck. Repeat this movement three to six times. Change and repeat on other side of neck-shoulder-arm.

Rock-a-Bye

With the heels of your hands on the upper part of the shoulders, rock the shoulders, depressing slightly downward toward the body and alternating hands, slowly stretching tense sternocleidomastoid and trapezius muscles (Figure 17–15).

ADVANCED BACK MOVEMENTS

These back movements are excellent for use in the application of products for back treatments.

Back Sweep

Starting at the waist, place your hands, palms down, on either side of the spine. Applying firm pressure, glide up along the sides of the spine to the top of the shoulders (Figure 17–16). Glide across the shoulders and down the client's sides to the waist. Repeat as needed.

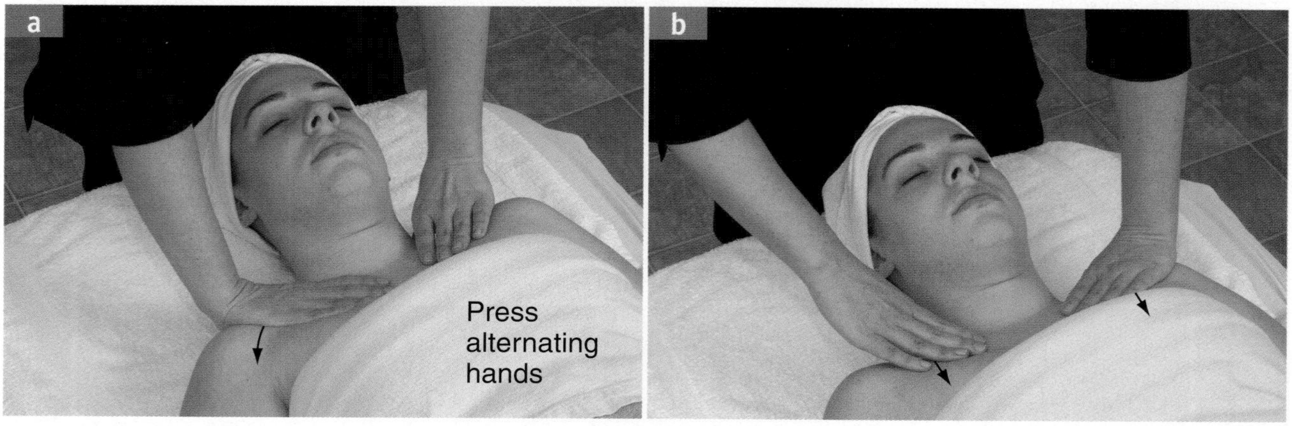

Figure 17–15 Rock-a-bye.

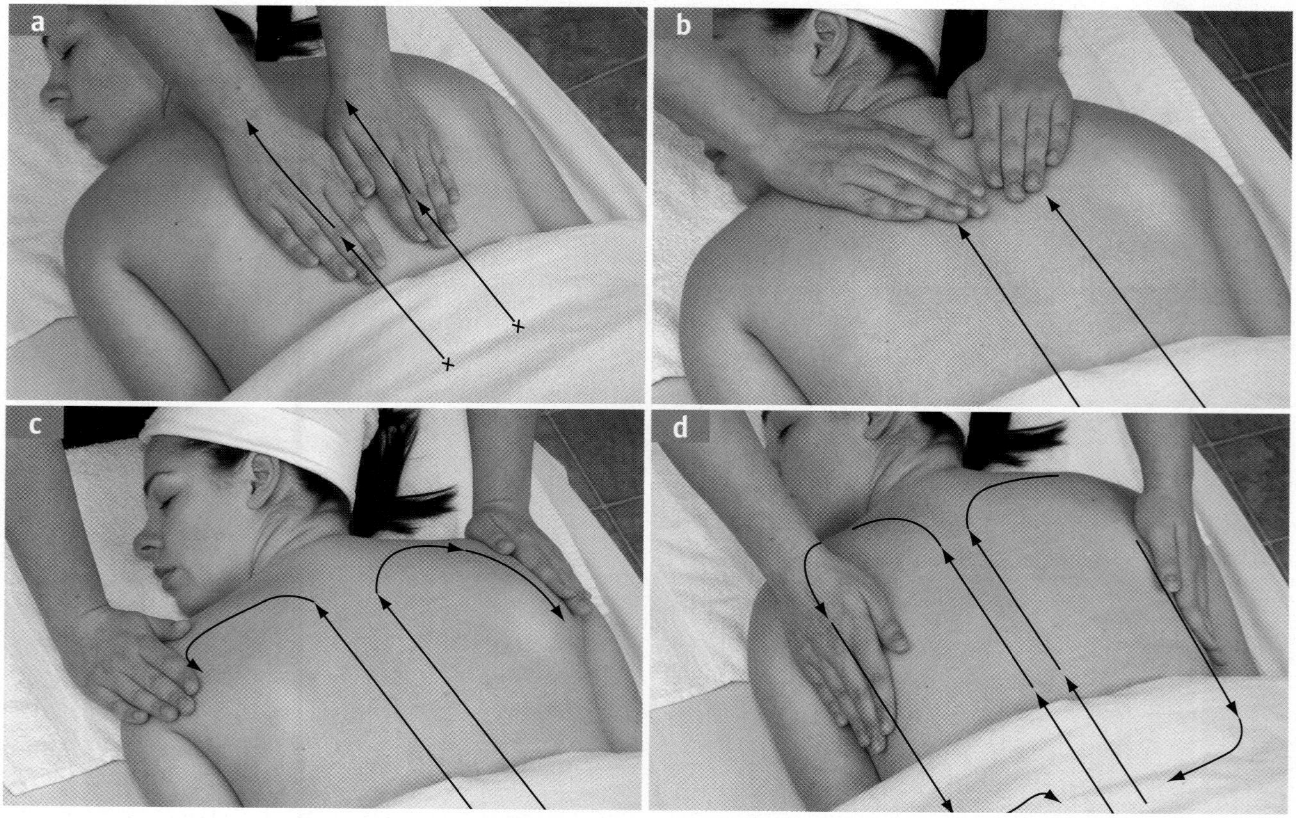

Figure 17–16 Back Sweep.

Spine Munch

With your thumb and index or middle finger, use a squeezing and pinching movement to work up along the spinal column from the waist to the neck (Figure 17–17). One hand leads the other as you progress upward. Repeat as needed.

Swim Up Back

With the flat of your hands, work up the client's back from waist to shoulders, performing large effleurage circle movements from the spine toward the sides of the body (Figure 17–18). Repeat as needed.

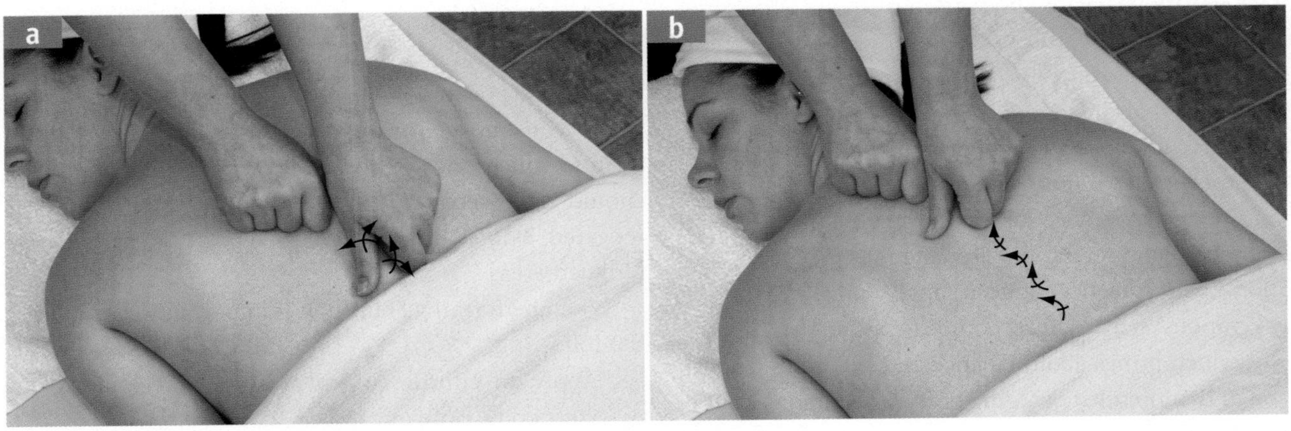

Figure 17–17 Spine Munch.

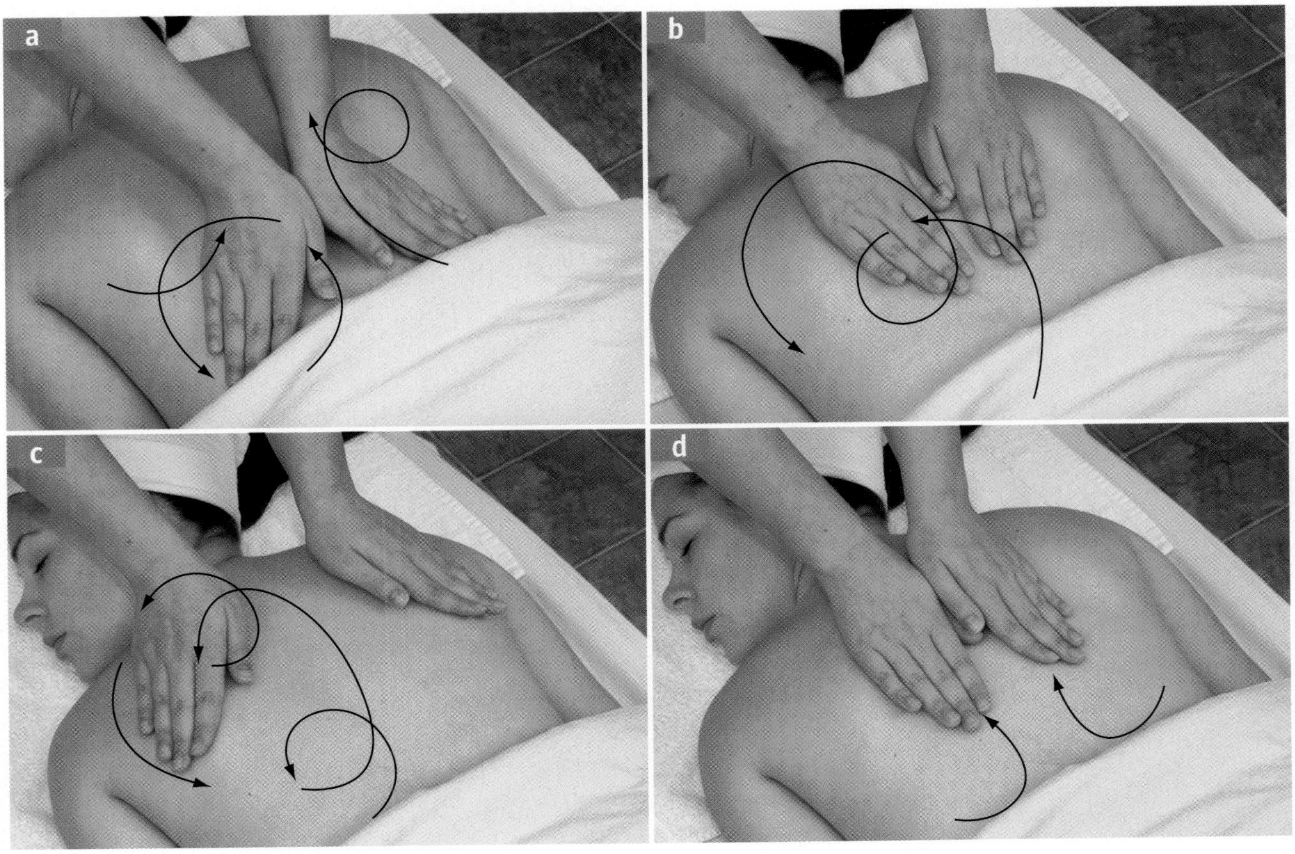

Figure 17–18 Swim Up Back.

SHIATSU MASSAGE FOR THE FACE

Shiatsu massage is a form of physical therapy for the body. This technique, which originated in Japan (the name means "figure pressure"), involves the application of pressure to **acupuncture** points found throughout the body. Acupuncture is a Chinese practice that is based on the belief that the body is made of energy pathways, which connect to various organs and parts of the body. A person's health is influenced by this flow of energy. When the flow of this energy is insufficient, unbalanced, or interrupted, the health of that organ, and potentially the entire body, can be adversely affected. While acupuncture has a long history, there is less scientific documentation on the effects of Shiatsu. The advantage for estheticians is that Shiatsu is easier to learn and safer to incorporate into practice.

Those who practice Shiatsu apply pressure to the body's various acupuncture points to assist the flow of energy, which brings about balance and promotes health. Although the intended outcome of these techniques is the client's relaxation, with no therapeutic benefits for the entire body, this facial massage still has benefits. The philosophy behind Shiatsu is that people carry a lot of energy in the head, and this leads to tension and stress, which shows up in lines and wrinkles. When you perform head and face Shiatsu, which consists of applying pressure to key points rather then along classical energy channels, you soothe and relax and release tension from the muscles.

Performing Shiatsu

Shiatsu can be performed at any time in a facial treatment; however, it is recommended as the close of a regular massage or in place of regular massage. Allow about 10 to 15 minutes for a complete Shiatsu treatment for the face.

Shiatsu is easy to learn; it requires no special equipment, supplies, or oils; and it can be performed as often as once a day. It is easily incorporated into any facial treatment. Each touch in Shiatsu is performed to the count of three:

1. Touch the skin.
2. Apply pressure.
3. Release pressure.

As you move through the steps, use this basic timing: Touch one, Press two, Release three. Each count should last 3 seconds and each point pressed should be repeated 3 to 5 times, with 10 repeats in particularly fatigued areas.

When performing Shiatsu, it is important to remember the following:

1. Apply an effortless, firm pressure that comes from your body, not your fingers, hand, or wrist.
2. Pressure that comes from within is relaxing to the client and technician. Pressure that comes only from your hand will create stress for both of you.
3. When applying pressure, use the pads of the fingers and thumbs, never the tips.
4. Learn to be sensitive and in tune to the areas of application and your client's needs.

With practice, you will develop the ability to recognize when you are performing a Shiatsu massage that benefits your client.

PROCEDURE 17-1 SHIATSU MASSAGE FOR HEAD AND NECK

IMPLEMENTS AND MATERIALS

- Typical facial lounge set up with linens and towels
- Best done with no massage vehicle

Preparation

1 Set up the facial lounge and prepare the room for the client.

2 Decant massage vehicle. (optional)

3 Before the client gets into the lounge, allow him or her to put on a gown.

4 Perform any portion of a facial prior to this massage.

Procedure

Starting with position number 7, repeat each move three times before moving to the next position.

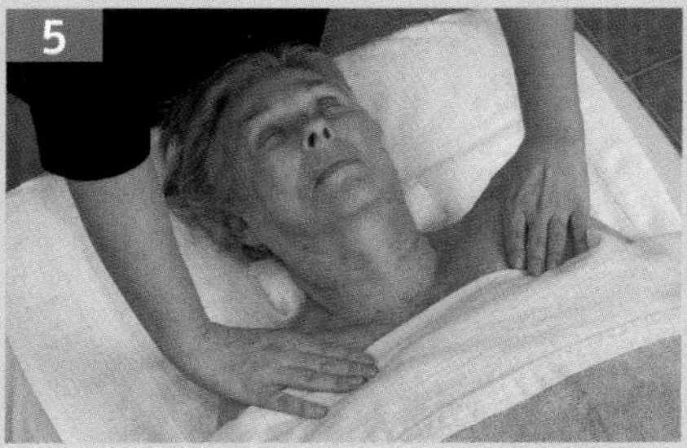

Start at shoulders.

5 Start with your hands resting quietly on client's shoulders to bond.

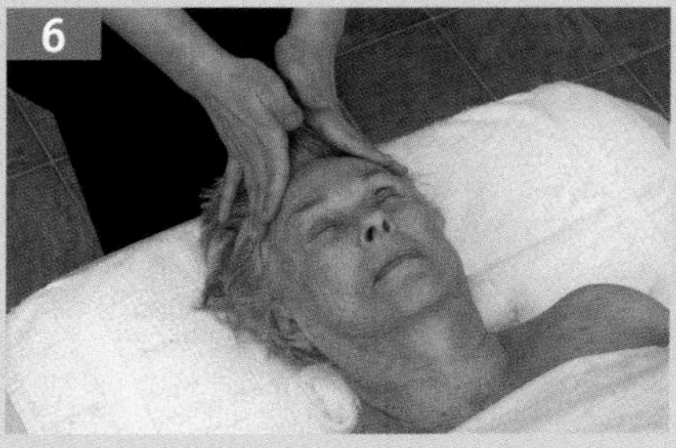

Glide up over face.

6 Glide your hands up over the face to the forehead.

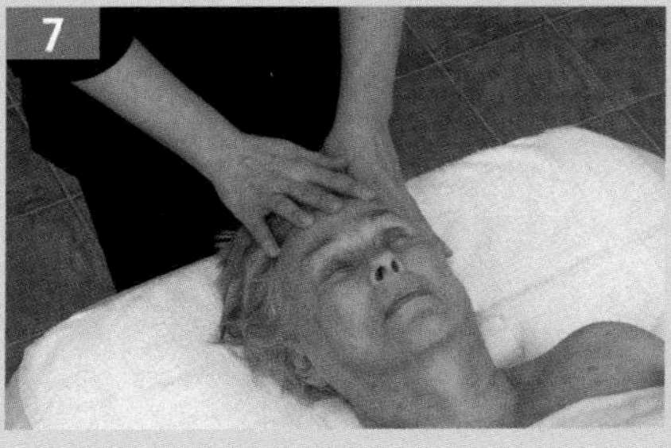

Begin at top of head.

7 Begin at the top of the head, running your fingers through the hair.

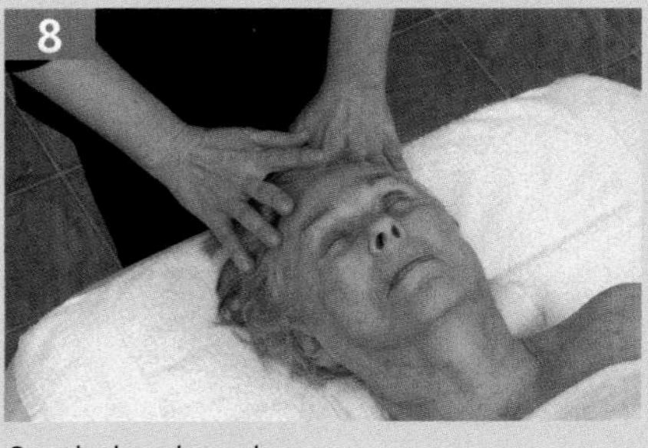

Gently brush scalp.

Running Water

8 Gently brushing the scalp, run your fingertips from the hairline back through the client's hair.

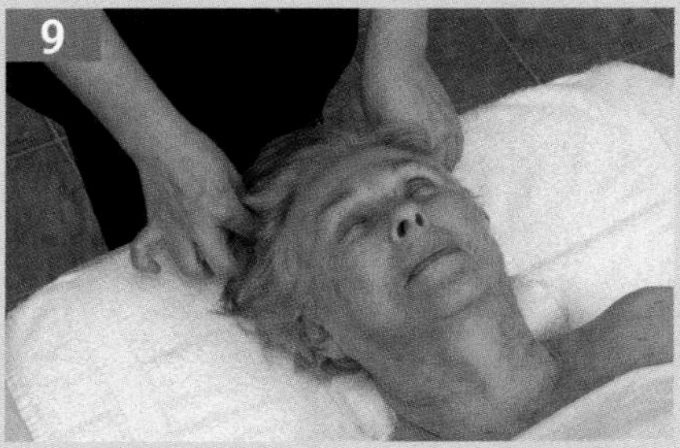

Gently pull sections.

Down River

9 Taking a small section of hair, gently pull small sections of hair, one at a time, all over the client's head.

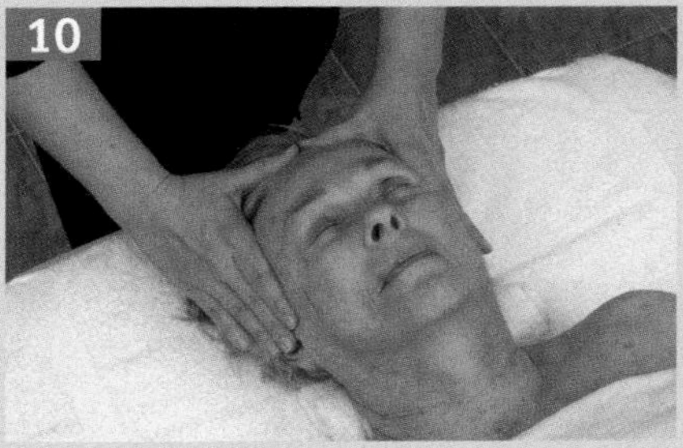

Hold head at sides.

Top of the Mountains

10 Overlap your thumbs and place them at the center of the hairline. With hands extended to hold the client's head at the sides, gently press. Repeat this

continues on next page

PROCEDURE 17–1, CONT. SHIATSU MASSAGE FOR HEAD AND NECK

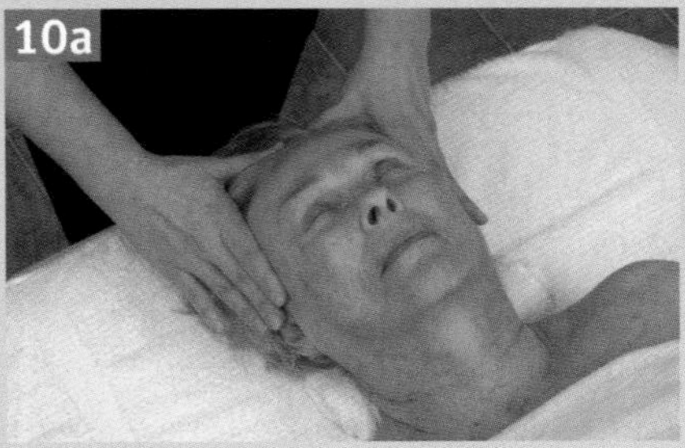

Repeat movement.

movement, shifting your hands back toward the crown at 1-inch intervals.

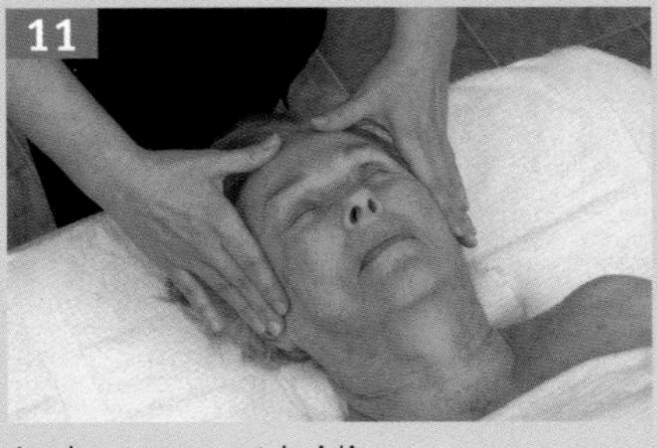

Apply pressure at hairline.

Step Wrinkle Erase

11 Using your thumbs, start at the center of the hairline directly above the nose. Gently apply pressure along the hairline.

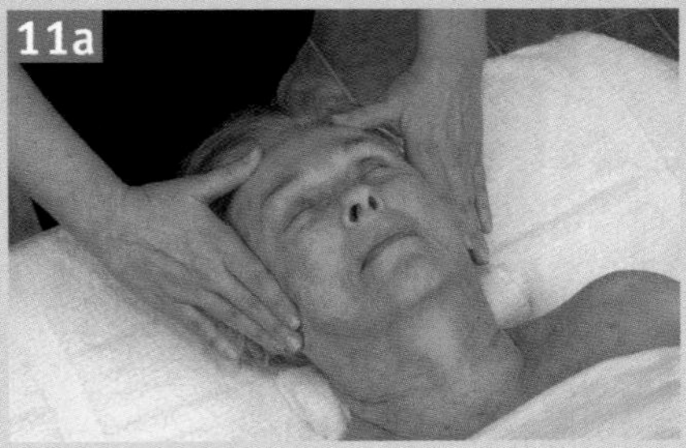

Shift toward temples.

a. Repeat this at ½-inch intervals as you shift your hands toward the temples.

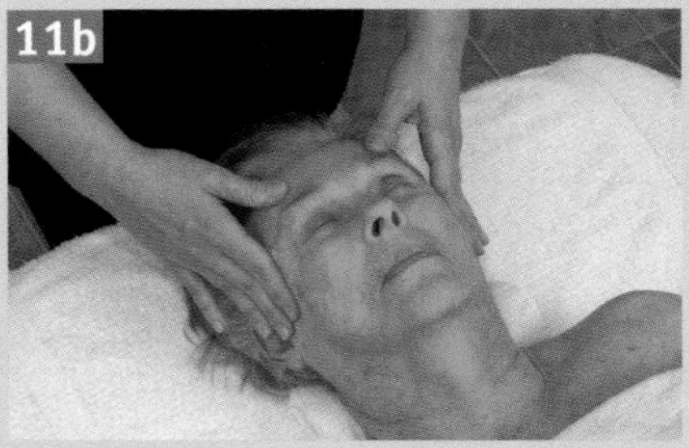

Shift to forehead.

b. Shift your hands to the center of the forehead and repeat.

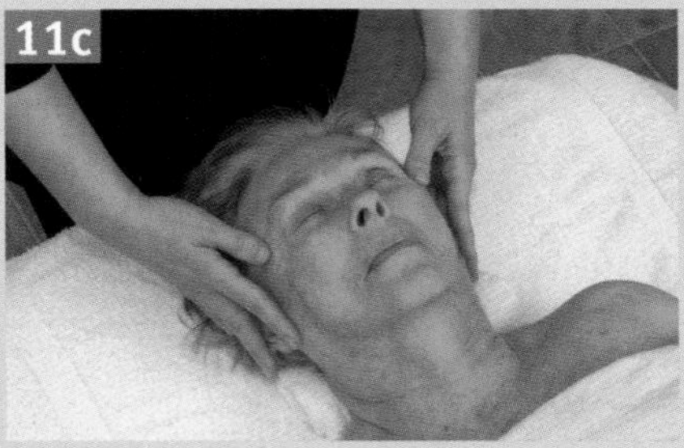

Shift toward temples.

c. As in step a, shift your hands toward the temples in ½-inch intervals, repeating the pressure-release movement.

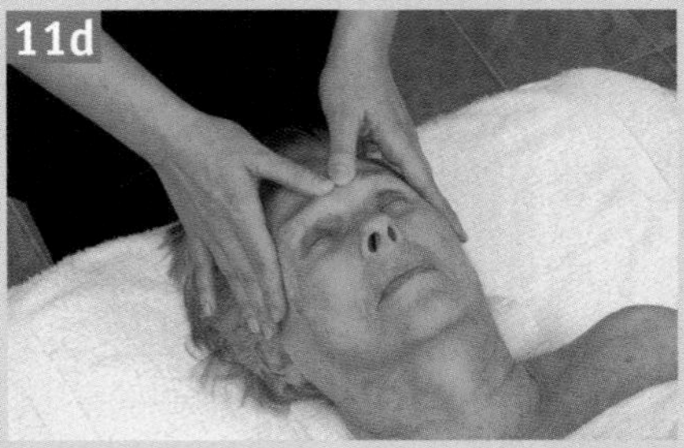

Shift to brow line.

d. Shift your hands to just above the brow line and repeat the pressure release.

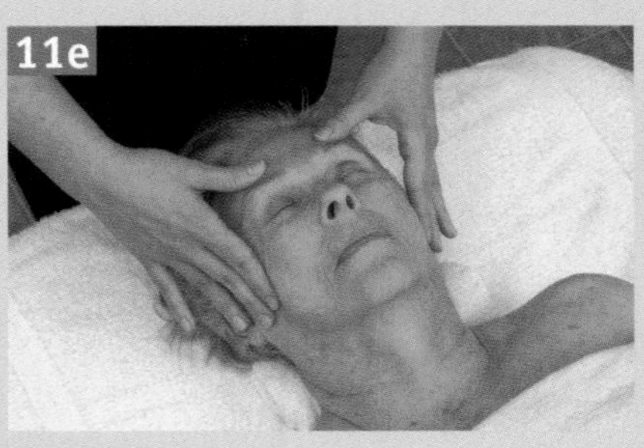

Repeat at temples.

e. As in step a, shift your hands toward the temples in ½-inch intervals, repeating the pressure-release movement.

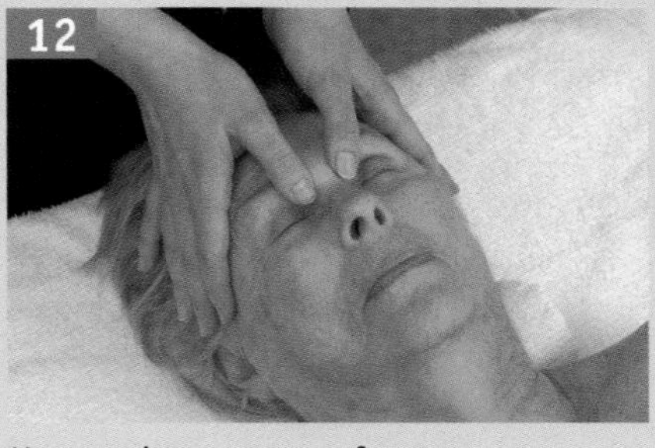

Move to inner corner of eye.

Bright Eyes

12 Move your hands to the inner corner of the eye and, with your thumbs, gently press the inner corner of the eye sockets for 3 to 4 seconds.

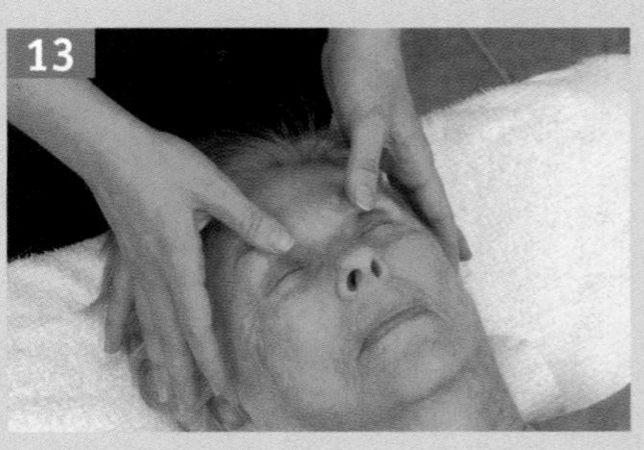

Press between brows.

13 With your thumbs, press the center between the brows.

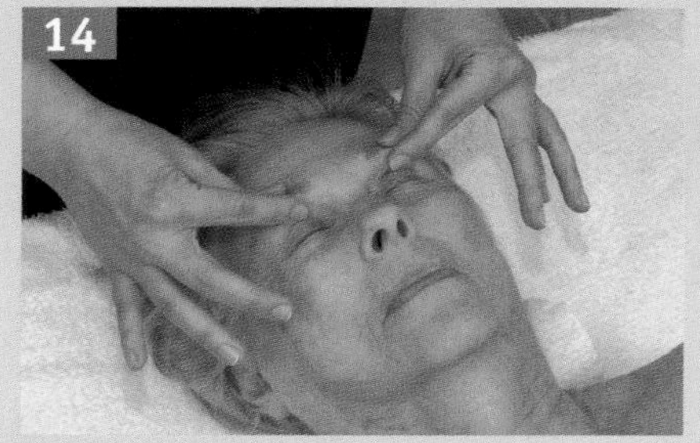

Pinch across brows.

14 With the finger and thumb, gently pinch across the length of the brow.

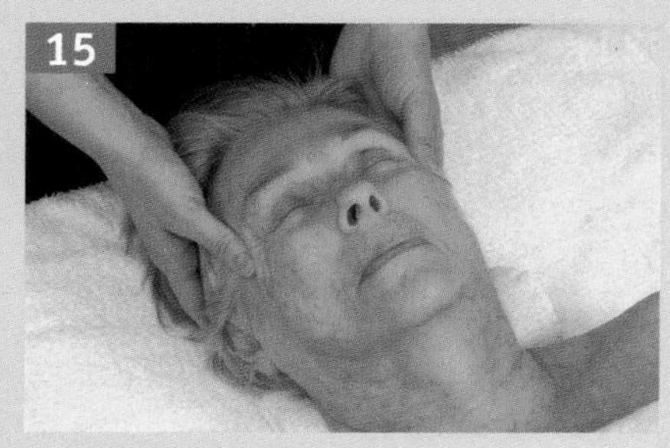

Press ridge of brows.

15 Placing your thumbs at the outer ends of the eyebrows, gently press the bony ridge and ends of the brows.

Mid-face Flush

16 Gently apply pressure at the temples, holding 2 to 3 seconds.

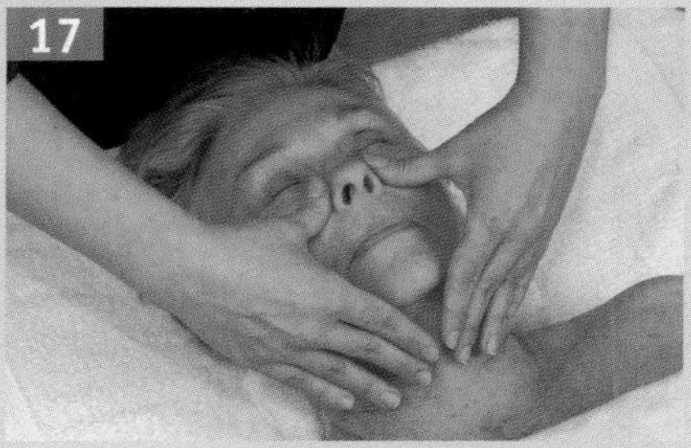

Apply pressure at sides of nose.

17 Glide to the sides of the nose.

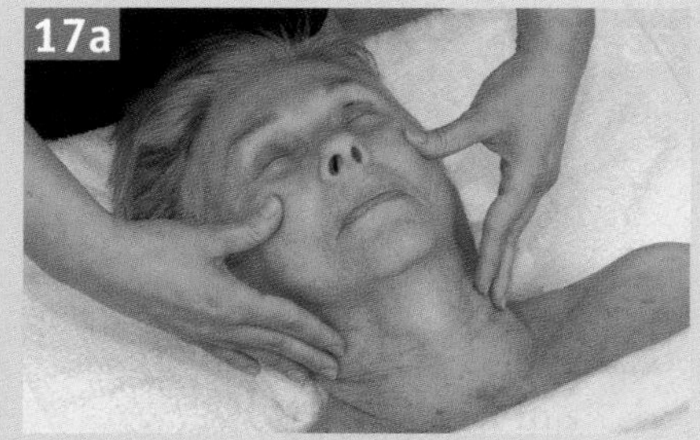

Move along zygomatic bone.

a. Gently apply pressure with your thumbs, starting at the sides of the nose.

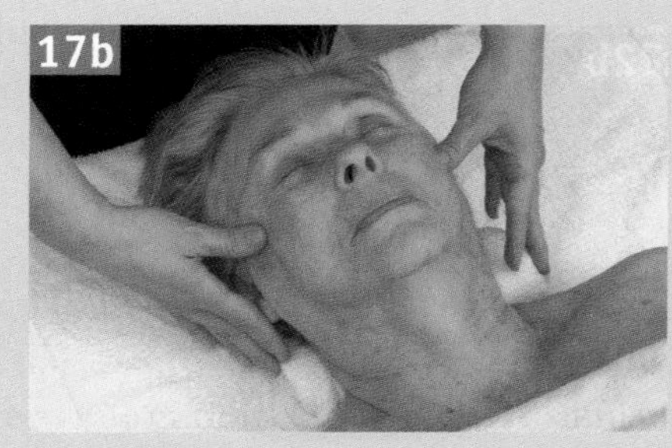

Move along zygomatic bone.

b. Repeat this movement, working at ½-inch intervals along the top of the zygomatic bone back toward the temples.

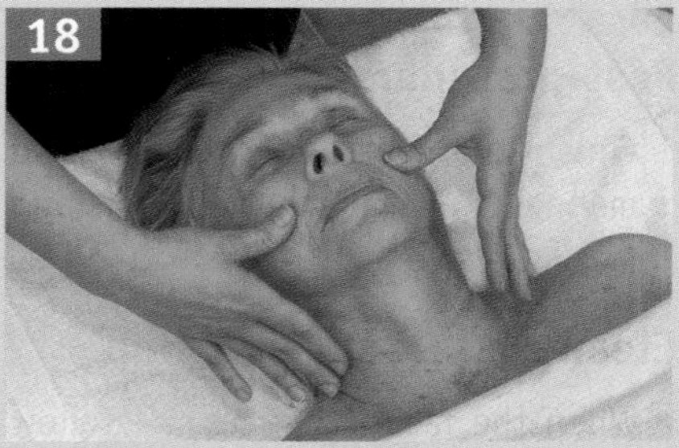

Repeat toward ear.

18 Glide back to sides of nose. Repeat this pattern, from the corners of the nose back just under the zygomatic bone toward the ears.

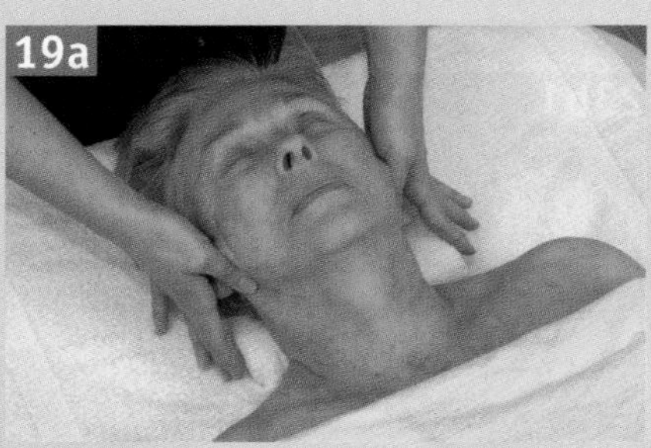

Apply pressure at center point.

19 From the ears glide in a straight line down to a small bundle of muscle just inside the jaw.

a. Apply light pressure at the center point of the bundle, and release.

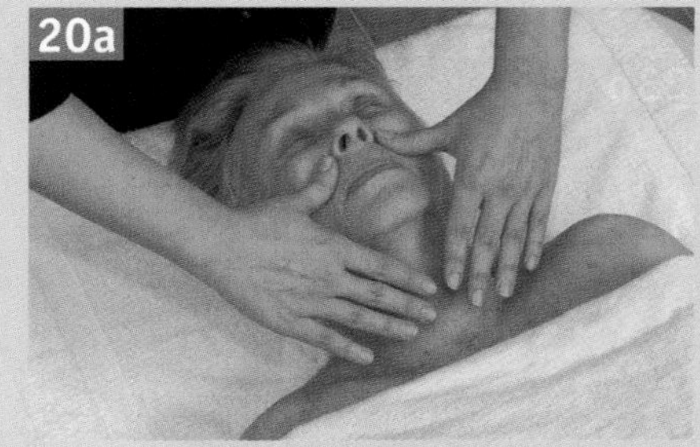

Apply at lower nostrils.

Mouthwash

20 Glide to the lower edge of the nostrils.

a. With your thumbs, apply pressure in the grooves at the side of the lower edge of the nostrils.

continues on next page

EAR REFLEXOLOGY

Reflexology is the art of massaging a reflex area in a location that corresponds with another location in the body. It promotes relief from aches and pains and aids in bringing about a natural balance to the body. If a body part is sore, rub it, even if you do not know which other part of the body this one corresponds to. This massage sends an electrical signal through the body to the corresponding location and helps restore energy flow. Every cell and every organ in the body responds to the electrical impulses.

Consider the size of the ear, which is small in comparison to other parts of the body. Do not let that small size fool you, though—the ear has more than 100 reflexes. It is impossible to pinpoint and stimulate each reflex individually, but a few exercises can stimulate as many reflexes as possible.

Performing ear reflexology consists of applying a firm but gentle pressure, a stroking or squeezing and pulling of the ear. Work both ears together using your thumbs and forefingers.

PROCEDURE 17–2 EAR REFLEXOLOGY MASSAGE

There are certain points on the ear that help to warm the body and are good to use when a client is cold. These can be performed at the beginning of a facial.

IMPLEMENTS AND MATERIALS

- Standard facial lounge setup with linens and towels
- Product supplies as needed for the facial
- Facial lounge

Preparation

1 Set up the facial lounge and prepare the treatment room.

2 Gather supplies needed for treatment.

3 When this procedure is part of the facial massage, prepare the client and perform the facial up to the point at which the massage will be performed.

4 Perform the facial massage.

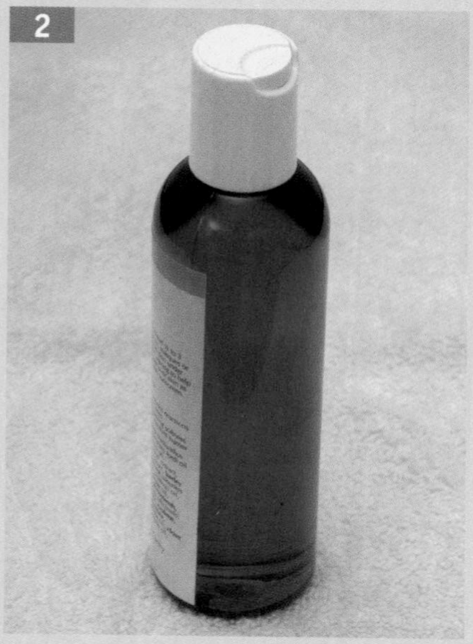

2 Gather supplies.

Procedure

Incorporate these steps into your facial massage as appropriate. Perform the following procedures doing both ears at the same time.

Ear-Pinch-Roll-Tug

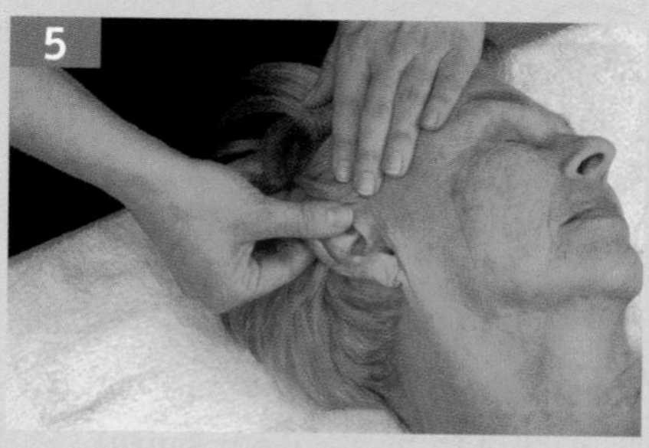

5 Pinch ears.

5 Starting at the top of the ears, pinch the ears.

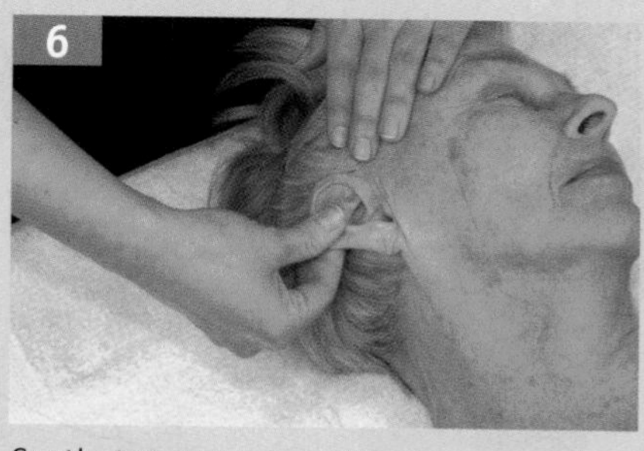

6 Gently tug ears.

6 Using a pinch-and-roll technique, gently tug the ears upward, followed by a pull outward from the head.

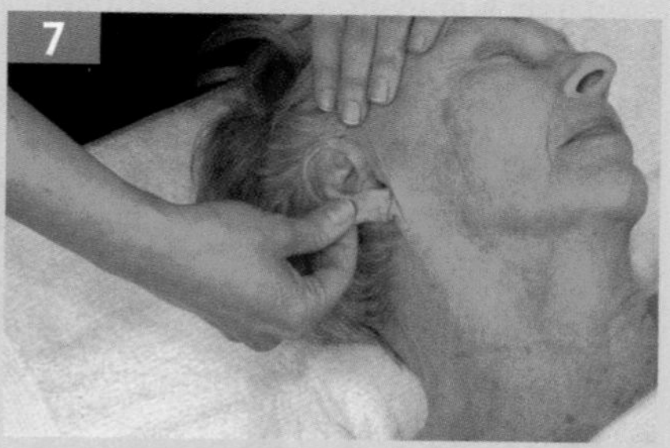

7 Down the outer ear.

7 Continue this movement down the outside of the ears, moving along about a ¼-inch at a time.

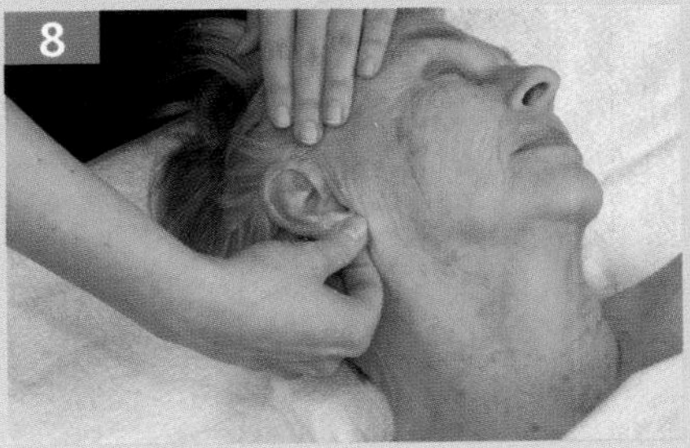

Continue to ear lobe.

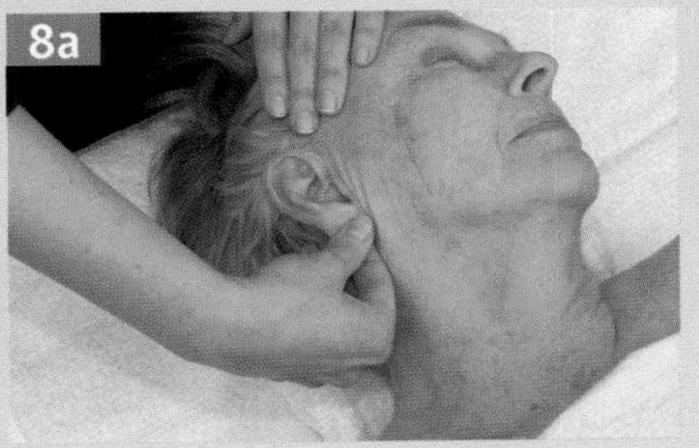

Pull the ear lobe.

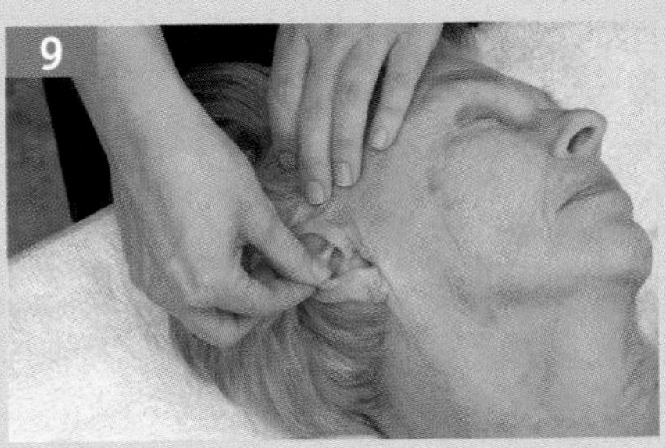

Slide up the ear.

8 Continue this movement to the ear lobes. While pinching the ear lobes, pull down and out on the lobes.

9 Slide your fingers up the outside of the ears and repeat the same pinch, roll, and tug upward and outward on the inside of the ears, working toward the ear lobes.

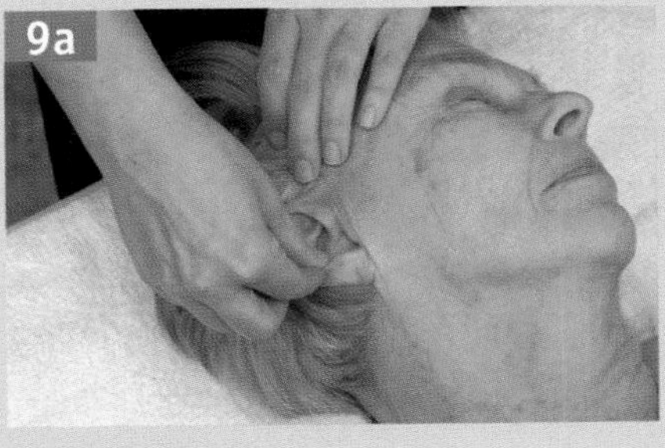

Slide up the ear.

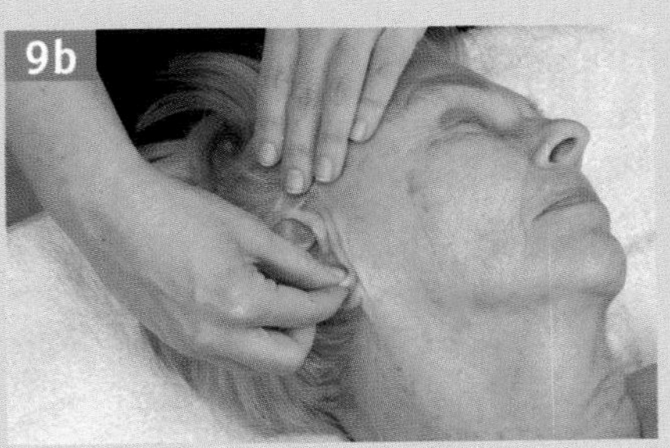

Slide up the ear.

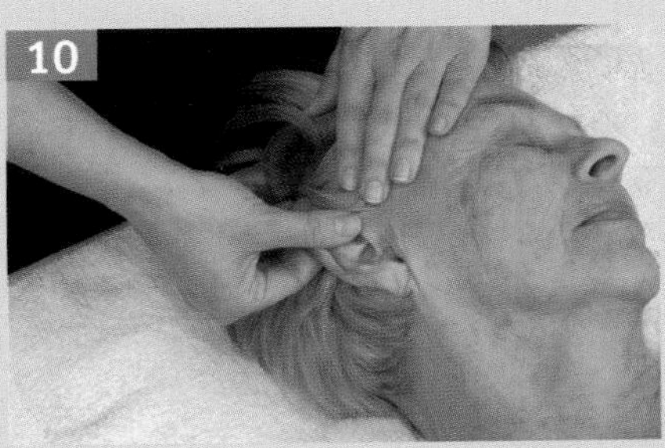

Pinch ear lobe.

10 Pinch the ear lobes; then gently pull down and out on the lobes.

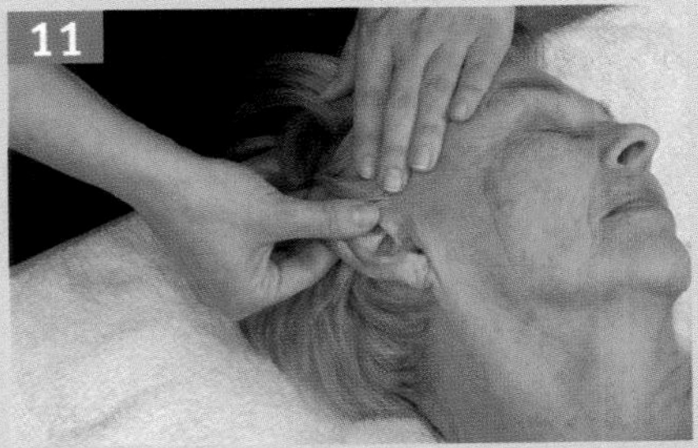

End at tragus.

Flap Pinch

End the massage at the tragus (the small flaps in front of each ear opening) by massaging and pinching these small flaps.

Post-procedure

Complete the facial massage and facial as desired for the client.

Clean-up and Disinfection

When the facial is complete, perform clean-up and sanitation as required following your state guidelines.

STONE MASSAGE FOR ESTHETICIANS

Heated and wrapped stones have been used throughout history in most parts of the world to warm and soothe. They have also found their way into various rituals and have been attributed with healing properties. It is known that rocks do have energy properties due to their makeup. While some specialty body massage techniques using stones have been developed and claim unique aspects, in the esthetic arena stones are used for their ability to de-stress and relax a client (Figure 17–25). Thermotherapy, or the use of heat and cold, is employed to trigger a circulatory response. Just as we employ hot towels or a steamer to transmit warmth to the face so we can use heated stones to transfer warmth.

The stones used in hot and cold therapies are found all over the world. Some stone specialists advocate the collection of stones only from uninhabited isolated regions, while others recommend gathering local stones that are in tune with residents' energy levels. Most technicians purchase their stones from suppliers that specialize in rocks of the most commonly used sizes and uniformities.

Warm Stones

Basalt composition is the preferred stone for heat retention. These **igneous** rocks are formed as a result of volcanic activity. Over millennia, pieces of basalt rock are broken off and washed down streams where the water smoothes, buffs, and refines them into the small, polished rocks valued for stone treatments. They are fine-grained and black to grey in color and should be nonporous and smooth (Figure 17–26). They transfer their heat to the body by means of **conduction.** The longer they are left in contact with the skin, the more heat is transferred and the deeper it penetrates. The exposure to the heat causes the skin to flush pink because of the increased circulation and inflammation to the area.

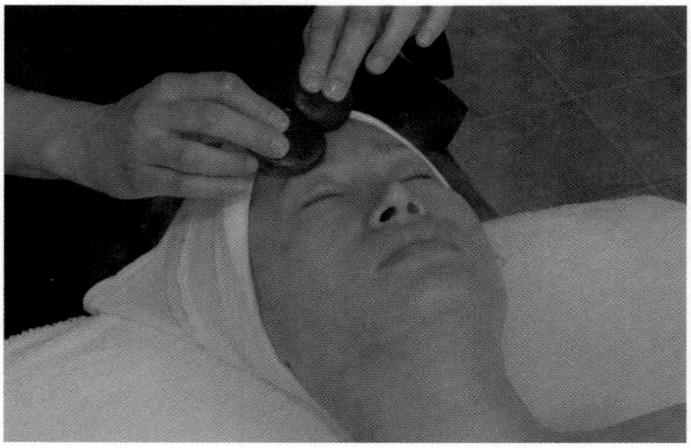

Figure 17–25 Stone treatment in process.

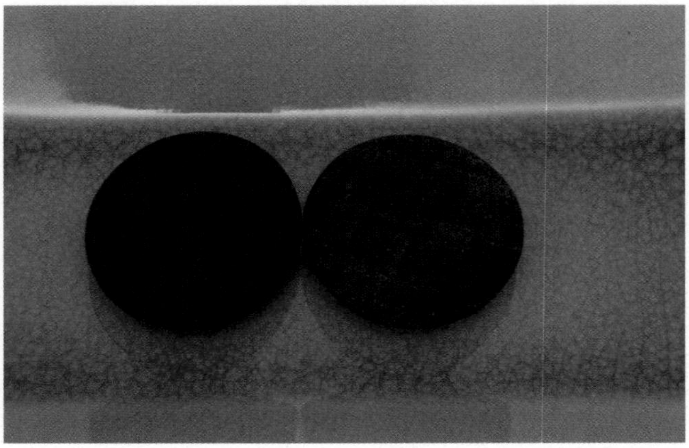

Figure 17–26 Basalt stones.

FYI

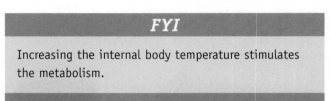

Increasing the internal body temperature stimulates the metabolism.

Cold Stones

Placing cold stones on skin triggers a vaso-constrictive effect, blanching the skin and reducing inflammation. There are two types of stones that are preferred for their ability to stay cold: marine **sedimentary** stones or marble, a **metamorphosed** form of sedimentary limestone (Figure 17–27). Marine stones are gathered from lakes, rivers, or oceans, although their origin is difficult to establish based on vendor information. Marble stones that are hand-cut and then sanded to a smooth texture

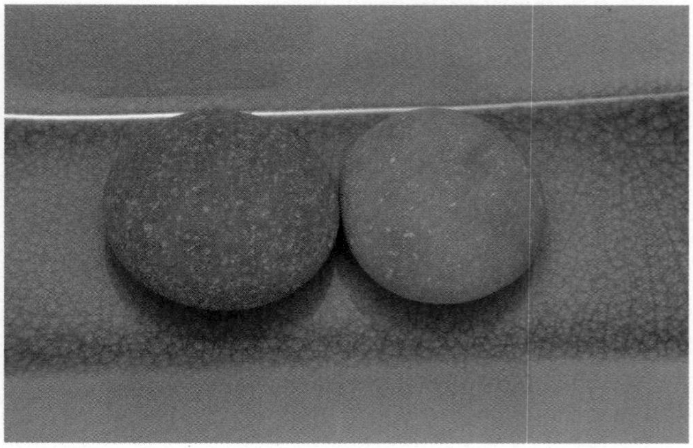

Figure 17–27 Cold stones.

Here's a Tip

Applying a cold stone to an area after waxing can reduce redness. Be sure to disinfect the stone before reusing it on another client.

as the pebble shapes are not found in nature, and, when frozen or chilled, they may change color.

Stone Handling

Prior to use and between clients, you should wash stones with an antibacterial soap and process them in a high-level disinfectant. Some technicians like to rinse them in water with sea salt added to clear their energy. After washing the stones, place them in the heating unit. At the end of the day, turn off the heater and remove the stones, washing them with an antibacterial soap, cold-sterilizing them, and laying them on a towel to air dry. Monthly, stones should be placed in an appropriate container filled about half full of sea salt and allowed to rest approximately 24 hours to re-energize them. Another way to reenergize stones is to place them in natural sunlight or moonlight and in direct contact with the Earth.

While some technicians like to use a slow cooker to heat their stones, most use a professional heater designed for this purpose to assure the maintenance of appropriate temperatures. Placing the stones systematically in the heater facilitates finding the right stone during the massage. Covering the bottom of the heater with a towel or gauze layers protects the heater finish from scratches. The water in the heater should cover the stones and be heated to about 120°F. Check this with a cooking thermometer and follow the manufacturer's directions. When handling the stones, carefully remove them from the water with a slotted spoon, tongs, or a net to avoid burns. Leave the hot stone on a towel until is has cooled enough that you can hold it comfortably.

You can store cold stones in a plastic bag in a refrigerator; during treatment, place them in a bowl of ice to retain their chilled temperature. It is important to have a towel available in the treatment area on which to place used stones. This allows for quick identification of the used stones and provides a place to quietly set them down as you are finished using them.

CAUTION!

Always check with your client that the temperature of the stones feels comfortable.

Stone Placement and Massage

Some estheticians like to place medium stones on the table with a towel over them and then have the client recline on them. Stones should be positioned on either side of the spine, not directly under it. Other technicians prefer to place stones under the shoulders and under the hands.

For facial manipulations small stones of less than 1½ to 2 inches in diameter work best; larger stones do not fit the facial contours well. For this treatment you use two stones simultaneously, one in each hand, in gentle effleurage movements following classical massage patterns.

Another technique involves holding a hot stone in one hand and a cold stone in the other. The hand with the hot stone leads and the hand with the cold stone follows in a sort of chasing pattern. As the stones lose their heat or cold, replace them with fresh stones. The tracing motion and the stones can have a rejuvenating effect on the client. You can offer this technique as a second massage or replace the standard massage in the treatment.

Contraindications

Avoid using hot stones on skins that are couperose, inflamed, irritated, or sensitive or that have a broken skin barrier. Do not use hot stones on post-surgical skin until it is completely healed. In general, do not use hot stones for any client who is not in good health or in situations in which hot temperatures are inappropriate. For example, clients who suffer from hot flashes will be more likely to enjoy the cold stone massage.

Here's a Tip

Practice handling stones so you can do it quietly and without dropping them. Clanking or dropping stones during a treatment can be very distracting to the client.

PROCEDURE 17-3 STONE MASSAGE FOR FACE

IMPLEMENTS AND MATERIALS

- Typical facial lounge setup with linens and towels
- Supplies for facial treatment
- Massage vehicle
- Hot and cold stones for treatment
- Stone warming unit
- Slotted spoon, tongs, or a net to lift hot stones out of water
- Extra towel on which to set used stones

Preparation

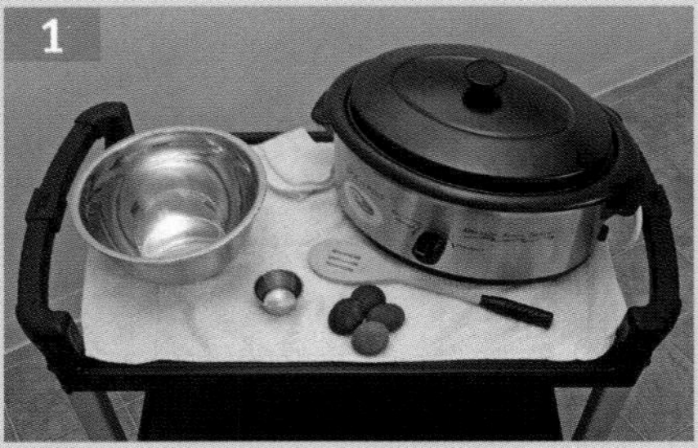

Prepare treatment room.

1 Set up the facial lounge in the typical manner and prepare the treatment room for the client.

2 Gather supplies for the facial treatment.

3 Place water and stones in the warming unit.

4 Turn on the stone warming unit and heat following manufacturer's guidelines. Ensure that the heat of the stones does not exceed 120°F.

5 Perform all massage steps of the facial before starting the stone massage.

a. Apply massage vehicle.

6 Check the stones to ensure that they are at the correct temperature.

7 Turn on the steamer if you choose to use it during the massage.

Procedure

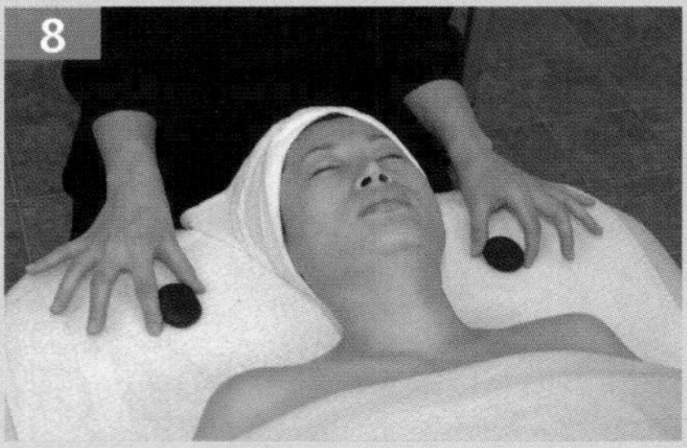

Remove two stones.

8 Remove two stones from the heater and place them on the towel.

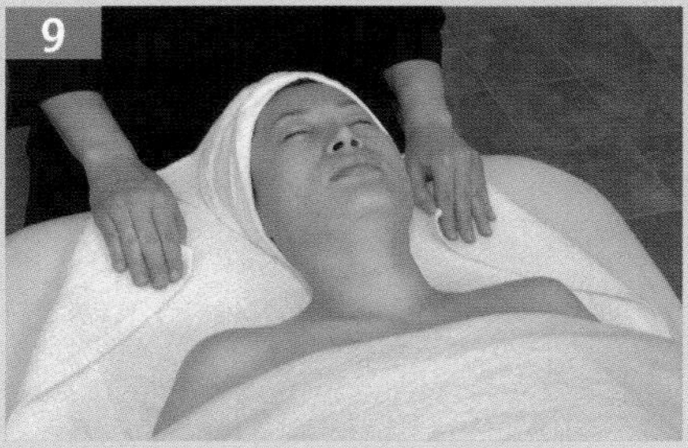

Test temperature.

9 Pat the stones with the towel and test the temperature to ensure that they are not too hot to hold in your hand.

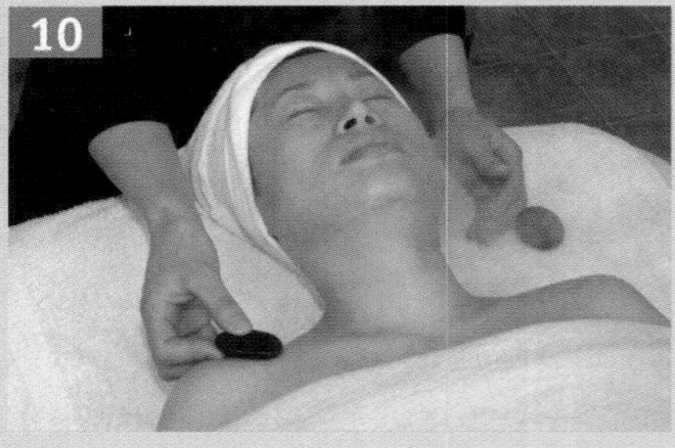

Assure comfort.

10 When stones feel comfortable to handle, test one against the client's skin to assure that the temperature is comfortable for the client.

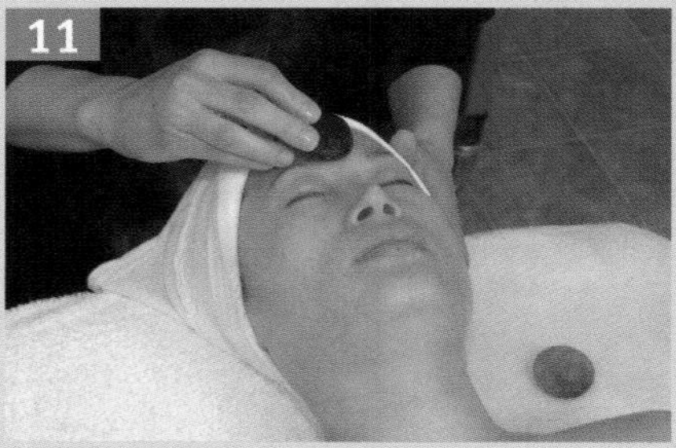

Start at corrugator.

11 Start at the corrugator muscle with one stone held between the thumb and first finger of each hand. *All movements are gliding, alternating hands and using stroking movements, unless otherwise specified.*

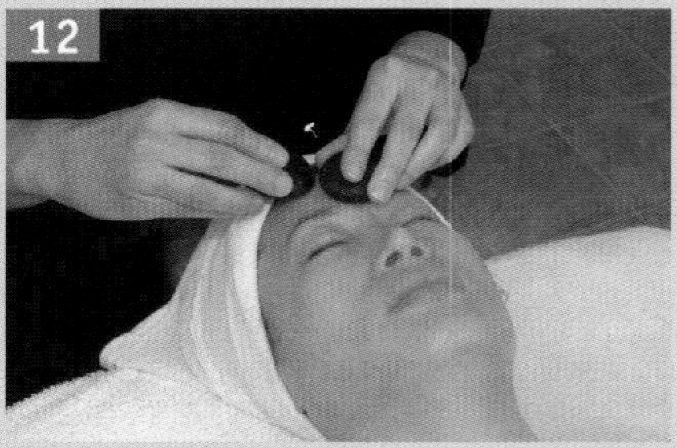

Glide to hairline.

12 Glide stones from the corrugator to hairline.

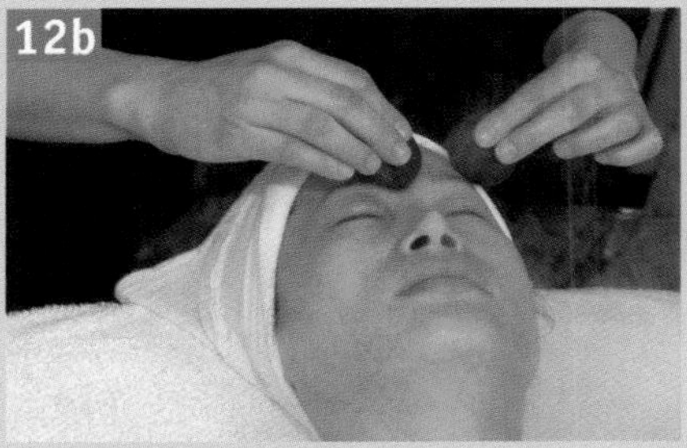

Move slowly from forehead to temple.

a. Repeat three to five strokes.

b. Repeat these horizontal strokes, slowly working from the center

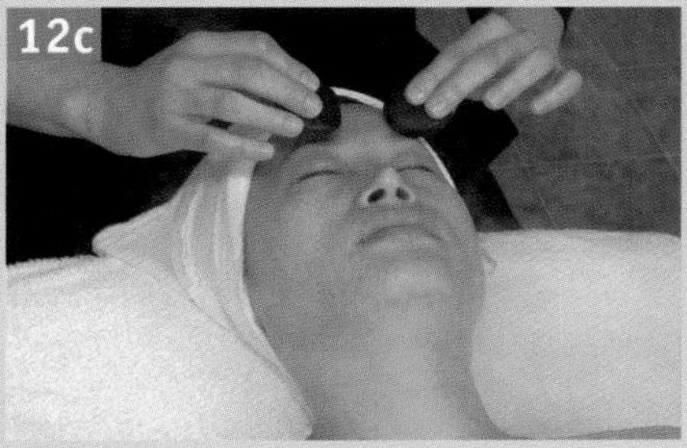

Go back to corrugator.

of the forehead to the temples using alternating hands.

c. Sweep back to the corrugator.

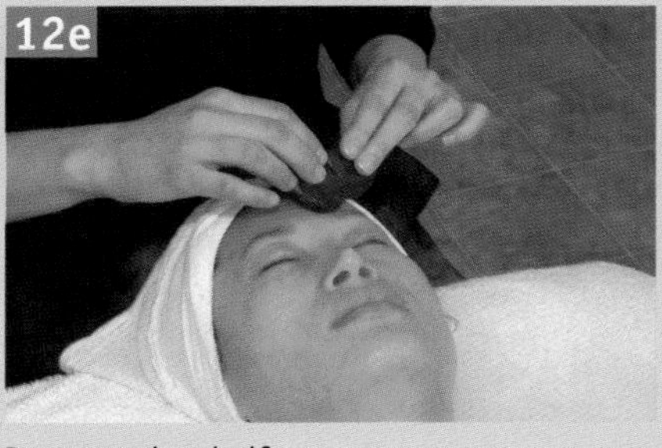

Repeat other half.

d. Repeat steps a, b, and c three times.

e. Repeat on other half of forehead.

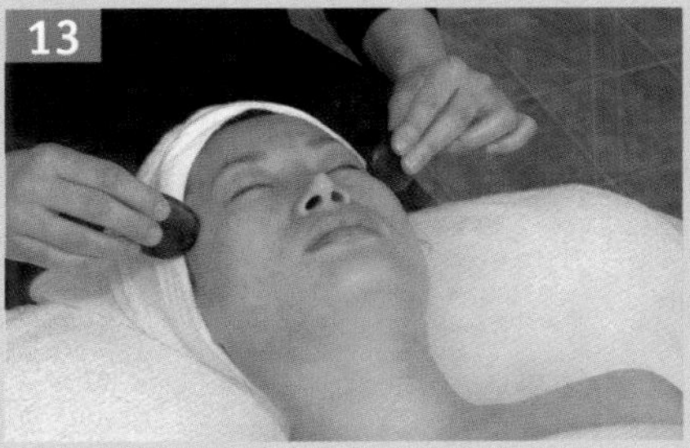

Circle over temples.

13 Glide stones simultaneously to the temples and perform five circles over the temples.

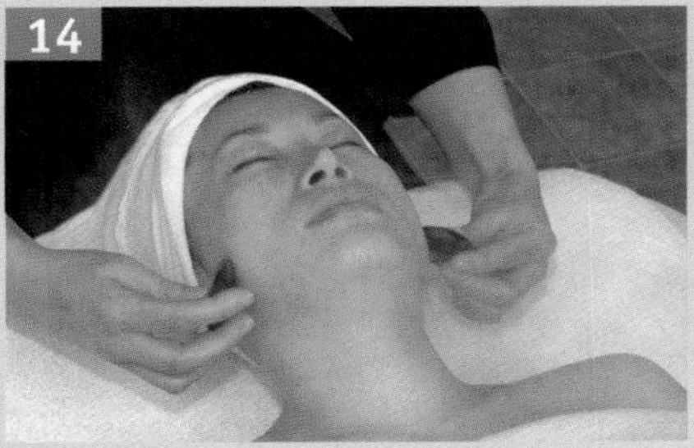

Meet at chin.

14 Glide stones along the perimeter of the face to meet at the center of the chin.

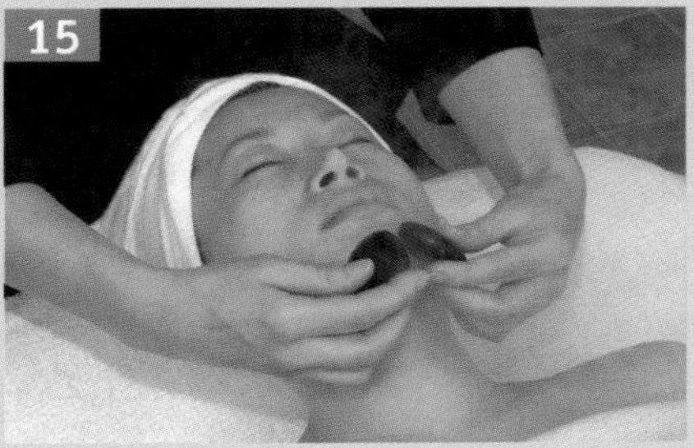

Circle the chin.

15 Perform five circles on the chin using both hands simultaneously.

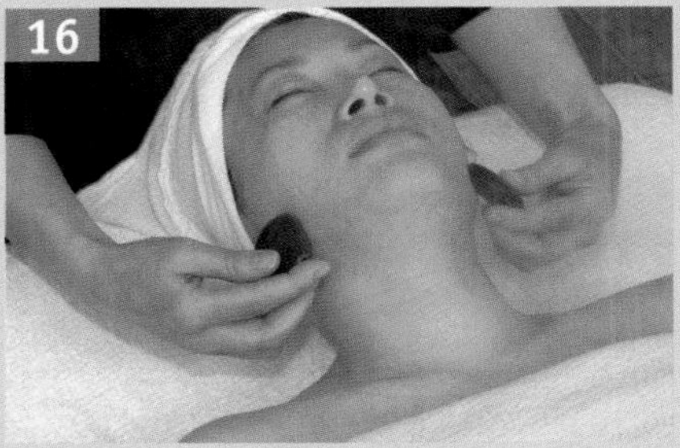

Move along toward ear.

16 Simultaneously perform circles, moving from the chin along the jawline to the ears.

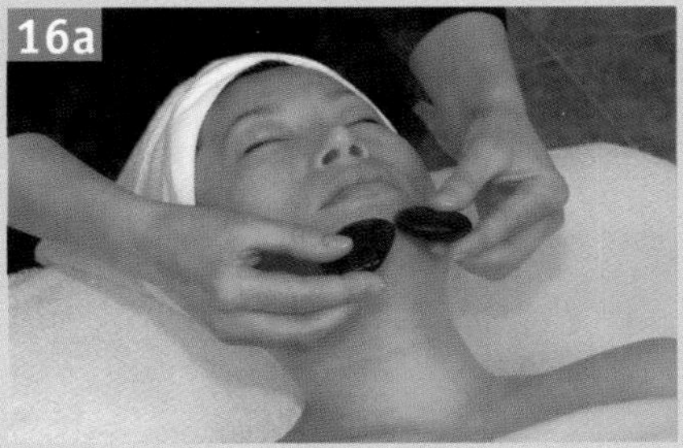

Glide to chin.

a. Glide back to the chin.

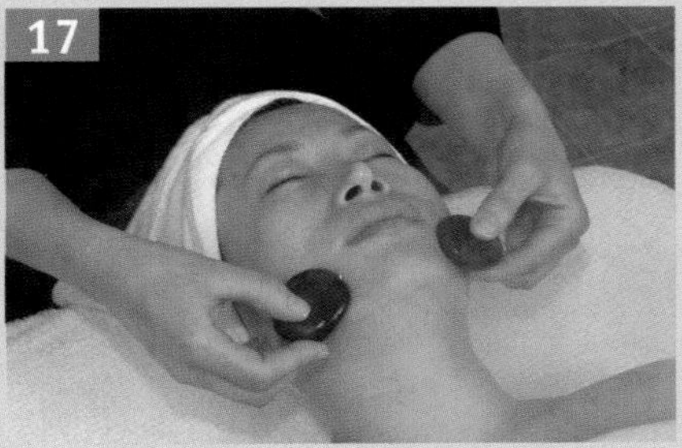

Move from chin to ear.

17 Using both hands simultaneously, glide up and repeat this process in the hollow above the jawline along the lower teeth, moving from the chin to the ears.

continues on next page

PROCEDURE 17–3, CONT. STONE MASSAGE FOR FACE

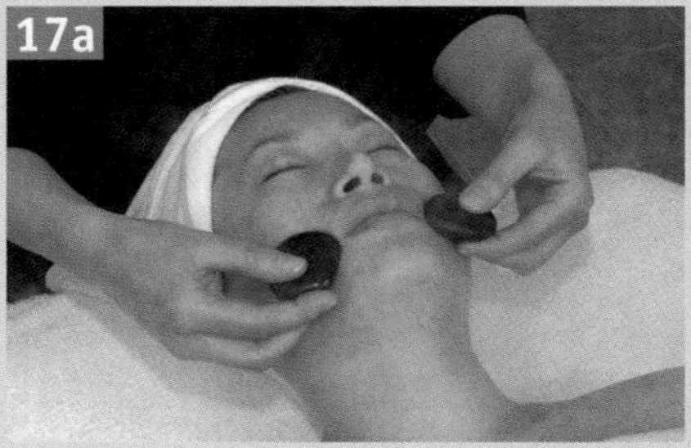

Move to corner of mouth.

a. Glide back to the corners of the mouth.

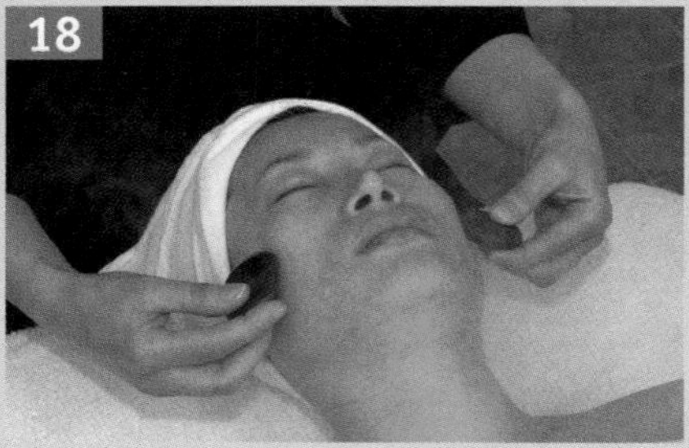

Circle to ear.

18 Simultaneously perform circles from the corners of the mouth to the ears.

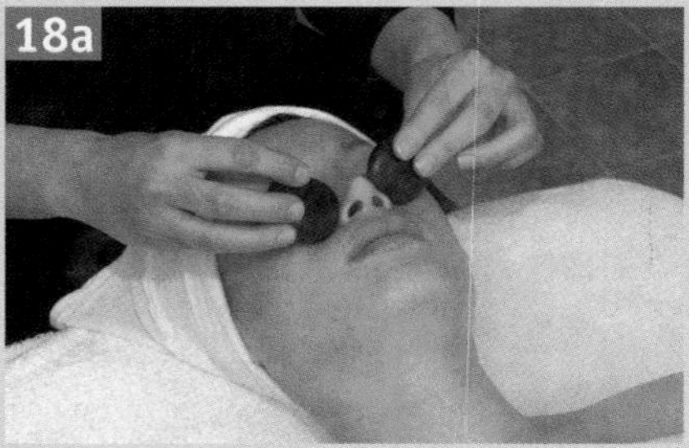

Go back to nose.

a. Glide back to corners of the nose.

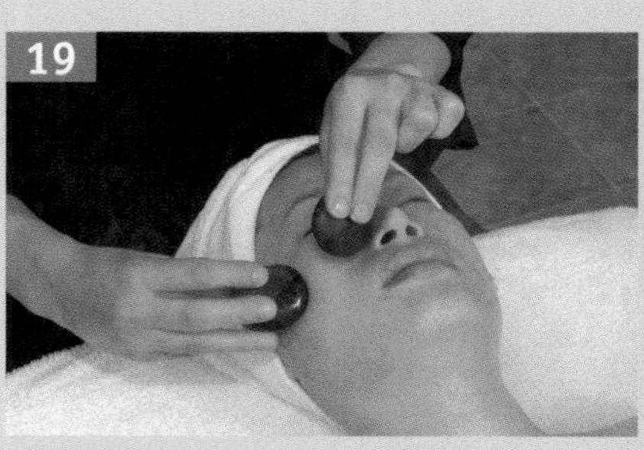

Stroke from cheeks to temples.

19 Using alternating hands, perform strokes from the corners of the nose, across the cheeks, and back toward the temples, starting on the right side of the nose.

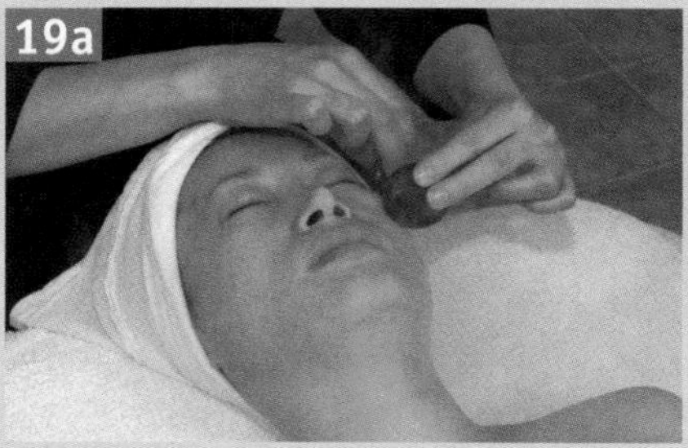

Repeat on left side.

a. Repeat on the left side of the face.

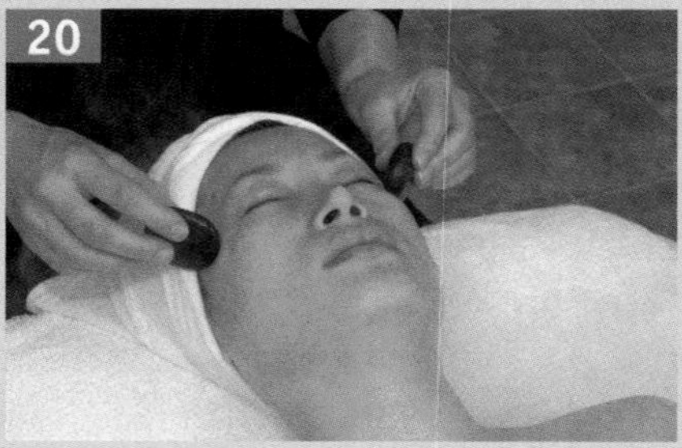

Glide to temples.

20 Repeat steps 18 and 19 three times, and then glide your hands to the temples.

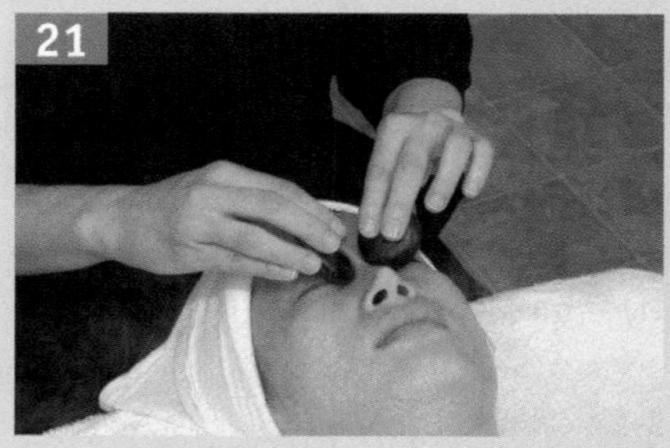

Move to inner eye.

21 Using both hands simultaneously, glide from the temples in a circle following the lower orbital bones to the inner corners of the eyes.

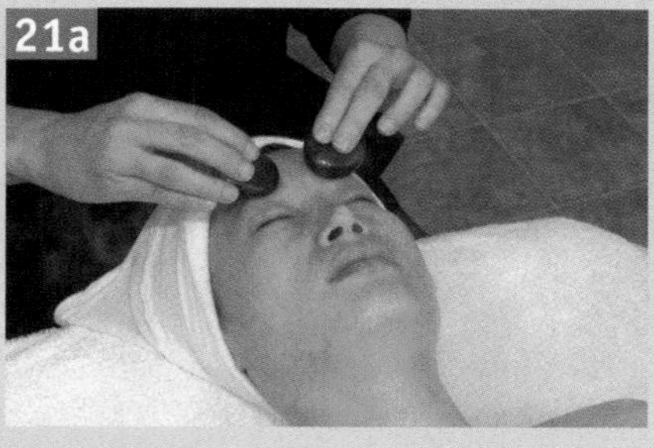

Go up and back to temple.

a. Move up over the brow and back to the temples.

b. Repeat five times.

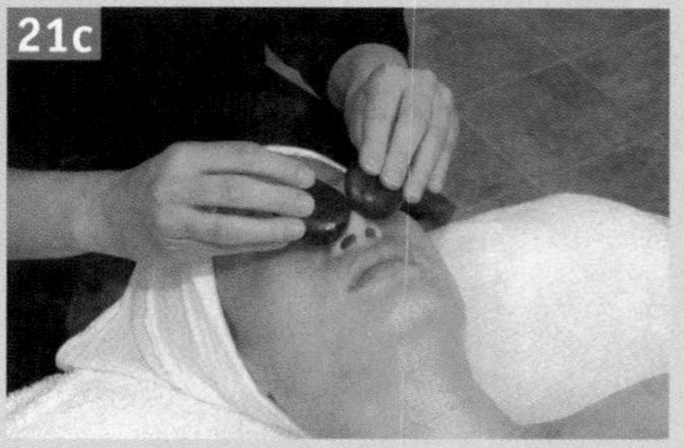

Move to tip of nose.

c. Glide from the temples to the tip of the nose.

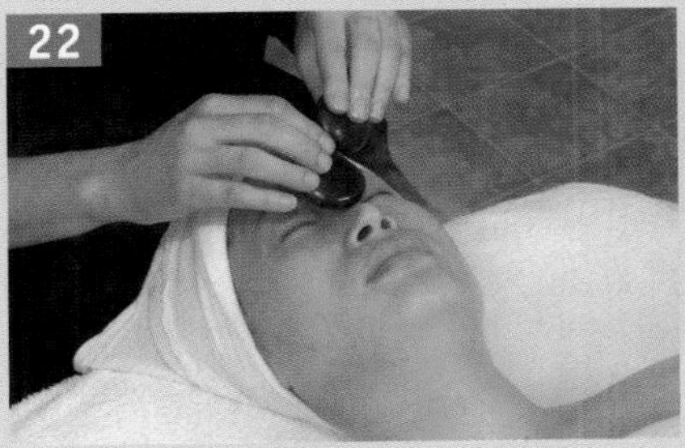

Stroke nose.

22 Stroke up the nose, alternating hands, eight to ten strokes.

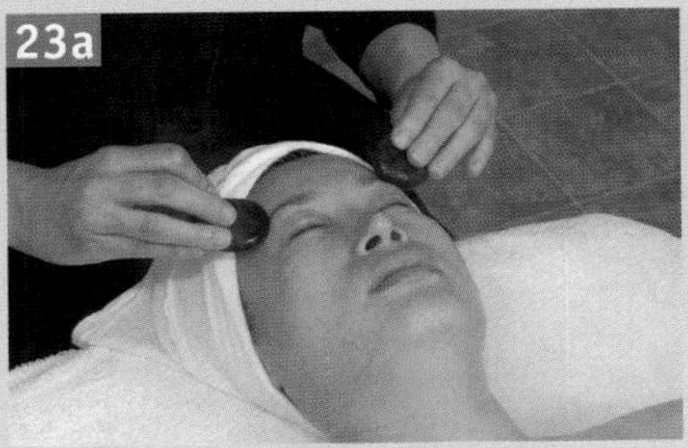

Glide to temples.

23 Moving both hands simultaneously, glide from the top of the nose up over the brow.

a. Continue glide to the temples.

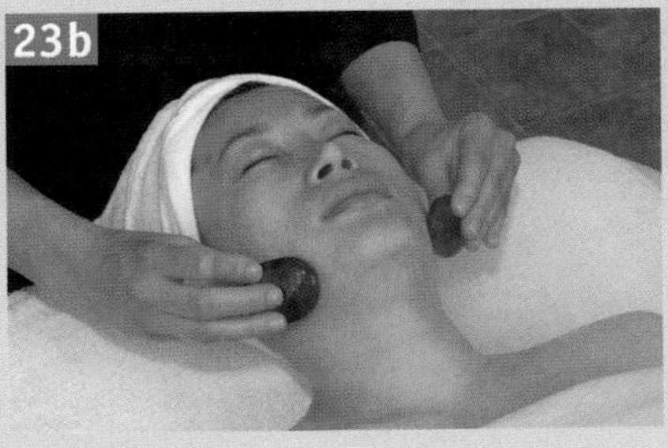

Glide to jawline.

b. Continue glide to the jawline.

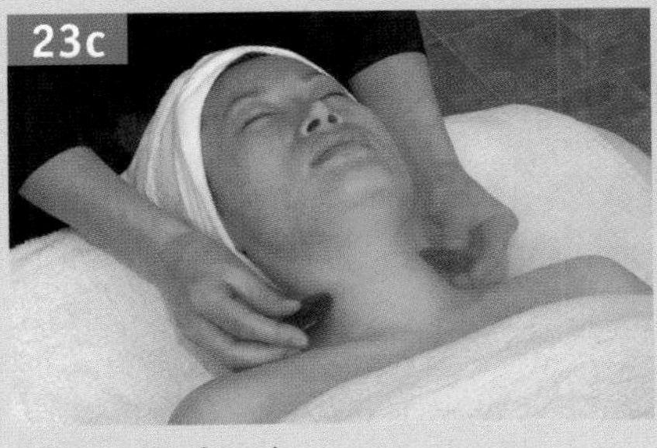

Down side of neck.

c. Continue down the side of the neck and bring your left

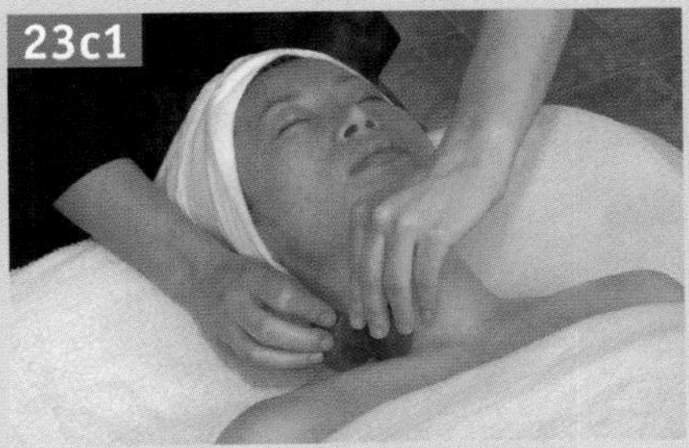

Down side of neck.

hand to join your right hand at the collarbone below the

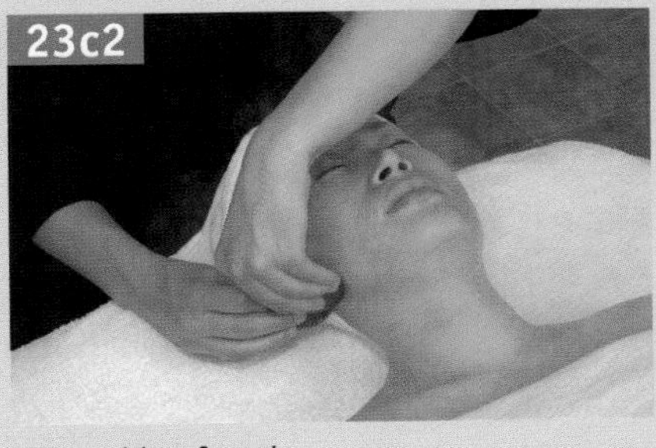

Down side of neck.

right ear, all in one continuous movement.

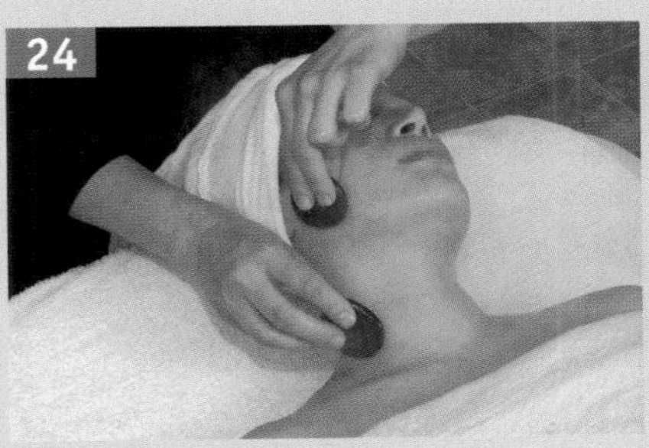

Up neck to jawline.

24 Alternating hands, stroke up neck to jawline starting on the right side of the face.

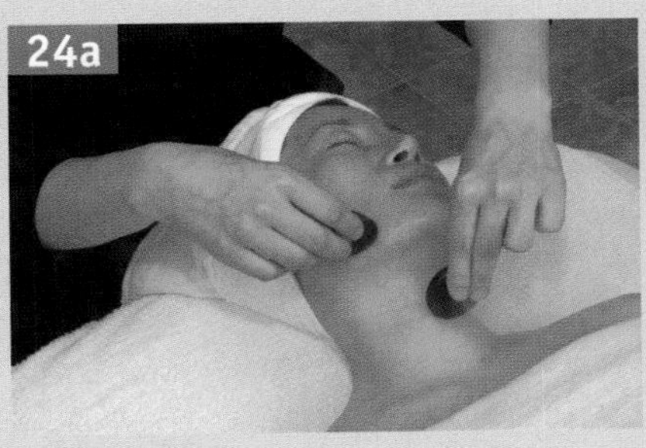

Repeat across neck.

a. Repeat movements across the neck.

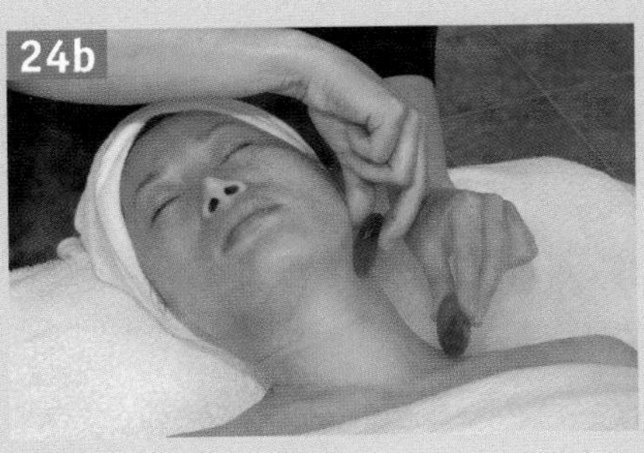

Up left side under ear.

b. Finish with strokes up the left side of the neck under the ears.

continues on next page

PROCEDURE 17–3, CONT. STONE MASSAGE FOR FACE

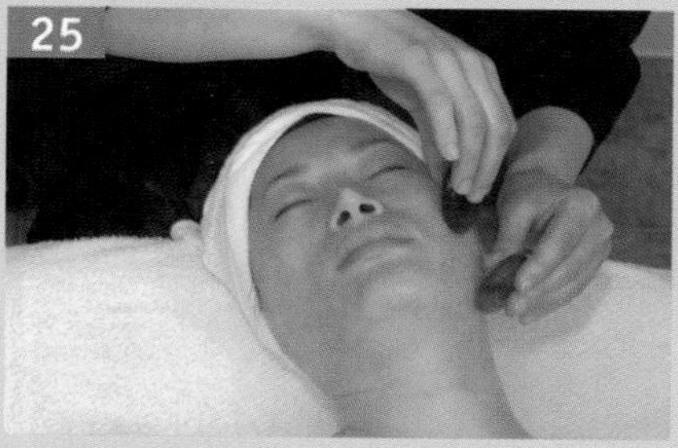

Up across toward mandible.

25 From the point just at the base of the ear on the left side of the face, stroke, using alternating hands, up across the face toward

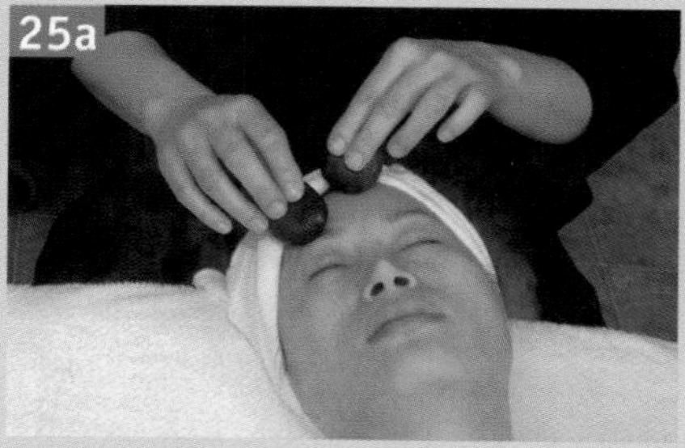

End at right temple.

the top of the mandible. With feathering strokes, repeat across the entire face, ending at the temple on the right side.

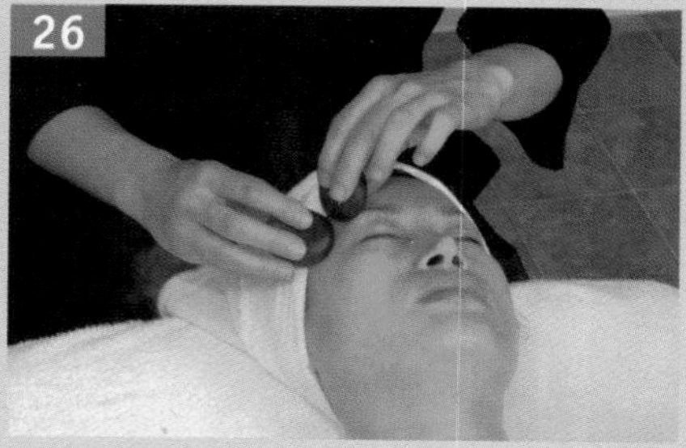

Feather across forehead.

26 From the temple on the right side, continue feathering strokes to the hairline. Repeat feathering strokes across the width of the forehead.

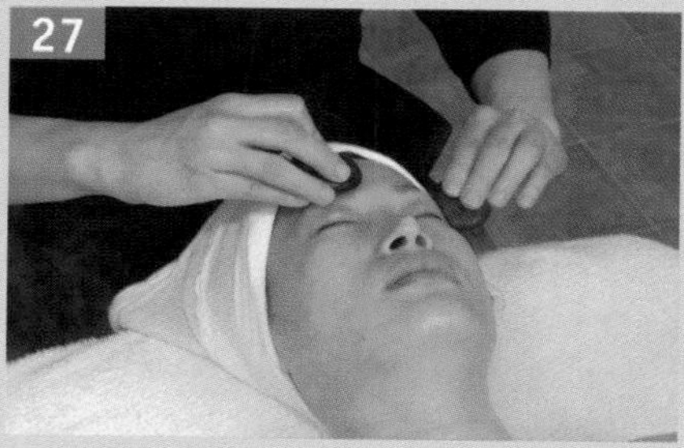

Feather face to temple.

27 Now shift feathering strokes from vertical to horizontal, stroking from the center of the face to temples.

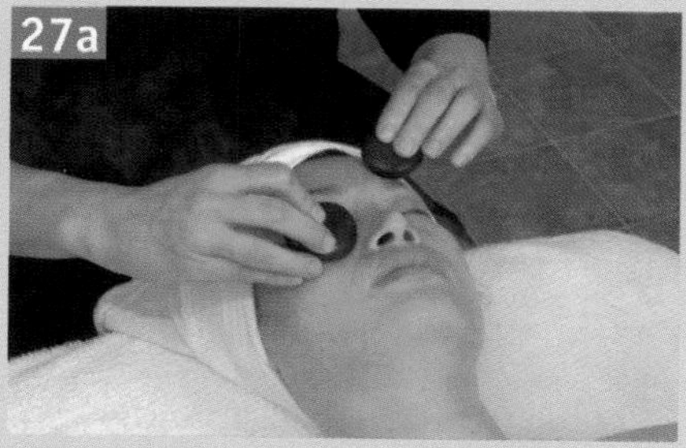

Start at hairline center.

a. Start these horizontal strokes at the center of the face at the hairline, using alternating hands.

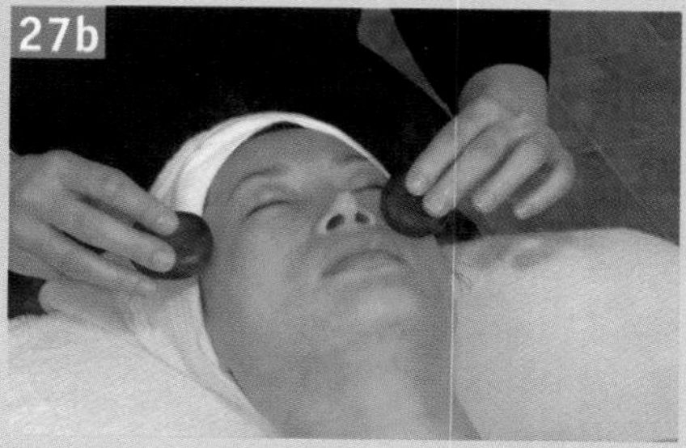

Down center to chin.

b. Repeat down the face to the chin, working from the center line to the sides of the face, bypassing the eye area.

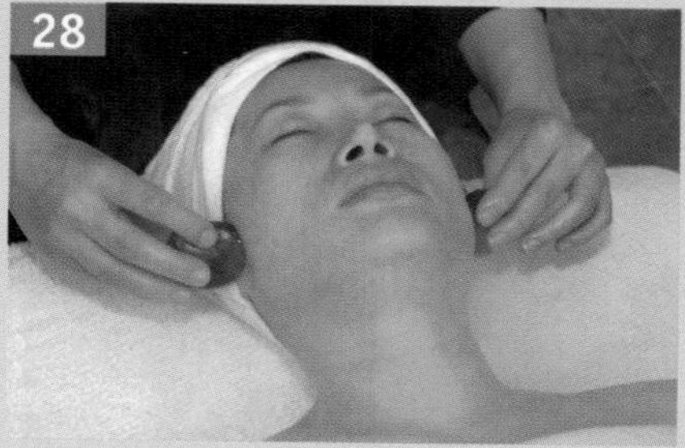

Glide to ear base.

28 Glide stones so each hand is positioned at the base of each ear.

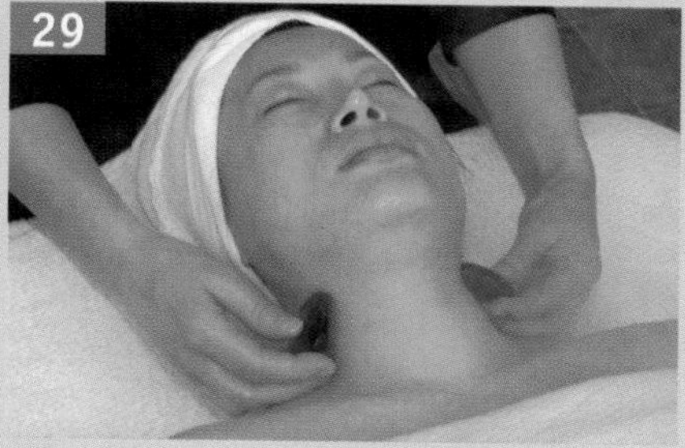

End at collarbone.

29 Use stones to simultaneously perform light downward lymph drainage movement, ending at the collarbone.

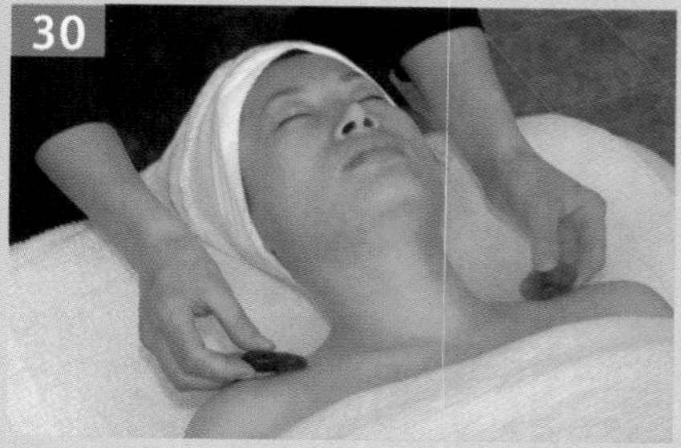

Glide off shoulders.

30 Finish by stroking stones simultaneously off each shoulder.

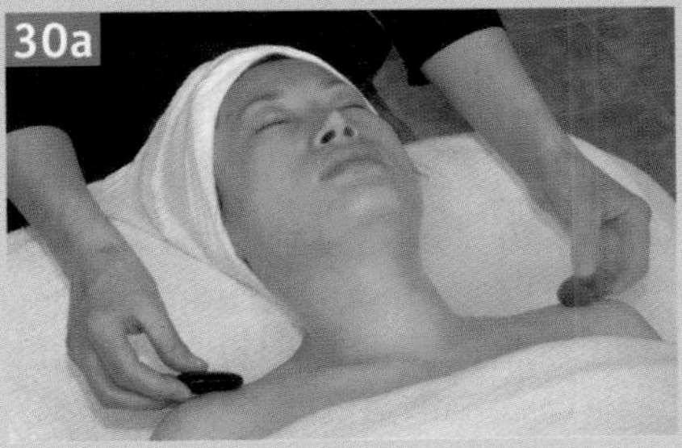

Glide off shoulders.

Post-procedure

Complete facial as desired.

Clean-up and Disinfection

When the procedure is complete, perform clean-up and disinfection procedures following OSHA or your state's guidelines.

LYMPHATIC MASSAGE FOR THE FACE AND NECK

Unless there is edema and/or scar tissue elsewhere in the body that needs attention, it is useful to give lymph drainage massage to a client's face and neck. Disease-causing organisms easily enter the body via the mouth, nose, and eyes and the body's immune system, including the lymph nodes of the head and neck, need to respond. Lymph drainage massage (LDM) stimulates the circulation of lymph and lymphocytes through the facial and cervical lymph nodes. Lymphatic massage is an advanced skill that requires practice. This section will introduce it to you, but additional training is recommended to enhance your proficiency. Modern lymphatic drainage techniques were originally developed by Dr. Emil Vodder to treat sinus conditions, enlarged lymph nodes, and problem skin in the late 1930s. While his techniques are probably the most widely known, other simpler-to-learn techniques have helped to make lymphatic drainage mainstream with estheticians and massage therapists.

★ REGULATORY AGENCY ALERT

Lymphatic or lymph drainage massage is not allowed in some states. Be sure to check with the regulating board in your state to assure that this form of massage is within your scope of practice!

Identifying Face and Neck Indications and Contraindications

LDM to the face and neck effectively reduces bruising and edema following injury or surgery, including dental and cosmetic surgery. Because blood clots are a concern after surgery, do not offer LDM until the client is released by the physician and requires no follow-up visits. Some physicians recommend LDM during healing. In that case, perform LDM according to the physician's instructions.

Facial edema can be the result of allergies, hormones, medication, fatigue, illness, infection, injury, excess salt in the diet, or weeping, among other causes. Because some of these conditions are contraindications, it is important to know the reason for the edema before proceeding. If the client is unsure and the edema persists, a medical examination may be in order before the client undergoes LDM. Once the client has a proper diagnosis and contraindications are ruled out, LDM may be used to reduce facial edema. LDM stimulates a sluggish immune system to more activity by increasing the circulation of lymph and lymphocytes. Those with this type of system may benefit from a series of LDM sessions at the beginning of cold and flu season. Recommend at least three sessions in a week, although up to seven sessions in a week would be more beneficial.

Similarly, LDM benefits clients with low energy. Low energy can result from stress, overwork, illness, or depression, any of which can depress the immune system. Stimulating immune circulation will help a fatigued client resist illness. In contrast, clients with high energy levels who work and exercise more than they should are prone to illness and injuries because they do not rest. LDM is deeply relaxing and may be used to help speed healing, as well as give overworked clients some rest.

Although LDM is focused on superficial tissues, the muscles underneath also respond to the light, skillfully directed touch and will relax. Pain due to muscle tension will reduce or disappear. For instance, LDM can help relax the muscles that cause muscle-tension headaches. When facial muscles relax, the facial expression softens and relaxes, which contributes to a more youthful and healthy appearance.

LDM carries microscopic organisms and the by-products of cellular metabolism away from the dermal tissues and allows increased nutrition to flow into the skin, improving the skin's condition. Regular LDM improves the complexion, causing the skin to glow with increased health. If, however, the skin is infected, or if there is inflamed acne, wait until the infection has cleared before proceeding with any kind of face massage.

Treating Chronically Swollen Lymph Nodes

Many people have chronically swollen lymph nodes, often from repeated infections and childhood illnesses. First, it is important to have the nodes examined to rule out more serious conditions. If no serious condition is causing the swollen nodes and no infection is present, regular LDM can help to reduce the size of the nodes and improve lymph circulation in the area. In this case, it is a good idea to teach the client to perform daily self-massage, which produces results faster.

A client who has had repeated infections and illnesses is sometimes prone to a healing crisis, or a flare-up of old symptoms, when receiving LDM. A healing crisis is not serious, but the therapist or esthetician should make the client aware of the possibility.

Keep lotion, oil, and aromatherapy oil out of the client's eyes. If using lotions, creams, or oils, consider placing a cotton pad over each eye. Use a warm, moist towel to clean the client's face before proceeding with the session. The towel has the added effect of relaxing muscles and stimulating lymph flow.

Locating Lymph Nodes on the Face and Neck

On the neck, lymph nodes are located in two triangles, one on each side of the neck, bound by the sternocleidomastoid muscle, the clavicle, and the superior border of the trapezius muscle (Figure 17–28). The apex of each triangle is immediately below each earlobe. Additional lymph nodes are below the mandible from the angle of the jaw to the chin and in the back behind the ears and along the base of the skull. On the face, nodes are in front of the ears, on the angle of the jaw anterior to the masseter muscle, and, occasionally, near the eyes, nose, and mouth.

Observing and Palpating Lymph Nodes on the Face and Neck

Before proceeding, and while the client is seated and facing you, look carefully at the client's face and neck. Look for symmetry, any swelling, or signs of inflammation in front of or behind the ears, under the eyes, along the jaw line, in the neck, and in the supraclavicular triangle (Figure 17–29). In a healthy person, the lymph nodes should not be visibly swollen or inflamed. When swelling or inflammation is present, discuss the condition with the client before proceeding. If the client does not know the reason for the swelling or inflammation and has never had it examined, do *not* proceed with the massage until a physician has ruled out serious health conditions. Swollen lymph nodes indicate infection, which is a contraindication for massage.

Some clients will have chronically enlarged lymph nodes due to a serious underlying health problem or to such chronic infections as sinusitis or tonsillitis. Lymph

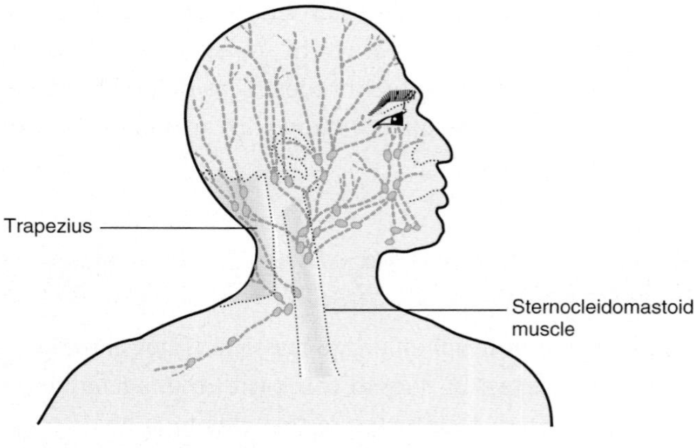

Figure 17–28 Locating lymph nodes.

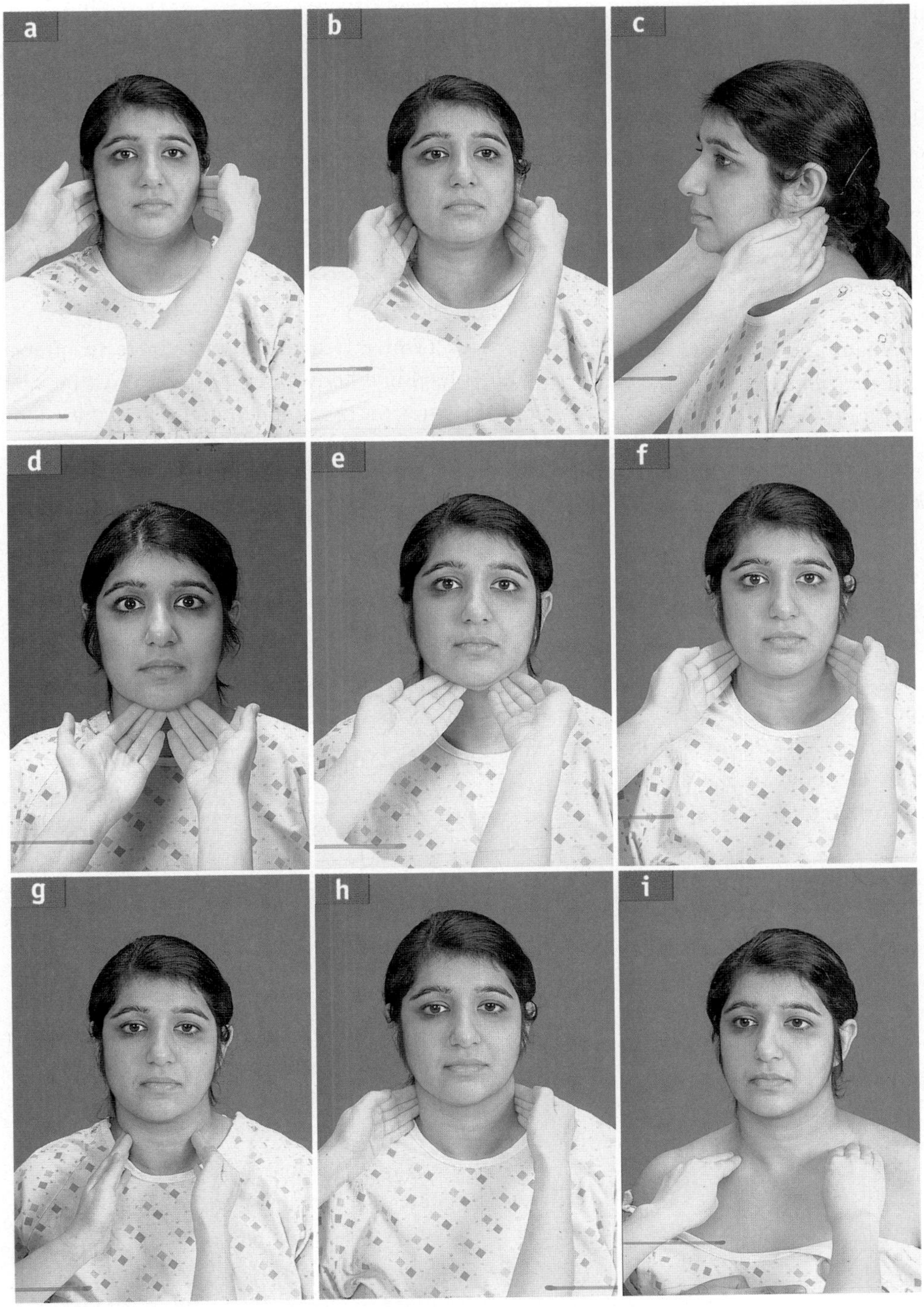

Figure 17–29 Guide for locating lymph nodes.

nodes can also be scarred by repeated infections and can remain enlarged after an infection has disappeared.

After observing the lymph nodes, the next step is to palpate the nodes. When the client is lying supine on the massage table, palpate the lymph nodes of the face and neck. Using medium to light pressure, massage in small circles over the areas where the lymph nodes are located, attempting to locate small, pea-sized masses that can be moved. Palpate the tissues behind and in front of the ears (post- and preauricular nodes), under the jawline from the chin (submental nodes) to the angle of the jaw (submandibular nodes), along the sternocleidomastoid muscle (anterior cervical chain), at the superior edge of the trapezius muscle (posterior cervical chain), and in the supraclavicular triangle.

In a healthy person, lymph nodes are generally quite small and cannot be palpated. If nodes are palpable, discuss this with the client before proceeding with the massage. Find out how long the nodes have been enlarged, whether the client is aware of any infection, whether the nodes are tender, and whether the client has seen a physician about the enlarged nodes. If the client does not know the history of the problem and has not seen a physician, do *not* proceed with the massage. Refer the client to a physician for examination to rule out serious underlying health conditions.

Establishing a Lymph Drainage Pattern on the Face and Neck

Lymph drainage on the face is usually divided into two areas. You can find these areas by drawing imaginary lines from the apex of the nose to the angle of the jaw on either side, creating a triangle (Figure 17–30). Inside the triangle, including the nose, mouth, chin, and jawline, lymph drains to the nodes under the mandible, then down through the anterior chain of nodes in the neck toward the lymphatic ducts at the medial ends of the clavicle.

Outside the triangle, including the forehead, temple, and cheeks, lymph drains to the preauticular nodes and the deep nodes on the neck below the earlobes before draining through the nodes in the neck toward the lymphatic ducts located near the medial ends of the clavicle.

Lymphatic vessels of the scalp drain posteriorly through the occipital nodes and then through cervical nodes. Lymph vessels on the back of the neck drain anteriorly toward the cervical nodes.

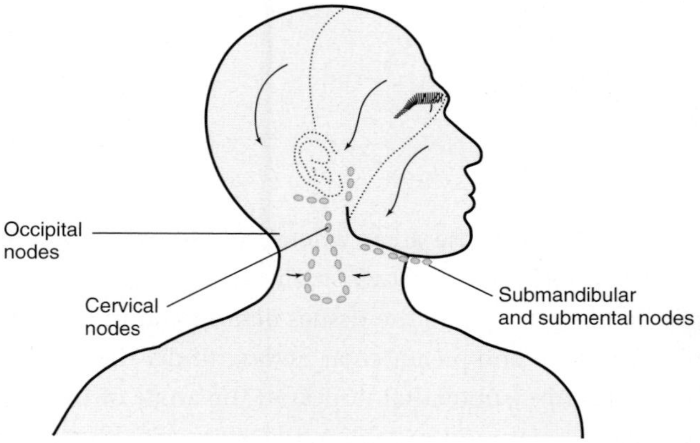

Figure 17–30 Direction of lymph drainage of the face and neck.

The basic pattern for the massage is to empty the lymph nodes on the neck and then to massage the entire neck before massaging the face. On the face, empty the lymph nodes first, then drain the lymph vessels on the face and scalp, draining the inner triangle first, then the remainder of the face and the scalp. Finish by draining the nodes on the neck again.

Extending Lymph Drainage Massage to the Face and Neck

Face and neck LDM is a nice add-on service to offer a client who is having a body wrap, but you must be sure the client does not become dehydrated. Offer the client water before the session begins, and have a glass of water with a flexible straw available during the session.

If the purpose of the treatment is to enhance the immune system during or before flu season, urge the client to have three to seven sessions in one week. While this frequency of sessions is beneficial, it is intense, and mind-body reactions or healing crises are possible.

When practicing this massage sequence, you may find that it can be tedious to keep counting the seconds and numbers of circles. However, the results are worth the

FOCUS ON: *Stationary Circles*

The basis of all LDM is the stationary circle (see Figure 17–31). The stationary circle has two important components: 1) a slight compression at the beginning of the movement and 2) a stretch of the tissues at the end of the movement. This move is called the stationary circle because it is important to remain stationary and repeat the movement 6 to 10 times before moving to an adjacent area.
To perform the stationary circle, use flat fingers and gently contact the skin, compressing slightly. Stretch the tissue in a circular movement, clockwise or counterclockwise. Lymphatic capillaries are very close to the surface of the skin, so there is no need for deep pressure.

KEEP IN MIND . . .

Manual lymphatic drainage is a technical procedure. It takes in-depth training to become proficient.

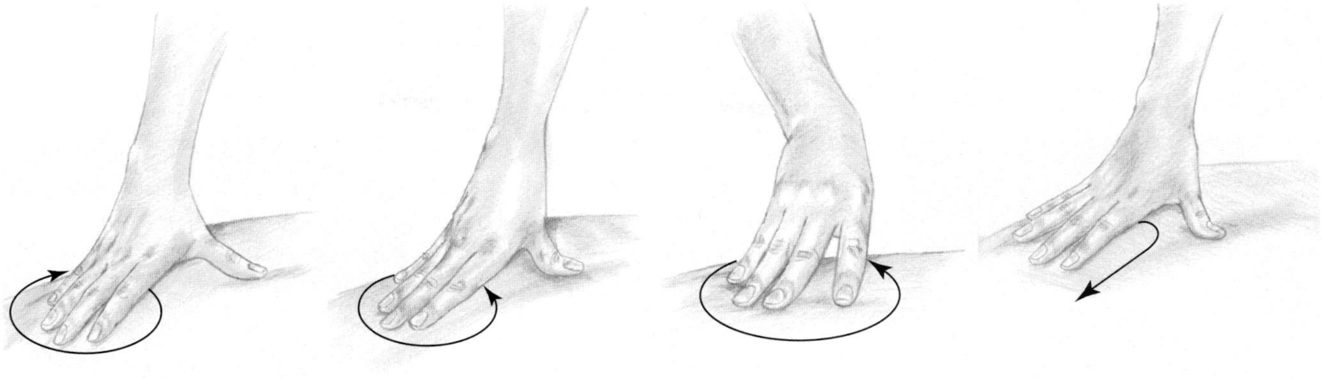

Figure 17–31 Using the stationary circle.

effort: This is a very delightful massage experience for the client. Not only does it stimulate lymph circulation, it is deeply relaxing. With appropriate music, soft lighting, subtle aromatherapy, and carefully selected emollient, as well as skillful, directed touch, the client perceives the work on more than one level and can find the experience profound.

LDM is performed on both sides of the neck and face at the same time, although the directions only mention one side. Use both hands and work both sides at the same time. *Unless otherwise indicated, use stationary circles. Each circle should last seven seconds, and the circles should be repeated for a full minute, for a total of at least seven circles* (Figure 17–31).

PROCEDURE 17–4 MANUAL LYMPHATIC DRAINAGE MASSAGE

IMPLEMENTS AND MATERIALS

- Standard facial lounge setup with linens and towels
- Cleansing product to remove makeup
- Massage lotion or oil (optional but recommended)
- SPF moisturizer to finish service

Preparation

1. Set up the facial lounge and treatment room.
2. Gather supplies.
3. Consult with the client to assure there are no contraindications to treatment and to complete all intake forms.
4. Assure the client has signed informed consent to service.
5. Have the client prepare for service in the standard manner.
6. Offer a bolster if the client needs one under his or her knees.

Procedure

This treatment is done in two phases—first the neck and then the face.

Treating the Neck

7. Sit or stand at the client's head.
8. Apply skin-cleansing agent.
9. Carefully drape a warm, moist towel over the client's face, leaving room for the client to breathe. Allow the towel to cool to room temperature.
10. As the towel cools, massage gently through the towel to relax the tissues. Before removing the towel, use it to gently wipe the face and to prevent massaging any cosmetics or environmental waste particles into the skin.
11. Apply warm lotion to the skin with smooth strokes, covering the face and the front and back of the neck.

continues on next page

PROCEDURE 17–4, CONT. MANUAL LYMPHATIC DRAINAGE MASSAGE

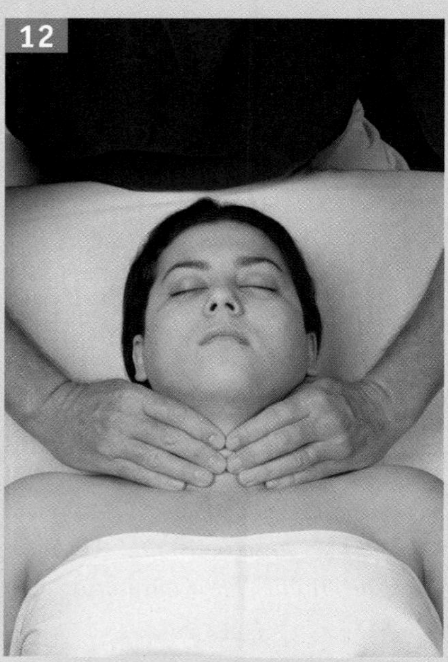

Twenty stationary circles over the supraclavicular nodes.

12 Begin with 20 stationary circles over the supraclavicular nodes, placing fingers above the upper margin of the clavicle. It takes about 3 minutes to massage the area.

13 Perform 20 stationary circles on the subauricular nodes, between the ears and the mastoid process, posterior and inferior to the ears. Use three or four fingers, flat against the skin, to stretch the skin gently in a circular direction, counting each circle carefully to keep the pace slow. This takes about 3 minutes.

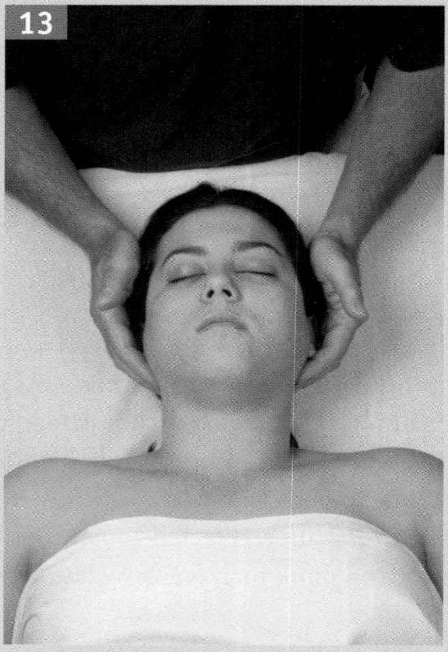

Twenty stationary circles on the subauricular nodes.

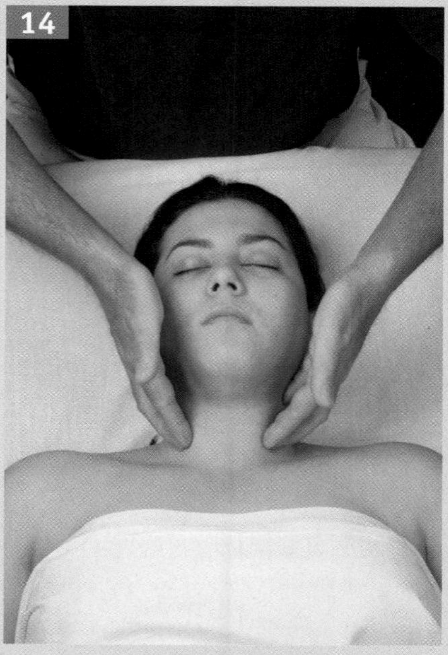

Drain the anterior cervical chain of nodes.

14 Drain the anterior cervical chain of nodes, along the region of the sternocleidomastoid muscle. Place all four fingers over the area from the bottom of the ears to the clavicle, and, very slowly, stretch the skin in stationary circles for about 3 minutes to massage the anterior cervical chain of nodes.

15 Repeat Step 6 on the posterior chain of cervical nodes.

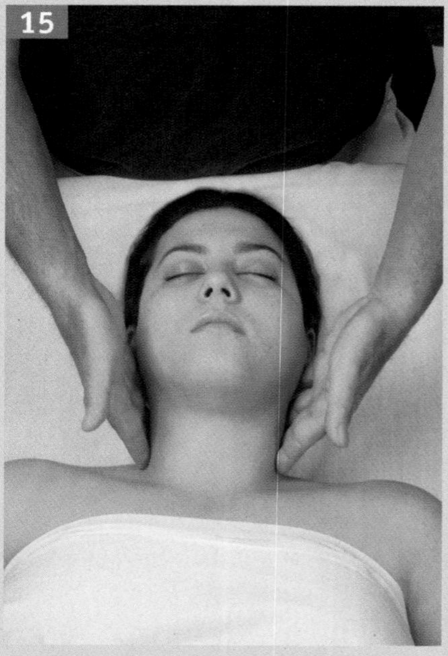

Repeat on the posterior chain of cervical nodes.

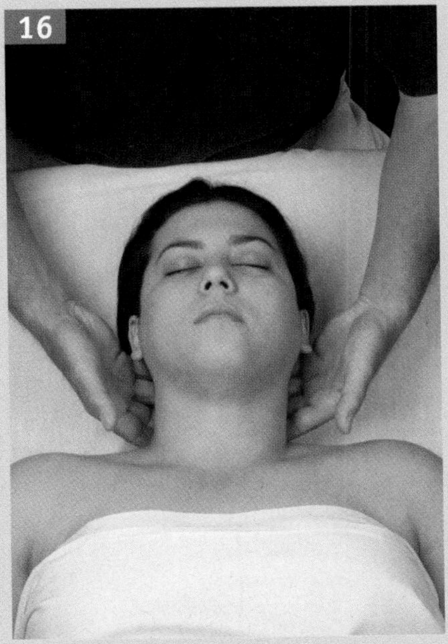

Move the skin on the back of the neck over the cervical vertebrae.

16 Slide the flat pads of fingers of both hands under the neck, covering the skin from the bottom of the neck to the hairline. Perform 7 stationary circles, moving the skin on the back of the neck over the cervical vertebrae.

17 Place the flat fingers on the sides of the neck, between the ears and the collarbone, and perform stationary circles on the sides of the neck.

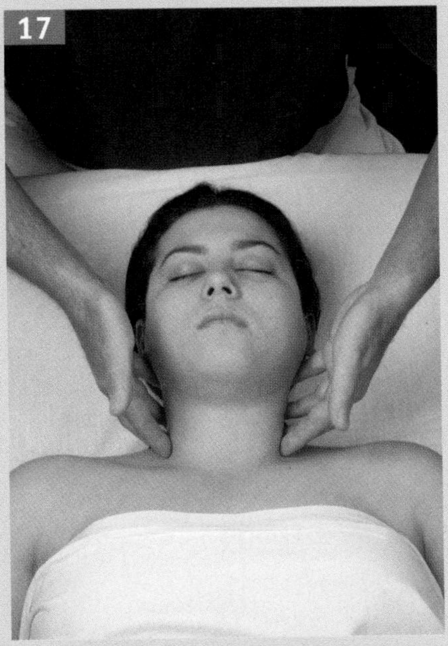

Perform stationary circles on the sides of the neck.

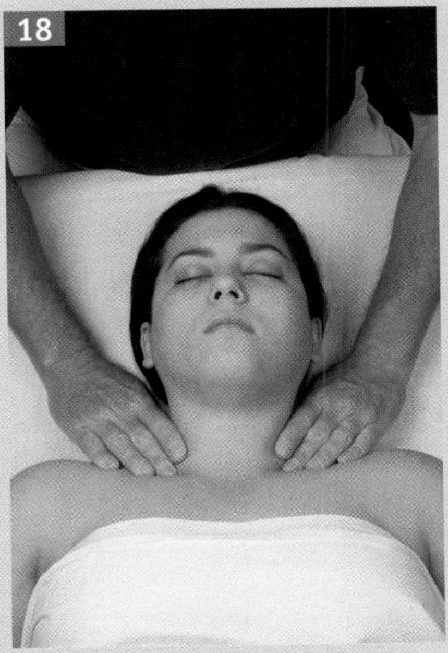

Place two flat fingers inside the triangle.

18 Place two fingers flat inside the triangle by the sternocleidomastoid muscle, the clavicle, and the scalene muscles, and again perform stationary circles for a full minute.

19 Move laterally to a position under the jawline (midway between the chin and the angle of the jaw), and massage in stationary circles for 1 minute.

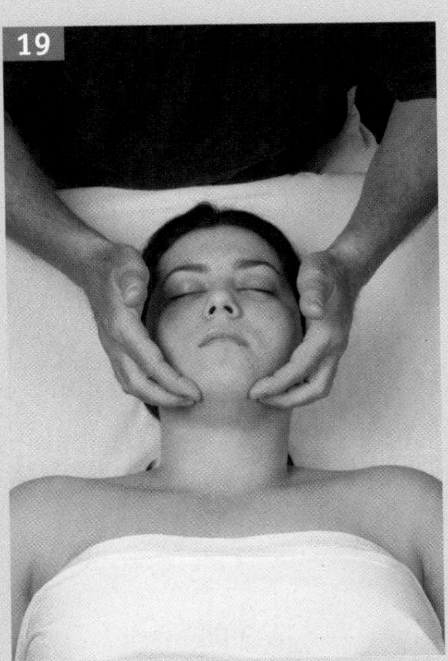

Move under the jawline.

continues on next page

PROCEDURE 17–4, CONT. MANUAL LYMPHATIC DRAINAGE MASSAGE

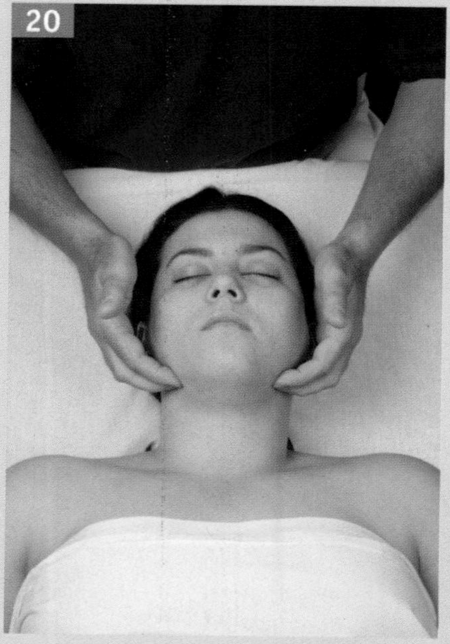

Place fingers on the neck immediately under ear.

20 Place fingers on the neck immediately under the ears with the fingers pointing toward the clavical, and massage in stationary circles for 1 minute.

21 Place flat fingertips in the depression between the thyroid cartilage and the sternocleidomastoid muscles, and perform rotary massage, using very light pressure.

> **CAUTION!**
>
> **Omit Steps 21, 22, and 23 (the front of the neck) for any client who has thyroid abnormalities.**

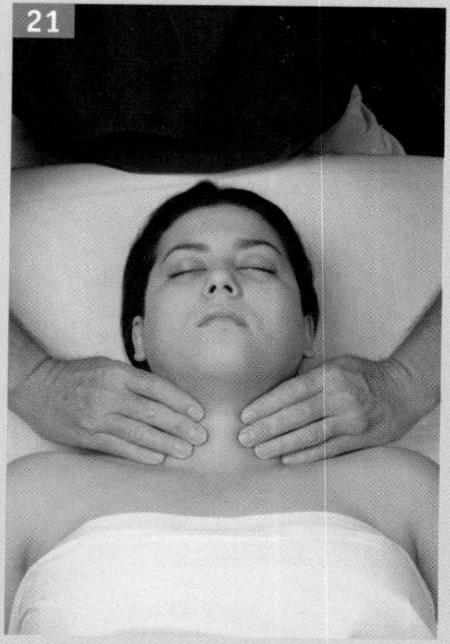

Massage between the thyroid cartilage and sternocleidomastoid muscles.

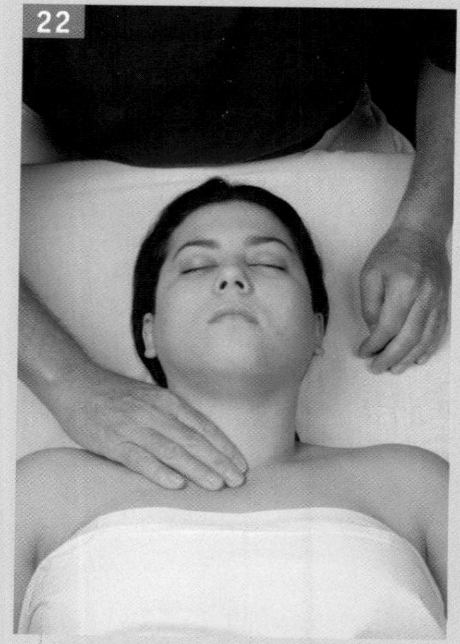

Massage at the bottom of the throat between the two sternocleidomastoid muscles.

22 Place the flat fingertips of one hand in the central depression at the bottom of the throat between the two sternocleidomastoid muscles, and do light rotary massage for 1 minute.

23 Use effleurage movements on the throat and the back of the neck. The direction of pressure follows lymph drainage.

Working on the Face

Note: The first section of the face takes about 15 minutes to complete.

24 Mist your hands with hydrosol or water (away from the client's face) to rehydrate the lotion or moisturizer. With warm hands, gently effleurage the face as an introduction to face work.

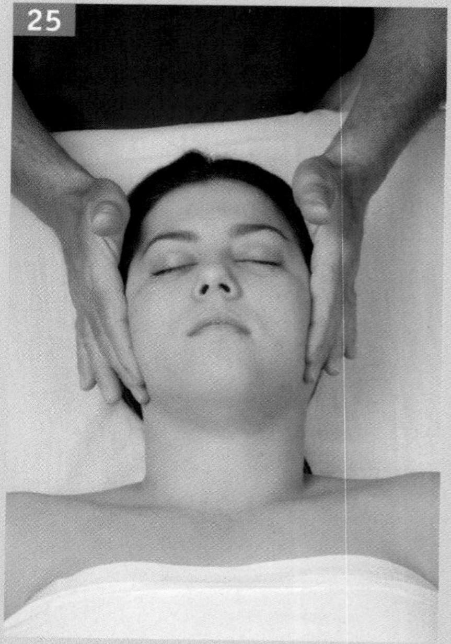

Massage masseter muscle.

25 Place pads of the fingers flat over the region of the masseter muscle, at the angle of the jaw. Perform 20 stationary circles (about 3 minutes at 7 seconds per circle).

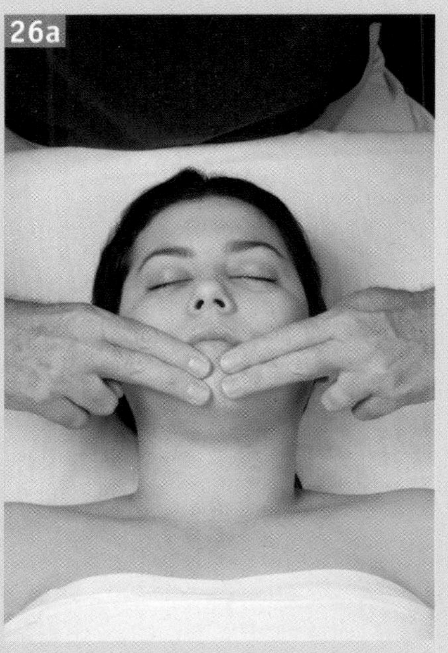

Perform massage on the chin, below the bottom lip.

26 Making pads of the fingers flat as much as possible, perform stationary circles in sets of 7 over the following regions, in order (each step takes nearly a minute):

a. On the chin, below the bottom lip.

b. Along the jaw line from the mouth to the angle of the jaw.

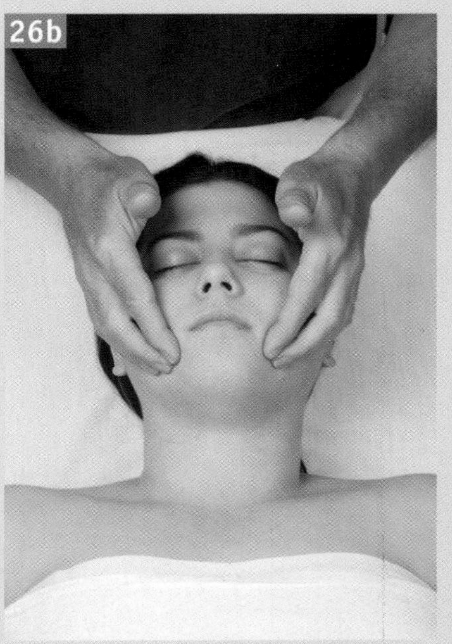

Massage along the jawline.

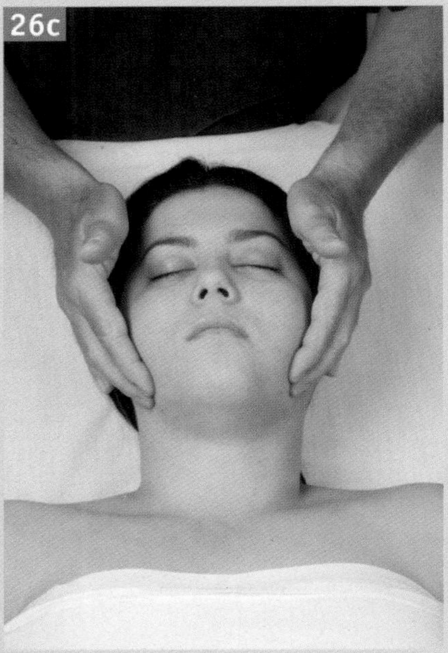

Over the angle of the jaw.

c. Over the angle of the jaw.

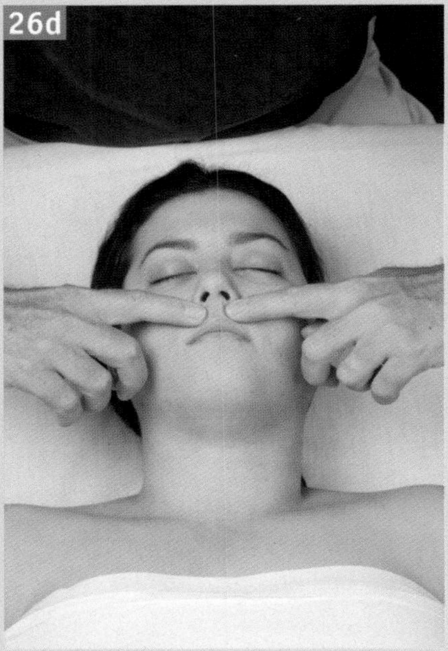

Over the upper lip, below the nose.

d. Over the upper lip, below the nose.

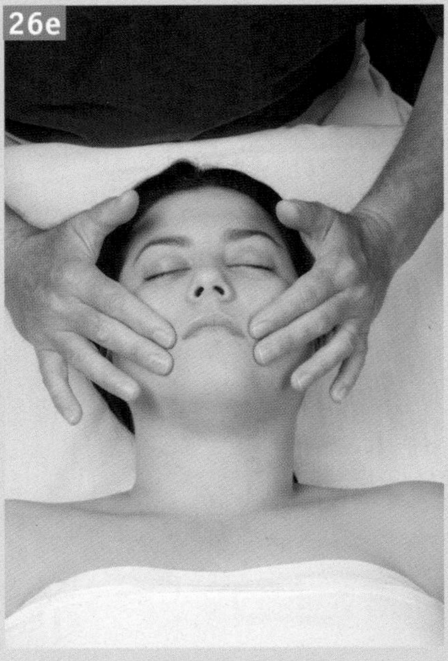

Over the corners of the mouth.

e. Over the corners of the mouth.

continues on next page

PROCEDURE 17–4. CONT. MANUAL LYMPHATIC DRAINAGE MASSAGE

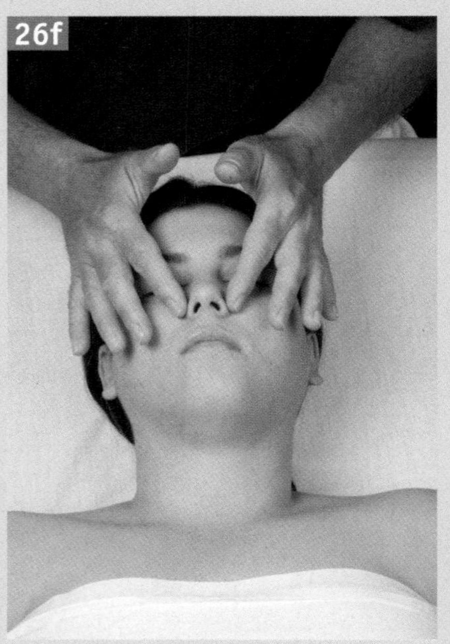

On the wings of the nose.

f. On the wings of the nose.

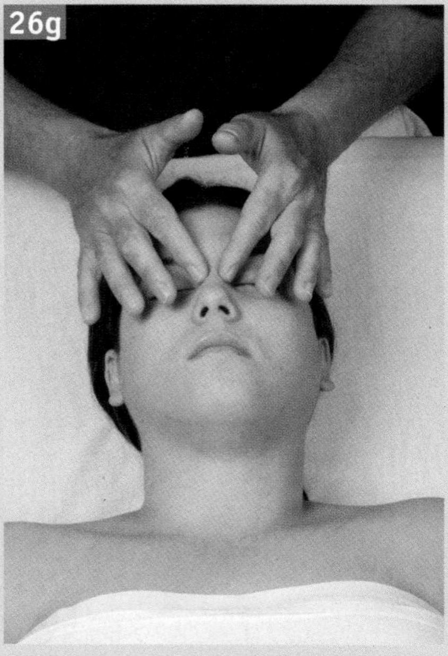

On the bridge of the nose.

g. On the bridge of the nose (over the bony area of the middle of the nose)

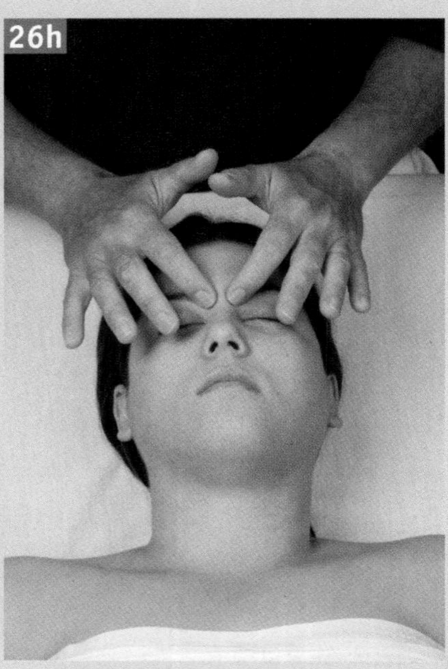

Root of the nose.

h. At the root of the nose (close to the eyes, but still on the bony protuberance of the nose)

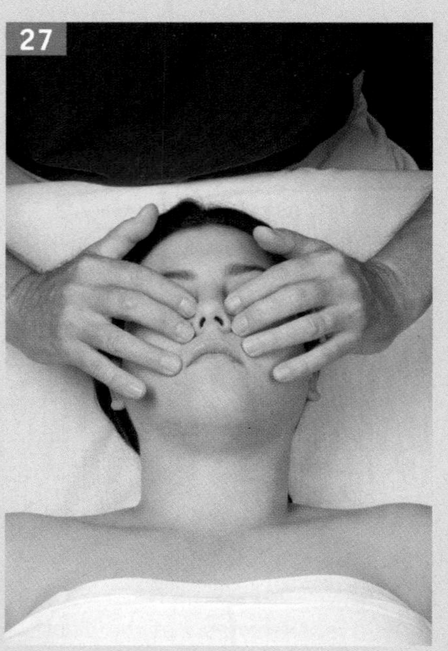

Follow the nasolabial groove or laugh lines.

27 Place the tips of all four fingers in a curve from the medial corners of the eyes to the bottom of the nose, following the nasolabial groove or laugh lines. Massage for 1 minute.

28 Place pads of the fingers flat over the region of the masseter muscle and massage 7 stationary circles, 7 seconds each.

Note: The second section of the face takes nearly 10 minutes to complete.

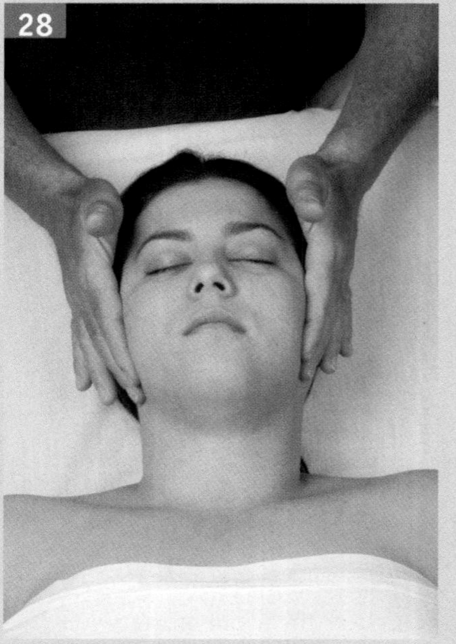

Massage masseter muscle region.

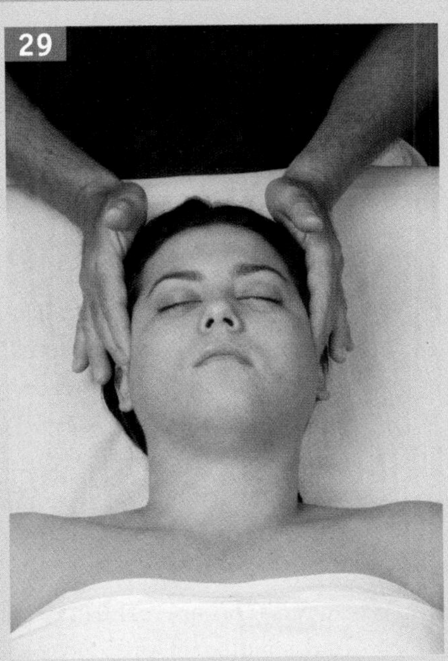

Place fingers in front of the ears.

29 Place pads of the fingers flat over the nodes, in front of the ears. Begin with 20 circles, which takes nearly 3 minutes.

30 Around the eyes, place the tips of one or two fingers in a semicircle below the eyes, as close to the tear ducts as possible, without touching the eyes. Massage for 1 minute.

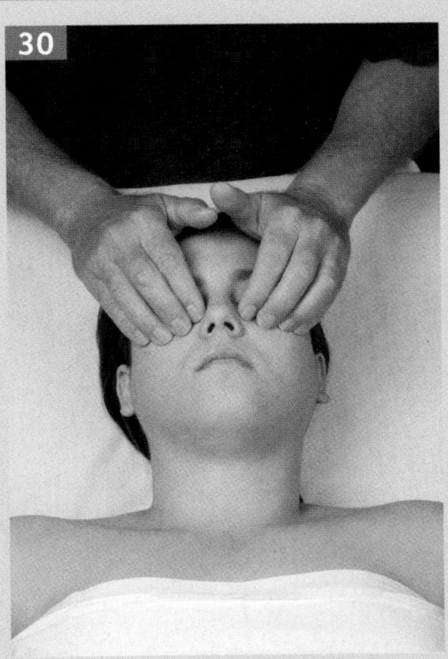

Massage around the eyes.

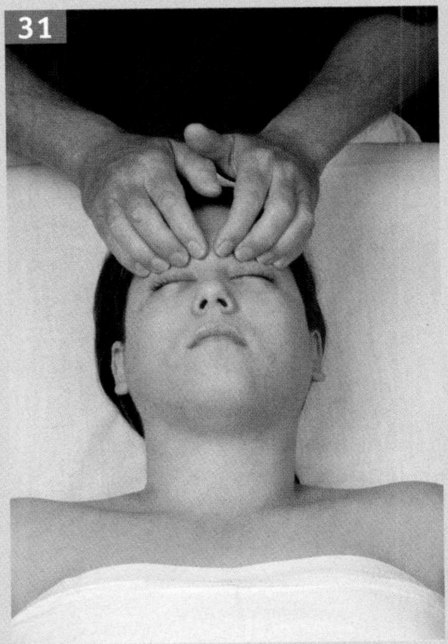

Massage the area above the eye socket.

31 Place the pads of the fingers flat over the eyebrows. Curl the fingertips down below the eyebrows to massage the area above the eye sockets as well. Massage for 1 minute.

a. Alternatively, in the Vodder method, you employ the thumb and flat pad of the index finger to press the eyebrow about five times.

32 Place the pads of the fingers of both hands flat on the forehead, and rest the palms of both hands on the scalp. Massage in larger circles, using the entire surface of each hand to move the skin of the forehead and scalp.

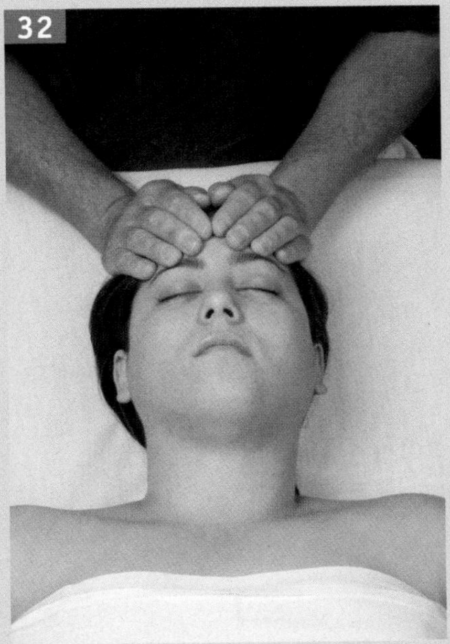

Massage forehead and scalp.

continues on next page

PROCEDURE 17–4, CONT. MANUAL LYMPHATIC DRAINAGE MASSAGE

33
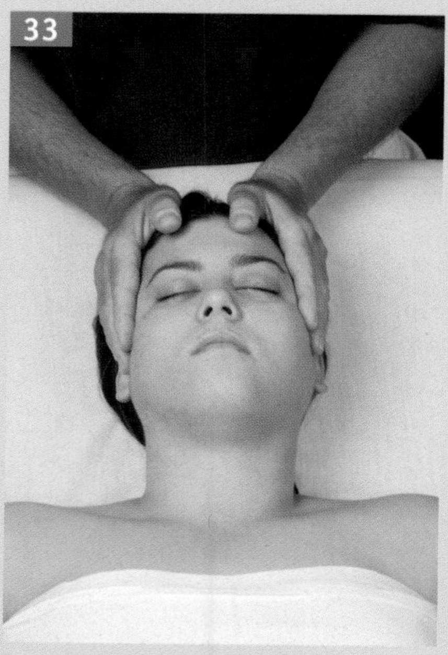
Cover the area between the eyes and ears.

34
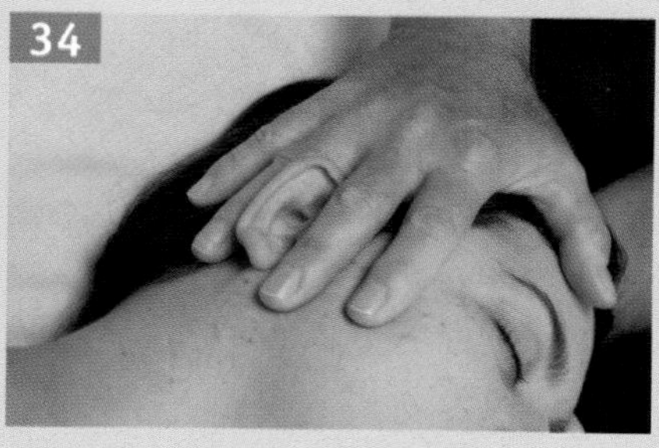
Place fingers in front of the ears and behind the ears in a forked position.

33 Place the pads of the fingers flat over the temples, covering the area between the eyes and ears, resting the palms on the scalp over the temporalis muscle. Massage for 1 minute, using the entire surface of each hand. It might be tempting to apply firmer pressure here, but maintain the correct pressure and speed.

34 Place two pads of fingers flat in front of the ears on each side, two fingers behind the ears in a fork position, and rest the palms of the hands on the scalp over the temporalis muscle. Massage for 1 minute.

35 Massage the scalp in large, gentle circles, moving the skin, for 2 or 3 minutes.

36 Massage each of the following areas for 1 to 3 minutes, until you can feel the lymph movement. If there are palpable changes in the tissues that show lymph drainage has increased, 1 minute will suffice. If lymph drainage is still sluggish or not palpable, up to 3 minutes on each location may be required.

36a
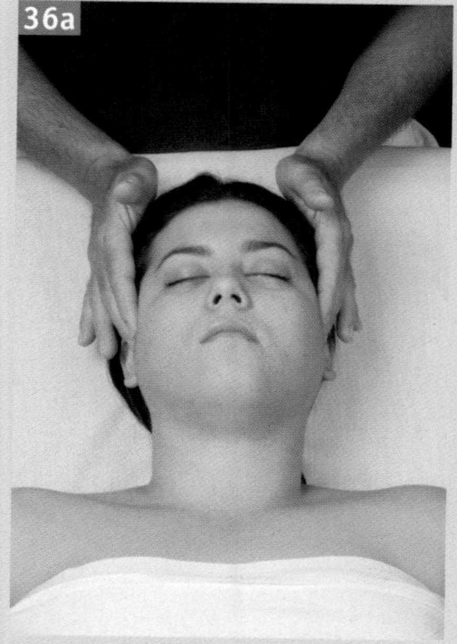
Massage preauricular node.

a. Preauricular nodes

36b
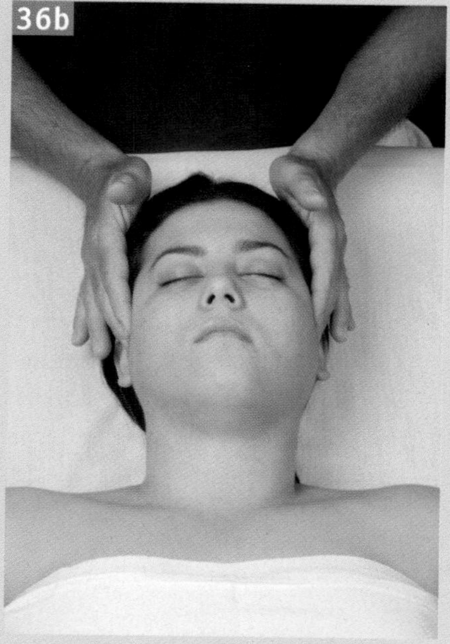
Massage angle of the jaw, over the masseter muscle.

b. Angle of the jaw, over the masseter muscle

36c
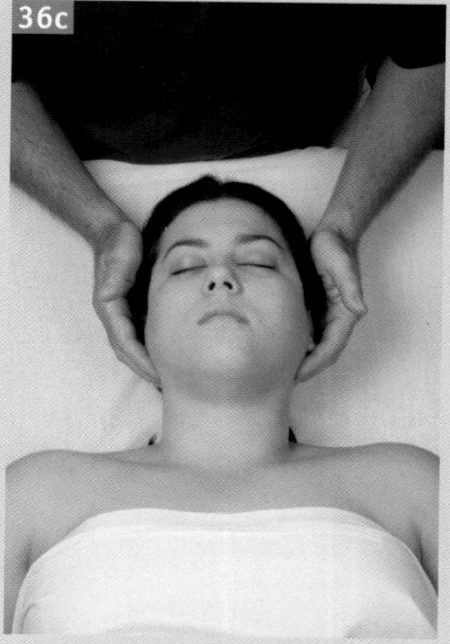
Massage posterior and inferior to the ear.

c. Posterior and inferior to the ear over the deep nodes

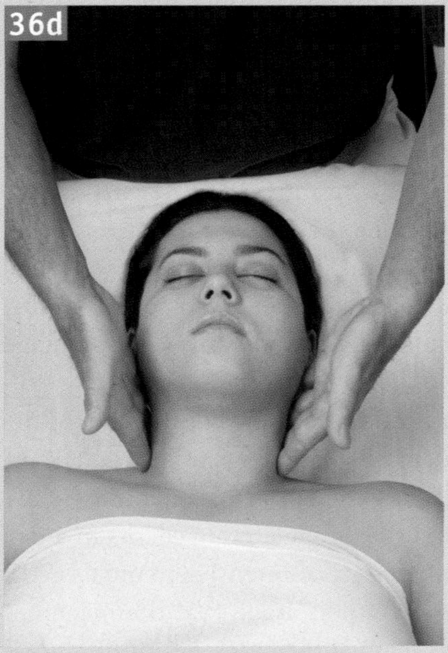

Posterior cervical chain.

d. Posterior cervical chain

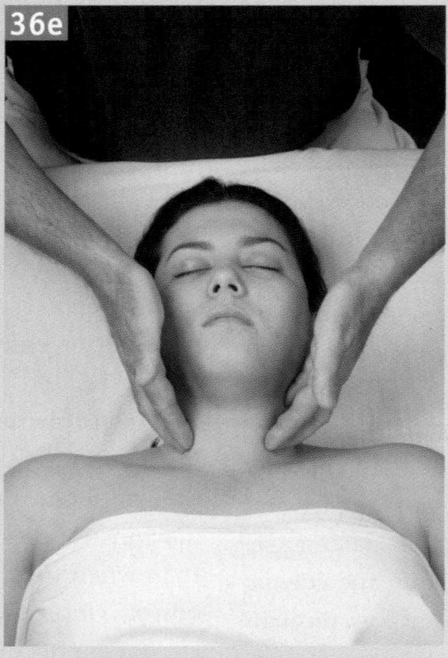

Anterior cervical chain.

e. Anterior cervical chain

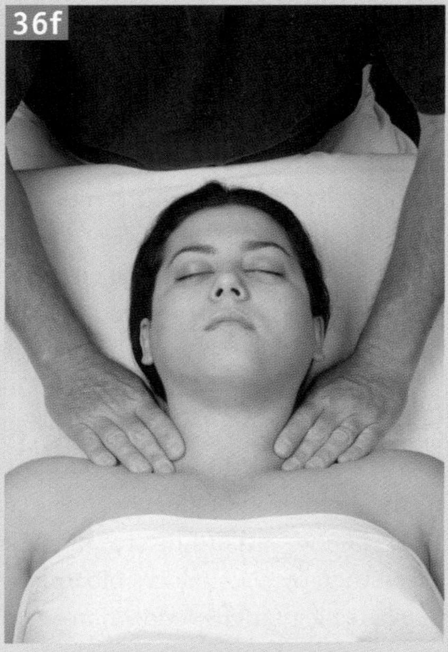

Along border of the clavicle.

f. Along the superior border of the clavicle

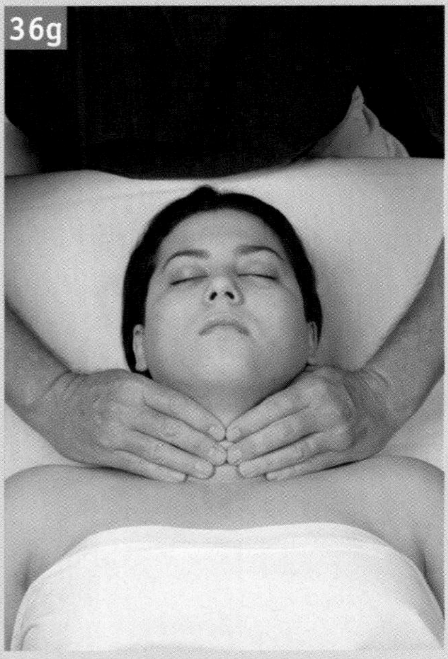

Above the medial ends of the clavicle.

g. Above the medial ends of the clavicle

37 Gently effleurage the face and neck.

a. Remove any excess massage product, tone, and apply SPF product.

38 Use scalp massage to begin to waken the client. Gently tell the client that the massage is over and that it is time to awaken. Ask the client to turn on the side in the fetal position to stretch the lower back briefly before arising.

39 Then, have the client sit on the table with legs dangling toward the floor to raise blood pressure and prevent fainting. Encourage yawning and stretching, which also stimulate lymph flow and raise blood pressure. After a few minutes, allow the client to stand.

40 Be sure to stand at the client's side as he or she slides off the massage table and stands.

Post-procedure

41 Offer the client water to promote hydration and internal cleansing.

42 Advise them to take it easy as their body readjusts from the deep relaxation.

Clean-up and Disinfection

43 When the procedure is complete, perform clean-up and disinfection procedures following OSHA or your state's guidelines.

44 Make appropriate notes in client's file.

45 Reset room.

MACHINE-AIDED LYMPHATIC MASSAGE TREATMENTS

Pressotherapy

Once only found in Europe as a treatment for cellulite, the Pressotherapy is a popular lymph drainage machine that has made its way to the United States. The Pressotherapy equipment comprises a compression system designed to increase the venous and lymphatic flow and enhance extracellular fluid clearance. Pressotherapy equipment includes a computer-controlled pump, which inflates the individual sections of the multi-chambered garment. The garment has five separate chambers, which are positioned around the limbs. The chambers focus on moving the venous and lymph flow, starting from the ankles and moving to the upper thighs. The pump inflates each chamber of the garment individually and in a preset sequence and time period, according to predetermined parameters. Pressotherapy also reduces bloating, swelling, and edema; alleviates leg fatigue; and improves oxygen flow through the entire body. Pressotherapy can be used in conjunction with seaweed wraps to detoxify, firm, tone, improve circulation, and increase lymph drainage (Figure 17–32).

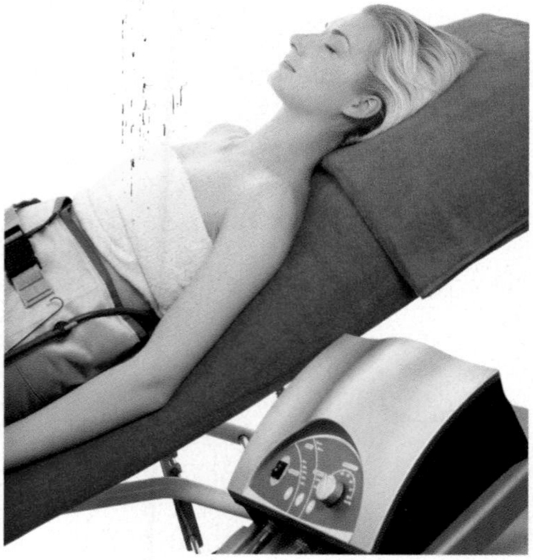

Figure 17–32 Pressotherapy in process.

Machine-aided Facial Lymphatic Massage

A typical vacuum/suction lymph drainage machine has a push-pull action, achieved with a computer-controlled pump or compressor. Some manufacturers offer a machine specifically made to achieve these results, but a typical vacuum apparatus (on a multi-function machine) combined with a rhythmic tapping (on/off action) on the vacuum hole of the glass attachment will achieve similar results. The intensity of the vacuum apparatus must be set on low for face and neck areas. Some companies make larger bell-shaped glass suction cups that can be easily adapted to the multi-function machine to mimic expensive lymph drainage machines.

The vac/suction action mimics the contractions made in the lymph vessels and assists the movement of the lymphatic fluid. Many therapists find that using these machines allows them to complete more clients in a day than when they use more labor-intensive manual methods of lymph drainage. Others argue that the machines are not as effective as manual therapies. Scientific studies tend to lean toward the greater effectiveness of a manual therapist, but these findings depend, of course, on the skill and knowledge of the therapist.

Basic Guidelines for Machine-aided Lymphatic Massage

Here are some suggested steps for machine-assisted lymph drainage. If you are using your vacuum system, it has only one hand piece, so you will need to work one side at a time. A lymphatic massage device has two hand pieces, allowing you to work both sides of the face at the same time.

If using the vacuum system, use one finger to tap–lift on the suction hole to replicate the pulses of the lymphatic device. The device moves during the lift, or non-suction, aspect of the pulse.

PROCEDURE 17-5 MACHINE-AIDED LYMPH DRAINAGE

IMPLEMENTS AND MATERIALS

- Standard facial lounge setup with linens and towels
- Basic cleanser
- Skin freshener
- Cotton pads, cloths, or wipes
- Lymph drainage device
- SPF lotion to finish

Preparation

1 Ensure that the treatment room is prepared and ready for use.

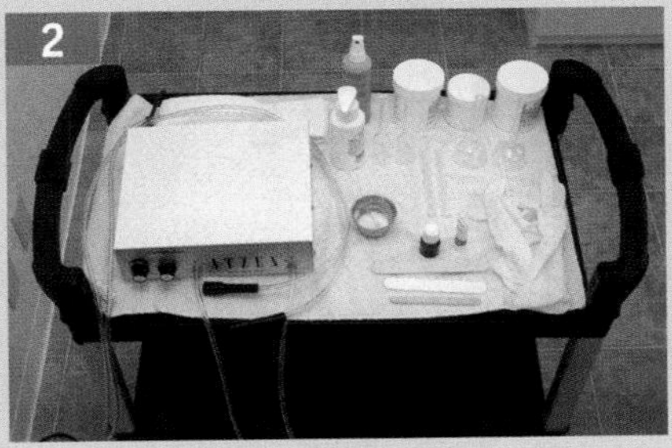

Gather supplies.

2 Gather supplies and decant products.

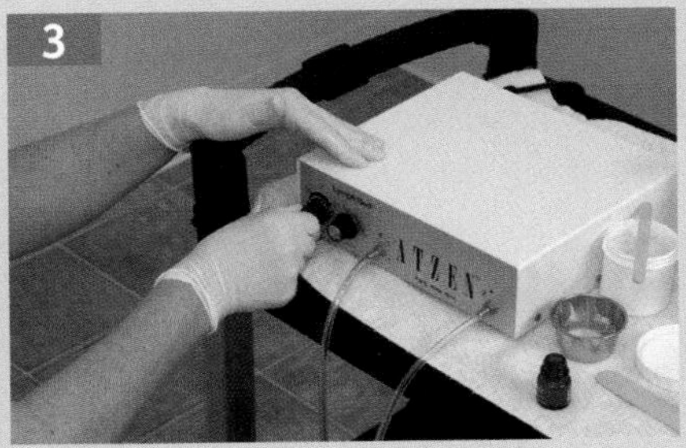

Test device.

3 Test the device for proper operation.

4 Council the client to assure that treatment is not contraindicated.

5 Advise the client as to what to expect following the treatment.

6 Have client prepare for the service.

Procedure

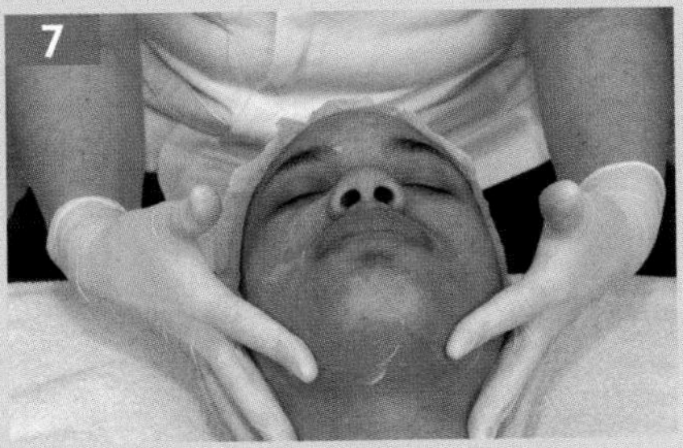

Pre-cleanse client.

7 Pre-cleanse the client's skin. Remove cleanser with cloths or warm towels.

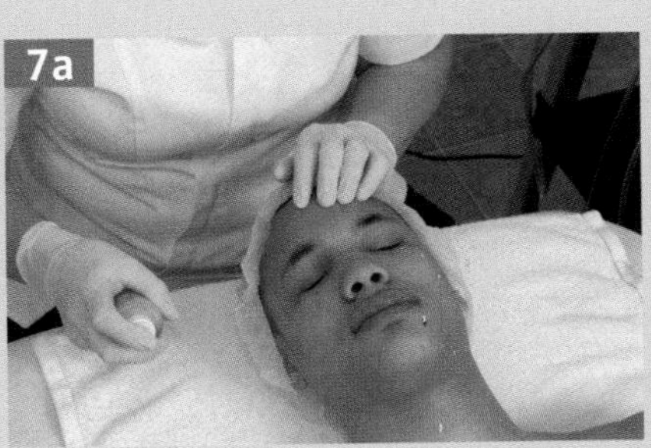

Apply products.

a. Apply treatment products per manufacturer's directions.

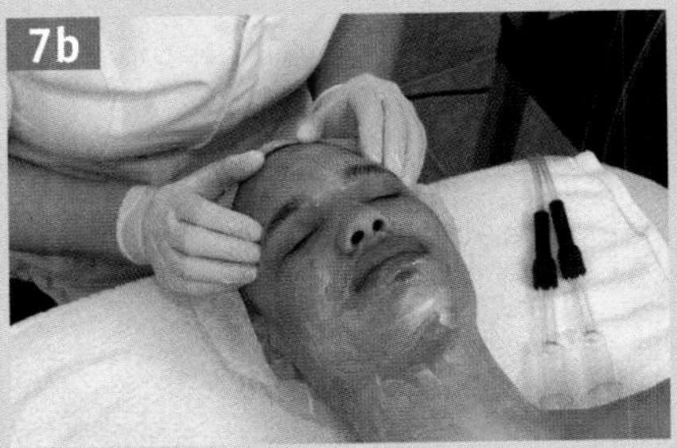

Effleurage across face.

b. Begin treatment with light effleurage movements stroking across the face.

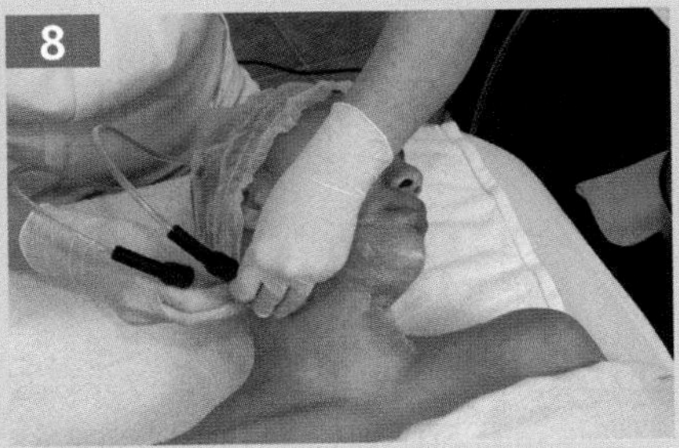

Place on postauricular area.

8 Have the client turn his or her face to one side and place the hand piece on the postauricular area (just behind the ear under the hairline).

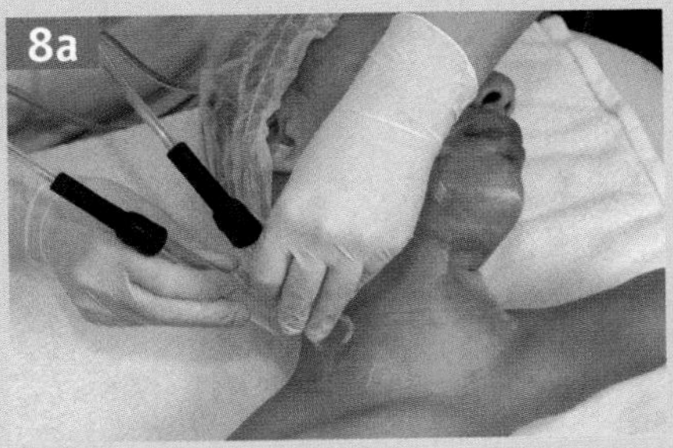

Move to clavicle.

a. Move the hand piece down the neck to the clavicle. Repeat the sequence 3 to 5 times.

continues on next page

PROCEDURE 17-5, CONT. MACHINE-AIDED LYMPH DRAINAGE

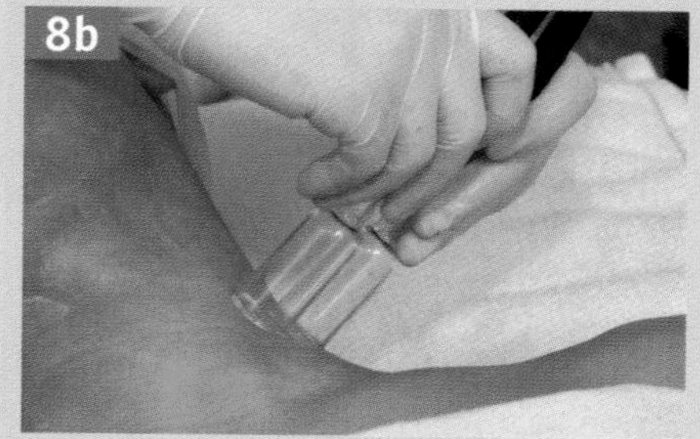

Repeat on opposite side.

b. Turn the client's head to the other direction and repeat on the other side of the neck.

9 Have the client straighten his or her head to a supine position.

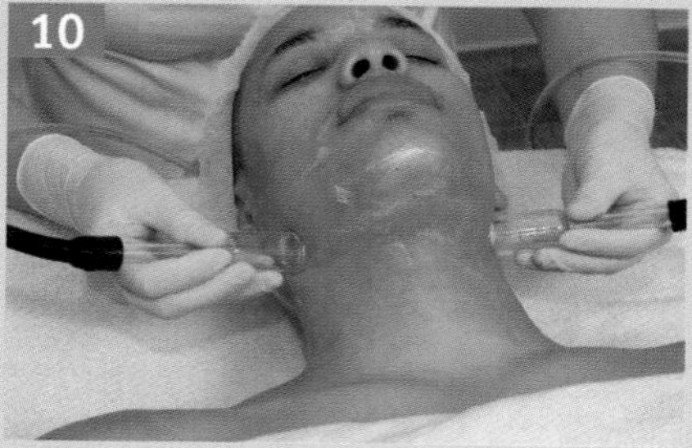

Place below preauricular area.

10 Separate hand pieces so that you have one in each hand. Place the hand pieces just below the preauricular area (in front of the ear) and move downward to the clavicle.

a. Repeat the sequence 3 to 5 times.

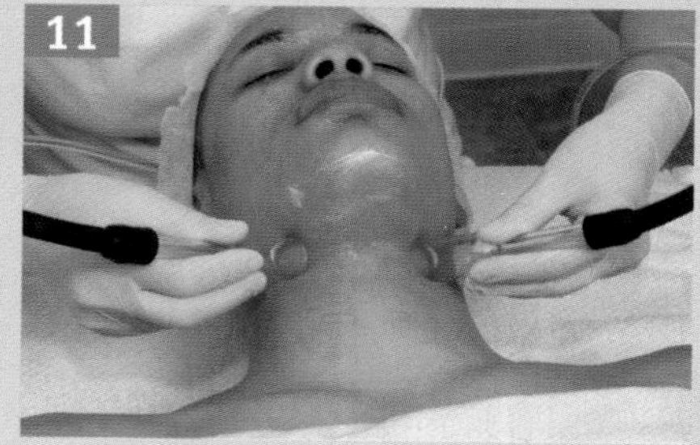

Move to clavicle.

11 With one hand piece in each hand, place the hand pieces on the submental area (under the jaw) and move downward to the clavicle.

a. Repeat until you have cleared the front of the neck, but exclude the trachea area. Repeat the sequence 3 to 5 times.

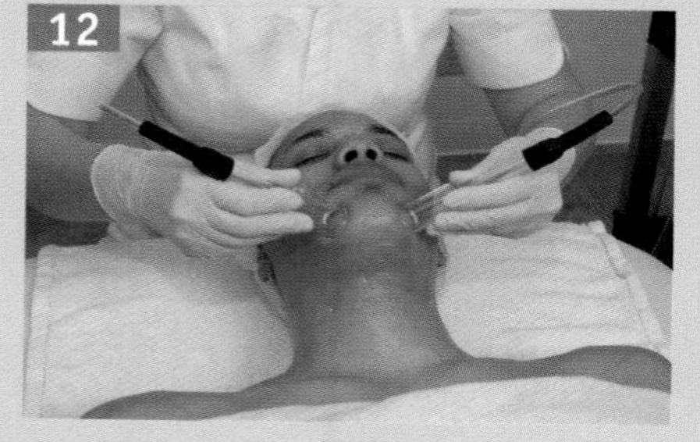

Move from submental to clavicle.

12 With one hand piece in each hand, place the hand pieces so that they are touching side by side on the top of the chin just above the submental area (above the jawline) and move downward to the clavicle.

a. Repeat the sequence 3 to 5 times.

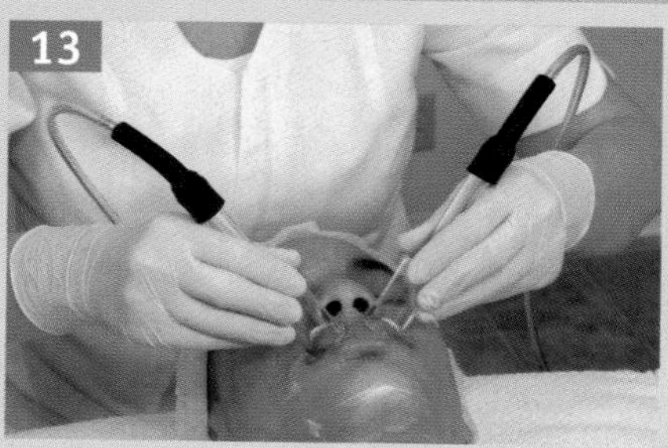

Place at top of lip.

13 With one hand piece in each hand, place the hand pieces so that that are touching side by side on the top of the lip, just below the nose, and move out to the ear area. Continue to move downward to the clavicle.

14 Repeat the sequence 3 to 5 times.

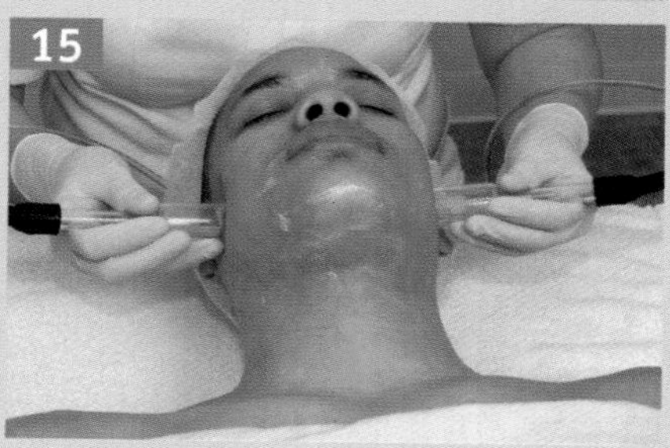

Move from ears to jawline.

15 With one hand piece in each hand, place the hand pieces on both sides of the face so that they are level with the top of the ears. Then move downward to the jawline.

a. Repeat the sequence 3 to 5 times.

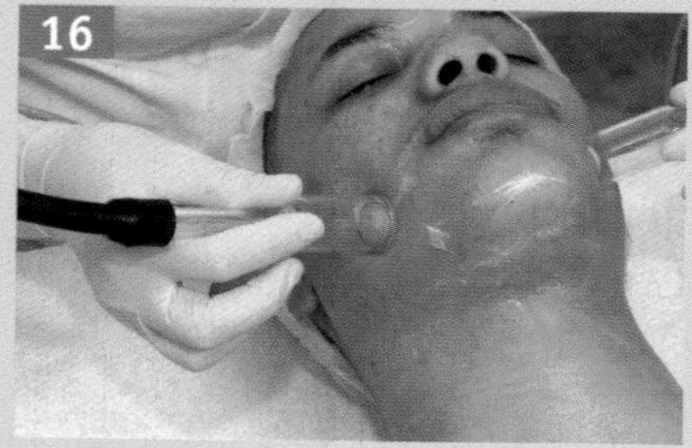

Place at sides of nose.

16 With one hand piece in each hand, place the hand pieces on either side of the nose and move out to the ear area. Continue to move downward to the jawline.

a. Repeat until you have moved progressively up to the area just

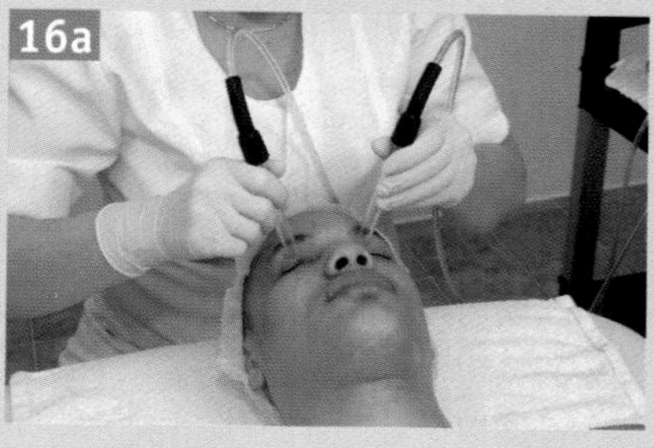

Just under eye.

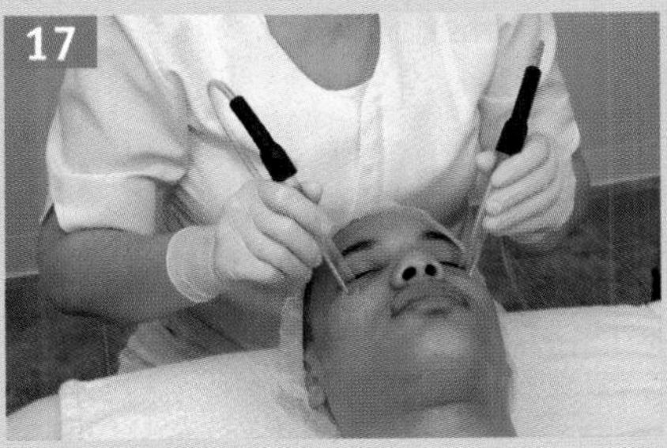
Move out to temples.

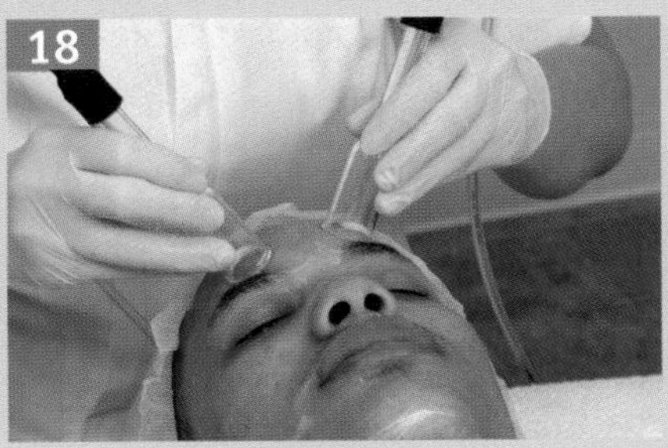
Brows out to temples.

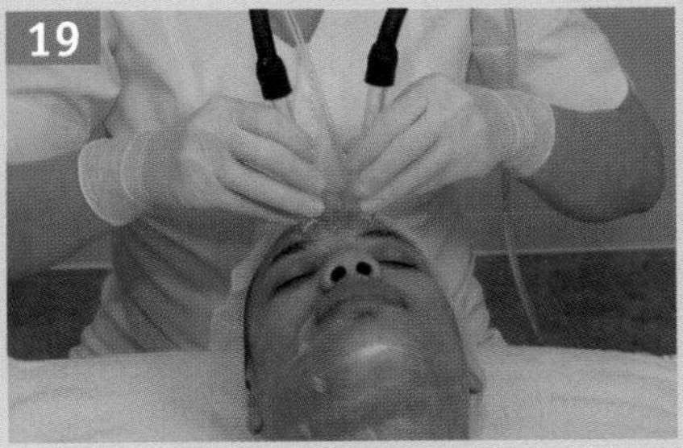
Forehead down to temples.

under the eyes. Typically this can be achieved with 3 points.

b. Repeat the sequence 3 to 5 times.

17 With one hand piece in each hand, place the hand pieces just under the eyes and gently move out to the ear area. Continue to move out to the corners of the eyes and to the lower temple area.

a. Repeat the sequence 3 to 5 times.

18 With one hand piece in each hand, place the hand pieces on the brow line and move out to the temples area.

a. Repeat the sequence 3 to 5 times.

19 With one hand piece in each hand, place the hand pieces on the forehead just above the brows and move outward to the hairline. Continue to move downward to the temples.

a. Repeat until you have cleared the middle forehead and upper forehead areas.

b. Repeat the sequence 3 to 5 times.

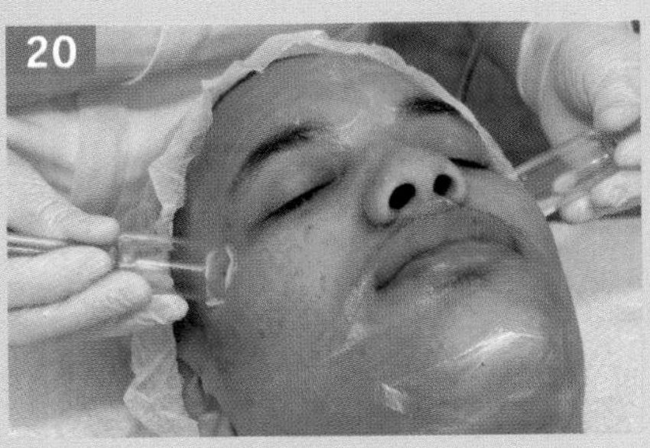
Proceed to clavicle.

20 With one hand piece in each hand, place the hand pieces superior on the either side of the temples. Continue to move downward to the jawline and proceed to the clavicle.

a. Repeat the sequence 3 to 5 times.

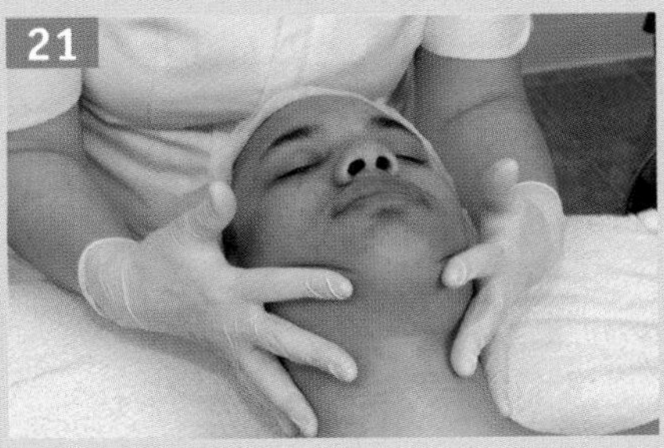
End with effleurange.

21 End with light effleurage movements.

Post-procedure

22 Remind client of any post-procedure directions.

23 Offer client water for rehydration.

Clean-up and Disinfection

24 When the procedure is complete, perform clean-up and disinfection procedures following your state's guidelines.

25 Disinfect implements following manufacturer and state guidelines.

FYI

With all of the massage techniques available to estheticians we can provide diversity and interest to our clients and customize treatments to achieve optimal results. Developing skills in additional techniques enhances the massage benefits we can offer our clients.

REVIEW QUESTIONS

1. Name three additional facial movements and discuss how you think they would be beneficial to the skin.
2. Discuss two advanced neck or décoletté movements.
3. Describe how you might incorporate the back movements into application for the cleansing process of a back facial.
4. If your client has mild rosacea, which of the new facial movements you have learned might be contraindicated?
5. Explain how and why you might include Shiatsu massage for your highly stressed client.
6. What is the pressure technique used in Shiatsu?
7. Are there any contraindications to Shiatsu? If so, what are they?
8. Describe ear reflexology and how it is performed.
9. What are the types of stones commonly used in stone therapy massage?
10. What are the temperature recommendations and guidelines for preparing, handling, and cleaning stones?
11. What type of massage movement is commonly performed with stones?
12. Are there any contraindications to using stones for massage? If so, what are they?
13. What are some benefits of lymph drainage massage?
14. What are contraindications of lymph drainage massage?
15. Describe the movement that is the basis for facial lymphatic massage.
16. Explain the basic process of manual lymph drainage.
17. Explain the basic process of machine-aided lymph drainage.
18. What are the pros and cons for manual lymph drainage and machine-aided lymph drainage?

CHAPTER GLOSSARY

acupuncture: the practice of inserting very fine needles through the skin to specific points to help relieve pain or cure disease. Origin: China.

basalt: a common grey to black fine grained volcanic rock.

conduction: the sharing or transfer of heat between objects.

igneous: rock that forms when magma (liquid rock) cools and solidifies.

metamorphosed: the result of a pre-existing rock form undergoing changes. The rock undergoes heat and extreme pressure, resulting in physical and chemical changes.

reflexology: based on the belief that working on areas or reflex points found on the hands, feet, ears, and face can reduce tension to the bodies corresponding organs and gland structures. Origin: extract origin is unknown.

sedimentary: a category of rock created by weathering actions of water, ice, wind, or other atmospheric actions, or by biological deposits.

Shiatsu massage: the application of pressure on acupuncture points found throughout the body to balance the body's energy flow and to promote health. Origin: a form of physical therapy from Japan.

CHAPTER OUTLINE

- THE PURCHASING PROCESS
- SKIN ANALYSIS DEVICES
- IPL FACIAL REJUVENATION
- LIGHT-EMITTING DIODES (LEDs)
- PHOTODYNAMIC THERAPY (PDT)
- MICRODERMABRASION
- ULTRASONIC TECHNOLOGY
- ELECTRODESSICATION DEVICES (RADIOFREQUENCY)
- MICROCURRENT "FACIAL TONING"
- MANAGEMENT OF COMPLICATIONS

CHAPTER 18

ADVANCED FACIAL DEVICES

LEARNING OBJECTIVES

After completing this chapter, you should be able to:

- Name the steps involved in purchasing cosmetic technology.
- Describe the technique for facial rejuvenation using an IPL.
- List the advantages of an LED facial treatment.
- Discuss the different types of microdermabrasion devices.
- Discuss the use of ultrasonic devices in the salon.
- Describe the steps used with advanced electrodessication devices.
- Discuss the technique for microcurrent treatment of the obicularis oculi.
- Know your scope of practice in a medi-spa environment.

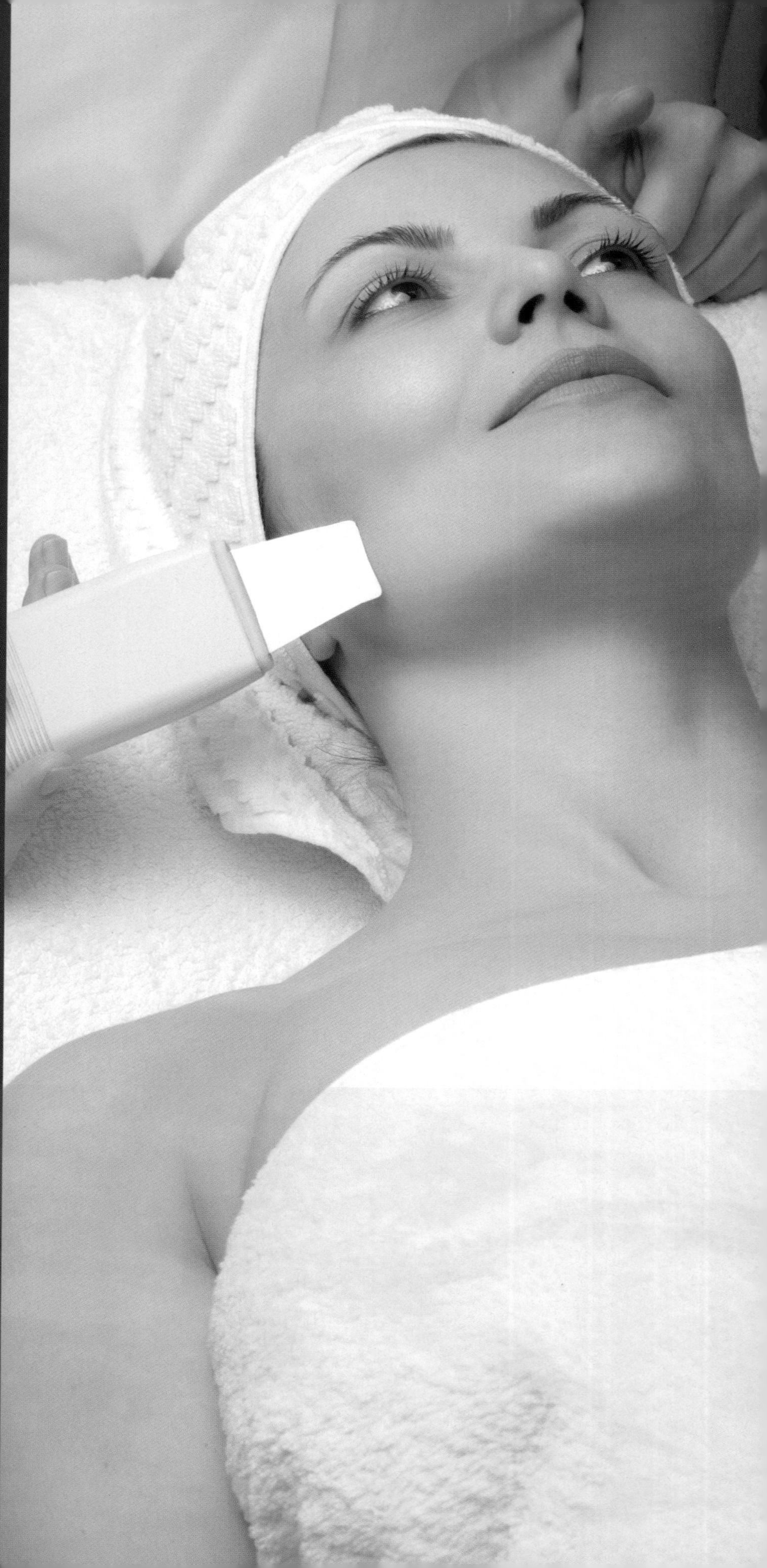

KEY TERMS

Page numbers indicate where in the chapter the term is used.

acetylsalicylic acid (ASA) 443
actinic keratosis (AK) 452
aerosolized 453
body dysmorphic disorder (BDD) 443
cellulitis 454
dyschromia 441
electrodessication 465
hydroquinone 442
impetigo 454
light-emitting diode (LED) 448
microampere 469
nonablative 440
photodamage 440
photomodulation 448
photorejuvenation 440
phototoxic 452
polychromatic 440
preventative maintenance (PM) 440

As you proceed to more sophisticated devices, you need to become even more astute about treatment benefits for clients versus documented risks and hazards. Each device presents many decision points in the research, evaluation, and purchasing process. Equipment models change, replaced by newer, more intricate devices. Some clients will be motivated to make cosmetic decisions based on the latest TV makeover or fashion magazine's recommendations. The media—be it print, Internet, or television—are flooded with advertisements of procedures and devices using false or inappropriate guarantees. That is why you, as the esthetician, must intervene as your client's advocate and recommend only those procedures and/or products that have shown clinical benefits and efficacy.

This chapter discusses what you need to keep in mind before purchasing any new equipment for a practice. Then it describes the different types of devices and offers some sample protocols for using each.

THE PURCHASING PROCESS

Before purchasing a piece of equipment, the owners of a practice or salon must decide who will be the technology experts in the practice. The practice's estheticians need to scrutinize state regulations and the FDA classification of devices for legality of use in their treatment environment. Decisions about products and treatments need to be made based on legalities, business goals, and financial opportunities. Within these parameters, owners and estheticians must decide about which leading-edge technologies are needed to make those products and treatments a reality in their practice. Following is a discussion of some of the important business issues to keep in mind, including analysis of your practice's needs and the necessary research required for product purchase and sales.

> **REGULATORY AGENCY ALERT**
>
> Contact your state licensing board and/or regulatory agencies to find out if the procedures you perform are within your scope of clinical practice. Some states require that estheticians be supervised by a medical provider or physician while performing particular treatments. Whether required or not, though, you should always seek and complete thorough training on equipment, including supervised clinical practice, before using any machine on a client.

Analysis of Your Practice Needs

Before jumping into the purchasing frenzy, you first must step back and analyze the needs of your individual practice. What is your business plan? Can you clearly define your client and his or her needs? What services do you presently offer? Will the client pay for this service? If you are not in an area where clients can pay the going rate for a particular service, it may not be a wise choice. Do you work in a salon, spa, medi-spa, or clinic? Answers to these questions will determine the complexity of procedures to be offered for facial rejuvenation and thus what type of device(s) to purchase. Finally, review the predominant skin type and demographic information of your clientele. This is an essential step, for some laser and light devices are only safe for a population with a particular skin type.

Equipment Options

After deciding on a specific type of equipment, find out which manufacturer offers the best device for your needs. Every device is built with its own specifications and you cannot rely on one research study conducted on a specific device to universally demonstrate that the competition will produce the same results. For example, look at cars. They all provide transportation, but they all are very different. The same is true for esthetic devices, so it is important to determine if the manufacturers you are considering can provide studies specific to a particular device. While this may not be as true for, say, microdermabrasion, it is certainly valid for some newer technologies. Before purchasing, be sure to look at a particular device's specifications, configuration, types of accessories, upgrade capabilities, training and support, indications and contraindications, appropriate FDA or ISO registration, clinical studies, manufacturing information, and any current patents. (Figure 18–1).

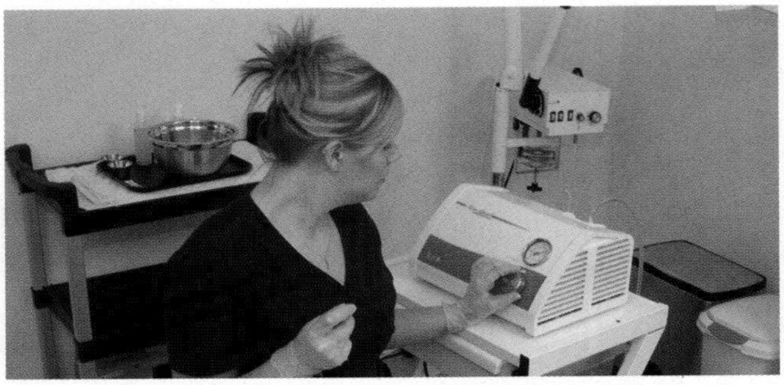

Figure 18–1 An esthetician using a device.

After thoroughly researching the equipment, negotiate with the sales representative and determine what is the actual price. Once you have that, crunch some numbers. How much can you charge for a procedure using this machine, and how many procedures do you think you can offer in a month's time? At that rate, how much money will you generate in three months' time? That's the benchmark: Can this device pay for itself in three months' time? For more expensive laser and light devices, one may be looking at six months or even up to a year in order to pay for the device.

New or Used Equipment Options

Should you buy a new machine from the manufacturer or a used device from a third-party vendor? There are advantages to both strategies. New pieces of equipment cost more but are under a service warranty from the company. New equipment guarantees the latest technology and is eligible for marketing tools and system upgrades. Usually, when you purchase new equipment directly from the manufacturer, you can negotiate some aspect of hands-on training and assistance in marketing.

Used equipment from a third-party vendor is obviously less expensive, but it may come with no training and no warranty at all. (Third-party sales may invalidate any company warranties.) In addition, there is no way of knowing if the equipment was serviced appropriately or how it functioned in the past. It could be a lemon! If you purchase a used device, make sure you negotiate a reputable maintenance and service contract along with the appropriate accessories, safety equipment, and manuals.

Financing Options

If you don't have the purchase price in cash, you need to decide whether to lease or finance your new equipment. Lease options may look very tempting to a cash-starved business. The process of leasing is easier, with quicker approval times, tax-deductible payments, and a lower monthly fee. However, be aware of the terms and what it will really cost you. What are the monthly payments? Do you need money up front? Do you have the right to refuse if the equipment is defective? Most importantly, what are the buy-out terms? Some lease contracts will require a payment at the end of the lease based on a certain percentage of the present market value. Will you owe thousands of dollars at the end of a five-year lease only to discover that the piece of equipment is worth nothing on the retail market? Are there any escape clauses to prematurely terminate the lease? What happens if the company goes bankrupt? Will you still be obligated for the balance of the lease? Often, this is the case. A lease must really be considered a purchase contract and once signed, you are committed for the entire price of the equipment.

Company Stability

Before purchasing your device, conduct extensive research into the manufacturer or third party's financial status. Take the time to research the company's history and financial reputability before purchasing a high-dollar piece of equipment. Make sure that they are not heading for bankruptcy or have pending lawsuits for infringement of patents on their devices. The FDA, the Better Business Bureau, your lawyer, and other estheticians can all assist with this process.

Legalities and Insurability

Before purchasing any equipment, it is important to contact your state regulatory agency to make sure the type of device in question is legal and within your scope of practice. Also get advice from a reliable source, such as legal counsel, as to whether this device is solely medical in nature rather than esthetic. There have been cases of physicians reporting an esthetician to the state medical board for working outside the esthetic scope of practice. The intended use statement of the equipment should help clarify whether it is esthetic or medical in nature.

Contact your insurance firm and ask about the cost of liability coverage for this equipment. If you cannot obtain liability coverage, it is a good clue that the machine is not within esthetic scope of practice.

Disposables or Reusables

The accessory issue is an essential component in the negotiating process with different vendors. One device may cost $50,000 less than one offered by its competition, but how many pulses is the disposable handpiece warranted for? What is the cost of the tips, conducting fluid, and treatment heads on a per-treatment basis? Most important, how many clients can you treat before you face expensive replacement? Investigate the total cost of all accessories before committing to a final purchase (Figure 18–2).

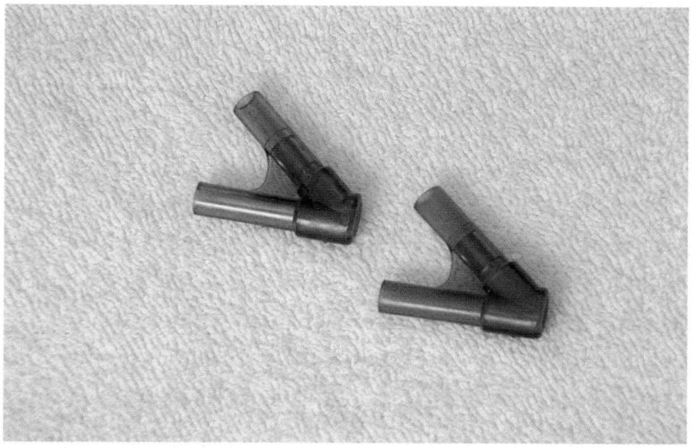

Figure 18–2 Disposable microdermabrasion tips.

Education

Training on a device can vary from a CD program, video, Internet webinar, or in-office lecture with hands-on training. Will training result in a certificate you can use to let your clients know you have been properly educated on this device? Obviously, the more sophisticated the piece of equipment, the more extensive the training should be from the manufacturer. Another factor that needs to be negotiated is who will do the training? Education from the company sales' representative is not always appropriate. If the trainer is not a skin care specialist will they be able to adequately answer your questions and provide the essential information needed for actual client treatments? It is always best if the trainer has experience in the field using the device in a working setting. Advanced training programs will offer you the theory behind the different types of equipment, but you may need to schedule time for supervised practical experience at a variety of clinics in order to receive a full, comprehensive education (Figure 18–3).

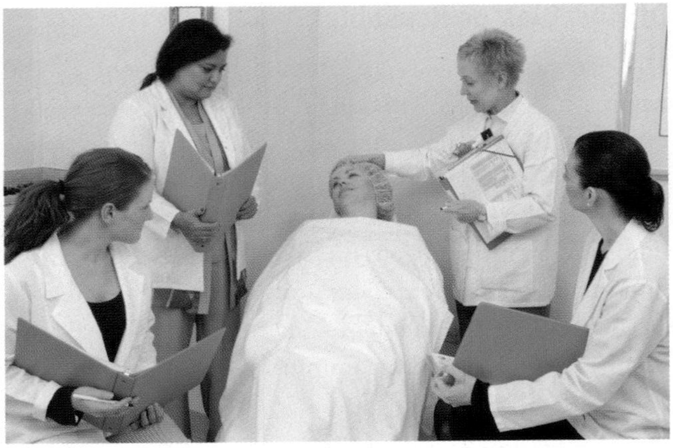

Figure 18–3 Estheticians being trained.

Warranties and Service Contract

If you purchase a new laser, IPL, or RF device, it usually comes with a one-year all-inclusive service warranty. This entails all costs for travel, time, and expense of the service technician, along with parts and software if the device fails. Investigate if the firm offers replacement or loaner backup equipment and what is involved in taking advantage of that option. To save yourself money in the future, try negotiating a second year before purchasing. Service contracts can exceed $10,000 per year for sophisticated IPL, laser, and RF devices. Make sure they include full parts, labor, and two **preventative maintenance** (PM) checks per year. When evaluating all other devices, ask about getting the service warranty in writing.

Device Labeling

The manufacturer can provide information concerning the equipment's FDA classification and/or, for a laser, the ANSI laser classification. These classifications help you determine whether you need physician supervision to use the equipment. In addition, the manufacturer's letter of intended use can clarify the device indications and under what supervision. Regulations differ from state to state, but, in general, many esthetic devices are considered Class I. While most states allow estheticians to use microdermabrasion, in some states a Class I device is illegal for estheticians. The regulations concerning FDA Class II devices vary with each device and state. They usually include most laser and light source equipment. Ablative capable devices are for use only by a physician regardless of classification. FDA Class III includes, many implanted and life-supporting devices and can only be used by a physician.

REGULATORY AGENCY ALERT

Be aware of your specific scope of practice under your state licensing board. Nationally, there are variations per state, device, and manufacturer. While NCEA (National Coalition for Estheticians, Manufacturers/Distribution & Associations) is seeking guidelines for clear interpretation, those guidelines have not yet been established.

SKIN ANALYSIS DEVICES

There are numerous devices that can enhance the skin analysis process and assist with client education. Some machines allow the client to view his or her skin, showing problem areas and levels of pigmentation. Other devices incorporate a camera that takes a client's image and projects it onto a computer screen, showing problems, concerns, and skin disorders. While these systems may be expensive, they do effectively assist in the documentation of results and client education. There is nothing like viewing an image of your own skin to enhance your desire to work toward resolution of any problems.

IPL FACIAL REJUVENATION

With more than a 33% increase in the last three years, photorejuvenation is becoming a very popular treatment that is commonly performed in a medi-spa or clinic environment. **Photorejuvenation** has been described as a nonablative process involving a laser or light device to treat the extrinsic and intrinsic signs of aging. All of the environmental and internal factors of aging can lead to superficial vascular and pigmented irregularities, along with a loss of elasticity and collagen. This procedure has been marketed under numerous names, depending on which manufacturer's device is used.

IPL facial rejuvenation has become the gold standard of photorejuvenation due to the **nonablative,** noncoherent, **polychromatic** flashlamp effects. During the procedure, intense white light is pulsed with wavelengths ranging from 500 nanometers (nm) to 1200 nm in the energy spectrum. (See Chapter 8 for a review.) Visible yellows and reds to the invisible wavelengths of infrared light are emitted instantaneously in a single white flash of light. These multiple wavelengths can together treat the numerous signs of **photodamage** (Figure 18–4).

Dr. Patrick Bitters, M.D., a prominent dermatologist, studied 49 patients who received four full face treatments

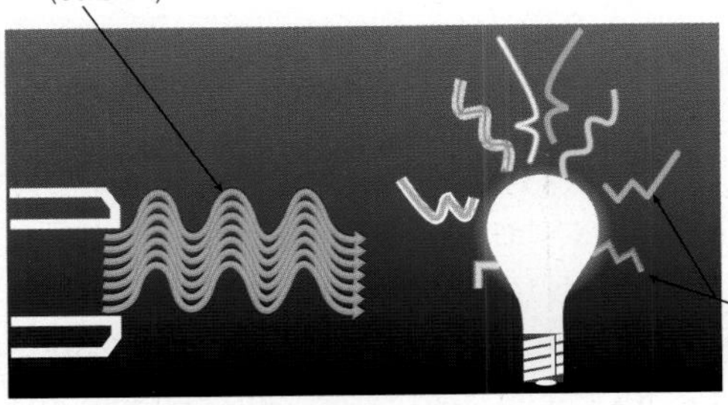

Figure 18–4 IPL devices are polychromatic white light compared to laser light.

spaced three weeks apart. More than 90% of the subjects reported a decrease of vascular and pigmented lesions and skin texture improvement, along with shrinkage of pore size. Dr. Brian Zelickson, M.D. showed an increase of epidermal collagen formation after a series of photorejuvenation treatments. Dr. Robert Weiss, M.D. studied 135 patients who experienced Poikiloderma of Civatte on their necks and chests. His subjects demonstrated a 75% improvement in pigmented and vascular lesions. Weiss also conducted a random five-year follow-up longevity study to analyze the long-term effects from photorejuvenation treatments. Five years after 80 patients received their treatments, more than 79% of the 80 patients still enjoyed benefits in reduction of **dyschromia**, telangectasias, and skin textural changes. It is good to be aware of these clinical studies in order to answer clients's questions concerning longevity of the photorejuvenation treatment's effects.

REGULATORY AGENCY ALERT

It is important to remember that IPL machines are Class II medical devices (Figure 18–5). Contact your state regulatory agency to determine your scope of practice in the use of these devices. Furthermore, if you will be per-forming IPL facial rejuvenation, prior to using any device, you need to first complete a thorough training course that includes clinical practice.

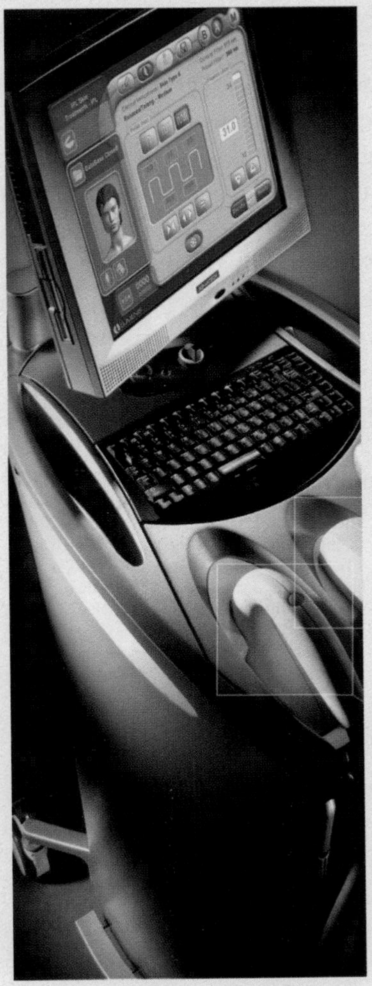

Figure 18–5 Lumenis Lume 1 IPL machine.

Indications for Treatment

Common conditions that can be treated with an IPL device and photorejuvenation include:

- Symptoms of rosacea, including diffusing erythema or redness, flushing, and papules
- Telangectasias or small spider veins
- Dyschromia or pigmented lesions
- Poikiloderma of Civatte
- Rhytids or fine lines and wrinkles
- Elastotic changes, including roughness, coarseness, or skin texture changes
- Enlarged pores

The Consultation

The consultation phase can be the most critical step in treating clients for facial rejuvenation. You must take a complete client history and skin assessment before initiating any procedure. No matter how expensive your device is, how educated you are, or what IPL experience you have, if your client selection is inappropriate or if your client has unrealistic expectations, then your procedure will fail.

During the consultation, your role is to assess the client's appropriateness as a candidate for the procedure, to educate the client, and to provide enough information so he or she can proceed confidently to the first scheduled treatment. In states where IPL use is restricted, the physician or medical practitioner may be required to be present during the assessment of the client prior to the first treatment. In those states, the physician or medical practitioners are responsible for reviewing client appropriateness, your treatment plan, and IPL parameters prior to treatment.

Following are steps to take during the consultation appointment:

- **Take a thorough medical history.** You must complete a consultation form that includes information about the client's allergies and medical conditions, such as heart disease, epilepsy, autoimmune diseases, and diabetes. Also, determine if the client has a history of outbreaks of the herpes simplex virus. The client may need a prescription of prophylactic antiviral medication before the first treatment. If the client has a history of bleeding disorders and is on anti-coagulant therapy, he or she may not be a candidate for treatment. Determination of a client's wound healing is also essential. Does the client easily hyperpigment after trauma to the skin? If yes, he or she may need to use an OTC bleaching cream such as 2% **hydroquinone** or a prescription formula for three to four weeks before their first treatment. Finally, review all his or her medications, including prescriptions for mental illness or depression, to determine if this is a suitable candidate for a procedure.

- **Evaluate the client's skin type.** Your assessment of the client's skin type will include the use of the Fitzpatrick Skin Scale to determine if he or she is a candidate for the treatment. Most IPL devices are cleared for Fitzpatrick Skin types I–IV (Figure 18–6). Skin type IV and Vs may be treated with some IPL systems but only with caution. One needs to check with the manufacturer for skin-type indications of the IPL device and the appropriate parameters for darker skin types. You can also use other skin-typing scales, including Glogau or Rubin's Classification of Photoaging to help with your skin type assessment. (Review Chapter 11.)
- **Determine the client's expectations and goals.** This is the point when the consultation can become difficult. When you ask the client, "What are your concerns and how can I help you?" listen to the client's response

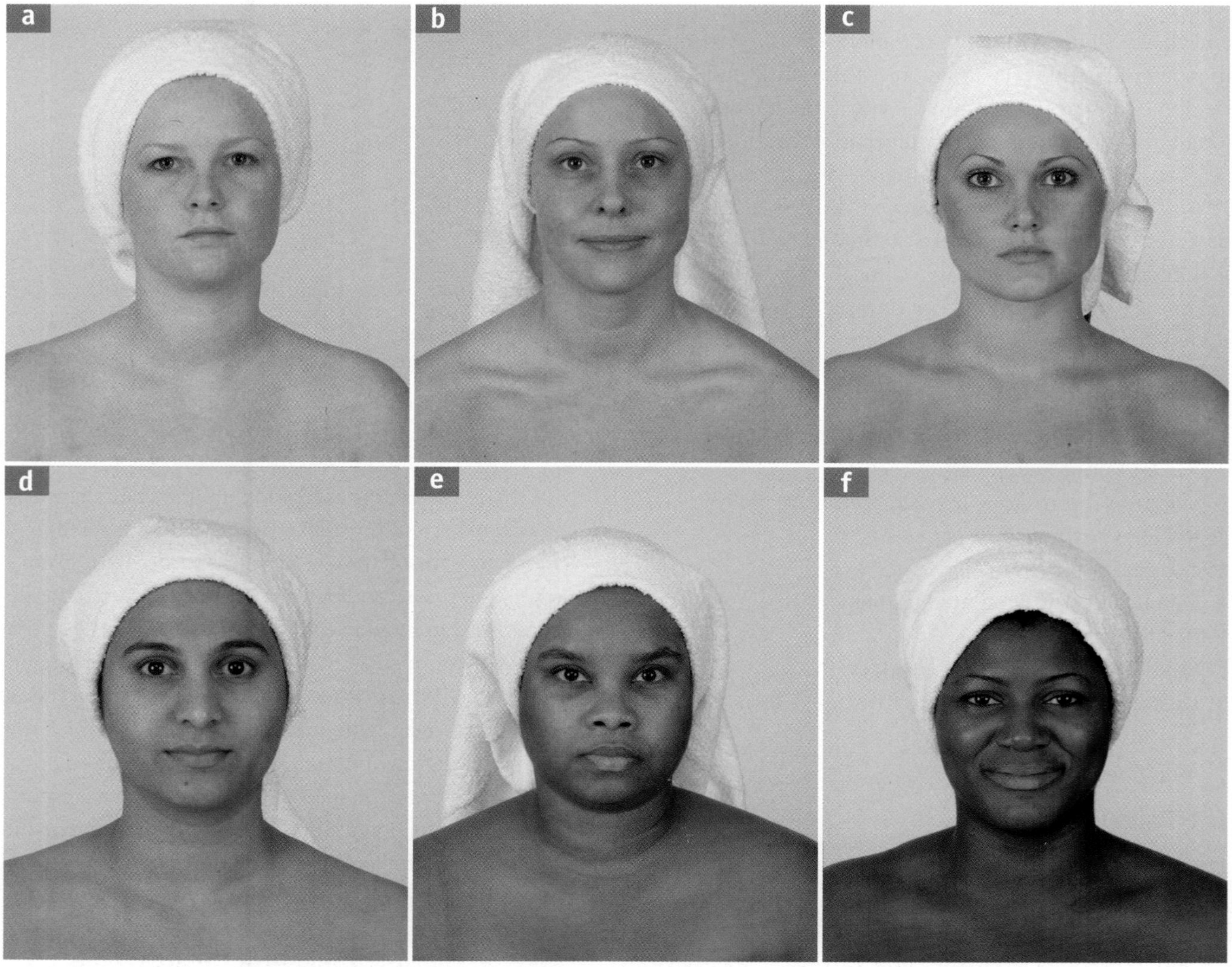

Figure 18–6 Fitzpatrick Skin Types.

carefully. You may be fixated on his large nasal telangectasias; however, the client may only be interested in a small lentigo on his left cheek. Through a detailed question-and-answer process, you can evaluate the client's expectations and idiosynosyncrasies, and you can determine whether you can offer a successful outcome. Here are some "red flags" that might come up during the consultation process:

- A client who gains all of her cosmetic information from Internet chat rooms or soap operas
- A client who wants to negotiate fees and compares you to the business across town
- A client who has **body dysmorphic disorder (BDD)** and is inappropriately fixated on her body. Signs can include history of multiple cosmetic procedures, acute obsessiveness, anxiety, depression, and acute stress.
- A client who demands the "extreme" makeover to look like his favorite Hollywood star
- A clients who chronically moves from clinic to clinic because of "dissatisfaction" with services

- **Evaluate the client's facial skin lesions.** This is the period during the consultation when you closely examine all vascular and pigmented lesions, along with evidence of solar elastic changes, enlarged pores, and rhytids. You must assess skin lesions and be able to determine if there are any that need to be seen by a medical professional prior to treatment. Nationally, there have been reports of clients filing malpractice suits because melanomas have been mistakenly treated with a laser or IPL device.

> **CAUTION!**
>
> **Remember that you are not allowed to diagnose skin disorders. If you see something that appears irregular or suspicious, refer the client to a medical professional for diagnosis before attempting to treat the area.**

- **Ask about medications.** You need to know what medications—both prescription and OTC—the client is currently using. Certain antibiotics can be photosensitizing, including tetracycline, doxycycline, and minocycline, which are commonly prescribed for rosacea and/or acne. (See Chapter 15 for a review.) In general, tell clients to avoid AHA, retinols, and glycolic acid products several days to a week before treatment. Also, before treating vascular lesions, advise clients to avoid **acetylsalicylic acid** (aspirin) and ibuprofen (Advil), if possible, for a week prior to treatment to reduce the chance of bruising due to the anti-coagulant effects of these OTC medications.
- **Ask about tanning history.** Due to the select absorption of melanin to IPL energy, any client who is actively tanning or has received active sun exposure should be rescheduled and not be treated. Clients should wait for four weeks after sun exposure and two weeks after synthetic "sunless" tanning solutions have been applied to avoid the risk of skin complications.

Contraindications

Do not treat clients who present with any of the following issues or conditions unless otherwise approved by a supervising medical provider.

- Photosensitivity to sunlight (for any reason)
- Accutane use within the last year
- Suspicious skin lesions, whether vascular or pigmented
- History of skin cancer in the area to be treated
- Photosensitizing drugs that may include antibiotics, OTC vitamins, or herbal supplements
- Current tan within the last four weeks, sunless tanning solutions within two weeks
- Medical conditions, including autoimmune disorders (HIV/AIDS, Hepatitis B, C, Lupus)
- Pregnancy and nursing
- History of keloid formation
- Psychological disorders (could affect the client's decision-making process)
- Recent or ongoing chemical peels or other exfoliating treatments

PROCEDURE 18-1 IPL PHOTOREJUVENATION

IMPLEMENTS AND MATERIALS

- Typical treatment lounge, client draping, and linen setup
- Disposable sponges, tongue blades
- Cleansing cloths and towels
- Gloves
- Disposable hair bonnet or head band
- Water and bowl or sink
- Gentle cleanser
- Post-treatment serum
- Sunscreen
- Gauze pads or cotton rounds
- Protective eyewear for client
- Protective eyewear for technician
- Water soluble cold gel

Preparation

Perform general treatment room setup (will vary depending on unit):

1 Prepare treatment lounge and client gown.

2 Assemble towels and disposables.

3 Set up products and protective devices.

4 Have ready the appropriate sign for the outside door.

30 minutes to 1 hour before the procedure:

5 Have client cleanse their face in a separate waiting area and apply topical anesthetic on the treatment site as directed and needed for the specific device. (Some devices require no anesthetics.)

6 Review client post-care instructions. These can be discussed while any anesthetic absorbs.

7 Close the doors, cover the windows, and hang the "IPL in Use" sign on door of the treatment room.

8 Hang the appropriate eyewear on the door for staff who may enter.

FYI

Light Speed® goggles or green eyewear with an OD (optical density) of 3 is appropriate for staff and operators. Prepare occlusive laser eye shields for the client if working on his or her face and neck. Obtain the appropriate IPL dark green goggles for client to wear if treatment is below the neck. (Always follow manufacturer's recommendations for specific IPL client eyewear.)

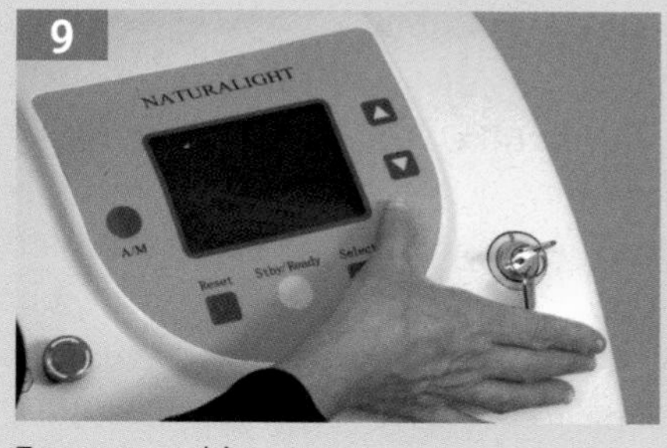

Turn on machine.

9 Turn on the IPL machine. Machine will undergo a self-test.

10 Perform machine calibration as the manufacturer recommends.

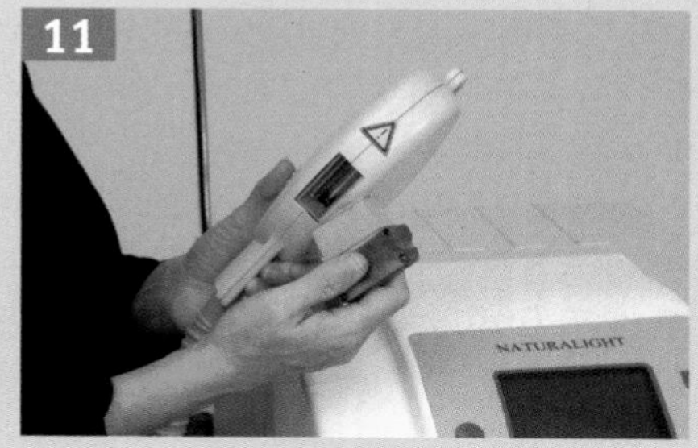

Replace pieces as necessary.

11 Replace any IPL handpieces or filters that need replacing.

CAUTION!

With topical anesthetics, follow manufacturer recommendations and apply in selected treatment zones, not over extensive areas. If in doubt, ask the anesthetic manufacturer or compounding pharmacist. Do not attempt to occlude areas, as it can increase the absorption and lead to toxicity and possible death.

Procedure

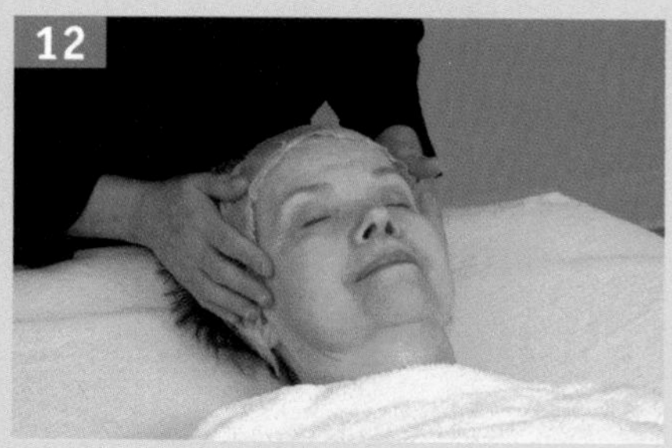

Secure client's hair.

12 Secure client's hair away from the face.

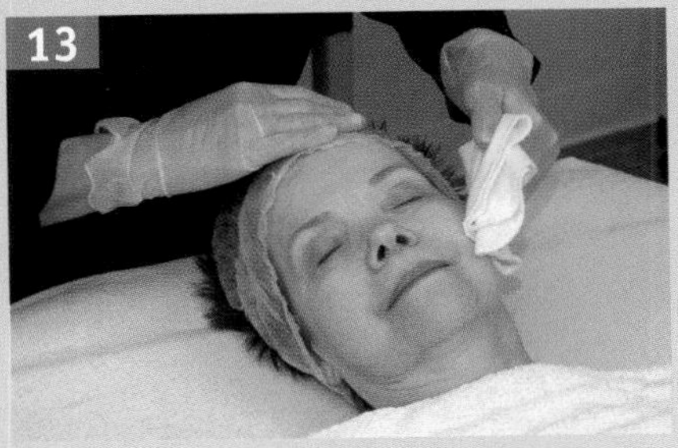

Pre-cleanse face.

13 Pre-cleanse and remove all makeup and anesthetics.

14 Assess the client as a Fitzpatrick Skin Type from I to V. (Some devices are only approved for clients skin types I-IV — check manufacturer's specifications)

15 Ask if the client has tanned recently or used self-tanner within the last month.

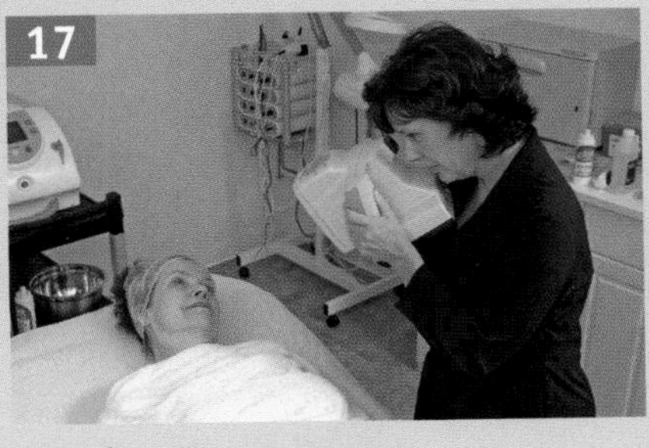

Take photos.

16 Reconfirm areas of treatment and the client's goals.

17 Take documentary photographs.

18 Enter the client's demographic data into the IPL system, if required by device.

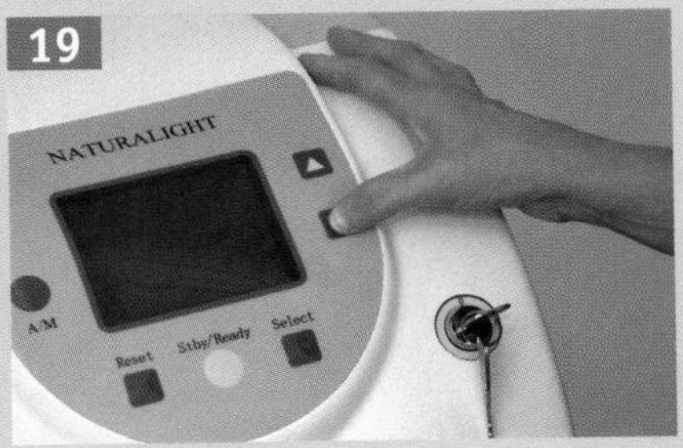

Select machine settings.

19 Select appropriate treatment mode, filter, and parameters on the screen and assure that the corresponding filter is inserted in the treatment head.

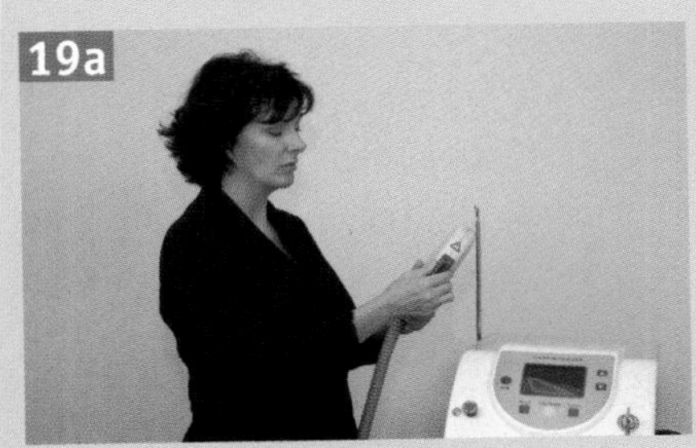

Assure appropriate filter.

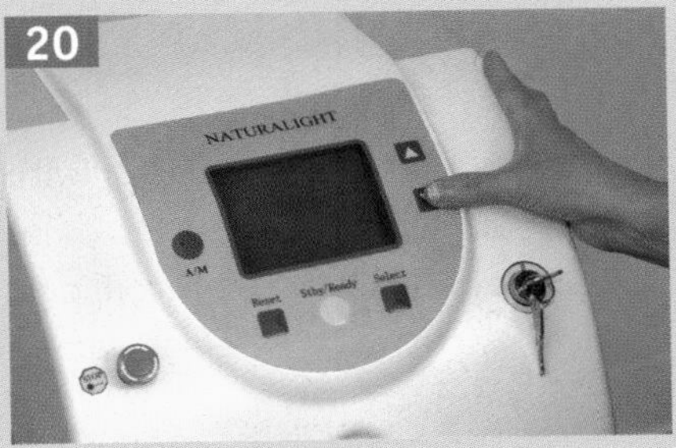

Double-check parameters.

20 Double-check all parameters before treating.

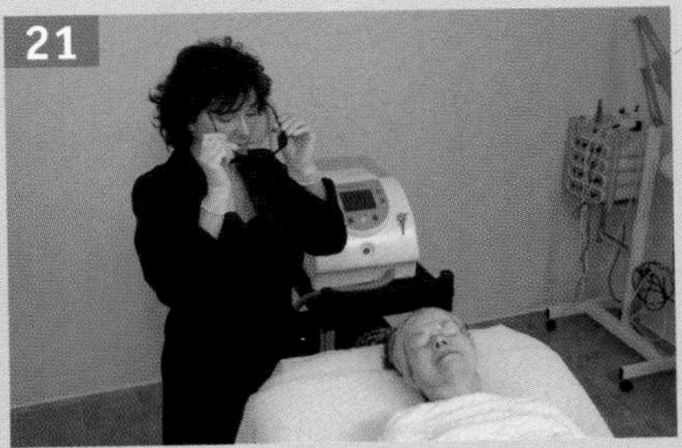

Put protective eyewear on yourself.

21 Place protective eyewear on the client and yourself.

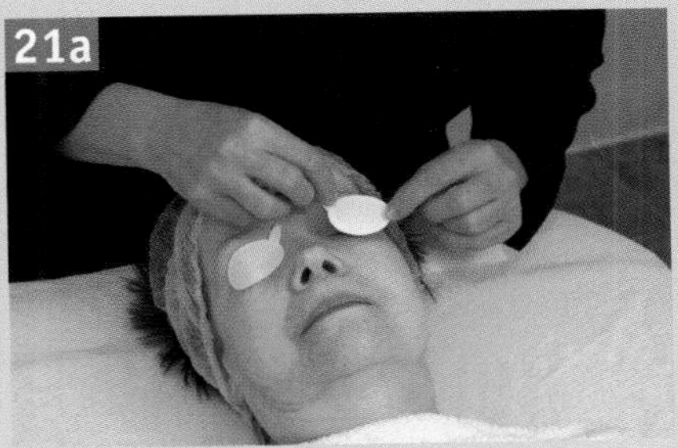

Put protective eyewear on client.

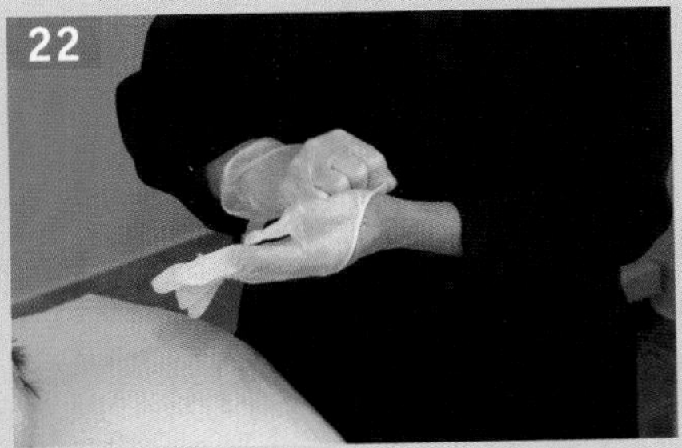

Put on gloves.

22 Put on gloves.

continues on next page

PROCEDURE 18-1, CONT. IPL PHOTOREJUVENATION

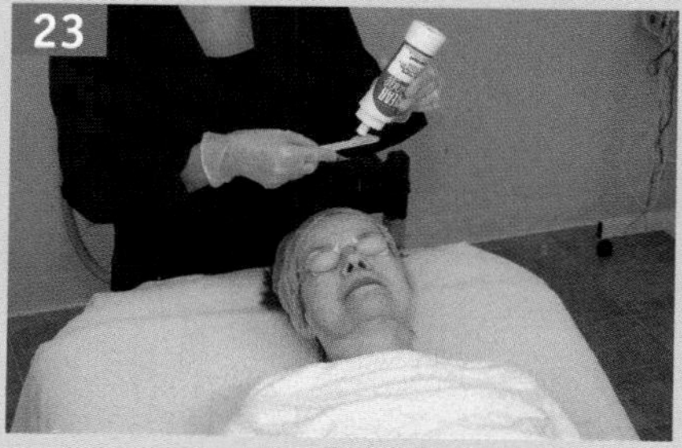

Apply coolant, if appropriate.

23 Apply gel coolant, if appropriate for device.

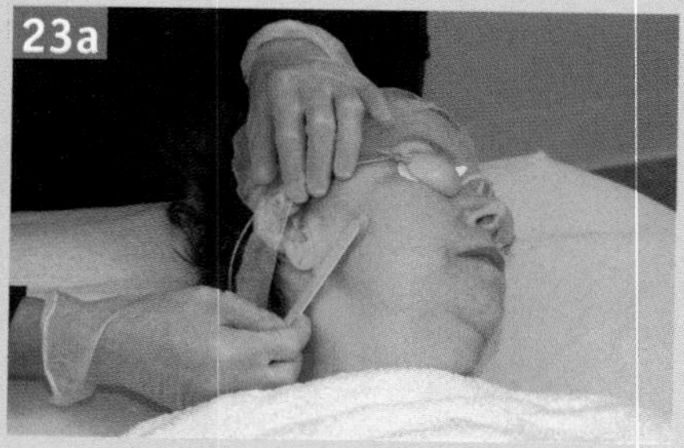

Apply coolant, if appropriate.

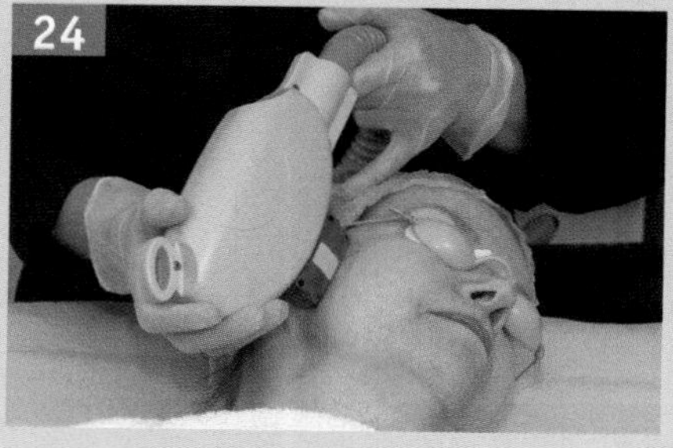

Spot test on side of face.

24 Test a spot on side of the face in front of the ear (pre-auricular area) following manufacturer guidelines.

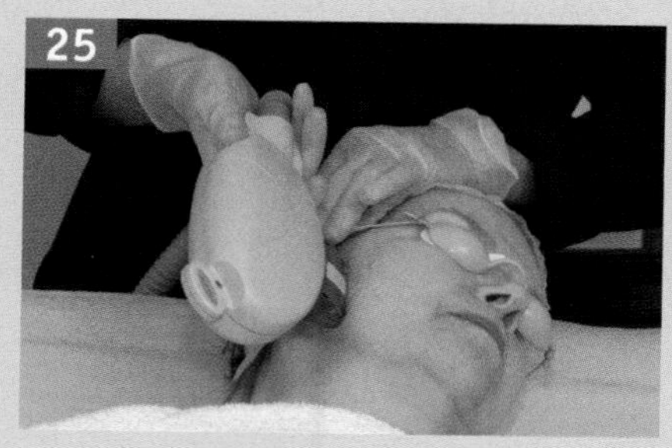

Floating will vary.

25 Float the filter in the gel if this is appropriate for your specific device. The degree of floating in the gel will vary based on the type of device and if the filter has a chilled sapphire window.

26 After testing the spot on the side of the face, assess clinical end points.

a. Observe for slight erythema.

b. Observe for darkening of a vessel or vasospasm.

c. Observe for darkening or redness of a lentigo.

27 If the test response is acceptable, continue treatment with the same settings. If not, raise or lower the joules accordingly or switch to a different parameter or filter.

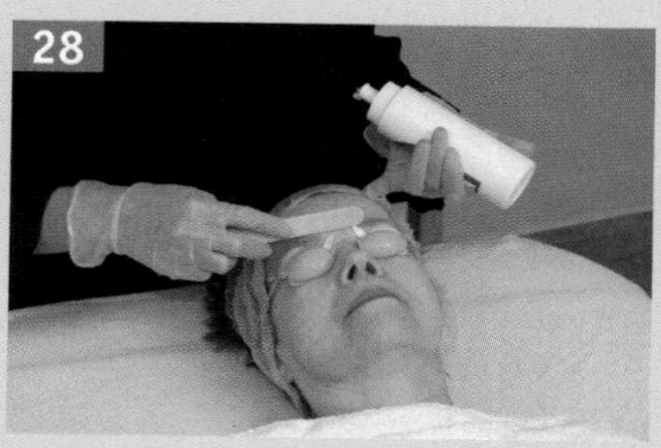

Start at forehead.

28 Start treatment with the forehead. Be careful of hair line and eyebrows. Protect them with a wet sponge, gel or tongue blade.

29 You can make single or multiple passes on treatment areas, depending on tissue response and device recommendations.

30 Place the handpiece perpendicular to the skin and floating in the gel, if one is required by the manufacturer.

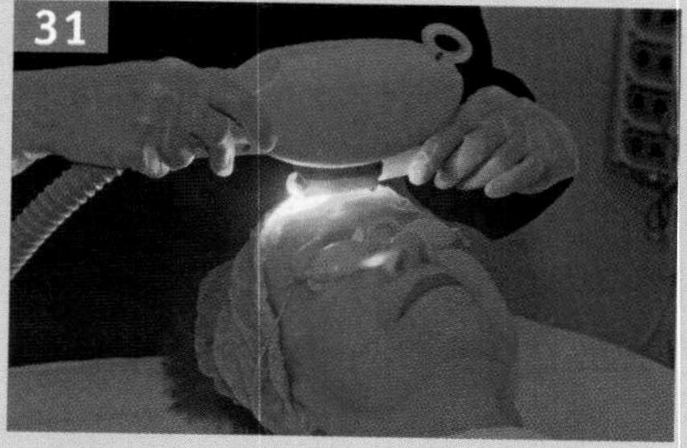

Fire trigger.

31 Fire the trigger.

32 Shift the handpiece to an adjacent area of skin with no overlap.

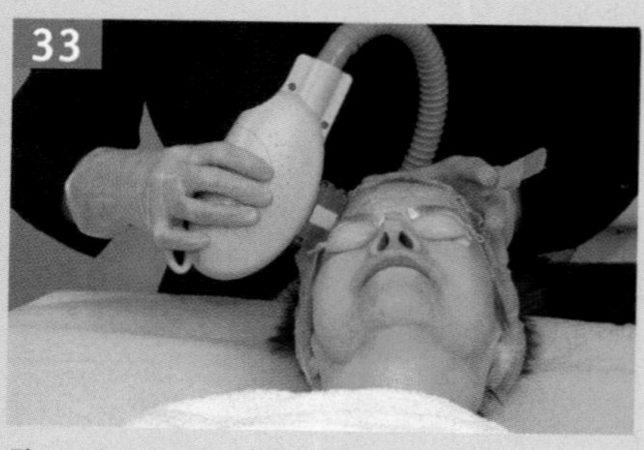

Fire trigger.

33 Fire the trigger.

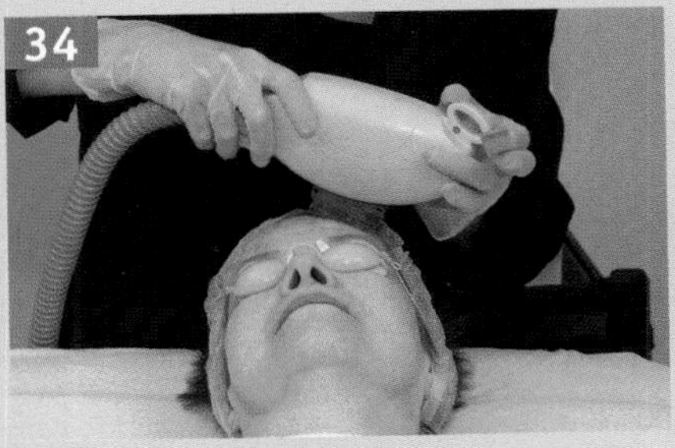

Repeat across forehead.

34 Repeat the process across the forehead, working in a systematic manner.

35 Continually assess the reaction and tolerance of the client's skin.

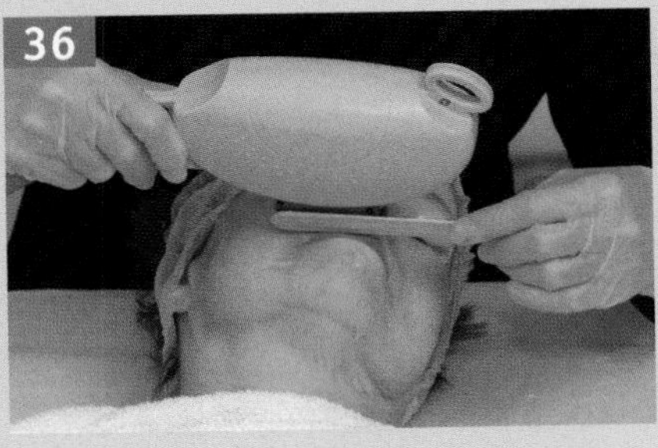

Move to nose, upper lip, and chin.

36 Move to the nose, upper lip, and chin in a systematic manner. Then move to below and above the lips, being careful not to work over lip vermillion.

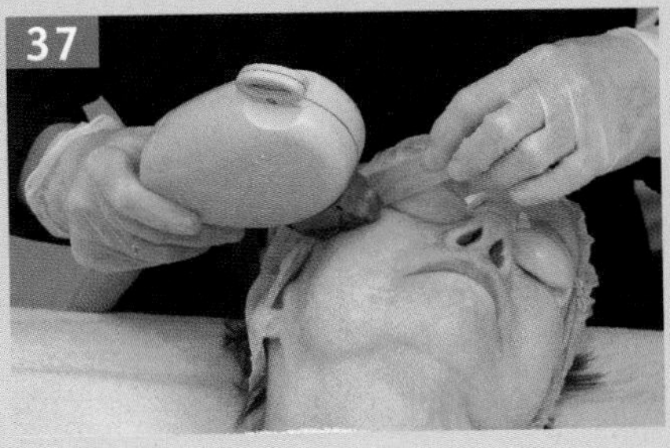

Progress to cheeks.

37 Progress to the cheeks and treat across the cheeks in a systematic manner.

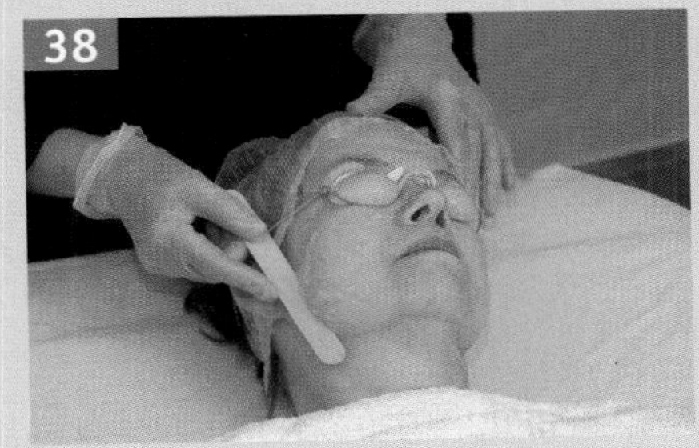

Remove gel.

38 Remove any residual gel.

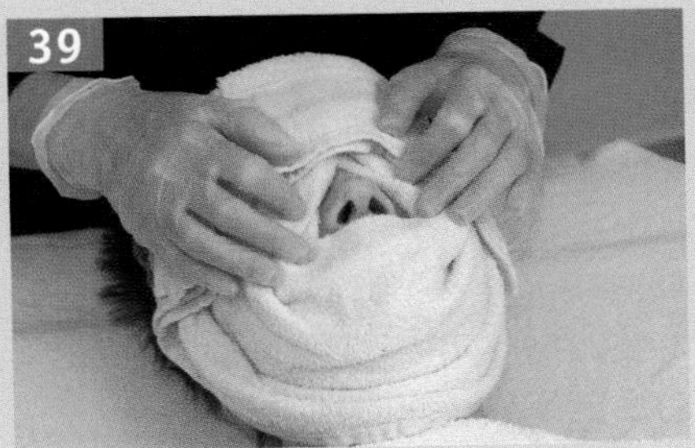

Cleanse skin.

39 Cleanse client's skin.

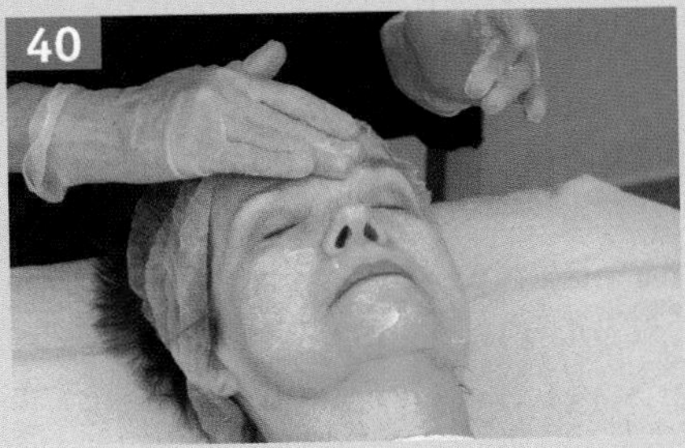

Apply products.

40 Apply soothing agent and protective sunscreen.

Post-procedure

41 Supply the client with an ice pack, if recommended or needed.

42 Escort the client to the front office for processing and scheduling of additional treatments and/or follow-ups.

43 Instruct the client to call the office to provide information on his or her condition the following day or if he or she has questions and/or concerns.

44 Complete the documentation on the procedure and place photos in client's file.

Clean-up and Disinfection

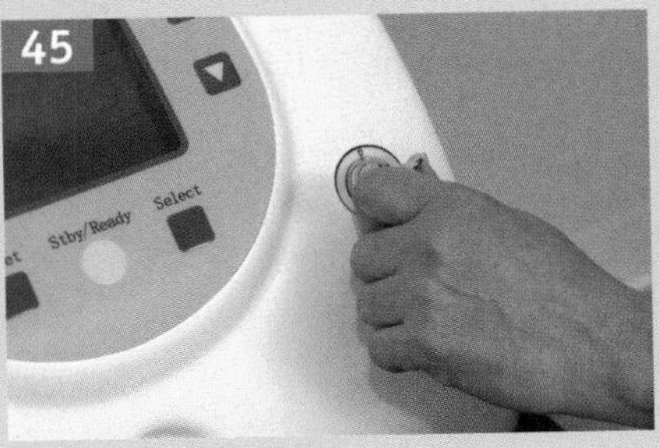

Turn off machine.

45 Turn off machine with the key following manufacturer guidelines.

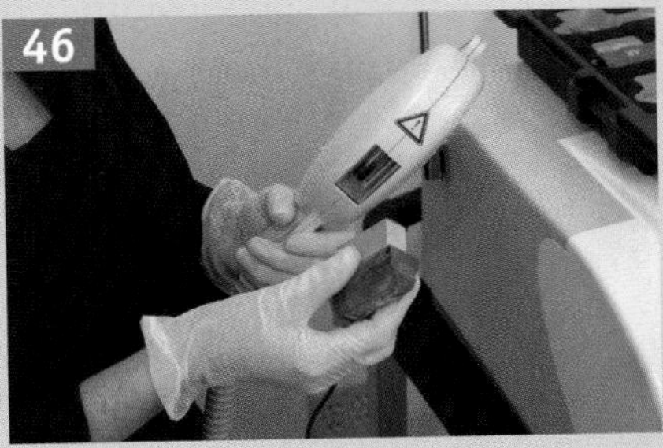

Wipe down machine.

46 Wipe down the machine with germicidal wipes.

continues on next page

PROCEDURE 18–1, CONT. IPL PHOTOREJUVENATION

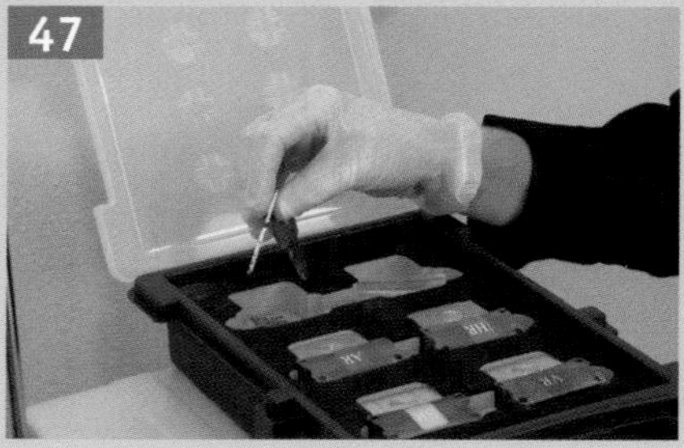
Remove and store key.

47 Remove and store the key.

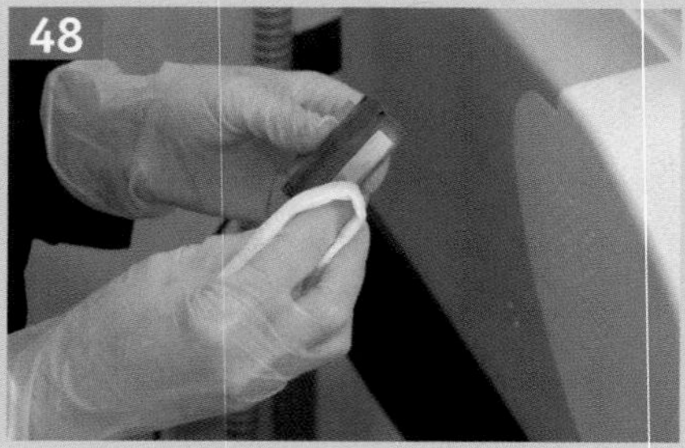
Clean handpiece and filters.

48 Clean the handpiece and filters with germicidal solution or 70% alcohol, per manufacturer guidelines.

49 Follow clean-up and sanitation procedures in accordance with OSHA and or state guidelines.

50 Reset and prepare the room for the next client.

As with all procedures, strict adherence to pre- and postoperative protocols defines client safety and treatment outcome. Parameters are device-dependent and supplied by the manufacturer. Procedures are scheduled every three to four weeks with an average of three to five treatments for maximum collagen stimulation and clearance of skin irregularities. Maintenance treatments are every six months to a year, depending on the client's daily use of sunscreen and whether or not the client is experiencing intrinsic diseases, such as melasma or rosacea (Figure 18–7).

LIGHT-EMITTING DIODES (LEDs)

Light-emitting diode (LED) technology involves the nonthermal, nonablative interaction of light delivered through tiny light-emitting diodes that activate skin cells. This process is called **photomodulation** or light-activated facial rejuvenation. This technology uses energy-producing packets of light to enhance fibroblast collagen synthesis and cause the production of new collagen. LED photorejuvenation equipment, rated by the FDA as Class I or II devices, depending on the model, uses one or more individual wavelengths of light delivered at a low level light intensity. These units come in two basic styles, handheld units and panels that may be handheld or free-standing. The handheld devices let you

★ REGULATORY AGENCY ALERT

Requirements regarding IPL devices vary from state to state. Check with your state regulatory agency to determine whether use of these devices is within your scope of practice.

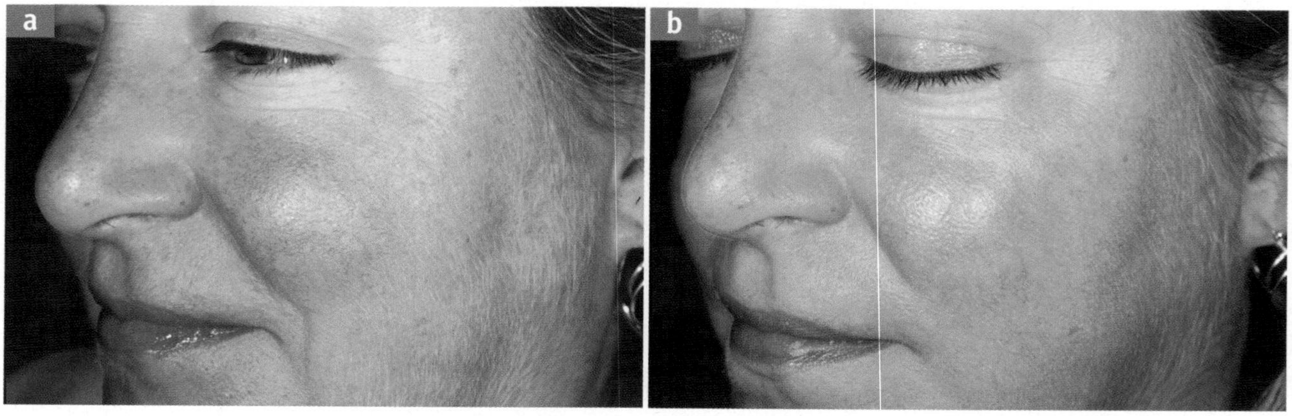
Figure 18–7 Before and after IPL treatment.

put the light head directly on the skin, allowing for less light scatter. The best panels place the light about 1 inch from the skin, minimizing light scatter and covering a broader area in a more systematic approach. Hands-free units allow you to treat other areas of the body, such as the décolleté, hands, or feet, while administering an even radiance of light. Check out both styles of equipment and read each firm's clinical studies to draw your own conclusions. Above all, make sure you are purchasing true LED technology, not just tiny light bulbs.

Treatment Guidelines

LED-device services are usually scheduled one to three times a week for eight to ten total treatments plus maintenance. Frequency is critical to maximize results. Treatments should be scheduled no closer than every other day. Plan your client's treatment in conjunction with laser or light source procedures in order to reduce erythema and promote skin healing. (See Chapter 8 for a more detailed discussion.) It can be used in conjunction with other types of treatments, such as peels, microdermabrasion, or microcurrent toning to enhance the goal of those treatments. Before treatment, screen for indications and contraindications and inform clients as to what to expect from the therapy.

Indications for Treatment

LED devices are commonly used to treat sun-damaged skin, mild to moderate acne, erythema from laser/light therapies, and sunburns and to promote collagen for improvement of skin tone and texture. LED therapy is also used clinically for pain reduction, stretch marks, eczema, and enhanced wound healing with various degrees of success.

Contraindications to Treatment

Clients with the following conditions are contraindicated for LED treatment.

- Current Accutane® (isotretinoin) users (must be off medication for at least one year)
- Clients with seizure disorders
- Clients with open or unidentified skin lesions
- Clients with autoimmune disorders (i.e., HIV/AIDS, Hepatitis B, C, Lupus)
- Clients using photosensitive medications (minocycline, erythromycin)
- Pregnant clients

PROCEDURE 18-2 LED SKIN TREATMENT

While the light color selection will change depending on whether the client is being treated for signs of aging, acne, or inflammation the basic steps will remain the same.

IMPLEMENTS AND MATERIALS

- Typical facial lounge, client draping, and linen setup
- Disposable sponges, cotton pads, or facial cloths
- Water and bowl or sink
- Cotton rounds or gauze pads
- Gloves
- Water-based cleanser
- Toner (degreaser)
- SPF protection
- Serums or ampoules based on skin conditions
- Eye protection as recommended by the manufacturer

Preparation

Perform general treatment room setup:

1. Prepare treatment lounge and client gown.
2. Assemble towels and disposables.
3. Set up products and protective eyewear.
4. Take a client history regarding conditions related to light sensitivity, irritant/allergic reactions, outbreaks of the herpes simplex virus (cold sores), and frequency of sun exposure or tanning bed use.
5. Review the client's concerns, indications, and contraindications for treatment; discuss the results that the client anticipates.
6. Have the client read and sign a consent form.
7. Take "before" photographs to use in showing the client's progress through the treatment series.
8. Assess and type the client's skin with Fitzpatrick skin typing.

continues on next page

PROCEDURE 18–2, CONT. LED SKIN TREATMENT

Procedure

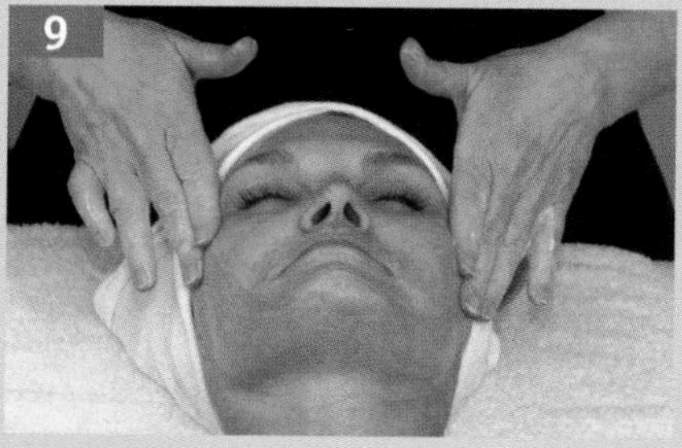
Pre-Cleanse skin.

9 Pre-cleanse. Remove client's makeup.

10 Degrease the client's skin or prep it with a stripping cleanser to remove all oils.

11 Thoroughly dry the skin prior to light treatments.

12 Perform gentle exfoliation with microdermabrasion or other methodology prior to LED treatment to increase absorption of the light.

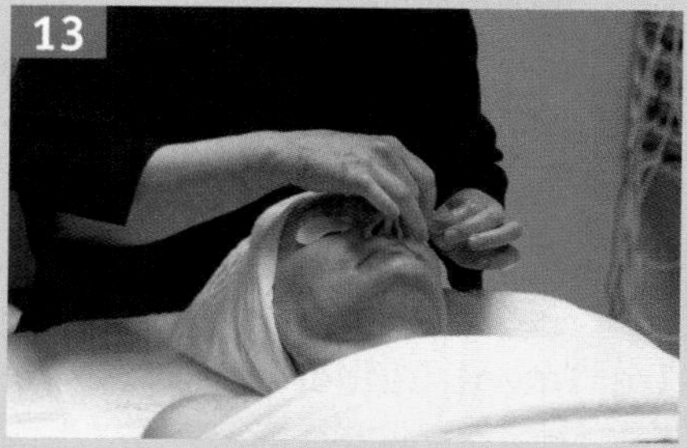
Apply protective eyewear.

13 Protect the client's eyes with appropriate eyewear following manufacturer's guidelines.

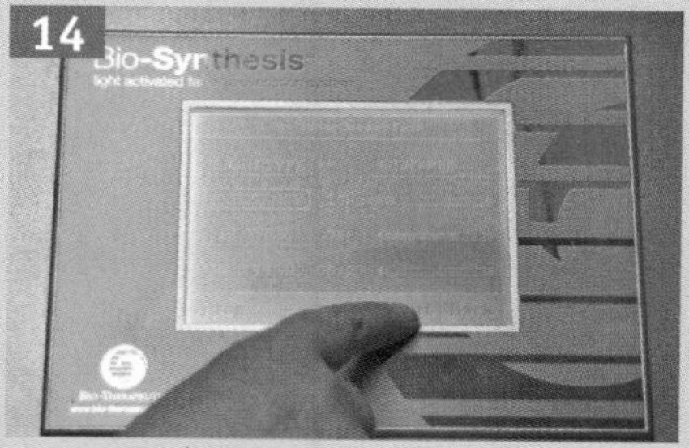
Program the unit.

14 Follow the manufacturer's protocol for performing the treatment. If you have an automatic panel device, program the unit for the treatment to be done, and then position the panels close to the client's face. Vary treatment or color selection following manufacturer guidelines.

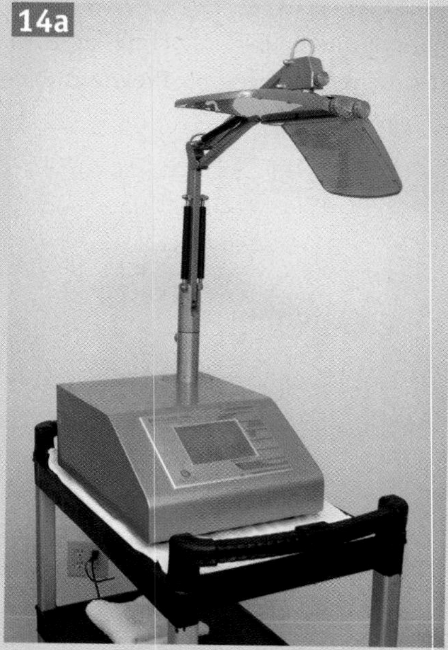
Position the unit.

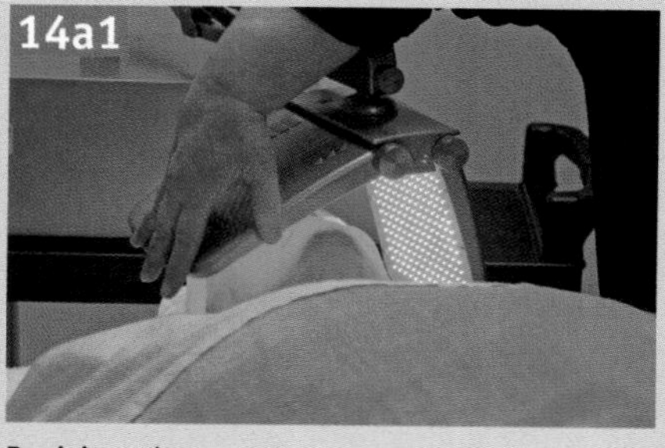
Position the panel.

ALTERNATIVELY: If you have a manual handpiece, work around the face holding the handpiece

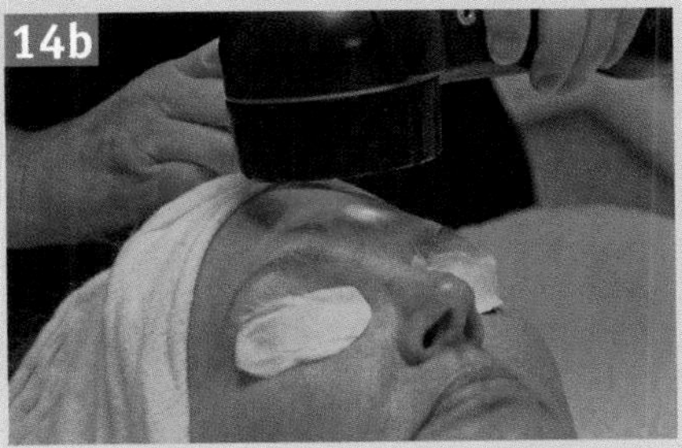

Hold for specified intervals.

so that the light strikes the skin. Hold it in position for specified intervals.

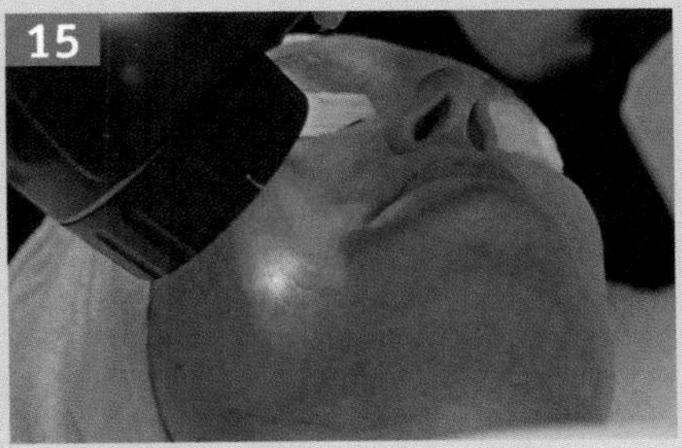

Move forehead to right side.

15 During the treatment, move from the forehead to the right side of the face, then to the left side of the face, and finally proceed to upper lip and chin area.

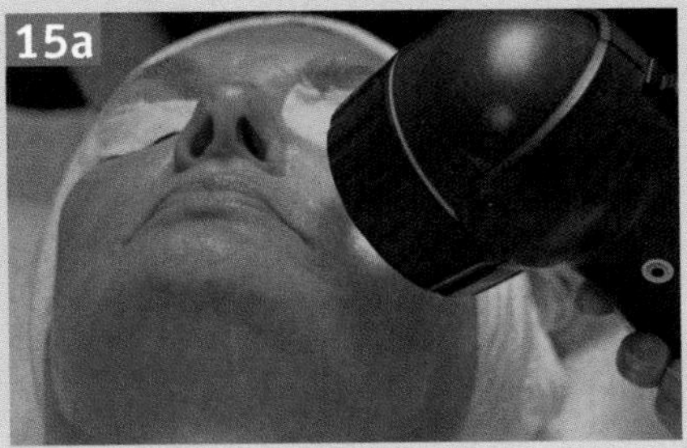

Move right to left side.

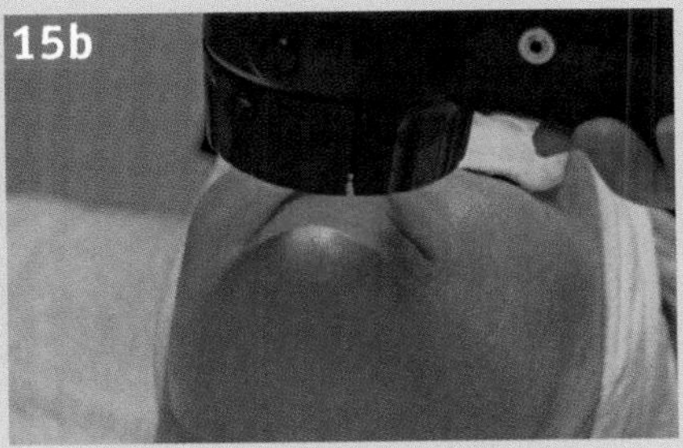

Move to the upper lip and chin.

16 Apply serum as needed to maintain moisture level, as recommended by the manufacturer.

17 End the treatment with serum appropriate to client's skin condition and sun protection. Another nice way to end this treatment is lymph drainage.

CAUTION!

All LED devices are manufactured differently. Treatment times may take from 2 to 16 minutes, depending on the device and application. Follow manufacturer's recommendations for time exposure and treatment protocols.

Post-procedure

18 Some devices may leave the client's skin feeling tender or with a sunburn sensation after light exposure. With others this is either not evident or redness may actually be diminished. In either case, use only soothing and hydrating products after the procedure.

19 Apply sunscreen along with post-treatment serums.

20 Include written instructions for home care use of gentle moisturizers and hydrating solutions along with daily use of sunscreen.

Clean-up and Disinfection

21 Perform clean-up and disinfection according to OSHA and or your state's regulations.

22 Wipe down the machine following the manufacturer's recommendations.

PHOTODYNAMIC THERAPY (PDT)

Photodynamic therapy is a stand-alone protocol, in a medical setting, using a photosensitizing drug enhancer, aminolevulinic acid (ALA) or Levelan. (Figure 18–8). Since ALA is a prescriptive drug, the treatment is performed only in a physician's office or medical spa. Initially used in the treatment of **actinic keratosis,** clinical trials and research have expanded the use of the therapy to include the treatment of acne and enhanced facial rejuvenation. For acne therapy, ALA (Levelan) is applied to the skin for a 30-minute to one-hour incubation period and fluoresced with light in the 380-nm to 440-nm range. ALA is absorbed by the sebaceous glands and when fluoresced with a specific light device, causes a **phototoxic** reaction, destroying *P. acnes,* bacteria which causes acne papules. After a series of treatments, there can be a reduction of sebaceous oil gland output and acne papules. At this time the drug, ALA, is only FDA approved for use in the treatment of actinic keratosis but off-label uses for acne and skin rejuvenation are widely accepted.

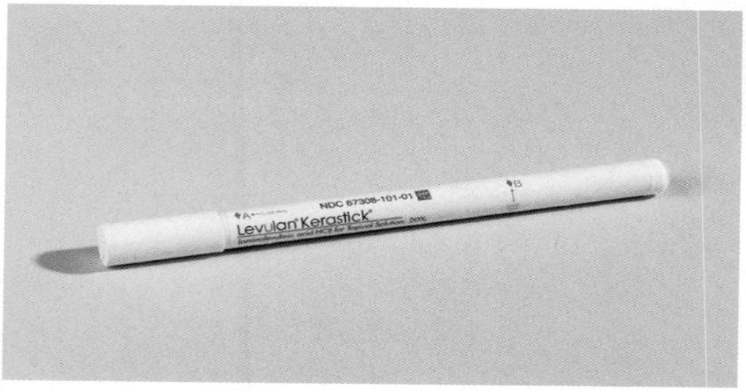

Figure 18–8 Kerastick which holds the ALA.

In a PDT treatment, ALA is painted on the client's skin and, after a period of resting time, the patient is exposed to the light sources. The duration of the exposure depends on which devices are used, IPL or LED, and the particular device settings. After the treatment, the client is photosensitive and cannot risk additional sunlight exposure. Activation of the ALA will continue even after the treatment, and an extreme sunburn and blistering could occur. Clients should stay inside out of daylight for two days following treatment (Figure 18–9).

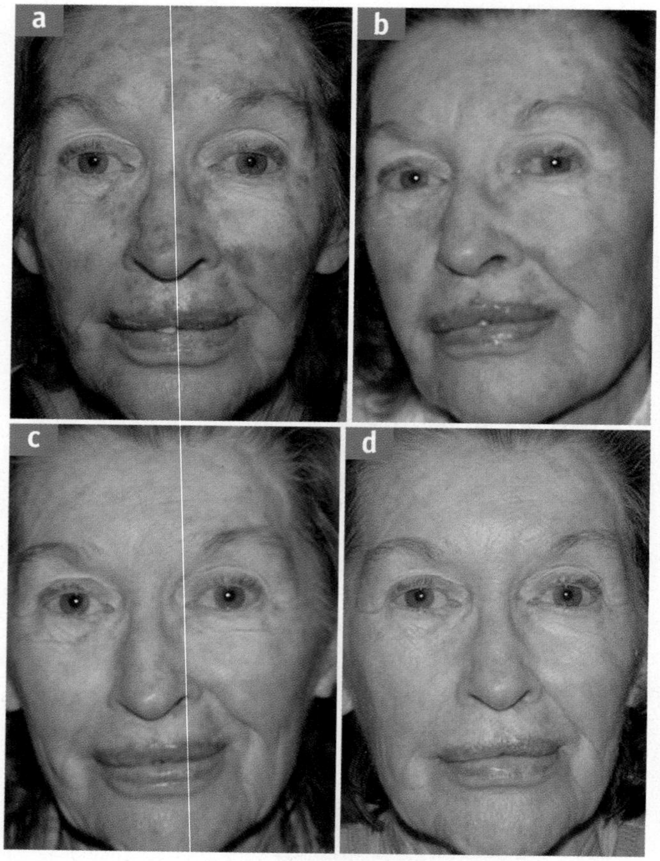

Figure 18–9 ALA/IPL treatment.

MICRODERMABRASION

Microdermabrasion is a process of physically exfoliating the skin. Estheticians use this method for clients who may not be suitable candidates for chemical exfoliation. Initially introduced in the United States in 1996 as a physical exfoliation treatment to improve skin tone and texture, the first treatments used a crystal spray and vacuum system. Now microdermabrasion uses crystals, diamond tips, or ultrasonic paddles to reduce skin irregularities found in early photoaging clients. Microdermabrasion has been documented to not only reduce pigmented lesions, superficial acne scars, and rhytids, but it also produces collagen, resulting in a supple skin tone and texture. A technique-sensitive procedure, the outcome varies with treatment techniques and settings.

As this book goes to press, there are more than 73 different devices from which to choose in today's cosmetic market. Most manufacturers sell two grades of microdermabrasion machines: esthetic models and physician models. Esthetic microdermabrasion machines have less force or vacuum capabilities while physician units are more aggressive. The medical units are capable of higher vacuum pressure and force and should be only used under the direction of a physician because damage to the skin can occur.

The depth of penetration and the degree of tissue exfoliation depend on several variables. The strength of the vacuum, coupled with the number of passes, speed of the passes, and pressure exerted by the operator play a role in the client's response. The size of the crystal being used is also a factor. Longer time spent in contact with the tissue produces deeper exfoliation or even an inflammatory response. A technique that is too aggressive can cause pinpoint bleeding as well as side effects, such as redness, infection, or hyperpigmentation.

Manufacturers offer a variety of accessory options and styles of handpieces. Opinions differ, but the 45-degree handpiece appears to cause less scraping of the skin than the 90-degree style. At this angle, crystals impact the skin and gently exfoliate the epidermis and the suction/vacuum returns the crystals to the system. Newer devices offer improvements, such as precision delivery systems, smaller sizes, and safety mechanisms, which provide better outcomes for the client. Some devices also offer ultrasonic attachments for increased product absorption. It is important to evaluate devices and decide which will offer your practice the greatest benefits.

Some estheticians perform an enzyme or salon chemical exfoliation prior to microdermabrasion, but manufacturers have different recommendations and it is critical that estheticians follow the guidelines for the devices. Soothing or rejuvenating masks, sonophoresis, iontophoresis, microamp therapy or LED therapy can be added for enhanced benefits and the reduction of redness or irritation. In addition, microdermabrasion is used with IPL/laser treatments and with ALA photodynamic therapies under a physician's guidance and supervision.

Crystal Devices

Following are descriptions of two types of crystal devices used in microdermabrasion (Figure 18–10). After learning about these options, make your own decision based on the uniformity of particulate size, airborne dust particulate, and clinical trials showing effectiveness.

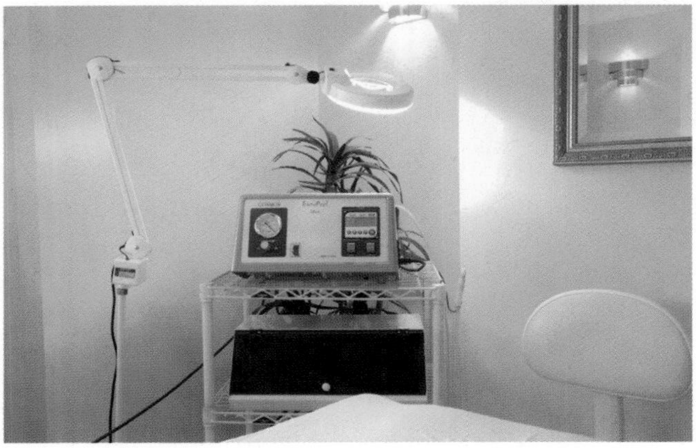

Figure 18–10 Crystal microdermabrasion device.

Aluminum oxide crystals (corundum) were chosen initially as a vehicle for exfoliating the stratum corneum. These inert crystals have proven to be stable and do not cause skin irritation. There are, however, disadvantages. Crystals cannot be reused due to the potential of cross-contamination between clients. Also, some machines allow **aerosolized** (microscopic airborne particles) crystals to leak into the room, which present an inhalation and ocular hazard to the esthetician. The World Health Organization considers aluminum oxide a "nuisance dust." Therefore, it is highly recommended that during microdermabrasion treatments the esthetician wear protective eye goggles and a filtration mask. Of course, the client's eyes are always protected.

Organic crystals are an alternative to aluminum oxide crystals for microdermabrasion procedures. Manufacturers claim salt crystal machines have many benefits, as salt is nontoxic and water-soluble. Salt crystals provide a deeper exfoliation and the client may need fewer treatments to reach an acceptable outcome. However, due to the irregular shape of the crystals, it may be more uncomfortable and potentially pose a higher risk for abrading the skin. Baking soda is another choice. There has been only one study on its effectiveness, but the clinical trials indicate it to be equivalent to the original aluminum oxide; however, the more random size of baking soda crystals and the enhanced "dust" create other considerations. Corn granules are also sometimes used, but there is little information available on this agent.

Non-Crystal Devices

Diamond crystal and diamond-encrusted machines represent an alternative in the field of microdermabrasion, especially for those who dislike dealing with the crystals or have issues with airborne particulate (Figure 18–11). They may also be more appropriate for more delicate or sensitive skins. This machine utilizes a variety of reusable wands with ball or straight tips. These wands work in conjunction with suction pressure to effectively exfoliate the stratum corneum. In addition to size, the wands have different gauges of roughness, ranging from coarse to fine-tipped. Some manufacturers also offer lymphatic wands for the eye area or larger wands for body treatments. The diamond machines eliminate the nuisance of crystals, but the wands must be cleansed and sterilized between clients. As with other devices, pressure settings

PROCEDURE 18-3, CONT. MICRODERMABRASION

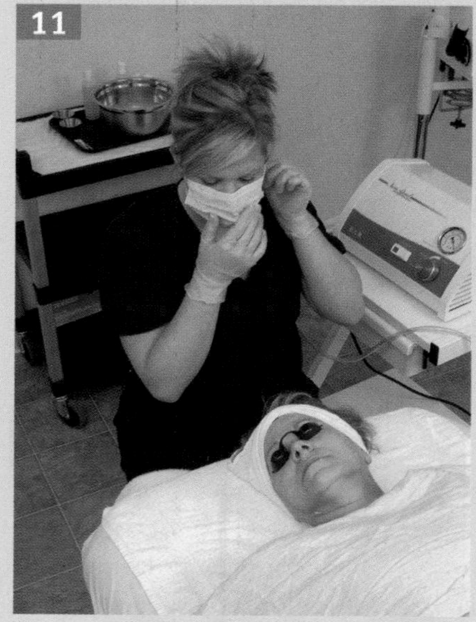

Apply protective wear.

11 Put on protective eye goggles, protective apparel, and gloves.

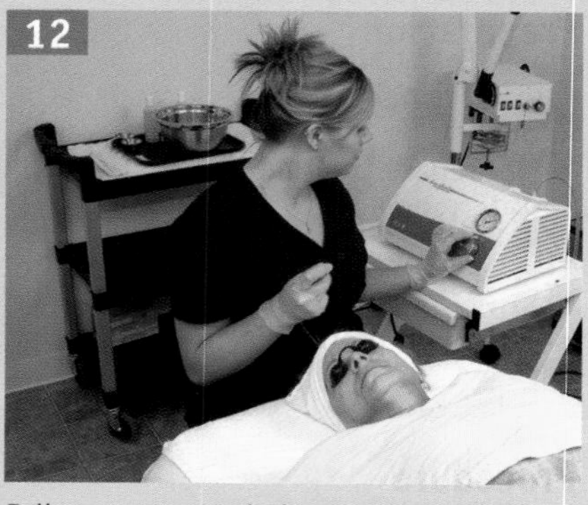

Follow recommendations.

12 Follow manufacturer's recommendations for pressure settings, time exposure, and treatment protocol.

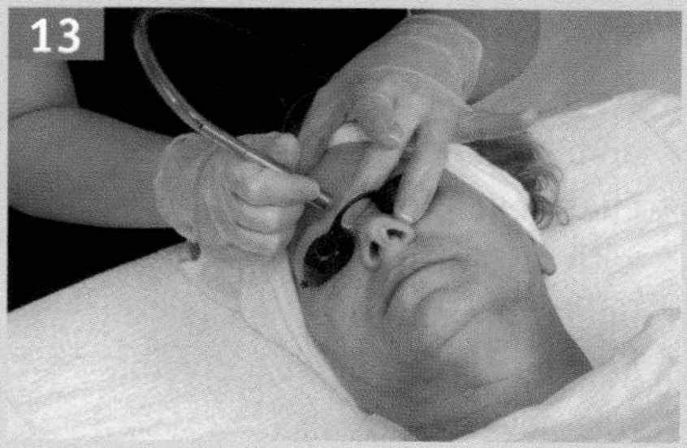

Conduct test pass.

13 Conduct a test pass adjacent to where the treatment is to be done.

a. Skin should be slightly pink and comfortable.

b. Using the medical pain response scale of 1 to 10 with 1 being no pain and 10 being the worst imaginable, client's response should never be higher than 5. Settings of 2 to 4 are comfortable and safe.

c. Start with settings low and increase as you determine how the client is tolerating the strokes.

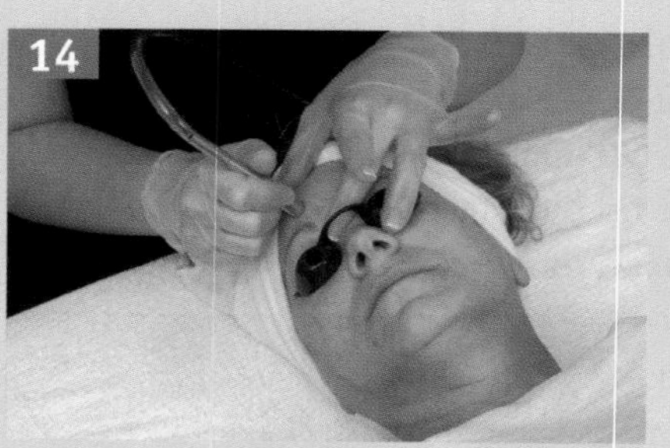

Begin at right side of forehead.

14 Start the procedure on the right half of the forehead. Using your non-dominant hand, hold the skin taut between your fingertips.

a. Make steady strokes with the device, maintaining constant pressure on the skin between the stretched fingertips.

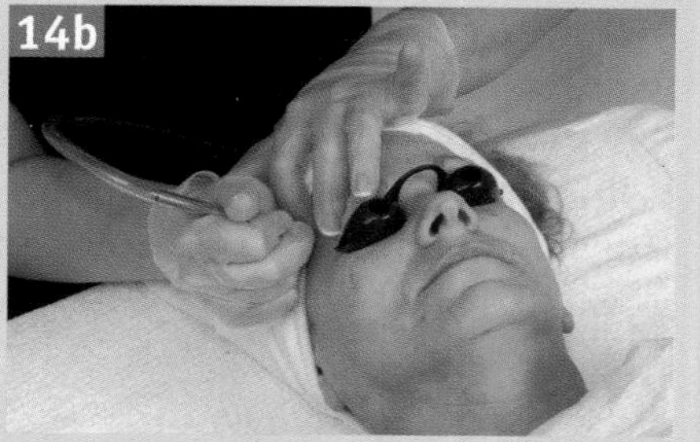

Begin strokes vertically.

b. Make vertical strokes on the entire width of the forehead, starting at the center just above the eyebrow and working toward the hairline above the temple. As you reach the side of the forehead, tip the

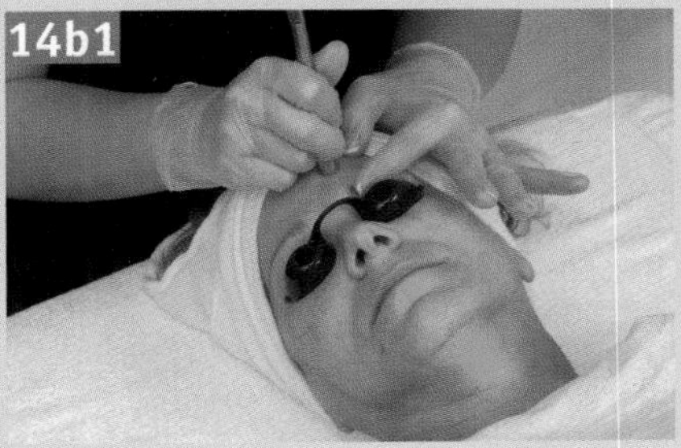

Slightly tip device.

end of the device slightly, loosening pressure contact for a smooth release.

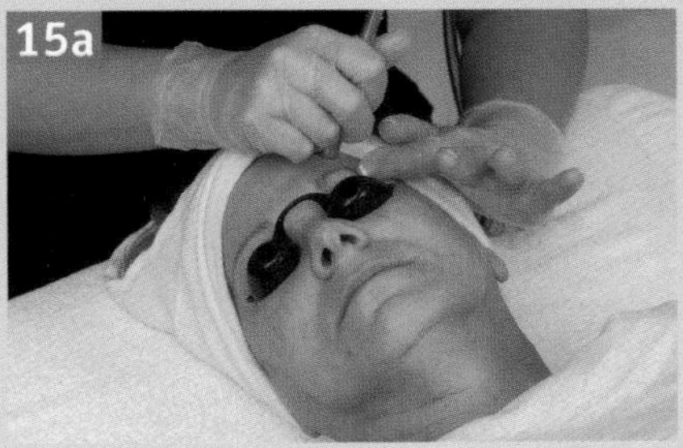

Work eyebrows to hairline.

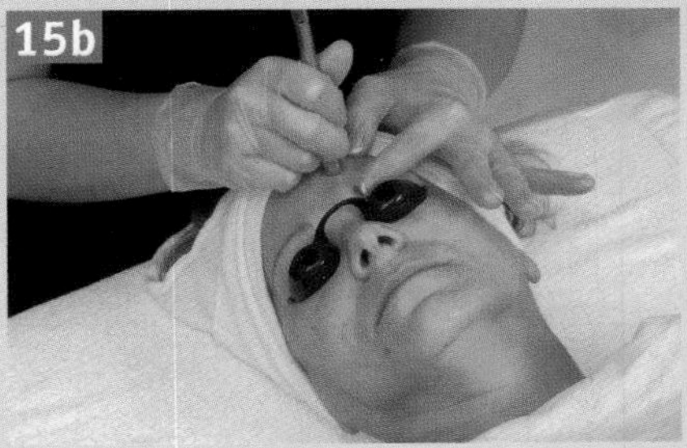

Rows up toward hairline.

15 The next set of passes should be a horizontal pattern perpendicular to the horizontal direction.

a. Holding the skin taut, work from eyebrows up toward the hairline.

b. Repeat this in adjacent passes, working in rows up toward the hairline.

c. Ensure that the pressure is comfortable for the client and appropriate for the skin type.

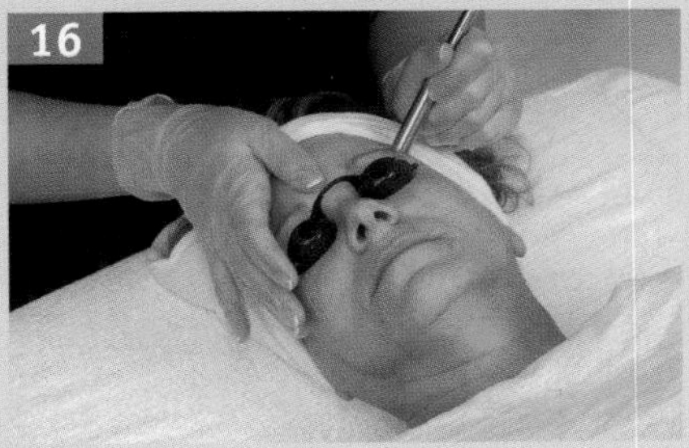

Repeat on other side.

16 Repeat both sets of passes on the other side of forehead.

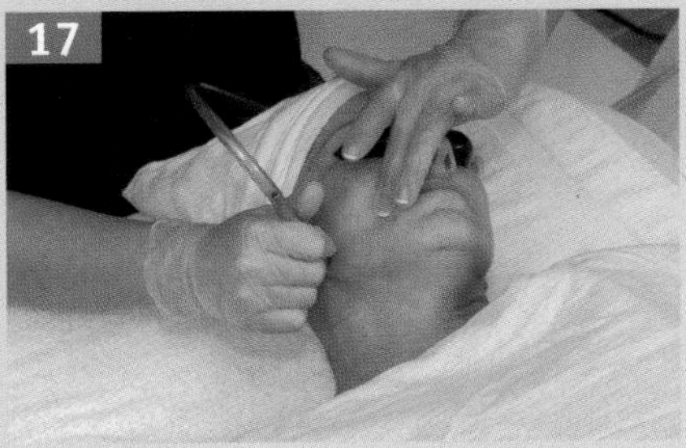

Repeat passes on cheeks.

17 Repeat both sets of passes on each cheek, working from the nose to jaw outward and from the orbital bone to the chin.

Here's a Tip

As you move to different quadrants of the face, pay attention to the characteristics of the skin. Note that the number of passes you make influences the degree of tissue effects, and individual devices may have guidelines about the number of passes required. Three passes are usually appropriate for normal to oily skin. Thinner, drier, more sensitive skin may require only two passes. Some companies recommend up to seven passes. With experience, you will determine the number of passes required to reach a desired end point.

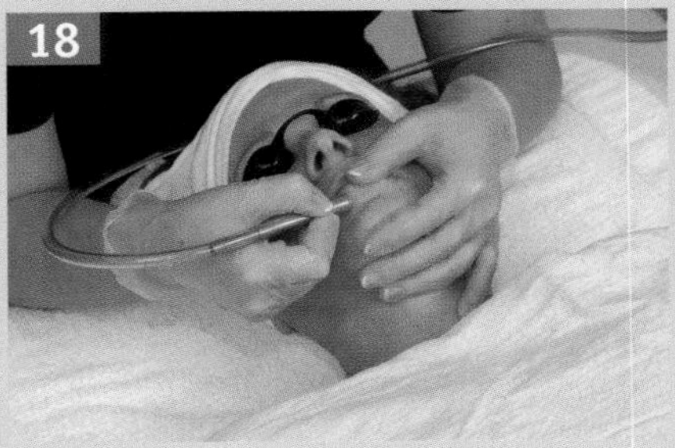

Repeat on chin.

18 Repeat both sets of passes on the chin.

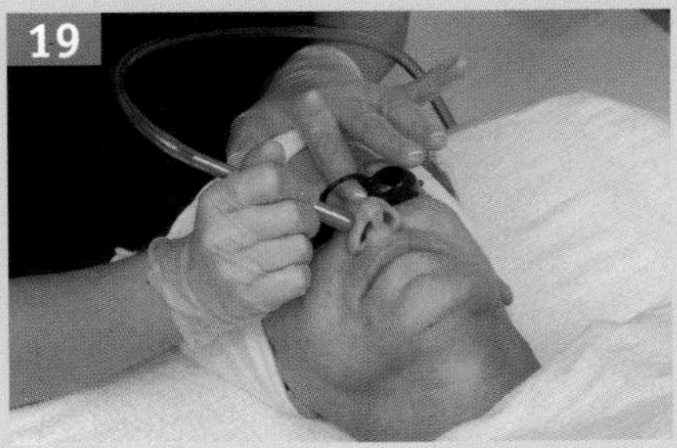

Perform on nose.

19 Perform passes on nose.

continues on next page

PROCEDURE 18-3, CONT. MICRODERMABRASION

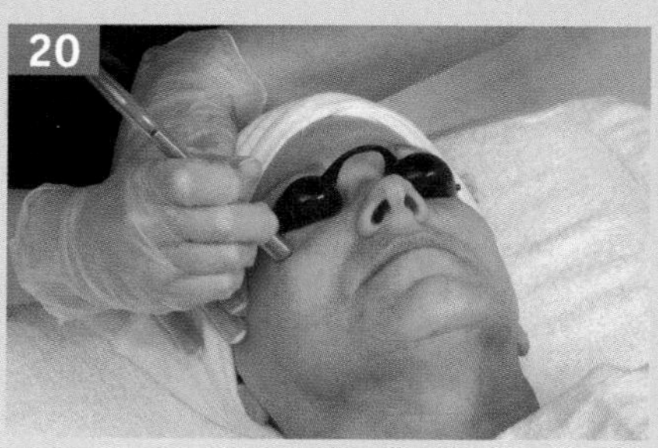

Move to lowest level for orbital area.

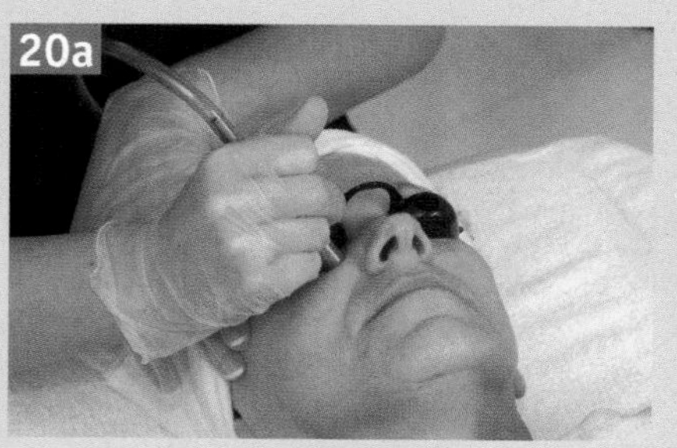

Use orbital bone as guideline.

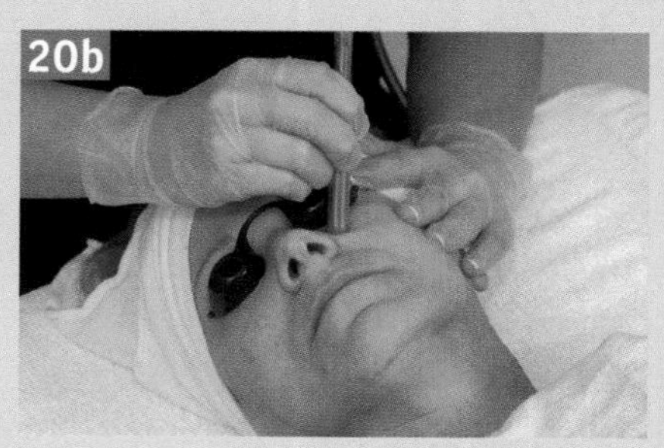

Make eye strokes according to machine.

20 Reduce the vacuum pressure to the lowest level in the orbital areas. Never work on the eyelid itself. Use the orbital bone as a guideline for how close to the eye to go. Eye strokes with crystal devices should be from the inner corner of the eye outward to prevent crystals from getting in the eye near the tear duct. Using non-crystal diamond wand devices, this stroke may be done from the outer corner toward the nose.

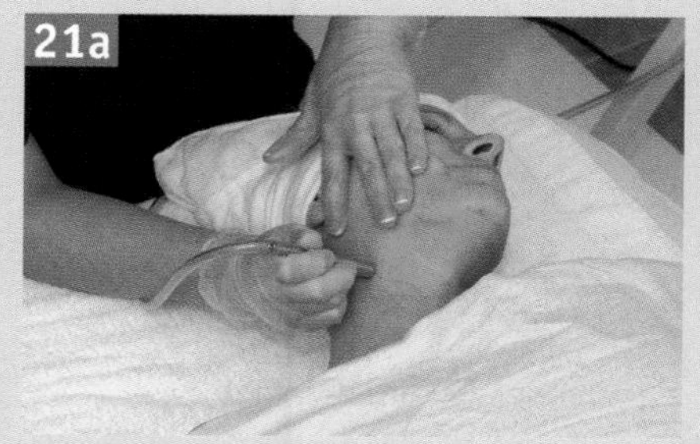

Pass vertically with lower pressure.

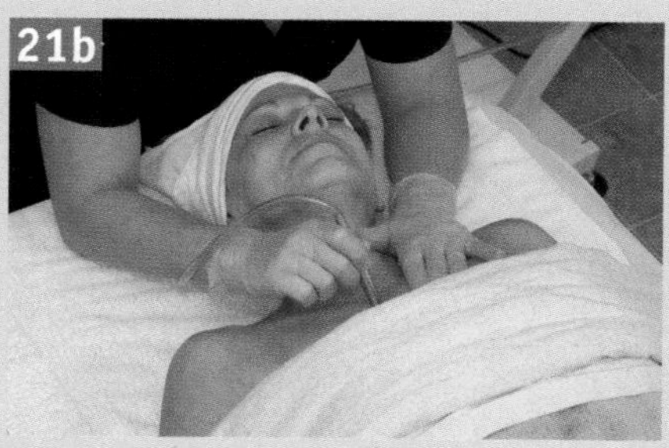

Begin décolleté in center.

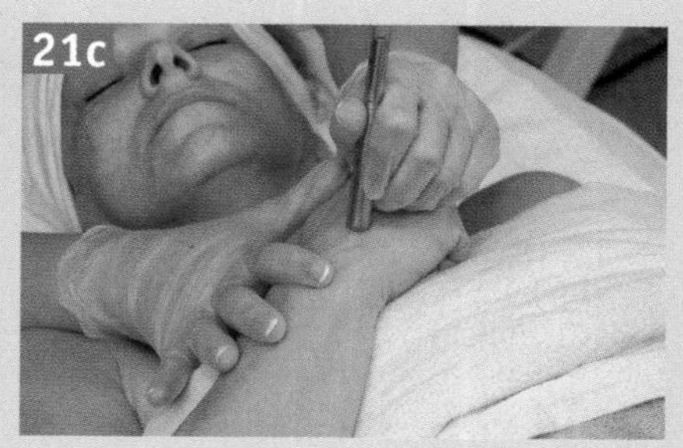

A fist to taut hands.

21 If making passes on other parts of the body, follow these guidelines:

a. Neck should be hyperextended with passes in a vertical direction and a lower pressure than used on the face. Start at the jawline and stroke down.

b. For the décolleté, start in the center of the chest and stroke outward, holding the skin taut.

c. Client should make a fist prior to treatment of the hands to produce a taut skin surface.

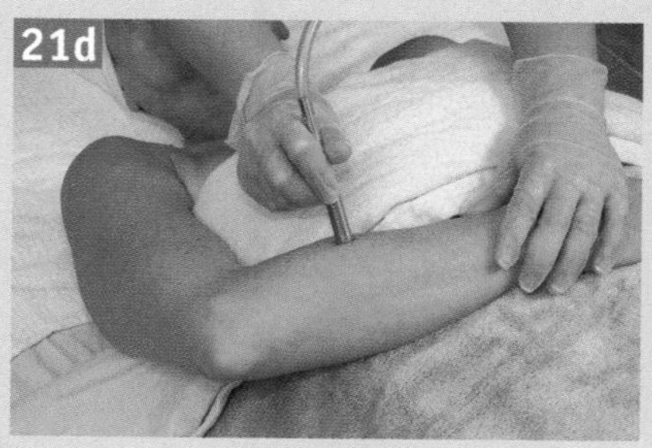

Pass on the forearms.

d. Passes on the forearms should be made in vertical direction, taking note of bony areas and skin thickness and texture.

22 After completing all microdermabrasion, brush away any loose crystals.

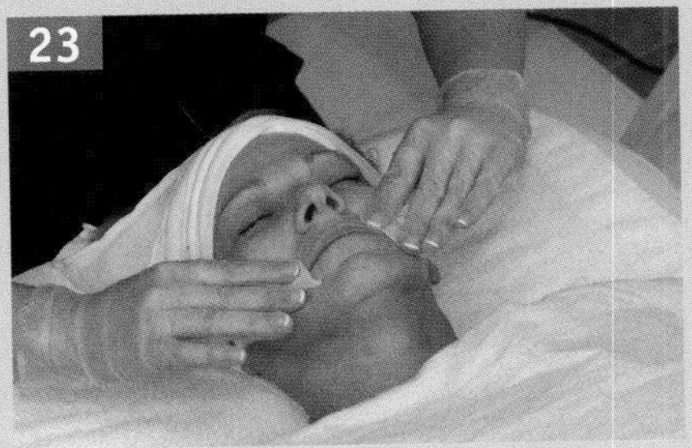

Rinse face.

23 Rinse the face to ensure that you have removed all crystals.

24 Follow with normal facial routine steps (mask, sonophoresis).

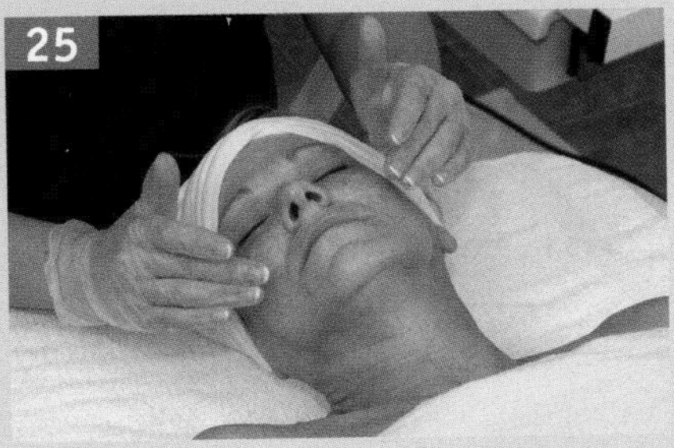

Apply products.

25 Conclude the treatment with soothing serum or lotion and sun protection.

Post-procedure

26 The client's skin may be tender or have a sunburned sensation after microdermabrasion. Remind the client to use sunscreen and protect themselves from direct sun exposure.

27 Give the client instructions for home care use of gentle cleansers, moisturizers, and hydrating solutions, along with daily use of sunscreen.

Clean-up and Disinfection

28 Perform clean-up and disinfection according to the guidelines of OSHA or your state's regulations.

29 Wipe down the machine following the manufacturer's recommendations.

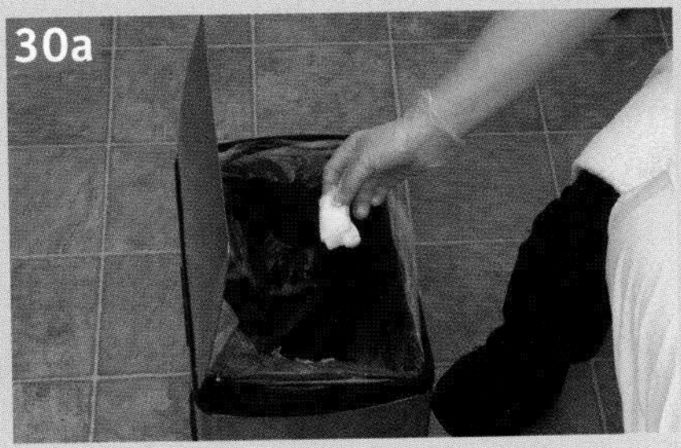

Dispose components.

30 Dispose of any disposable components.

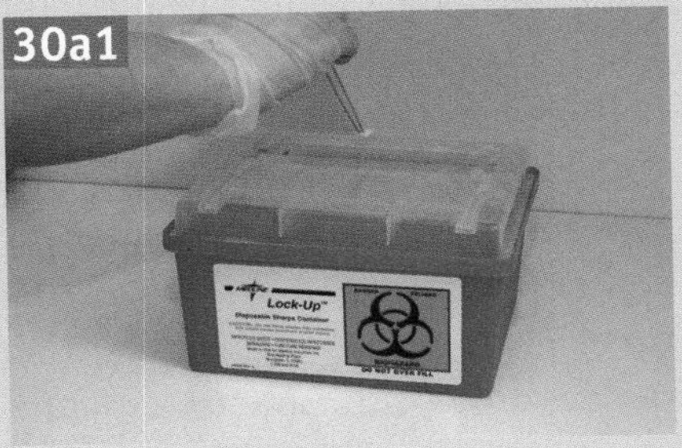

Dispose components.

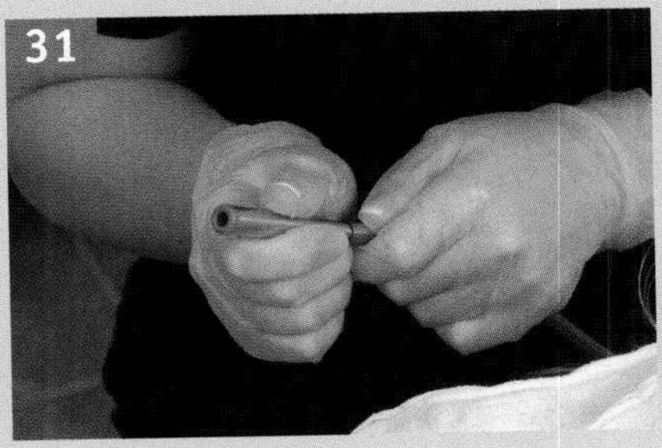

Check filters and tubes.

31 Check the device's filters and tubes per the manufacturer's directions.

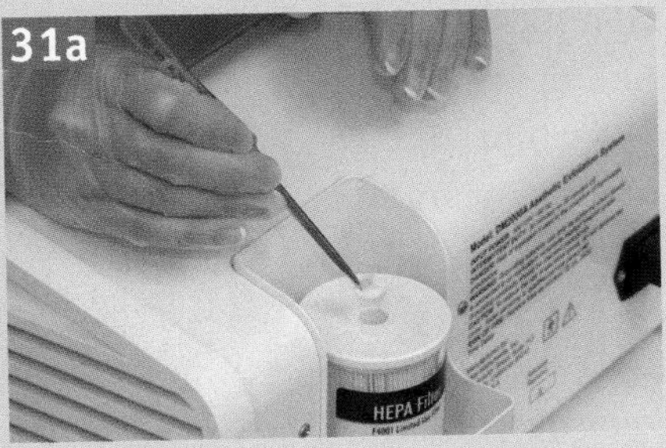

Check filters and tubes.

32 Sterilize any reusable components per the manufacturer's instructions.

33 Vacuum the floor to remove any crystals.

> **? Did You Know**
>
> Clients may notice improvement after one treatment; however, a series of microdermabrasion treatments will offer a better outcome. Usually 4 to 8 procedures are recommended, scheduled every 2 to 4 weeks. Maintenance treatments are also recommended to promote long-term improvement of skin tone and texture.

ULTRASONIC TECHNOLOGY

In a physical therapy setting, ultrasound is used to stimulate blood flow, increase metabolic rate, and warm up tissues to promote temporary pain relief. Estheticians use ultrasonic technology, not ultrasound devices, to provide cleansing exfoliation treatments called *cavitation*, penetration of products using sonophoresis, and in some units, micro-amp therapy to promote homeostasis. The depth of tissue penetration depends on frequency, not intensity. Most ultrasonic energy with a 3-megahertz frequency will be absorbed in superficial tissue, making this application more appropriate for esthetic uses. In contrast, a slower, 1-megahertz frequency will heat tissue up to 3 to 5 centimeters deep. One-megahertz frequency devices are not suitable for esthetic use but are used by physical therapists to treat muscle trauma.

For cavitation, the device includes a spatula-like handpiece that is used in conjunction with water, water-based cleansers, and/or steam to perform a deep cleansing. While this is an electric device, the technology uses sound waves, not electrical current, to exfoliate, dislodge any surface contaminates, and loosen impurities embedded in the follicles (Figure 18–13). The minute vibrations loosen stratum corneum cells and some manufacturers claim up to a 35% reduction of the stratum corneum in one treatment.

For sonophoresis, an esthetician uses the reverse side of the ultrasonic's blade or a circular flat handpiece in conjunction with serums and ampoules for deeper penetration of performance ingredients. Some manufacturers claim that their devices provide up to 10 times more penetration than manual massage.

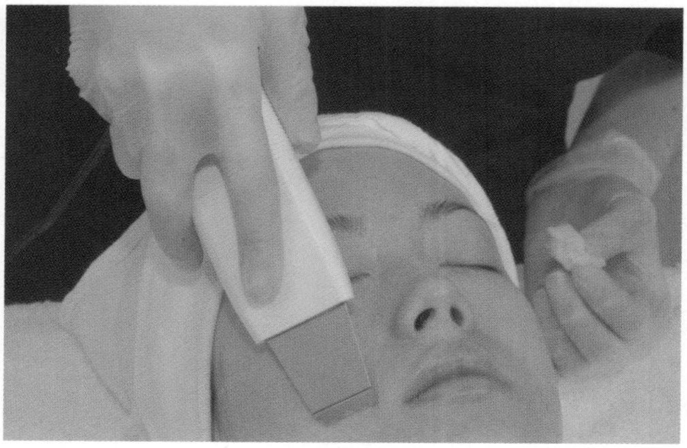

Figure 18–13 The use of an ultrasonic device in a facial.

During treatments, it is important to maintain constant movement of the handpiece on moist skin. If you leave the handpiece on one section of skin for too long, there will be excessive heat buildup, causing unstable cavitation. In addition, never use the handpiece near the eye area or on thin, fragile skin.

Due to its gentle, nonabrasive nature, this treatment is more suitable for clients with rosacea than are microdermabrasion or other exfoliating services. Depending on the device used and protocol followed, even sensitive skin clients will not experience any red appearance to the skin. As gentle as it is, though, there are clients who are not good candidates for this therapy: clients with heart conditions or pacemakers or electrical implants, pregnant women, or clients with diabetes. Just as with other procedures and treatments, always obtain a thorough health history and written consent from a client before proceeding.

> ***Here's a Tip***
>
> The blade of the ultrasonic device is made of very thin metal. It is fragile, so you should always place it in its protective cap or cradle before setting it down. Follow manufacturer's guidelines for cleaning and handling to prevent nicking or pitting the blade which will need to be replaced.

PROCEDURE 18–4 ULTRASONIC FACIAL

IMPLEMENTS AND MATERIALS

- Typical facial lounge setup, client draping, and towel setup
- Gloves
- Gauze pads or cotton rounds
- Disposable sponges or facial cloths
- Water bowl
- Eye pads for client
- Ear protection for client (such as ear plugs or cotton)
- Water-based cleanser
- Treatment mask (optional)
- Massage cream
- Toner
- Specialty serums or ampoules
- Moisturizing sunscreen (SPF15 minimum)

Preparation

Perform general treatment room setup:

1 Prepare the treatment table with linens.

2 Check the device for proper operation.

3 Gather and set up disposables and products.

Procedure

Part I: Peel Modality (Cavitation)

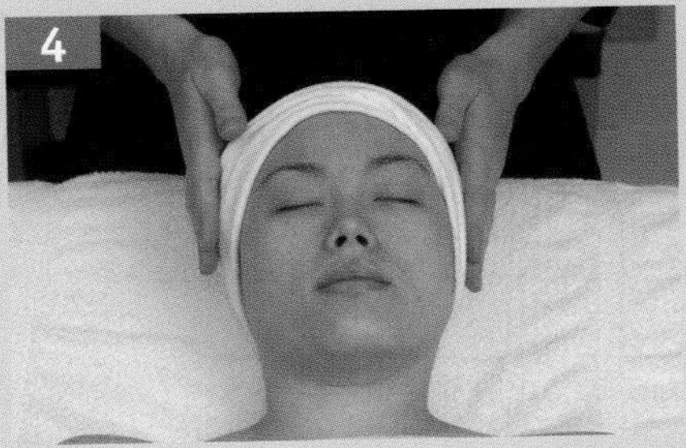

Drape client.

4 Drape the client and secure hair away from the face.

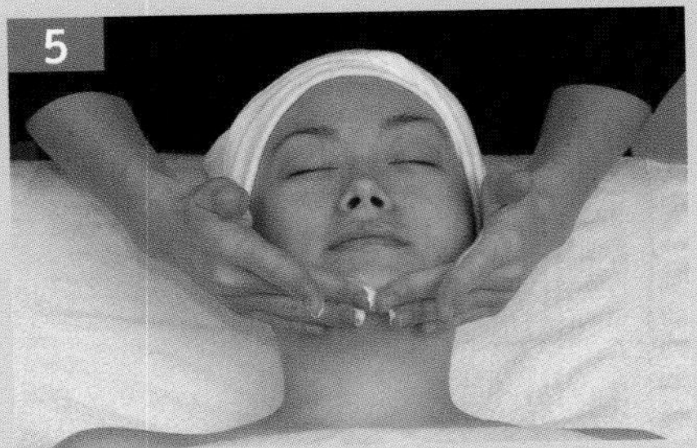

Pre-cleanse client.

5 Pre-cleanse and remove makeup using a water-based cleanser.

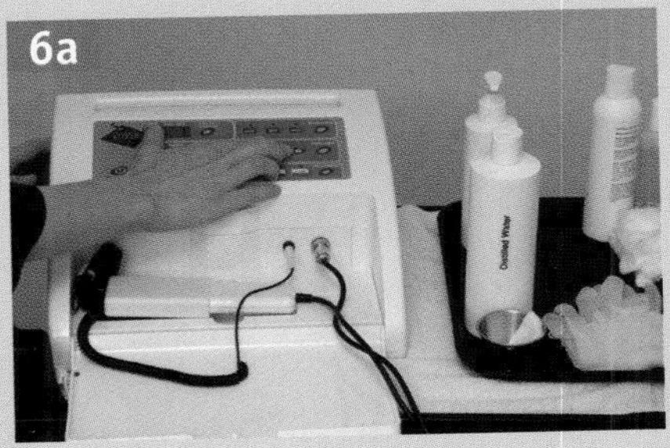

Adjust setting.

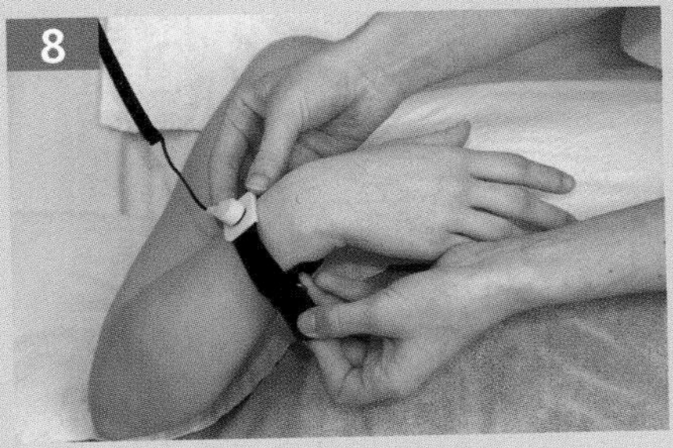

Attach wristband to client.

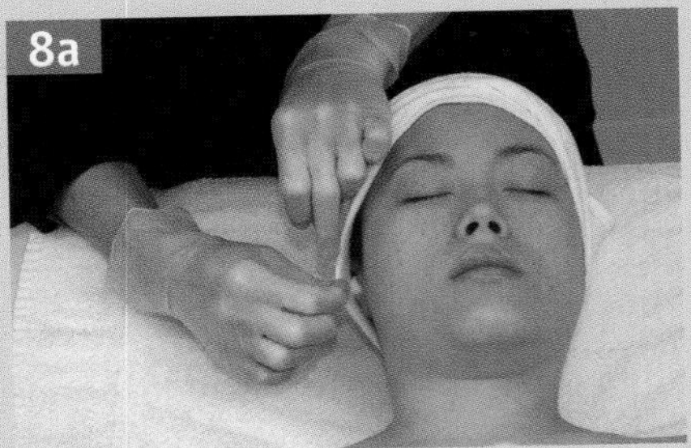

Insert eye and ear pads.

6 Adjust machine settings per manufacturer instructions and based on client skin type.

7 Apply cleanser, combined with a small trace of water for moisture, and apply to the client's face in small circular motions, leaving that area slightly wet. Use a mild desincrustation fluid on severely oily and congested skin types.

8 Attach the wristband to the client and insert ear pads and eye pads for protection, if required by your state regulations.

continues on next page

PROCEDURE 18–4, CONT. ULTRASONIC FACIAL

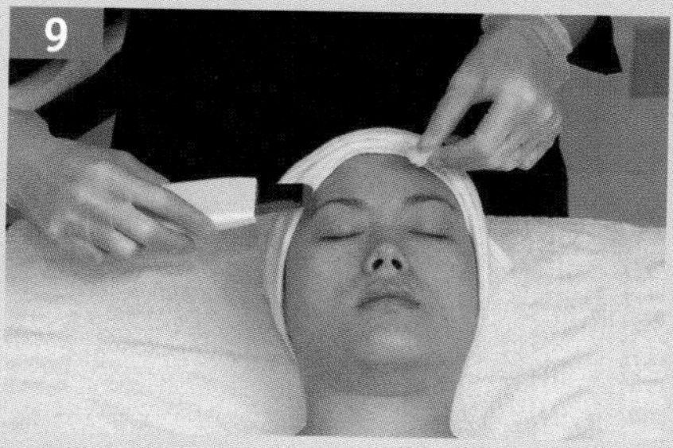
Rewet as needed.

9 You can use steam to maintain moisture at this time. Alternatively, use a gauze pad or sponge dipped in distilled water or manufacturer wetting solution to rewet the skin as needed. Work only on moist skin.

10 Adjust settings or discontinue treatment if the client feels any discomfort at any time.

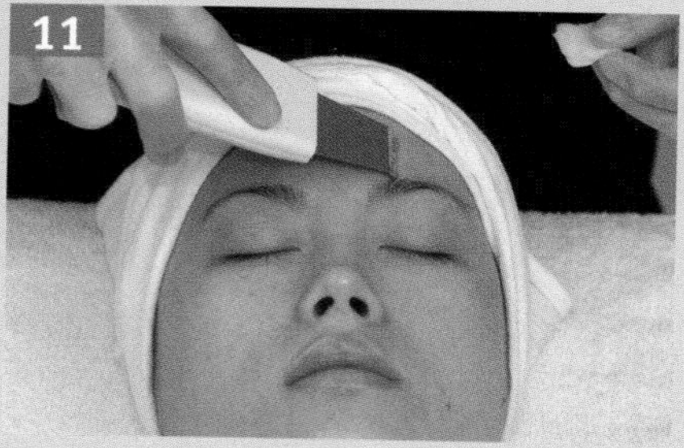
Face blade downward.

11 Starting with the forehead, gently secure/stretch the skin to be treated between your thumb and pointer finger, just as when you perform a microdermabrasion treatment.

a. Hold the ultrasonic blade at a 45-degree angle with the blade tip facing downward.

b. Gently glide the handpiece across the skin surface in a light forward movement and using no pressure. The wand should almost float across the skin on the water or hydrator. It is the water and the vibration that do the work. A proper stroke will yield a fine forward arch of moisture droplets spraying from where the blade touches the skin.

c. Increase or decrease intensity as indicated by the manufacturer.

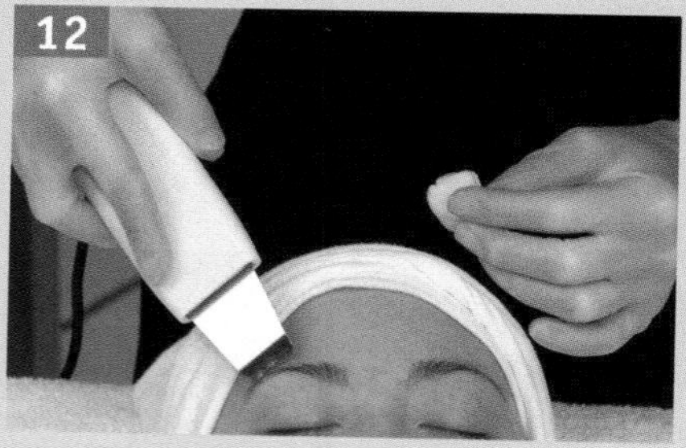
Begin horizontally on forehead.

12 Stroke first in a horizontal pattern across the forehead and then from the brows upward toward hairline.

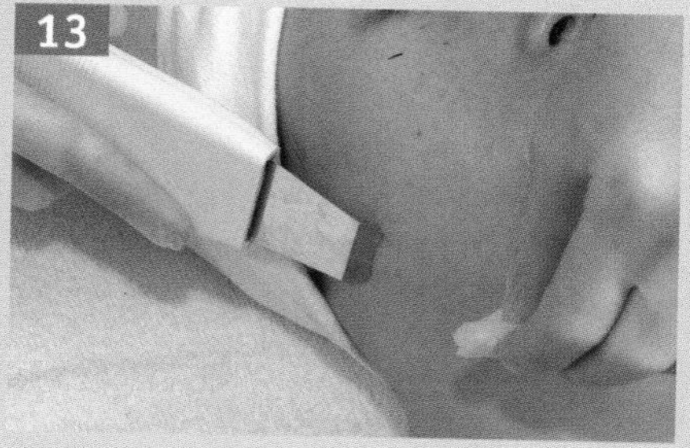
Move to right cheek and repeat.

13 Move to the right cheek and repeat movements.

a. Start from the nose toward the perimeter of the face and from the upper cheek to the jawline.

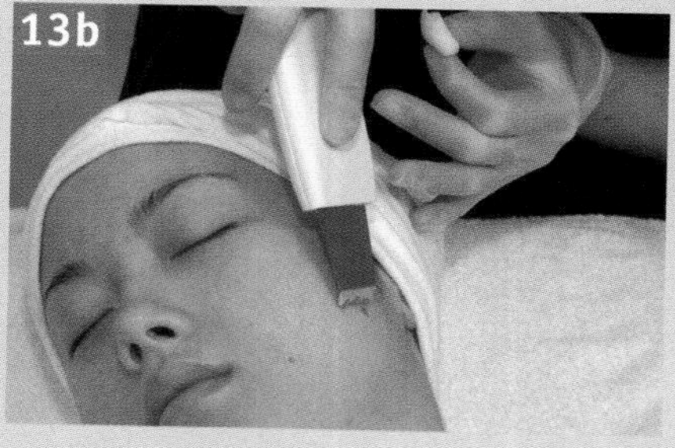
Repeat on left cheek.

b. Repeat on the left cheek.

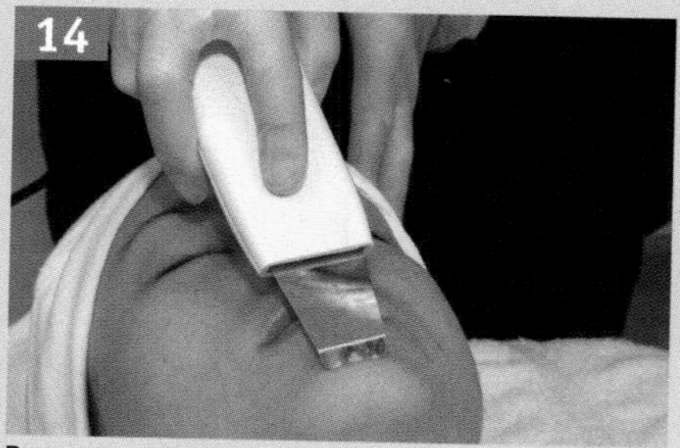
Repeat on chin.

14 Repeat this procedure on the chin.

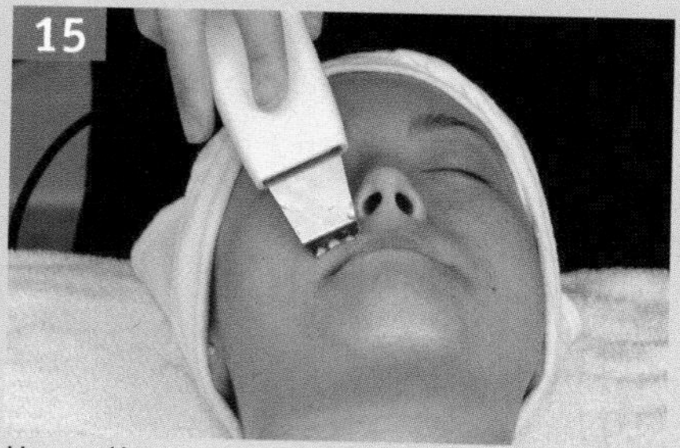
Have client compress lips in an *M*.

15 Ask the client to hold his or her lips in a compressed "M" while you stroke across and downward from the nose toward the upper lip. Do not stroke upward toward the nose because spray can enter the nostril.

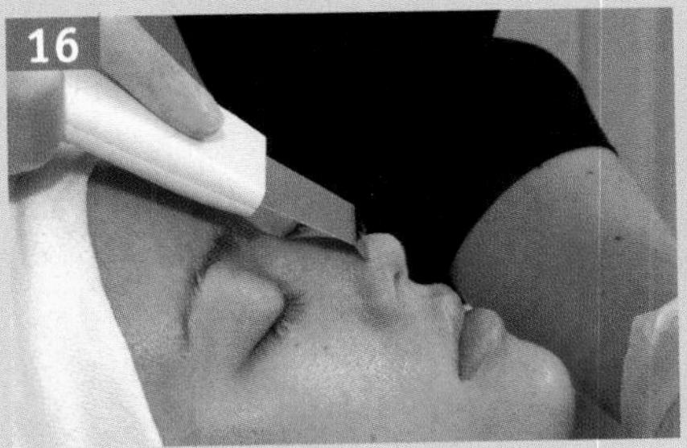

Stroke nose downward.

16 Stroke downward on the nose.

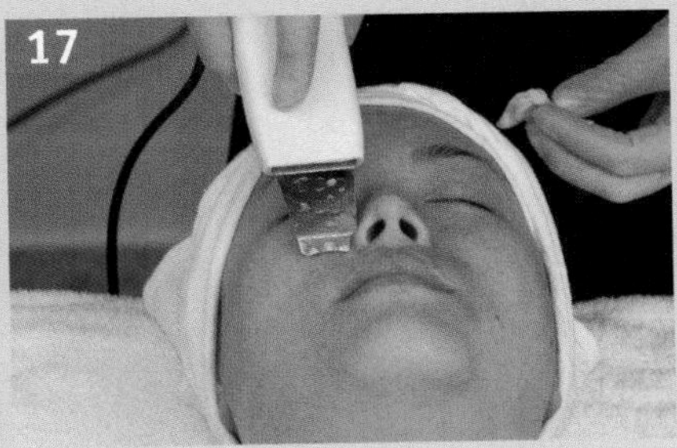

Use blade for nasal flare.

17 Use the corner of blade to stroke around the nasal flares.

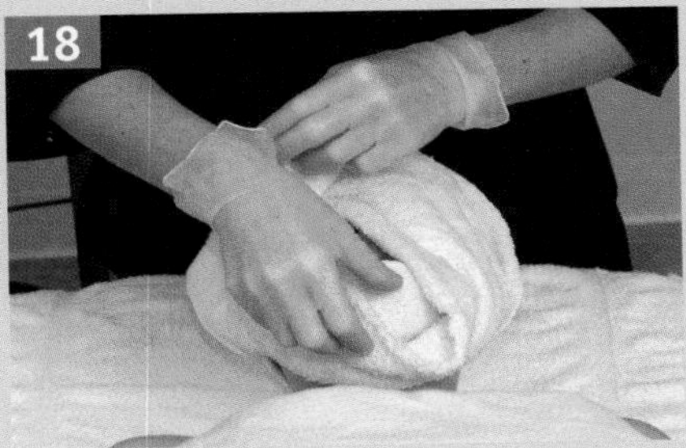

Rinse.

18 Rinse with sponges and/or a warm towel.

Part II: Hydration and Penetration of Serums for the Facial Area

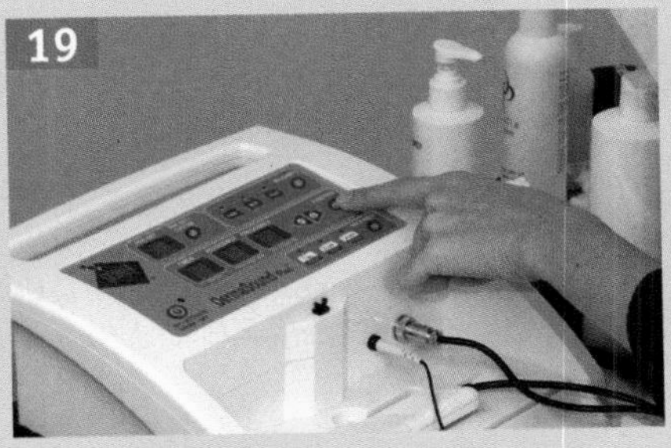

Adjust settings.

19 Adjust machine settings as the manufacturer recommends. Some units have a round penetration handpiece with a flat head that is used in circular motions as directed by the manufacturer.

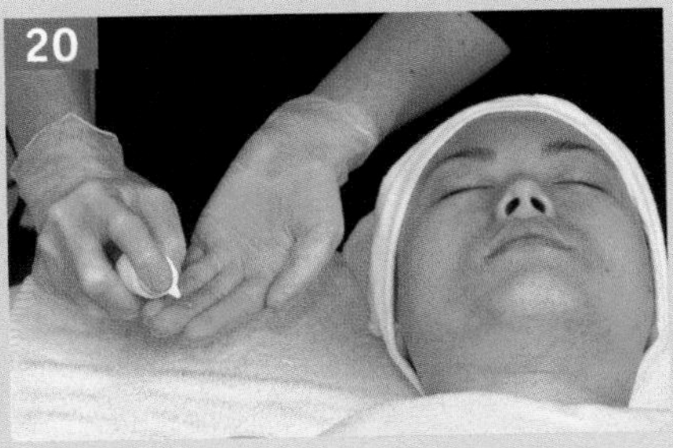

Apply products.

20 Apply product to be penetrated in accordance with manufacturer guidelines. If your device uses iontophoresis rather than sonophoresis adjust the settings according to the pH of the product being used following manufacturer guidelines.

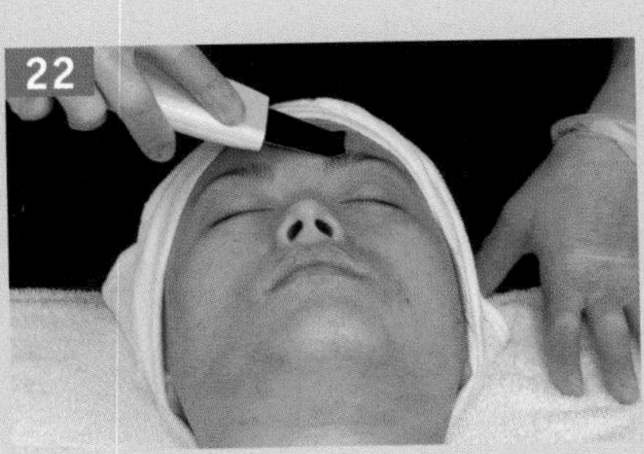

Turn blade over.

21 As in Part I, start with the forehead. If the skin shows signs of laxity, isolate areas in the same manner.

22 Turn the blade over, holding it at a 30° angle with the blade tip facing upward.

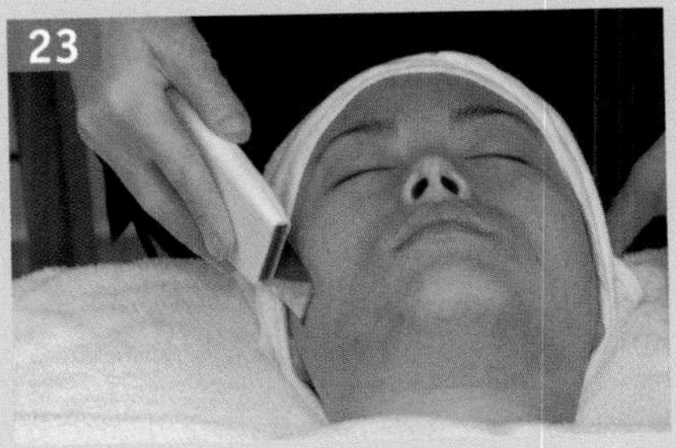

Gently glide without pressure.

23 Gently glide the handpiece across the skin surface in a light gliding movement with *no* pressure. (Think of it as gently ironing the lines away and helping performance ingredients penetrate.)

24 Increase or decrease intensity as indicated by the manufacturer.

25 Apply additional serum as needed to maintain moisture level.

continues on next page

PROCEDURE 18–4, CONT. ULTRASONIC FACIAL

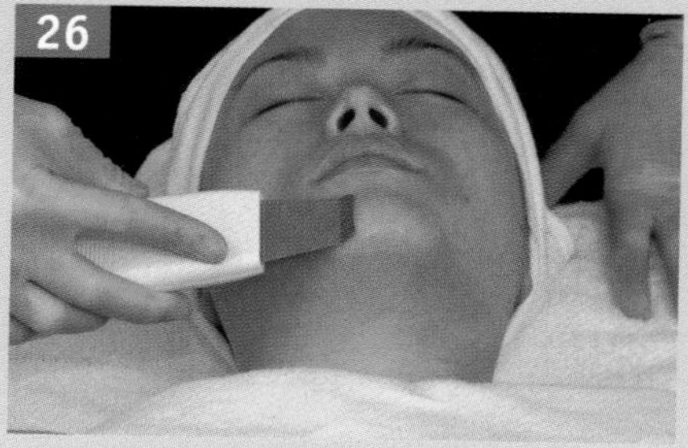

Move both horizontally and vertically.

26 Make strokes in both horizontal and vertical directions, as in Part I.

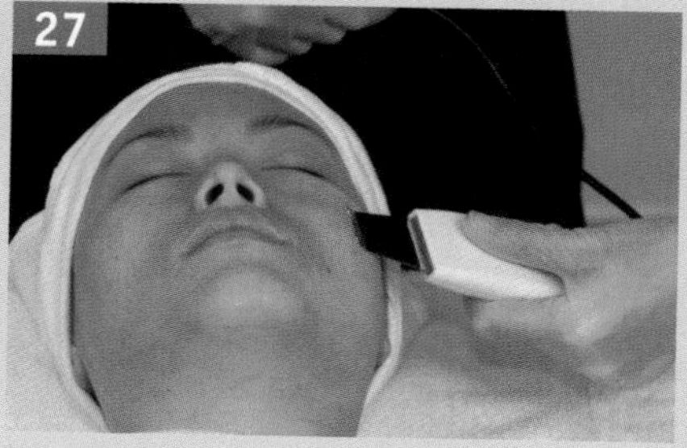

Move over cheeks, chin, and center.

27 Move to the cheeks, chin, and the center of the face, repeating the process.

28 When you have treated the entire face, either move to the micro-amp phase of unit operations or conclude with a moisturizer and sun protection.

Part III: The Micro-amp Phase

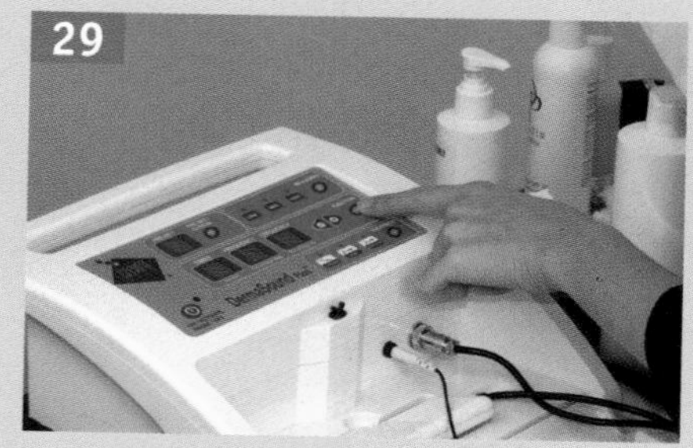

Adjust settings.

29 Some ultrasonic units have settings specifically for the micro-amp or homeostasis phase. See the manufacturer's recommendations for those settings.

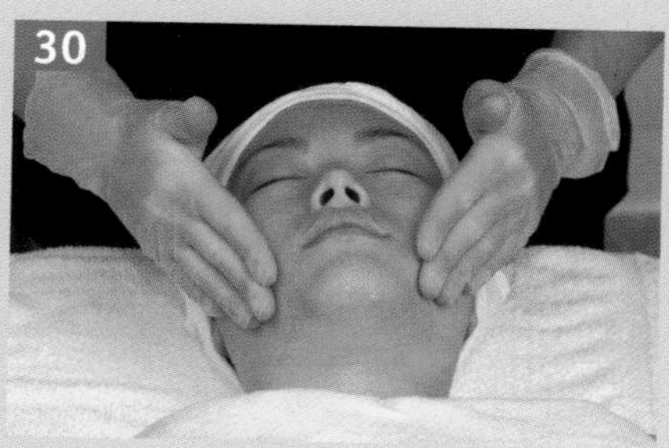

Apply gel.

30 Apply conductive gel as recommended.

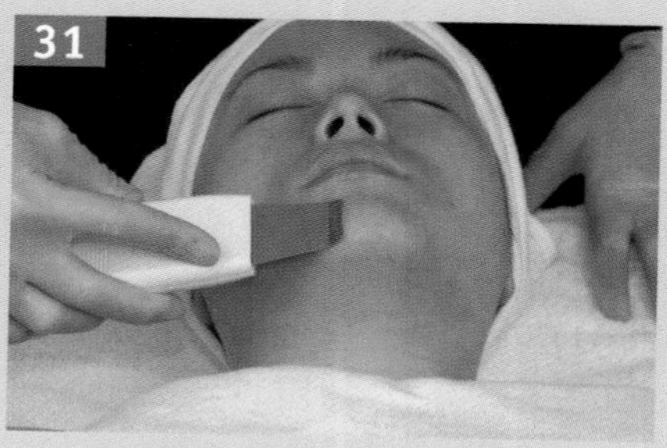

Blade tip facing up.

31 As in Part II, use the blade with the tip facing up.

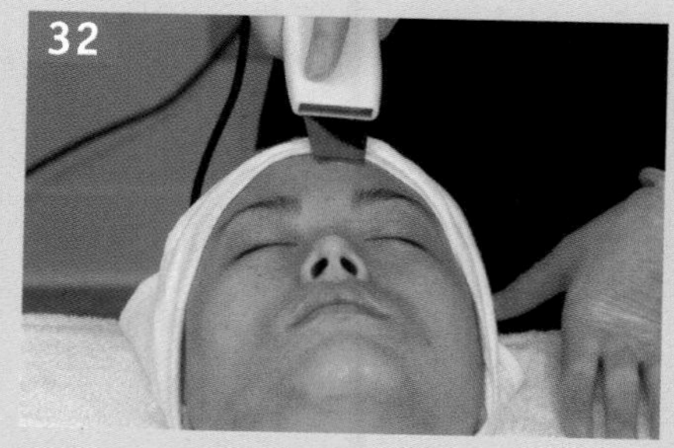

Work systematically around face.

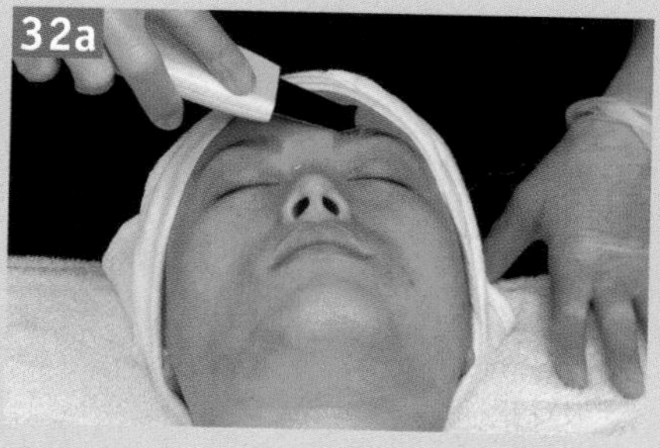

Both horizontal and vertical.

32 Following the same protocol as in Part II, work systematically around the face performing horizontal and vertical strokes.

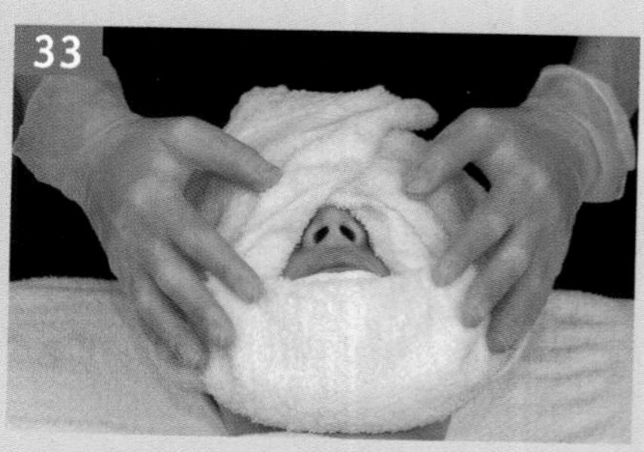

Follow the same protocols.

33 Rinse off excess gel with warm, moist towel.

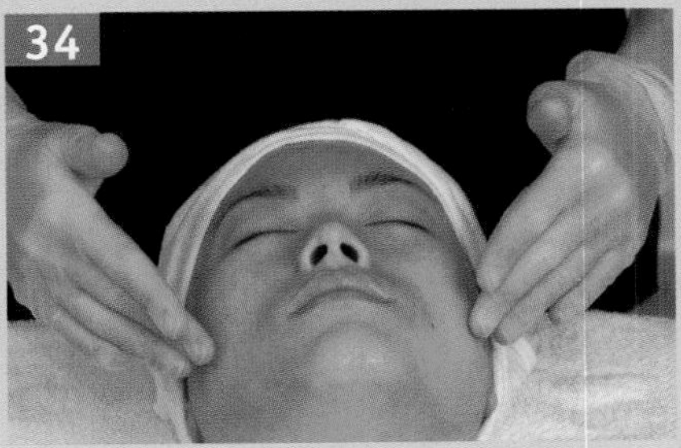

Apply products.

34 Apply moisturizer and sun protection as needed.

Post-procedure

35 Inform the client about appropriate home care.

36 Reschedule his or her next visit.

Clean-up and Disinfection

37 Perform clean-up and disinfection according to OSHA or your state's regulations.

38 Disinfect the device and implements according to the manufacturer's recommendations.

ELECTRODESSICATION DEVICES (RADIO FREQUENCY)

Electrodessication comes for the Latin word *desiccare,* meaning "to dry." An electrodessication device (Figure 18–14) uses low-level radio-frequency current to create heat that evaporates cellular fluid and causes either blanching of the target, vasospasm, or results in a dark, coagulated vessel. The treatment is specific and results in minimal skin reaction or collateral tissue damage. The units use an external probe and gel to conduct the energy on the surface of the skin. The probes vary in size—smaller for the facial area and larger for the body areas.

Units have been developed for clinic and medi-spa settings using low-level radio-frequency current to help remove unsightly minor skin irregularities (Figure 18–14). Units may be classified as Class I or Class II medical devices and may be subject to medical supervision or may not even be in your scope of practice. Numerous devices on the market integrate low levels of radio-frequency and high-frequency current, which arch onto the skin and attract moisture from the skin lesion. Too much heat can lead to lateral tissue damage with possible scarring and hypo- or hyperpigmentation. (See Chapter 8 for more information.)

Before performing any services with these devices, make sure you have had thorough hands-on training and knowledge of your state regulations. If you are working without medical supervision, you can use only over-the-counter topical anesthetic agents. If a treatment requires the injection of anesthetics as opposed to topical agents, injections must be performed by a properly licensed

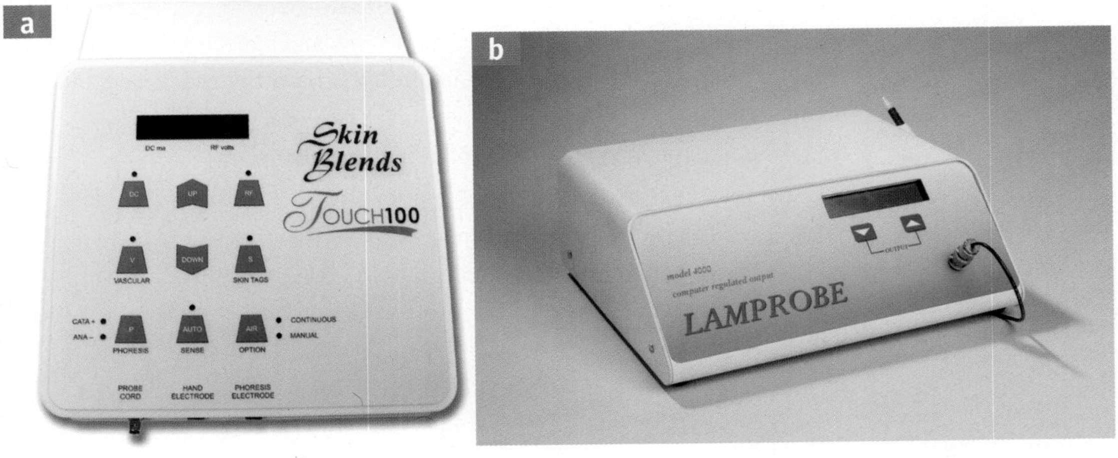

Figure 18–14 Electrodessication units.

> **★ REGULATORY AGENCY ALERT**
>
> Keep in mind that in the majority of states, estheticians are not allowed to perform any ablative procedure, which includes anything that cuts, vaporizes, or removes skin tissue. Check with your state agency before purchasing or performing electrodessication procedures unless you work under direct medical supervision. Even then this procedure may not be in your scope of practice as an esthetician.

medical practitioner. If the services are performed under a physician's supervision, then prescription-strength superficial topical anesthetics may be used.

Indications for Treatment

Candidates for electrodessication services include those with common cosmetic lesions, such as milia, sebaceous hyperplasia cysts, telangectasias, skin tags, cholesterol deposits, and cherry angiomas. Most of these procedures will be performed under medical supervision, so follow the protocols provided by those medical professionals for all electrodessication services.

> **★ REGULATORY AGENCY ALERT**
>
> Because electrodessication changes the skin or blood vessels in it, your state may define this type of procedure as needing to be medically regulated. Check with your state regulatory agency to determine whether these treatments fall into your scope of practice.

Contraindications to Treatment

If a client comes in with a suspicious-looking lesion, refer him or her to a medical provider for consultation. Clients who are not candidates for electrodessication are those with open wounds, high blood pressure, pregnancy, a heart condition, a pacemaker or pacemaker leads, a muscular disease, epilepsy, advanced diabetes, and autoimmune disorders (because of a reduced ability to resist infection). If a client has any metal implants or other contraindications, refer him or her to a physician for written approval for the service.

> ***FYI***
>
> Never attempt to diagnose a skin lesion. Refer all such cases to a physician for diagnosis.

PROCEDURE 18–5 ELECTRODESSICATION TREATMENT FOR SKIN TAG

IMPLEMENTS AND MATERIALS

- Typical facial lounge, client draping, and linen setup
- Disposable sponges or 4 × 4 gauze squares
- Water and bowl
- Cotton rounds
- Oil-free cleanser to degrease skin
- Antiseptic solution
- Anesthetics (pre-applied per manufacturer's guidelines)
- Conductive gel
- Plastic tweezers (disposable)
- Sharps container for any nondisposable items
- Sterile implements as suitable for the specific device and treatment
- Gloves (nytril or vinyl)
- Antibiotic ointment (if appropriate)

Preparation

Perform general treatment room setup:

1. Prepare the treatment table with linens.
2. Check the device for proper operation.
3. Gather and set up disposables and products.
4. Review the client's concerns, medical history, and indications for treatment, along with discussion of anticipated results. Have the client read and sign a consent form.
5. Take photographs prior to and following the treatment.
6. Have the client remove all metal and jewelry.
7. If recommended, apply topical anesthesia to the area and reapply it 30 to 60 minutes before the procedure.

Procedure

8. Wash your hands and put on gloves.

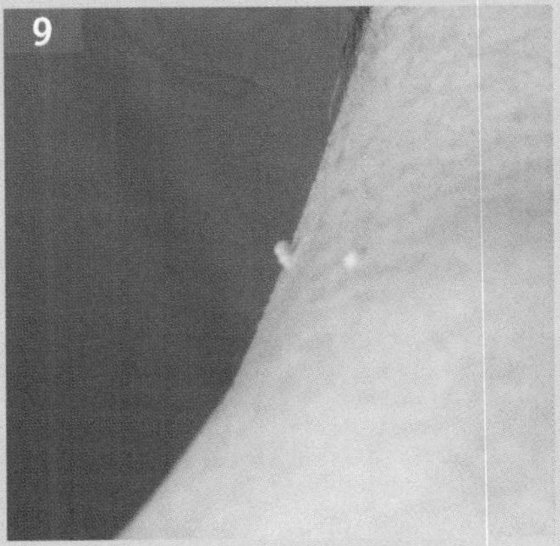

Pre-cleanse entire area to be treated.

9 Pre-cleanse entire area to be treated.

10 Wipe the client's skin with antiseptic solution on a 2 × 2 gauze pad and allow it to dry completely.

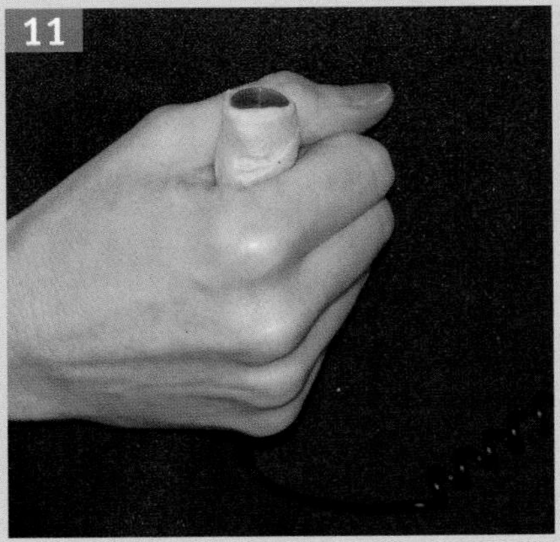

A client may be required to hold a ground.

11 Your manufacturer's directions may require the client to hold a ground, as with galvanic facial therapies. Treatment parameters vary by device; follow the manufacturer's recommendations.

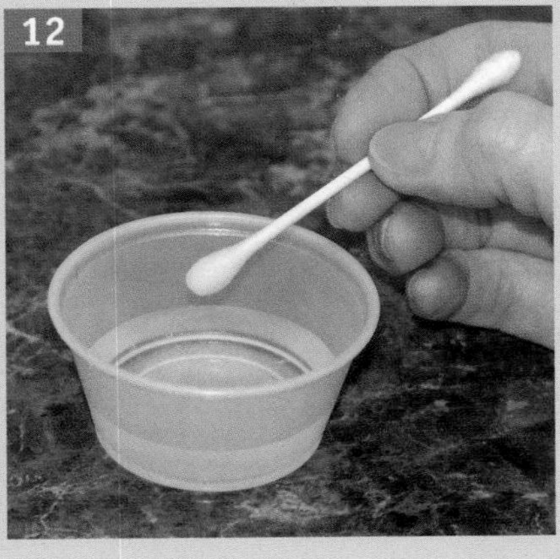

Apply conductive gel.

12 Apply conductive gel with a cotton swab to target area.

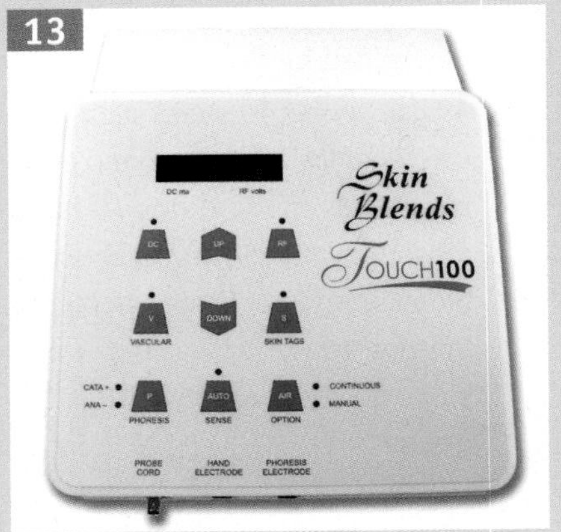

Treatment parameters per device will vary depending on manufacturer.

13 Place a sterile probe on the surface of the skin at the target area.

14 At low-level radio-frequency/direct current pass through the probe to the vessel or target lesion.

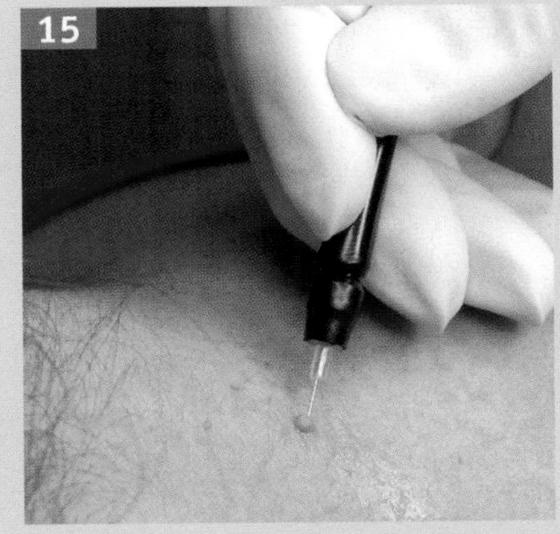

Start at the base of the tag just above the skin surface.

15 Use these steps to remove skin tags; the target is the base of the tag just above the skin surface. Look for blanching or coagulation of the vessel or targeted lesion.

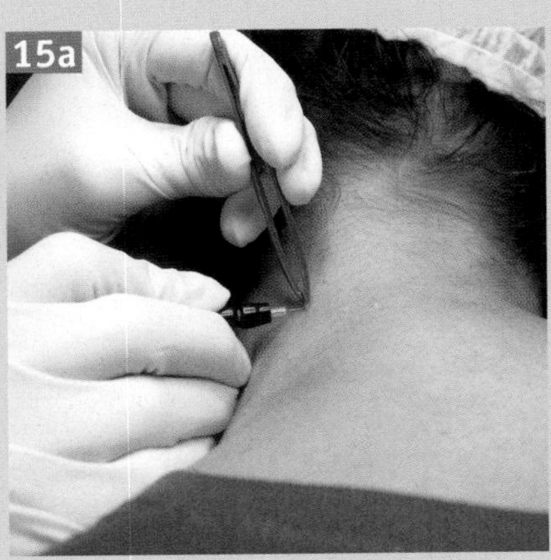

Use plastic tweezers to extend the tag.

a. Use plastic tweezers to extend the tag.

b. Use radio-frequency current only.

continues on next page

PROCEDURE 18-5, CONT. ELECTRODESSICATION TREATMENT FOR SKIN TAG

15a1

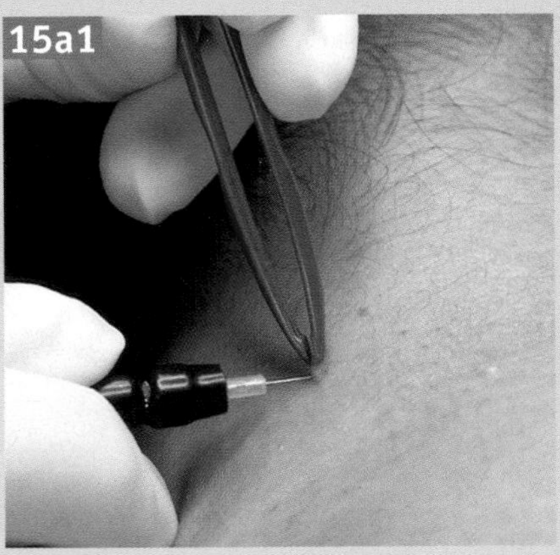

Use plastic tweezers to extend the tag.

15c

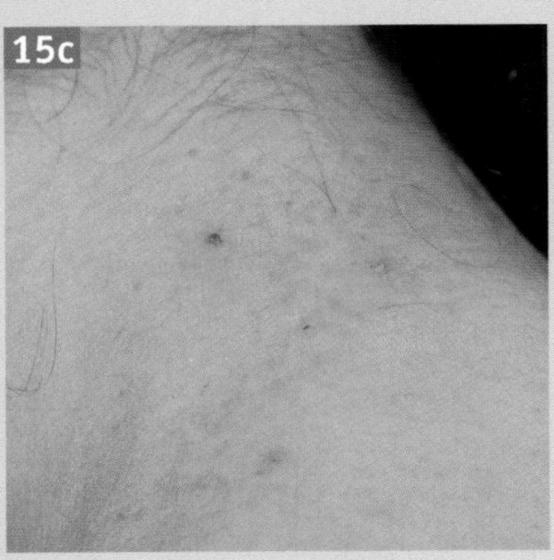

Close up 30 minutes after treatment.

Note: The treatment causes a disruption of blood flow, resulting in the tag dropping off in several days to a week.

15c1

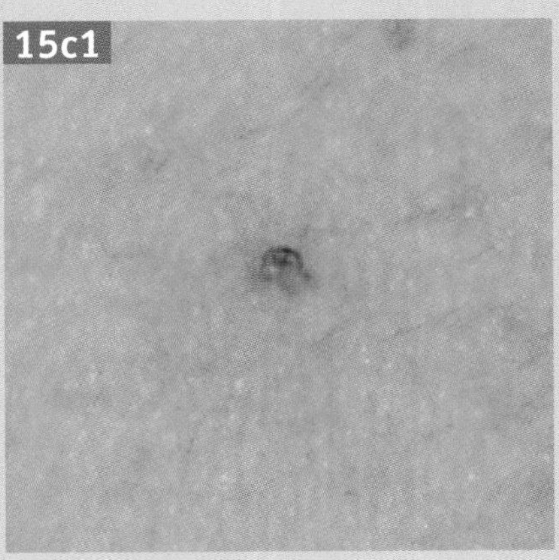

30 minutes after treatment.

15c2

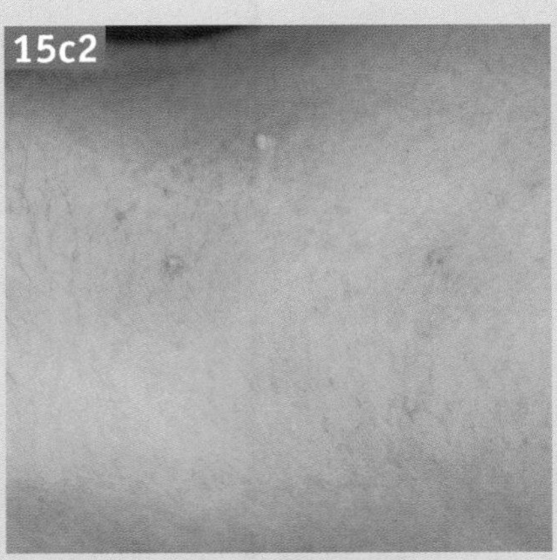

After treatment

Post-procedure

16 The client's skin may be tender after treatment. Tell the client not to disturb lesions or vessels for 24 hours.

17 If the manufacturer or supervising physician recommends it, apply an antibacterial ointment to the treated area.

18 Use only soothing and hydrating products.

19 Apply sunscreen along with a post-treatment cosmeticeutical as recommended by the manufacturer.

20 Advise clients to avoid sun exposure, saunas, steam rooms, exercise, and rubbing the treated area. Any activity that raises blood pressure may cause an inferior result and could cause blood to resume flow within the treated area.

21 For treatments in the facial area, advise the client to abstain from washing, rubbing, or patting the face for the first 12 hours.

22 Document the equipment settings used for the client's treatment in treatment record sheets.

Clean-up and Disinfection

23 Perform clean-up and disinfection according to OSHA or your state regulatory agencies.

24 Dispose of any sharps directly into a sharps container.

25 Disinfect and sterilize probes per the manufacturer's guidelines.

MICROCURRENT "FACIAL TONING"

Microcurrent technology is used in the treatment of loss of muscle tone in the face due to the effects of aging, genetics, sun, and gravity. Microcurrent devices operate on a very low level of current called the *microampere*. (The symbol for the microampere is "A.") The **microampere** is a current of .001 ampere or less, which is generally defined as the cosmetic current level. Microcurrent treatments typically use a combination of galvanic and faradic current. The galvanic current is a direct current (DC) and utilizes the iontophoresis mode for penetration of an ionized solution into the surface tissue. The faradic current is a DC galvanic interrupted current that is used to affect the tone of the muscles through microcontraction muscle sequences. The unit usually has an Hz (cycles per second) setting, which allows for changes in frequency and in whether the muscle will be relaxed (lengthened) or tightened (shortened).

Microcurrent units typically come with two handpieces or probes that may have electrodes on the ends. These may be single electrodes or double-pronged units (Figure 18–15). The probes culminate in metal electrodes or in hollow tubes that allow for the insertion of cotton swabs soaked in a conductive medium. The cotton swabs are less conductive than the metal probes and may be more suitable for some clients. Some devices include gloves with sensors in the fingertips that the technician wears to perform the service. Special glove liners ensure the current goes to the client, not the technician. These gloves conduct the least current and are more suitable for areas where you want minimal penetration or for clients who are very sensitive to electricity.

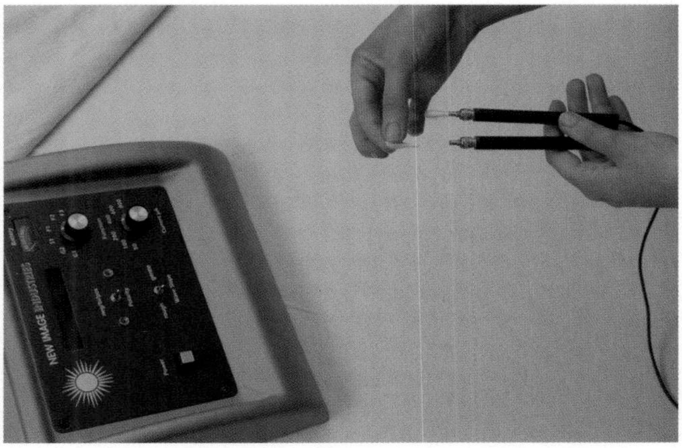

Figure 18–15 An example of microcurrent machine with single probe.

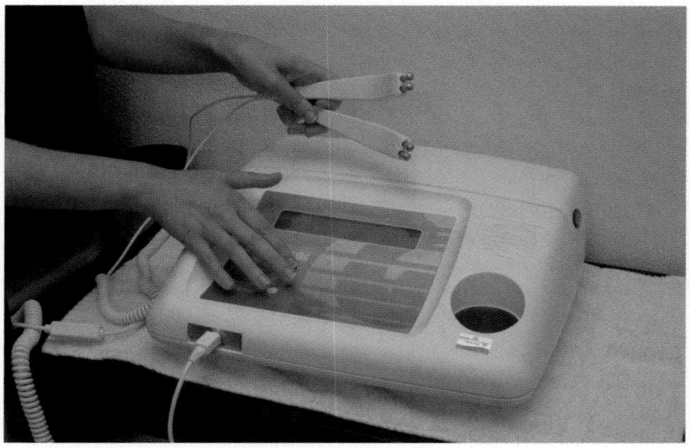

Figure 18–16 Microcurrent with dual metal probe.

The probes are applied to the treatment area and moved with distinct and very precise directional movements to strengthen or relax facial muscles. The protocol for relaxation of the muscle is to position the probes at the base of the muscle (also called its *belly*) and move them toward the origin and insertion. This movement results in relaxing and lengthening of the muscle (Figure 18–16). The protocol for lifting, strengthening, or tightening the muscle involves positioning the probes at the muscle origin with a steady movement toward the muscle. There are various other movements that can be administered, depending on the area and issue to be addressed, but relaxing and tightening are the most often performed with microcurrent technology.

Many microcurrent devices also offer micro-amp therapy. This allows for penetration of products into the skin or for cellular stimulation, with the goal being enhanced ATP output at the cellular level without the use of massage. (Massage is contraindicated following facial toning services.)

Indications for Treatment

Microcurrent parameters and techniques can be combined to enhance the deep penetration of therapeutic serums for hydrating dry skin while stimulating tissue circulation and nourishment uptake. Microcurrent treatments are beneficial for reducing facial laxity, raising brows, tightening jawlines, and reducing submental chin laxity. Microcurrent treatments may result in toning of facial muscles, decreasing the look of sagging lines and skin laxity prevalent with aging (Table 18–1).

Contraindications to Treatment

Before a microcurrent treatment, screen clients for evidence of open wounds, cancerous lesions, a heart condition, pacemaker or pacemaker leads, muscular diseases,

Table 18–1 Microcurrent Treatment of Various Muscle Groups

DESIRED TREATMENT	MUSCLE GROUP	TECHNIQUE
Reduction of eyelid hooding and brow drooping	**Obicularis oculi muscle** closes the eyelid and compresses the lacrimal sac (tear duct)	Lifting, strengthening, and tightening
Reduction of jawline laxity and skin drooping	**Temporalis muscle** elevates and closes the jaw, retracts the mandible	Lifting, strengthening and tightening
Reduction of furrowing and lines between brows	**Corrugator muscle** brings the eyebrows together in the glabellar area	Relaxing and lengthening
Reduction of furrowing and lines between brows	**Procerus muscle** depresses and move eyebrows together	Relaxing and lengthening
Reduction of forehead lines and laxity	**Frontalis muscle** lifts the eyebrows and causes forehead transverse wrinkle lines	Relaxing and lengthening
Reduction of marionette lines	**Risorius muscle** retracts the mouth	Lifting, strengthening, and tightening
Reduction of marionette lines	**Zygomaticus major and minor muscles** raise the mouth upward and backward when one smiles	Lifting, strengthening, and tightening

epilepsy, advanced diabetes, hemophilia, and pregnancy. A medical practitioner or physician needs to assess clients with newly injected fillers, Botox, and/or implants.

Because the treatment is dependent on proper positioning, it is important to review muscle location, origin, and insertion. Improper placement could result in no improvement or an undesired result such as further relaxation of an already lax muscle.

Client Protocol

As the movements are complex and lengthy, this chapter will only address the use of microcurrent on the obicularis occuli area (Figure 18–17). Each manufacturer uses slightly different movements based on the configuration of the device. The manufacturer of your device should provide complete training with the device and list the protocols appropriate for that unit.

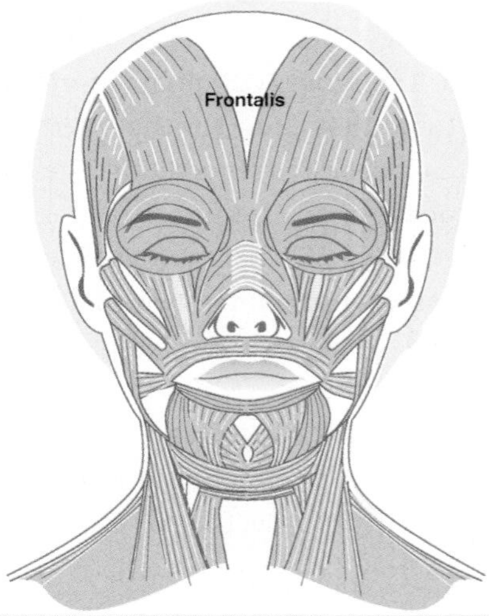

Figure 18–17 Facial muscles.

PROCEDURE 18-6 MICROCURRENT FOR OBICULARIS OCCULI

IMPLEMENTS AND MATERIALS

- Typical facial lounge, client draping, and linen setup
- Bowl and water
- Disposable sponges, 4 × 4 gauze squares, or facial cloths
- Cotton swabs with paper shaft or presterilized metal probes
- Gentle cleanser
- Ionized ampoule or serum
- Conductive gel
- Moisturizer and sunscreen

Preparation

1 Perform general treatment room setup:

a. Prepare the treatment table with linens.

b. Check the device for proper operation.

c. Gather and set up disposables and products.

2 Review the client's concerns, indications for treatment, and anticipated results.

3 Have the client read and sign a consent form.

4 Take photos—both full-face and profile views—before and throughout the treatment process,.

Procedure

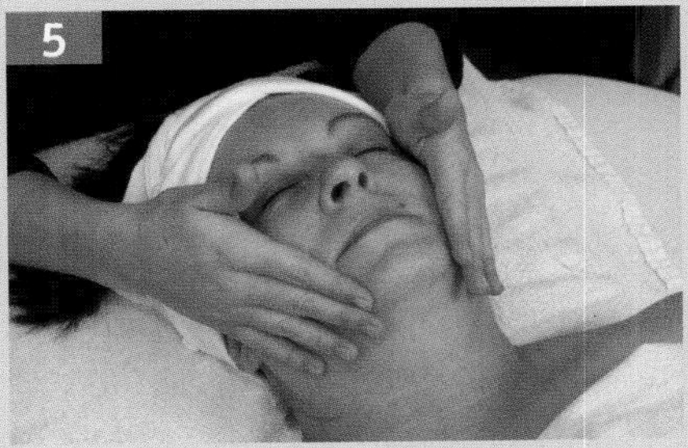

Cleanse the skin.

5 Cleanse the skin using a gentle, water-based cleanser. Rinse and remove.

6 Apply the conductive gel or manufacturer's lotion along the area that you will be treating.

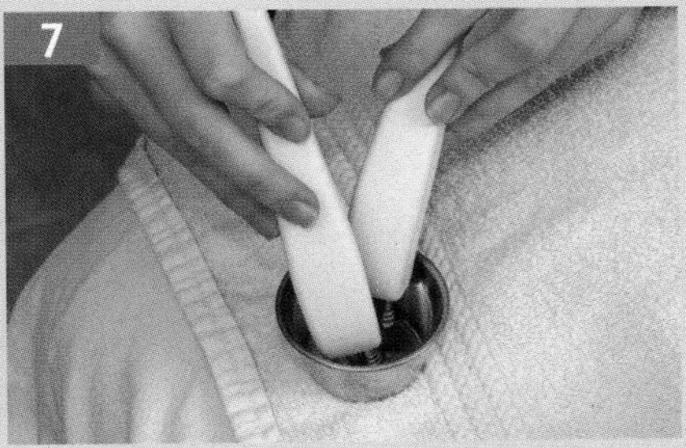

Moisten applicators.

7 Moisten the metal conducting probes or cotton swabs that are inserted into the conducting probes with manufacturer's recommended product.

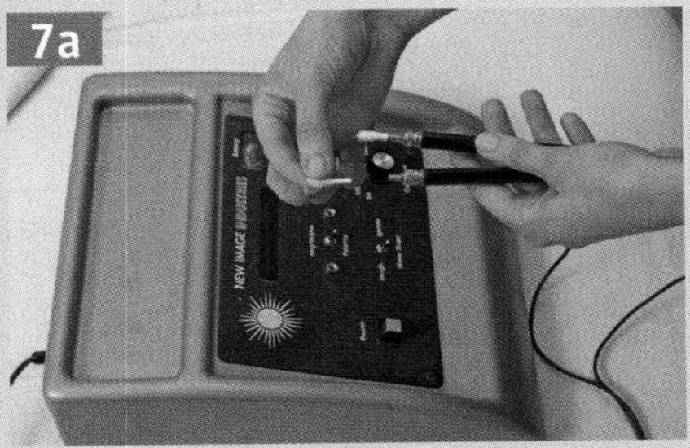

Moisten applicators.

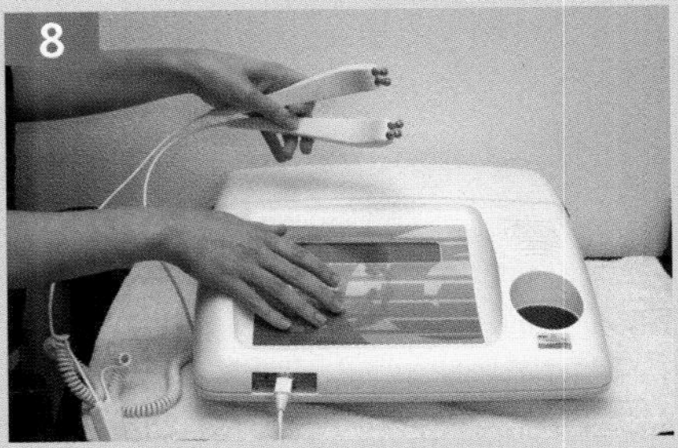

Set currents.

8 Set the machine currents to the levels recommended by the manufacturer for the eye area.

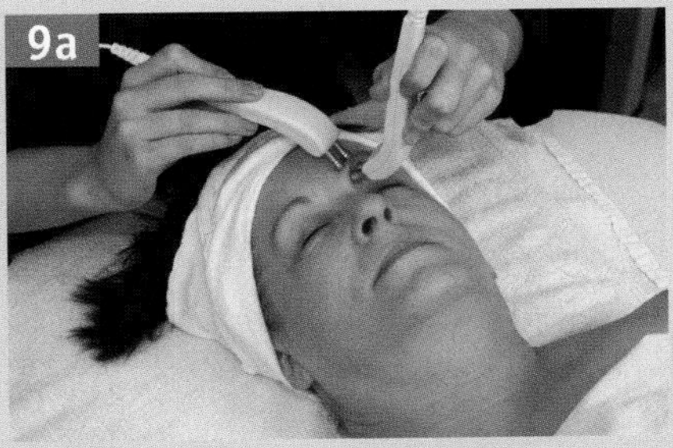

Place one electrode at brow.

9 Starting at the end of the brow closest to the nose, systematically move toward the brow end closest to the hairline.

a. Place one electrode at top edge of eyebrow hair at the start of the brow.

b. Place the other electrode directly below the brow.

continues on next page

PROCEDURE 18–6, CONT. MICROCURRENT FOR OBICULARIS OCCULI

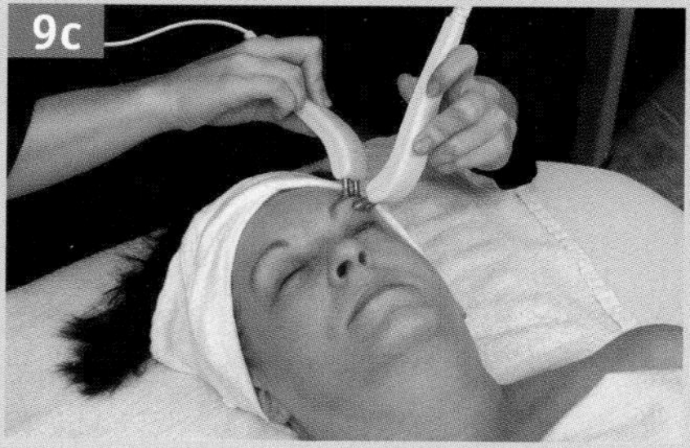

Use a compression-like movement.

c. Move the lower electrode toward the stationary electrode to pinch together a ½-inch fold of tissue with a compression-like movement.

d. Hold for 4 seconds (or the time specified by the manufacturer).

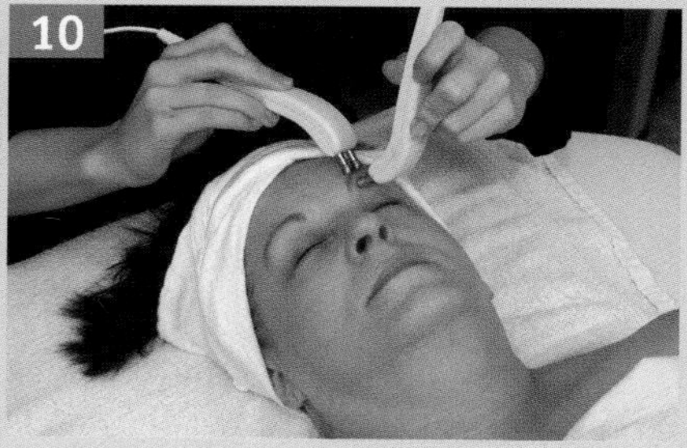

Move along the brow, toward hairline.

10 Move a scant 1/3 inch out along the brow toward the hairline (or as directed by manufacturer). Compress and hold for 4 seconds.

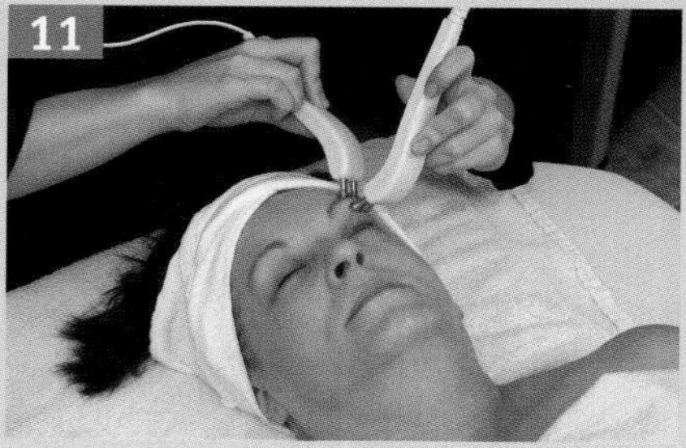

Continue entire length of brow.

11 Continue the same process in 1/3 inch-increments until you have completed compression movements along the entire length of the brow.

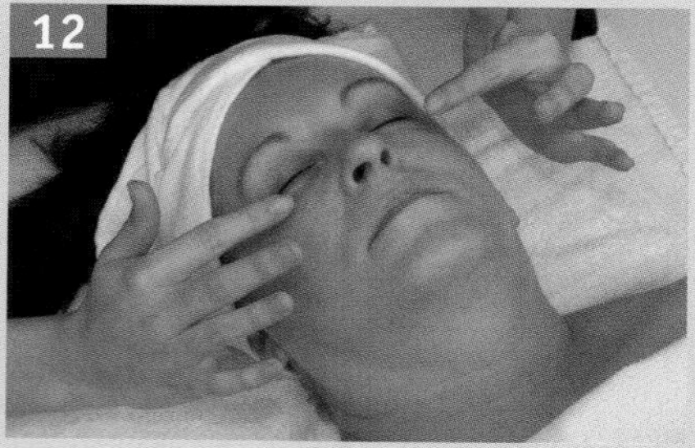

Apply products.

12 Apply eye serum and SPF protection.

13 Do not perform additional massage on the client.

Post-procedure

14 Tell the client that he or she can resume normal home care and daily activities.

Clean-up and Disinfection

15 Perform clean-up and disinfection according to your state's regulations.

16 Disinfect and sterilize the probes per the manufacturer's guidelines.

CAUTION!

Each unit is programmed differently. Follow the guidelines for settings and duration of each movement provided by your unit's manufacturer.

FYI

For effective results, microcurrent treatments are scheduled two to three times per week for an average of 10 treatments. Depending on the client's age, he or she may need monthly maintenance treatments.

MANAGEMENT OF COMPLICATIONS

Even though you are a competently trained and educated esthetician, clients will occasionally experience complications. They are a part of the cosmetic business. If a client experiences a side effect or complication, the protocol to follow is very straightforward:

1. Have the client discuss the problem with you.
2. Then have them come to your work area so you can do a visual assessment. Document your assessment and interventions.
3. Finally, seek intervention by a physician or medical provider.

Documentation is essential for quality assurance and risk management purposes along with photographs of the problematic area. It is important to maintain your client-esthetician relationship and follow the client throughout the healing phase. It is also important for the client to know that you are attentive and supportive and want him or her to achieve the best possible outcome. Table 18–2 shows possible side effects that a client may experience, no matter what device is being used.

As technology advances, new systems and techniques are being accepted as standardized esthetic practice. Procedures are becoming more aggressive and complicated and are being combined with other rejuvenating treatments. It is important to take the time and undergo the appropriate training under direct supervision before treating your own customers. Do not be shy. Ask questions of your physician, manufacturer representatives, and peers. Seek out the opportunity to network on a local and national level. Finally, trust your own judgment and always proceed cautiously when initiating a new procedure or working with a new client.

Table 18–2 Interventions for Possible Complications

SIDE EFFECT	POSSIBLE INTERVENTIONS
Excessive swelling	Apply ice packs and advise the client to sleep with extra pillows. Occasionally, oral antihistamine medication can be helpful.
Excessive redness or skin reaction	Immediately apply and reapply cold compresses and soothing skin preparation, such as aloe vera. Physician may prescribe topical steroid administration to the injured site.
Blistering or crusting	Keep the area covered, apply antibiotic ointment, and do not pop the skin if blistered. Physician may order steroids or antibiotics.
Hyperpigmentation	Physician may prescribe bleaching creams (hydroquinone) along with the constant use of sunscreens.
Hypopigmentation	This hopefully will resolve itself in 6 to 24 months.
Infection	Physician may order antibiotic, antiviral, or antifungal medications.
Scarring	Collagen rebuilding laser treatments to reduce the appearance of the scar (1,320 nm, 1,550 nm, 1,450 nm lasers)

REVIEW QUESTIONS

1. List six steps involved in the purchase of a cosmetic device.
2. Describe the two types of crystals used in microdermabrasion.
3. What is the facial technique for using a microdermabrasion device?
4. What are the components of a successful consultation?
5. Why do you not want to treat a recently suntanned client with IPL?
6. What safety measures should you enforce during an IPL treatment?
7. What are the benefits of an IPL facial rejuvenation treatment?
8. What types of skin can benefit from treatment with an LED device?
9. Describe three procedures that can be performed with electrodessication.

LEARNING OBJECTIVES

After completing this chapter, you should be able to:

- Discuss the importance of safety and disinfection procedures.
- Describe basic threading techniques and their uses.
- Discuss sugaring as an alternative technique.
- Employ advanced facial waxing techniques.
- Build speed-waxing techniques.
- Perform Brazilian waxing.
- Perform male waxing services.
- Discuss the basics of laser and IPL hair removal.
- Describe liability issues related to hair removal.

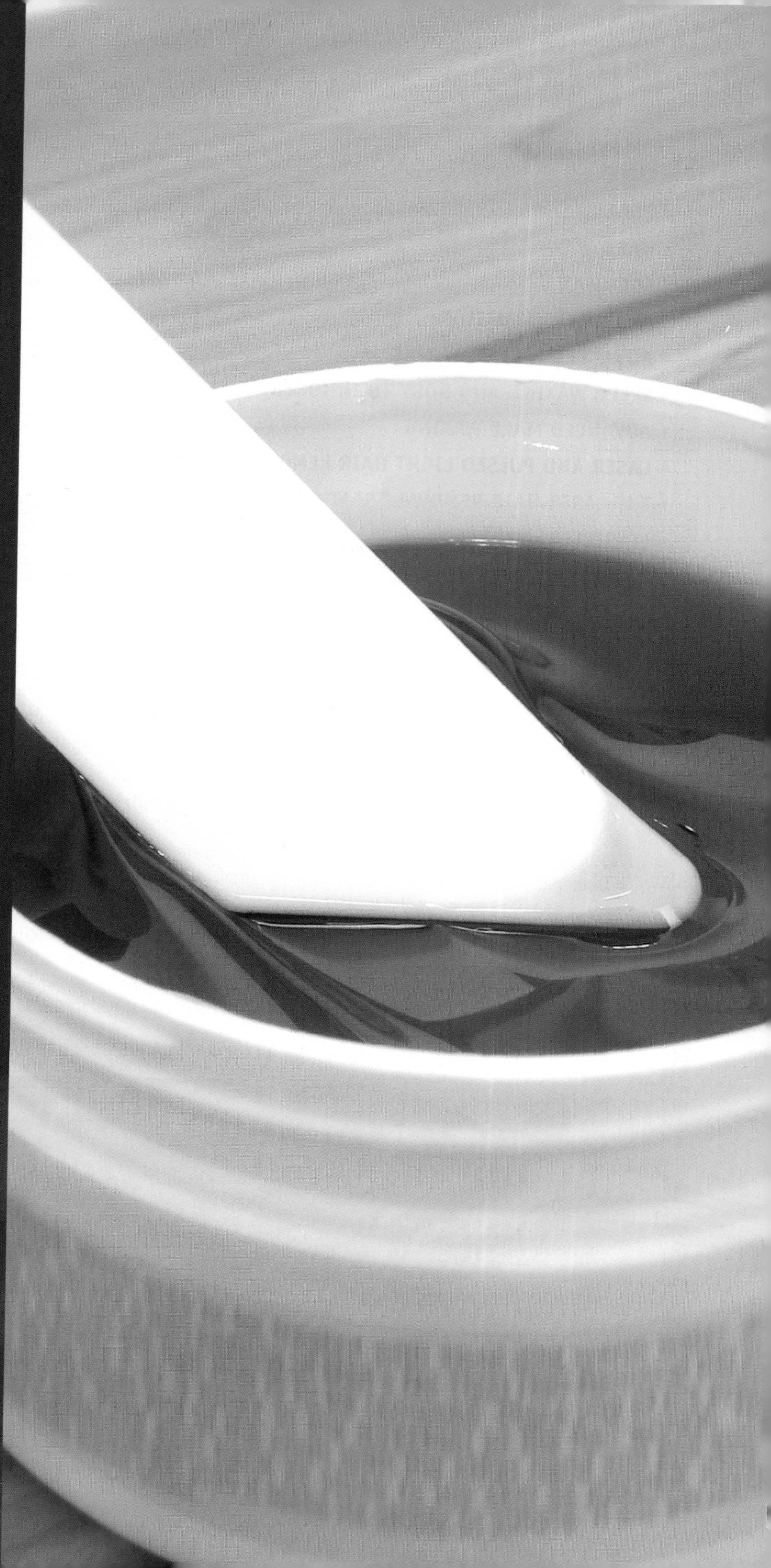

KEY TERMS

Page numbers indicate where in the chapter the term is used.

chromophore 503
dermal scattering 513
energy fluence 510
fatlah 478
human papillomavirus (HPV) 478
hydroquinone 515
joules 513
khite 478
monochromatic 503
Nikolski sign 509
oxyhemoglobin 512
polychromatic 504
pulse duration 510
pulse width 513
selective photothermolysis 504
splattering 515
thermal storage 510
threading 478

Hair removal is big business. A client's personal preference and budget will dictate whether he or she seeks temporary hair removal, permanent hair reduction, or electrolysis. Whatever technique you use in your clinic, client safety and disinfection are paramount. Your skill and knowledge of multiple hair removal techniques will allow you to better serve and educate your clients.

? Did You Know

Each hair follicle has the potential to grow more than one hair. This is why hair may reappear even after permanent hair removal. A new hair will grow from the follicle in which another was destroyed.

SAFETY AND DISINFECTION FIRST

As you learned in basic waxing, safety and disinfection precautions are important. This cannot be stressed enough. Times have changed and old practices have been retired because of risks to you and/or your client. Just as your physician and dentist have changed their techniques to more modern, sanitary ones, so must you, the esthetician.

CAUTION!

Always wear gloves during procedures and replace them if they become compromised.

When hair is extracted from skin, there is a *real potential* for blood, lymph, or body fluids to come to the surface. This means two things for you. First, wear gloves during all hair-removal procedures, such as waxing, tweezing, and sugaring. Second, take care to avoid cross-contamination of product or applicators from client to client. As you do more intimate waxing, such as the Brazilian, it is critical to keep in mind the possibility of herpetic breakouts or genital warts, along with other health issues. The more hygienic your practice, the more comfortable clients will be with coming there for intimate waxing services.

Herpes Simplex Breakouts

A herpes simplex virus (HSV-2) breakout presents as an ulceration on the penis or the mucous membrane of the vulva, vagina, and cervix. Recurrent breakouts usually occur in the genital and buttock regions. Tingling, itching, or burning will usually result in clusters of vesicles on a red platform. Infections usually heal within 7 to 10 days. Mild fever, pain, and swollen lymph nodes sometimes accompany recurrent HSV-2.

Clients with HSV-2 are acutely aware of the virus and its patterns of breakout. You will discover this when you take a thorough health history during the pre-treatment consultation. Counsel these clients to obtain antiviral medication from a physician, which they should use prior to hair removal treatments. Under no circumstances should you perform hair-removal services on a client experiencing a herpetic breakout.

Genital Warts

Genital warts are visible signs of a cutaneous viral infection—the most common sexually transmitted disease—caused by the **human papillomavirus** (HPV or genital herpes). Scientists have identified more than 100 different types of HPV, and by some accounts as many as 80% of people worldwide have been infected by at least one type of HPV. Most people do not even know that they have been infected with genital warts. Because infection can go unnoticed, transmission is easy. If during waxing you find any unidentified lesions in the pelvic area, abort the procedure and refer the client to a physician for diagnosis and treatment.

Pregnancy

Pregnant women, particularly those in the third trimester, should not have hair removal procedures in which the client has to lie flat for more than 20 minutes. Many clinics require a pregnant client to obtain permission from her physician that hair removal is suitable for her. For the pregnant client an option to hair removal is a tidy bikini "trim" performed with rounded nose safety scissors. This takes less time and can be done while the client lays from side to side. Figure 19–1 offers contraindications for hair removal.

THREADING

Threading, also known as "banding," is a method of hair removal in which the technician maneuvers a looped and twisted cotton thread with his or her fingers. The most common area for threading is on the face. Although not as common as other means of hair removal, threading is worthy of mention because it is a fast, inexpensive method of mass tweezing that does not cause trauma to the skin. It is a method of hair removal worth considering for individuals who have skin treatments or use products that prohibit waxing. Threading is a technique that is difficult to self-teach, and hands-on training is recommended.

The History of Threading

Threading has been used for centuries in Middle Eastern countries such as Iran, Turkey, India, and Pakistan. In Arabic, threading is known as ***khite;*** in Egyptian, it is **fatlah.** It is an inexpensive method of hair removal that is gaining popularity in many parts of the United States. For many clients, finding an experienced and skilled "threader" is like "finding gold."

The Benefits of Threading

In the hands of a master threading practitioner, threading moves at a much faster rate than tweezing and does so without waxing's trauma to the skin. Because it does not affect the skin, threading is a good choice for individuals who cannot tolerate waxing on the face due to use of prescription medications and other products (such as Retin-A, Differin, Accutane, and alpha hydroxy acids) or who have had facial treatments that cause negative reactions when waxed. The level of discomfort during threading is usually less than electrolysis but is similar to tweezing. Because the hairs are snagged faster than tweezing, the plucking sensation is more tolerable. Threading requires only the use of strong household cotton thread, an antiseptic pretreatment, and soothing aftercare. The effects of threading closely resemble the effect of waxing and last about the same length of time. And the final benefit: The speed of an experienced and skilled technician with the minimal product overhead equates to a good profit margin.

Preparation of Equipment and the Treatment Area

To begin, use a new, clean thread for each client. As thread can wear when working, make sure you have several strands of pre-cut thread available. Place the client in the treatment chair lined with a fresh sheet, towel, or paper.

Preparation of the Client

Protect the client's hair by wrapping it to avoid snagging hairs on his or her head. After the hair is wrapped, thoroughly wash your hands. Cleanse the area to be treated of any make up, wipe it with a mild liquid antiseptic, and allow it to dry. Avoid creams, as they will remain on the hair and reduce the gripping effectiveness of the threading.

Threading Technique

The most popular areas for threading are the eyebrows, the area above the eyebrow (up to the hairline), sideburns, sides of face, upper lip, chin, and under the jaw. The thread should be a strong cotton household thread. Maintain

Contraindications

Contraindications of Waxing

- **Blood and circulatory disorders**—Blood and circulatory disorders, particularly those that cause easy bruising (e.g., thrombosis) are contraindicated.
- **Cancer treatments**—Chemotherapy and radiation may cause increased sensitivity. It would be productive to wait until 6 weeks after the last cancer treatment.
- **Epilepsy**—Epilepsy is contraindicated unless it has been controlled for a long period and with medication that does not cause easy bruising. A physician's approval must be attained before the waxing service. The technician should receive a physician's note and have the client sign a release.
- **Diabetes**—The client with diabetes should consult with the physician for the degree of severity and the degree of healing and sign a release.
- **Fractures and sprains**—The area of fracture or sprain should not be waxed until it is completely healed.
- **Hemophilia**—Clients with hemophilia should not be waxed, because bleeding can occur, especially when removing a high percentage of anagen hairs. The removal of anagen hairs breaks the cycle of blood flow to the dermal papilla and causes bleeding in the follicle.
- **Herpes, herpes simplex (cold sore)**—Clients with herpes should not be waxed during active outbreaks. Prophylactic medication should be taken before waxing.
- **Inflamed or irritated skin**—Inflamed or irritated skin should not be waxed.
- **Lack of skin sensation**—The lack ofskin sensation can be due to circulatory problems arising from heart disease, diabetes, or multiple sclerosis. There can be an increased risk of burning, injury, or infection. These clients should not be waxed.
- **Lupus**—Those with mild forms of lupus and not presenting with the rash on the areas to be waxed can be waxed, but it is not advisable. At the very least, these clients should seek referrals from physicians and sign waivers.
- **Moles, skin tags, and warts**—All moles, skin tags, and warts should be avoided. Any mole that looks suspicious; has any of the precancer signs of size, shape, and color; or has hair growing out ofit should not be waxed without the permission of a physician. Hair-removal specialists offer a valuable service when they recognize suspicious moles and refer their clients to physicians.
- **Pregnancy**—There is nothing intrinsically wrong with waxing the bikini area or any other area on the pregnant client, but a judgment should be made by both parties jointly and a release form should be signed. If the pregnant client is considered high risk, has high blood pressure or anxiety, it is better to avoid waxing. If the areas to be waxed take more than 20 minutes of the client lying flat on her back, then the client should wait until after the birth of the baby. Prolonged time flat on the back could deplete oxygen to the fetus. Even though there are no recorded cases of infants being harmed because their mothers received wax service, it leaves open the possibility of a lawsuit. The bottom line is to get a physician's permission and have the client sign a release form.
- **Scar tissue**—No scar tissue, including keloids, should be waxed over.
- **Sunburn**—Sunburned areas should not be waxed. Any such area must have healed completely.
- **Skin disorder conditions**—Skin disorder conditions like eczema, seborrhea, and psoriasis maybe waxed depending on severity. Minimal flakiness of dead skin cells can be waxed, but not i fthe skin is broken. Double dipping should be avoided. In mild cases, the skin may benefit from the exfoliating properties of waxing, but in more advanced stages, broken skin could result, so it is imperative that the technician receives asigned release from the client before waxing.
- **Varicose veins**—Technicians must not w ax over varicose veins (Figure 9–3) but they may wax surrounding areas.
- **Sensitive areas**—Never wax eyelids, inside the ears or nose, or the areola of the breast.
- **Any uncertain situation.**

Figure 19–1 Indications and contraindications.

lengths of thread in a sanitary environment and dispose used thread after each client. Thread length should range from 24 inches to 30 inches. Shorter lengths are easier to control when learning and developing the skill and are better for technicians with smaller hands. As you become more skilled, you will be able to manage a larger loop of thread.

Knot the two ends of the thread together, forming a loop. Place your forefingers, middle fingers, and thumbs through each end of the loop in a "cat's cradle." Twist the loop at one end approximately a dozen times. Then coax the twists into the center of the loop, making sure the knot is at one end near the fingers so it does not interfere with the twisting. To start threading, place the upper end of the twist under the unwanted hairs so that they hang over the twist, then quickly manipulate the twist upwards by spreading the lower fingers, thus entrapping or snagging the unwanted hairs and plucking them out (Figures 19–2 and 19–3). This is followed by quickly spreading the upper fingers, thus moving the twist toward the lower fingers, dropping some of the plucked hairs. Move quickly to another area of unwanted hairs. The fingers must move rapidly at a rate of one movement approximately every quarter of a second.

As the twist becomes congested with hair, it inhibits the rapid movement of the twisting, so twist a new part of the loop or use a new thread used (Figure 19–4). After the service is complete, apply a soothing lotion to the skin.

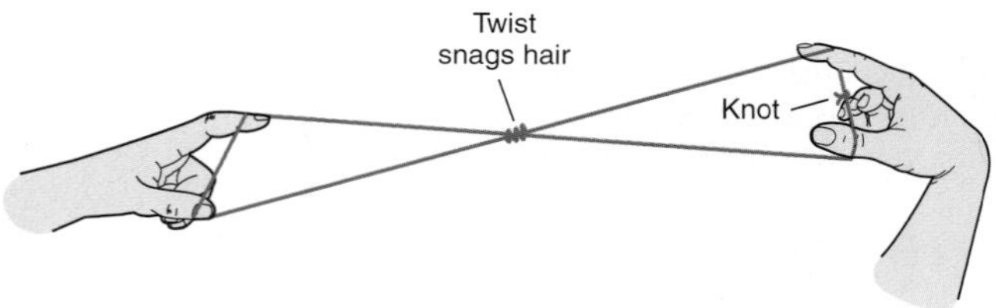

Figure 19–2 Two-handed threading.

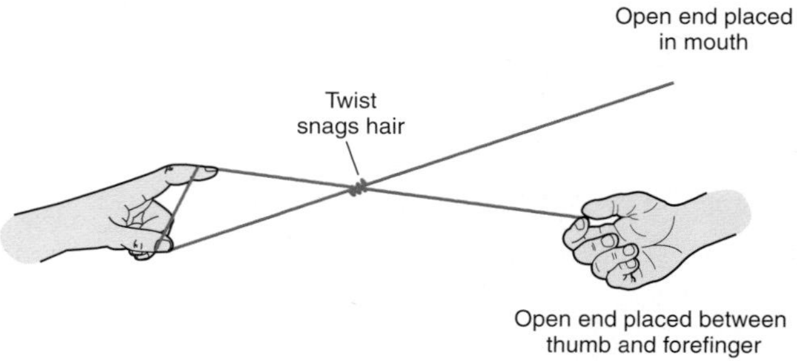

Figure 19–3 Traditional hand and mouth threading.

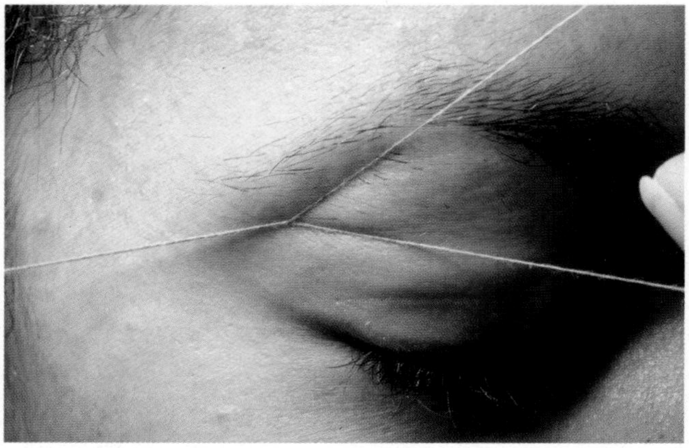

Figure 19–4 Threading.

A second, more traditional technique that many threading practitioners use is to put one end of the loop of thread in the practitioner's mouth gripped between the teeth and maneuvering the loop from one end. This method is usually applied by threading practitioners on themselves. While the idea of this method may seem unhygienic to many, there has been no data to suggest that it is harmful to a client. However, before trying it, check with your state's cosmetology or esthetic regulatory board.

SUGARING

Like threading, sugaring is an ancient method of hair removal that has found its way to North America and has become increasingly popular. Customers like the idea of an ancient, well-utilized technique, and they like that the sugar paste is 100% natural (Figure 19–7). As ancient as this method is, it is still employed in its original form around the world; however, the technique has evolved in the Western world with different aspects and consequences.

The original sugaring formulas, made without resins, required only a warm, moist cloth for aftercare. Manufacturers who have jumped on the sugaring bandwagon have attempted to distinguish themselves by altering the original formulas with additives and promoting the faster method of using fabric strips to remove the hair and sugar paste. With these alterations what was once a somewhat slow method that caused little distortion to the hair follicle is now applied in the same way as the strip method of soft waxing (applied with a spatula, covered with a fabric strip, and removed by pulling in the opposite direction of growth).

Threading Indications

- The most popular areas for threading are the face, including the eyebrows; between the eyebrow and hairline; the upper lip; and the hair along the jaw, under the chin, and on the sides of the face.

Threading Contraindications

- broken, irritated skin
- active eczema and psoriasis
- active herpes lesion
- sunburned skin

Figure 19–5 Pros and cons of threading.

Pros & Cons

Pros of Threading

- good alternative for those unable to tolerate waxing on the face due to prescription and other product use (e.g., Retin A, Differin, AHAs) or facial treatments that cause negative reactions when waxed
- inexpensive, requiring only the use of strong household cotton thread, an antiseptic pretreatment, and soothing after-care
- minimal product cost service and, when administered by an experienced practitioner, achieved quickly (faster than tweezing) for a high profit
- discomfort level is usually less than electrolysis and waxing, similar to tweezing, but because it is faster than tweezing, the plucking sensation is more tolerable

Cons of Threading

- ineffective for large parts of the body
- can be uncomfortable because the hairs are snagged out of the skin faster than tweezing but more slowly than waxing
- when not done with care and accuracy, the practitioner may unwittingly remove vellus that was not problematic and in doing so encourage the vellus to grow back irregularly or become terminal hair, thereby aggravating the hair-growth situation
- because some follicles will become distorted due to the pulling, the regrowth hair may stand in a wispy fashion where it once lay flat on the skin
- as the hair grows back, folliculitis, pustules, and inflammation that can cause pigmentation problems may increase

Figure 19–6 Threading indications and contraindications.

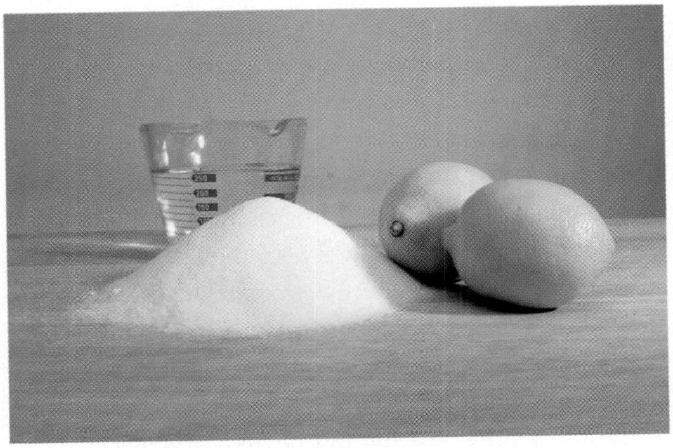

Figure 19–7 Key sugaring ingredients.

Sugaring any facial skin is not a choice for those clients using Retin-A or AHAs unless they have stopped using the product for at least five days prior to treatment. Their skin will be thinner and is more prone to irritation; thus caution is advised.

The History of Sugaring

Used for centuries in the Middle East, North Africa, and the Mediterranean, sugaring is believed to have been discovered as a form of hair removal in ancient times, possibly quite by chance, when sugar paste was used to treat a wound, to dress a burn, to prevent infections from developing, and to aid in healing. Removing the paste removed the hair while leaving the skin with little irritation.

Ancient Egyptians believed that body hair was unacceptable and unclean. Women removed all of the hair on the body except for brows and the hair on the head. They shaved or used tools like tweezers to remove the hair. Sugaring was a faster, less painful, and more effective method that also exfoliated the skin, leaving it smoother and without stubble. Because of the way sugaring removes the hair, the regrowth is softer and finer; thus, it is understandable why sugaring became a lasting and preferred method of hair removal around the region.

While sugaring techniques have remained basically unchanged in many regions, the technique began to evolve dramatically when it arrived in the United States. Today, there are two very different types of sugaring: the applicator-applied/strip removal method and the hand-applied/non-strip method. These techniques have very different effects on the skin and hair.

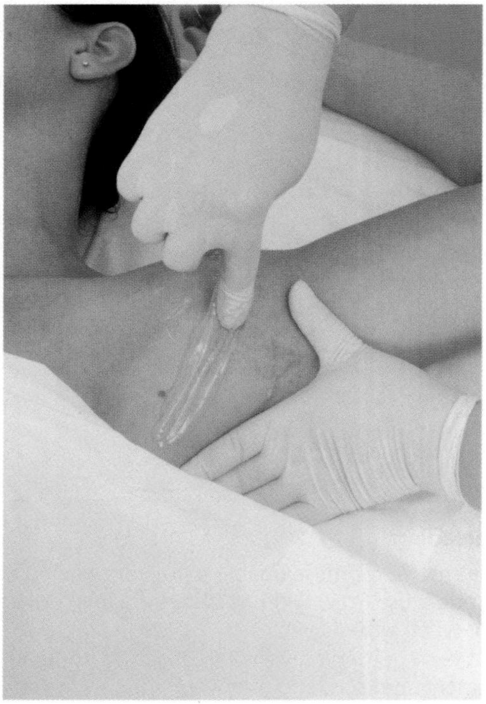

Figure 19–8 Client being sugared.

The Benefits of Sugaring

Sugaring's benefits are determined by the method used—either the hand-applied method or the spatula-applied method. Neither method carries a risk of burning the client because both use material at body temperature. In addition, the traditional formulas without resins do not adhere as tightly to the skin. This means there is a minimal risk of bruising and less discomfort during removal. Because of the temperature and adhesion qualities, the same area can be treated more than once without risk of irritation or trauma. Another benefit is that the sugar paste has natural antiseptic properties, which inhibit bacterial growth, cause less irritation, and reduce possible breakouts in the days following the treatment. The final benefit is that the sugar paste is water-soluble, therefore making the clean-up for the client easy and gentle, with no sticky residue left on the skin. In addition, the technician can wipe down all equipment, walls, floors, and treatment tables with hot water, followed by the usual disinfectant. Last, the regrowth hair is often lighter, softer, and less dense.

The Hand-Applied Method

The foremost benefit of the hand-applied method of sugaring (Figure 19–8) is that there is no risk of burning because it is applied at body temperature. (Always check the temperature of the sugar paste before application.) You can use the hand-applied sugaring method safely on dry psoriasis and dry-itch eczema. Due to its temperature, and the fact that the sugar paste does not adhere to the skin like waxes containing resins, this treatment is considered safe to use on areas with varicose veins or spider veins. However, use caution, common sense, and good judgment with regard to these conditions. In addition, because of the lower risks, this method is considered safe for individuals with diabetes, but those clients should still seek a physician's approval and sign a medical release before treatment.

Virginal (previously untreated) hair only need be 1⁄16 inch in length for removal. You can perform hand sugaring of the face, neck, and backs of hands and arms quickly because you do not have to keep dipping, applying product, and pulling a strip. You can sugar one area and immediately move on to the next.

The original hand method was done by applying the sugar paste down the hair, in the direction of hair growth; one company now teaches estheticians to apply the hand sugar paste against hair growth for removal. Both methods have been found to be effective in removing the hair from the follicle without irritation or damage to the follicle or surrounding skin. Classical hand sugar is pliable and not stiff (meaning that the sugar is soft enough that you cannot roll it into a ball), and you can handle it for effective hair removal. Hand sugar pulls up from the jar in a long strand

and will *bend with the hair* as it is being flicked; thus, it cannot *break off* the hair inside or near the follicle opening. The ball method uses a sugar that is stiffer and can be rolled into a ball.

While there are many benefits to the hand-applied sugaring method, there are a few significant downsides. First, this method is slow and time-consuming to perform, especially on larger areas. It is not a preferred method for larger body areas like the legs and back. There is some minimal discomfort similar to—but not as uncomfortable as—waxing. Folliculitis and ingrown hairs may result; however, the risk of these conditions is less with the sugaring methods than with waxing methods. Some technicians report a variation in consistency between batches of sugar paste, which affects effectiveness. This may be product-related or it may be technique-related. With the ball method the firmer product can make it more difficult to catch all the hair, as it has a harder time "flowing" around the hair.

The Spatula-Applied Method

Unlike the hand-applied method, the spatula method is much faster, therefore making it more practical for treating larger areas. As with the hand method, the spatula-applied method can be used safely on dry psoriasis and dry-itch eczema, but *only* if the sugar paste is a resin-free formula. There is some discomfort with this method, similar to waxing, but if you prepare the skin properly and do the strip technique with precision, the client will have few problems with folliculites and ingrown hairs. Many clients who have ingrown hairs from being waxed find the problem disappears if they switch to the sugar method.

Sugaring Paste

The sugar paste is made of 100% natural raw sugar, which is heated until syrup forms (Table 19–1). The sugar-paste mixture for hand-applied methods should be a consistency that can be rolled into a ball. For sugaring using a spatula or strip, the paste can be thin but not too runny, similar to molasses. Most sugar paste made and used in the Middle East is 100% natural black. The classical formula is considered hypo-allergenic and is not irritating to the skin. If you use a brand of sugar paste that has added gums and resins along with fragrances, it it not considered a true sugaring product and may even be more irritating to the client's skin. It is important to read the product labels to check the ingredients.

THE DIFFERING BENEFITS OF SUGARING TECHNIQUES

- **Minimal risk of bruising because of lower adhesion.**
- **Due to the application temperature and the fact that it does not adhere to the skin like waxes containing resins, sugaring is considered safe to use on areas with varicose veins or spider veins. However caution, common sense, and good judgment should be used with regard to these conditions.**
- **Because the sugar paste does not adhere as tightly to skin cells, the paste will only remove the hair and exfoliate the loose cells of the stratum corneum with minimal discomfort and trauma to the skin and can be used safely on dry psoriasis and dry-itch eczema.**
- **Because of the temperature and adhesion qualities, the same area can be treated more than once without the risk of causing irritation and trauma.**
- **As there is no risk of burning or tearing the skin, sugaring is considered safe to use on individuals with diabetes. However, a physician's approval should be obtained and a medical release signed.**
- **The hair length only need be 1⁄16 inch in length for removal for previously untreated hair.**
- **Re-growth hair is lighter, softer, and less dense.**
- **Easy clean-up of the equipment, walls, floors and treatment table, because the sugar paste is water-soluble.**
- **Easy clean up for the client.**
- **Natural antiseptic properties, which inhibit bacterial growth.**
- **Hygienic because the sugar paste is not re-used on other clients.**

Table 19–1 Recipe for Sugaring Paste

RECIPE FOR SUGARING PASTE
Ingredients
2 cups sugar
¼ cup lemon juice
¼ cup water
All ingredients sould be combined and cooked slowly over low heat. The mixture should not be heated above 250° F. A candy thermometer should be used to read the temperature accurately. The mixture should be allowed to cool in a glass jar. It should be used at body temperature when applied by hand or with a spatula.

Application Techniques for Sugaring

After you have spent time observing both application techniques for sugaring—by hand and with a spatula—you can decide which method you prefer. Before using either on a client, especially one who has not had a sugaring treatment before, it is a good idea to perform a patch test. As we have learned there are two distinctly different sugaring methods: (1) application and removal by hand (Figure 19–9) and (2) application by spatula (Figure 19–10) and removal with a strip. While the techniques for spatula-applied sugaring are similar to those of spatula-applied waxing, the hand-applied sugaring method is unique.

The Patch Test

A patch test is a way to gauge a client's reaction to the service and to find out if the client should have the treatment within a day or two of an important engagement. Any reaction, particularly a histamine reaction, will appear almost immediately; if microorganisms have been introduced to a vulnerable area, small white pustules or a small red rash may appear up to 48 hours after the treatment, especially if resins have been added to the sugar paste used for the spatula method. A client with known skin sensitivities or who has an important event coming up will want to know if he or she will experience any reaction to the sugar paste. Do the test on the face but in an area that is not noticeable (e.g., toward the front of the ear).

Application by Hand

Before the treatment begins, wash your hands and apply gloves. Hand sugaring with gloves takes practice, but you can master the technique, providing protection to both you and the client. Cleanse the area to be treated with an antibacterial cleanser, creating totally clean skin that

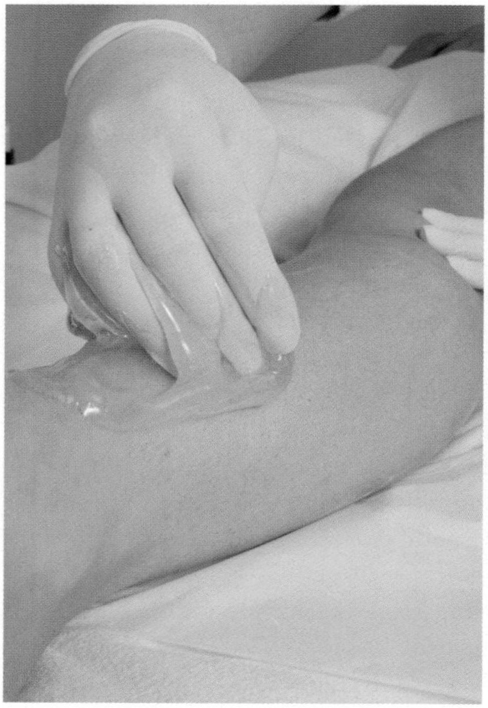

Figure 19–9 Hand method of sugar application.

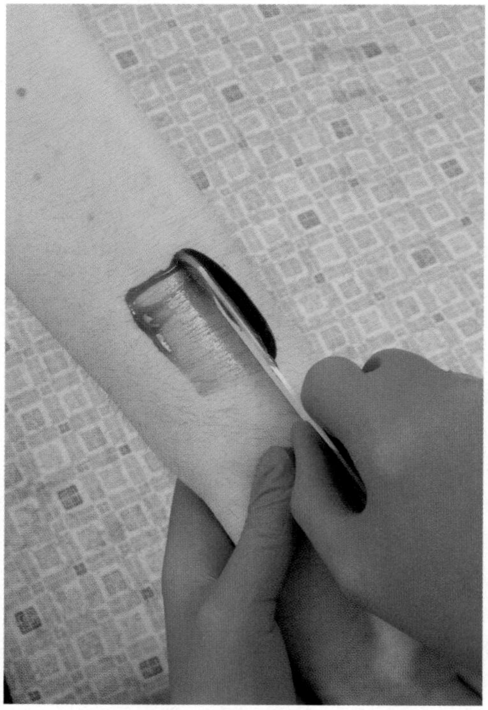

Figure 19–10 Spatula method of sugar application.

is free from makeup, oils, and lotions. If the skin is not completely clean, the sugar will not adhere properly and will not be as forgiving in removal. The skin should feel warm to the touch for a more effective and comfortable treatment. If the skin is cool and goose bumps are causing the hair to stand upright, this may increase discomfort and cause some of the hairs to snap.

Next, lightly dust the area with a fine-grained powder that is free from chemicals, perfumes, and aluminum that could irritate the skin post-treatment. The powder will absorb any residual moisture, which will help make the treatment more effective. If you apply too much powder, the sugar will not adhere well.

Manipulate the sugar paste between the fingers; it should be easy to manage. Press and push the paste against the hair growth and back over the top, followed by a quick flicking motion that is parallel to the skin, pulling the sugar paste off in the direction of hair growth (Figures 19–11 and Figure 19–12). If any hair remains behind, reapply the sugar paste to the same area.

When the area is cleared, you can use the same sugar to remove hair on the adjacent area, and so on, until the service is complete or until the sugar becomes so congested with hair that it is rendered ineffective. In that case, you will need a new amount of sugar paste. You can use the same sugar paste on the face and later the body, but for sanitary reasons the reverse is not true. Never use one client's sugar paste on another client. When the service is finished, roll the sugar inside the glove and thrown it all away.

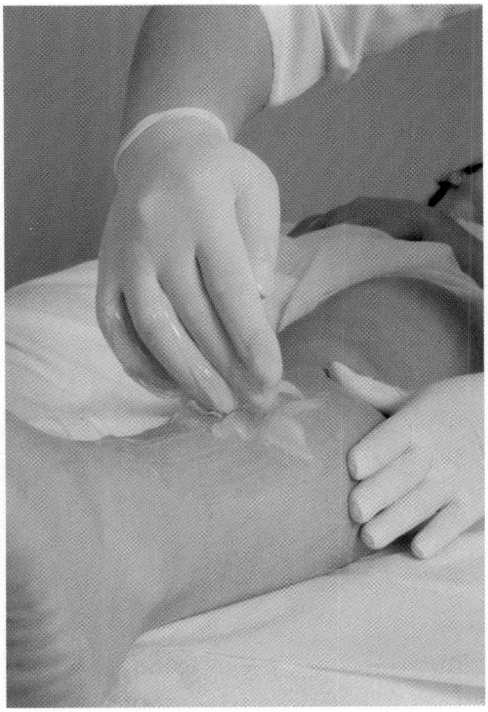

Figure 19–11 Manual removal of sugar paste.

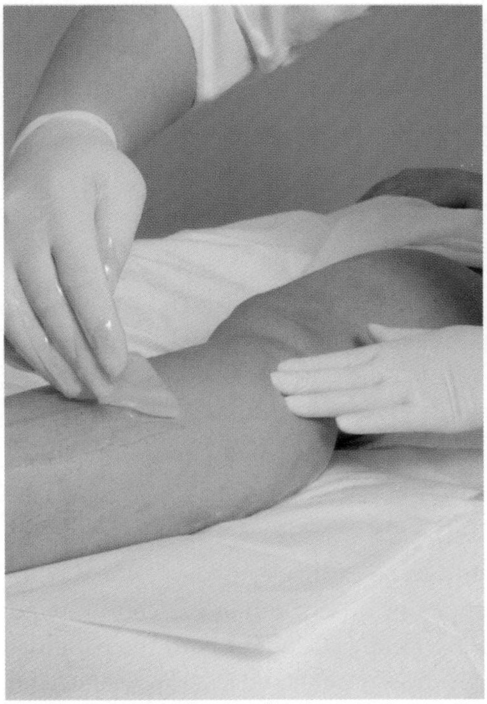

Figure 19–12 Manual removal of sugar paste.

Application by Spatula with Strip Removal

Application by spatula is done in the direction of hair growth; then you apply a muslin strip over the top, rub in the direction of hair growth, and quickly pull away against the growth, keeping close and parallel to the skin and using the opposite hand to keep the skin taunt. (Figure 19–13).

Some sugar paste formulations, especially those with added resins, require the temperature to be hotter than that of the ancient hand-applied method and are therefore more like hot wax. (Read further in this chapter for the guidelines, concerns, and contraindications of using wax.) Warm strip sugar does not adhere well to pellon (the strips used to remove wax) and tends to "bleed" though the softer pellons. Regular-weight pellons used for waxing are too stiff to use with sugar; they do not allow for a quick "pulling" action. Muslin strips allow the sugar to bind to the fabric fibers and is as flexible as the sugar, allowing for a smooth and effective pull.

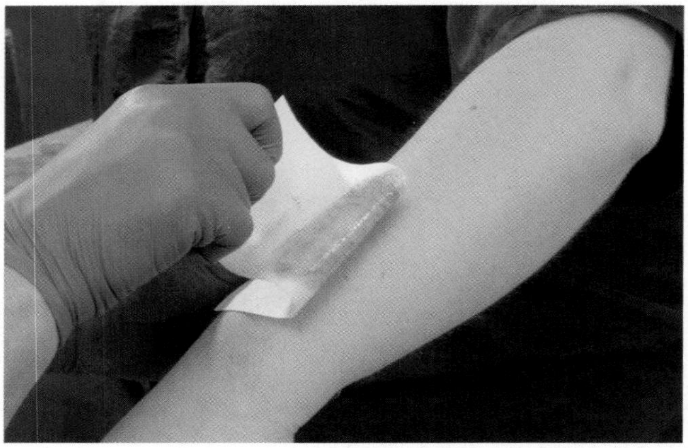

Figure 19–13 Strip removal of sugaring.

Post-Treatment Care

The client's skin can be easily cleansed of natural 100% sugar paste with a warm washcloth or wet cotton round; clients never leave feeling sticky. For both the hand and the strip method, the service should leave the skin feeling clean and dry. Applying creams to the depilated area after sugaring is not necessary.

Clients can usually go 6 to 12 weeks between treatments, although this will vary between individuals and depend on the parts of the face and body treated. Sugaring technicians often say that if a client uses sugar as his or her only method of hair removal, the time between each treatment may increase.

Every form of hair removal has its fans. Your research, practical experience, and daily hands-on experience will be your best guide. For more information about sugaring, refer to *Milady's Aesthetician Series: Advanced Hair Removal* by Pamela Hill and Helen Bickmore (Clifton Park, NY: Delmar Cengage Learning, 2007).

HARD WAX

Hard wax was the original depilatory wax that vanished into relative obscurity when the quick and efficient soft wax came to the forefront in salons. Although soft wax with the strip is quicker and more practical for large body areas, in recent years hard wax has made a strong comeback, in part because of advances in skin care. As clients seek advanced anti-aging and anti-acne skin care treatments from estheticians, dermatologists, and plastic surgeons, new concerns about facial waxing and the effect of waxing on exfoliated or treated skin have arisen. Home skin care regimens that effect more dramatic changes in the skin are causing concern for those who provide facial waxing. With the increase in clients' home use of retinoids and AHAs has come an increase in incidents of skin lifting during an eyebrow, lip, or other facial waxing services. It has become apparent that the hard wax of decades past caused fewer injuries to clients receiving specialized skin treatments because it does not adhere to the skin. This is a time to be more vigilant than ever when waxing a client's face. However there are now gentle but effective waxes formulated for strip waxing that are available for use on delicate skin.

Hard wax should be soft in the pot and easily spreadable without burning the skin. Once on the skin it should quickly solidify without becoming brittle. For all this to take place, the melting point of a depilatory wax must be greater than 98°F/37°C but less than 165°F/73.9°C. Because the body temperature is around 98.6°F/38°C, if the melting point were lower, the wax would not solidify. In addition, the wax must be sufficiently firm to grip the hair. Therefore. the temperature for hard wax should be between 125°F/51.6°C and 160°F/71.1°C. Wax cools rapidly, at approximately 7°F/3.9°C per second, so a technician needs to work quickly to achieve maximum efficacy from the wax. As no one wax meets these criteria, depilatory waxes are often combined with beeswax, candelilla wax, and carnauba wax to modify their melting points and increase strength (Figure 19–14).

Strip (soft) wax is much hotter and is more liquid on application than hard wax, so it more readily runs to the base of the hair shaft. Because the application temperature of hard wax is somewhat lower and therefore thicker, it sets faster when applied. Applying most hard waxes initially in the opposite direction of hair growth gives the

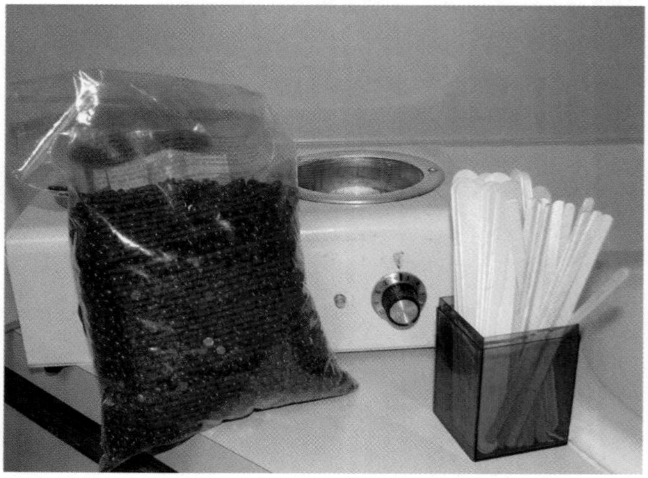

Figure 19–14 Hard wax requires a variety of supplies.

wax the chance to get to the base of the hair while the wax is still warm. The wax then starts to shrink as it cools and sets. Gliding the wax back over the top of the hair, like frosting a cake, allows for thorough coverage of the hair shaft. Thorough coverage around the hair shaft means a good, tight grip on even the coarsest hairs. Although the wax is usually removed against the hair growth, hard wax can also be removed in the direction of hair growth, especially when it is used on fine non-colored vellus hair, without distorting the hair follicles.

SOFT WAX

Soft wax—also called strip wax because the technician removes it using a strip of fabric— is currently the most popular method of hair removal and has been since its inception in the 1970s (Figure 19–15). However, as mentioned previously, with the ever-evolving skin care treatments, products, and regimens, it has posed problems, particularly on the face. Therefore it is important to know when soft wax is the client's preference and when it may not be the most suitable method of hair removal.

This wax, which has a liquid-honey consistency, is popular because it is a much faster method of removing hair than hard wax and is more effective in the hair it removes, clearing virtually every hair of the appropriate length in its path. In addition, when used correctly, soft wax causes limited discomfort.

Larger body areas such as legs and the back benefit from being waxed with soft wax because of the speed and effectiveness. Manufacturers are now recognizing the concerns of clients whose skin is more sensitive, particularly on the face, because they are using more sophisticated treatments and products. As a result, companies are producing many other types of soft wax for more sensitive skin and skin that sports the stubbly coarse hair that still requires the soft wax strip method. These new waxes have a more opaque, creamier texture and can achieve a thin, liquid consistency at a lower temperature. They may also contain azulene, chamomile, or tea tree oil for their soothing and calming properties.

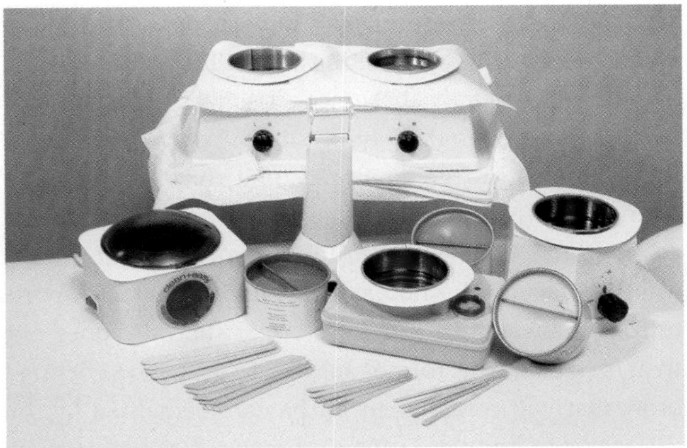

Figure 19–15 Different soft waxes and wax heaters.

One of the side effects of soft waxing is an increase in ingrown hairs. This occurs mostly in the bikini area; however, many people are prone to ingrown hair regardless of how they have hair removed. There are many good products available to help keep ingrown hairs to a minimum. These products usually contain a percentage of AHA or salicylic acid. Many ingrown hairs can also be removed manually. It can be a long and tedious process to remove a lot of ingrown hairs in the salon, so it is a good idea to ask the client to release—*but not remove*—as many hairs as possible at least four days before the waxing service. The client should release the hairs as close to the follicle opening as possible using sterile needle-pointed tweezers; the hair should not be tweezed away but left sticking out of the opening, allowing time for the follicle to heal and normalize around the hair. If the skin is broken and the hair is completely removed, the opening will scab over, a new anagen hair may become trapped under the scab, and it will become ingrown, perpetuating the problem.

If the ingrown hair looks like a blackhead (this is particularly apparent in the bikini area), then it usually has a follicle opening and the client can extract it gently and easily before the service. If you are going to remove the ingrown hair(s), wear gloves and wipe the pre-waxed area with an antiseptic first. Gently squeeze the "blackhead" using the *sides* of both forefinger nails, *not* the nail tips, until the hair extracts (Figures 19–16 and 19–17). Once the hair is extracted, you can wipe it away. Because the skin was not broken, the follicle opening was not compromised and it does not need time to heal and normalize.

For embedded hair that is visible under the skin as a thin line, you can release the hair after the waxing service. With gloves on, wipe the area with alcohol and use sterile, sharp-pointed tweezers. A magnifying lamp can make this procedure much easier. The tweezers should be sharp enough to break the skin as minimally as possible. Slide the tweezers' point underneath the hair as close as possible to where the follicle should be. Once the hair is lifted, use a different pair of tweezers with flat, slanted tips, as the sharp-pointed tweezers can actually cut the

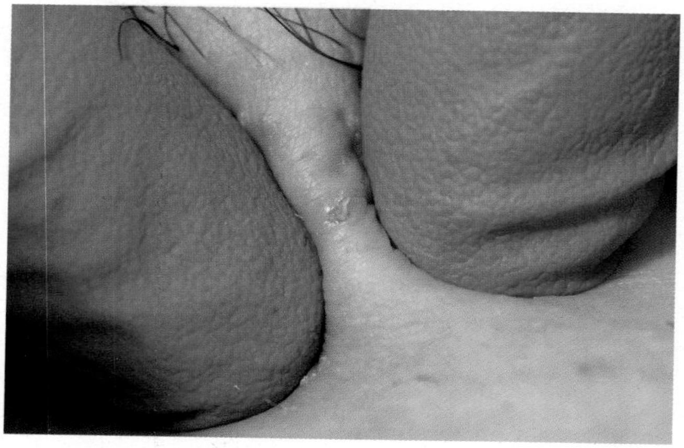

Figure 19–16 Extraction of the blackhead type of ingrown hair.

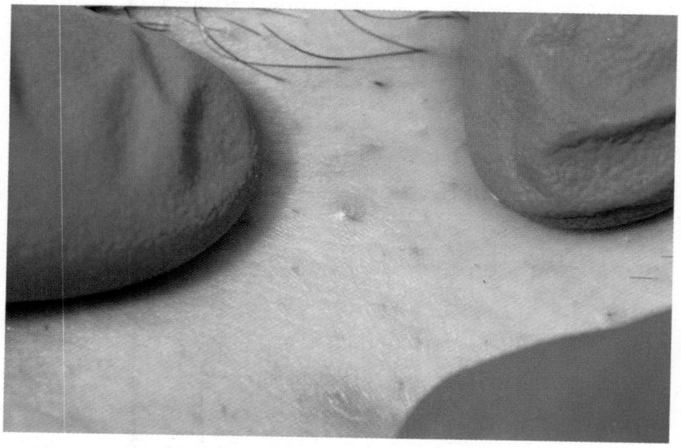

Figure 19–17 Sample blackhead type of ingrown hair.

hair in half during removal. Instruct the client to leave the hair protruding for as long as possible, up to four days, allowing the follicle to heal and normalize around it. He or she can then tweeze the hair away. The needle-pointed tweezers or lancets used to break the skin must be treated as surgical instruments and sterilized.

> **REGULATORY AGENCY ALERT**
>
> Check with your state licensing board on the use of tweezers and lancets. Their use is prohibited by some state licensing boards.

PRODUCT EVALUATION

There are many good hair removal products on the market and it may take some experimenting to find your personal preferences. Every product has its own "personality" and needs practice to obtain optimum results. Keep this in mind as you try a new product as it may not behave exactly as the one you had used previously. If you are going to be treating the full body, you will need more than one product as each has its specialized use.

ADVANCED FACIAL WAXING

Brow Design

Waxing of the eyebrows is not simply about the removal of unwanted hair, as it is for most other parts of the body; it is also about aesthetics. Understanding shape, balance, and artistry are all important in shaping eyebrows. To create the perfect shape takes a good eye. Your knowledge of the basic rules of eyebrow and face shapes will benefit your client greatly.

If a client is coming in to get her eyebrows waxed and shaped for the first time, take notice as she initially enters the room. Her appearance and image can affect the look she wants her eyebrows to reflect. Is she sophisticated or sporty? Well-groomed individuals generally appreciate more precise and defined eyebrows whereas sporty or more casual individuals may be comfortable with a more natural look that just requires a little "clean-up." The sophisticated client who comes in on a day off may be dressed down, so while you wash your hands, ask a few polite questions to hone in on the client's image. Another consideration is hair length. Is the hair long or short? Short and/or fine hair suits a thinner, more defined brow; conversely, thick and/or longer hair may suit more substance to the brow. The age of the client is also an important consideration. The sophisticated, thin eyebrow of a woman in her forties may not be right for a teenage girl. A more mature woman may benefit from a more obvious arch, especially if her eyelids are starting to droop, because it gives the illusion of lift and opens the eyes more. Generally speaking, a younger female should sport a more natural eyebrow shape. As a woman ages, the eyebrows can gradually become thinner and more defined but this client may have thick and unruly white or grey hairs that will need to be removed or trimmed. Another factor is whether the client generally sports full face makeup on a daily basis or typically does not wear makeup. The former may opt for a more defined brow that will complement or be complemented by the eye makeup, and the latter may prefer that the brow be natural and not too thin. If it is the client's first eyebrow

Table 19–2 Waxing Problems and the Potential Causes

HARD WAX	
Problem	**Cause**
Hard wax broke during removal process.	1. Wax was too old or was not "refreshed" with new wax. 2. Wax may have been overheated or kept hot for 24 hours or more. 3. Wax may have been allowed to get too cold during application. 4. Wax may have been applied too thinly.
Too many bits of wax were left on the skin after removal.	Wax was not applied with clean, even borders.
Client experienced small pustules a few days after a lip wax.	Area was not sufficiently cleansed of makeup and dirt. Massaged-in aftercare lotion transported microorganisms into the vulnerable follicle or client failed to observe home-care instructions properly.
SOFT WAX	
Skin lifted off during eyebrow or lip wax.	1. Client used a skin-altering product like Retin A. 2. Poor waxing technique—the strip was pulled up too high during removal, rather than parallel to the skin, and the skin was not held taut.
Wax stayed on the skin and did not come off with the strip.	1. Client's skin may have been damp. 2. Client's skin may have been dry. 3. Client's skin may have been too cold. 4. Client's skin was not held taut. 5. Technician did not rub wax strip properly.
Client experienced bruising in the bikini area.	1. Wax was applied over the femoral ridge, and not up to it, crossing two planes. 2. Skin was not held taut.
Too much hair was removed in the eyebrow.	1. Too much wax was applied, which "bled" into the brow line when the strip was rubbed. 2. Hairs growing downward at the point of arch may have accidentally got caught in the wax and been removed. 3. A strip with wax already on it may have been reused.

wax, communication is key to helping her achieve the desired look.

In addition to the *image* factors listed above, there are other factors to be considered when assessing the shape of an eyebrow, so position the client in a semi-reclined position and hand her a mirror for viewing the desired shape and any irregularities. Take her hair back off her face so that you can both assess her face shape and eye placement and also so her hair stays out of the way of the wax.

For clients with a round or broad face (Figure 19–18) or wide-set eyes (Figure 19–19), bring the point of the arch to the inside of the iris as the client looks straight ahead, creating the illusion that the face is narrower or that the eyes are closer together. For narrow faces (Figure 19–20) or those with close-set eyes (Figure 19–21), place the point of the arch to the outside of the iris as the client looks straight ahead, creating the illusion that the face is wider or the eyes are more in balance with the face.

When defining the eyebrow shape, use the following guidelines and Figure 19–22, bearing in mind that these

FYI

Make sure the client is aware that constantly removing eyebrow hairs may inhibit regrowth. The client should not overtweeze the brows to accommodate a fad or fashion.

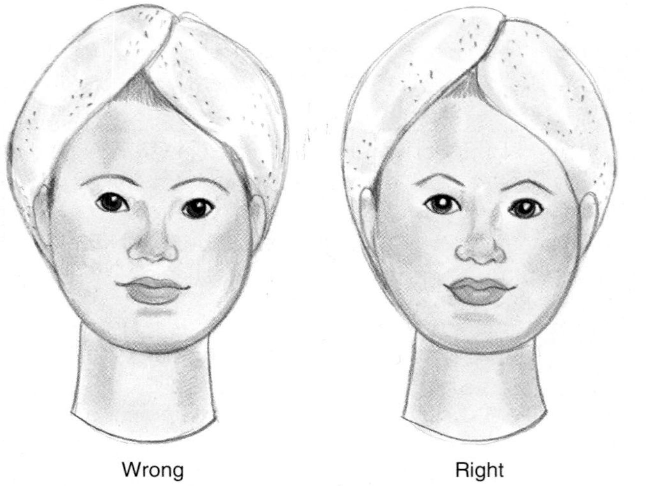

Figure 19–18 Eyebrows on a round face.

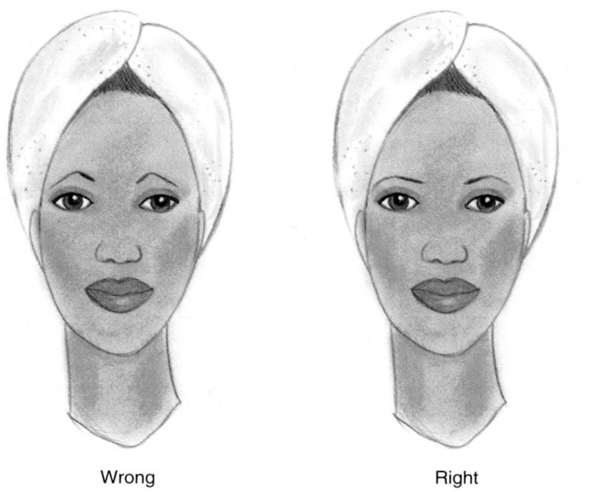

Figure 19–20 Eyebrows on a narrow face.

guidelines are applied to a perfect oval-shaped face with eyes that are positioned in perfect balance and proportion to that face shape. The start and point of the arch can be changed with subtle adjustments to create that desired illusion of balance and proportion.

1. **Start:** Identify the first point of reference, the point 1, by resting a thin, wooden applicator orangewood stick or pencil along the side of the nose, just above the nostril, in the cleft of the nose and straight up to the inner corner of the eye. Some clients have wider nostrils than others, which could affect the start line, so placing the stick just above the nostril gives a more accurate start point. The point above the inner corner of the eye where the stick passes determines where the eyebrow should start. Remove any hair to the outside of the stick, unless the eyes are wide-set, and fill any space on the inside with an eyebrow pencil unless the eyes are too close together.

2. **Point of arch:** Use the second point of reference, point 2, to locate the arch; it is the arch that can also be slightly adjusted to correct brow proportions. To find the correct point of the arch, the client should be looking straight ahead. For a normal face shape and eye placement, place the stick at the base of the nose and angle it so that it crosses in front of the pupil. The point at which the stick touches the eyebrow is where the point of the arch should be (Figure 19–22). With broad faces and with the client looking straight ahead, you can bring in the arch slightly to just above the pupil. Conversely, with narrow faces you can adjust the arch further to the outside of the pupil.

3. **End:** The final point of reference, point 3, allows you to locate the correct ending of the brow. To do this, slide the stick, still at the base of the nose, farther around so that it crosses over the outer corner of the eye. The point

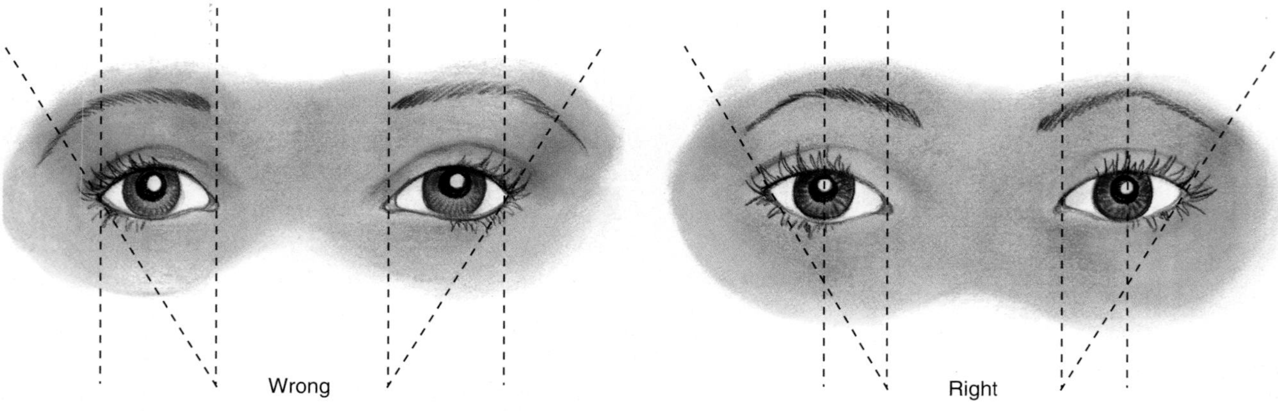

Figure 19–19 Eyebrows showing arch position for wide-set eyes.

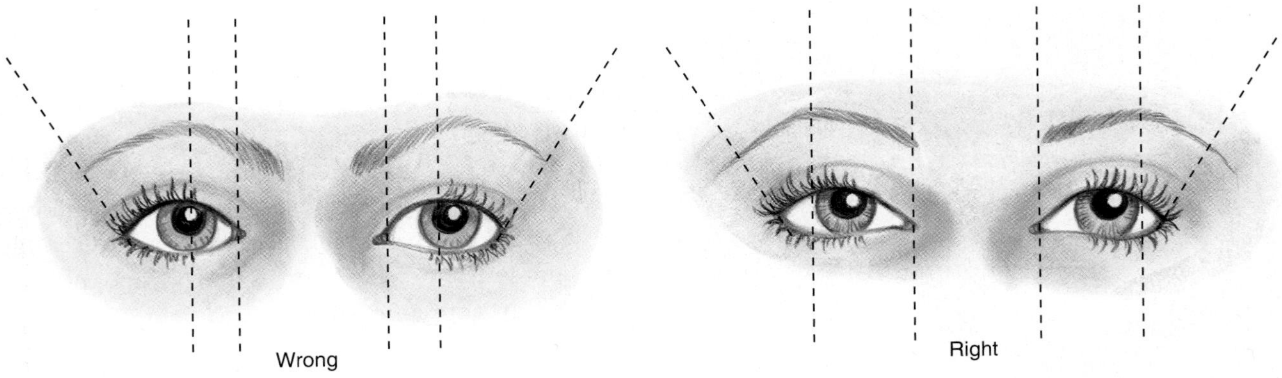

Figure 19–21 Arch position for close-set eyes.

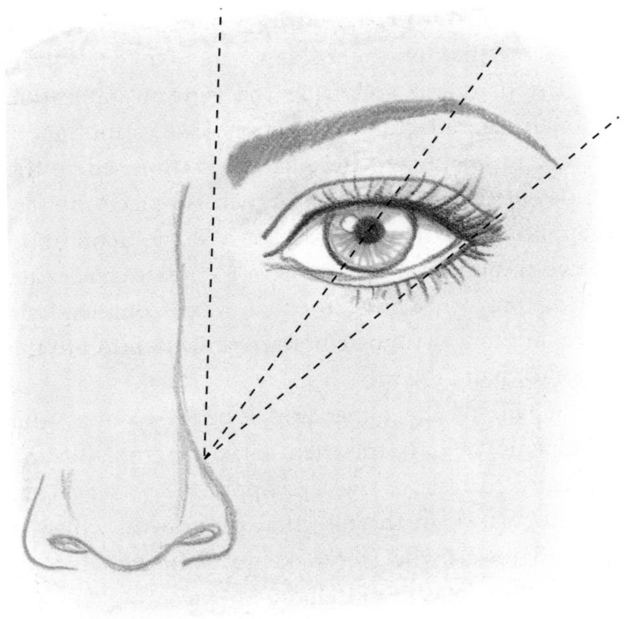

Figure 19–22 How to determine brow shape.

at which the stick meets the brow is where the brow should end. Remove any hair that goes beyond the stick, and pencil in any space on the inside of the stick. If the end is too short and not penciled in, the client may look like she does not have an eyebrow when seen in profile.

Overall, there should be a clear ascent from the start to the point of arch and a clear descent from the point of arch to the end. The line should be gradual and tapered without going from too thick on the ascent to too thin on the descent.

The Sides of the Face

Waxing the sides of the face or the chin can create problems for the client because this skin can respond with irritation. However, some female clients choose it as their best option. If the hair is visible but minimal in quantity, suggest electrolysis as the first choice. If there is a significant amount of hair, and the client rates favorably in the Fitzpatrick Scale, then laser hair removal may be a good option. For male clients, laser or IPL is the best option. The terminal hairs on a male client's face are not well suited for waxing. If neither electrolysis or laser/IPL are options your female client wants to explore, then hard wax is more desirable than strip wax because the hard wax won't distort the follicles and it better grips the stronger hairs of the sideburn with less skin irritation. If the hair is not too strong, sugaring is also an option. Discuss the pros and cons of each option with your client and be certain that he or she understands those options.

SPEED WAXING AND BODY TECHNIQUES

Speed waxing involves applying soft wax to an entire area and removing it rapidly with the same strip or a small number of strips (Figure 19–23). Developing a good speed-waxing technique will be financially more profitable for you because you'll have shorter treatment times and can book more clients. It is also beneficial for the client to receive the service in a more timely manner and with a shorter period of discomfort. He or she will be more inclined to rebook.

To be an effective speed waxer, you must be well organized and have the service protocols thoroughly worked out. Placement of the treatment table with easy access to the wax is also important. Avoid drips and spills, because the time it takes to clean up the threads and drips of wax is time that you could be working on clients. To be an effective speed waxer, you must know the start point and follow the same rehearsed routine for each body part with each client. Thinking about where to go next is time

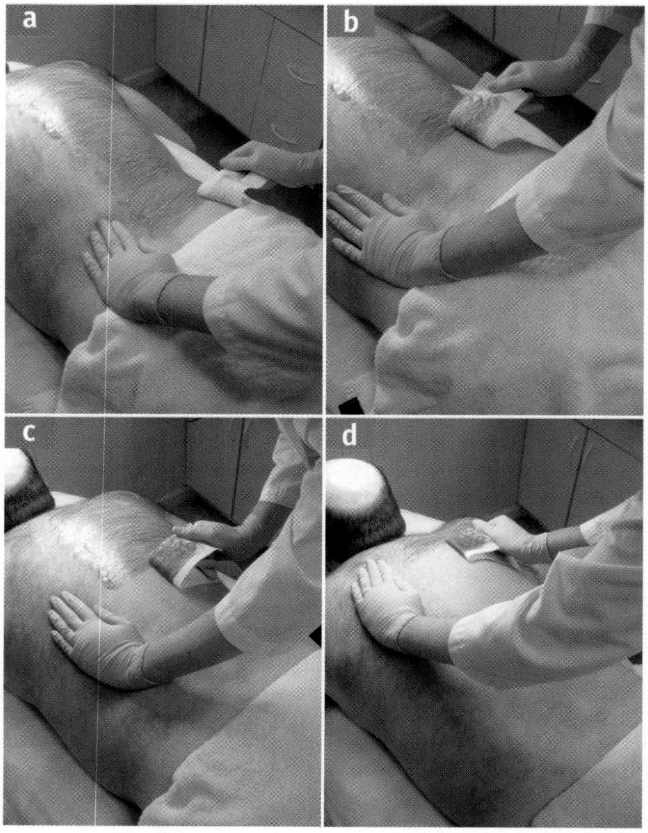

Figure 19–23 Speed waxing.

lost. The same is true for the application of pre-care and aftercare products.

To start a treatment, mist the fronts of both legs once, top to bottom, followed by a quick wipe-down with a paper towel in each hand. To save time, you can ask the client to raise his or her legs, one at a time, so you can mist and prep the backs at the same time as the fronts. Sprinkle dusting powder quickly and rub again with both hands in unison. These protocols save considerable time. When speed waxing the legs, apply the wax down one side of the front of the leg, knee to ankle, and removed it quickly along the entire length with the strip. Only one or two firm rubs with the strip is necessary. More rubbing than that is a waste of "valuable" time.

Arms

Strip wax is the fastest, most effective way to remove hair from the arms. However, because of the pulling direction against the growth of the hair, the hair may start to grow back in an unruly fashion, sticking up. Hard wax or sugaring prevents unruly regrowth, particularly if it is a client's first time for an arm wax and the client is getting the service for a special occasion but doesn't see it being repeated in the near future. However both hard wax and sugaring methods are slower methods than strip wax.

For hair removal of the forearm, give the client a gown or apron to protect the clothing. Have him or her sit on the treatment table, legs dangling over, while you stand in front of the client. Spray or wipe the forearm with an antiseptic solution, and then dust it with powder.

Arms and Hard Wax

For a hard wax treatment, have the client hold the arm outstretched with the palm facing up. Begin by waxing any unsightly hair on the inside where there is less hair. Apply the hard wax following the general application rules or the manufacturer's directions. We cannot apply hard wax to an immediate adjacent section where the two sides of the section would touch, so place the second application with the space of a single application in between, and treat the in-between area treated after removing the other two strips of wax. Complete the forearm all the way to the elbow, paying attention to the direction of hair growth.

If the hair of the upper arm is more obvious and requires removal, have the client relax the arm, allowing the forearm to rest on the lap. Apply the wax against, then immediately in the direction of, growth, which is downward toward the elbow. Remove the hair in sections, starting toward the elbow and working upward toward the shoulder, blending,or feathering if necessary, at the top by picking up a few additional hairs on the strip of wax that has just been removed.

Arms and Soft Wax

In a soft wax treatment, apply the wax thinly and downward, because the hair grows downward toward the wrist. Continue up the lower half of the inside arm, toward the wrist. Apply the strip over the wax, leaving enough of a free edge to grab. Rub and remove in the usual manner. The next section should be just above the previous section. After completing the inner arm, ask the client to turn the still-outstretched arm so the palm faces downward. Holding the arm firmly in place and starting down at the wrist, apply the wax across the top of the arm from the inside (thumb side) to the outside (little finger side), the width of the strip. Remove in the usual manner. Continue in strip-sized sections all the way up the forearm to the elbow. Next, have the client hold the arm straight upward, bent at the elbow, and apply the wax to the side that follows down from the little finger. You can do this in two sections. The hair grows downward, toward the elbow. Apply the wax to the first section, starting near the wrist, working up, toward the elbow. Proceed in the usual manner.

Most often, the upper arm has just a few hairs right above the elbow. If you are using soft wax, you can often remove these hairs with the wax that is already on the strip. The strip will remove the more obvious hairs, leaving some shorter hairs behind. This technique is known as blending or feathering, because it produces a gradual link between complete hairlessness and more dense hair.

Hands

After completing the lower and upper arm, proceed to wax the knuckles and hands, if necessary.

Hands and Hard Wax

To wax the hand with hard wax, take the hand and apply the wax in the usual manner. The hair growth is usually downward, toward the fingers, and angling out, toward the little finger. You can do the entire top of the hand, not including the fingers, at one time. On the fingers, the hair grows toward the middle knuckle, so take one finger at a time, starting at the thumb, and work toward the little finger. Apply the wax in the usual manner. Once you have applied the wax to all fingers, it should be set and ready for removal. Begin again at the thumb and quickly pull with hair growth. After removing all of the hair, take the hand in a handshake grasp and apply a soothing lotion along the topside, toward the elbow (and shoulder, if you waxed the upper arm) and down the underside to the hand. If you waxed the hand, finish by massaging the lotion into the hand and fingers. Massage the thumb and little fingers simultaneously, followed by the ring and index finger and finishing with the middle finger and thumb a second time.

Hands and Soft Wax

Soft wax is preferred for hands. Take the hand and apply the wax with the growth, which is usually downward, toward the fingers, and angling outward, toward the little finger. You can do the entire top of the hand at once, not including the fingers. Have the client form a fist, tucking the fingers under, because this tightens the skin. Apply the strip over the entire area, and rub in the direction of growth. It is important to have a good grip of the hand when removing the wax, which means that you cannot apply pressure after the pull, because both of your hands will be occupied. If the fingers have a slight amount of hair that needs removing, you can often use the wax that is already on the strip. The hair grows toward the middle knuckle, so take one finger at a time, press the wax onto the hair, rub in the direction of growth, and quickly pull off against the growth. If this doesn't work, complete the process by applying more wax. After removing all of the hair, take the hand in a handshake grasp and apply a soothing lotion along the topside, toward the elbow (and shoulder, if you waxed the upper arm) and down the underside to the hand. If you waxed the hand, finish by massaging the lotion into the hand and fingers in the manner described above.

Bikini Variations

Bikini waxes can be classified in three ways, according to how much hair should be removed: American (or standard) bikini wax, French bikini wax, and Brazilian bikini wax. You must communicate with the client so she clearly understands what will be removed and what will be left with each type of bikini wax.

American

An American wax removes hair that is visible at the top of the thighs and just under the navel when the client wears a regular bikini bottom. A regular American bikini wax can be performed using either strip or hard wax. The standard style wax works well, but cream wax also works well for hair that is not too coarse or too short and stubbly. If the client is wearing her own swimsuit or briefs, protect the fabric with a paper towel, placing one corner placed down the crotch area and tucking two corners into the sides and the remaining corner over the top. Using a small applicator, pull out from under the panty line any hair that must be removed, leaving the remainder tucked in behind the panty and giving a clean, even line to both sides of the bikini area. If the hair is so long that it curls, trim it to 1/2 inch. For a small amount of hair, use scissors; for a more considerable amount of hair, use an electric shaver. Cleanse the area with an antiseptic cleaner and pat it dry. Then dust the area with powder. Have the client leave one leg straight and bring the sole of the other foot to the level of the knee. If you are working first on the right side of the client's bikini area, have her place the *left* hand firmly on the paper, fingers straight downward. Ask her to keep her hands on the paper at all times to avoid getting wax on them. She should place her free hand on the outer edge of the thigh to help pull the skin taut.

Working on the bent leg, apply the wax with the edge of a wax applicator in the direction of hair growth. The first application should be to the section farthest away and only up to the femoral ridge. Hair growth is usually downward, following the panty line. However, toward the denser hair on the pubis bone, the hair grows more horizontally and inward, toward the center. Place the strip over the wax, leaving space to grab the free edge. Rub twice in the direction of growth, and then place that same hand firmly at the end of the strip with the free edge. The client should help hold the skin especially taut in this area. Grab the strip and pull backward in a swift, continuous manner, as close to the skin as possible. Do not cut the movement short; follow through with the movement, even slightly beyond the placement of wax. Lifting too soon will make the client uncomfortable and could cause bruising. Apply immediate, firm pressure to alleviate the discomfort.

Once you have removed all hair from all sections leading up to the panty line, you can remove the hair that grows down from the femoral ridge. Ask the client to bring the sole of the foot a little higher to just above the knee. Apply the wax just two-thirds of the way down in the downward direction of hair growth, leaving enough space at the bottom for the client to place her hand to hold the skin taut. Place the wax strip over the area, again leaving enough of a free edge to grasp. Rub twice, vigorously, and then, holding the skin as taut as possible, quickly pull the strip straight upward, as close to the skin as possible. Follow by quickly placing the hand firmly on the area for relief. Finally, to finish that side, have the client lift the leg to the chest, grasping the ankle with the opposite hand and drawing the leg across the body. This should expose the last remaining third of the hair that was too near the table for you to apply the wax. This position also ensures that the skin is nice and taut. Apply the wax as before, downward, and pull upward.

If the client is going to have a full leg wax or an upper leg wax and she can maintain this grasp for a little longer, this is an excellent position from which to remove the hairs from the top and back of the thigh, while the skin is tight. Halfway down the back of the thigh, the hair changes direction and grows across from the outside in; it should not be removed in this position. Always complete one side of the bikini area before going to the other side.

French

Named for the high-cut French-style thong, this style involves the removal of all hair, including that of the anus and labia, except a strip of hair in the front on the pubis. Follow all directions for a regular American bikini wax (see above), paying special attention to the cleaning and powdering of the areas to be waxed. Hard wax is preferred for removing the hair on the labia, because it grips the strong hair in this area while reducing the risk of injury to the delicate skin. Because the hair grows inward toward the vaginal opening, you cannot apply the rule of soft wax, removing against the growth, but hard wax can be effectively removed in this area.

There are two positions that clients can assume to facilitate the removal of hair from the buttocks. The first position involves the client lying flat on the back, raising the knees to the chest and turning the soles of the feet in together (Figure 19–24). The client can grasp the feet between the legs with one hand, leaving the other hand free to move the panties aside. Although hard wax may be preferred in this area, strip wax can be used successfully. You apply the wax downward to a small section on the lowest, inside part of the buttock. You place the strip over the wax, give two firm rubs, and remove it in the usual manner. Then apply the wax to the next section above and so on until the area on that side of the inside buttock is cleared of hair. The client should then switch hands, moving the panties to the opposite side, and grasp the feet with the other hand. Remove the hair in the same manner.

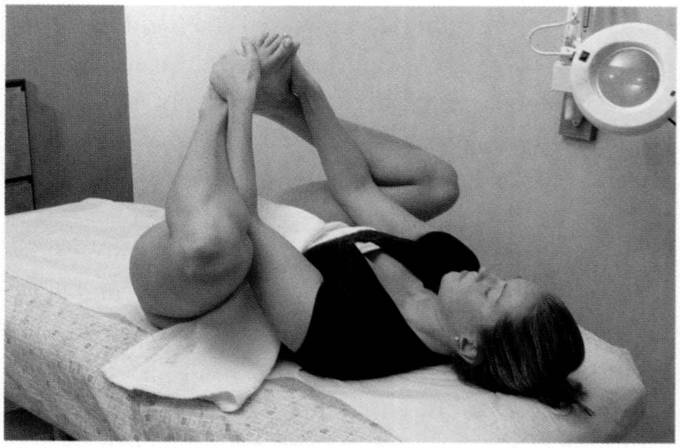

Figure 19–24 First position for French and Brazilian bikini wax.

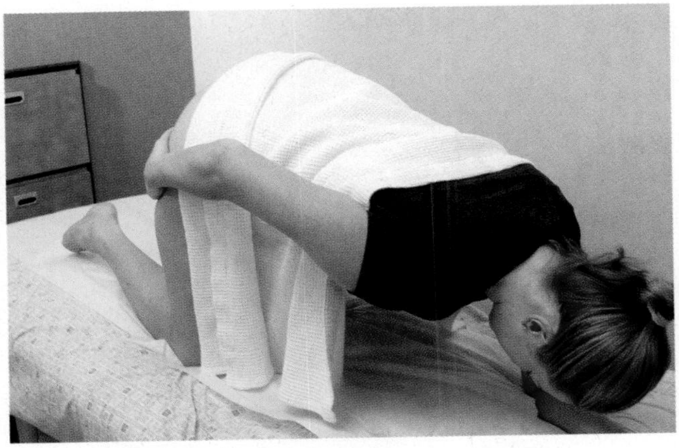

Figure 19–25 Second position for French and Brazilian bikini wax.

The second position for French bikini waxing involves the client turning over and kneeling (Figure 19–25). With one forearm resting on the table in front of her, the client has a free hand to move the panties to one side and to help separate the buttocks. Wax the area in the same manner as for the previous position, except for one point: Apply the wax from the side of the anus toward the vaginal opening. The client must switch hands when you are ready to switch to the other side of the inside of the buttocks.

The final part of the French bikini wax is the removal of the hair around the labia (Figure 19–26). This area should only be waxed with hard wax and the application strips should be kept small, approximately 1 by 3 inches. (There are experienced technicians who successfully use gentle soft waxes on the labia with small muslin strips, but training and experience is crucial before attempting it as a *paid-for* service on the general public.) Because the direction of hair growth on the labia is inward, the pull in this direction cannot be outward, against the growth, so you pull the strip upward. A swift outward pull on the labia majorum *against* the hair growth could result in a laceration in the crevice between the labia majorum and labia minorum, which is distressing for the client and for you and can result in possible litigation.

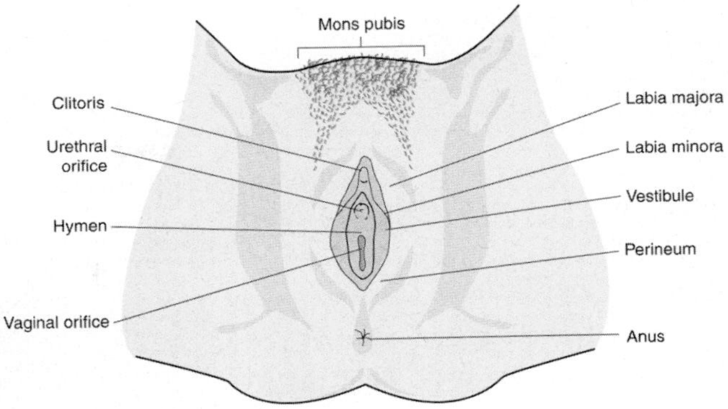

Figure 19–26 The vaginal opening.

Brazilian

The Brazilian bikini wax involves the removal of absolutely everything. The hair is removed as for the French bikini wax, including the area between the buttocks and the labia. In addition, the hair on the pubis is removed. Because of the direction of hair growth, the coarseness of the hair, and the delicate skin of the labia, hard wax should be used for this area. Explain to the client that blood spots may appear and are to be expected. With any first-time bikini wax, advise the client to return within three weeks for a follow-up wax. After that, the client should space waxing service every four to six weeks.

Remove all traces of wax at the end of the service, using plenty of soothing antiseptic lotion. You can apply a product containing salicylic acid with cotton, but it may sting uncomfortably if applied to the labia; it can be applied the next day. This helps remove any redness and bumps and reduces the risk of ingrown hairs.

CAUTION!

Keep in mind that you should never, ever, double-dip an applicator into a wax pot, regardless of the area being waxed. The temperature of wax is not adequate to kill pathogenic organisms.

PROCEDURE 19–1 BRAZILIAN WAX

While each technician develops his or her own preferred routine, this is a basic starting protocol. The client's front will be waxed first, follow by the client turning over for waxing the rear area. Prior to treatment, evaluate the client and discuss alternate positions and the wax to be used.

MATERIALS AND IMPLEMENTS

- Facial lounge, disposable client draping, and set for waxing
- Client modesty towel (disposable)
- Gloves (change as necessary)
- Disposable apron for technician (protects clothing from wax and OPIM)
- Wax heater
- Hard wax
- Adequate quantities of disposable single-use wax applicators
- Disposable bikini thong
- Blunt-tipped scissors
- Disinfectant lotions
- Powder (non-talc)
- Soothing antiseptic lotion
- Wax remover
- Wax solvent

Preparation

1

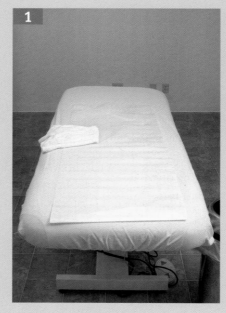

Set up treatment table.

1 Set up treatment table.

2

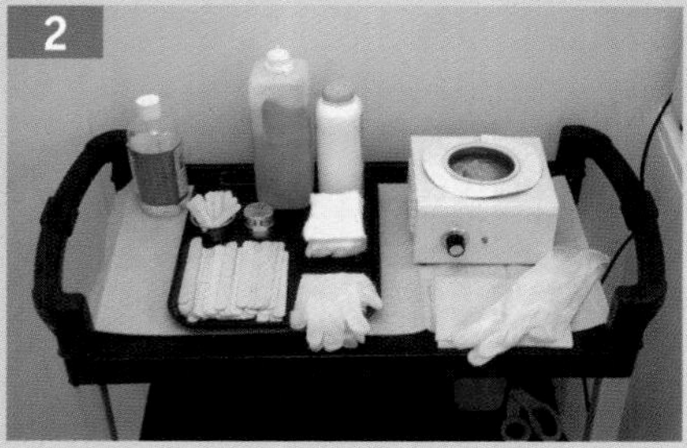

Check wax.

2 Check wax supplies to ensure you have an adequate amount to perform the treatment.

3 Talk to the client to assure that there are no contraindications to the treatment and to review the extent of the hair she wants removed.

4 Have client sign informed consent (minors may require parental consent).

5 Have client remove her lower garments and don the disposable bikini thong.

Procedure

6 Wash your hands and put on the gloves and apron.

7 Help the client onto the bed and ask her to assume a supine (face up) position.

8

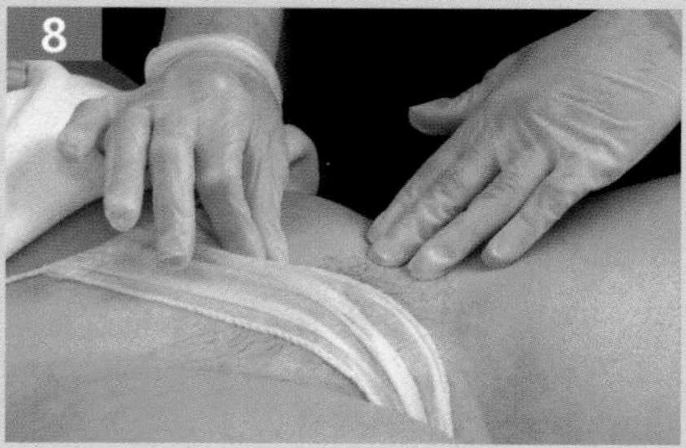

Trim hair to 1/2-inch length.

8 Evaluate the hair length. If the hair is so long that it curls, it should be trimmed to 1/2 inch using scissors or a clipper, if your state regulations allow.

9

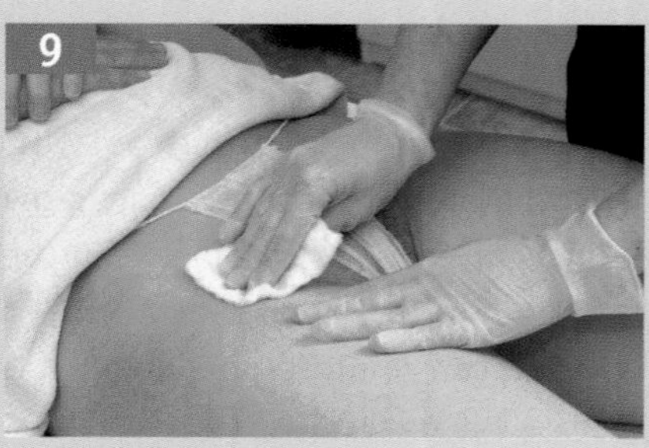

Cleanse area and pat dry.

9 Cleanse the upper leg and the bikini area with an antiseptic cleaner and pat dry.

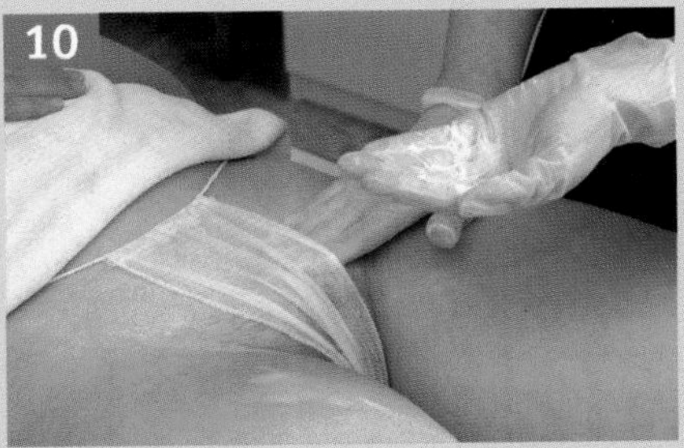

Dust area with powder.

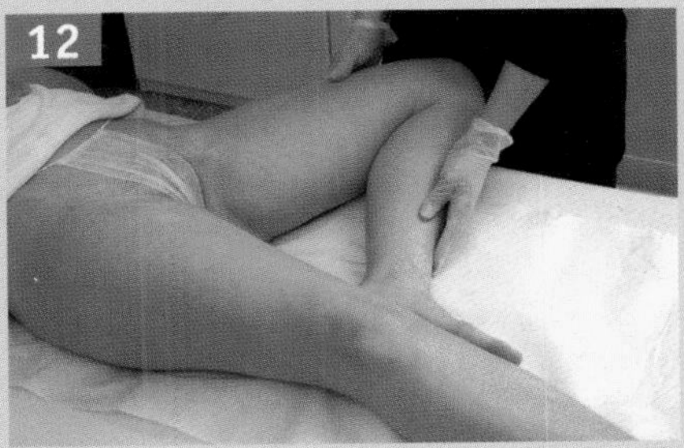

Position client.

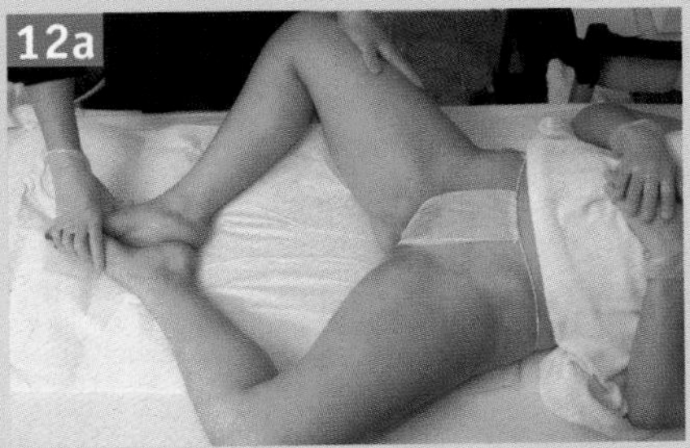

Have client bring both feet together in a "frog" position.

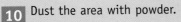

10 Dust the area with powder.

11 Offer the client gloves.

12 Have the client leave one leg straight and bring the sole of the other foot to the level of the knee. Alternatively, have the client bring both feet together in a "froggy" position.

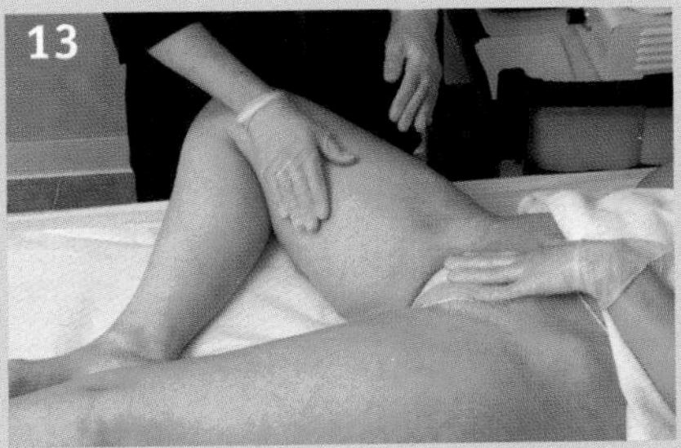

Start on the right side of the client's bikini area.

13 Starting first on the right side of the client's bikini area, have the client place the *left* hand firmly on the skin, stretching with fingers straight downward. Client should wear gloves when assisting with the stretching. Some technicians prefer to work on the leg "across" from them, standing on client's right side and working on left leg, and then vice versa. This may minimize the wax you get on yourself.

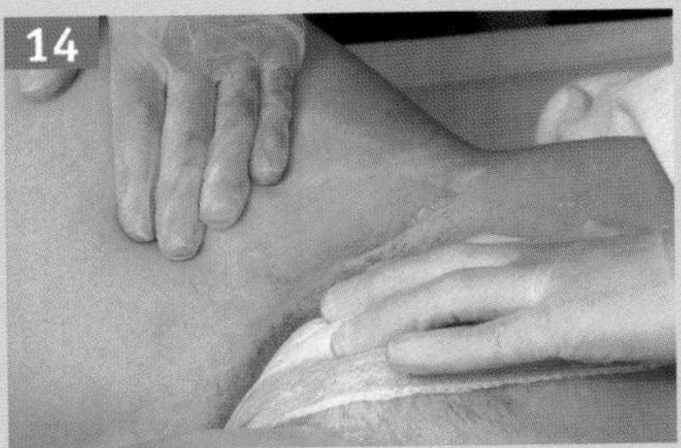

Pull skin taut with free hand.

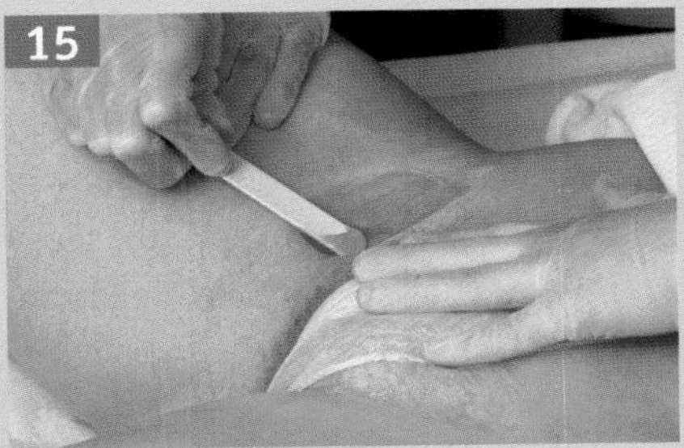

Apply the wax in the direction of hair growth.

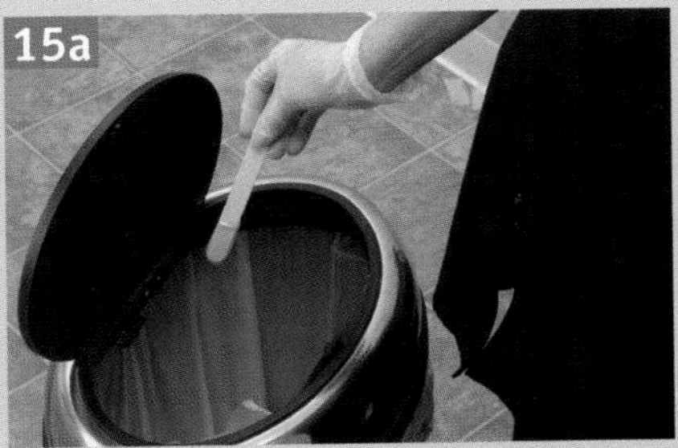

Never double dip.

14 Have the client place her free hand on the outer edge of the thigh to help pull the skin taut.

15 Working on the bent leg, apply the wax with the edge of a spatula in the direction of hair growth. The first application should be to the section farthest away from the bikini line and only up to the femoral ridge, following the downward direction of hair growth. Remember: Never double dip. Dispose of each applicator after you have used it.

continues on next page

PROCEDURE 19-1, CONT. BRAZILIAN WAX

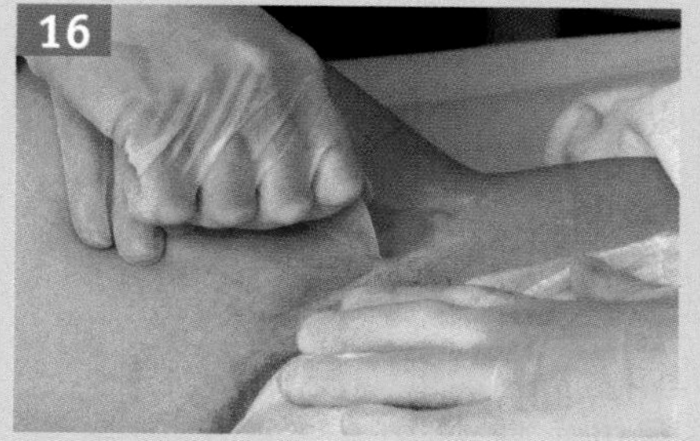

Remove wax off backward in a swift, continuous manner.

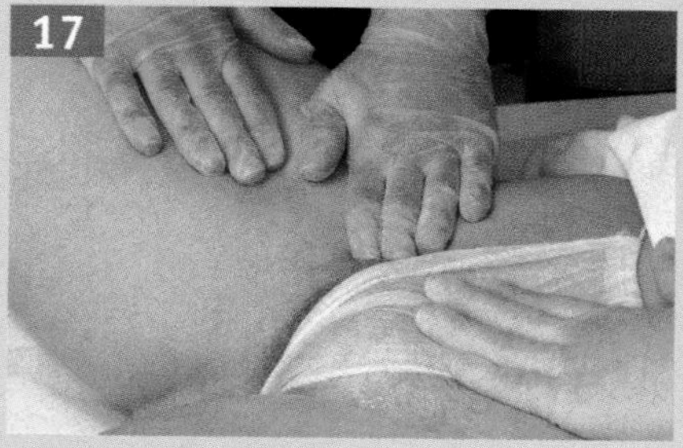

Apply immediate, firm pressure.

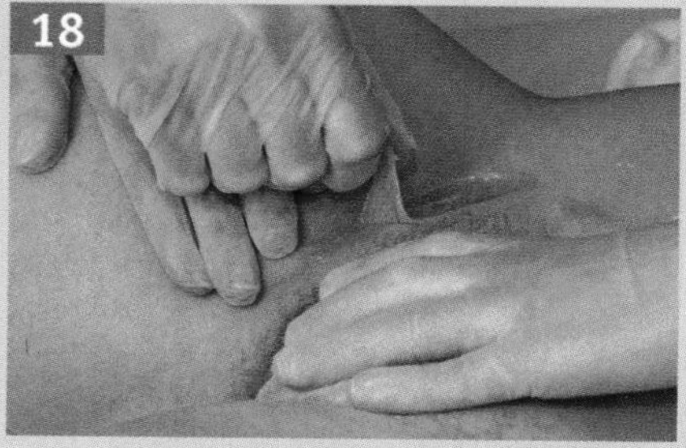

Continue to work toward the bikini line.

16 As soon as the wax has set, flick the free edge to loosen it. Grasp the free edge with one hand and stretch the skin taut with your free hand. Remove the wax backward in a swift, continuous manner, as close to the skin as possible.

17 Apply immediate, firm pressure to alleviate the discomfort.

18 Repeat this process, working toward the bikini line.

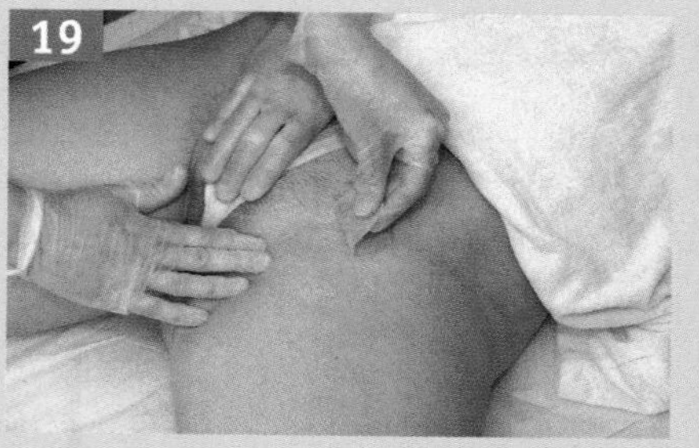

Repeat on left side of clint's bikini.

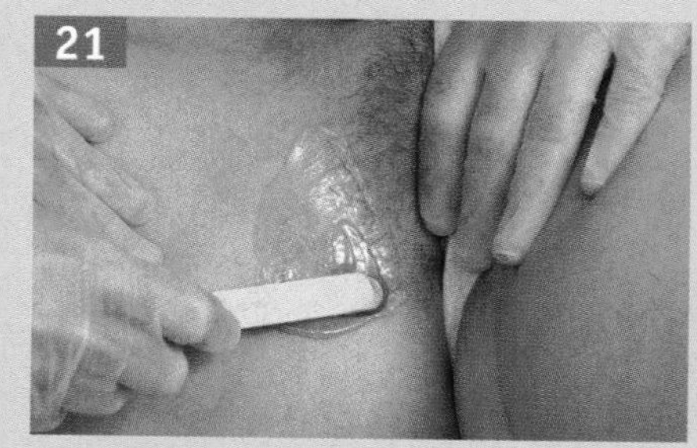

Apply wax two-thirds of the way down.

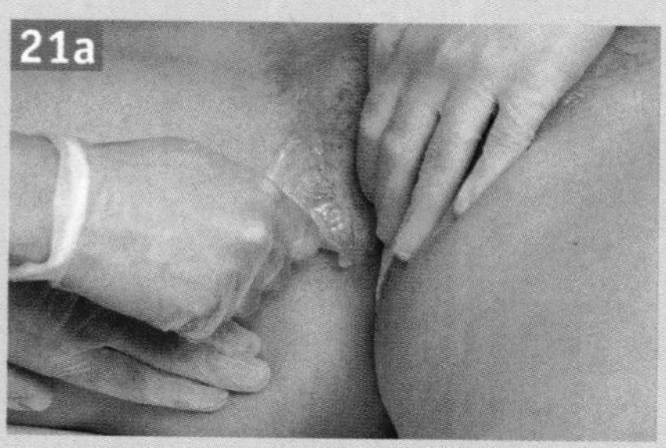

Remove hair and apply pressure for relief.

19 Repeat on left side of client's bikini.

20 Move to the hair that grows down from the femoral ridge.

21 Apply wax two-thirds of the way down in the downward direction of hair growth, leaving enough space at the bottom to place your client's hand to hold the skin taut. Allow the wax to set. Take hold at the free edge, using the other hand to hold skin taut. Remove hair and follow by quickly placing your hand firmly on the area for relief.

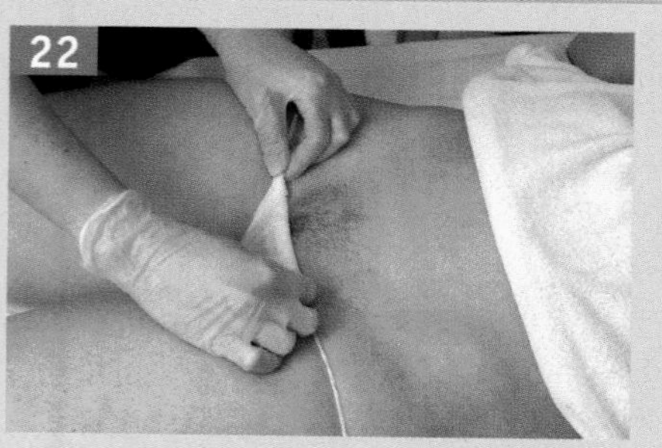

Move to the pubis.

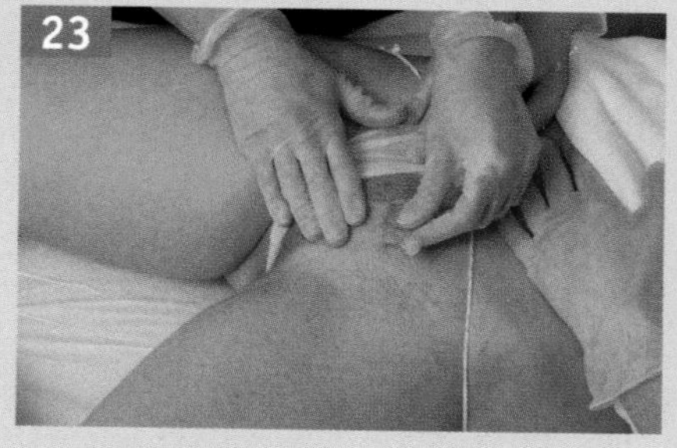

Allow wax to set.

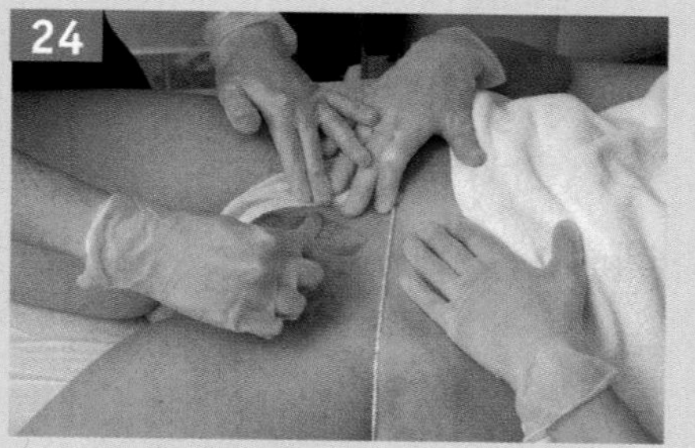

Repeat across pubis until all hair is removed.

22 Move to the pubis and remove hair. Apply wax in direction of growth in 1- by 3-inch segments.

23 Allow wax to set and remove it, followed by pressure.

24 Repeat this process across the pubis until you have removed all hair.

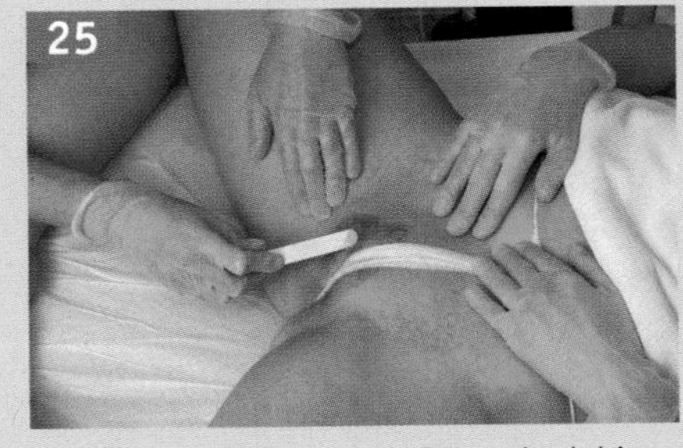

Proceed to remove the hair on the labia.

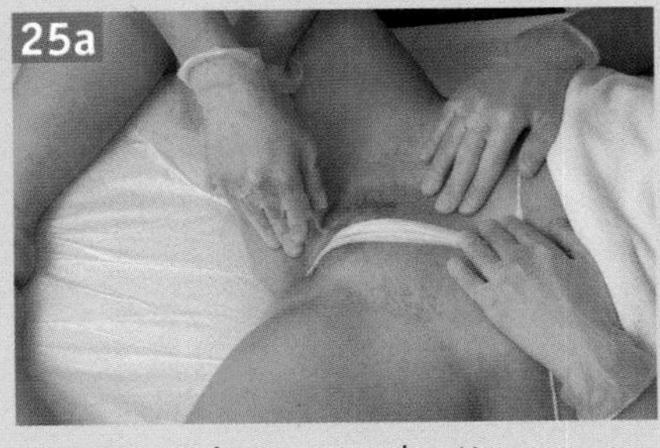

Remove wax in an upward pattern.

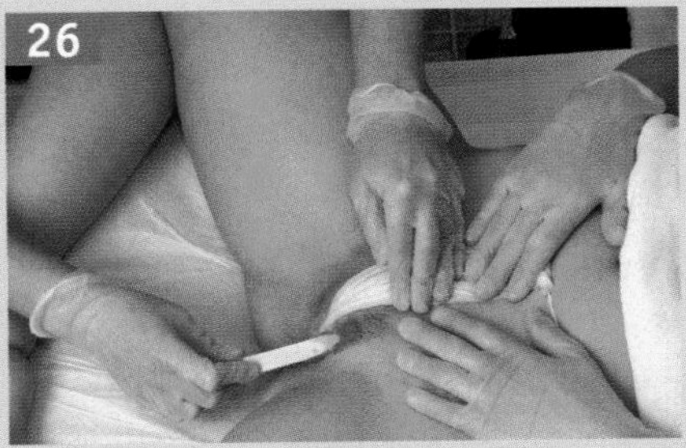

Work in small sections to remove hair on both sides of the labia.

25 For removing the hair on the labia, apply the wax in the direction of growth in a 1- by 3-inch section. Allow the wax to set and remove it in an upward, *not outward,* pattern.

26 Repeat until you have removed all hair on both sides of the labia, working in small sections to minimize client discomfort.

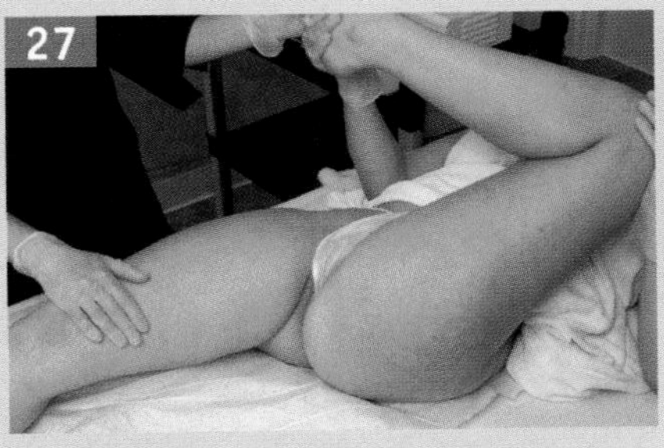

Have the client lift one leg toward her chest.

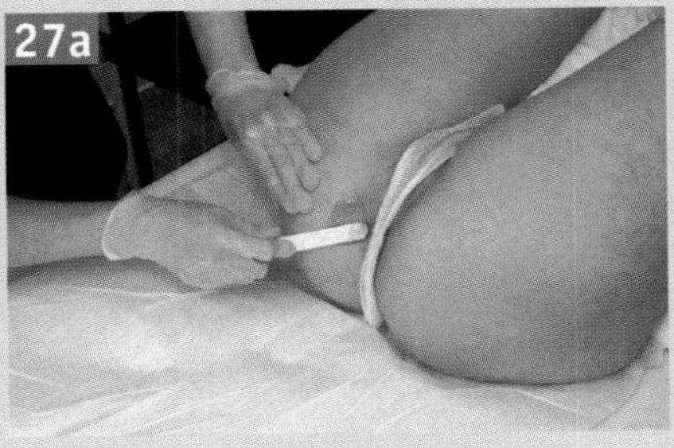

Apply wax downward, and pull upward.

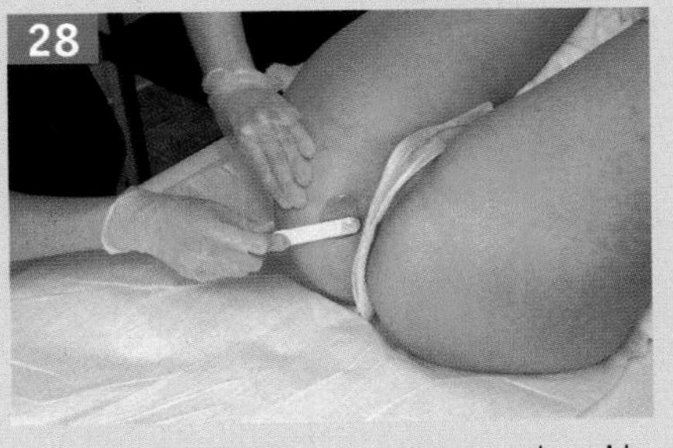

Have client reverse legs; repeat on other side.

27 Have the client lift one leg toward her chest, grasping the ankle with the opposite hand and drawing the leg across the body. This should expose the last remaining third of the hair that was too near the table to apply the wax. This position also ensures that the skin is nice and taut. Apply the wax as before, downward, with the pull upward.

28 Have the client reverse her legs and repeat on the other side. To speed the process and if the client is flexible enough, have her bring both legs up at the same time.

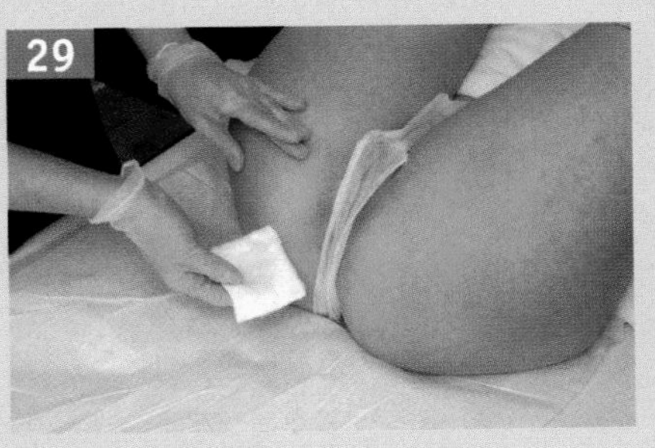

Use soothing antiseptic lotion.

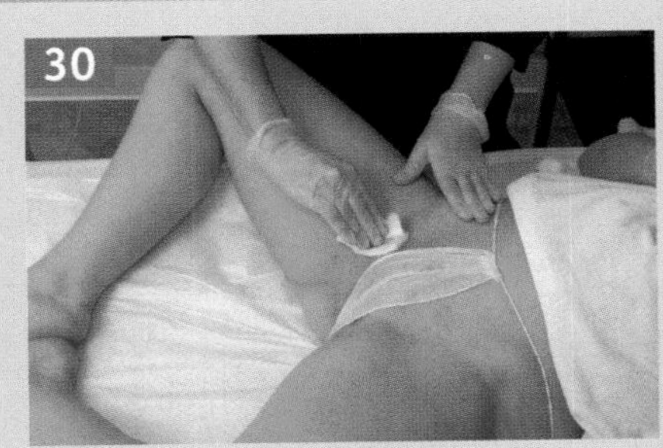

Remove any traces of wax.

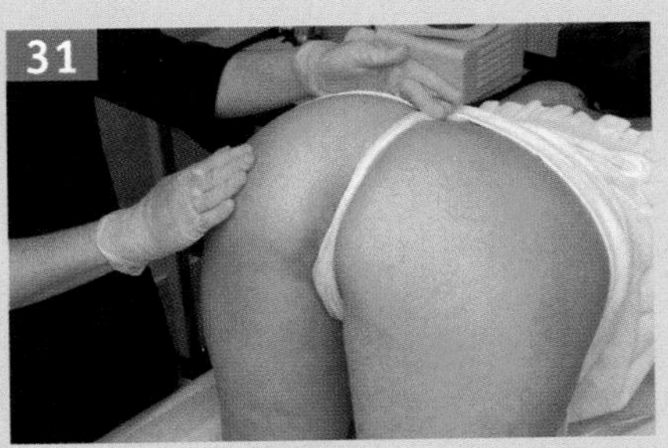

Have client turn over into a kneeling position.

29 Use soothing antiseptic lotion on the entire area that has been waxed.

30 Remove any traces of wax from area that has been waxed.

31 Have the client turn over into a kneeling position with one

continues on next page

PROCEDURE 19-1, CONT. BRAZILIAN WAX

forearm resting on the table in front of her. This allows the client a free hand to move the panties to one side and to help separate the buttocks. Some technicians find that if the client brings her legs to her chest and grabs the ankles, the technician does not have to turn the client on the side or stomach. This may vary with the client.

32 Use preparatory disinfectant on the area and apply powder.

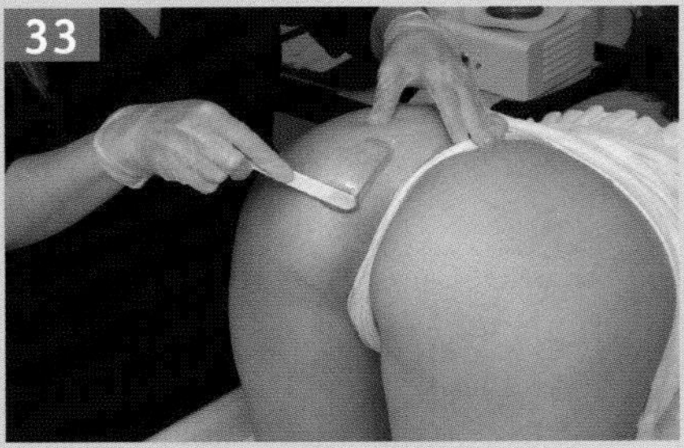

Apply wax starting at the rear of the buttocks.

33 Starting at the rear of the buttocks, apply the wax in 1- by 3-inch strips in the direction of hair growth toward the anus, enlisting the client's assistance to make the area available to wax.

34 Allow the wax to set, and then remove against growth.

35 Follow removal with pressure.

36 Repeat these steps, working from the rear toward the vaginal opening until all hair is removed.

37 Repeat on the other side of the buttocks, having the client switch supporting arms and making her other hand available to assist with making the area to be waxed more available.

38 When you have removed all hair, use soothing antiseptic lotion and ensure that you have removed any residual wax.

Post-procedure

39 While a warm shower is not contraindicated, suggest that the client avoid extremely hot water for at least 24 hours. She should also avoid vigorous exercise and tanning beds or sun.

40 Ensure client has any home care products that may assist in reducing or preventing ingrown hairs.

Clean-up and Disinfection

41 Follow state guidelines for clean-up and disinfection of the treatment room and any nondisposable implements used.

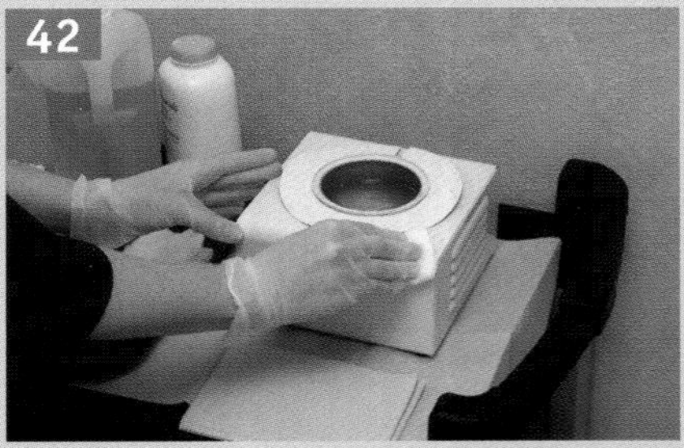

Use wax solvent to clean up and disinfect.

42 Use wax solvent to ensure that the wax pot and surrounding area are free of any wax drips. Then disinfect the pot following state guidelines.

While some technicians like to use a warm towel for clean-up, they must then treat the towel as if it were contaminated with potentially infectious material requiring special handling. Using all disposable materials simplifies risk management and clean-up.

ADVANCED MALE WAXING

The areas male clients most commonly choose to have waxed are the back, the shoulders, between the eyebrows, and the outer ear. Some, especially swimmers or body builders, have the chest and legs waxed, too. There are also those who dislike any body hair and want full Brazilian waxing. Occasionally, male clients enter the salon dressed as women and request more extensive waxing. Men requesting sex-change operations are often required to go through psychiatric testing and are asked, before having major surgery, to live and dress as women for a period of time. Eventually, these clients may opt for hormone therapy, laser treatments, and/or electrolysis prior to male-to-female transgender surgery. Until then, however, they may choose to have much of the torso hair waxed away, along with the arm and leg hair. You may find these situations awkward, but they are also awkward for those requesting the services. Your confidence, compassion, and professionalism are paramount. Ascertain from clients what hair removal services they want and clearly explain what can and cannot be done and what they can expect.

Many athletes are turning to waxing as an alternative to shaving the entire body. The removal of body hair offers less water resistance or drag for swimmers and is more comfortable for wrestlers, who then have no hair to drag or catch on the mat. Ask the client to wear swimwear that is slightly smaller than his competitive sports attire, and then remove all exposed hair. Protect the swimwear with a paper towel as you wax in this area.

Eyebrows

Most men simply want the glabellar area, often called the "unibrow," waxed (Figure 19–27). Occasionally, a little tweezing under the brow is warranted. Often, the brow hairs are long and unruly, and trimming them with scissors can make a big difference in their appearance.

Men's eyebrows should not be waxed in the same way women's eyebrows are waxed. Men do not want a feminine sophisticated look and do not expect or want high arches. They generally prefer a more natural look that is simply well groomed. To wax and groom men's eyebrows, cleanse, pre-treat, and powder the client's eyebrows in the usual manner. Offer the client a handheld mirror and discuss the shape as well as what should be

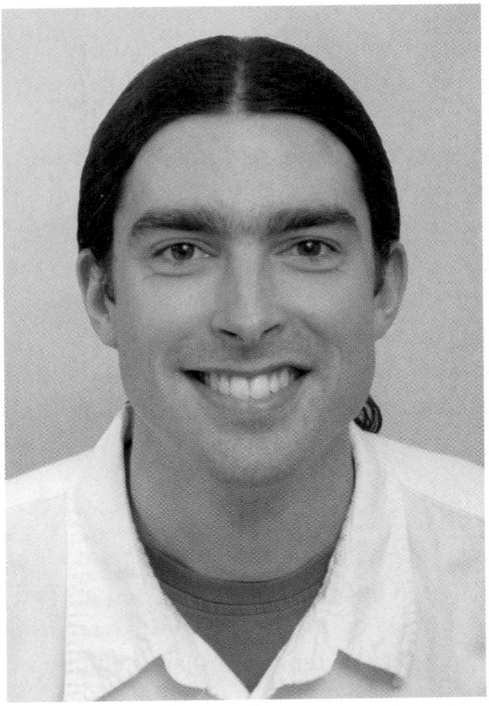

Figure 19–27 Male eyebrows, before.

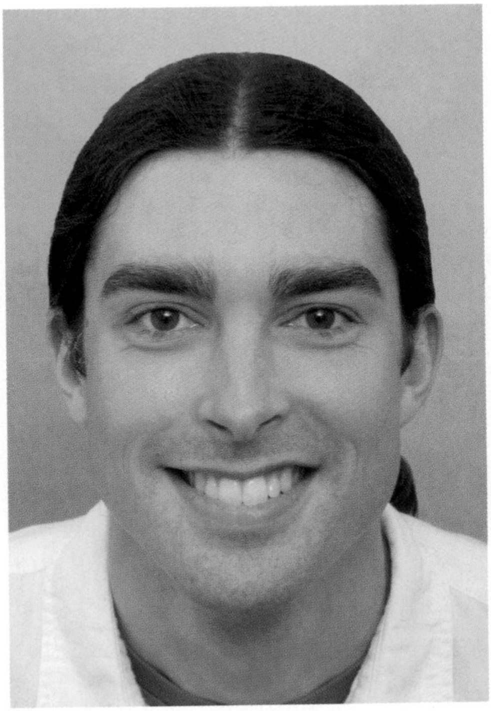

Figure 19–28 Male eyebrows, after.

removed and what should stay. Using a small amount of wax on the end of a thin, wooden applicator, isolate the hairs under the brow that should be waxed. Apply the wax in the direction of growth. Apply the strip, also rubbing in the direction of growth, and quickly pull away, against the growth. After completing both eyebrows, move to the center. A man's eyebrow should always start just to the inside of the corner of the eye; everything else in the glabellar area can be waxed away. Most of the hair in the glabellar grows upward, but there may also be a significant amount of hair at the top of the nose that grows downward and should also be removed following the appropriate rules (Figure 19–28).

Back

When men book back waxes, they generally want all of the hair removed from just below the waistband upward. If the client is wearing a business suit and will be returning to work, suggest that he remove his pants and upper clothing. Provide a hanger on which to hang the clothes and a towel or drape to place around the waist. Leave the room while the client changes. If the client does not need to remove his pants, have him at least remove the belt from his pants for comfort, then have him lie prone on the table. His arms should be upward, with the elbows sticking outward. The client should rest the side of the face on the tops of the hands. Place two paper towels along the top edge of the client's pants. If the hair is longer than ½ inch, trim it (Figure 19–29). Stand on the same side on which you are going to apply the wax, changing sides after that half is completed. Warn the client that he will feel a cold spray, and then spray the area with a mild antiseptic solution. Wipe off any excess moisture with a paper towel, and dust with powder.

Soft wax is the preferred wax for this area due to its speed and effectiveness. Begin the hair removal at the area just above the waistband of the pants. The first application of wax should begin from the outside edge of the torso where the hair growth starts (Figure 19–30). Using a large spatula, dip into a full pot of wax until one-half to two-thirds of the spatula is covered. Remove the spatula, scraping its underside on the side of the pot or on the scraping rim provided. Using the edge of the spatula, glide inward, following the direction of hair growth toward the base of the spine, allowing a thin layer of wax to cover the area. Apply the strip, leaving a 1-inch free edge at the farthest end. Rub the strip twice in the direction of growth, and then, with the free hand placed over the base of the spine and holding the skin taut, quickly pull backward and downward against the growth and as close to the skin as possible. It is important to follow through with the movement, in a downward motion, to where the hair growth started. Quickly apply firm pressure with the free hand. Make the following application right next to the preceding one. If the length of the strip is too long to do in one try, remove the strip on the outside first. The second strip should be toward the middle, the third strip to the side of the first, and the fourth strip above the third, going to the middle. Continue in this manner until reaching the top. At the top, the hair starts to grow downward in the center, along the spine. Complete the removal on that side by following the waxing rules and directional changes.

At this time, if the client would like, include the back of the shoulder. When that side is complete, move to the other side of the table and repeat the process. Apply plenty of soothing antiseptic lotion to the area that you have waxed. Be careful not to extend beyond

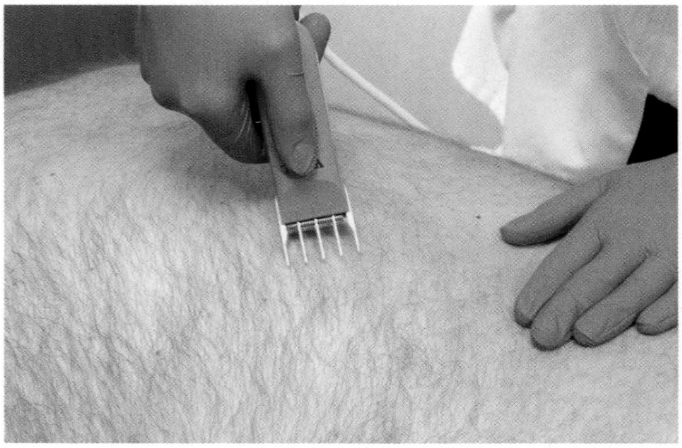

Figure 19–29 Preparation of client for back waxing.

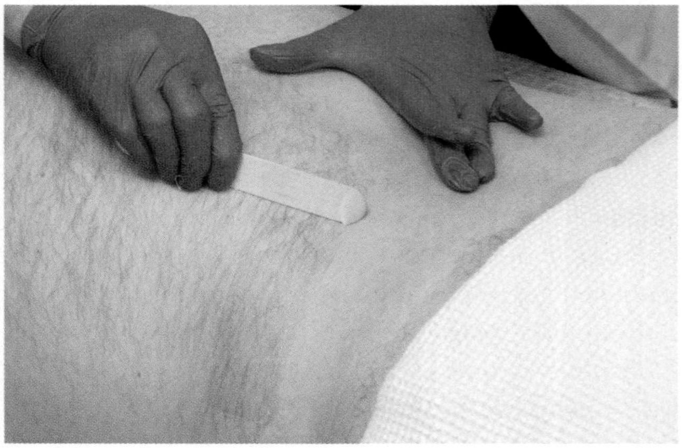

Figure 19–30 Initial wax application to back.

that, because there may be a few more strips to do with the client sitting up. You can also apply a cool compress soaked in a baking-powder solution. It is not unusual for hives to develop in this area. They will subside in an hour or so, and applying an OTC salicylic acid product will help reduce the redness and bumps. Because the client cannot see his back, let him know when the blood spots have diminished and when it is safe to get dressed. Do not let him risk getting blood spots all over his clothing.

The client should now sit on the edge of the table, facing you. At this time, with arms at his side, you can wax the rest of the shoulder area and do any blending toward the front, making sure both sides are balanced and even. Wax the shoulders in a manner similar to doing the knees, one surface area or plane at a time; do not attempt to round a curve with the strip. The hair on the shoulder usually grows inward to the center of the shoulder from the back and inward toward the center from the front. Waxing the front is considered a separate service (part of the chest wax), but blending a little with wax already on the strip is acceptable.

Chest

Before waxing a man's chest, have the client sit on the side of the table and discuss which areas the client would like cleared of hair. Some men book this service wanting abdominal hair or hair in front of the shoulders removed right up to the chest area but leaving the hair on the chest (i.e., above and between the breasts) intact. Make sure the you clearly understand what he wants. For this service, the client should be lying supine. Stand at the side to be being worked on, changing sides after that half is completed.

If the client's chest hair is longer than ½ inch and curly, trim it to ½ inch long. When trimming the hair with an electric trimmer, trim well away from the wax, or cover the pot, because the hair will "fly" into the wax pot. After trimming the hair, warn the client that he will feel a cold spray. Spritz or wipe the entire area with a mild antiseptic solution. Wipe away any excess with a paper towel, and dust the area with powder. Soft wax is the preferred wax for this due to its speed and effectiveness. Begin the first application of wax on an outer edge, working upward and inward, toward a denser area. Always apply the wax in the direction of hair growth, rubbed in the direction of the hair growth, and remove it against hair growth. Use a large strip. As the area becomes dense, make the wax applications in smaller strips, applying immediate pressure after each pull. On completion, soothe the entire area with the aftercare lotion.

Ears

The hair on the outer rim and lobes of the ear can be waxed but not hair inside the ears. Men often trim earlobe hair with scissors, leaving it bristly. Waxing the hair results in much softer regrowth. To wax the earlobes and ear rim, have the client lie supine or assume a semi-reclined position. Cleanse and dry the area. Both hard and soft waxes are effective for this task. With hard wax the applications are small, following the usual rules for hard wax, or the manufacturer's recommendations, starting at the top of the rim. Hold the top of the rim for the removal downward. With soft wax the wax is applied to the lobe in a downward direction with a narrow stick, then a small strip placed over the area. Hold the earlobe taut with the free hand and pull upward quickly. Proceed to the area above. Apply the wax in a downward motion along the rim. Apply the strip, again rubbing downward. Holding the top portion of the lobe taut, pull upward quickly, against the growth. After completing the second ear, soothe the area with lotion, massaging both earlobes simultaneously for a more pleasurable end to the service. When you have mastered this wax service, 10 minutes should be more than enough time.

Male Brazilian

The process of removing hair for a male bikini or Brazilian wax service is accomplished in much the same way as for a female with the exception of handling the male genitals. The client should be enlisted to hold the penis and scrotum out of the way so that you can wax the bikini line. The skin on the genitals is very thin and easily torn. Waxing this area can be very risky. Even very experienced technicians state that injuries do occur. Do not attempt to wax male genitals without proper training with a live model and a signed client consent form.

LASER AND PULSED LIGHT HAIR REMOVAL

Monochromatic Light

Monochromatic literally means "single color." In this case it describes a type of laser light. Laser light has its own color, which determines its single wavelength. During hair removal, the color of the laser light determines how the laser will react with the pigment in the hair and skin. All lasers react to different **chromophores**, depending

Table 19–3 Lasers and the Efficacy on Hair Removal

LASER OR LIGHT	SKIN TYPE	HAIR COLOR	TYPE OF HAIR
Pulsed Diode	I–IV	Black to light brown	Prefers coarse
Ruby	I–III	Black to light brown	Fine and coarse
Normal mode Nd:YAG	I–VI	Dark	Prefers coarse
Q-Switch Nd:YAG	I–VI (temporary removal only)	Black to light brown	Fine and coarse
Alexandrite	I–IV	Black to light brown	Fine and coarse
Intense Pulsed Light	I–IV	Black to light brown	Prefers coarse

on the wavelength. This is why there are so many different lasers; each has a different purpose (Table 19–3).

Intense Pulsed Light

Intense pulsed light (IPL) is **polychromatic** and broadband. The clinical use of polychromatic light is achieved through filters that affect the wavelength. Typically, the wavelength is between 400 nm and 1000nm. The filters that are used create wavelengths that selectively target different skin structures—hair, pigment, or vessels. Intense pulsed light, while not a laser, does behave like a laser from the perspective of **selective photothermolysis,** or the use of color focused light to destroy hair. Lasers treat one chromophore with one monochromatic light, while intense pulsed light can target multiple chromophores. It is the head or filter on the IPL device that determines the type of service for which it is effective.

Some IPL devices have demonstrated efficiency in hair reduction. The client selection process, safety issues, and procedure techniques are similar for both pulsed light and laser devices. These procedures are gaining popularity because they are nonablative, more comfortable, faster, and less expensive for both the client and the practitioner.

Safety in the Laser Treatment Room

Before the client enters the treatment room, the technician must survey the room with safety and legal considerations in mind. First, even if the room used for laser treatments or IPL treatments is used for other treatments, this treatment room must be set up following the strictest guidelines associated

BENEFITS OF LASER OR IPL HAIR REMOVAL VS. OTHER TREATMENT MODALITIES

- **Offers a fast, long-lasting hair reduction**
- **May produce some permanent or complete results**
- **Can treat large body areas with greater speed by treating multiple hairs at once, unlike the hair-by-hair method of electrolysis**
- **Offers no risk of disease transmission via blood; treatments are non-invasive compared to electrolysis**
- **Not considered as uncomfortable as electrolysis, though that is subjective**
- **Regrowth can be finer and lighter**

DRAWBACKS TO LASER OR IPL HAIR REMOVAL VS. OTHER TREATMENT MODALITIES

- **Costly, requiring an average of six to nine or more treatments**
- **Safety and effectiveness concerns over the long term**
- **Ineffective on light and nonpigmented hair, like blonde, red, or gray/white**
- **Generally ineffective on dark or tanned skin (A few lasers now bypass this concern.)**
- **Safety concerns for the eyes necessitate protective eyewear**
- **Mild discomfort**
- **No guarantee of satisfaction**
- **Inadequate and inconsistent state regulatory controls and guidelines**

> **? Did You Know**
>
> Lasers used in hair removal target the melanin. This is why it is easier to treat dark-haired, fair-skinned individuals.

with laser equipment. While IPL devices do not have the nominal hazard zones associated with laser, precautions concerning closed doors, signage, and goggles are pertinent. The room used for hair removal should have no windows or the windows should be blacked out with protective coverings. In addition, no large mirrors or artwork housed in glass should be hung on the walls of a room where laser is performed. This will minimize the risk of unwanted reflective damage. The laser treatment room should have a door that can be kept closed during the treatment and a warning light or sign (Figure 19–31) outside indicating treatment in progress or warning others not to enter. Protective eyewear should be available for the client and for individuals to put on before entering a treatment room.

Any technician performing laser hair removal treatments should be well trained and qualified in the use of the device. Technicians should also be protected by insurance in case of accident or malpractice claims. Prior to conducting a hair removal treatment, the technician and client must remove all reflective clothing and jewelry and should be dressed sensibly and professionally with a lab coat and comfortable shoes (preferably with closed toes). The technician, client, and other individuals in the room must wear ANSI-approved protective eyewear to prevent risk of laser blindness, and the eyerwear must stay in place throughout the treatment. At the conclusion of the treatment, the technician should make sure the key is removed from the laser equipment. The key should *never* be in the equipment when it is not in use. The technician should also make sure the laser tip is regularly cleaned to prevent carbon buildup and contamination.

The treatment room itself ought to be well ventilated, because vaporized hair shafts smell of sulfur. In large quantities, the smell can irritate the respiratory tract. Having proper ventilation is beneficial to both client and technician.

Client Selection

There are four main categories of excess hair growth: hypertrichosis, hirsutism, hair-bearing flaps, and, finally, cosmetic concerns. Hypertrichosis is increased hair growth that is not androgen-dependent. Typically it is a result of medications or disease. Hirsutism is androgen-dependent and can be accompanied by other diseases (Figure 19–32). Hair-bearing flaps are the result of surgeries in which skin flaps have been used in the reconstructive process. While, surgeons try to be careful about turning flaps with unwanted hair, it can still happen. Then a patient may seek hair removal laser to remedy the situation. A cosmetic concern is by far the most common reason for seeking hair removal. Primarily this is an issue of unwanted hair in areas such as the legs, bikini line, face, and back.

An important consideration in client selection involves client expectations. Managing a client's expectations ensures an optimal outcome for both you and the client. The first and most important conversation should be about permanency. Clients that seek laser hair removal should know the difference between temporary hair removal, permanent hair reduction, and complete hair removal.

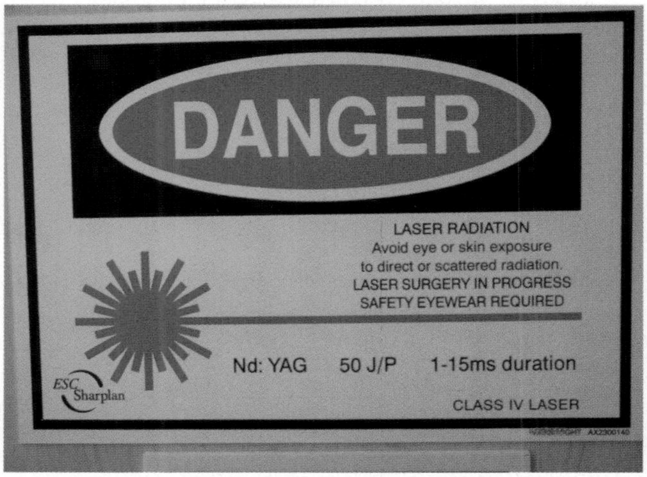

Figure 19–31 Laser sign on treatment door.

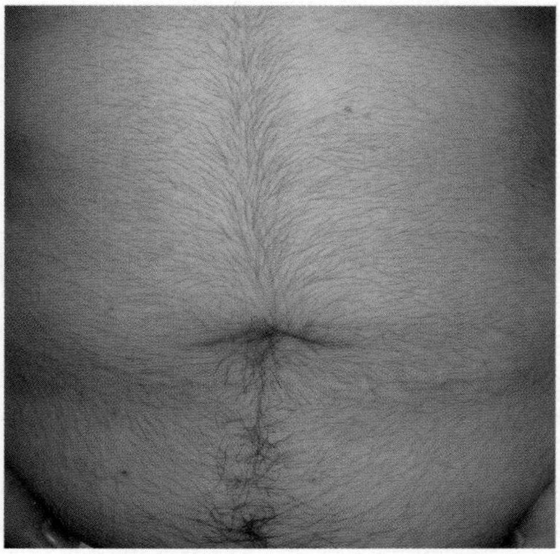

Figure 19–32 Excessive hair growth.

Temporary hair removal is a short-term (up to three months) reduction in hair. Permanent hair reduction is longer termed, but there is a great probability of the hair follicle recovering. Complete hair removal involves the obliteration of the hair follicle beyond recovery. While it is a possibility that some candidates will experience complete hair loss, most will only experience permanent hair reduction. Once you have educated a client about the topic of permanency, you can evaluate their suitability as a candidate for hair removal. The best candidate is light-skinned and dark haired, with no tan and a normal endocrine status, who does not wax or tweeze the area (Table 19–4). Furthermore, a potential client should understand and accept the possible risks and complications that can occur with laser hair removal treatments.

As you evaluate a client for laser hair removal, know the contraindications (Table 19–5). These conditions include open wounds in the area to be treated, pregnancy, and epilepsy. In addition, clients taking photosensitizing medications are not candidates for these services. Most important, learn to recognize a herpetic breakout and refer clients with this skin condition to a doctor for pre-treatment with an antiviral medication.

Table 19–4 Skin Type and Laser Hair Removal

FITZPATRICK SKIN TYPE	DESCRIPTION	LASER HAIR REMOVAL CONSIDERATIONS
Type I	Very fair skin accompanied by blonde or light-red hair and blue or green eyes; never tans, always burns	May not be good candidates because of lack of contrast between hair and skin color
Type II	Fair skin accompanied by light-brown or red hair and green, blue, or brown eyes. Occasionally tans, always burns.	Good candidates for laser hair removal
Type III	Medium skin accompanied by brown hair and brown eyes; often tans, sometimes burns	Good candidates for laser hair removal
Type IV	Olive skin, accompanied by brown or black hair and dark-brown or black eyes; always tans, rarely burns	Good candidates for laser hair removal. Best done by experienced practitioners.
Type V	Dark-brown skin accompanied by black hair and black eyes; rarely burns	May not be good candidates because of lack of contrast between hair and skin color. If performed, use only Yag lasers run by experienced practitioners.
Type VI	Black skin accompanied by black hair and black eyes; rarely burns	May not be good candidates because of lack of contrast between hair and skin color. If performed, only use Yag lasers. Best done by experienced practitioners.

Table 19–5 Partial List of Contraindications for Laser Hair Removal

PARTIAL LIST OF CONTRAINDICATIONS FOR LASER HAIR REMOVAL
Pregnancy
Epilepsy
Tanned or sunburned skin (or any previous thermal injury resulting in hypo- or hyperpigmentation)
Open wounds
Birthmarks, moles, or beauty spots on the area to be treated, unless treatment is approved by a physician
History of keloid scarring
Certain oral and topical medications known to cause photosensitivity or photoallergic reactions (especially oral antibiotics used to treat acne, such as doxycycline or minocycline)

Effects of Laser on Skin Type

While all skin types have a great deal in common, such as the number of hair follicles (whether or not they actively produce terminal hair), thickness of the epidermis and dermis, and components found in layers, they have other characteristics that set them apart. As previously discussed skin color is important in the candidacy of a potential client. Following is a discussion of some of the many different skin types defined by the Fitzpatrick Scale along with a description of the skin type's relationship to laser hair removal.

Caucasian European

Caucasian Europeans have the most varied skin type and hair and eye color variations, as determined by heredity. In most cases this ethnic group has lighter skin but the hair can range from very light (Norwegians) to darker (Germans). Typically, this is a good ethnic group for laser hair removal.

Eastern Asian and Pacific Islander

Eastern Asians include the Chinese, Japanese, and Koreans. This group of people generally have the least amount of facial and body hair. In terms of laser hair removal, they are good candidates due to their dark hair. Their skin can be dark so take care when treating these individuals to avoid skin injury.

Middle Eastern and Mediterranean

Middle Eastern and Mediterranean people tend to have the darkest and coarsest hair on the face and body. Skin color varies from dark white to medium brown. Individuals with lighter skin are the best candidates for laser hair removal. There is an increased risk of causing hyperpigmentation on the skin of this ethnic group.

Treating Ethnic Skin

With dark brown skin, African, African-American, African-European, and African-Caribbean peoples are typically poor candidates for laser hair removal. This is because the laser light absorbs into the skin pigment before it reaches the hair follicle. Unfortunately this can cause burns and scars, including keloids if the client is predisposed to them. However, newer hair removal lasers used on the proper settings can safely treat these clients with only minimal risk. When treating a patient with this ethnic background, proceed slowly.

The Consultation

The primary objectives of the consultation are education and the determination of candidacy. After it is determined that the client is a good candidate for laser hair removal, give him or her a brief, basic overview of laser hair removal, including the variables affecting treatment. It is important that the client understand the three stages of hair growth, which has an impact on the number of treatments. In particular, make sure the client understands that hair grows at different times and in different follicles in the same area. Generally, three to nine treatments are needed for optimal, long-lasting reduction.

Make the client aware of the time commitment and the financial commitment before entering into a treatment relationship. In particular, be sure the client understands the expense involved in the number of agreed-upon treatments. Because it is considered cosmetic, laser hair removal is not covered by insurance. Each laser treatment is separate and usually incurs a separate charge unless a specific treatment package is arranged.

Discuss post-treatment considerations and the fact that there may be increased discomfort if the procedure is performed just prior to or during menstruation. Inform the client of risks of hyperpigmentation for a particular skin type and in relation to the device being used. Clients may have questions about information that they have researched on the Internet or read about in magazines. It is your role to debunk the inaccurate or misleading information.

Make sure the client understands that he or she must cease all methods of hair removal other than shaving or depilatory creams at least four to six weeks before laser hair removal treatment. Removing the hair from the follicle by tweezing, waxing, or electrolysis eliminates the chromophores that the light-based hair removal depends on for effective destruction. Shaving or clipping may be done up to two days before treatment. This is important so that you can ascertain the percentage of growing hairs and then shave the area before the treatment.

Overall, at a consultation for laser hair removal, the client should receive the following:

- A detailed and thorough consultation, including information about cost and possible number of treatments
- Pre- and post-care instructions
- Information that adequately describes the benefits and risks of treatment
- Instructions to remove all reflective clothing and jewelry

If possible, if the client indicates the wish to move forward with treatments, have him or her read and sign the consent at the consultation (Figure 19–33). If the laser is available at the time of the consultation, do a patch test and analyze it (see "Patch Testing" in Figure 19–34). When the client arrives for his or her first treatment, treatment can proceed without delay.

Laser Hair-Removal Consultation/Record Form

Name ______________________________ Date ___/___/___

Address ______________________________

Telephone Home (___)______________ Work (___)______________ DOB ___/___/___

Attending physician ______________________________

Medical History:

- Allergies ______________
- Infectious diseases ______________
- H/L blood pressure ______________
- Hormone therapy ______________
- Herpes ______________
- Epilepsy ______________
- Diabetes ______________
- Lupus ______________
- Scleroderma ______________
- Keloid scars ______________
- Cancer/melanoma ______________
- Heart disease/pacemaker ______________
- Thyroid condition ______________
- Nervous disorders ______________
- Laser resurfacing ______________
- Pregnant ______________
- Vitiligo ______________
- Other ______________

OB/GYN History ______________________________

Medications and herbal supplements currently and recently taken ______________________________

____

Area(s) to be treated ______________________________

Natural color of hair: ☐ brown ☐ blonde ☐ red ☐ gray/white Hair pelosity: ☐ coarse ☐ medium ☐ fine

Skin tone

☐ Very fair: Always burn, never tan, blue eyes
☐ Fair: Mainly burn, sometimes tan
☐ Medium/olive: Mainly tan, rarely burn
☐ Dark: Never burn, dark hair, dark eyes

☐ Tattoos or permanent makeup
☐ Gold and salt injections

Previous Hair Removal

Temporary means of hair removal______________ Frequency ______________

Permanent means of hair removal ______________________________

Date began ____________ Last treatment ____________ Approximate number of treatments ____________

I, the undersigned, do hereby certify that the answers to the above questions are correct to the best of my knowledge.

Signature ______________________________ **Date** ____________

Signature of parent/guardian if under 18 years of age______________________________

Date	Laser Device	Area(s) Treated	Fluence	Pulse Width	Spot Size	Additional Comments

Figure 19–33 Laser hair-removal consultation/record form.

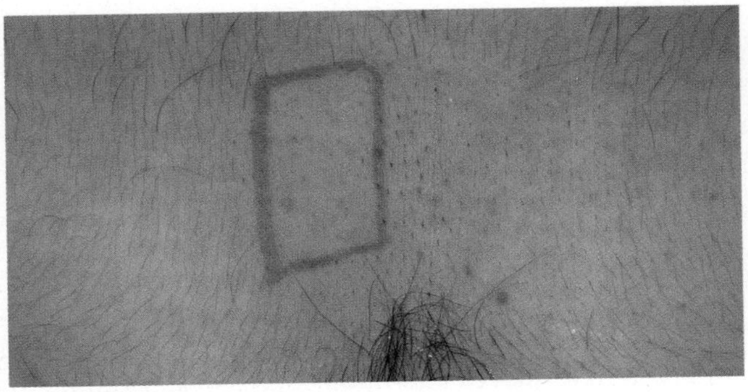

Figure 19–34 Patch test.

Patch Testing

A patch test is important for two reasons (Figure 19–34). First, it gives the technician an opportunity to gauge a client's tolerance to the treatment and to select the appropriate fluence levels. Second, it gives clients an opportunity to experience the laser and to perhaps relieve some of the anxiety that might be associated with the treatment. An initial, single pulse should be performed at a test site near the treatment area and observed for damage to the epidermis. The clinical manifestations observed are perifollicular edema, erythema or blistering, or an epidermal, separation caused by lateral pressure on the skin, called the **Nikolski sign.** If the client has a reaction, lower the fluence by 5 j/cm^2 to 10 j/cm^2. Record the test results on the record form.

THE LASER HAIR REMOVAL TREATMENT

At this point you have had the consultation with the client, who has decided to move ahead with the treatment. The client has read and signed a consent form and you performed a patch test; the results of that test, along with your assessment of the client's skin and hair color, indicated that the client is a good candidate for the treatment. You have informed the client to keep from tweezing or waxing before the treatment. You have prepared the treatment room with safety and legal considerations in mind. Now it is time for the client's treatment appointment.

Table 19–6 lists the first steps you should complete before beginning the treatment. Hopefully, the client has complied and the area to be treated has only been shaved. The next step is skin cleansing, preparation, and numbing of the skin, if required. The client's skin should be clean and free from oils, perspiration, deodorants, perfumes, and cosmetics that could impede the laser or aggravate the skin post-treatment. The cleanser should be mild and gentle and have the capacity to rinse away cleanly, leaving the skin dry, non-irritated, and unstimulated. To clean larger body areas, the client can shower before the appointment with a simple antibacterial soap.

Skin Preparation

The client's skin should be close-shaven; however, if the client has opted to use a topical anesthetic, then shaving ought to be done a day or two prior to treatment to allow any superficial scrapes or irritations to resolve themselves. This can be done prior to the appointment, particularly for the first treatment. However with subsequent visits, you may choose to assess the hair growth pattern and have the client come to the office unshaven.

Topical Anesthesia

With today's laser devices, cooling heads, and gels, anesthesia of any kind is often unwarranted and unnecessary for most clients for most treatment areas, but there are exceptions. For those individuals that have difficulty with the pain of laser hair removal, there are choices of anesthesia. However, complete pain blockage is not appropriate, because feedback from the client helps determine if the treatment power is too high. Typically, clients can purchase a numbing cream from the clinic or be supplied with a prescription from a physician, who should instruct the

Table 19–6 Steps to Complete Prior to Treatment

STEPS TO COMPLETE PRIOR TO TREATMENT
Instruct the client to remove all necessary clothing, and provide a gown and drapes. Leave the room, and knock before reentering.
Take photos, if none were taken during the consultation.
Cleanse and free the area of lotions, deodorants, perfumes, and cosmetics.
Shave the target area.
Cool the skin before treatment to help reduce side effects.
Give the client the safety goggles to wear.

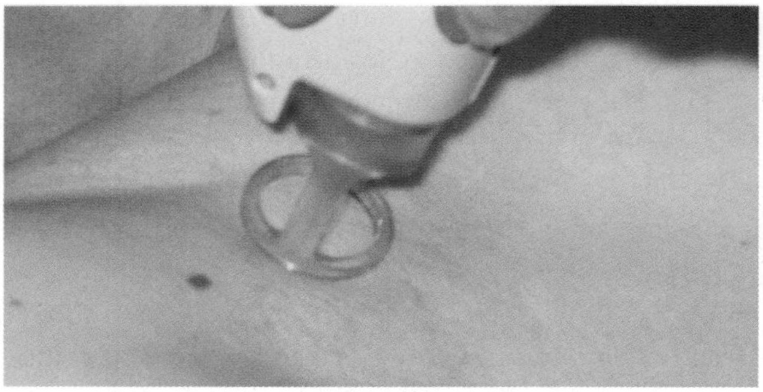

Figure 19–35 Client undergoing laser treatment.

client on the use of the numbing cream. These are powerful medicines and can have harmful adverse side effects. In the United States, the most popular prescription-required topical anesthetic used by clients is a mixture of local anesthetics. It is important to note that topical anesthetics cause vasoconstriction in the area where applied, making the area look blanched. If you do not see the blanching in advance, you may misinterpret the status of this client's skin.

Over-the-counter products from the first-aid section in your local drugstore usually contain 2% lidocaine and come in a cream, spray, or gel. An esthetician can offer OTC numbing agents or creams, liquids, gels, and sprays or provide retail products like LMX™, or Topicaine™. (Clients must sign off on receiving these on the consent form.) If the client obtains this directly from a physician, the medication may only be used on that client. These drugs usually contain 4% Lidocaine or 20% Benzocaine as the active ingredient. Do not use these products around the eyes, and avoid the inner corners of the mouth, as these can seep in and make the tongue and throat numb. Do not use liquids and sprays around the ears, and do not use spray anesthetic on the face unless the eyes are well protected. Instead, spray cotton until it is well saturated with the numbing solution and apply it to the area. When using any numbing cream, caution the client to follow the manufacturer's directions and understand the warnings.

Topical anesthetics can be dangerous and can cause death and injury. These medications should not be handled frivolously. Numb large areas in sections and never occlude them as this can increase absorption and the risk of serious side effects. If for some reason the skin blisters and is open or potentially open, *never* reapply numbing cream to the area. The medications can be absorbed systemically, causing severe problems. In short, be careful with numbing cream and always follow the manufacturer's directions. If you have questions or concerns, bring them to a qualified pharmacologist.

CAUTION!

Use extreme caution with topical anesthetics. Make sure that the client knows the importance of following a physician's instructions for the use of these medications.

Laser/IPL Treatment Parameters

Once you have shaved and numbed the area, it is time to begin the treatment. Some clinicians use a treatment grid to ensure that they have covered the treatment area evenly with the laser. It is important to use a specific pattern to avoid missing spots, or worse yet, double treating spots in the area. When doing the forehead, place your index finger over the client's eyebrow to ensure you stay out of this area and prevent brow hair loss. Refer to the patch test before starting the treatment. Examine the area and discuss it with the client to get any relevant feedback.

Remember, each machine has varying wavelengths, **pulse durations**, fluence, and other considerations that will affect the outcome of the treatment. Several technical issues will have an effect on the overall result of the hair removal process. Among these issues are: spot size, **energy fluence**, cooling the skin, pulse duration, **thermal storage** coefficient, (the amount of time the tissue retains the heat, and thermal relaxation time, the amount of time it takes for that heat to dissipate. While many lasers today are computerized and there is no need to look for this information, you should have an understanding of the theories and processes used to achieve hair removal. As such, the following provides a brief review of each.

Cooling the Skin

Cooling the skin allows for a higher and more effective fluence, as discussed in Chapter 8. There are different means of cooling the skin during treatment, all of which help prevent epidermal tissue damage but also reduce the discomfort of the treatment. The use of ice packs on the area about three minutes prior to the treatment is a good idea. Some laser devices include a forced-air technology to cool the skin.

Spot Size

The spot size, measured in millimeters, is the size or width of the beam effecting treatment. The larger the laser beam's spot size, the less fluence. A spot size of 12 mm to 18 mm is considered acceptable for laser hair removal. Spot sizes smaller than 12 mm lose depth of penetration,

PROCEDURE 19-2 PERFORMING LASER OR IPL HAIR REMOVAL TREATMENTS

Follow all treatment steps in their entirety for a safe, effective, and comfortable treatment. Communicate with the client throughout the treatment to monitor his or her level of comfort.

IMPLEMENTS AND MATERIALS

Whether these clients dress down will depend on the area to be worked on. With lasers, do not use linens so as to minimize fire hazards, and keep a fire extinguisher handy.

- Laser or IPL unit
- Key to laser or IPL unit
- Treatment lounge
- Pre-treatment cleansing product
- Paper towels
- Topical anesthetic (if recommended by manufacturer)
- Laser or IPL "In Use" sign, following OSHA guidelines
- Protective eyewear for client
- Protective eyewear for technician
- Protective eyewear to hang outside room
- Soothing lotion
- Disinfecting lotion
- Gloves (as recommended)

Preparation

1 Set up the treatment room per manufacturer's guidelines.

2 If using a laser device, cover windows and all reflective surfaces.

3 Test equipment for proper operation.

4 Gather and set up supplies.

5 Remove jewelry and have the client remove all jewelry.

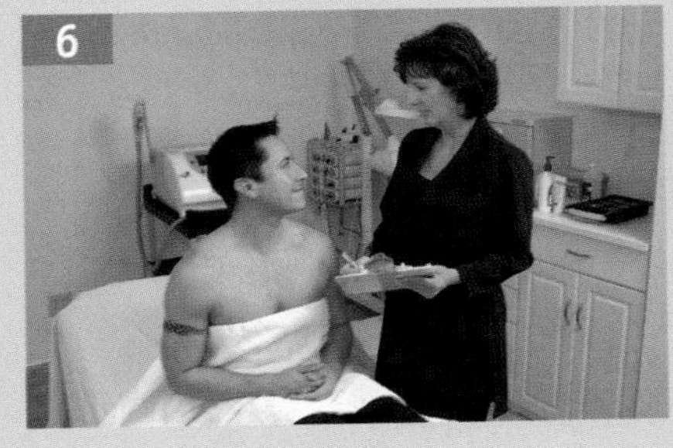

Perform client consultation.

6 Counsel the client and ensure his or her suitability for the procedure.

7 Have client read the home-care instructions and sign informed consent.

8 Apply topical anesthetic if recommended by the equipment manufacturer.

9 If needed, have the client put on the appropriate treatment gown.

Procedure

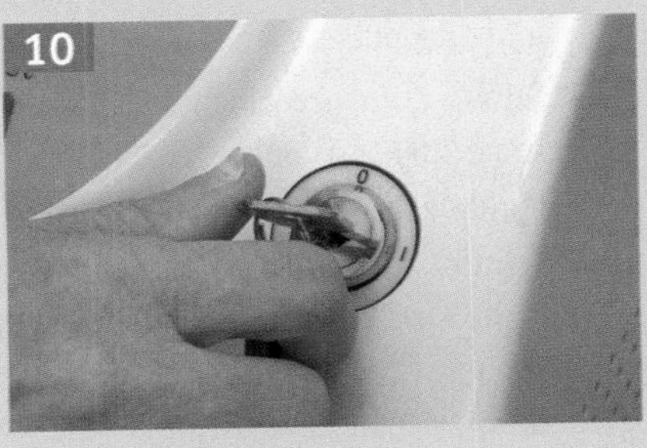

Unlock the laser device.

10 Unlock the laser device.

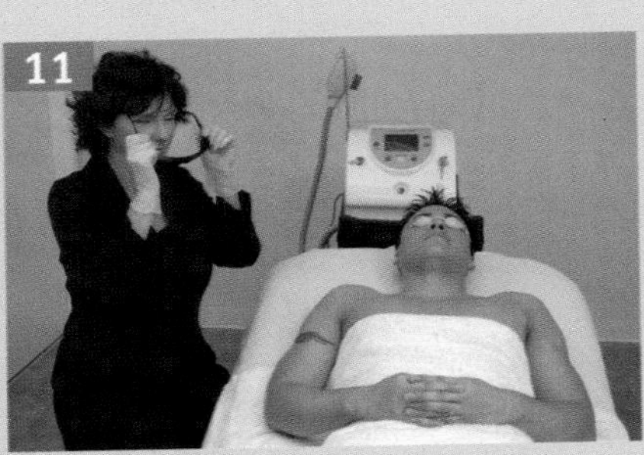

Put on safety goggles and gloves.

11 Put on safety goggles and gloves.

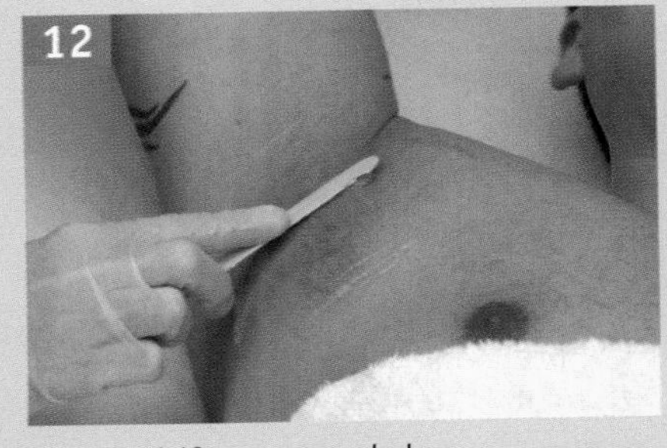

Apply gel if recommended.

12 Apply gel if recommended by manufacturer.

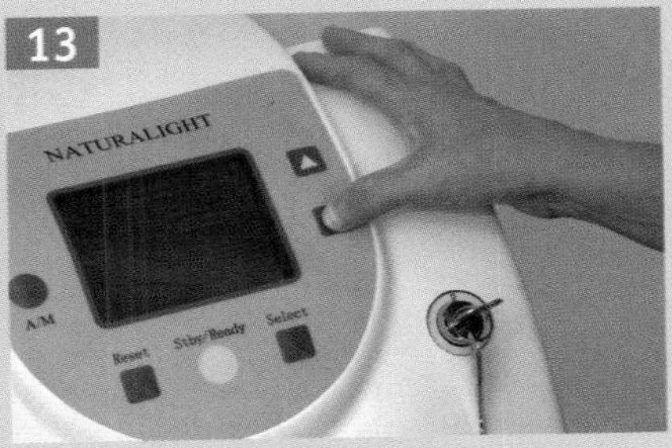

Set the treatment parameters.

13 Set the treatment parameters according to manufacturer's guidelines or charted settings from previous treatment for the area, hair, and skin and according to the response at the test site.

continues on next page

PROCEDURE 19-2, CONT. PERFORMING LASER OR IPL HAIR REMOVAL TREATMENTS

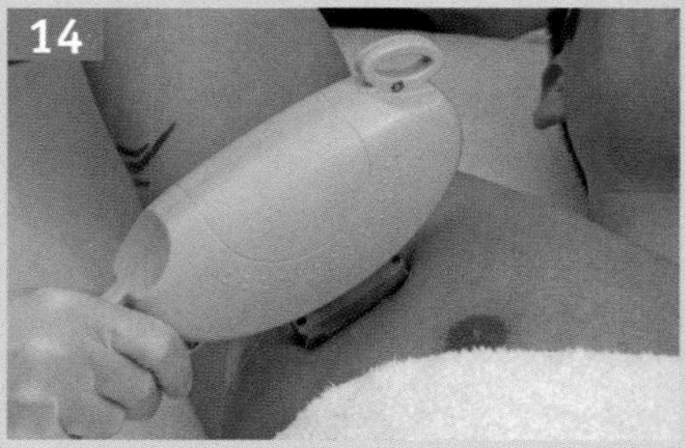

Perform the treatment.

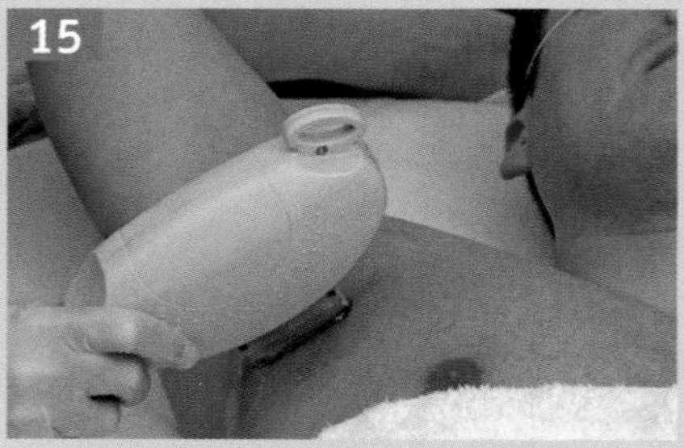

Compress the skin firmly with the handpiece.

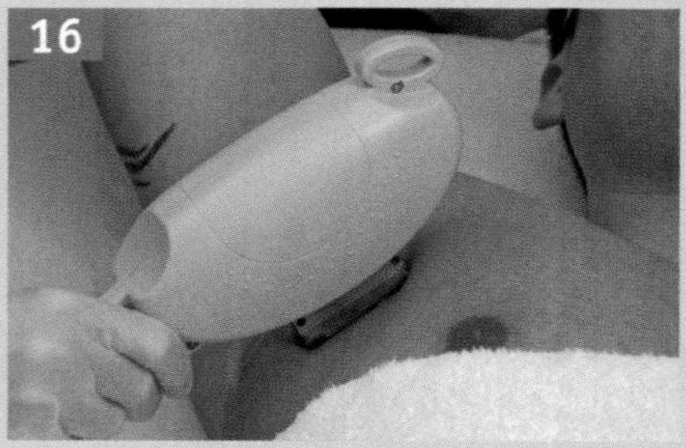

Select a starting spot and do a test pulse.

14 Perform the treatment at the highest fluence the skin can tolerate and in accordance with the manufacturer's recommendations for the most effective hair reduction. The time needed to cover the area depends on the spot size of the beam and the scanning pattern of the handpiece.

15 Compress the skin firmly with the handpiece to disperse the **oxyhemoglobin** (a chromophore that competes with melanin) away from the treatment area. Doing so allows for greater absorption of the laser light and reduces the risk of epidermal damage, as well as maneuvers the dermal papilla closer to the surface, which makes for a more effective treatment.

16 Select a starting spot and do a test pulse to ensure that the client can tolerate fluence.

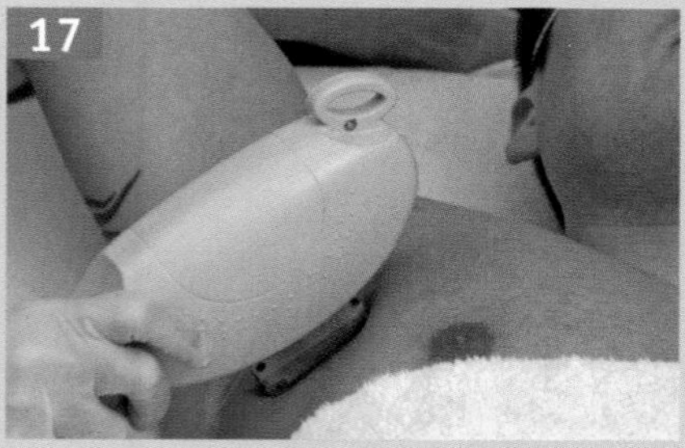

Administer a single pulse per area.

17 Following a well-defined pattern, work across the area where hair is to be removed, administering a single pulse per area.

18 During the treatment, between some of the pulses, clean the handpiece with a mild cleaning solution to free it of the carbonized hair that collects on the window. The buildup makes the window feel hot and impedes the flow of the laser beam. Some laser device manufacturers recommend the use of ultrasonic gel on the skin to prevent accumulation of burnt hair on the laser lens.

19 Read the skin. If topical anesthesia and cooling remedies have not reduced the client's discomfort, make adjustments.

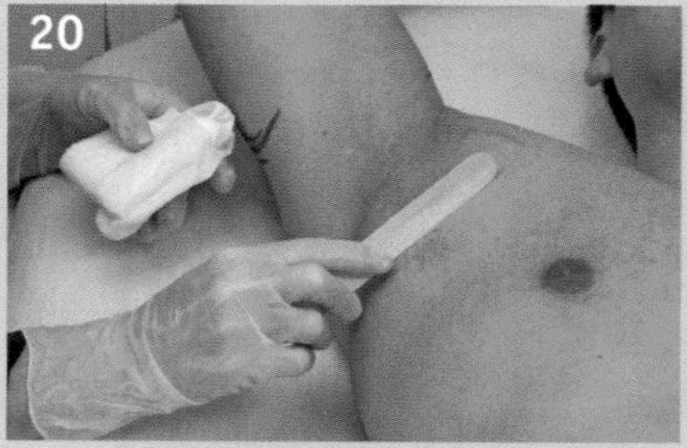

Remove any gel that you used with the device.

20 Remove any gel that may have been used with the device.

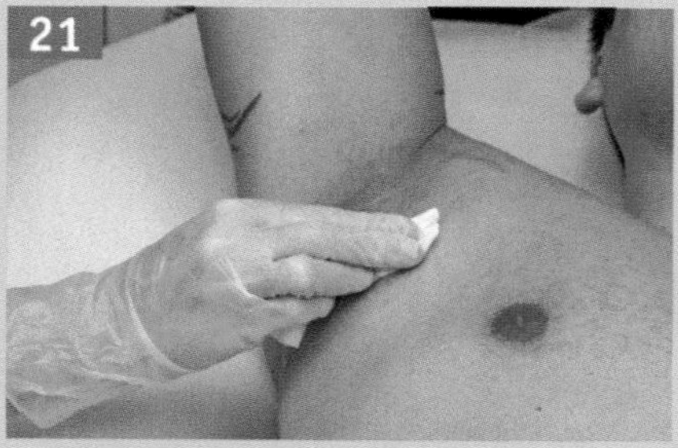

Wipe the skin with antiseptic lotion.

21 After treating the entire area, wipe down the skin with soothing antiseptic lotion.

Post-procedure

22 At the end of the treatment, turn off the laser device and remove the key.

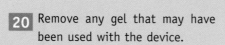

23 Provide client with home-care guidelines.

24 Schedule the client for a follow-up visit.

Clean-up and Sanitation

Because the handpiece contacts the skin, wipe it clean with a disinfectant between treatments or soak the distance gauge in disinfectant according to manufacturer's directions.

causing less controlled damage to the hair follicle and yielding a poorer result. The spot size can be affected by **dermal scattering,** how the light scatters or spreads within the skin tissue, which affects the relationship of the spot size deeper in the tissue due to its size on the skin's surface. (I.e., deeper in the tissue, the spot size is smaller, and it gradually becomes larger on the surface.) The spot size also affects penetration depth.

Wavelength

Described in nanometers (nm), the wavelength of a laser is on a spectrum ranging from 400 nm to 1200 nm. Recall that the greater the wavelength, the deeper the penetration. As discussed in Chapter 8, the wavelength is specific to the light source used, and each will have a different effect on the skin tissue and how the light is absorbed. For example, a diode laser has a wavelength of 800 nm, whereas an Nd:YAG laser has a wavelength of 1064. (See Chapter 8.) The optimum wavelength for hair removal is that which is highly absorbed in the melanin of the hair.

Energy Fluence

Choosing the highest tolerable energy fluence ensures the best results. Used in pulsed lasers, energy fluence is measured in **joules** per square centimeter (j/cm^2); (Figure 19–36). The larger the laser beam's spot size, the more fluence that is necessary to produce the same effect. Lower fluences have been observed to cause higher rates of double hairs in regrowth. Fair-skin Types I to III traditionally can take a fluence level of 25 to 40 j/cm^2. As noted above, by cooling the epidermis you can make a higher fluence possible and consequently achieve a better result.

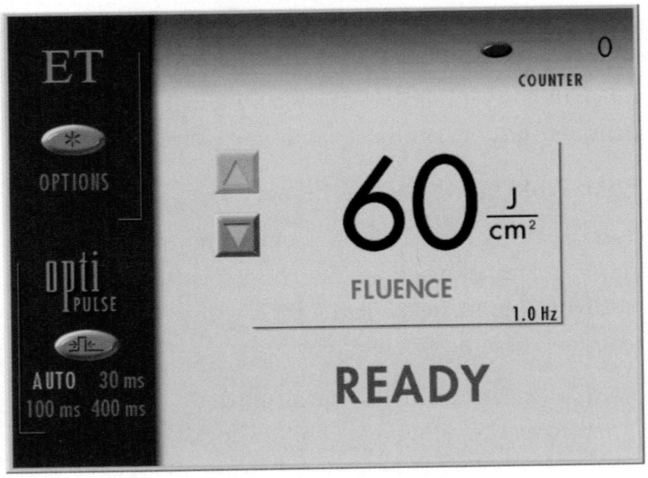

Figure 19–36 Laser machine showing the settings.

Thermal Storage Coefficient

The thermal storage coefficient (Tr_2) is the storage of heat in a chromophore. When a chromophore is heated beyond its Tr_2, the heat spills over and is diffused into the surrounding tissue. Hair has a higher Tr_2 than the epidermis. Coarse hair has a higher Tr_2 than finer hair. To minimize damage to surrounding tissue by not exceeding the Tr_2 of the chromophore, you should understand this principle and follow the recommended guidelines of pulse duration and energy fluence.

Pulse Duration

Pulse duration (or **pulse width**), which is measured in milliseconds (ms), is the timing of light energy, or how long the laser is actually on the skin. The pulse duration should match the fluence needed to damage the target hair follicle. A longer pulse duration is generally required for melanin in the hair than for fragile capillaries in the epidermis. Typically, coarser hair requires a longer pulse duration. Longer pulse widths are considered more effective with fewer side effects, because they allow for more skin types to tolerate higher fluences. This is particularly true of dark skin. The pulse should also be longer than the thermal relaxation time of the epidermal tissue but shorter than the thermal relaxation time of the hair follicle, keeping the heat in the hair follicle. This is aided by the use of cooling agents or mechanisms applied to the epidermal tissue. Use caution when treating areas with dense hair and a longer pulse width. Thermal conduction can occur between the closely adjacent hair follicles.

Thermal Relaxation Time

Thermal relaxation time (TRT) is the time it takes for 50% of heat energy to be dissipated from the target tissue. It can be registered in microseconds (ms). For skin it is between 600 ms and 800 ms. Because the TRT of the hair follicle depends on the follicle's diameter, the laser source must have a range of pulse widths capable of damaging different size follicles. Knowing the TRT and making the necessary adjustments in the treatment of different-sized follicles in different areas minimizes collateral thermal damage to the dermal tissue, or skin tissue not at the surface of the skin.

Post-Treatment in the Clinic

Post treatment procedures help minimize client discomfort and prevent adverse post-treatment reactions. A client should never leave the facility without being informed of appropriate aftercare.

1. Use ice in a vinyl surgical glove for aftercare. Use cold packs, aloe vera, chilled metal rollers or any other cooling preparation to ease temporary, mild burning.
2. Apply a sunscreen (SPF30 or greater) if the area will be exposed to ultraviolet light.
3. Apply makeup as long as the skin is not broken. Makeup also serves as additional sunscreen. Use new, uncontaminated makeup product, and apply it with a clean sponge.
4. Advise the client to return within 4 to 12 weeks or in the length of time it takes for the telogen stage of hair growth for that area of the face or body. For some areas, the optimum time may be six to eight weeks, so discuss this with the client to establish the best return schedule. Ensure that any hair follicles that were in the resting stage during the initial treatment are in a growing stage at the time of follow-up.

At-Home Care

Encouraging the client to follow the recommended home-care guidelines will promote faster healing and prevent adverse reactions like hyperpigmentation and hypopigmentation. Make sure that the client fully understands his or her responsibility in following the guidelines.

1. The client can take quick, warm showers. If areas other than the facial area are treated, advise no hot baths for 24 to 48 hours.
2. Place additional clean, cold packs on the treatment area. Bags of frozen peas wrapped in a clean cloth, work well.
3. Have the client apply a soothing, healing ointment like Aquaphor™ and keep the area lubricated to prevent tissue crusting or scabbing.
4. In the event of blistering, the client can apply a topical antibiotic cream or ointment and cover with a nonadhering dressing. Have the client notify you and/or the physician overseeing the laser treatment.
5. Advise the client to avoid the sun for one to two weeks following Nd:YAG treatments and four to six weeks following Alexandrite or diode treatments to avoid hyperpigmentation. Also advise him or her to avoid tanning if planning to have follow-up treatments.
6. The client can apply a sunscreen of at least SPF30 to any area that could be exposed to ultraviolet light as long as there is an erythema. If further treatment is needed, have the client commit to staying out of the sun. Sun exposure creates certain minor complications, which should be discussed fully.
7. He or she can apply makeup and lotions the next day or when signs of irritation or erythema have subsided and if the skin is not broken. The client should use uncontaminated makeup, and apply it with clean fingers or a new, clean sponge.
8. Instruct the client to contact the facility and you or a physician if there are any concerns or questions.
9. For areas prone to friction, like the abdominal area or inner thigh area, advise the client to avoid tight clothing to prevent infection and irritation.

Spacing the Return Visit

The spacing for a return visit depends on the client's previous methods of hair removal. If the area has been previously waxed, forcing the telogen stage, you can anticipate when the new anagen hairs will come through based on the telogen stage of the hair follicles in that area so schedule the follow-up session accordingly. The key is to treat a high percentage of terminal hair in the anagen (preferably early anagen) stage. Depending on the area to be treated, you may ask the client to return every three to eight weeks.

When to Stop Treating

A few clients have little or no success with laser treatments. These clients are called nonresponders, and there is no way to predict which clients they will be. Even with all optimal conditions, such as hair in the anagen phase and melanin in the hair shaft, laser is still unpredictable. If after several treatments the client does not respond, discontinue the treatments. (That said, it may be that the hair is returning but at a slower rate.)

Treatment Consequences

Treatment consequences are a predictable outcome of the procedure that occurs in a reasonable percentage of people having the procedure. In the case of laser hair removal, treatment consequences might include erythema and perifollicular edema. Clients should expect to see tiny black spots in the follicles over a few days. These "singed" hairs, called **splattering,** will gradually and naturally expel from the skin and can be wiped away (Table 19–7).

Side Effects and Complications

Side effects are an action or effect other than that desired. In the case of laser hair removal care, a side effect might be crusting, temporary redness (lasting longer than two hours), or skin discoloration (hyperpigmentation). Hyperpigmentation may be treated with prescription-strength formulas of **hydroquinone** (Figure 19–37). Clients must strictly adhere to follow-up instructions for their comfort and protection and to minimize these potential problems (Table 19–8).

Complications are infrequent untoward events that occur following a normally applied procedure. For example, a patient has a peel and a scar results. In the case of laser hair removal, a complication would be defined as epidermal separation or blistering (Figure 19–38). Other complications include hypopigmentation, scarring, intense itching, and hives. It has been noted that respiratory irritation can occur if the plume of smoke secondary to the hair is significant. Failure to recognize and respond to a negative or adverse reaction is negligent and could result in serious repercussions, including a possible malpractice lawsuit. In the event of an adverse reaction, end the treatment immediately and call in appropriate medical intervention by a qualified medical professional (Table 19–9).

LIABILITY CONCERNS

Regardless of the hair removal technique you decide to offer clients, it is important to cover all bases, in terms of liability, before you begin. Always have the client read and sign an informed consent form, which confirms that the

Table 19–7 Treatment Consequences of Laser Hair Removal

TREATMENT CONSEQUENCES OF LASER HAIR REMOVAL
Erythema and edema, most of which subsides within 20 minutes to a few hours
Longer wavelengths produce tiny bumps resembling goose bumps, also known as perifollicular edema and additional edema, which should subside in a matter of hours.
Singed hair, called *splattering*

Table 19–8 Side Effects of Laser Hair Removal

SIDE EFFECTS OF LASER HAIR REMOVAL
Herpes Simplex
Bacterial Infection (very low risk)
Crusting
Extended Redness
Hyperpigmentation

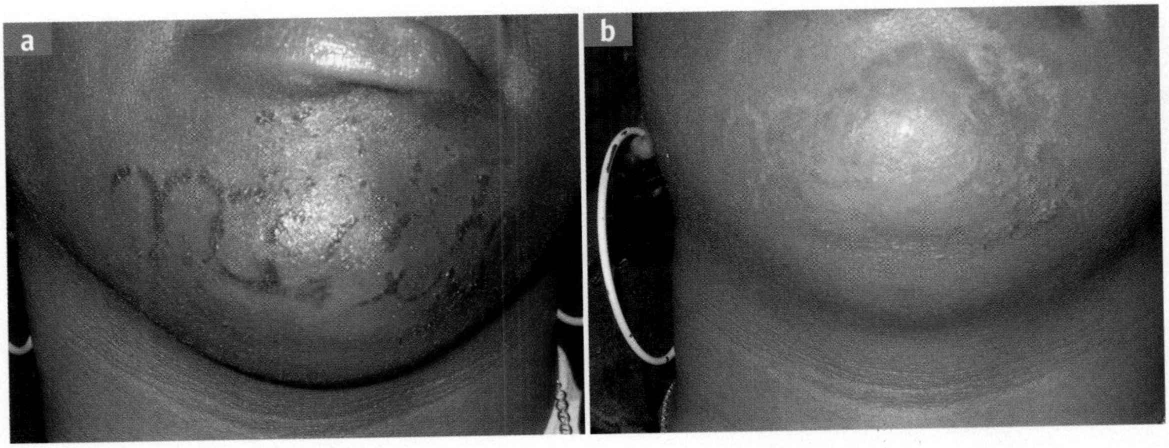

Figure 19–37 a) Hyperpigmentation following laser hair removal, and b) Hyperpigmentation following laser hair removal after a period of fading.

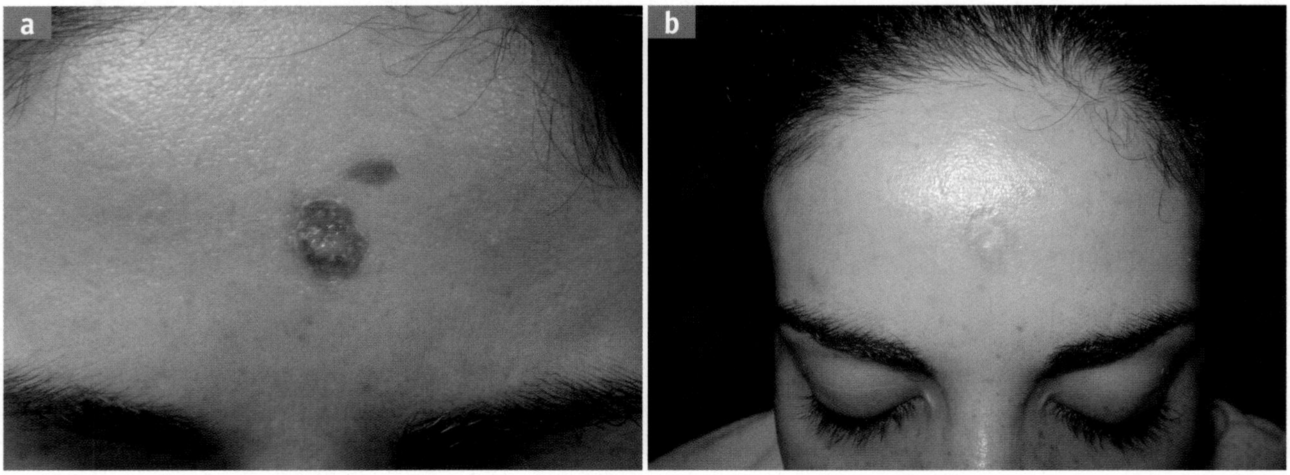

Figure 19–38 The result of epidermal separation or blistering.

REGULATORY AGENCY ALERT

Licensure requirements vary a great deal of variation between states. Some states require only cosmetology certification to operate a laser device for hair removal, whereas other states require that a physician operate a laser device. Most states allow estheticians to operate laser devices for hair removal although it may be only under a doctor's supervision. Consult your state's regulatory agency to find out the specific requirements for laser or pulsed light device operation. The rules and regulations for licensure not only vary, but they are also subject to frequent revision. Therefore, staying abreast of legislative amendments affecting your practice within your state will help you stay within the boundaries of the law.

client wants the procedure and has divulged all relevant information. Finally, check with your insurance provider to determine that they will cover you for the services you want to perform. Some insurance policies specifically exclude Brazilian waxing. Some require documentation of special training to cover laser or pulsed light equipment. Most importantly, your insurance will only stay in effect as long as all products and equipment are used following manufacturer's guidelines and state regulations.

The diverse choices available to the esthetician for hair removal ensures that you can find one to best suit the needs of your client base and your treatment goals. The choices and technicques will continue to evolve and change so it is important that we stay abreast of these alterations to our industry.

Table 19–9 Complications of Laser Hair Removal

COMPLICATIONS OF LASER HAIR REMOVAL
Blistering
Hypopigmentation
Scarring
Intense pruritus and urticaria
Respiratory irritation due to inhalation of plume

REVIEW QUESTIONS

1. Discuss the two techniques of threading and how they differ.
2. Discuss the two techniques of sugaring and their pros and cons.
3. Hard wax is best used for what services and what are its key attributes?
4. Soft wax is best used for what services and what are its key attributes?

5. Outline the protocol used for brow design.
6. Outline the steps for Brazilian waxing.
7. What is the difference between American and Brazilian waxing?
8. Discuss three key factors to keep in mind when waxing male clients.
9. What is the difference between laser and IPL hair removal units?
10. What are the contraindications for laser or IPL hair removal?
11. What are safety precautions that must be observed for laser or IPL hair removal?
12. Define energy fluence.
13. What is thermal relaxation time?
14. Which clients are most suitable for laser or IPL hair removal?
15. Which clients are least suitable for laser or IPL hair removal?

CHAPTER GLOSSARY

chromophore: responsible for a molecular color. Elements that laser light is attracted to; melanin, hemoglobin, water, protein, or dye particles.

dermal scattering: how light scatters or spreads within the skin tissue.

energy fluence: the energy level of a laser, measured in joules.

fatlah: egyptian word for threading.

human papillomavirus (HPV): a cutaneous viral infection commonly caused by sexual transmission and exhibited by genital warts.

hydroquinone: a topical medication that is used for bleaching or reducing excessive melanin lesions in the epidermis.

joules: units of energy or work. In thermodynamics, joules are defined as a unit of heat energy used to measure the energy change in an object as it warms or cools from temperature T1 to temperature T2. 1 joule = 1 watt per second.

khite: arabic word for threading.

monochromatic: light consisting of one wavelength that is typically emitted from a laser system.

Nikolski sign: an epidermal separation caused by lateral pressure on the skin.

oxyhemoglobin: hemoglobin in red blood cells that has been oxygenatal; a protein in red blood cells.

polychromatic: multiple wavelength light, appearing as different colors, as exhibited in Intense Pulsed Light emissions or seen with visible sunlight.

pulse duration: the duration of an individual pulse of laser light; usually measured in milliseconds. *See* pulse width.

pulse width: The period of time in which a pulse of light is emitted. *See* pulse duration.

selective photothermolysis: treatment utilizing an appropriate wavelength, exposure time, and pulse duration, with sufficient energy fluence to absorb light into a specific area; allows damage to targeted tissue without involving the surrounding area.

splattering: singed hair.

thermal storage: measure of heat stored in a chromophore.

threading: hair removal using strands of thread.

CHAPTER 20

ADVANCED MAKEUP

CHAPTER OUTLINE

- SEMIPERMANENT EYELASH EXTENSIONS
- MINERAL MAKEUP
- MINERALS FOR CAMOUFLAGE
- AIRBRUSH MAKEUP
- AIRBRUSH CAMOUFLAGE TECHNIQUES
- PERMANENT COSMETICS

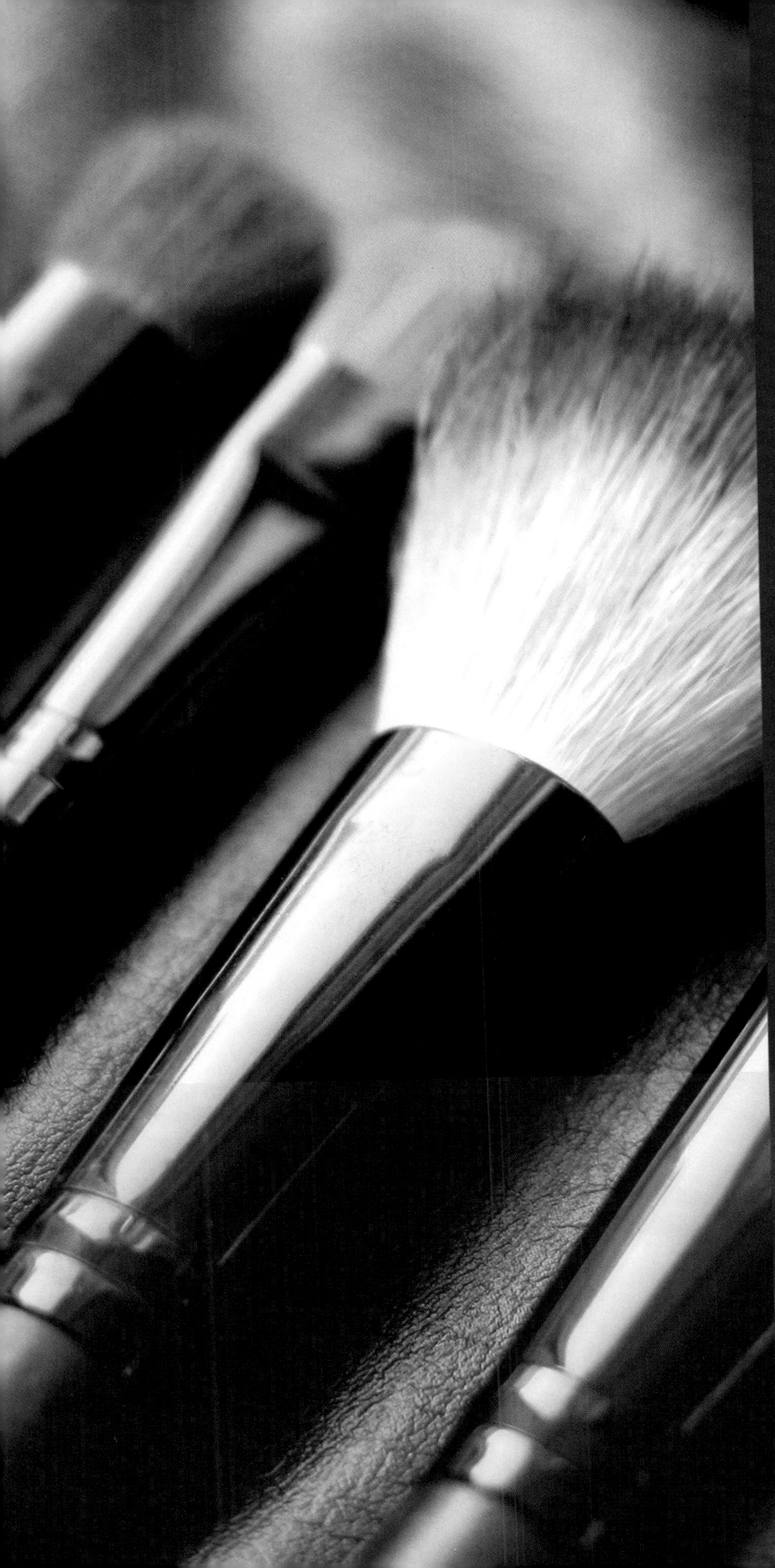

LEARNING OBJECTIVES

After completing this chapter, you should be able to:

- Apply different forms of lash enhancements.
- Describe techniques for lash perming.
- Define and evaluate mineral makeup.
- Use mineral makeup application techniques.
- Use mineral makeup camouflage techniques.
- Identify products and equipment used for airbrush makeup.
- Master the techniques needed to achieve a desired look.
- Complete a beauty makeup application.
- Accomplish maximum coverage makeup.
- Design and create custom stencils for fantasy makeup and body painting.
- Explain basic permanent cosmetic procedures and training protocols.

KEY TERMS

Page numbers indicate where in the chapter the term is used.

airbrush makeup 546
airbrushes 548
back bubble 550
stencils 554

Makeup artistry goes beyond the knowledge of skin tones, face shapes, and product application. In recent years the industry has undergone dramatic changes with new products and techniques flooding the market and offering Hollywood enhancement to everyday clients. Women have moved from false temporary eyelashes to semipermanent extensions. The demand for natural healthy-skin products has triggered a boom in mineral makeup. While classical camouflage techniques are still in use, more natural minimization using mineral makeup and camouflage using airbrushing are becoming the new standards. Clients with challenges or busy schedules are increasingly asking for permanent cosmetics. It is important for today's artist to be knowledgeable in all of these areas.

SEMIPERMANENT EYELASH EXTENSIONS

Semipermanent eyelash extensions are different from traditional false eyelash strips, clusters, or individual lash tabbing. These recently invented synthetic eyelash extensions are single lashes applied one by one to your natural lashes for longer, fuller, more natural-looking eyelashes (Figures 20–1, 20–2). With the right combination of products, adhesive, and proper application, semipermanent lashes can last for up to two months. Clients can enjoy eyelash extensions year round by following simple maintenance and care instructions along with retouch applications every two to four weeks. With growing popularity, semipermanent eyelash extensions are becoming a standard in the esthetics industry and creating an additional profit center for salons and spas.

Consultation

Twenty-four hours before applying lashes for a client, have her come in for 15 minutes to talk about what she can expect during her appointment. Examine her eye area; if you see any redness, swelling, itching, or crusted areas, recommend that she be seen by her physician or eye doctor before you apply the lashes.

Preparation, Health, and Safety

Since this service is so close to the eye, safety is your number one priority. Follow all sterilization and disinfection guidelines for your equipment. In addition, incorporate as many single-use disposable components as possible and set these up within easy reach. Wash your hands thoroughly before starting.

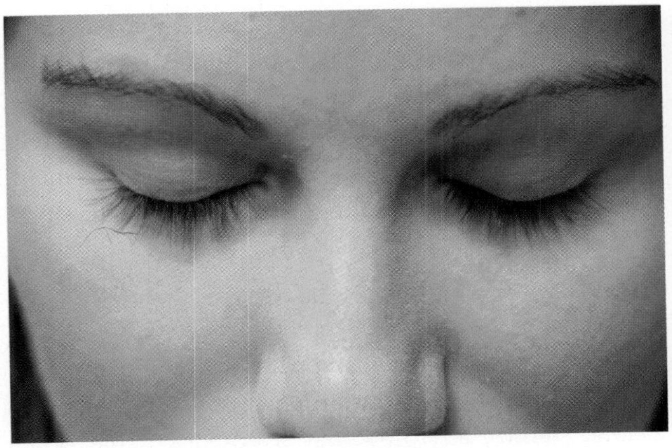

Figure 20–1 Client before lash extensions.

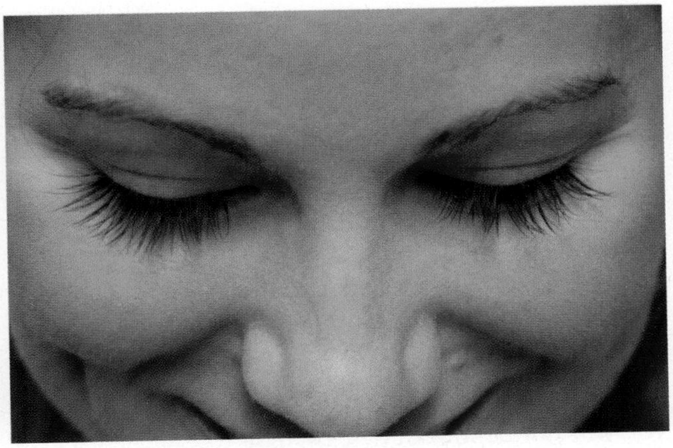

Figure 20–2 Client after lash extensions.

CAUTION!

Clients with the following conditions should not seek lash extensions:

- Pregnancy
- Eye irritations
- Eye allergies
- Blepharitis
- Glaucoma
- Excessive tears
- Thyroid problems affecting lash growth or hair loss
- Asthma (Client may be sensitive to the adhesive odor.)

? Did You Know

Many estheticians use magnifying visors or glasses to enhance their vision for lash application.

Here's a Tip

Clients who wear contact lenses may want to bring a pair of glasses to the appointment. If their eyes are at all irritated after the process, they can leave contacts out and wear glasses.

Some adhesives may have fumes that can cause a burning sensation to the eyes. During your consultation you will be able to determine if sensitivity may be an issue for your client. If this is the case you can test by applying one lash to each eye 24 hours prior to the application to check for reaction.

Have the client remove contact lenses prior to the procedure. Make sure you have a good light source, as this is important for proper application. Make sure there is a saline or water close to your workstation in case you need to irrigate the eye for any reason. If adhesive should get in the eye, immediately flush with plenty of water and contact a physician. Adhesive should not come in contact with the skin. If this should occur, remove it immediately, but gently, with a small amount of adhesive remover, and then rinse thoroughly with water and pat dry.

Disinfect all tools before the procedure to ensure that you will not be introducing bacteria to the client's eyes.

CAUTION!

The client should keep her eyes closed during the entire procedure and at no time should adhesive be allowed to enter the eye. If this happens follow emergency eye cleansing protocol: Flush with sterile eyewash solution, then assist the client in washing her eyes with warm water for at least 15 minutes. Then seek medical attention immediately.

Handle tweezers only by the handle, never the tip, and always have extra pairs of tweezers available so you can disinfect a pair between clients. When removing lashes from their container, use clean tweezers rather than your fingers. Dispose of leftover lash extensions, and do not reintroduce potentially contaminated lashes back in with the clean ones.

Client Comfort

Provide a comfortable place for your client to recline, with the neck and head well supported. Make sure she is relaxed and comfortable, and be ready to offer her a blanket. This procedure can last up to two hours, and you want your client to be as comfortable as possible during that time.

Eyelash Growth

The main purpose of the eyelash and eyelid is to protect the eye from harmful substances or objects. It is important to know the stages of the growth cycle when selecting lashes for extensions placement (Figure 20–3). You should avoid the lashes that are in the anagen stage, or new growth. Application at this stage tends to weigh down the natural lashes, which can result in premature detachment; also, the lash will look unnatural once it reaches full growth. The ideal lash stage for extension placement is the catagen stage, the time when the lash has just finished growing. Lashes at this stage will last longer and tend to look more natural. The telogen or resting stage is also an appropriate stage for lash placement, but lashes at this stage will be the first to be shed.

Procedure Notes

Disposables

Use as many disposables as possible to speed clean-up and minimize the sterilization process. Before every procedure, sterilize anything that is not disposable. Some

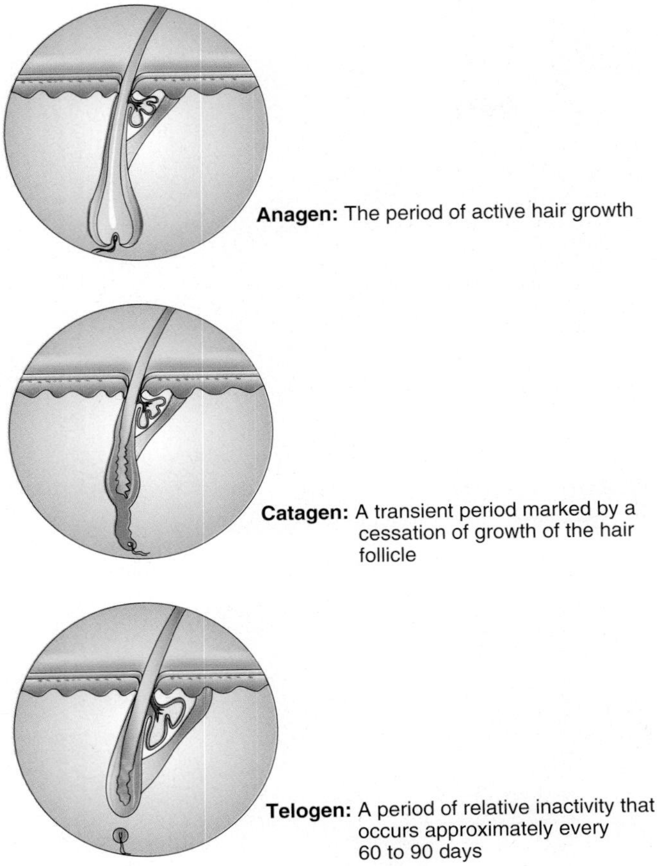

Anagen: The period of active hair growth
Catagen: A transient period marked by a cessation of growth of the hair follicle
Telogen: A period of relative inactivity that occurs approximately every 60 to 90 days

Figure 20–3 Natural life cycle of the eyelash.

manufacturers recommend the use of a jade stone to hold the adhesive; this, too, must be sterilized between clients. An alternative is to apply two strips of tape side by side on the jade stone or use a disposable adhesive holder and follow manufacturer's directions for its use.

Tools

TWEEZERS Some manufacturers recommend using only straight tweezers while others recommend both straight and curved; whichever you prefer, you will need two pairs for each procedure.

FORCED AIR You may prefer using something to aim air at the lash to stimulate drying of the adhesive. Always blow from the top of the lash down toward the nose. Remember that when you blow air into the client's eye, you run the risk of drying the cornea.

MAKEUP REMOVER You want absolutely no oil on the lashes during the procedure because it interferes with adhesion. Ideally, you want the client to come to the appointment wearing no mascara or eye makeup. If she does arrive wearing makeup and you must remove it, use an oil-free eye makeup remover, which minimizes eye irritation.

THE EYE GEL PAD AND SURGICAL TAPE Trim the bottom quarter of the gel pad and set aside. Place the gel pad directly over the lower lashes up to the lash line. Do not come into contact with the inner eye rim. Apply white surgical tape to cover any exposed lashes. The surface of the eye gel pad is made with a very fine-fibered fabric. The fibers near the upper curved line may become loose during the procedure, causing the upper lashes to stick to the fibers. covering the upper edge of the pad with white surgical tape will also prevent this from being an issue. (Figure 20–4). Some estheticians do not use any eye pad but place the tape directly on the lower lashes and the skin. Others feel that removing the tape from the skin causes skin irritation, even tearing of this delicate tissue. (Figure 20–5). Consider how the different approaches

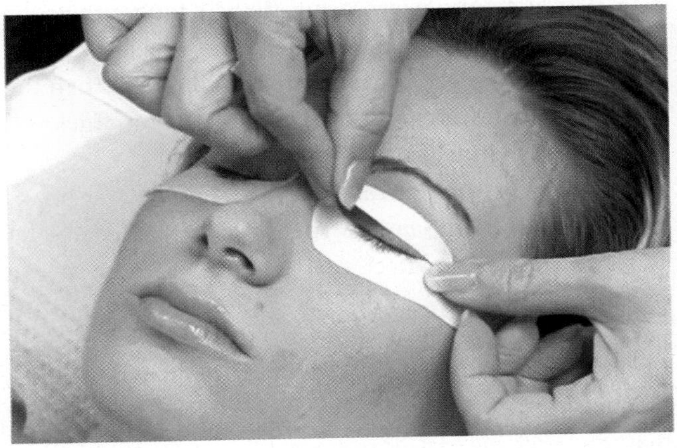

Figure 20–4 Under eye with lower lashes taped to pad.

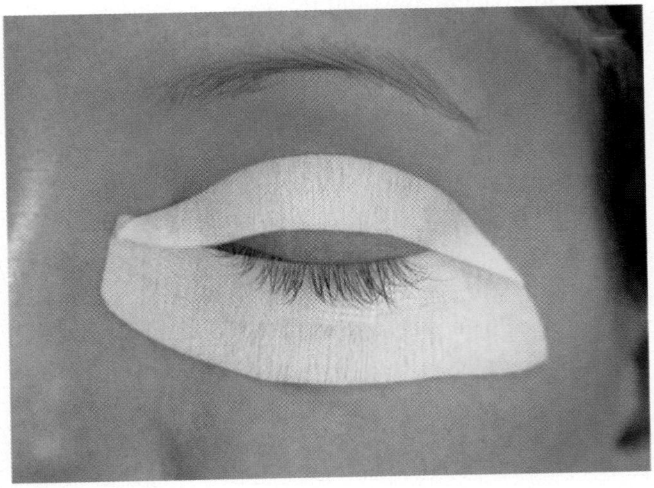

Figure 20–5 Under eye pad over lower lashes.

CAUTION!

Many people are sensitive to the tape. The less tape applied directly to the skin the better.

work and client safety as you select the technique you will employ.

Lash Selection

Lashes may all be the same length or varied for a softer look. Depending on your training and the manufacturer's style, you may use from three to seven different lengths of lashes. (Before dealing with variations, however, first learn basic lash selection and application techniques.) Check the client's natural lash length and then select lashes based on her goal for the finished look.

- **Natural Look:** Select lashes slightly longer than the client's lashes. (This makes the lashes appear fuller.)
- **Feminine:** Select lashes about a third longer than the client's lashes increase diameter to .20 for thickness and flair slightly longer at outside corners.
- **Dramatic/maximum:** Select lashes half again as long as the client's lashes. Try using .20 to .25 diameter for thickness and effect.

Practice

Before you attempt this service on a client, you need to practice your technique under trained supervision. One manufacturer has developed a very clever way to allow you to practice. You will need the following supplies:

1. Plastic-type mannequin head
2. Set of upper false eyelashes
3. Set of lower false eyelashes and adhesive
4. Colored electrical tape

Prepare your mannequin by applying the lower lashes to the lower rim of the mannequin eyelid (Figure 20–6). Next apply the eye gel pad as directed in Procedure 20–1 (Figure 20–7). Take the upper eyelash strip and set it on your mannequin along the brow bone. Carefully place a strip of colored electrical adhesive along the lash line of the false upper lashes (Figure 20–8). Pick up the strip adhered to the tape and reposition on the mannequin to simulate a client with closed eyes (Figure 20–9). You are now ready to practice lash extensions on a live subject (Figure 20–10).

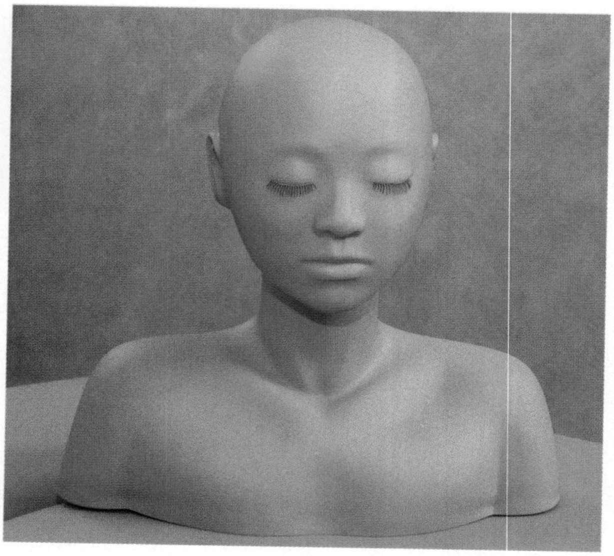

Figure 20–6 Applying lower lashes on a mannequin.

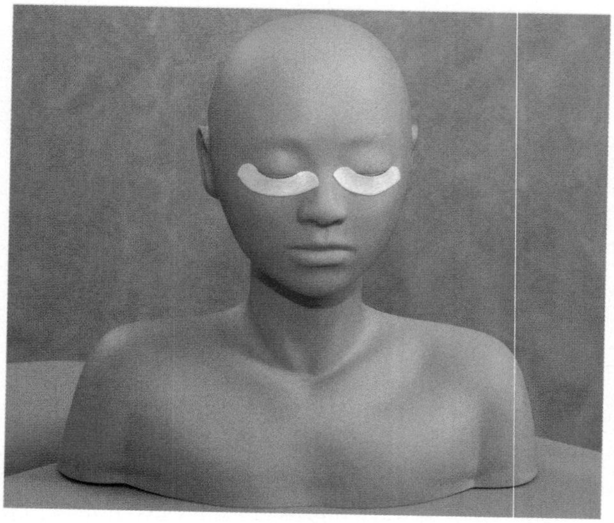

Figure 20–7 Apply eye pad over lashes.

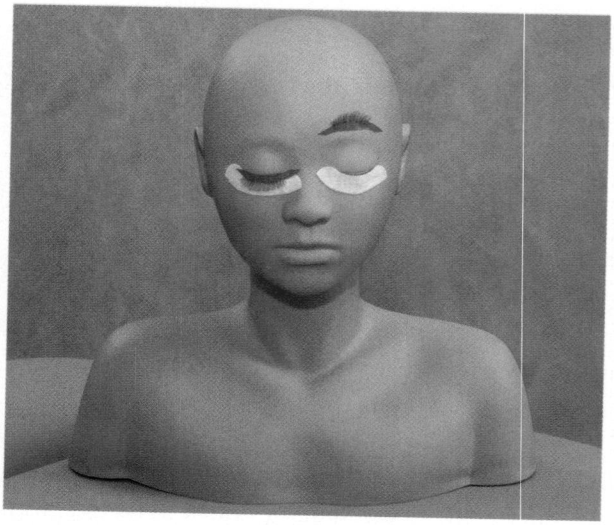

Figure 20–8 Upper lashes adhered to electrical tape.

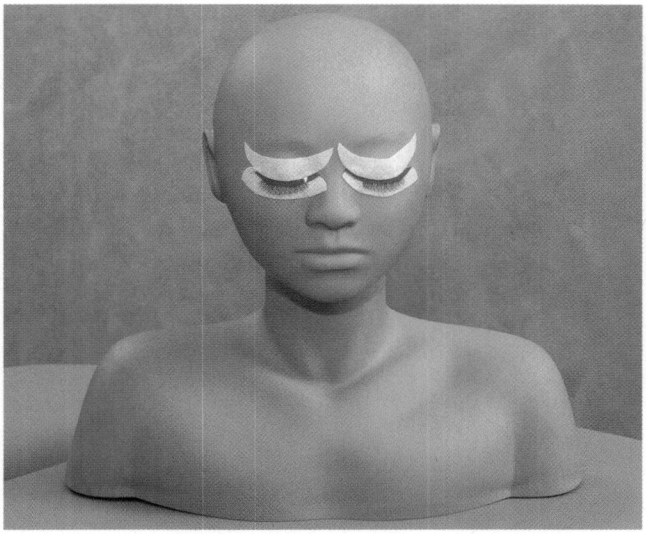

Figure 20–9 Upper lashes positioned to simulate closed eye.

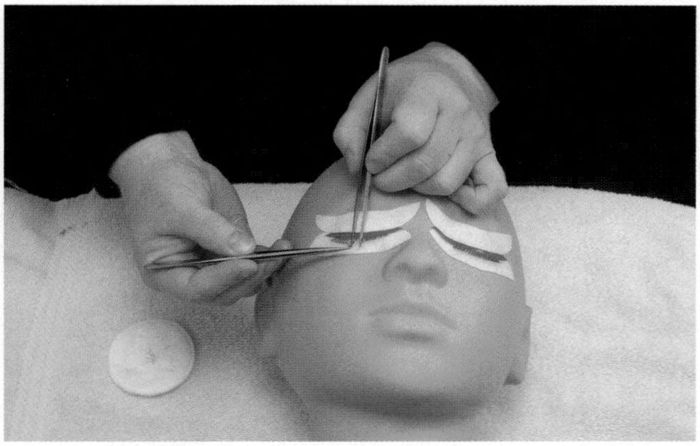

Figure 20–10 A mannequin ready for practice.

PROCEDURE 20–1 APPLYING SEMIPERMANENT EYELASH EXTENSIONS

IMPLEMENTS AND MATERIALS

- Headband or hair clip
- Magnifying lamp or light
- Adhesive (for professional use only)
- Adhesive remover
- Assortment of individual synthetic eyelashes
- Under-eye pads (single-use, disposable)
- Tweezers, straight pointed tip (must have)
- Tweezers, curved (optional, but you need two pairs of tweezers)
- Adhesive holder (sterilized or disposable)
- Bulb syringe or mini-fan (optional)
- Eye makeup remover (non-oil)
- 3M clear surgical tape
- Lash comb/brush (disposable)
- Micro swabs (disposable)
- Cotton or sponge-tipped swabs (disposable)
- Manicure scissors
- Paper towels

Optional Supplies

- Moisture barrier lash coating
- Heated eyelash curler (optional)

Preparation

1 Set up facial lounge and treatment room. Most clients do not dress down for this procedure.

2 Gather supplies.

3 Review the client's history with her and have her read and sign a consent form.

4 Review the client's expectations and the procedure.

5 Confirm that she has removed her contact lenses.

Procedure

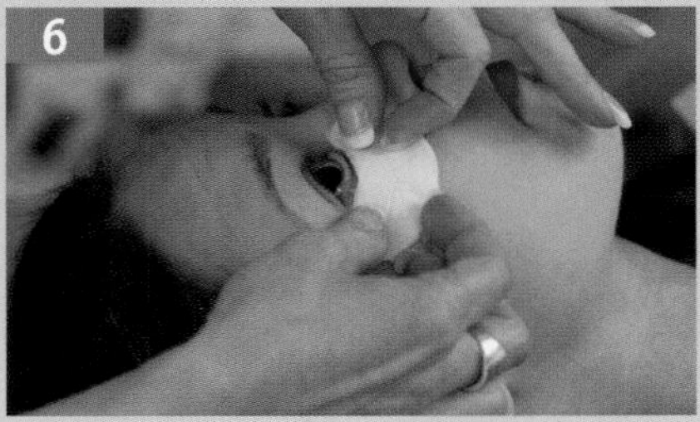

Place gel pad.

6 Trim lower quarter of the soothing eye pads, saving the extra pieces. Standing behind the client's head, have the client open her eyes and look upwards toward you. Remove the gel pads from their protective backing and position them under each eye covering the lower lash line, being careful not to let the eye pad come into contact with the client's inner eye rim. Check for comfort, then apply white surgical tape to cover any exposed lashes and fibers.

7 Have the client close her eyes. Apply the remaining section of the eye gel pad at the crease of the upper lid. This helps to remind client to keep eyes closed during the procedure.

continues on next page

PROCEDURE 20–1, CONT. APPLYING SEMIPERMANENT EYELASH EXTENSIONS

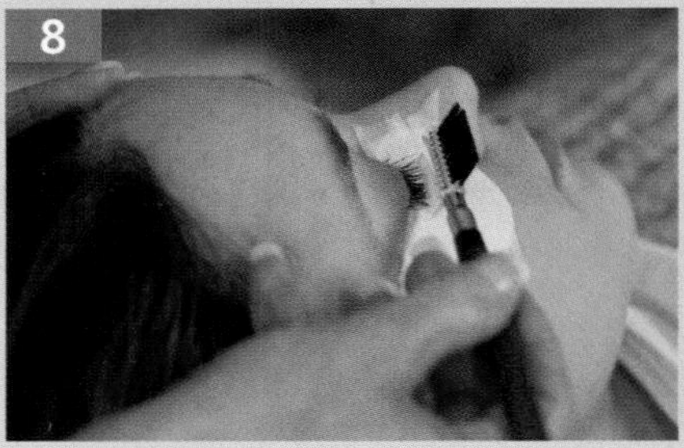

Gently comb through lashes.

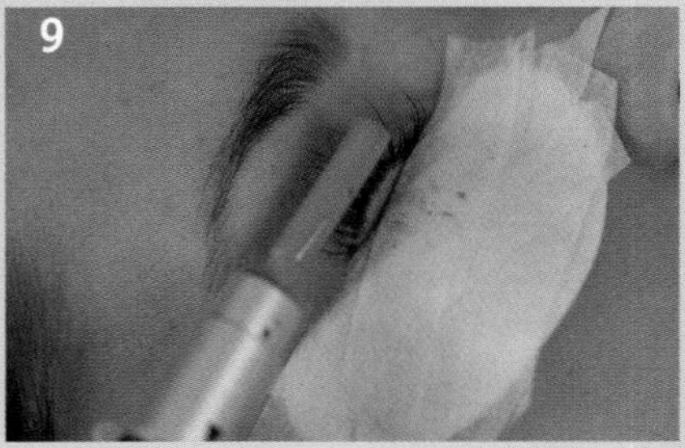

Use a heated eyelash curler for straightening lashes.

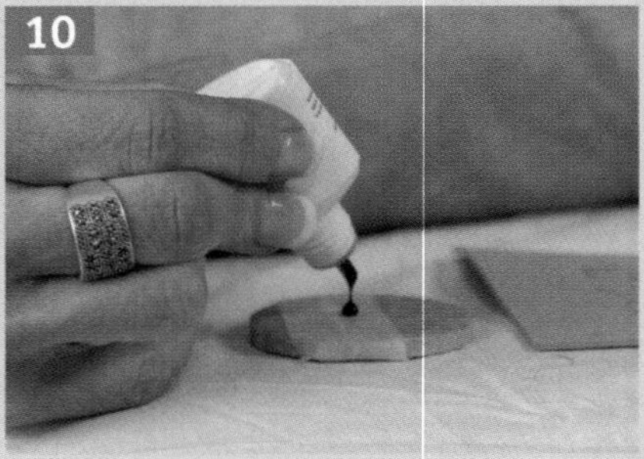

Place a small drop of adhesive on jade stone.

8 Optional: Gently comb through the lashes to straighten and remove any loose lashes.

9 Optional: You may want to use a heated eyelash curler for straightening lashes that may be curled or twisted. Keep in mind that this effect is only temporary and will not have an impact on the natural lash growth pattern.

10 Place a drop of adhesive onto the taped and sterilized jade stone or disposable container. Choose the lashes that suit your client best and place them onto the lash pad.

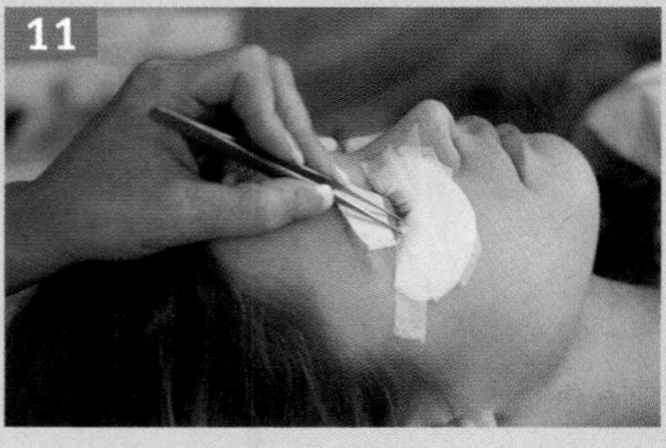

Isolate a single lash.

11 Isolate a natural single lash, beginning with the outside corner of the eye and using the curved or straight tweezers in your nondominant hand.

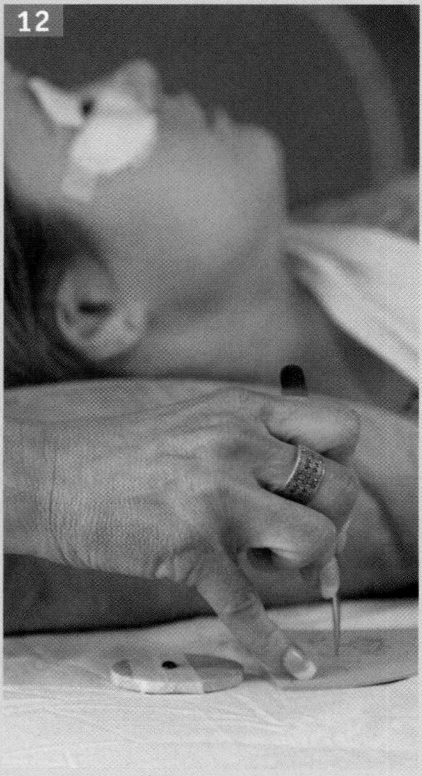

Pick up lash at tapered end.

12 With the tweezers in your dominant hand, pick up a lash extension by the tapered end of the lash.

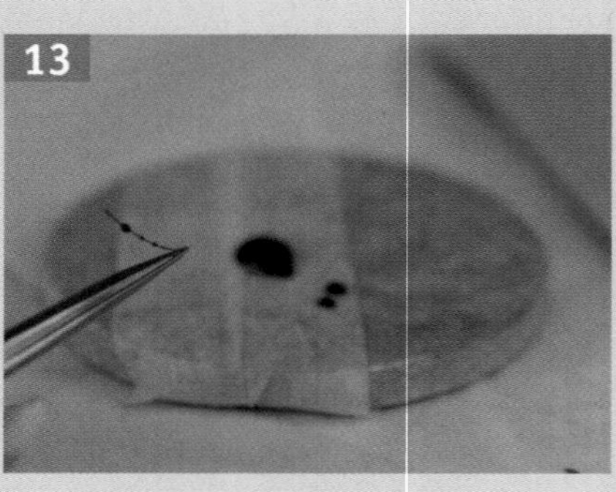

Lash should have tiny droplets of adhesive.

13 Gently swipe about two-thirds of the thick end of the lash through the adhesive, blotting any excess adhesive off of the lash but leaving enough so you can see tiny droplets along the length of the lash extension.

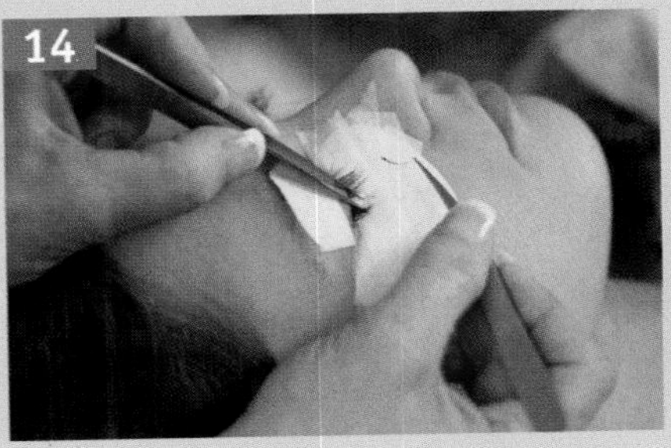

Place adhesive-dipped lash on isolated lash.

14 Apply the lash extension to the isolated lash. For best results, hold the lash and tweezers at a 45-degree angle. Place the extension on top of the lash roughly .05 mm to .1 mm from the base of the lash. Do not apply it at the base of the lash because this can cause skin irritation or breakage. Leave a space of 0.5 mm to 1.0 mm between the base of the lash and the extension.

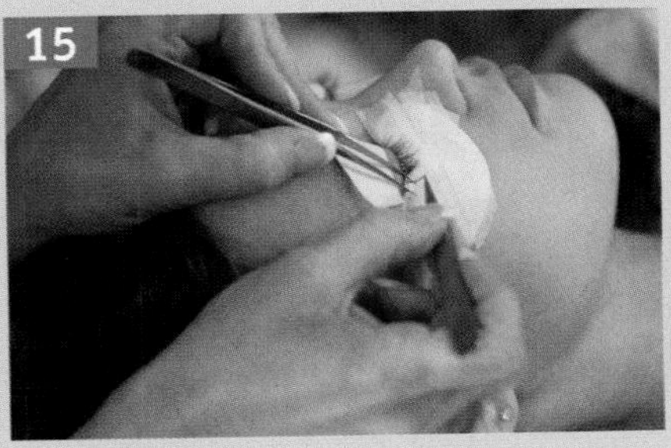

Smooth excess adhesive along lash.

15 Using the backside of the tweezers, gently spread the adhesive and smooth out any excess droplets to ensure a natural, flawless appearance. The J curl (lashes curved in the shape of a J with the blunt end at the bottom and the tapered end at the top) should be curved in the direction of the natural lash. Allow 5 to 10 seconds for the adhesive to dry.

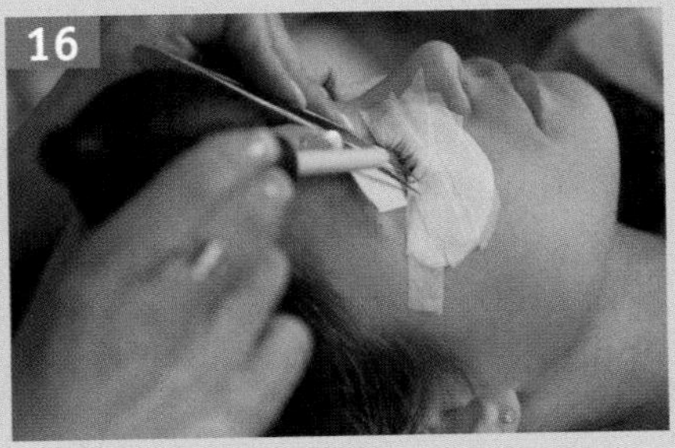

Dry with gently puffs of air.

16 Optional: To prevent sticking to adjacent lashes or clumping, dry the lash with gentle puffs of air with a bulb syringe or a mini-fan while the lash is still isolated.

17 Repeat this process on the opposite eye, alternating between the eyes to ensure proper drying time between extensions. Placing lashes at spaced intervals is another good way to avoid sticking or clumping and will help to even out the lash line.

CAUTION!

Keep the adhesive from coming in contact with the skin or the eye.

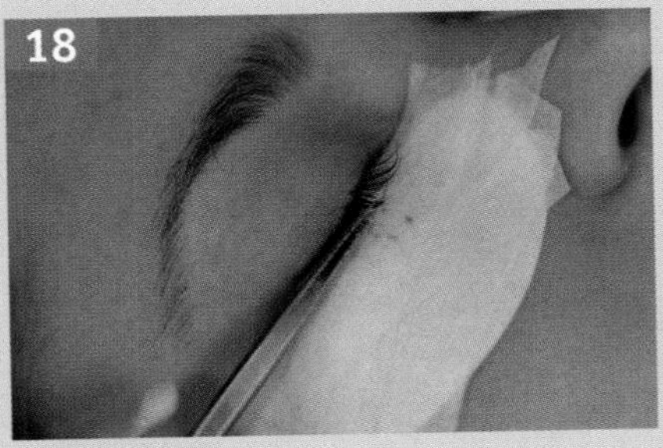

Grasp a section of lashes.

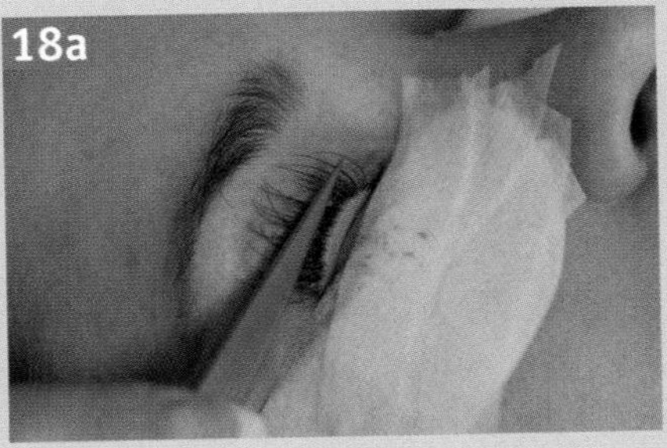

Check for sticking by gently pulling back the lash line.

18 Check for sticking by grasping a group of lashes with the tweezers. Turn the lash line back just enough to expose the inside of the lash line. You should check for sticking several times during the procedure.

continues on next page

PROCEDURE 20–1, CONT. APPLYING SEMIPERMANENT EYELASH EXTENSIONS

19 If a client's lashes are stuck together, use a clean micro swab to gently separate them. You may need to use a small amount of lash adhesive remover on the swab to break the bond. Alternatively, you can use your tweezers to gently pull stuck lashes apart, if possible, or remove them using the removal technique and reapplying.

CAUTION!

Once the lashes are in place, if any trimming is necessary do so with great care. Position your client in a reclined position with her eyes closed. Trimming can be kept at a minimum by selecting the proper lash lengths before application.

20 Once all lashes are in place, wait 10 minutes for the adhesive to completely set up and then apply a coat of the protective coating solution with a disposable brush. Allow this to dry completely—at least 5 minutes—before moving to the next step.

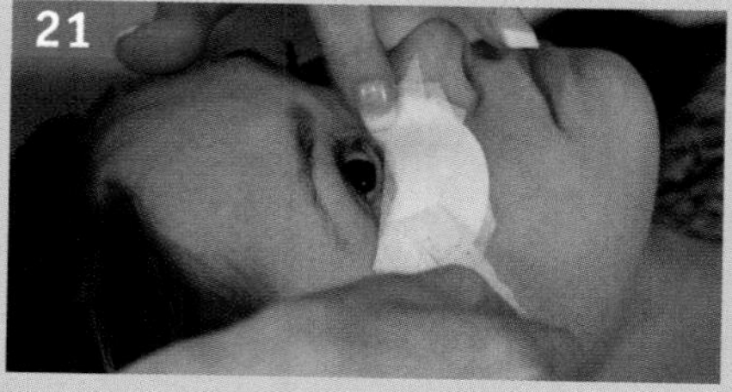

Remove tape first.

21 If you used the technique that tapes the lower lashes to the gel pad, remove the pad now.

Here's a Tip

Many manufacturers suggest coating the lashes with a special solution that acts as a moisture barrier for the first 24 hours. Before applying the solution, be sure to allow the adhesive to set up at least 10 minutes after lash placement.

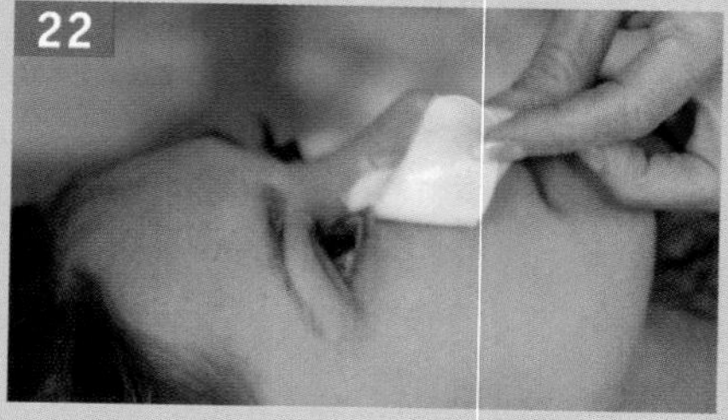

Gently remove under-eye pad.

22 Gently remove the gel pad, removing strips of tape first and the gel pad last to avoid pulling out any lower lashes that may be tucked between the pad and tape.

Post-procedure

23 Review home care with the client, reminding her to avoid getting the lashes wet for 24 hours to ensure maximum lash life.

24 Remind the client not to use waterproof mascara; removing it can result in loss of lashes.

Clean-up and Disinfection

25 Throw away all disposable items.

26 Follow state guidelines for clean-up and disinfection of the treatment room.

27 Sterilize any tools or implements that will be used on the next client.

Technique Variations

Use different lash lengths to achieve different looks. Following are some suggestions for variations.

1. To make the eyes appear wider, apply three to five different lengths of eyelash extensions.
2. For a more almond eye:
   - Use the longest extension at the outside corner of the eye.
   - Use the medium length to fill the center portion of the lashes.
   - Use the shortest extensions at the inside of the eye. Example: 12 mm/11 mm/10 mm/9 mm.
3. For a larger more open-eyed look:
   - Use medium-length extensions at the outer portion of the eye.
   - Use the longest extensions to fill in the center. Example, 8 mm/10 mm/12 mm/10 mm/8 mm.
   - Use the shortest lash extensions at the inner corner.
4. To create a thick, lush, glamourous look (Figure 20–11):
   - Apply long lash extensions evenly across the eye.
   - Use a longer lash extension for every second or third lash; for example, alternate 12 mm/14 mm.

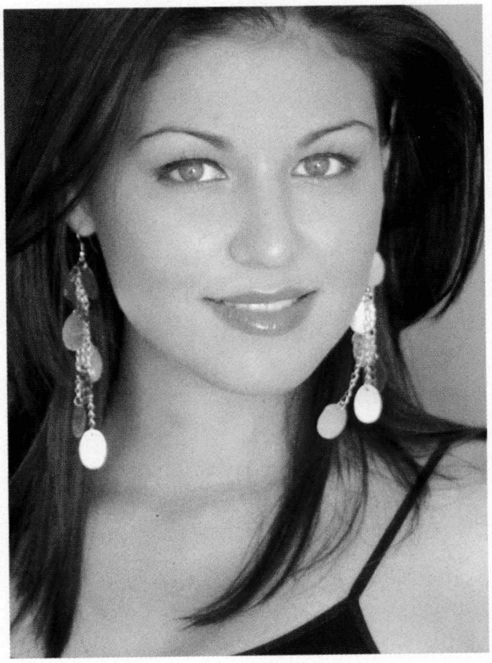

Figure 20–11 The glamour look.

? Did You Know

Lashes are available in 0.10-mm, 0.15-mm, 0.20-mm and 0.25-mm thicknesses and lengths from 6 mm to 17 mm.

Application Variations

Procedure 20–1 describes how to apply lashes by rotating from one eye to the other and from the outside in. Another method involves applying lashes to one eye at a time. To do this, start with the centermost lash application. Then move to the outermost lash then halfway between these two and then halfway between the center lash and the inner corner of the eye. Once these are in place, go back to the center and start adding an adjacent lash next to each of the existing ones, rotating across the eye. Repeat this step until you have applied all of the lashes. Then move to the other eye and repeat the process. Using this technique allows you to offer the client a break when you have completed one eye.

Lash Removal

When removing lash extensions, take care to protect the eyes from the removal solution and to avoid taking natural lashes in the process.

PROCEDURE 20-2 LASH EXTENSION REMOVAL

MATERIALS AND IMPLEMENTS

- Headband or hair clip
- Magnifying lamp or light
- Adhesive remover
- Under-eye pads (single-use, disposable)
- Adhesive remover holder (sterilized or disposable)
- 3M clear surgical tape
- Cotton swabs or micro swabs (disposable)
- Paper towels

Preparation

1 Set up facial lounge and treatment room. Most clients do not dress down for this procedure.

2 Gather supplies.

3 Review the client's history with her and have her read and sign a consent form.

4 Review the client's expectations and the procedure.

5 Confirm that she has removed her contact lenses.

Procedure

General procedure:

6 Ask your client to sit upright for the procedure to prevent adhesive remover from entering the eyes and so that you can clearly see the lash line and the extension.

7 Clip her hair back.

8 Protect the under-eye area with gel pads.

9 Saturate two large swabs with adhesive remover. Gel type remover is preferred but if you are using liquid type, blot off any excess liquid with a paper towel.

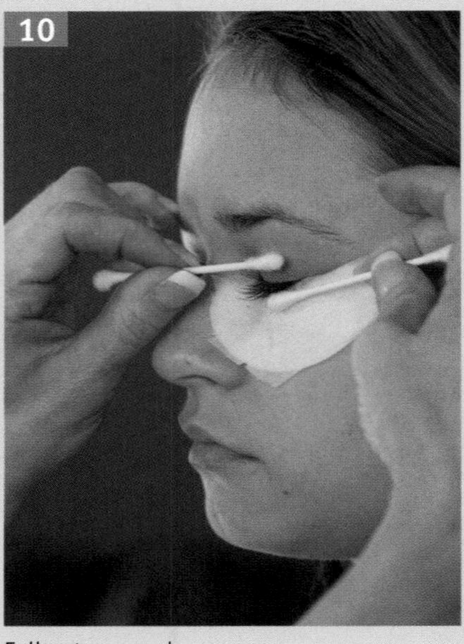

Full-set removal.

10 Gently hold the swabs on both sides of the lash for approximately 60–90 seconds, and then stroke the lash in a gentle outward motion until the lash is completely removed.

11 Repeat step 4 until the bond is dissolved and you have removed all eyelash extensions have been removed.

For single-lash removal:

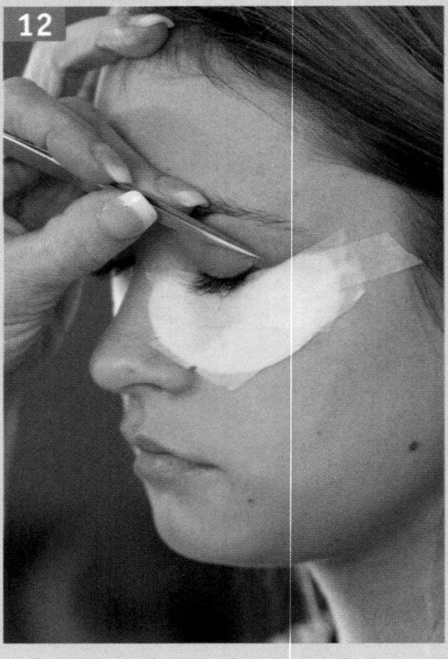

Isolate single lash to be removed.

12 Grasp the eyelash extension at the tip with the forceps, pulling it back gently from the surrounding lashes.

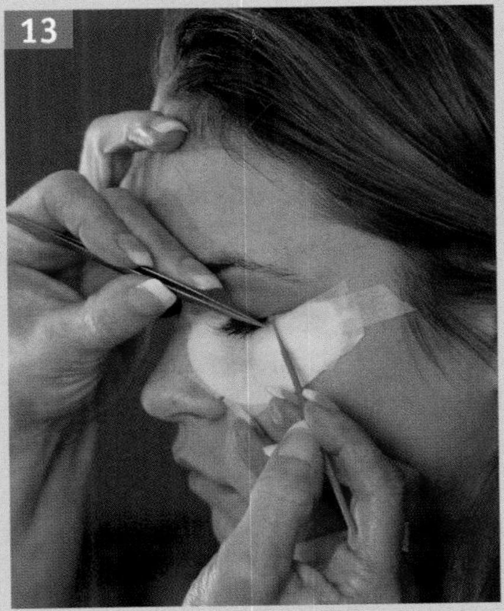

Stroke lash with micro swab dipped in remover.

13 Dip a single micro swab in lash adhesive remover. With the swab, gently stroke the eyelash extensions to be removed in an outward motion until the bond dissolves and lash can be removed.

14 Clean off any residue with gentle cleanser, lash toner, or a protein remover pad.

FYI

You may need to clean the lashes with a fresh remover swab to remove any adhesive residue left on the lash.

CAUTION!

If lower lashes are taped to the gel pad and you do not remove the tape before removing the gel pad, the client may lose lashes.

Post-procedure

Give the client any home-care instructions in writing.

Clean-up and Disinfection

15 Follow state guidelines to clean and disinfect the treatment room and work area.

16 Disinfect and sterilize any reusable implements.

After the Procedure

Home-Care Instructions

Following is a list of aftercare instructions for the client. Always follow manufacturer's guidelines if they vary from this list, but these items are a good starting point.

1. You can maintain your regular cosmetics and cleansing routine, but avoid contact with water, moisture, makeup, removers, and so on, for a period of 24 hours after application.
2. Avoid hot steam or swimming for 48 hours.
3. Avoid using any product on the bonded area of your new lashes and avoid using oil-based products of any kind near the eyes.
4. Do not rub your eyes or pick at the lashes.
5. *Do not use waterproof mascara.* However, you can use water-based mascara on the tips of your lashes for a more dramatic look.
6. Do not use mechanical eyelash curlers. These can damage lash extensions and break the bond of the adhesive.

Common Reasons Lash Extensions Fall Off

1. Mascara residue on eyelashes compromise the contact area between eyelashes and the extensions.
2. Actual eyelashes fall off due to lash life cycle.
3. The esthetician used poor technique with inadequate lash bonding.
4. Lashes come in contact with water too soon after the procedure.

Eyelash Perming

Permanent eyelash curling involves the use of specially formulated products that keep eyelashes curled for long periods of time without the use of eyelash curlers. Permanent eyelash curling can make the eyes look more open, giving the lashes a longer, more youthful look that lasts for several weeks.

Some clients may want to combine other services with eyelash perming, such as eyelash extensions or eyelash tinting. Unless otherwise indicated by a manufacturer, perform these procedures after you have permed the lashes according to the following guidelines. When adding semipermanent eyelash extensions, wait a minimum of 48 hours to ensure that no residue from the perming solution remains on the lashes. Also, use larger rollers to avoid overcurling, as it is difficult to adhere lash extensions to tightly curled lashes. Eyelash tinting should be performed no sooner than 24 hours after eyelash perming. Clients who have had permanent eyeliner procedures should wait a minimum of two weeks for any other procedures; the eyes need to be completely healed to avoid loss of lashes, irritation, or heightened risk of infection.

Consultation

Twenty-four hours before applying lashes for a client, have her come in for 15 minutes to talk about what she can expect during her appointment. Examine her eye area; if you see any redness, swelling, signs of conjunctivitis, or flaking, recommend that she be seen by her physician or eye doctor before you apply the lashes. Clients with glaucoma, sensitivity to perming solutions, or thyroid conditions that affect lash growth are not candidates for eyelash perming. Clients with recent vision correction surgery should have clearance from their physician or wait until their eyes return to feeling normal. To avoid an allergic reaction to the perming products, do a patch test. Follow manufacturer's recommendations for this process and refer any reaction to the client's physician. Do not perm lashes that appear weak or brittle. As with any products that you use on or near the eyes, be sure to follow manufacturers' recommendations carefully. Failure to do so can result in ocular damage or blindness.

Preparation, Health, and Safety

Advise the client not to wear mascara or eye makeup to the appointment because removing mascara can irritate the eye. Wash your hands thoroughly before starting. Client's contact lenses should be removed prior to the procedure. Clean lashes very thoroughly with an oil-free makeup remover and allow to dry completely to ensure rods will adhere to the lids. Your client should be lying in a reclined position for this treatment.

PROCEDURE 20–3 EYELASH PERMING

IMPLEMENTS AND MATERIALS

- Clean towel
- Hand mirror
- Oil-free makeup remover
- Cotton pads
- Cotton swabs
- Bowl of warm water
- Timer
- Perming lotion
- Setting lotion
- Conditioning lotion
- Glue
- Cleanser
- Pre-glued eyelash rollers
- Applicator sticks
- Toothpicks

Preparation

1. Set up facial lounge and treatment room. Most clients do not dress down for this procedure.
2. Gather supplies.
3. Review the client's history with her and have her read and sign a consent form.
4. Review the client's expectations and the procedure.
5. Confirm that she has removed her contact lenses.

Here's a Tip

Pre-curl the lashes with a lash curler to help adhere lashes to the roller.

CAUTION!

Do not use hair perming solution on or near the eyes, as this can cause blindness and damage to the skin.

Procedure

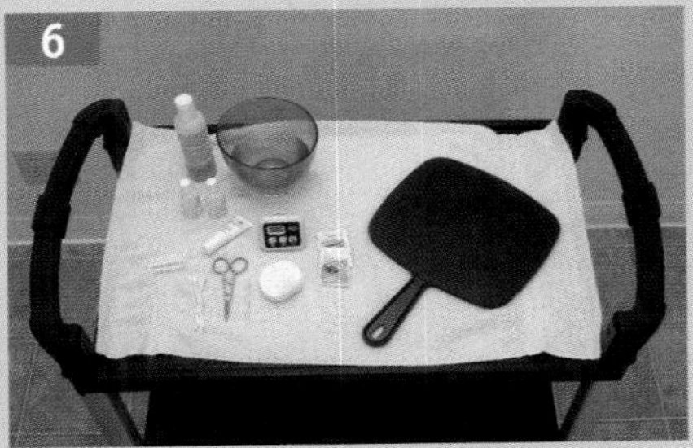

6 Lash perming materials.

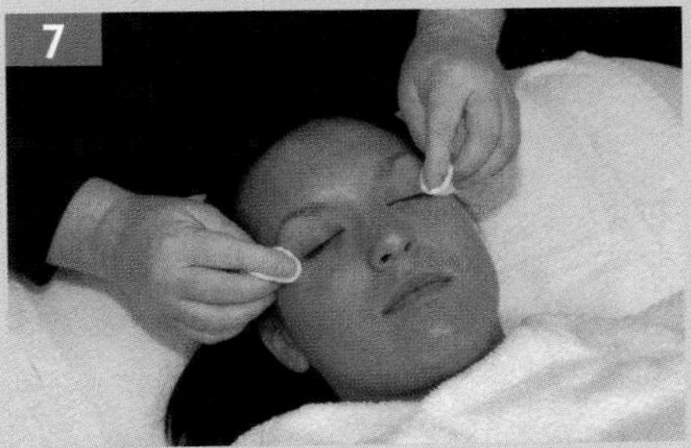

7 Clean the lashes.

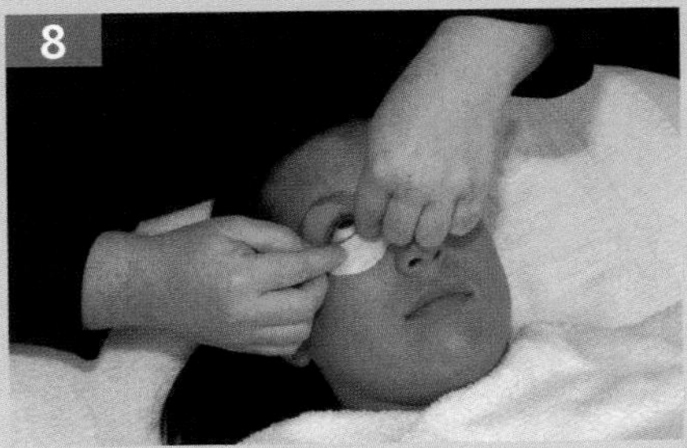

8 Protect lower lash line with damp cotton pad.

6 Use the following guidelines to select the roller size:

- Smaller rollers are best for shorter eyelashes or if a tighter curl is desired.
- Medium rollers are the most commonly used for a good all-around curl.
- Large rollers are best for the longer lashes or a looser curl.

7 Cleanse the eyelashes, removing all eye makeup.

8 Place a damp cotton pad on the lower lid to prevent fumes from entering the client's eyes.

Here's a Tip

For very coarse lashes, apply perming solution to lashes for 3 to 5 minutes before starting the procedure. Rinse and remove and then start the perming process.

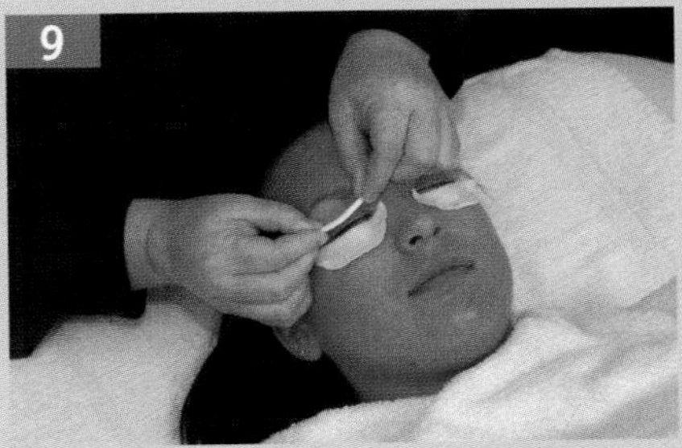

9 Bend the roller.

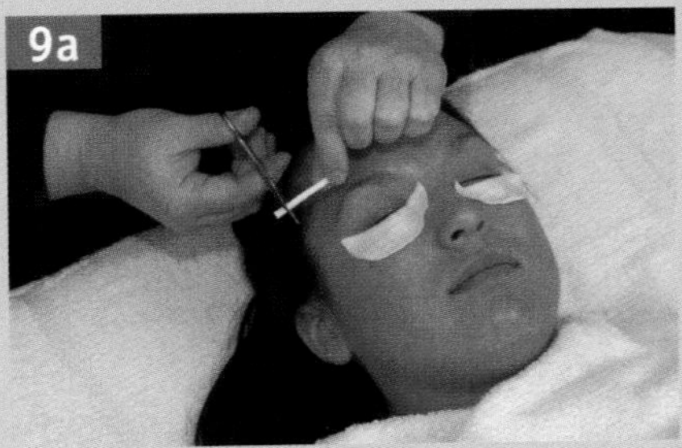

9a Measuring and trim roller to fit.

9 The rollers are self-adhesive so be careful to handle them only at the tips. Bend the roller slightly to fit the shape of the eyelid and trim the rod to the appropriate length of the eyelid.

continues on next page

PROCEDURE 20-3, CONT. EYELASH PERMING

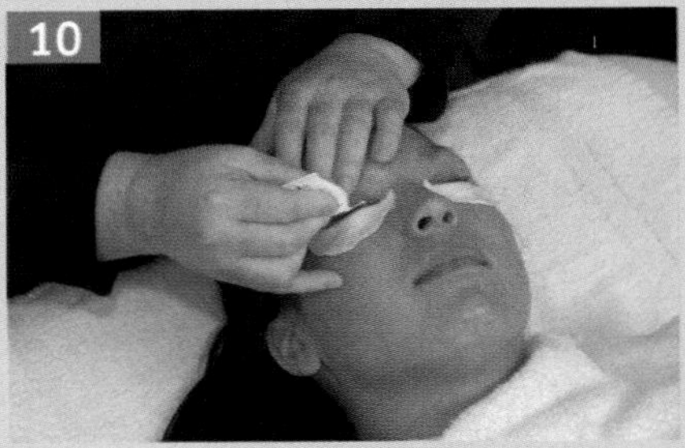

Apply perm glue to eyelid at base of lash line.

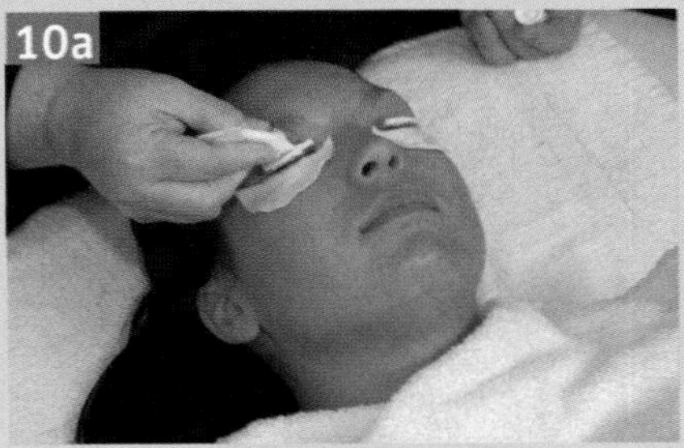

Place roller at base of lash line and apply more glue on top.

10 Apply eyelash perming glue in a line at the base of the lashes and position the roller as close as possible to the base of the lashes. After positioning the roller, add more glue on the top of the roller.

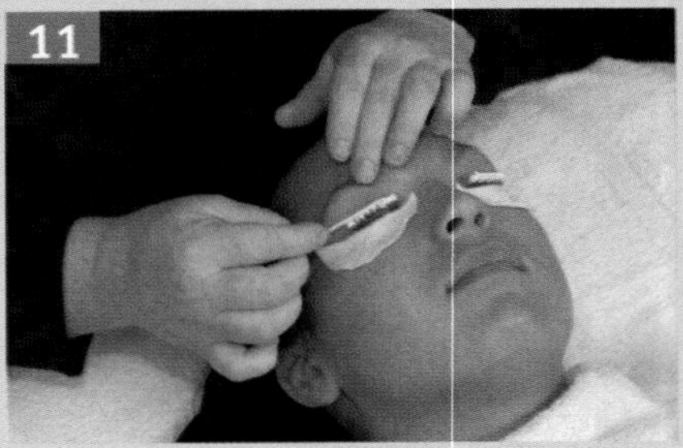

Using wooden applicator, place lashes on roller.

11 Using the wood applicator, carefully press the lashes on the roller one at a time to avoid overlapping or crossing of lashes.

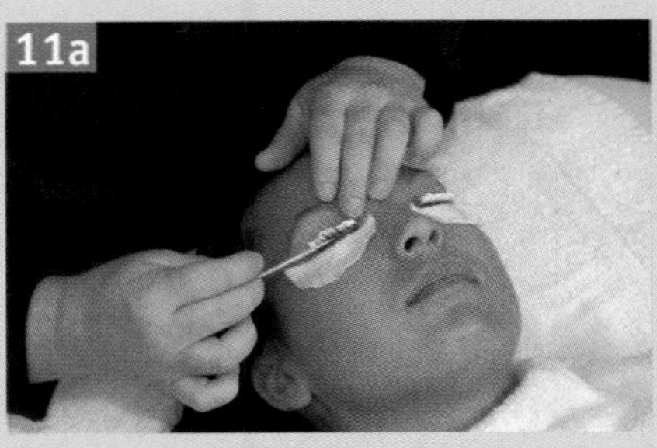

Application steps incorporate a small brush or wooden applicator.

Make sure that the lower lashes are not curled onto the rod.

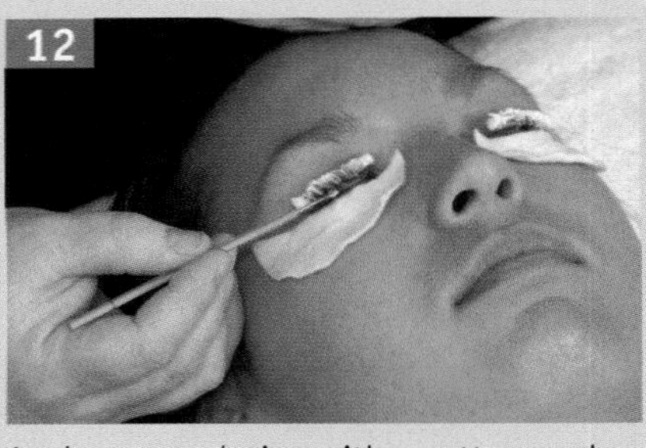

Apply perm solution with a cotton swab.

12 Apply perm solution with a cotton swab or manufacturer's applicator across the lashes adhered to the rod. Avoid contact with the skin. Carefully follow manufacturer's instructions for processing; depending on the kit, timing ranges anywhere from 8 to 15 minutes.

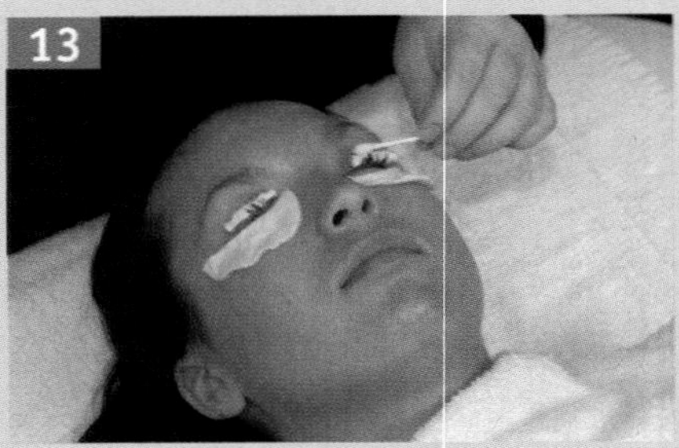

Check for desired curl.

13 Check lashes by separating one or two from the roller with a toothpick. If you do not yet see the curl you are trying to achieve, leave the lashes on the roller for 2 to 3 minutes longer. Wipe off any excess perming lotion and rinse thoroughly following manufacturer's guidelines.

Here's a Tip

If you have a facial steamer, use it after step 7 to aid in creating heat, but keep it well away from the client.

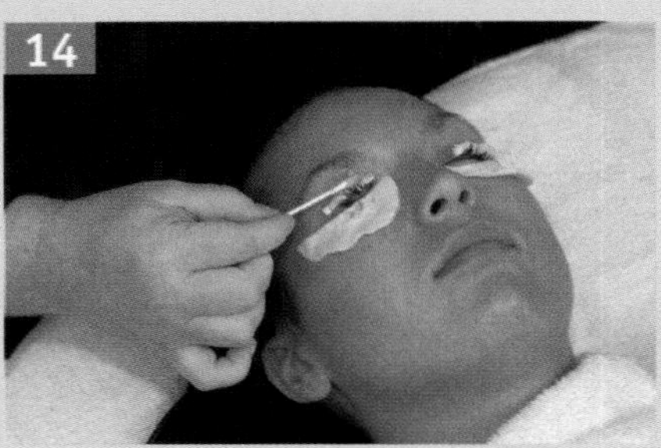

Apply setting or neutralizer lotion to lashes with application stick.

14 Apply setting or neutralizer lotion to lashes with the application stick. Leave neutralizer on according to manufacturer's instructions, generally 5 to 10 minutes.

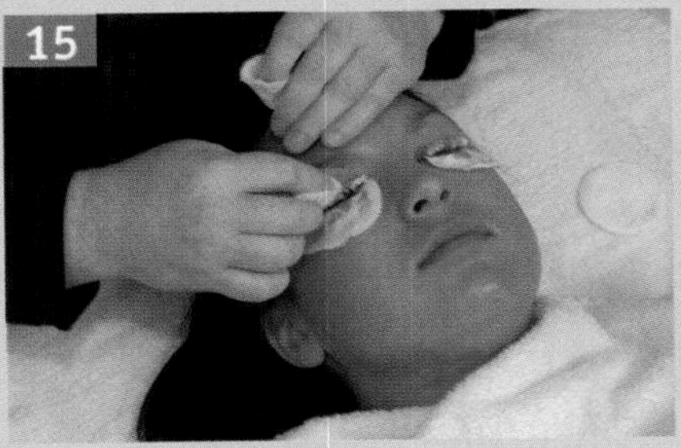

Remove setting lotion.

15 Remove setting lotion with wet cotton-tipped swabs or wet cotton rounds, rinsing thoroughly.

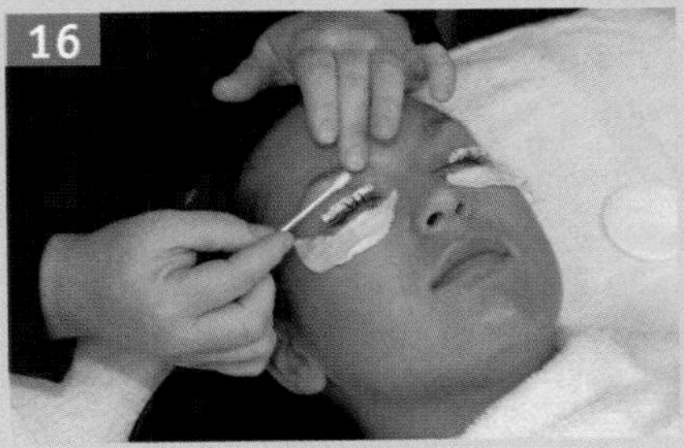

Apply post treatment lotion.

16 If the kit includes a post-treatment lotion, apply it now with an applicator stick or cotton swab. Let lotion set for 5 minutes or according to manufacturer's instructions.

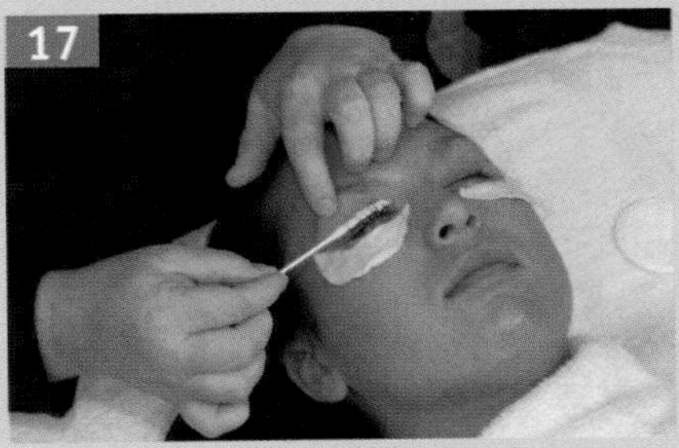

Use cleanser.

17 Use cleanser and gently swipe the upper part of the roller, touching the eyelid. Using a damp cotton-tipped swab, clean the eyelid from side to side. Slowly roll the rod downward with the cotton swab, freeing the lash from the rod.

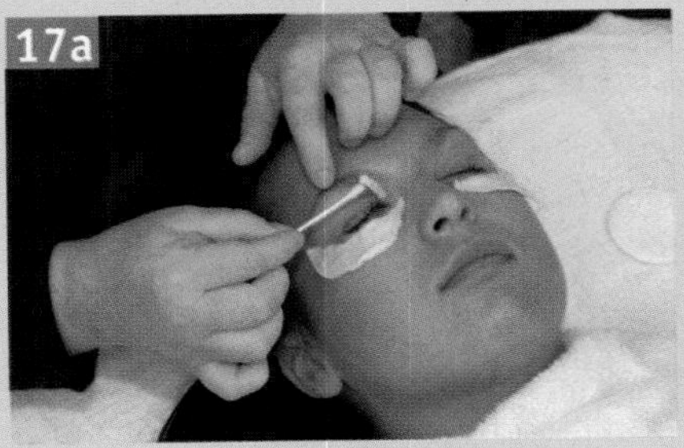

Remove perm rollers.

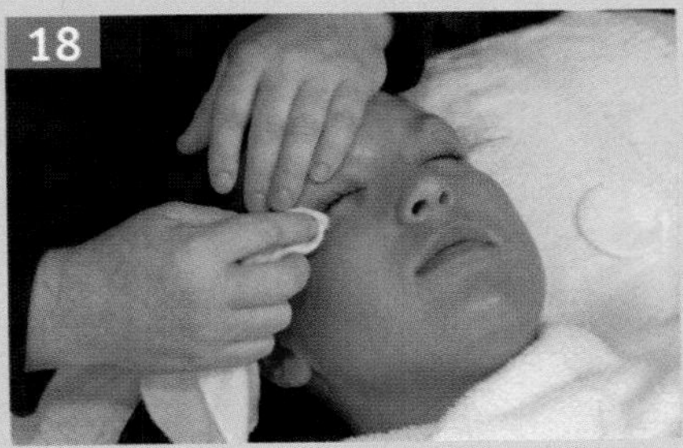

Clean eyes and lashes.

18 Clean lashes with a warm, damp cloth.

Post-procedure

Provide client with home-care instructions. It is best to let the lashes rest for 24 hours prior to applying mascara.

Clean-up and Disinfection

19 Clean the work area and dispose of used perm rods and all disposable items.

20 Disinfect work surfaces and sterilize any nondisposable implements, such as tweezers, following state guidelines.

CAUTION!

Do not let any perming solution enter the client's eyes or touch her skin.

MINERAL MAKEUP

The term "mineral makeup" was coined in 1994 to describe a concentrated pigment powder that was unlike the widely used, predominantly talc-based formulae found throughout the cosmetic world. Traditionally, color cosmetics—base, blush, and eye shadows—contain 70% to 90% talcum powder, a finely powdered magnesium silicate, and are colored with synthetic colorants (FD&C dyes). Mineral powder, on the other hand, contains no talc or FD&C dyes. Instead, it is pure pigment that provides a foundation, powder, concealer, and, in some instances, a sunscreen all in one. It blurs the line between makeup and skin care.

Here's a Tip

A good mineral makeup will always have an SPF of at least 15. Regulations require that this be published on the label and any box packaging.

Typical Ingredients in Mineral Makeup

Mineral makeup usually comprises a selection of titanium dioxide, zinc oxide, mica, bismuth oxychloride, boron nitride, and iron oxides. (You will sometimes see sercite listed. This is a type of mica.) All of these ingredients contribute something to the final look, feel, and performance of the finished product. However, not all minerals are created equal. There are many grades and particle sizes as well as coatings that all play a significant part in the efficacy of the final product. There are no federal guidelines for what ingredients or percentages must be present in order to classify a product as a mineral powder. There may be as little as .00001% of some listed ingredients. The practice of using trace amounts is most common in inexpensive mass-marketed products that use the inclusion of the ingredient for marketing purposes.

Following is a discussion of some of these minerals and their benefits. These minerals should be in the top positions on the ingredient labels of any mineral makeup.

FYI

Minerals used in powders are inert substances. *Inert* describes something that cannot support bacterial life. Minerals have no relationship to mineral oil, which is a liquid petrolatum, a by-product of petroleum.

- Titanium dioxide (TiO_2) is a naturally occurring oxide of titanium. This white substance is found in three minerals: rutile (beach sand), anatase, and brookite (relatively rare). Titanium dioxide is one of the two ingredients approved by the FDA as physical sunscreens. It not only gives some mineral makeup its sun protection factor, but it also provides opacity. It is only used raw and in small percentages when it functions as a pigment. Raw titanium dioxide oxidizes and creates free radicals which attack the skin's cells. This is why it is usually coated to eliminate the oxidation process and to increase its ability to refract UV rays. Dimethicone is commonly used as a coating to increase the light-scattering properties of TiO_2.
- Zinc oxide (ZnO) occurs in nature in the mineral zincite. Zinc oxide is the other ingredient approved by the FDA as a physical sunscreen. This pure white mineral is also known for its anti-inflammatory and antimicrobial properties.
- Mica—a naturally occurring mineral—gives slip and glide to the finished product. It can be used in a larger particle size to provide shimmer to the finished product, or it can be used in a much smaller particle size which will render it absorbent with a matte finish. Mica can also be used as a colorant.
- Bismuth oxychloride is a synthetically prepared iridescent white or nearly white powder. Its metallic sheen has led it to being called synthetic pearl. It adds color, coverage, and adhesion to the finished product.
- Boron nitride (BN) is a white, silky powder that gives smoothness, coverage, slip, and sheen to the finished product. It is also known as the "soft focus" mineral because of its light refraction qualities.
- Iron oxides (Fe_2O_3), commonly known as rust, are primarily used as colorants. The mineral form is hematite and is mined as the main ore of iron. However, iron oxides used in cosmetics are not obtained from this source. They are synthesized under strict laboratory processes because iron ore in nature is contaminated with heavy metals. Apart from colorants, iron oxides can have the effect of boosting sun protection by working synergistically with zinc oxide.

There is a misconception that minerals used in mineral powders come directly from the earth. In fact, most minerals are either extracted from the original rock and manipulated extensively in the laboratory or manufactured in their entirety. This is the only way to abide by FDA guidelines and ensure that minerals are not contaminated with heavy metals and other toxic materials.

Remember that the most common ingredient in standard makeup is talc. You will not find talc in a true mineral makeup. Other ingredients that are not found in an authentic mineral makeup are synthetic preservatives, FD&C dyes, and synthetic fragrance. All three ingredient groups are known sensitizers.

Benefits of Mineral Makeup

Coverage

Mineral powders are a foundation, concealer, and powder all in one. If the label indicates an SPF, they are also a sunscreen. Because they are concentrated pigment, undiluted by talc, they give excellent coverage with very little product. It is the way minerals interact with light that creates the illusion of perfection rather than a layer of product hiding imperfections underneath. Minerals interact with light in complicated ways:

- They allow light to pass through the particles so it bounces off the skin and reflects back some of the skin's hue, literally taking on the color of the skin.
- They reflect, refract, and diffuse light, creating a soft-focus effect that minimizes imperfections.
- They create a luminous look to the skin, imparting a healthy, youthful glow.

This interaction with light makes color-matching the skin easier than with traditional makeup. In fact, you will rarely see where minerals end and the skin begins. Because of this interaction with light and the subsequent ability to blend with the skin, it is important to try minerals on the skin to test for color and not to make a decision based on the color in the jar.

Adherence

Mineral makeup is made up of a variety of particle sizes. When applied to clean, moisturized skin, these particles cling together and create a surface tension that overcomes gravity and holds the minerals tightly to the skin. The result is that they resist running, creasing, and smearing and can only be removed with a cleanser. (No special cleanser is required.) There is far less transference with mineral makeup compared to traditional makeup.

? Did You Know

The look, adherence, and payoff of a mineral makeup will differ from manufacturer to manufacturer, depending on the quality and type of minerals used as well as the blending techniques.

Sun Protection Factor (SPF)

The sun protection factor of mineral makeup can be an important part of its benefits. If a client is wearing a chemical sunscreen underneath her makeup, she runs the risk of being sensitive to the chemicals as well as reacting to the occlusive nature of many formulae. A chemical sunscreen also creates a difficult base for makeup application. A mineral makeup with an SPF can eliminate the need for a chemical sunscreen.

Titanium dioxide and zinc oxide are physical sunscreens and give broad spectrum protection (UVB and UVA). It is important to read the ingredient list to see if one or both minerals are included. Only mineral powders that have been tested on 20 human subjects in an FDA certified lab can claim sun protection, and this must be listed on the label. If you do not see it, then you can assume that the mineral powder does not give protection.

FYI

The SPF rating refers to the measured UVB protection only.

Feel and Look

If minerals are applied properly, they should feel weightless on the skin. Some wearers even report that for the first time in many years they can actually feel air on their skin. Indeed, minerals allow the skin to breathe and function normally, a boon to all skin types but especially to those with acne and rosacea.

If minerals feel heavy or look cakey, then it is probably an application problem and not the minerals themselves. The look should be sheer and luminous, although if minerals are being applied for camouflage, then they can look more opaque. If minerals are properly applied, they will mimic the look of a young, healthy skin.

Application

To apply minerals, you generally need two things: a good quality brush and the knowledge that "less is more." For example, foundation that is too dark will exaggerate fine lines and accentuate pores. Skin of Fitzpatrick values V or VI need a powder that is slightly lighter than the skin tone to minimize any ashy tendency. On some clients, you may need to use two colors; these clients' faces may have distinctly different color in the center than around the perimeter.

Mineral powders come in two forms: loose and pressed. Each needs a slightly different application technique.

Applying Loose Mineral Powder

Most loose mineral powders are packaged in two ways: a jar with a sifter, which requires a separate brush, or a cylinder, which dispenses mineral powder through a brush at the end of the cylinder (Figure 20–12).

Jar with Sifter

Remove the seal from the sifter or puncture holes in the seal for a more controlled flow. Do not remove the sifter. Replace the lid, turn the jar upside-down and tap the bottom of the jar. A small quantity of the minerals will now be available in

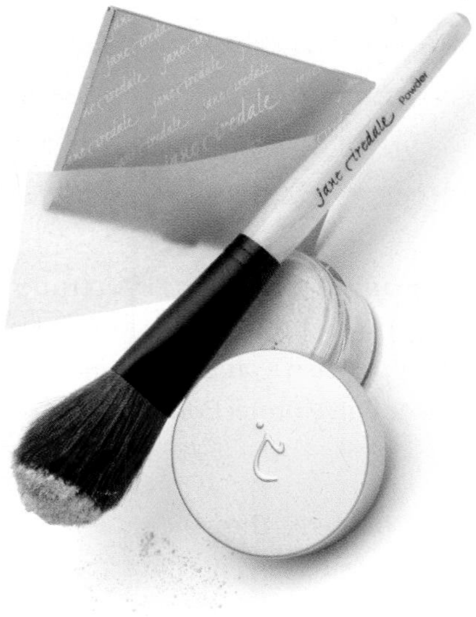

Figure 20–12 Jar with brush.

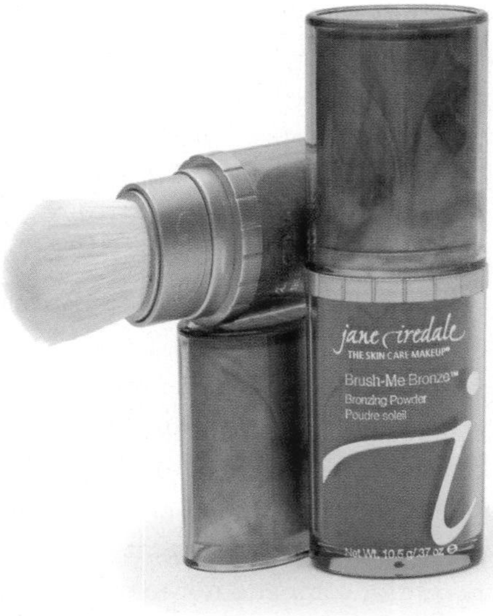

Figure 20–13 Powder-dispensing brush.

the sifter. If you are working person-to-person, tip the minerals from the sifter into a receptacle such as a shallow dish.

Cleanse the client's face and moisturize. Allow the moisturizer to absorb. Pat off any excess. To choose the correct color, test a little on the jawline. Try to do this in natural light, if possible. Minerals are more forgiving than conventional makeup; one shade suits a wide variety of skin tones because of the interplay with light.

The best tool for loose mineral powder is a kabuki or chisel powder brush. Do not use a brush with a large head, which will scatter the minerals. Look for a brush that can be used in smaller areas such as the eyes and nose. Lightly dip the brush into the minerals, tap off any excess, and use the lid of the container or a dish to work the powder into the brush so it is evenly distributed. The minerals should cling to the bristles all the way around the brush and not just on the ends.

Treat the face in quadrants and apply one brushload to each quadrant. Apply the minerals in thin layers, finishing with downward strokes. If you have applied too much, use a sponge with a nap (a flocked sponge) to remove any excess. If you need additional coverage in specific areas spot with a sponge. It is easy to overdo when you first work with mineral powders because they are concentrated pigment. Layering is the preferred technique.

Powder-Dispensing Brush

When starting a new brush, run it over your knuckles or a tissue so that you can see when the powder begins to disperse and judge the amount of product you want to use (Figure 20–13). Have a receptacle nearby so that you may trap any excess powder as it begins to work its way

Here's a Tip

To "pull" out the center of the face and give the same flattering effect as highlighting, use a lighter base in the aesthetic triangle and a darker one on the perimeter (Figure 20–14). This is especially useful when working with Asian faces, which have a flatter plane.

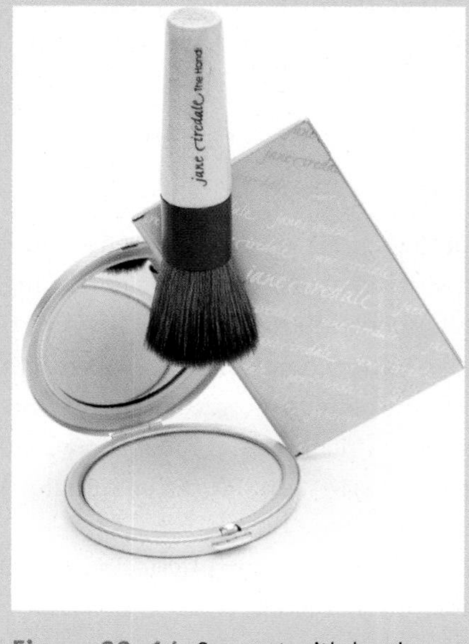

Figure 20–14 Compact with brush.

Here's a Tip

Traditional cosmetic sponges do not allow you to blend minerals. Because of the way they adhere to the skin, you will need a sponge with a surface flocking.

Here's a Tip

If the minerals look powdery, wait a few minutes for the skin's natural oils to emerge, or you may speed the process by using a facial spritz. Gently pat the moisture into the skin.

through the bristles. Begin on the area of the face that needs the most coverage, moving in circles.

Clean the brush by wetting a tissue or paper towel with a brush-cleaning fluid. Clean the tips of the brush first and then run the entire brush across the dampened towel from the bottom of the brush to the top. This will help to maintain the shape of the brush. Lay the brush flat and allow it to dry. If the brush has a cap, do not replace it while the brush is wet.

Applying Pressed Powder

A natural-hair flat-ended brush is preferable when working with pressed mineral powders. Swirl the brush around the cake and tap off any excess. Cover one quadrant of the face at a time, finishing with downward strokes. Add more coverage with the brush or a flocked sponge if needed. Spritz to hasten setting. Layer your minerals; do not try to cover everything at once.

PROCEDURE 20–4 APPLYING MINERAL MAKEUP

MATERIALS AND IMPLEMENTS

- Mineral powders
- Brushes
- Sponges
- Client drape to protect clothing
- Metal spatula
- Disposable or metal pallet from which to work
- Gloves (optional but required if you use the back of your hand as a pallet)
- Makeup area with adequate lighting
- Facial cleanser
- Moisturizer
- Cleansing cloth or pads
- Towel
- Tissues
- Brush cleaner

Preparation

1 Set up the makeup application area.

2 Talk to the client to assess the skin and goals for the application.

Procedure

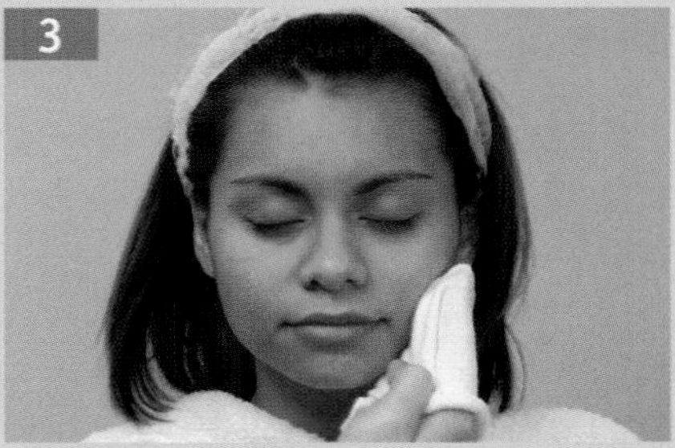

Pre-cleanse client's skin.

3 Pre-cleanse the client's skin and pat dry.

continues on next page

PROCEDURE 20–4, CONT. APPLYING MINERAL MAKEUP

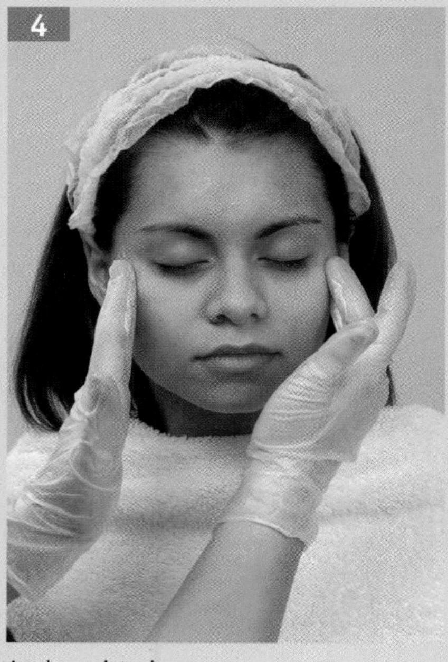
Apply moisturizer.

4 Apply moisturizer.

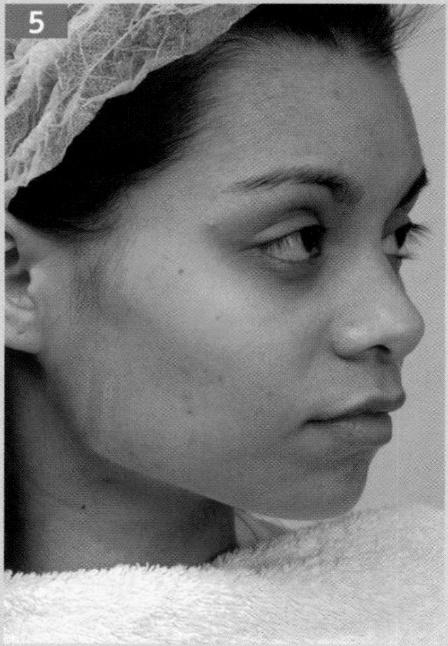
Test makeup along jawline.

5 Select the correct makeup tone for client's skin. Test along the jawline.

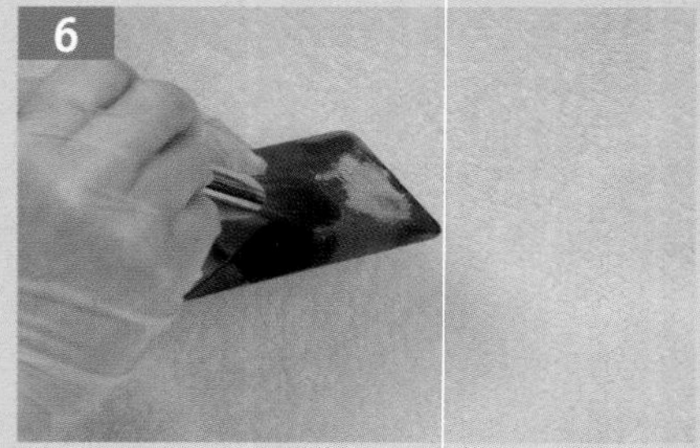
Dispense minerals onto a working pallet.

6 Dispense some of the minerals onto a working pallet.

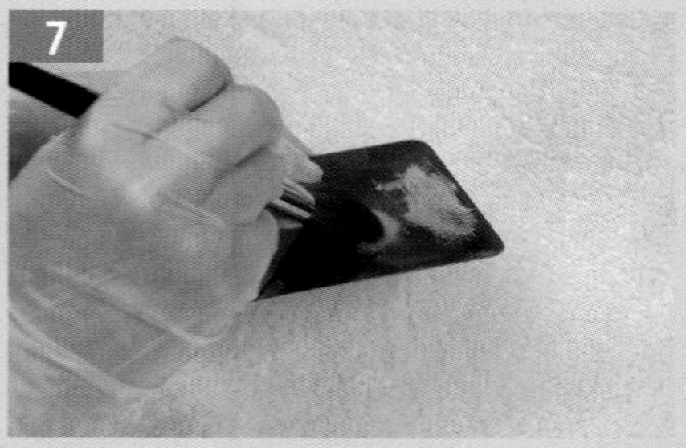
Load brush, tapping on pallet to remove excess.

7 Load the brush, tapping it on a pallet to remove excess.

8 Divide the client's face into quadrants, starting with the forehead. Apply one brushload to each quadrant. Do not apply too heavily; light coats are best.

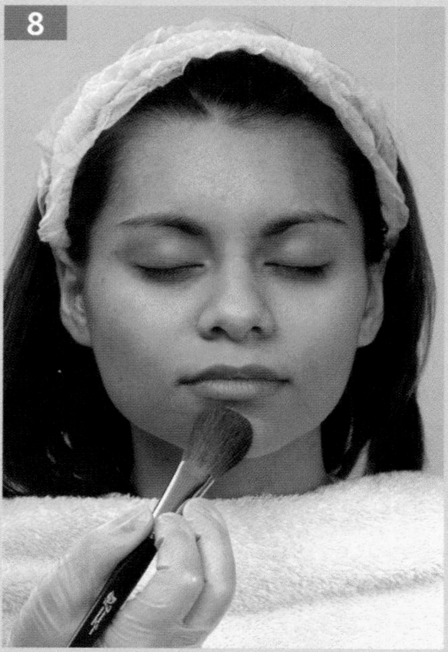
Apply one brushload to each quadrant.

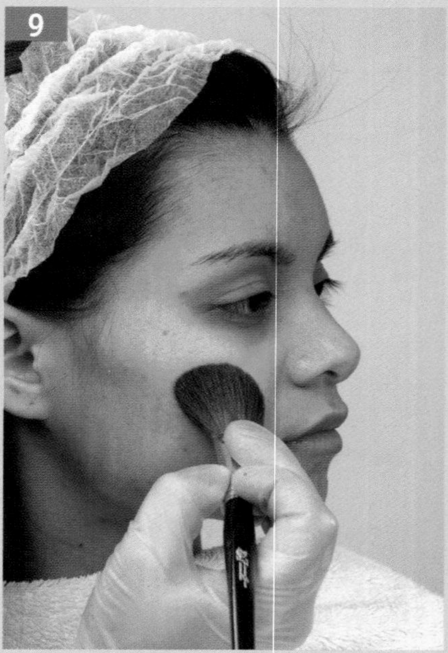
Finish strokes in each area in a downward motion.

9 Finish strokes in each area in a downward motion.

10

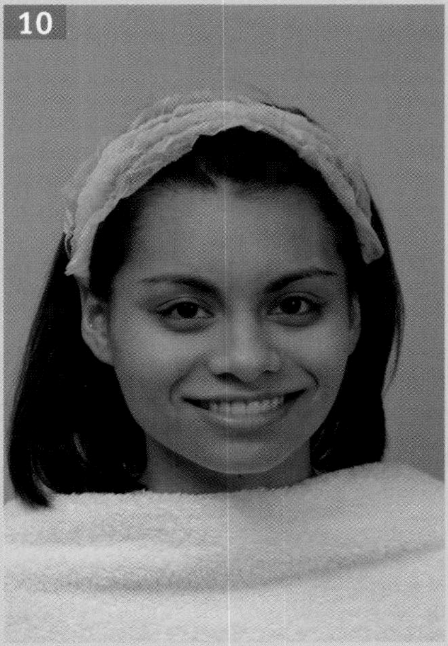

Apply thin additional coats.

10 If additional coverage is required, apply thin additional coats.

Post-procedure

Complete makeup process following classical guidelines:

a. Apply blush.
b. Apply eye makeup.
c. Apply lip color.

Clean-up and Sanitation

11 Clean up the work area following state guidelines.

12 Clean and disinfect brushes using a professional brush cleaner or warm soap and water.

13 Lay brushes on a paper towel to dry.

Application Problems

Once you understand the pure pigment nature of minerals and the amount of coverage, you will find application fast and easy. Following are some tips to help you.

1. **Too Much Shine:** Layering too thickly and pressing into the skin with a sponge tends to separate the individual minerals. This pulls the mineral that creates the glow to the surface. Avoid this by applying the minerals in thin layers in downward strokes with the brush. Keep adding layers until you reach the desired coverage.
2. **Accentuates Pores or Fine Lines:** Try using a pressed powder; loose tends to be more luminescent. Spray with a facial spritz and pat dry. If the under-eye area is lined, pat a small amount of moisturizer around the eye on top of the minerals.
3. **Uneven and Blotchy:** This condition happens when the minerals have been applied before the moisturizer has absorbed or because the moisturizer is too occlusive. Always wait for the moisturizer to absorb and blot any excess.

In addition, some unevenness can be attributed to sponge applicators that do not move the product on the skin. If you use a sponge, try a flocked sponge because it blends the powders without dragging on the skin.

MINERALS FOR CAMOUFLAGE

Because of the concentrated pigment nature of mineral powders, these are good tools for camouflaging the effects of certain conditions, such as acne and rosacea. You will need additional mineral camouflage for other conditions such as bruising (Figure 20–15).

Do not expect to get camouflage right on your first or second attempt. Practice your technique on fellow students, models, or friends until you feel confident. A client will understand if you ask for another chance to achieve a better result. You will build credibility with a client if you are honest about what you expect to be able to

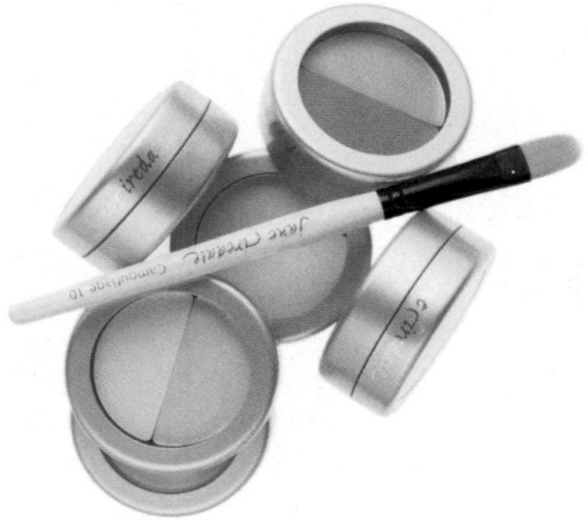

Figure 20–15 Concealer with camouflage brush.

> **? Did You Know**
>
> Due to strategies for enhanced safety and cross-contamination prevention, many professional makeup artists now wear clear, unpowdered gloves while applying makeup. It allows them to use the back of one hand as a pallet without having to clean bare skin, and it shows a level of concern for keeping the area sanitary. If the client has any redness or skin that is in the process of healing, she will feel more comfortable and confident about your care of her.

> **FOCUS ON:** ***Time Spent on a Process***
>
> Clients want a simple and quick process and complete understanding of the steps you took to achieve the result. If the process is too long and complicated, your client will be discouraged and look elsewhere.

> **CAUTION!**
>
> **Never attempt camouflage on a client who has just had a medical procedure; refer the client to the attending physician for written permission.**

accomplish. *It is rare that you can make a facial distraction completely invisible.* Your goal is to normalize your client's appearance as much as possible so that she does not draw attention to herself.

Covering Redness

In the world of makeup, the color green has been the tool used to cover redness; the theory is that green and red are complementary colors and, therefore, cancel out each other. This technique works well on an artist's canvas, but it does not always work as well on human skin. Sometimes a greenish tinge emerges, requiring further concealment or makeup repair. Yellow-toned mineral bases will cover redness effectively and require less concern for subsequent color changes.

To find the color that will cover redness on a client's skin, first ask the client to sit in natural light. Test for the complexion color on the jawline. If the chosen color is yellow, it is all you need to neutralize the red in the skin. If the correct base shade has a pink tone and the redness in the skin is not pronounced, try the base on a small section of the client's face to see if it covers sufficiently. You may not need the help of a yellow tone. If it does not cover sufficiently, your first layer should be a yellow base of the same value as the complexion shade. You will brush the complexion color over the yellow base at the end of the application.

Before applying any makeup, cleanse the client's face and moisturize. Allow the moisturizer to absorb. Pick up loose or pressed mineral powder and apply as you would for a normal makeover. Then use a flocked sponge to pick up additional powder and work it into the sponge to ensure even distribution. Now, with a roll press motion, apply the makeup to areas that need more coverage. When you have sufficient coverage, run the brush or sponge down the client's face to remove any excess. Spray with a facial spritz to set the minerals (Figure 20–16).

Hiding Circles Under the Eyes

This is the biggest beauty complaint from women, but men and women both worry about under-eye circles, believing that they add age to the face as well as a look of fatigue. Among other things, circles can be the result of:

- Genetics: usually grey pigment that is apparent below and often above the eye
- Allergies: usually blue/grey
- Lack of sleep: usually grey
- Smoking: usually purple/grey
- Hyperpigmentation: brown to grey
- Thinning of the skin so that the capillary network of the muscle can be seen: blue/purple
- Shadows caused by retention of water or a slipped fat pad

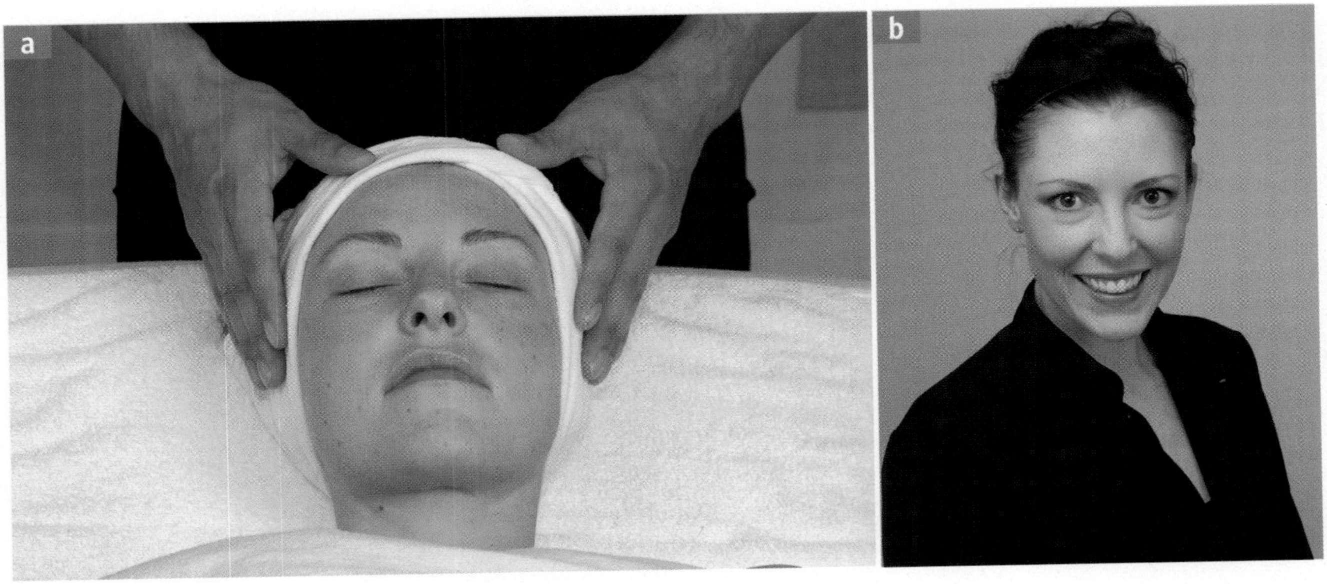

Figure 20–16 Covering redness on a client with rosacea.

> **? Did You Know**
>
> Bletharoplasty (eyelid surgery) is the number one plastic surgery procedure.

Circles come in many different colors, shapes, and sizes and, therefore, require different products, application techniques, and colors. Mineral concealers work with light prisms to camouflage these circles, and your concealer doubles as a highlighter. One of the most common mistakes estheticians make when choosing a concealer is to choose one that is too light. The darker the circle, the darker the concealer should be. A concealer that is too light will only leave an unattractive ashy effect, and if there is a puff involved, it will look more pronounced. To avoid this, test the color of the concealer *over* the foundation. If it disappears, it is the right color. This is especially easy to do when using a mineral foundation.

> ***FYI***
>
> Minerals conceal so effectively that you may not need to use a special concealer. Apply the base first and bring it up under the eye to see if that gives you enough coverage. If it does not, you can then apply a concealer.

The Corrective Color

Cream mineral under-eye concealers usually come in a variety of yellow and peach tones. Do not be afraid to try a yellow shade on one eye and a peach shade on the other to see which one works best. Sometimes you can be surprised at the results. Peach will almost always add an attractive brightness to the under-eye area.

Brown is a mixture of colors so has no complementary color. It is the hardest color to conceal. It is important here to experiment. Try a beige concealer first and then add orange/peach or yellow, depending on the color that seeps through.

Try a concealer with two colors so that you may mix the exact shade; the intensity of circles changes from day to day. Always apply with a camouflage brush. It will give you the most natural coverage and allow you to reach small areas such as under the lashes.

Pick up some of the concealer with a spatula and transfer it to a stainless steel palette or the back of your gloved hand. Mix the color with the camouflage brush. Begin application on the innermost color of the eye (the most recessed area of the face), and with light patting strokes spread the color under the lashes and over the discoloration. Be careful not to sweep the color too far out as this will fall into and accentuate wrinkles (Figure 20–17).

Do not only use horizontal strokes when applying concealer. The skin is not a piece of plastic. A criss-cross motion will ensure that the concealer covers all of the skin area, including indentations. Upward strokes also give a lift to the face. Use a combination of all three.

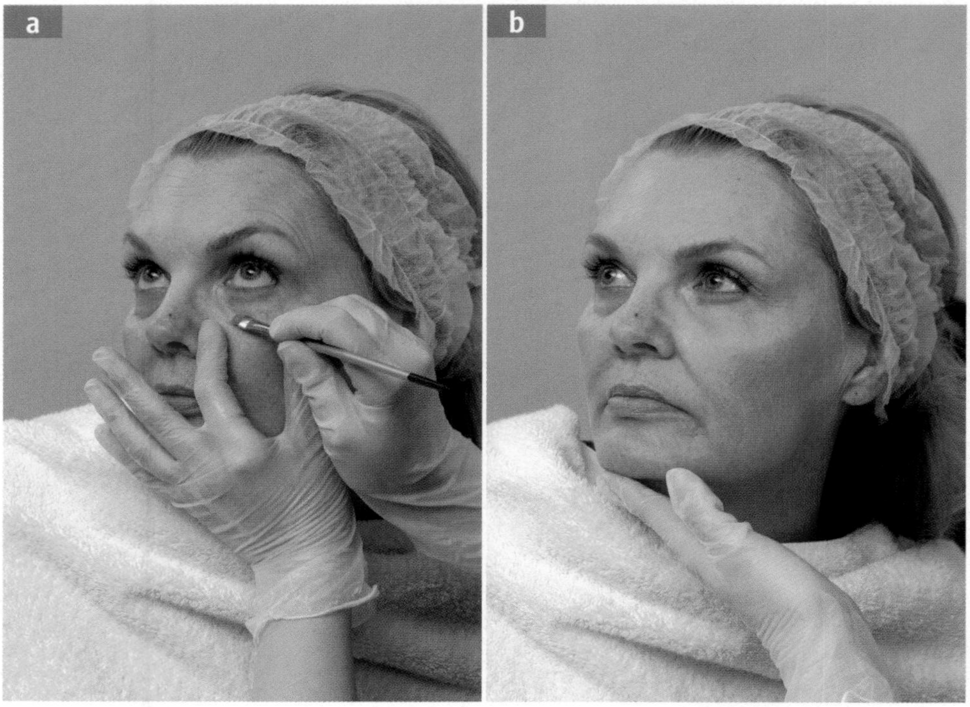

Figure 20–17 Concealing under-eye circles on a client.

Your ring finger is the weakest finger you have, so use it to blend the edges of the concealer. It will ensure that you do not use too much pressure, and the warmth from your finger will melt the concealer into the skin. You may now add a layer of minerals over the concealer, but do not do this if the under-eye area is lined. The less product used on the delicate skin around the eye, the better.

Be sure to neutralize the upper lid, which can often be red. A layer of mineral powder will serve as a good base for shadows. You may also use a concealer, but be sure that you only apply it in a thin layer or it will cause the shadows to crease. Use your ring finger for that, too. It is more difficult to regulate pressure on this sensitive area with a brush.

Liquid Mineral Under-eye Concealers

Liquid mineral under-eye concealers come in a tube with a brush on the end. Liquid concealers (Figure 20–18) have a lighter texture than their cream counterparts and so are especially useful on a mature eye, where they lessen crepey areas; add a highlight and do not fall into lines.

Twist the bottom of the tube to force the concealer through the brush. At home, your client may use the brush directly on the eye. As a professional, you want to use a spatula and a camouflage brush. The application

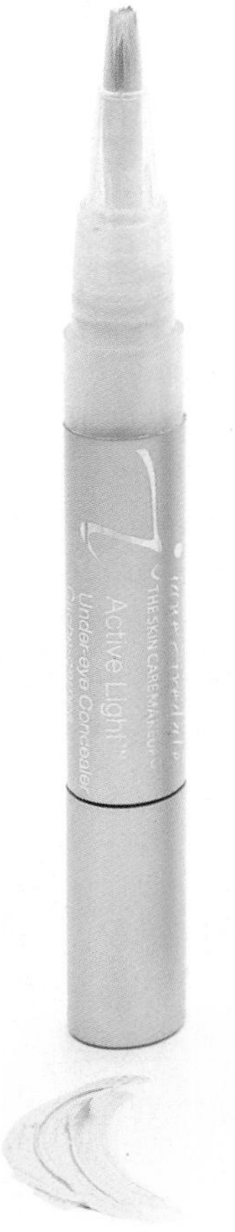

Figure 20–18 Liquid mineral under-eye concealer.

techniques for this type of concealer are the same as for the cream concealer. However, this concealer will also double as a highlighter. Run the concealer down the nasal labial folds, between the brows to lessen furrows, on top of the cheekbones, around the mouth—any area that you want to "pull out." Always blend the edges with your ring finger.

Concealing a Puff

You can minimize a puff under the eye by graduating the color from light at the edges to darker in the middle (Figure 20–19). This will have the effect of pulling out the corners of the eye and diminishing the center of the puff. To minimize the shadow created by the puff, use a clean eye shadow brush to apply a mineral powder that is a shade lighter than the foundation shade directly underneath the puff where the shadow occurs. The light-diffusing nature of the minerals will help to conceal the shadow.

Hyperpigmentation and Vitiligo

You will probably need to try a variety of techniques to cover these distractions. No one technique works for everyone. Try one or more or a combination of the suggestions below.

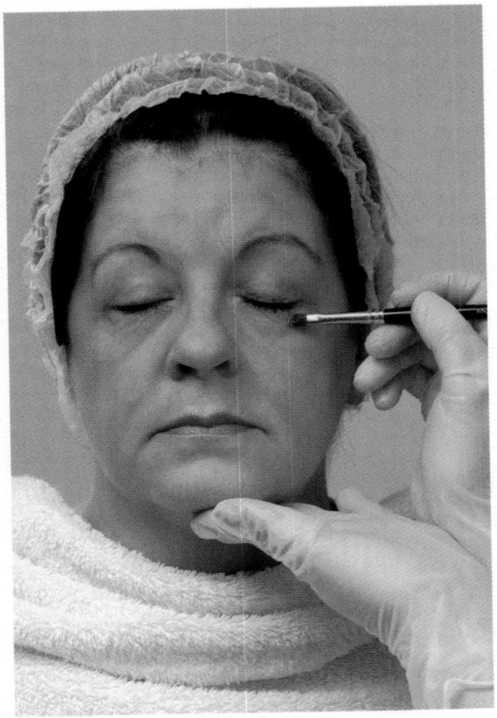

Figure 20–19 Eye with a puff showing where the concealer is applied.

White-Washing

Spritz your flocked sponge with a facial spray. (Three spritzes are usually sufficient.) Press the wet sponge into loose minerals, and use a palette to further press the minerals into the sponge. With long strokes, layer the minerals over the area to be covered. The minerals will look lighter in the beginning, but they will dry to their normal color. Smooth out with the sponge or a foundation brush. You may brush dry minerals on top.

This is a particularly effective technique for vitiligo, for which it is better to find a color between the dark and light areas and apply a wash in order to blend the two together. It is usually unsatisfactory to try to match the white areas to the darker pigmentation. Apart from how time-consuming it is, there will almost always be a dark border around the areas where there is no pigment. Most vitiligo patients would rather find a fast way to minimize the contrast between the two areas, thereby lessening the impact of the contrast. You can accomplish this with minerals because of their light-diffusing qualities.

Orange

Orange can effectively neutralize the brown from hyperpigmentation. It has to be used judiciously, but it will stop the ashy bleed-through common when covering dark pigment. First, match the skin tone to the correct mineral base shade. Then, with a spatula, pick up some of the cream concealer and transfer it to a stainless steel palette. With a camouflage brush, work some of the concealer into the brush. Pat the concealer onto the patches of darker pigmentation.

With a flocked sponge, pick up some of the mineral powder and roll-press it onto the areas you are camouflaging. With your powder brush, layer minerals over the entire face. Set with a facial spritz. If you need more coverage on the pigmented areas, you may add another layer of the orange concealer and roll-press the minerals again. This layering technique is more effective than trying to cover everything at once. You will have a more natural result.

Concealer

Match the skin tone to the correct mineral foundation shade. Then, use a heavily pigmented mineral concealer. Choose a shade that matches the flesh tone. Transfer some of the concealer to a stainless steel palette and with a camouflage brush, stipple over the hyperpigmented areas. While the concealer is still tacky, roll-press the foundation minerals over the area with a flocked sponge. If there is ashy bleed-through, pick up a matte orange blush with a clean eye shadow brush, and press it on the grey areas. With a powder brush, brush the mineral foundation all over the face. Spritz with a facial spray to set.

Scarring

Scars are areas of fibrous tissue that replace normal skin after destruction of some of the dermis. Scar tissue is not the same as the tissue it replaces. It is less resistant to UV rays, and it does not contain sweat glands and hair follicles.

Mineral powders that contain SPF protection are ideal for covering scarring. They provide the much-needed protection from UV rays and adhere better to the shiny scar tissue than traditional camouflage.

Because scars contain no sweat glands and hair follicles, it is more difficult to obtain adherence of product, but it can be done if you use a layering technique. Minerals will also conceal the redness common in new scarring. Mature scars are usually raised, so it is important to match the mineral base to the surrounding tissue or even use a shade darker. A shade darker is especially important if you are concealing a hypertrophic scar, which will look like a red lump on the skin.

Prepare the skin by moisturizing heavily. Blot off any excess. With a cream-based concealer and a camouflage brush, stipple the concealer onto the scarred area. Wipe the brush and use it to pick up mineral powder. Stipple that onto the scarred area. Use your flocked sponge to press it into the scar. If you need more coverage, repeat the process. Then apply the base as usual.

Bruising and Tattoos

Bruising and tattoos offer your biggest challenge in camouflage. You will need to try different techniques until you find the right combination of products that camouflage to your client's satisfaction.

For covering the blue/purple in bruises and tattoos, yellow will once more be your best friend. Cleanse the face and moisturize. Choose a two-toned cream concealer, and on a stainless steel palette mix a shade that has the density you require. With a camouflage brush or a sponge, press the mixture over the bruise or tattoo. Pick up loose or pressed mineral powders with a flocked sponge and roll-press it over the area you are concealing. Both bruises and tattoos tend to throw off a greenish cast through the camouflage. Try layering the concealer and mineral powders again. If discoloration is still visible, pick up a peach blush with a sponge and press it on top. This will usually neutralize the ashy/green color. Apply the mineral base, as usual.

> **FYI**
>
> Some bruises and tattoos respond well to techniques described in the section on hyperpigmentation.

The act of tattooing damages underlying tissue, so as you work on the tattoo, expect it to swell. This will be evident once you have the tattoo covered, because it may look slightly raised. After a time, the tattoo will flatten. You may need to layer a tattoo a number of times until it is concealed sufficiently (Figure 20–20). Do not be afraid to continue the layering process. Because of the light-refracting ability of minerals, it will not look heavy and caked. The different texture may be visible to the human eye, but it will not be visible with a camera.

> ***Here's a Tip***
>
> Be sure to feather the edges of the camouflage or it will look like a patch.

When a bruise is in its final healing stages, it will look yellow. This yellowness can exist for a number of days and will need to be neutralized. A lilac concealer is often helpful, and you can simplify the process by using a pink-based mineral powder. Cleanse the face and moisturize. Match a mineral base to the skin tone. Pick up a pink mineral base with a flocked sponge and roll-press it over the yellow discoloration. Brush the complexion shade over the entire face. Repeat if needed. Spritz to set.

Practice a mix of techniques to ensure your success in distracting the eye from skin imperfections.

AIRBRUSH MAKEUP

Airbrushing makeup is a precise and effective method to apply foundation. With the advent of high-definition television and digital photography, flaws in the skin are being exposed like never before. The solution is **airbrush makeup** with the correct product and technique. From natural beauty makeup, camouflaging tattoos, and hyperpigmentation to fantasy body designs, airbrushing is the most versatile technique in makeup artistry, complementing traditional makeup techniques.

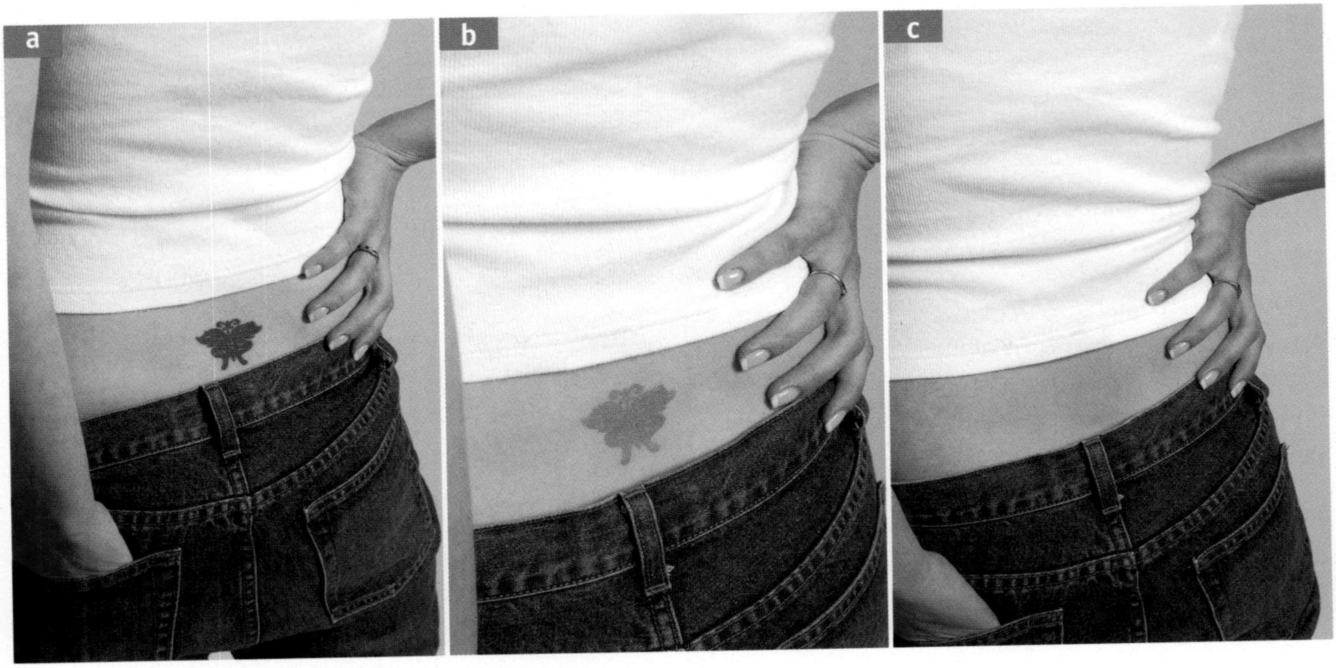

Figure 20–20 Before, during, and after tattoo camouflage.

When makeup is airbrushed onto the skin (Figure 20–21), it lands in microdroplets, mimicking the tonality of perfect skin. This atomization process sprays ultrasheer layers onto the skin. When the layers are applied consecutively, they produce sheer to maximum coverage. The result is a seamless beautiful blend.

Airbrush foundation was designed to enhance traditional makeup techniques. This type of application is faster and uses a minimum amount of makeup with maximum results. Airbrushing is preferred because of its high detail, high-precision accuracy. It can be used alone or in conjunction with traditional makeup techniques. The objective is to create a three-dimensional makeup look that appears like true skin, especially in front of high-definition and digital cameras.

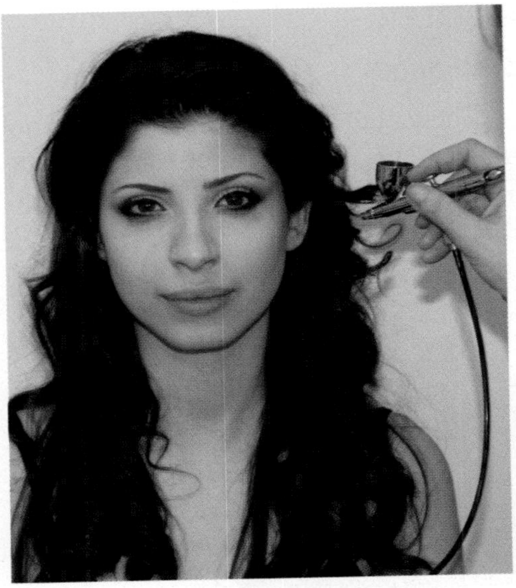

Figure 20–21 Makeup model being airbrushed.

The Foundation

There are two preferred airbrush makeup formulations: water-based and alcohol-based. Both are designed to appear like skin.

Water-based Formulation

The most beneficial water-based liquid airbrush foundations contain humectants, vitamins, oil absorbers, and color pigments. When airbrushed, it can be layered to provide coverage ranging from ultrasheer to maximum opacity. When applied with a foundation brush or sponge, it provides a moderate amount of coverage. Using setting powder provides a smudge-resistant surface.

Alcohol-Based Formulation

Alcohol-based airbrush makeup was created for maximum endurance. Alcohol is an essential ingredient, acting as a vehicle, which, when combined with air, evaporates rapidly, activating the ingredients and binding them together to create a waterproof and smudge-proof surface. Like the water-based formula, the alcohol-based makeup provides coverage ranging from ultrasheer to maximum opacity.

CAUTION!

Alcohol-based products dry quickly and are to be used only with an airbrush.

Airbrush Tools and Equipment

Airbrushes

Airbrushes come in a variety of models and sizes. A dual-action airbrush is recommended for all airbrush applications. A dual action airbrush works by pressing down on the lever to release air while simultaneously pulling back on the lever to release air and makeup. The different styles are listed below.

Smaller airbrushes usually work at a low pressure designed for makeup on the face. Larger ones are great for doing makeup on the body as well as airbrush tanning. While the techniques discussed in this chapter will teach you how to control an airbrush, the size of the airbrush also affects the desired result.

Airbrushing Beauty Makeup

This type of airbrushing requires an airbrush with a small- to medium-sized needle/nozzle configuration (.2 mm to .35 mm). This allows you to use a minimal amount of product and keep the makeup spray pattern focused and detail-oriented.

Airbrushing Body Makeup

This requires an airbrush with a medium- to large-sized needle/nozzle configuration (.3 mm to .5 mm). This allows you to airbrush a larger area within a faster time frame.

Airbrush Tanning

Airbrush tanning requires an airbrush with a large-sized needle/nozzle (.5 mm). This covers the body with broad strokes and allows for a smooth and even spray pattern of tanning solution.

TOP-FED AIRBRUSH A top-fed airbrush is also called a *gravity feed airbrush* (Figure 20–22). The makeup is placed in the cup that sits on top of the airbrush. This allows the makeup to gravitate to the tip of the airbrush. These airbrushes are generally low-pressure devices designed for beauty makeup application.

BOTTOM-FED AIRBRUSH A bottom-fed airbrush is an airbrush with the cup mounted underneath (Figure 20–23). It is larger than the top-fed airbrush and has the capacity to hold more makeup and cover large areas without having to reload the cup. Bottom-fed airbrushes are preferred for body makeup and tanning.

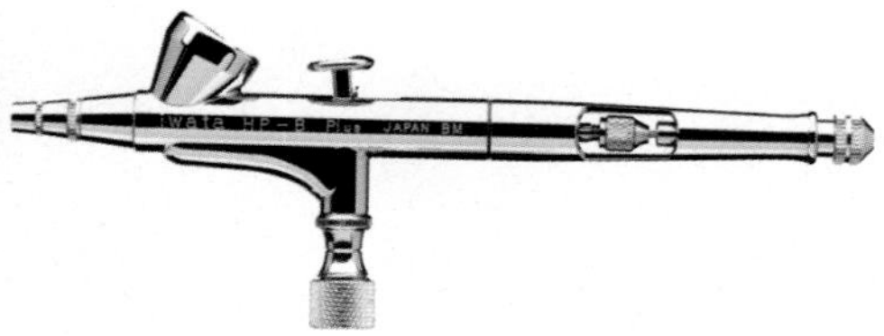

Figure 20–22 Top Fed Airbrush.

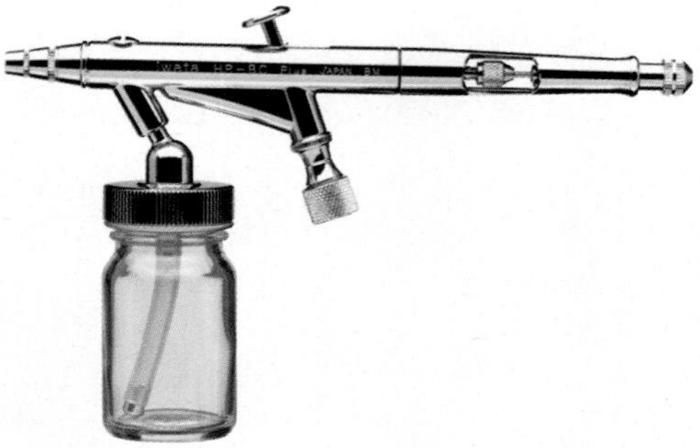

Figure 20–23 Bottom Fed Airbrush.

AIR SOURCES An airbrush is used in conjunction with an air source, such as a compressor, motor or electronic pump (Figure 20–24). Each of these takes in atmospheric air and releases it through a hose connected to the airbrush. The features of these air sources and their applications are evaluated according to two factors:

LPM: Their intake capacity, which is measured in liters per minute.

PSI: Maximum air pressure they create, which is called pounds per square inch.

Airbrush Techniques

The most important feature of airbrushing is total control of the airbrush. It is imperative that you manage this control. All spray patterns are based on distance. The closer the airbrush is to the subject ,the narrower the

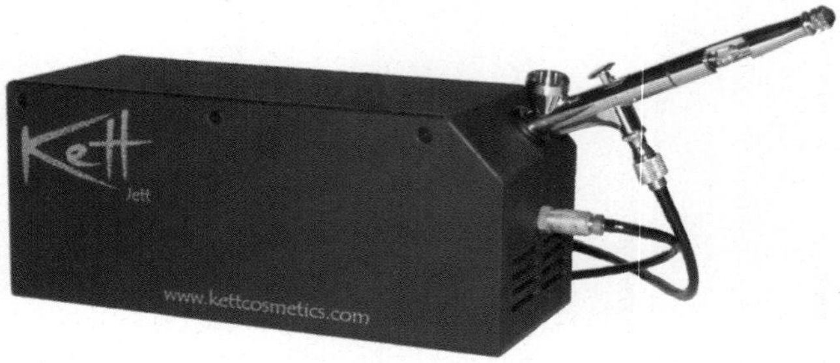

Figure 20–24 Kett Jett.

FYI

For the face, sufficient pressure is 6 psi to 8 psi. Higher pressures can be dangerous around the face and can cause eye injury.

For the body, sufficient pressure is 9 psi to 15 psi.

spray pattern The further the airbrush is from the subject, the wider the spray pattern. To control the width of the spray pattern, increase or decrease the distance between the airbrush and the surface.

The Point & Shoot/Dot Method

Pressing down on the lever will release only air and will cause an indentation on the skin at close range. This is a perfect indication of where the makeup will be applied. (Figure 20–25). Pressing down (for air) and then pulling back gently on the lever will release air and makeup on the skin. While maintaining downward pressure, gently move the lever back to the forward position to stop the flow of makeup. You must increase or decrease pressure gently without lifting your finger off the lever. If you do this incorrectly or abruptly, spatter is bound to happen.

The Dash Method

A dash is a long brushstroke that is used to create a contour on the cheek. It is also used at a distance to blend foundation on the entire face. Correct dashes should have ends that fade away (Figure 20–26).

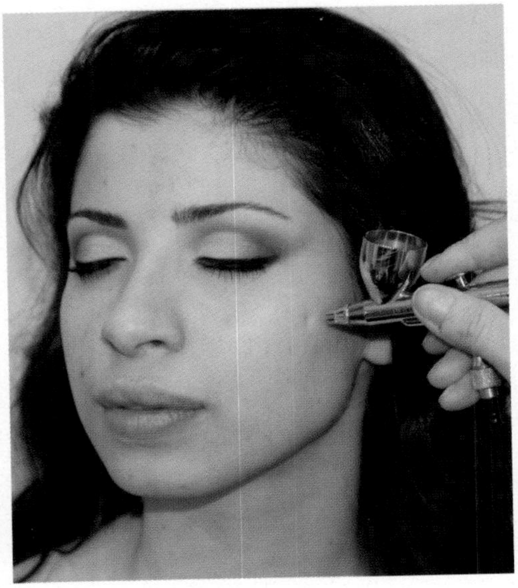

Figure 20–25 The dot method.

Figure 20–26 Narrow spray pattern.

Narrow Spray Pattern

Distance from the skin: ¼ inch to 3 inches. This method is used for fine detail work, such as concealing imperfections. (Figure 20–27)

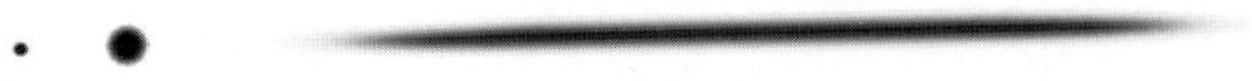

Figure 20–27 Small dots, narrow dash.

Wide Spray Pattern

Distance from the skin: 3 inches to 6 inches. This method is used for the application of foundation on the face and body when less detail and more coverage of a large area is required.

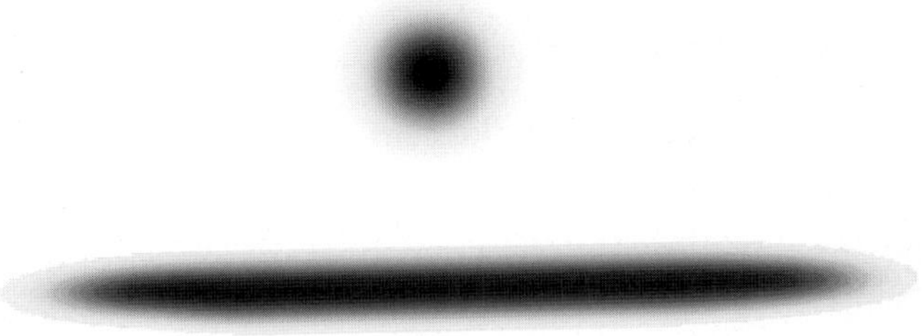

Figure 20–28 Large dot, wide dash.

FOCUS ON: *Airbrushing*

A single pass of the airbrush creates a veil of makeup. Use multiple passes to build opacity.

Cleaning Method

Clean the airbrush between each color with the appropriate cleaning fluid. Water cleans water-based makeup. Alcohol cleans alcohol-based makeup.

Back Bubble Cleaning Technique

Fill the cup half way with the appropriate cleaning fluid. With your finger, use a tissue to block the tip of the

Very important:

Water cleans water base; alcohol cleans alcohol base.

airbrush. This prevents the air from escaping. Pull the lever backward and you will create a **back bubble** effect that will loosen the makeup in the cup (Figure 20–29). Remove your finger from the tip and spray the tissue. Pour out the excess fluid onto the tissue and repeat this step until the fluid sprays clear. Finish by using your finger with a tissue to remove any excess residue that might remain in the cup.

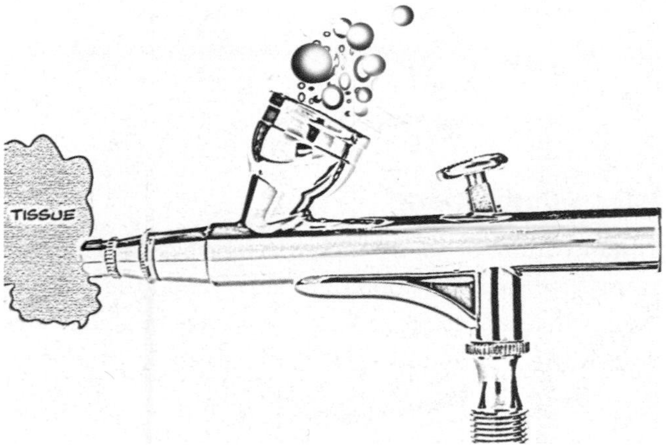

Figure 20–29 Back bubble.

Airbrush Beauty Breakdown

All skin colors, whether light or deep, are enhanced in the same way. Ideally, four tones are suited well to match, highlight, contour, and color the complexion. (Figure 20–30).

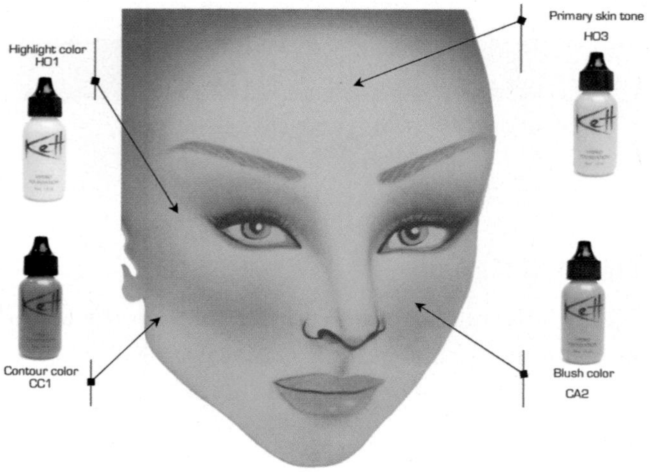

Figure 20–30 Airbrush beauty breakdown.

> **CAUTION!**
>
> Apply concealer manually. Airbrushing close to the under-eye area will cause a client to squint, creating an undesirable aging effect.

Select the primary skin tone color by using the standard technique of placing a swatch of makeup on the jaw line. Once you have determined the primary color, choose one shade lighter for the highlight. Using the primary skin tone color, utilize the point-and-shoot method to conceal imperfections and neutralize unwanted colorations (rosacea, blemishes, etc.). Once you have achieved this, apply foundation to the rest of the face as needed. Increase the amount of passes to build coverage.

Using the utmost control with product and air pressure, apply the highlight color to the upper cheek bones, blending it upward to meet the concealer applied earlier. For this type of makeup application, the contour should look like a shadow on the face. Choose a medium to dark neutral brown color. Using the dash method, start at the hairline, adding the contour color toward the apple of the cheek and tapering off near the middle of the eye and no lower than the top lip (Figure 20–31a and Figure 20–31b).

The final step is applying blush to the cheeks. After choosing the desired color, apply blush using the dash method at a distance. Each layer will build color and depth. Finish the application by setting the foundation with powder. Once you have completed these steps, convert to traditional products to finish the makeup (Figure 20–32a and Figure 20–32b)

Maximum Coverage Makeup

As a makeup artist, you will be faced with the challenge of covering undesired colorations on the face and body and sometimes even tattoos. The following procedure is an exercise in color theory neutralization and applying multiple layers of makeup.

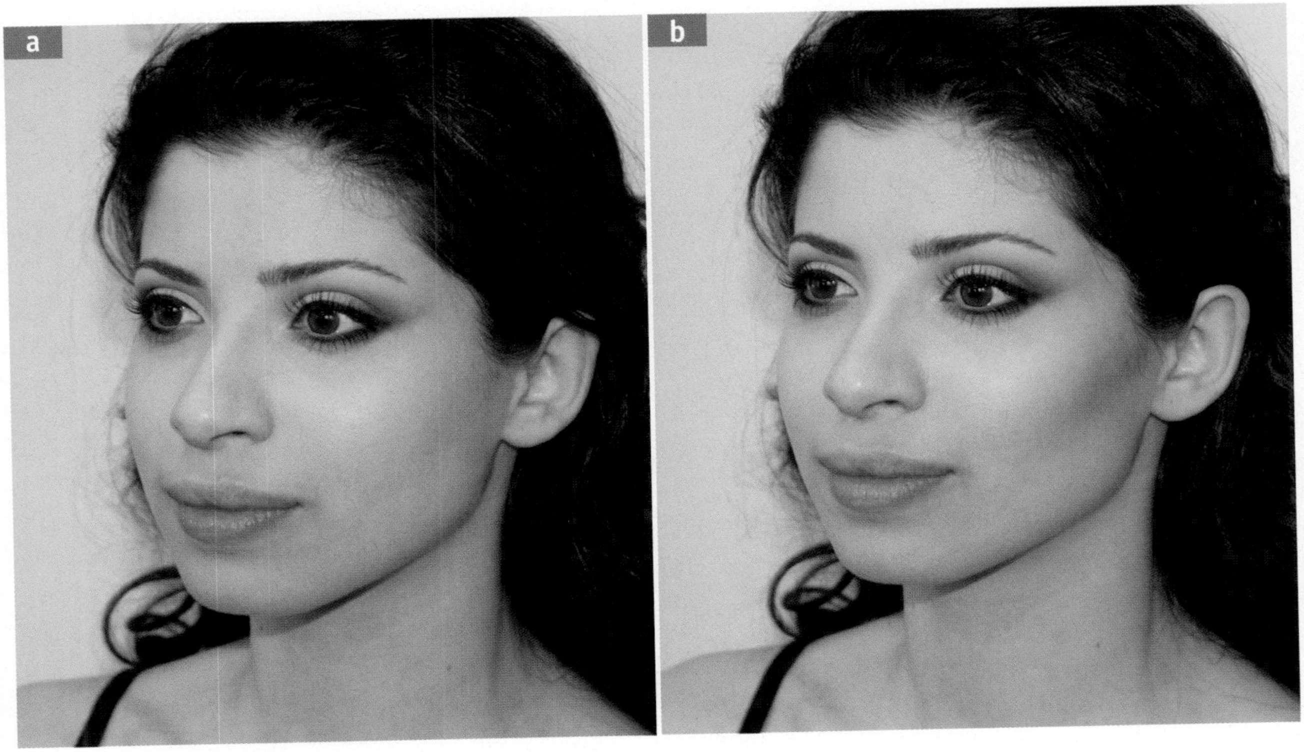

Figure 20–31 Coutour before and after.

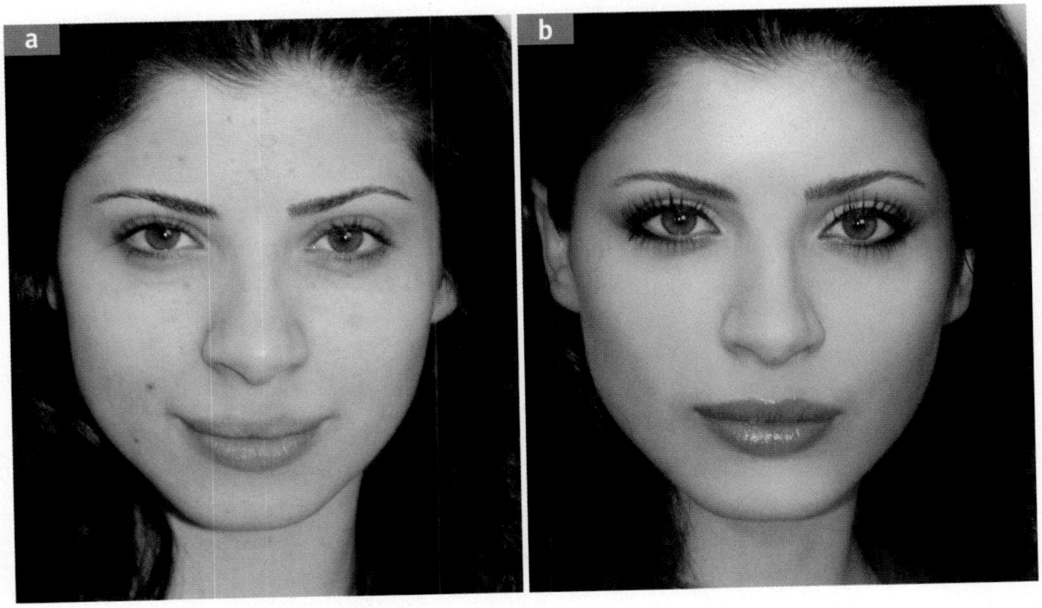

Figure 20–32 Beauty before and after.

PROCEDURE 20-5 MAXIMUM COVERAGE AIRBRUSHING

MATERIALS AND IMPLEMENTS

- Airbrush equipment
- Airbrush foundations
- Disposable sponges or makeup brush for applying powder
- Disposable Razor if needed for tattoo coverage
- Setting powder (colorless)
- Drape to protect client's garments
- Headband to protect client's hair, if working on the face
- Disposable cup containing water
- Frisket for freckle replication, if needed
- Water or alcohol for cleaning

Preparation

1 Prepare the work area for makeup application.

2 Test the airbrush with water to ensure it is operating properly.

3 Gather supplies.

4 Review the client's history with her and have her read and sign a consent form.

5 Review the client's expectations and the procedure.

Procedure

6 Seat the client and cover the clothing surrounding the area with tissue.

7 Disinfect your hands.

8 If covering a tattoo, shave the area of all invisible hairs. Use colorless powder instead of shaving crème.

9 Using a water based makeup, select a foundation color that matches the primary skin tone surrounding the discoloration. Keep this color aside. You will use it for the final layer.

10 Now select a foundation shade with the undertone intended for neutralization. Foundation skin tones are easier to work with and more adaptable than primary or secondary colors.

11a

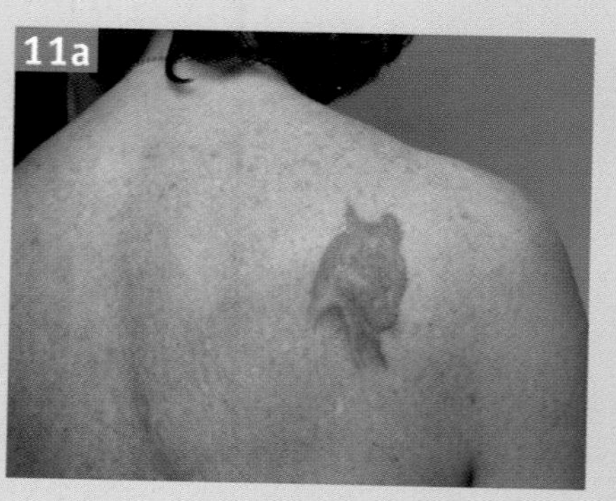

Before photo of tattoo to be covered.

11 Use the neutralizing color with a light touch targeting the natural shape of the hyperpigmentation or the design of the tattoo.

a. Apply a thin coat to the area, staying within the shape the tattoo or hyperpigmentation. Try not to go outside of the lines with the neutralizing color.

11b

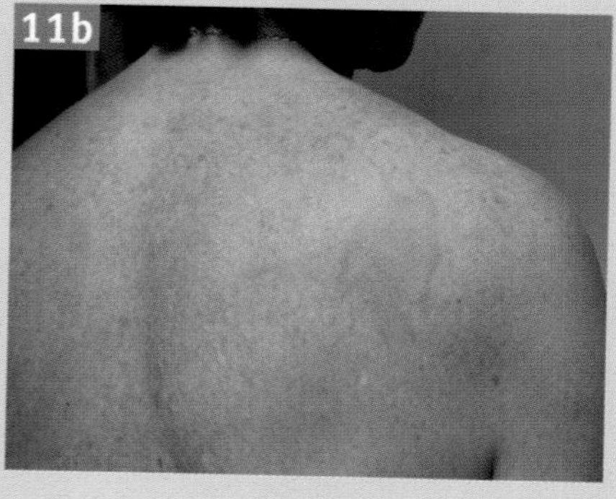

Apply a coat of setting powder.

b. Apply a generous layer of setting powder to the area using a soft fiber large powder brush.

c. Repeat these steps to achieve coverage.

d. When using alcohol-based makeup, it is not necessary to powder in between layers.

e. Step back and view your results as you work to check your progress. It will look different from a distance than it does up close.

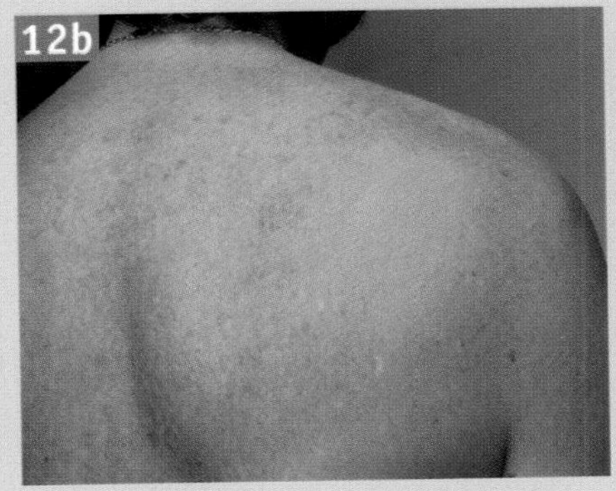

Introduce the primary skin tone shade.

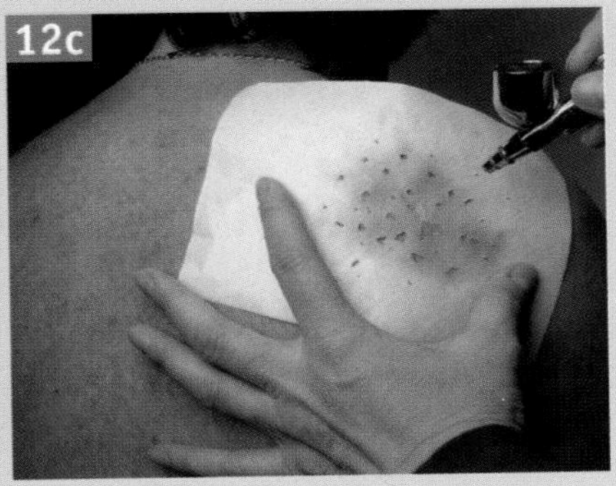

Create a stencil with frisket film to recreate freckles.

12 When you have achieved 90% coverage and neutralization:

a. Rinse the airbrush to remove excess makeup.

b. Now introduce the primary skin tone shade selected in step 1. Use this shade in broad sweeping dashes extending out onto the surrounding skin.

c. Create a stencil.

13 If the skin's surface has freckles, you will need to reintroduce them.

14 Create a stencil with frisket film. It can be pierced with a pin to create odd-shaped holes, recreating freckles (For more details on frisket film, see the section later in this chapter on fantasy makeup.)

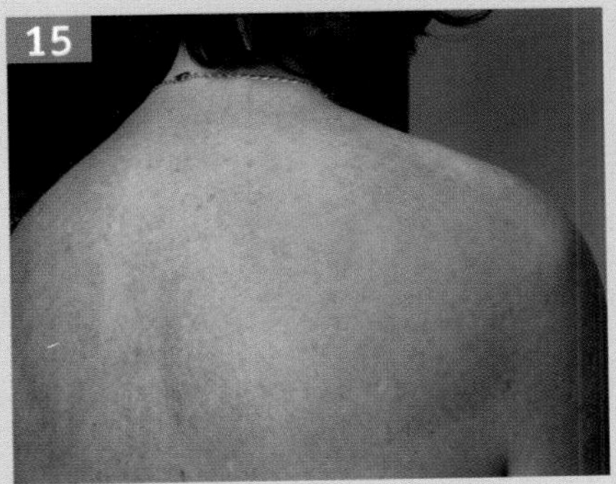

Apply freckle tone and re-powder.

15 Using the freckle stencil, apply the freckle tone. Rotate the stencil and reapply. Repeat this process until the freckles match the surrounding area.

16 Finish with no-color setting powder.

17 When complete, rinse airbrush cup to clean the foundation from it.

Post-procedure

18 If using a water-based product, advise the client to avoid rubbing the area.

19 If using an alcohol-based foundation, provide the client with instructions for removal of makeup, as this is waterproof.

20 If working on the face, proceed to complete makeup in the classical manner.

Clean-up and Disinfection

21 Clean up the work area following OSHA or state guidelines.

22 Clean the airbrush unit.

23 Dispose of any sponges and clean and disinfect any brushes used.

> **? Did You Know**
>
> Frisket film is the slightly tacky plastic film that is used by airbrush artists to create templates (stencils). It is readily available at art supply stores.

Fantasy Makeup

Amazing fantasy looks, body art, and temporary tattoos can be achieved by using **stencils** (Figure 20–33).

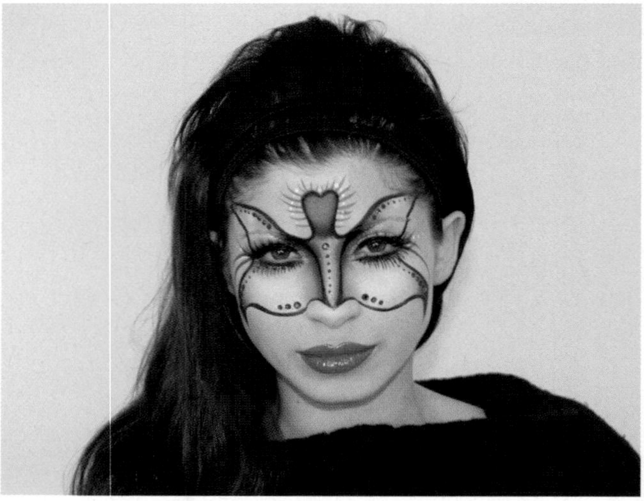

Figure 20–33 Complete fantasy look.

Inspiration can come from fabric designs, art, or even nature. You can choose ready-made stencils or, if you want to get realy creative, custom design your own. Custom-made stencils can be created by using frisket film, an X-acto knife, and a light box, all found at your local art supply store.

Here are the basic steps for creating a stencil. All it takes is a time and experimentation.

1. Ask someone to assist you.
2. Place the stencil on the desired location. Have your assistant hold the stencil in place (Figure 20–34). (Lifting or moving the stencil will create underspray that will ruin the design's edge.)
3. Introduce the airbrush makeup directly onto the design using the dash method while following the stencil-designed pattern. Pass over the design consecutively until the desired opacity is achieved creating the background color.
4. Powder with a no-color setting powder (Figure 20–35).

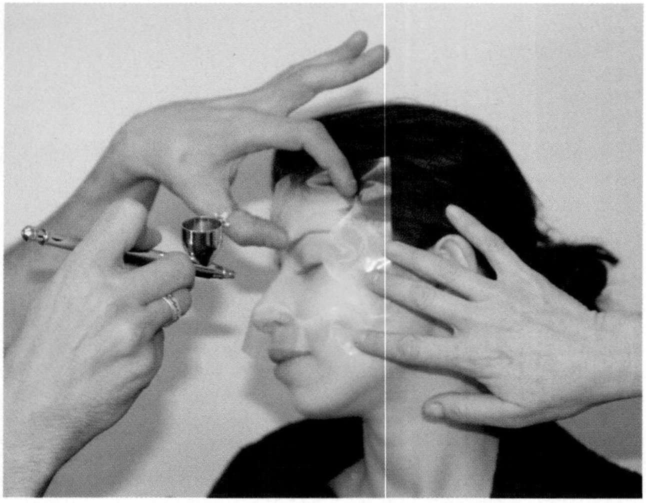

Figure 20–34 Place the stencil on the desired location.

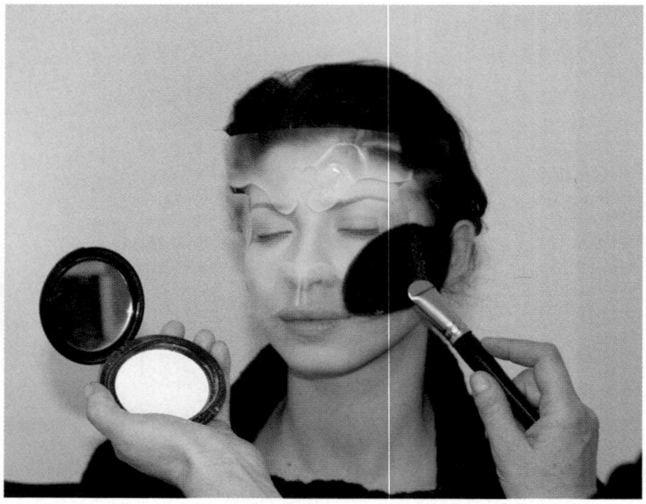

Figure 20–35 Powder with a no-color setting powder.

5. Now add secondary and tertiary colors until the design is complete (Figure 20–36).
6. Paint details by hand, if necessary (Figure 20–37).
7. Carefully lift the stencil from the skin's surface to reveal the design.
8. Powder with no-color setting powder.

PERMANENT COSMETICS

While called by different names, *permanent cosmetics* is the term used by the majority of professionals to describe the implantation of pigment into facial skin (Figure 20–38). It is a cosmetic tattoo that can replace missing eyebrow hair, enhance eyes, or give lips more color. The majority of clients are women, but men also seek these professional services. Visual impairments, unsteady hands, busy

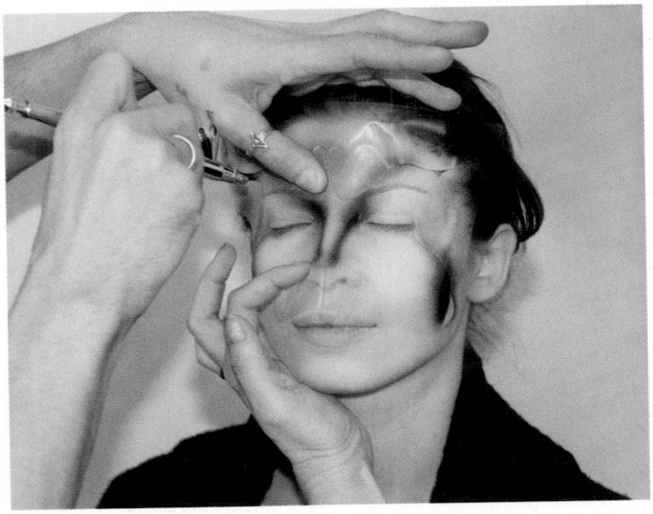

Figure 20–36 Add secondary and tertiary colors.

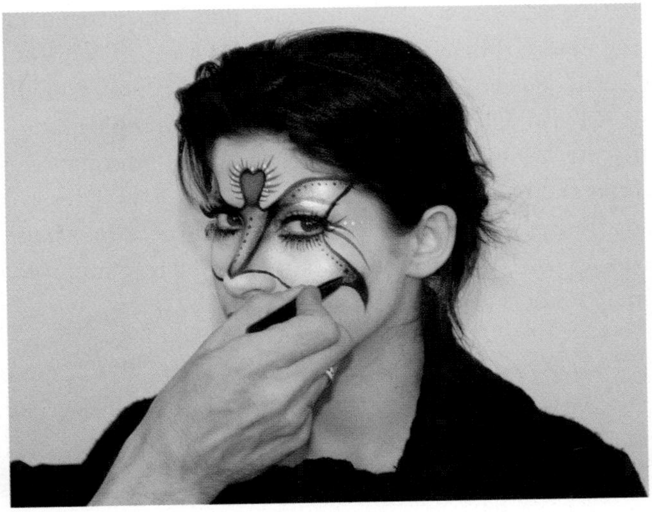

Figure 20–37 Paint details by hand.

lifestyles, stress, clean-room work environments, changes in hair growth due to hormonal changes or medications, and allergies are all reasons given by those requesting these services.

FYI

The Society of Permanent Cosmetic Professionals (SPCP) Vision 2006 study shows that 36% of all permanent cosmetic technicians are also estheticians.

Regulations and Training

The application of permanent cosmetics appears to be a rather simple process. Nothing could be farther from the truth. It requires in-depth training and lots of practice to get the pigment implanted into the correct layer of the skin and deal with what can be a tense or nervous client. In 2006 the governor of Oklahoma signed a bill legalizing tattooing and permanent cosmetics so it is now recognized and legal throughout the United States. In Oklahoma it is called *medical micropigmentation* and is controlled as a practice of medicine. Beyond U.S. borders, few countries

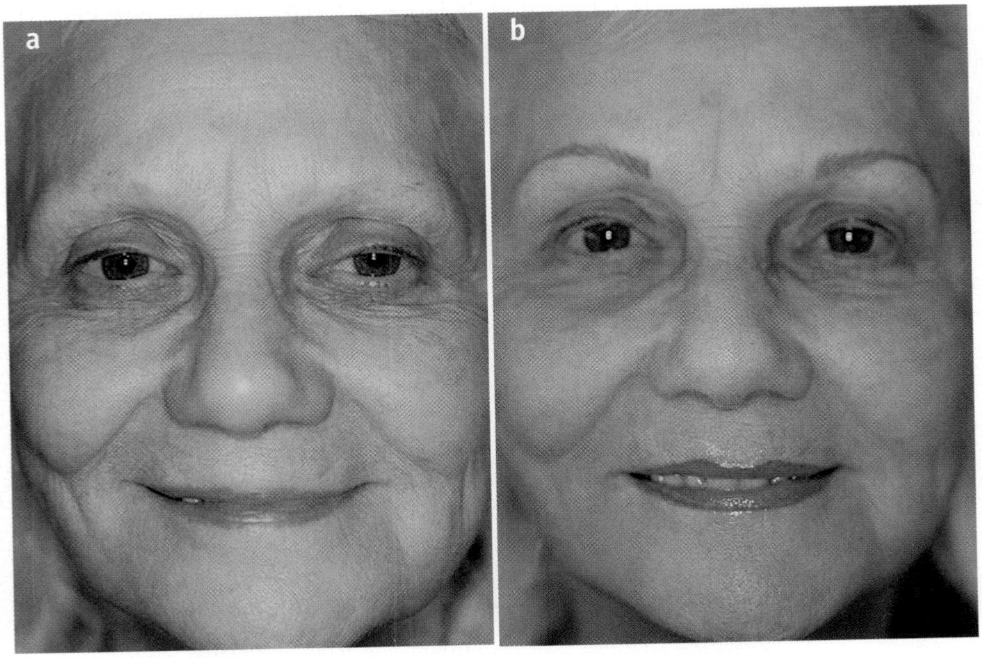

Figure 20–38 Permanent makeup before and after.

have guidelines for tattooing, but more are recognizing the need for this based on the demand for these services.

The Society of Permanent Cosmetic Professionals (SPCP) is the largest nonprofit organization in this industry. Its Web site, http://www.spcp.org, has informational links and complete regulatory guidelines for all states. For many states the only requirement may be a minimum age for the client, but others have detailed regulations for practitioners and training.

Laws differ from state to state. Check with your regulatory agency.

Unfortunately, many experts think that training in this field is still inadequate considering its permanent nature. State standards range from no training or regulatory requirements to intensive programs of 300 to 600 hours followed by licensure. International certification is available through the SPCP.

Training and Trainers

Those wanting to learn permanent cosmetics should recognize that this is a skill that can only be achieved with hands-on training and lots of practice. There is no way to safely and adequately learn this craft with home-study and a video. Seek a well-experienced trainer who participates in continuing education, has national certification, and who is willing to work with you as you undergo the extensive learning curve. It is important to be able to return to the trainer for continuing support after the initial training class. The training program, if short (under 100 hours), should focus on only one type of device. In 2008 the trainer members of the Society of Permanent Cosmetic Professionals agreed to increase their minimum training requirements to 100 hours.

Once a student becomes proficient on one type of equipment during basic training, he or she can explore others. A basic or fundamental program should include training in eyebrows, eyeliner, and an introduction to lipliner. Full lip color is considered an advanced procedure, as is areola repigmentation, cheek color, eye shadow, or scar camouflage.

Common Modalities

Common types of equipment include the manual method, rotary or digital rotary, and coil. The manual method is done with a hand tool, which has no motorized components. The coil is the classical tattoo device. Rotaries emerged in the late 1980s and quickly became popular as they were smaller, lighter, and less intimidating than the coil and had disposable components. At least one manufacturer sells a rotary that looks like a coil and performs like a coil, but has a closed housing that is lighter and quieter than the traditional coil. In recent years the digital rotary has emerged and has a devoted following based on its enhanced power, simplified component structure, and precision. Each type of device has its own group of advocates, but it is the skill of the technician, not the device, that determines quality work and the longevity of the tattoo (Figure 20–39).

? Did You Know

SPCP guidelines for fundamental training include:

- Introduction to Permanent Cosmetics
- Client Consultation and Management
- Office Setup
- Disinfection and Sterilization
- Client Preparation
- Color and Pigment Theory
- Skin Anatomy
- Machine Theory
- Needles
- Photography
- Aftercare
- Procedure Experience
- Business Setup

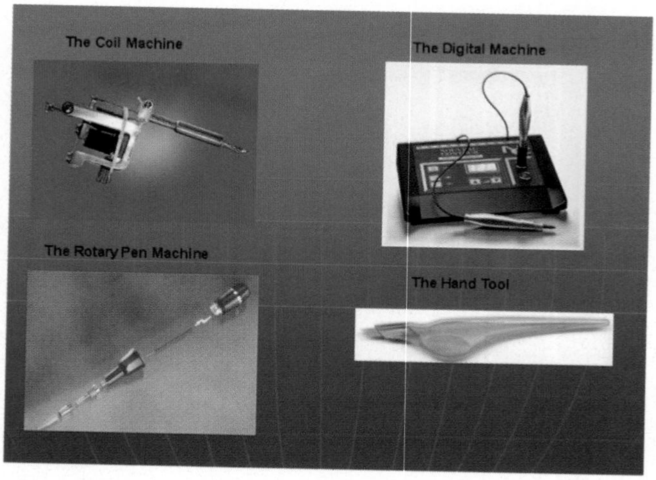

Figure 20–39 Tattoo equipment: coil, digital, rotary, and manual.

Eyebrows

Eyebrows are one of the most commonly requested procedures. Aging clients find that dexterity and vision challenges can make applying conventional cosmetics tedious and time-consuming. The skilled permanent cosmetic technician can fill in missing eyebrow hairs or create a brow where none exists. A powder-fill application looks like a powdered brow makeup product has been applied. The hair-stroke technique implants what looks like fine individual hairs. The natural brow should not be removed but rather the pigment placed behind/between what exists. The brow should be placed where the natural brow belongs anatomically. To protect the healed eyebrow, the client should use topical SPF products daily and minimize UV exposure. Fading will still occur and the brow color will need to be refreshed periodically. As the color that has been implanted in the skin fades, the undertone of the pigment used will emerge. Since yellow is the weakest of the colors, it is the first to disappear from the skin. If you have a client whose eyebrows have taken on an odd color, maybe appearing more orange or more ash than is desired, refer them back to their technician; it is past time for a color re-enhancement. This does not mean there was an error in the tattooing process or color selection. It means the permanent makeup color has been affected by casual exposure to UV light. Caught early, it is very easily corrected in a color re-enhancement process.

Eyeliner

Eyeliner is another commonly requested procedure (Figure 20–41). Tiny dots or a line are placed in and/or just beyond the lash line. For safety reasons the line should never be placed on the mucosal tissue or completely encircle the eye. Industry guidelines recommend the line should start and stop where natural eyelashes do. You can select from a variety of styles for the client, but keeping to a classical natural look withstands the test of time. Some technicians use fashion colors but most clients opt for classical browns to blacks. Recommend that the client wear dark glasses when in the sun to ensure optimum life for the tattoo.

Lip Coloration

While lip lining is an option, the client may find it necessary to wear lipstick to make the line blend in with the lip. Most technicians prefer to do a full, soft, natural lip finish, giving the client optimum cosmetic choices. Clients who suffer from herpes simplex need to obtain antiviral medication from a physician first; this medication will prevent an outbreak as a result of the tattooing process. If the client wants larger lips, refer her to a medical professional for lip-enhancing injections following the lip color application, as this will result in the best finished appearance (Figure 20–42).

Areola Work

Areola repigmentation is the implantation of color in a manner to restore the nipple of the breast to a natural appearance (Figure 20–43). This procedure helps the client during the healing process following breast cancer surgery or breast reduction and gives the client enhanced self-esteem. It incorporates numerous techniques depending on the type of surgical procedure that was involved. If you have clients who have survived breast cancer, refer them to the best, most experienced technician you can locate in your area. It takes a combination of professional skills and permanent color skills to achieve the best results.

Other Areas

Cheek color and eye shadow are much less popular than other permanent cosmetic applications. Clients who are most apt to seek cheek color are active, outdoors-type people. However, those who have this procedure must

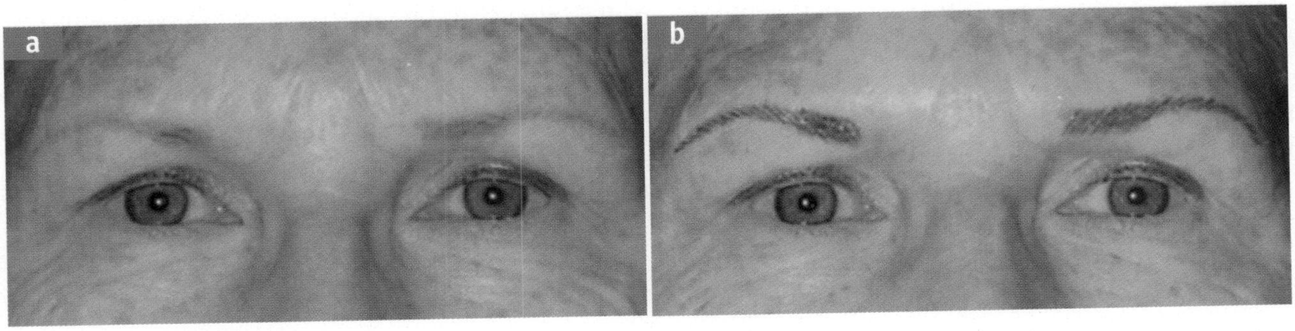

Figure 20–40 Eyebrows before and after.

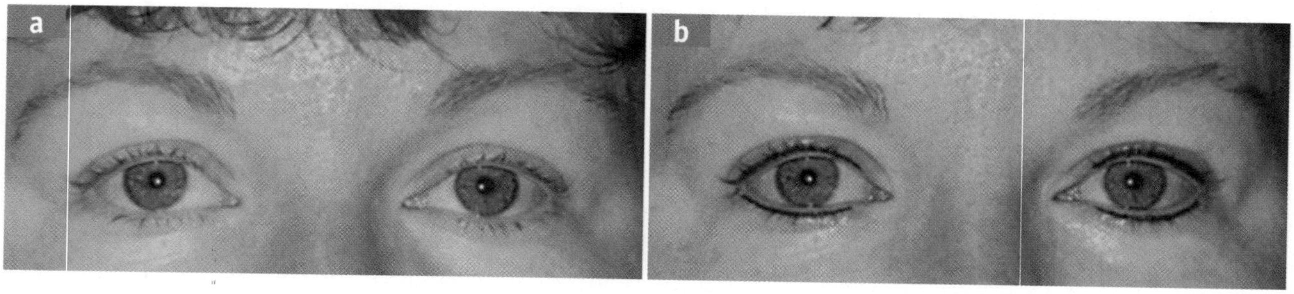

Figure 20–41 Eyeliner before and after.

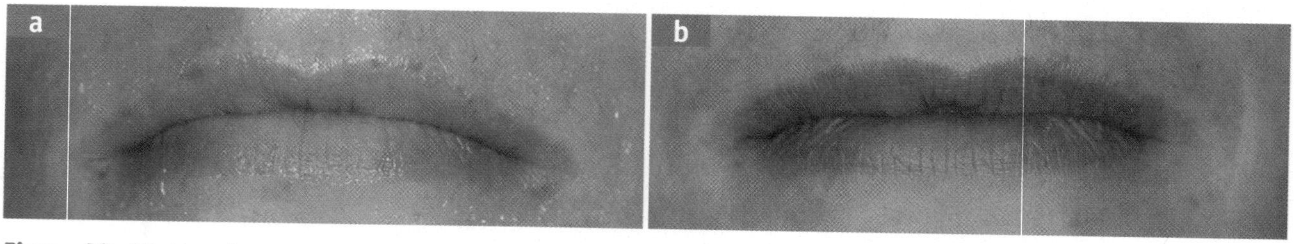

Figure 20–42 Lip color.

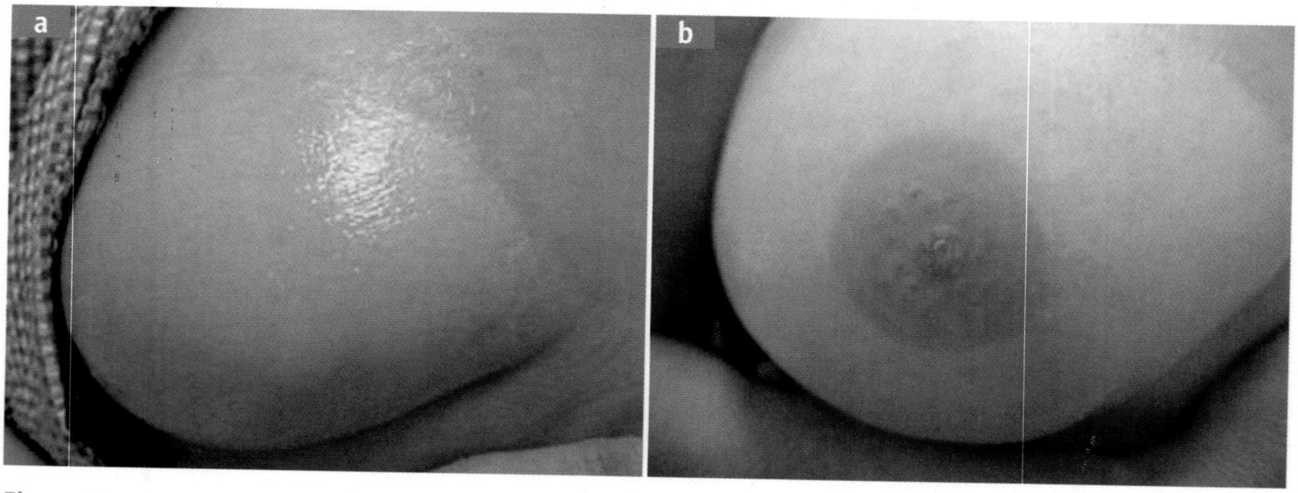

Figure 20–43 Areola reconstruction.

stay out of the sun, so this makes them very poor candidates. Clients who have cheek color must also avoid antiaging acids, light therapies, and most other age-fighting treatments. As these are popular therapies, this procedure is offered less frequently.

When properly done, eye shadow is very soft and natural. If done too heavily, it will age the eye rather than enhance it. Commonly the client will have a black eye (bruising) following this procedure.

Scar camouflage should only be performed by the most experienced permanent color technicians. These clients have already experienced emotional trauma, and poorly executed work can exacerbate it. Often these clients want back the skin they had before the trauma. This is not possible, but a deftly applied layer of color can break up small, light-colored scars. No form of cosmetic tattooing is effective on darker-than-skin-tone discolorations. It will only make the problem worse. In some cases the best option for a body scar is an artistic tattoo, as this will direct the eye away from the problem. Find technicians who live near you so that you can make an appropriate referral, if needed, to your client.

Client Care

A client interview is a two-way street. The client should be sure he or she is comfortable with the technician by reviewing the portfolio and asking questions about training, experience, and style, as well as safety and

REGULATORY AGENCY ALERT

Be sure to follow OSHA and CDC guidelines for setup and clean-up of permanent makeup procedures.

disinfection. Technicians need to determine if the client is suitable for the procedure. They need to feel they can achieve the client's goals and that expectations are realistic. If the client has medical conditions that might have an impact on the healing process, the esthetician must direct the client to consult a physician for a medical release before the procedure is performed. Clients should be educated as to the process of the tattooing procedure, the use of topical anesthetics, and care for their new permanent cosmetics. Photo and written documentation are integral parts of all procedures. The industry's standard of care dictates that every client is seen for at least one follow-up appointment approximately one month after the initial procedure. This allows for fine-tuning or adjustment work or for the technician to validate that the client is pleased with the result.

Regardless of the equipment or device used for the permanent makeup process, needles and pigments are considered single-use. Any products decanted for the procedure are disposed of following OSHA and CDC guidelines. Use of barrier film, plastic tubing, and covers as are commonly used in the dental hygiene setup are considered a standard requirement for the permanent cosmetic industry.

Estheticians wanting to augment their skills by adding permanent color to their repertoire need to do their research, locate a skilled trainer, and be committed to ongoing education in this field. It takes time and practice to become proficient. In some states permanent color cannot be performed within a salon setting and in Oklahoma it must be done under a doctor's supervision.

An alternative to training is to locate a well-qualified permanent makeup technician with whom you can refer clients back and forth. Look for someone whose work appeals to you as a makeup artist. Does it naturally enhance the client's features? Is it a style that will stand up to the test of time and aging? Does it look realistic? The goal is that no one will know what the client has done, only that he or she looks great.

Permanent makeup technicians will appreciate your eyebrow design and shaping skills, which will make their jobs easier, as many are not estheticians. Likewise, clients with profuse blonde or grey eyebrows may be better suited to brow tinting rather than permanent brow color. If the client's skin is in optimum shape, this will also enhance the permanent makeup process. Networking and teamwork can create the best possible results—happy clients.

REVIEW QUESTIONS

1. Name three safety precautions for lash extensions.
2. What is the best stage of lash growth to apply lash extensions?
3. What are the guidelines for lash extension selection?
4. How can the client remove lash extensions?
5. Discuss the safety precautions for lash perming.
6. What are key attributes for mineral makeup?
7. Name three ingredients common in mineral makeup.
8. Discuss techniques for applying mineral makeup.
9. Describe the process for camouflaging with mineral makeup.
10. What color undertone is used to most successfully camouflage redness?

REVIEW QUESTIONS

11. Discuss the key types of strokes used for airbrush makeup application.
12. How would beauty makeup be different from spray tanning in application?
13. What is the difference in clean-up after using a water-based airbrush makeup product and an alcohol-based product?
14. Describe the use of a frisket.
15. What air pressure is safe for airbrush makeup? Why not more?
16. What are the most popular areas of permanent makeup application?
17. What are key factors to look for in a training program?
18. What are the most common types of equipment used for permanent cosmetics?
19. What would you look for in a technician when referring your clients for permanent cosmetic services?

CHAPTER GLOSSARY

airbrush makeup: the process of applying makeup to the skin using an airbrush device.

airbrushes: small, air operated tools that spray liquid such as makeup.

back bubble: the bubbling of liquid and air into the holding bowl of the airbrush during the mixing and cleaning processes.

stenciling: use of a template or stencil to prevent color from being applied beyond a certain area.

PART

5

SPA AND ALTERNATIVE THERAPIES

Chapter 21 Spa Treatments
Chapter 22 Alternative Therapies
Chapter 23 Ayurveda Theory and Treatments

CHAPTER OUTLINE

- UNDERSTANDING SPAS AND THEIR SERVICES
- PREPARING THE CLIENT
- THE POPULARITY OF BODY WRAPS AND MASKS
- TYPES OF BODY WRAPS
- HYDROTHERAPY AND OTHER SPECIALTY TREATMENTS

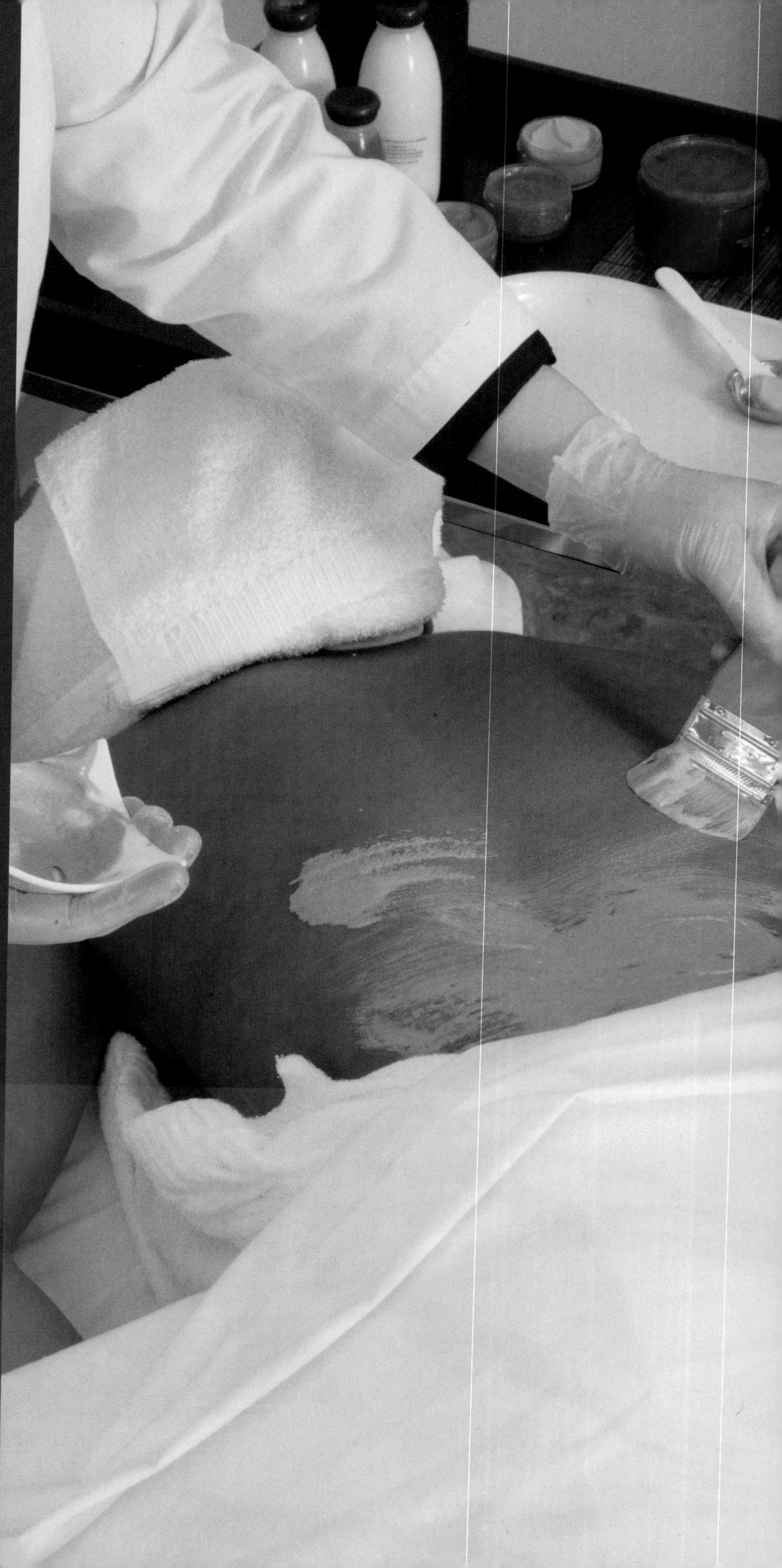

CHAPTER 21

SPA TREATMENTS

LEARNING OBJECTIVES

When you complete this chapter, you should be able to:

- Discuss the differences in spa types and services.
- Select the table that best suits your needs.
- Handle client preparation, treatment suitability, and confidentiality and privacy issues.
- Discuss types of wraps and mask options.
- Discuss the supplies and equipment needed for spa treatments.

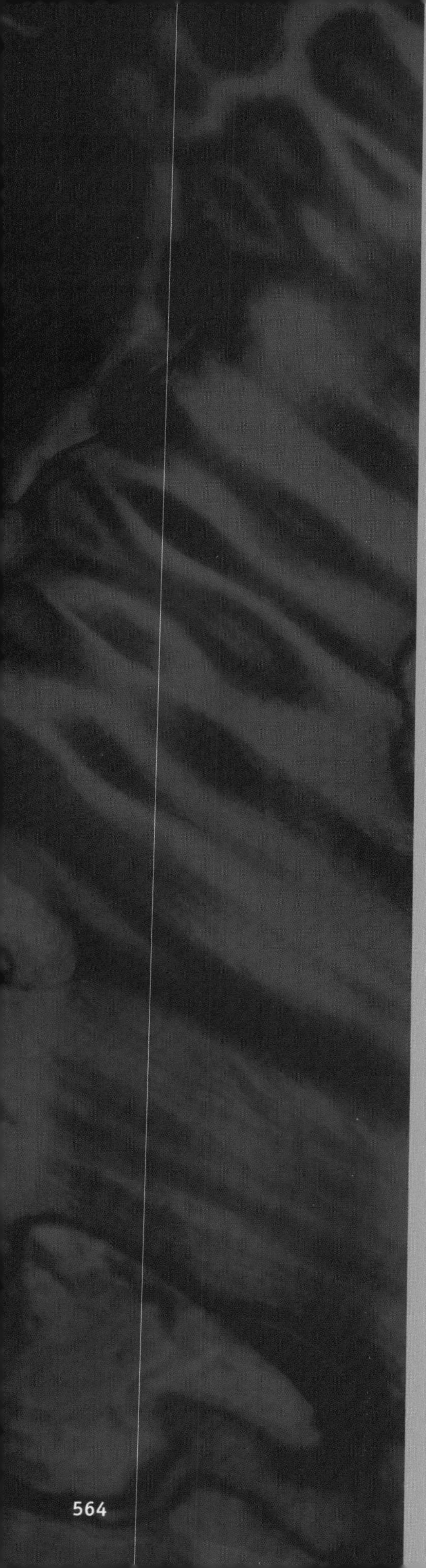

KEY TERMS

Page numbers indicate where in the chapter the term is used.

blanket wraps 590
body mask 576
cellophane body wrap 590
diaphoretic 584
elastic wraps 578
herb wraps 584
hydrocollators 584
hydrotherapy 589
Kneipp body wraps 591
moist heat unit 584
Scotch hose 596
seaweed wraps 579
thalassotherapy 589
Vichy shower 567
wet room 567

The spa industry is now big business. Busy, stressed consumers are looking for relaxation and rejuvenation (Figure 21–1) and are willing to travel to find the right spa. In many cases they want to achieve this in a limited amount of time. The most popular spa treatment is massage. With typical treatment times of 50 to 80 minutes, a client can achieve a relaxation/rejuvenation goal in far less time than it takes to play a typical round of golf. This may be one reason that some of the most recent industry figures show golf revenues down and those of spas up.

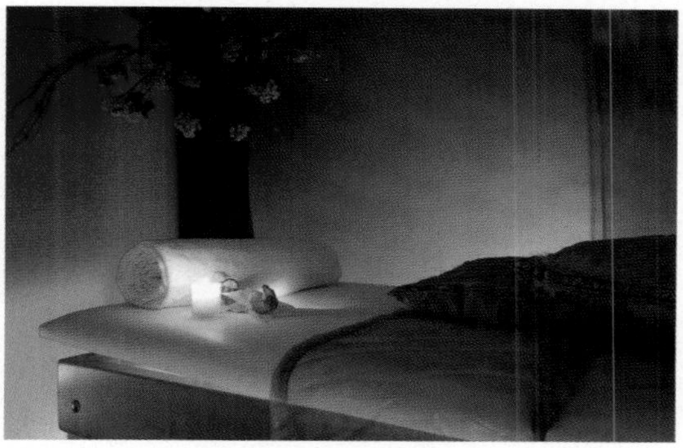

Figure 21–1 Massage room at luxury spa.

UNDERSTANDING SPAS AND THEIR SERVICES

Today's esthetician must be well informed on the different types of spas and treatments offered and be able to counsel clients who may be considering a visit to a spa when they travel. Clients who are considering spa services will appreciate guidance and referrals. Estheticians who become skilled in a number of services can find their employment options expand greatly.

Spa Types

There are seven types of spas. Spa clients select a spa type based on personal goals of health and wellness or relaxation and pampering.

> **Activity**
>
> Do an Internet search for spa guides, which help clients find a particular type of spa.

Day Spas

A day spa is a facility with or without a beauty salon and/or fitness component. It can be owner-managed or part of a chain. Day spas are operated and located in hotels, resorts, retreats, malls, cruise ships, or freestanding buildings. Spa experiences are created with specific treatments in certain time frames, such as a half day or full day (hence the term *day spa*).

Destination Spas

Destination spas usually thrive in warm climates with beaches, oceans, mountains, or deserts. They offer more extensive spa experiences with longer time frames, such as 5 to 14 days. Clients of these spas usually desire a more holistic approach to their well-being with a more physical, philosophic, and spiritual component. Accommodations usually include meals (specific to the spa concept), body treatments, fitness facilities, exercise classes, medical evaluations, and outdoor activities. Pools, thermal waters, and sea water are often available.

Resort Spas

The resort spa is an amenity available to guests who are staying at a resort, usually in a warm climate or at a ski resort. The facilities can be separate from the resort or incorporated into the resort facility. Clients can purchase different packages; some are included with accommodations and meals and others are à la carte.

Medical Spas

Classified as the next generation of the spa industry, medical spas fall into a specific classification that may be sited in a day spa, destination spa, or resort spa setting. The International Spa Association defines the primary purpose of a medical spa as providing comprehensive medical and wellness care in an environment that integrates spa services with conventional and complementary therapies and treatments. Usually these spas include on-staff medical doctors, plastic surgeons, dermatologists, and/or naturopaths who will perform health examinations or different forms of cosmetic and laser surgery, peels, and cosmetic injections. Plastic surgeons and dermatologists have been joining day spas and expanding their practices, offering higher-level spa services and care. Pharmaceutical companies are designing products solely for medical spas. Hospitals and health insurance companies are even recognizing these spas as alternative medical care and offering coverage.

Fitness/Health Clubs

Fitness/health clubs are integrating spas into their facilities to expand well-being treatments for existing clientele. This is a great meld, if there is enough space to separate the two modalities. Excellent soundproofing is required; The upbeat atmosphere required for a gym differs dramatically from the soothing ambiance needed for relaxation in the spa. Resorts often handle this problem by placing each in its own building or in separate areas of the same building so that not even locker rooms are shared.

Hospital and Rehabilitation Centers

Hospitals and rehabilitation centers have begun offering physical therapy, water therapy, and specialized exercise programs. As the medical profession recognizes the health benefits of spa treatments, more treatments and services are being made available to patients.

Wellness Centers

Wellness centers—which have naturopaths and chiropractors on staff—offer yoga, Pilates, personal development seminars, and weight-loss clinics and sell homeopathic, vitamin, mineral, and nutritional supplements. These centers are now jumping on the bandwagon and offering spa services and treatments. They also tend to offer a wide selection of retail items, such as spa products, books, videos, and other health and wellness aids.

Body Treatments

A body treatment is simply a facial for the body. Though the concerns that body wraps and facials address may differ (i.e., cellulite versus rejuvenation), there are many similarities between the two. Both include cleansing, exfoliation, targeted skin treatments, and metabolic stimulation. In addition, body treatments offer many additional benefits, such as hydration, detoxification, and relaxation. Certain treatments may also reduce the appearance of cellulite or sun damage.

While the long-term efficacy of body wraps for such conditions as cellulite reduction is a subject for debate, it is well known that body wraps are a superb means of promoting healthy skin all over the body. They are also an excellent means of pampering and achieving a state of relaxation (Figure 21–2). Following is a list of factors involved in performing body wraps.

Confidentiality and Privacy

One of the core tenets of your facility and practice is client confidentiality. Your clients should be able to trust that you will handle all of their personal information according to HIPAA guidelines. This means that you will safeguard all personal information, keeping it in a safe place and withholding it from individuals who are not involved with the treatment plan. In addition, you will not discuss any client's personal information in the presence of nonessential staff or other clients.

In the course of providing spa services to a client, you may find a need to exchange information about that client with other estheticians or spa personnel. These discussions are often necessary for client care and are an

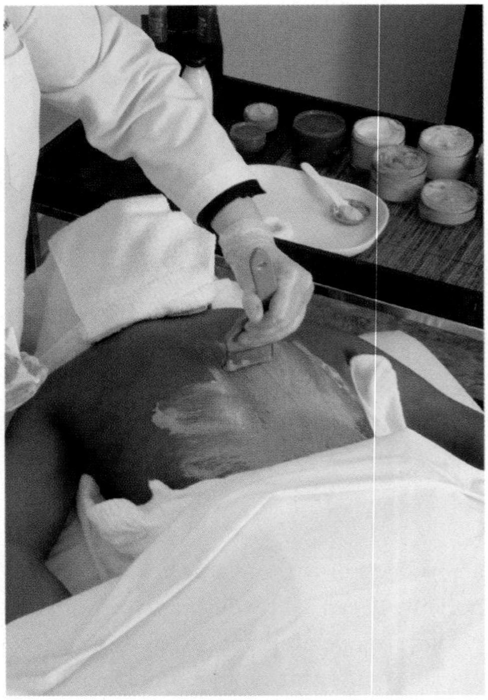

Figure 21–2 A client enjoying a body treatment.

integral part of ensuring the optimal outcome of the treatment. This disclosure is justifiable as long as you take precautions to limit others from hearing or seeing confidential charts and information. Never discuss a client's information in a public place.

There are two exceptions to rules about disclosure. First, you may speak to proper authorities if you must do so to protect individuals from any serious threat of harm, as in the case of abuse or domestic violence. Second, if you know a client has an infectious disease, you are required to tell public health authorities.

By respecting clients' privacy and creating a trusting environment, you promote an open and comfortable place in which your clients will feel safe and respected. It is important that they feel comfortable disclosing the most personal information with you because it may be something that can affect the outcome of a treatment. Even the smallest plastic surgery, application of a filler, or injectable can be contraindicative to a treatment's results.

Health Screening, Indications, and Contraindications

As with any esthetic service, you must assess a client's suitability for treatment. When applying products to large areas or on the entire body, the risk of a client having an allergic reaction or complication increases substantially. For this reason, you must be thorough in obtaining information during your client intake interview and asking questions on assessment forms. Be certain that the client has completed all of the necessary paperwork, including a thorough health history as well as a skin history (Figure 21–3). In addition, make sure that the client has signed and dated all documents. Go over the client's answers with him or her and complete any portion left undone. Determine if the treatment is appropriate and look for responses that might indicate that the client is not a candidate for the treatment. Follow up any concerns (for instance, consult with the supervising physician, if one is on staff). The importance of this step cannot be overstated; you must review a client's health history information every time he or she returns to your facility and document any changes.

As with any treatment, product manufacturers provide a list of conditions that are specific contraindications for particular procedures. Following is a list of conditions that generally indicate a client should not have a treatment:

- Pregnancy
- Open wounds
- Varicose veins
- High or low blood pressure
- Medications for high or low blood pressure
- Heat sensitivity
- Heart problems
- Diabetes
- Lupus
- Raynaud's disease
- Chemotherapy
- Bust surgery or mastectomy within the last two months or as indicated by physician
- Plastic surgery within the last two months, or as indicated by physician
- Pre- and post-surgery, as indicated by physician
- Numbness, or loss of sensitivity
- Allergies to products being used
- Claustrophobia

Beds and Table Options

One of the most important pieces of professional equipment you will use as an esthetician is the treatment table, which is especially vital to performing body wraps. Treatment tables ought to be durable, functional, and comfortable for both your client and you (Figure 21–4).

For body treatments, you may want to consider a table that has a cut-out for the client's face when he or she is lying in the prone position. In chairs without cut-outs, clients must lie with their heads turned to the side for extended periods of time, a position that clients would hardly find relaxing. Another option is a massage table. In addition to being comfortable for the client, the massage table allows you to adjust the table height, which will make you more comfortable as you work. Some manufacturers offer a hydraulic table that you can adjust easily.

Some spas or clinics have a **wet room,** generally a tile lined room with drains, where shower or hose treatments are performed. Wet rooms require tables that are modified versions of massage tables, with waterproof legs and a durable, waterproof material covering the cushion. Other options include wet tables, which have a composite or plastic base and are covered with a waterproof removable pad. These tables are often found where overhead **Vichy showers** or hoses are used. Vichy showers have from five to seven heads and cascade a large amount of water over clients to rinse their skin.

a

Confidential Health History—Body Treatments

PLEASE PRINT

Today's Date____________________

First Name ____________________ Last Name ____________________ Date of Birth ____/____/____

Street ____________________ Area # ________ City ____________ State ________ Zip ________

Phone: Home ( ) ____________________Work ( ) ____________________ Mobile ( ) ____________________

Physician/chiropractor ____ Phone ( ) ____________________

Emergency Contact ____ Phone ( ) ____________________

Your occupation ____E-mail : ____________________

Referred by ❑ Friend ❑ Mailer ❑ Walk-by ❑ Yellow Pages ❑ Gift Certificate ❑ Other________________

Technician's Name ____

---

1. Is this your first body treatment ❑ Yes ❑ No
2. What is the reason for your visit today?
   ____
3. What other body treatments have you had?
   ❑ Massage ❑ Salt glow ❑ Seawead wrap
   ❑ Moor mud ❑ Body scrub ❑ Other ________
4. If yes, was it a good experience?
   ____
   ____
5. Are you presently under a physician's care for any current health problem? ❑ Yes ❑ No
6. What? ____________________________________
7. Are you pregnant? ❑ Yes ❑ No
   If yes, how many weeks?
   ____
8. Are you taking birth control? ❑ Yes ❑ No
9. Hormone replacement ❑ Yes ❑ No If so, what?
   ____
10. Do you wear contact lenses? ❑ Yes ❑ No
11. Do you smoke? ❑ Yes ❑ No
12. What is your stress level? ❑ High ❑ Medium ❑ Low
13. Are you now using or have you ever used Accutane?
    ❑ Yes ❑ No
    If so, when and for how long? ____________________
14. Do you have any allergies to cosmetics, foods, seaweed, shellfish or drugs? ❑ Yes ❑ No
    Please list ____________________________________
15. Are you presently taking medications – prescribed or over-the-counter, including aspirin?
    ❑ Yes ❑ No
    If so, please list ____________________________________
    ____
16. What products do you use presently? ❑ Soap
    ❑ Cleansing milk ❑ Toner ❑ Scrubs ❑ Mask
    ❑ Creams ❑ Sunscreen ❑ Shower gels
    ❑ Body lotions

Please Indicate if you are affected by or have any of the following:

Asthma	Heparitis	Metal bone pins or plates
Broken bones Where?	Herpes	Pacemaker
Cardiac problems	High blood pressure	Phlebitis, blood Clots, poor circulation
Eczema	Hysterectomy	Psychological
Epilepsy	Immune disorders	Sinus problems
Fever blisters	Lower back or back problems	Skin diseases What?
Headaches, chronic	Lupus	Urinary or kidney problems

Head and/or neck injury? Where & how long ago?

Figure 21–3 A confidential health history questionnaire.

b

Please explain above problems or list any other significant health concerns or issues:

____

____

____

____

Please list areas of the body that are of concern.

____

____

____

____

____

____

____

If having massage, what type of pressure do you prefer:

❑ Light? ❑ Medium ? ❑ Deep tissue?

I understand that the services offered are not a substitute for medical care, and any information provided by the therapist is for educational purposes only and nor diagnostically prescriptive in nature. I understand that the information herein is to aid the therapist in giving better service and is completely confidential.

SALON POLICIES

1. Professional consultation is required before initial dispensing of products.
2. Our active discount rate is only effective for clients visiting every 4 weeks.
3. We do not give cash refunds.
4. We require a 24-hour cancellation notice.

I Fully understand and agree to the above spa policies.

Signed ______________________________ Date ______________

Figure 21–3 *continued*

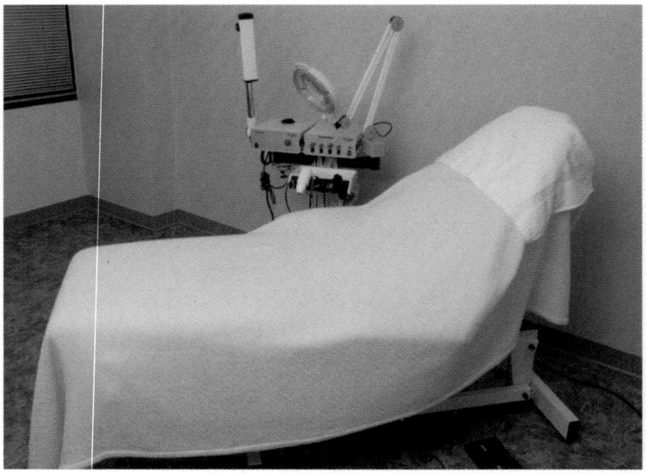

Figure 21–4 Treatment bed that can be used for spa treatments.

Preparing the Room for a Body Wrap

A body treatment requires a little more preparation than a standard facial does. First, be sure the room is extremely clean and is the proper temperature. This will help put the client at ease. Next, you must prepare the table with materials you will need for the treatment. Keep in mind that the outermost layer of materials represents the first treatment you will perform. Following is a checklist for preparing the room (Figure 21–5):

- Cover the table with a sheet.
- Cover the table with a wool or insulating blanket.
- Cover the table with a thermal blanket.
- Cover the table with a plastic sheet. (Depending on the treatment, you may want to cover this plastic sheet with a cotton sheet, which will be more comfortable for the client.)
- Provide an additional sheet or large towel for the client to slide under to maintain proper draping during the procedure.
- If the client will not be wearing disposable undergarments, provide two modesty towels for women and one for men.
- Adjust the table height for your comfort.
- Provide a bolster for under the client's knees, if needed.

PREPARING THE CLIENT

Now that you have prepared the treatment room, you are ready for the client to arrive. Always greet him or her in a professional manner; your professionalism will put your client at ease. Then, before you start the treatment, follow the steps outlined below.

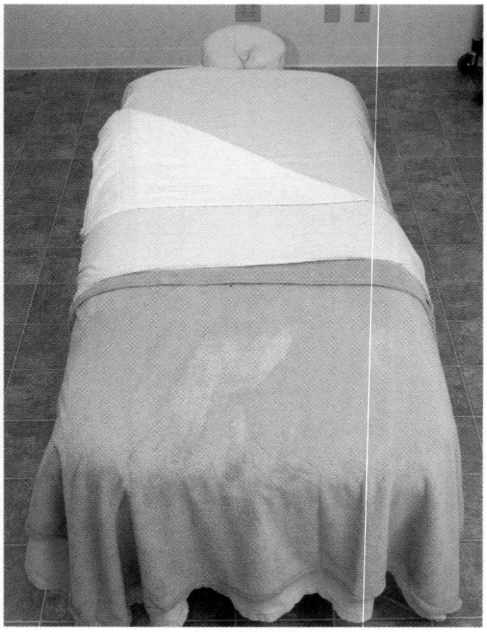

Figure 21–5 Treatment bed set up for a spa service.

General Client Preparation Procedures

Once the treatment room is fully prepared, bring the client into it. Take some time to review the client's health history to ensure that nothing has changed since you first spoke to him or her about the treatment. Reviewing health history is not only important for your purposes, but it conveys to the client that you are concerned about his or her well-being, thus making him or her more comfortable.

It is equally important to discuss modesty with your client. Advise him or her of the steps you will be taking and what is required from him or her (Figure 21–6). Remind the client to be comfortable and ask if he or she has any concerns. Be open to any suggestion the client may have that won't impede the treatment. Your goal is to make him or her as comfortable as possible. Otherwise, the treatment might not have the desired results. Be sure to let the client know that you will keep the entire body draped except for that part you are treating. Usually body treatments are performed on nude clients or those wearing disposable undergarments provided by the spa. Ask the client if he or she has a preference. While some people are very comfortable in the nude, others are very shy.

Once you ascertain that it is safe to proceed with the treatment, follow these general steps:

- Give the client instructions that include the removal of all jewelry. If the client indicated that she or he wants the disposable undergarments, set those out. Indicate the proper place to store all personal items.

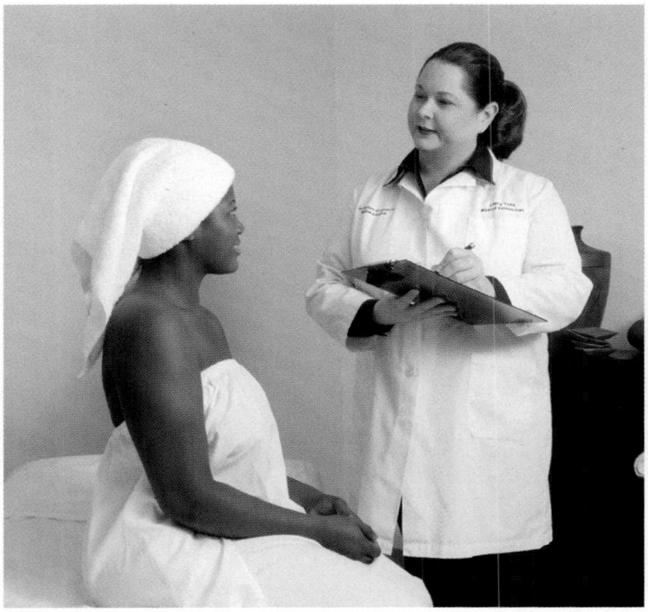

Figure 21–6 Client needs to understand the process of body treatments.

CAUTION!

Never leave a client unattended during a body treatment. Leaving someone unattended for any amount of time can be dangerous, as problems need to be addressed quickly. For example, if the client is allergic to sulfur/iodine, which is commonly found in some body treatment masks, a simple spa treatment can result in anaphylaxis, a serious and rapid allergic reaction. If the reaction is severe enough and the affected person does not receive immediate medical attention, he or she could die.

- Instruct the client on how to get onto the treatment table and into position. Keep in mind this may be his or her first treatment, so be sure all of your instructions are clear and that your client understands. This is also the time to indicate the additional sheet he or she can slide under to help maintain proper draping. Before leaving, inform the client that you will knock on the door before reentering the room.
- When you return, drape the client's hair to protect it from any creams or muds, just as you would with a facial. A disposable cap or a hair protector works well for this. This is also a good time to check on the client's comfort level. If necessary, add an additional blanket or fold up the layered ones on which the client is lying; it is important that he or she does not get chilled or overheated during the treatment.
- If the client has chosen not to wear the provided undergarments, properly drape him or her with the modesty towels. The client is now ready for the treatment.

Comfort

The key to the success of every treatment is relaxation. In order for the client to relax, he or she must be comfortable. During the relaxation response, breathing, heart rate, and blood pressure all slow down. The long-term effects of this response include improved concentration and increased energy, and the body becomes less responsive to stress hormones.

Quiet leads to relaxation. To keep noise to a minimum, be prepared for the treatment and perform your duties as quietly as possible. For example, wear soft-soled or rubber shoes, and avoid running water in the sink while the client is relaxing. Some people have differing thresholds for temperature comfort, so be sure to ask the client if the temperature setting is appealing. Other important comfort factors include lighting and sound. Bright lights can be annoying. Last, avoid unnecessary conversation and keep surrounding sounds, such as doors slamming and garbage cans rattling, to a minimum. Remember, quiet is the key to relaxation!

Proper body temperature and hydration are important too (Figure 21–7). Watch for signs of dehydration, especially if your client is using a heated blanket. Always have plenty of drinking water on hand. Monitor the client's body temperature, continually checking to ensure that he or she is never cold. Some clients may be claustrophobic; your intake form should include questions about how to address a client's particular comfort zone.

Ensure your client reaches a full state of relaxation by using the treatment's processing time for hand and foot massages. Add heated mitts or booties and a scalp massage, when possible. Always look to your client for feedback, letting him or her know that comfort is one of your top priorities.

Remember that modesty is another important aspect of the client's comfort. Many spas provide robes for clients when they are moving from the locker room to their designated treatment room or for use when they are relaxing in a meditation room between treatments.

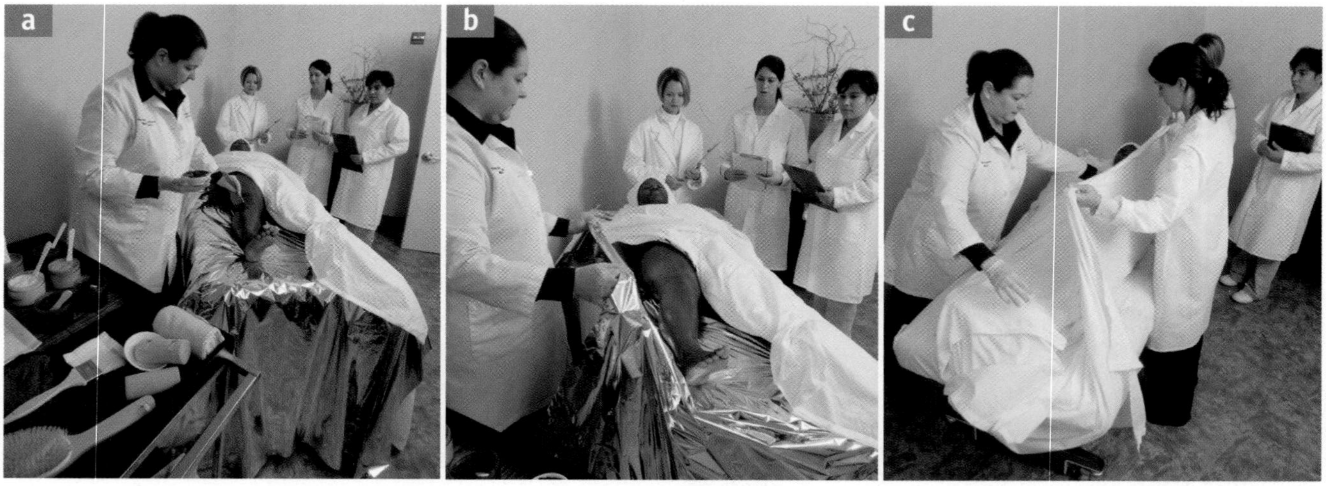

Figure 21–7 A Client having a body wrap.

Many clients may be spending the whole day at your spa and will find comfort in wearing a robe. When a client is removing or putting on a robe, always step out of the room and knock before reentering.

You can help clients overcome modesty issues by describing the treatment and explaining the draping protocol used during the treatment. For proper draping, place two modesty towels on women, one on the pelvic area and one on the bust; use one towel for men, on the pelvic area (Figure 21–8). Drape the towel and fold back the sheet. Address the area to be treated and then re-drape the sheet.

When it is time for the client to roll from a prone or supine position, or vice versa, ask him or her to roll over. Lift the towel or sheet horizontally, extending your arms over your head holding the linens between you and the client to ensure the client's privacy. Cover the client with added blankets or large bath towels. When performing treatments that include the application of foils or plastic after-treatment products, close and secure the foil or plastic and replace the modesty towels immediately, as this makes the client feel more secure.

Help clients off of the treatment table slowly to avoid injuries, as they may be unsteady after lying down for an extended period of time. During some treatments, you may escort or help your client into the shower. Before a client showers, check the water temperature, setting it to cool, then tepid to help slowly lower his or her body temperature. If your treatment involves the use of foils or plastic, remove these and re-drape the client so that they do not slip and fall from the materials.

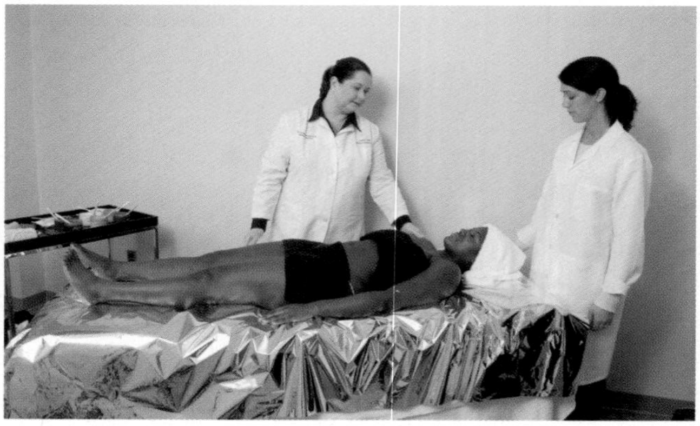

Figure 21–8 Using modesty towels is important for client privacy.

Towel Techniques for Product Removal

If you do not have access to a wet room, removing muds and body masks will be messy. One technique that has proven effective is using moist towels heated in a hot towel cabbie. First, use spa exfoliating gloves to break up the mud/seaweed and then use hot towels. Begin at the ankle and place the towel so that it covers the lower portion of the client's leg (Figure 21–9). Gently press the towel to the ankle, and begin pushing the towel upward with some pressure to "carry and remove" product from the skin as you work upward to the end of the towel. If you are using the right amount of pressure as you move along, the towel will gather and continue to remove about 99% of the product. Do not press too hard on bony areas, which could cause the client discomfort. Once you reach the end, fold the towel in half, ensuring that the clean areas of the towel are exposed as the outer

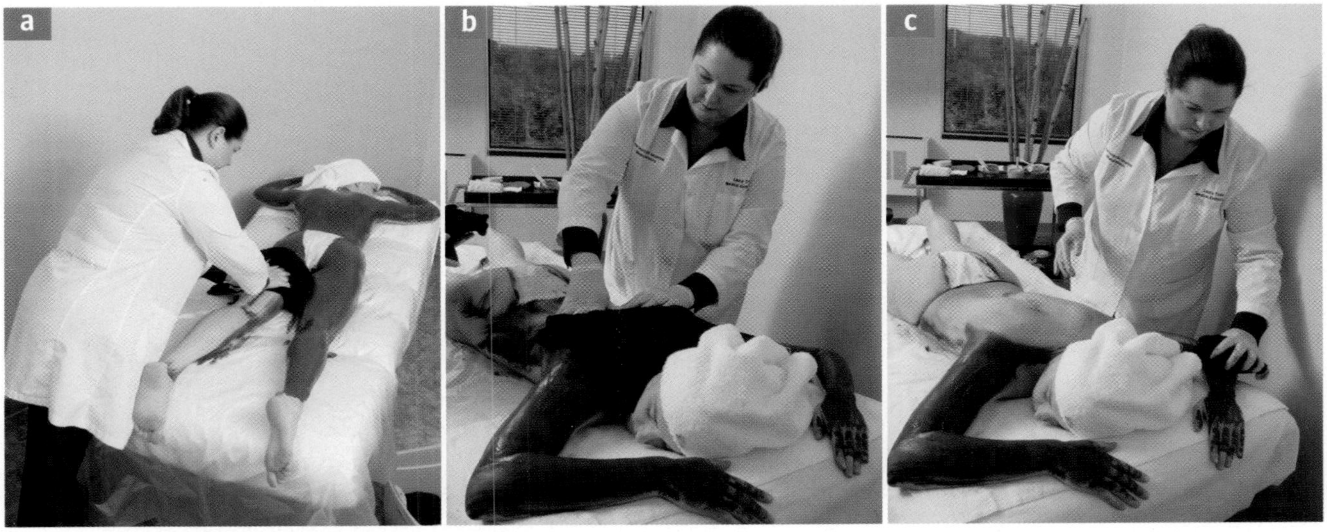

Figure 21–9 Towel method for the removal of masks.

portions. Use both sides as necessary to remove any residual product. Place a new towel at the knee in the same fashion, covering up to the upper thigh, and use the same press-push-slide technique. It may take 10 to 12 towels to remove product from the entire body. You may need to practice, but this is the best way to remove stubborn products. This technique can be applied to any portion of the body. Some technicians add moistened and warmed towels over products for further benefits. For added client comfort, heat dry towels in the cabbie and add drops of essential oils to provide further relaxation.

Facial for the Body

When performing a facial for the body, use the same approach as for a facial for the face, neck, and décolleté. For whole-body facial, however, you will cover more area and you will need to treat both sides of the body.

PROCEDURE 21–1 STEPS FOR A BODY SCRUB WITH HYDRATING PACK/MASK

IMPLEMENTS AND MATERIALS

- Facial lounge
- Plastic sheet (or drop cloth)
- Blankets
- Linens
- Towels (standard size and bath sheets)
- Hot towel cabinet
- Lucas or spray applicator
- Cleansing product
- Exfoliating scrub or granules
- Large, wet, disposable sponges or other product applicators
- Handheld brush or brush machine
- Gloves (optional)
- Oil or lotion
- Hydrating mask
- Body lotion

Preparation

1 Prepare the table with the materials you will need; remember that the outermost layer of material represents the first treatment.

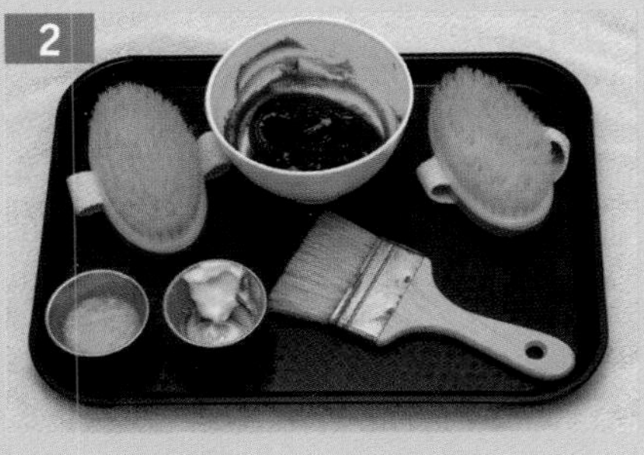

Gather supplies.

2 Gather supplies.

3 Prepare hot, wet towels and place them in the towel cabinet.

4 Review client health history to ensure that the client is still a candidate for this treatment.

5 Situate the client on the table in a prone or supine position according to treatment plan; allow for the least amount of movement by the client.

6 Discuss modesty; keep the client's entire body draped except for the part you are working on.

continues on next page

PROCEDURE 21–1, CONT. STEPS FOR A BODY SCRUB WITH HYDRATING PACK/MASK

Procedure

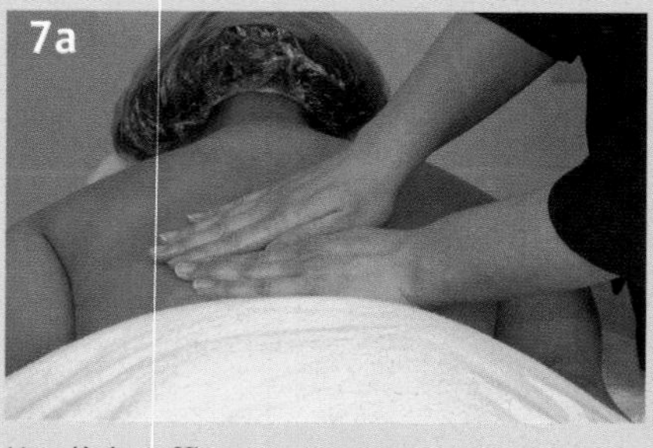

Use light effleurage movements.

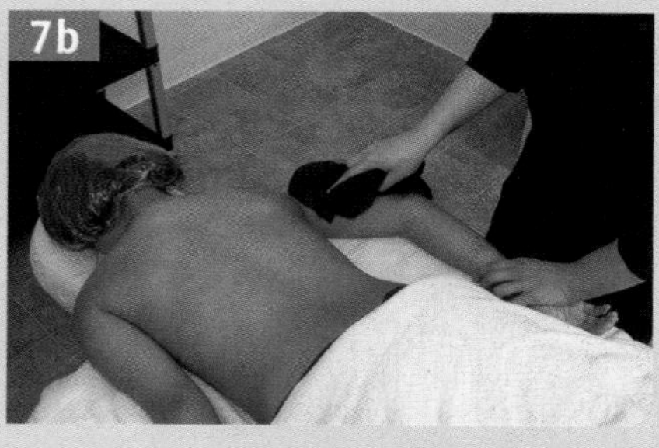

Rinse.

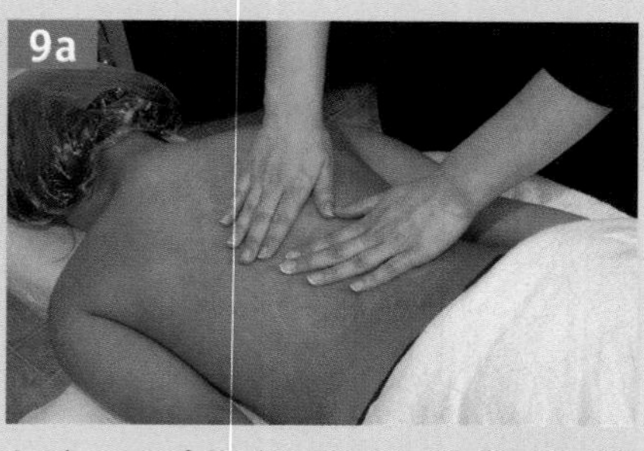

Apply an exfoliating scrub and massage in circular motion.

7 Prepare the body with a cleansing gel or lotion, depending on the client's skin type.

a. Use light effleurage movements over the entire body.

b. Rinse with large, wet sponges. For a more luxurious feel, use hot moist towels.

8 Spray appropriate toner with the Lucas or other spray applicator of your choice.

9 Apply an exfoliating scrub or granules by hand or with a brush.

a. Massage in a circular motion.

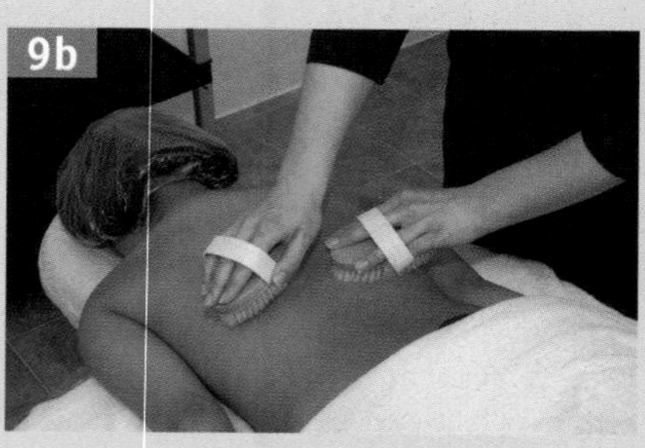

For enhanced exfoliation, use a handheld or machine-aided brush.

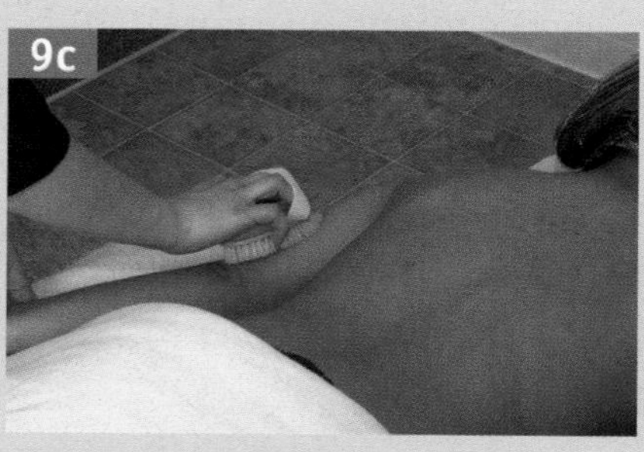

For sensitive skin, opt for dry brushing or wet brushing with a cleansing gel or lotion.

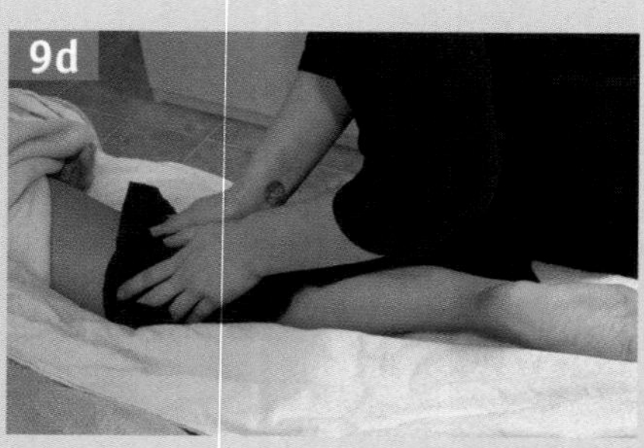

If a granular scrub is used, rinse with large wet sponges or hot moist towels.

b. For enhanced exfoliation, use a handheld or machine-aided brush.

c. For clients with sensitive skin, or if they have just shaved, waxed, or been in the sun, you may omit the exfoliation product and opt for light dry brushing or wet brushing with a cleansing gel or lotion. This is also an appropriate time to use a steamer. For a stand-alone steamer, move it up and down the body, focusing on the area being exfoliated.

d. If a granular scrub is used, rinse with large, wet sponges or hot, moist towels. Remember to maintain proper draping, exposing only the area being worked on.

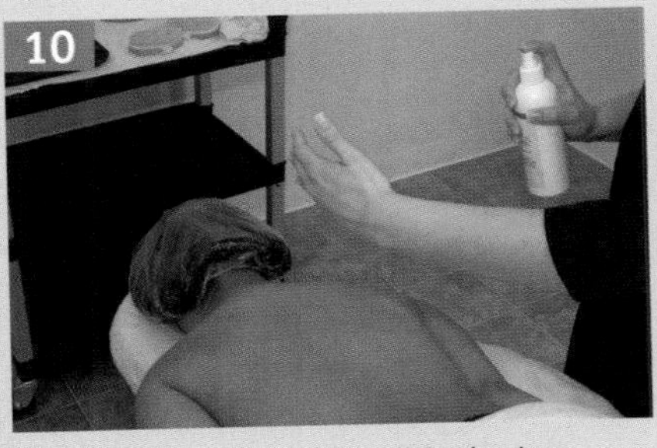

Spray appropriate toner with the Lucas spray applicator.

10 As in step 2, spray appropriate toner with the Lucas spray applicator of your choice.

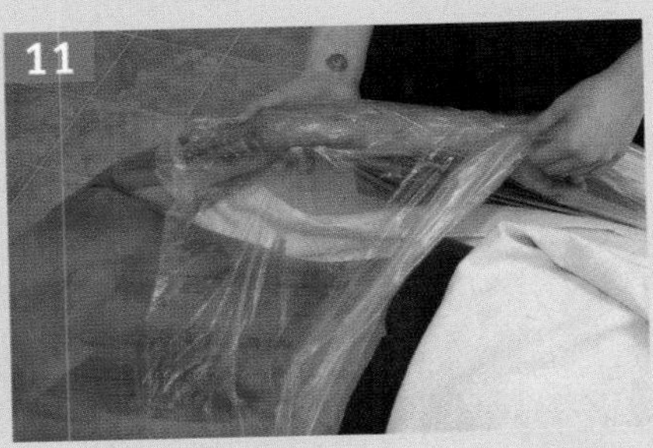

Generously apply the appropriate mask.

11 With a large brush applicator, generously apply the appropriate mask. Cover the client with plastic and blankets to keep him or her warm. Allow the mask to process the appropriate length of time. Cover the client well during the mask as he or she may feel cool during the process time. If working on the back of the body, take this time to do a scalp massage. If doing the front of the body, use this time to give the client a hand or foot massage or treatment.

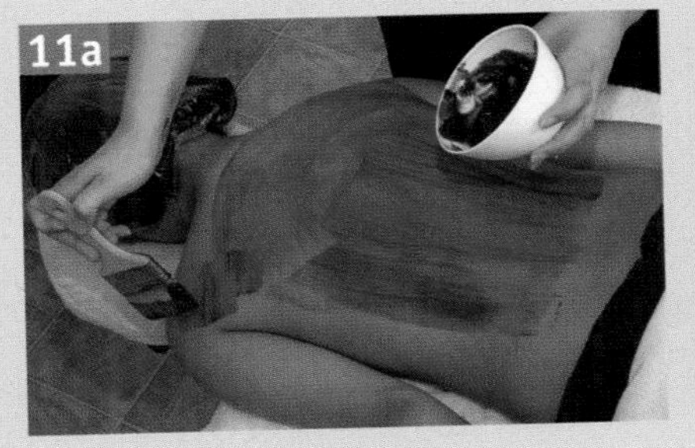

Allow the mask to process.

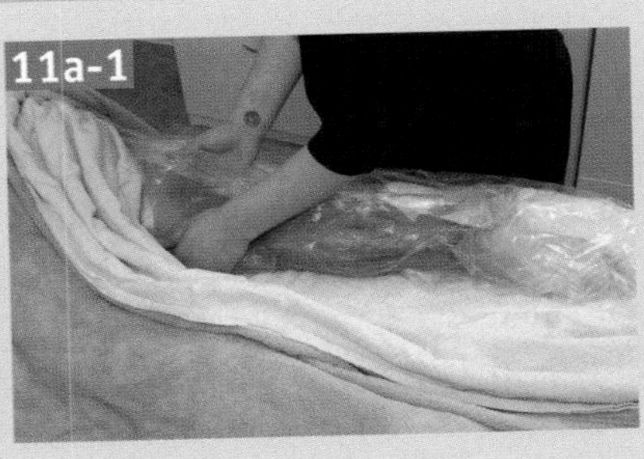

Cover the client well.

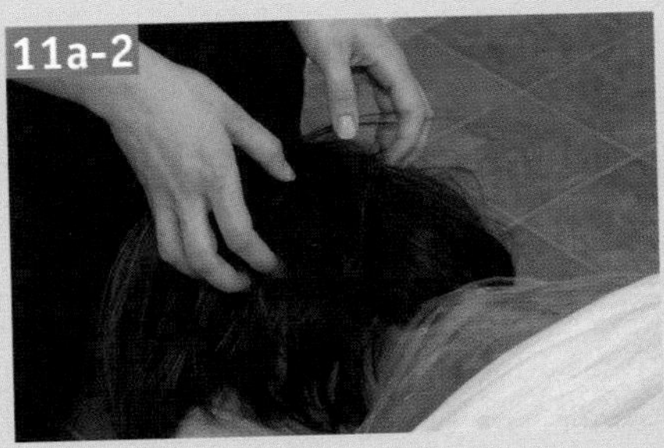

Use this time to give the client a massage.

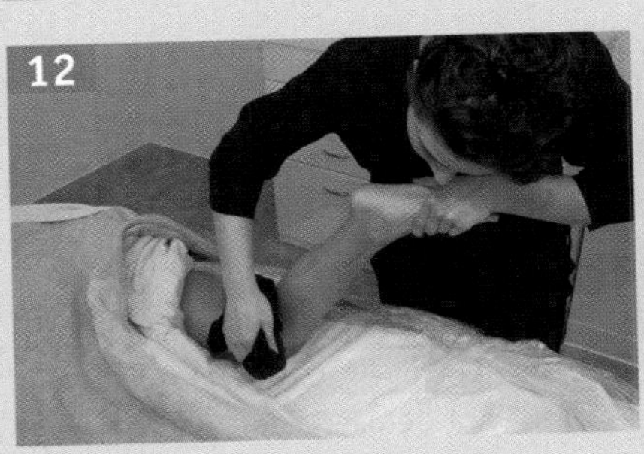

Rinse and remove mask one body area at a time.

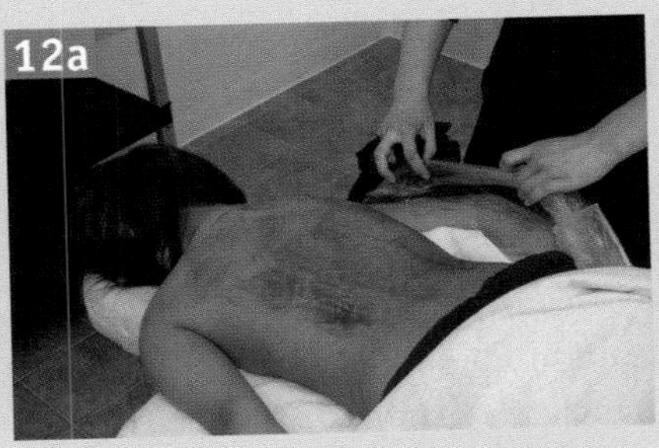

Rinse and remove mask one body area at a time.

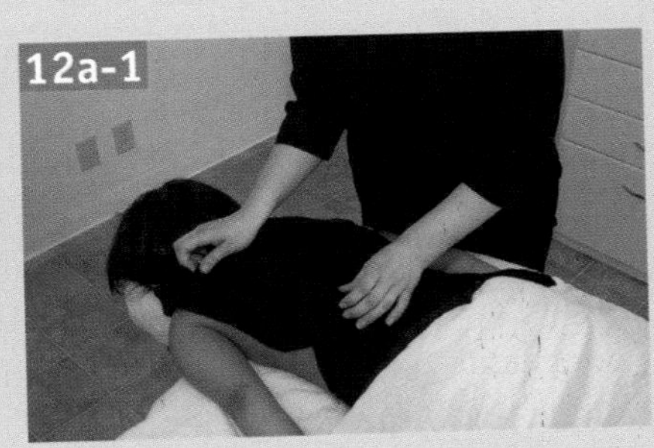

Rinse and remove mask one body area at a time.

12 Rinse and remove the mask, one body area at a time, with large, wet sponges or hot, moist towels.

continues on next page

PROCEDURE 21–1, CONT. STEPS FOR A BODY SCRUB WITH HYDRATING PACK/MASK

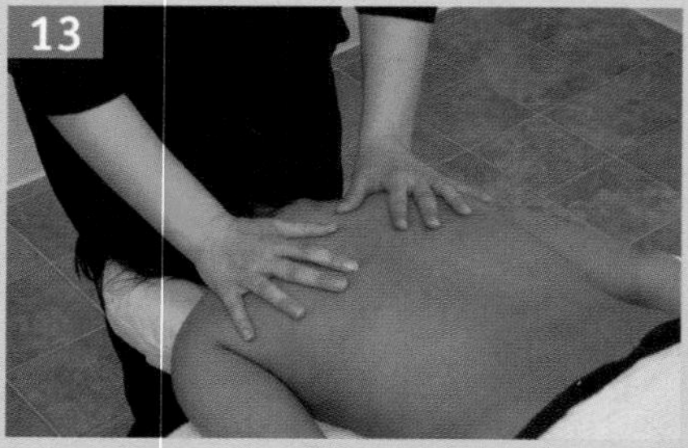

Apply a finishing massage cream or oil.

13 Apply a finishing massage cream or oil to the body, using light effleurage movements.

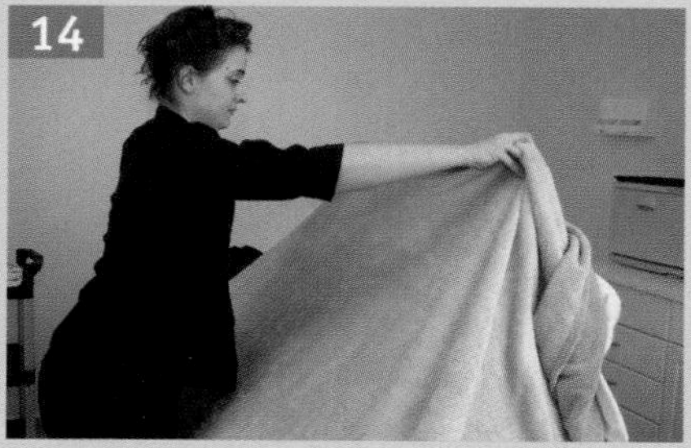

Help the client turn over.

14 Help the client turn over, maintaining the appropriate draping protocols. Repeat this entire process on the other side of the body.

Post-procedure

15 Help the client get up off bed carefully.

16 Offer the client water to drink.

Clean-up and Disinfection

17 Follow clean-up and disinfection procedures in accordance with OSHA or state guidelines.

18 Disinfect implements according to OSHA or state regulations.

THE POPULARITY OF BODY WRAPS AND MASKS

Body wraps and masks are growing in popularity, as is demonstrated by the increased number of requests for them in today's spas. One theory for this is that consumers are becoming more educated on the benefits of treating the body as a whole. As a result, many of today's savvy clients are opting for body wraps and masks to combine the relaxation of a massage with the added benefits of a skin treatment (Table 21–1). These body treatments range from salt glows and sugar rubs, to full-body herbal wraps and detoxifying paraffin cocoons, to Sedona and French red clay body masks—all of which work to create truly invigorating spa body treatments for your clients (Table 21–2). Spas work diligently to develop unique and tantalizing-sounding treatments to encourage the client to experiment and indulge (Figure 21–10).

FYI

Body wrap: A body treatment that integrates linens or elastic bandages infused with ingredients to reduce the appearance of cellulite or to hydrate the skin.

Body mask: A body treatment involving the application of an exfoliating, hydrating, detoxification mask to the entire body.

These treatments are easy to learn; they are based on your fundamental knowledge of performing a facial.

Many of the following ingredients are the same ingredients you already use in your treatments; however, many spa products are sold in large quantities because of the amount used per client. Masks are often sold powdered; you rehydrate them with warm water when you are ready to use them. This provides a nicer feel for the client and makes the product less expensive to ship.

ALPHA HYDROXY ACID (AHA): These are a common skin care ingredient. They may come as an ingredient in an exfoliator or you may do an AHA body peel. Caution the client not to shave or wax legs within 24 hours prior to having this treatment done, as stinging can result.

BETA HYDROXY ACID (BHA): You are also familiar with salicylic peels. While they are excellent for acne conditions, keep in mind they should not be used for full body peels due to the increased risk of a salicylic reaction which can have serious health effects in some clients. They are quite suitable for facial peels or for acne back facials, but never do both on the same client on the same day.

CAFFEINE: A stimulant present in coffee, tea, and soda beverages, caffeine is also useful to soothe puffy eyes. It is commonly used in cellulite creams.

CAMPHOR: An anti-infective agent with a unique taste and smell, camphor cools and refreshes itchy skin. It is commonly used to stimulate circulation and refresh the skin in foot treatments.

Table 21–1 Seaweeds and Their Uses

MAIN GROUP	GENERAL GROUP PROPERTIES	SUBGROUPS	PROPERTIES	RECOMMENDED BODY CONDITION AND TREATMENT
Algae (alginates)	Aids in skin firmness, cell renewal, and moisturization			
Chlorophyta (green)	Softening, antibacterial, anti-inflammatory	*Lichen moss*		Dry skin, irritation
Cyanophyta (blue-green)	High nutritional group, rich in vitamins A, B, C, E; stimulates cell metabolic rate	*Spirulina*	Rich source of beta-carotene, total food source, sugars (moisturizing), antioxidant	Detox, cellulite, softening, and conditioning
Phaeophyta (brown)	Probably the strongest group for blood and metabolic stimulation	*Laminaria digita*	Sugars (moisturizing); vitamins (antioxidants, etc.); provitamins (carotenoids, vitamin D, etc.); minerals (iodine, etc.); antibacterial, metabolic stimulation	More active treatments using heat and stronger stimulation, detox, cellulite, moisturizing and conditioning, revitalizing.
		Fucus	Similar to *Laminaria digita*	Similar to *Laminaria digita*
		Fucus vesibulosus		
Rhodophyta (red)	Contains highly balancing emollient algae	*Chrondrus crispus*	Highly viscous (thick and stabilizing), balancing, emollient (soothing)	Moisturizing and conditioning
		Carageenan	Highly viscous (thick, slippery), emollient (soothing)	Moisturizing and conditioning

Table 21–2 Muds and Clays

GROUP	PROPERTIES	SUBGROUP	PROPERTIES	USE
Kaolinite	Fine powder	China clay		Drawing, tightening, toning
Illite/chlorite (sea mud)	High in minerals, magnesium, potassium			
Smeetites (volcanic ash)	Rich in minerals. Used to congeal thinner clays; stimulating, vasodilation	Fango mud	High volcanic content; used in Italian hot spring spas	Mask: remineralizing, detoxifying; combine with paraffin for greater benefit. Mud easier to remove when combined with paraffin
Moor (peat) mud	Obtained from bogs rich in decayed plant material, essential oils, minerals			Masks: face, body hydrotherapy

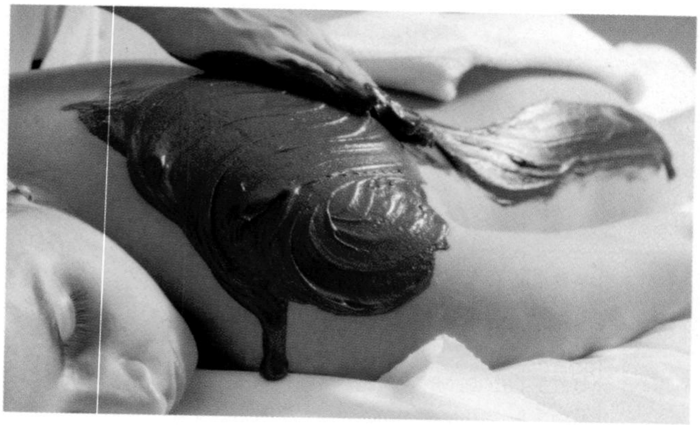

Figure 21–10 Cocoa (cacao) body mask being applied.

COLLAGEN: Collagen is added to topical creams for its moisturizing benefits.

ELASTIN: A protein in the dermis, elastin is added for its moisturizing effects.

GRAPE SEED EXTRACT: This is a botanical extract known to increase the effectiveness of vitamin C by acting as a vehicle and a restorer of oxidized vitamin C.

GREEN TEA EXTRACT: This derivative from decaffeinated green tea contains catechins, which are effective antioxidants, and is a soothing agent to irritated skin.

HYALURONIC ACID: Also known as *cyclic acid*, this is a powerful moisturizing agent.

JOJOBA OIL: Jojoba oil is used for its humectant and lubricating properties.

KAOLIN: Also called *China clay*, this fine clay is white in color. Kaolin is often used in facial masks and powders that absorb oil.

SHEA BUTTER: Shea butter is a rich moisturizing agent used for its conditioning properties.

SULFUR: Used for its soothing properties and ability to kill bacteria, sulfur is found in many masks, especially body treatments products.

THEOPHYLLINE: The tea extract version has been useful in treating cellulite. Its chemical structure is similar to caffeine.

VITAMIN A: Vitamin A is used in skin care products because it improves aging skin and firms skin texture. It can also dry out acne. It must be used in conjunction with sunscreens.

VITAMIN C: Vitamin C is used to boost collagen synthesis and its ability to enhance sun protection.

VITAMIN D: A moisturizing agent, Vitamin D is sometimes helpful for psoriasis.

VITAMIN E: Vitamin E is an oil-soluble antioxidant and is used to speed healing and in products that soften skin.

TYPES OF BODY WRAPS

With all of the different types of body treatments that are available today, manufacturers are constantly vying to set their product apart from the competition. Spas are also doing this through the use of ingenious marketing techniques and partnerships with brand names that complement their products and services. Despite all of these efforts, most body treatments are similar in technique. It is their ingredients, target, or the benefit desired that sets them apart. You as the clinician can distinguish yourself by your personal touch with each treatment.

Body wrap basics involve a wrapping treatment that is applied on top of a mask or treatment. This wrap helps to intensify the treatment by working on the principles of occlusion. The wrapping technique prevents the client from becoming cold and allows the product to remain in place. This protocol can be used with most body treatments. The difference would be in the type of wrapping agent or modality used, such as **elastic wraps** or bandages that are wrapped around an individual's legs, arms, and torso or a full cotton sheet (Figure 21–11) that wraps the client like a mummy or as if in a cocoon.

The wrapping results in increased body temperature and circulation and dilation of the blood capillaries, which

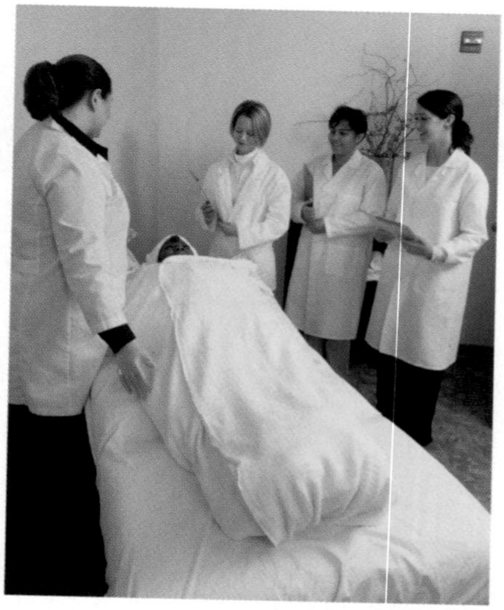

Figure 21–11 Client in the cocoon of a body wrap.

allows absorption of the therapeutic ingredients through the pores and hair follicles. The increased body temperature also relaxes tense muscles and increases perspiration and waste elimination. Adding ingredients such as clays or muds gives clients the added benefits of drawing out toxins. Elastic wraps are used frequently when clients are going for a temporary slimming effect. The elastic wraps are soaked in a slimming agent or mixture (Figure 21–12) and pre- and post-treatment measurements are recorded. Take care during the measuring process that you take the "before" and "after" measurements in exactly the same positions to ensure accuracy.

Seaweed and Algae Wraps

Seaweed wraps are popular, not only for relaxation purposes, but to stimulate circulation and rid the body of toxins. It is said that seaweed wraps may also address cellulite by providing vitamins and minerals, such as copper, iron, potassium, zinc, and iodine, which can help break up the body's fatty deposits. The overall benefit of seaweed wraps is that the skin looks and feels supple and smooth. The wraps' ingredients comprise micronized algae that can be mixed with warm water. Because the algae have a strong odor, some manufacturers include an additional additive for the client's comfort. You may premix this just prior to escorting your client into the treatment room. Store it in a hot towel cabinet to keep it at a comfortable temperature.

First, exfoliate or dry brush the client's body to stimulate the circulation, and then apply the algae. To dry brush the skin, stroke a handheld brush or loofah across the skin in brisk sweeping motions (Figure 21–13). Then apply seaweed paste all over the body (Figure 21–14). Next, wrap the area with cellophane or warm thermal sheets and let it process for approximately 45 minutes. After the seaweed has fully processed, remove the sheets. Have the client shower off the seaweed; or you can remove it with warm moist towels.

Advise the client that because the wrap removes toxins from the skin, it is important to drink extra water for 24 hours before and after the wrap. General contraindications for this treatment include allergies to fish, shellfish, or iodine, which can be major components of the mineralized seaweed powder.

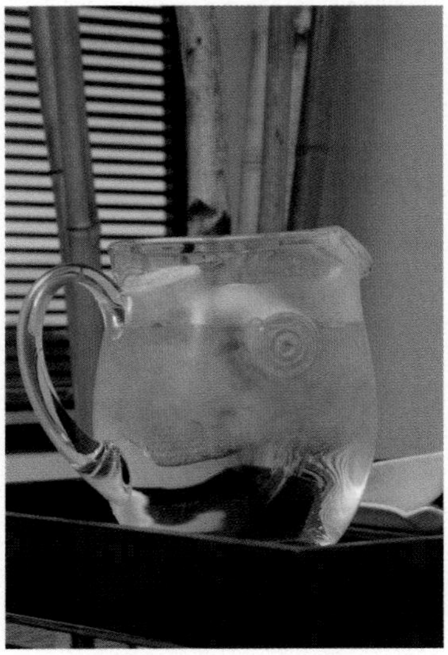

Figure 21–12 Elastic wraps soaking.

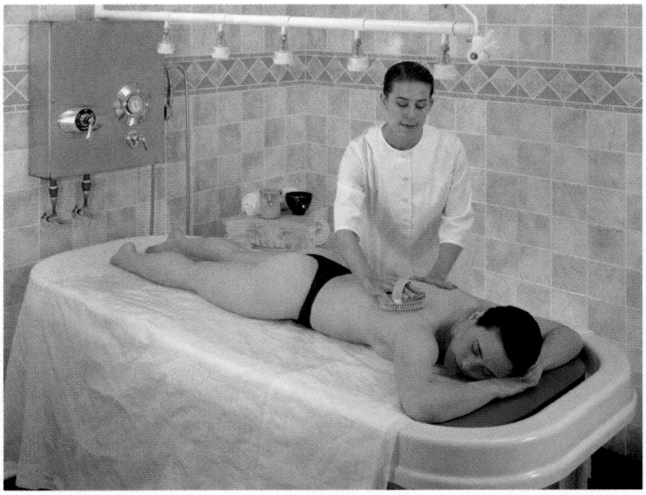

Figure 21–13 Dry brushing is an excellent exfoliation by itself or as part of a treatment.

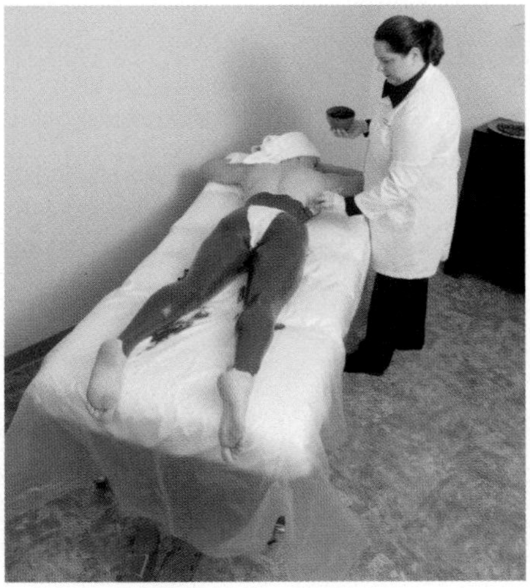

Figure 21–14 Application of seaweed mask.

PROCEDURE 21–2 APPLYING AND REMOVING SEAWEED WRAP

MATERIALS AND IMPLEMENTS

- Spa treatment lounge setup with linens and towels
- Towels or sponges for product removal
- Cleanser and toner of choice
- Seaweed product
- Moisturizer
- Water
- Thermal blanket
- Oversized brush

Preparation

1

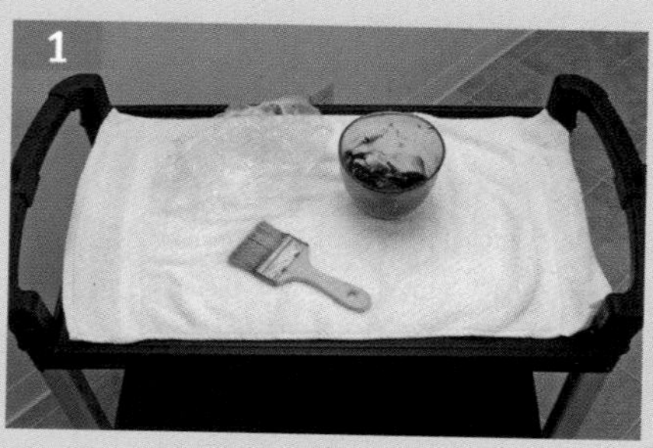

Prepare treatment table.

1 Prepare the treatment table with a protective covering (such as a sheet, plastic protector sheet, wool blanket, cellophane sheet, or space blanket, and a top sheet or towel).

2 In a bowl, combine the seaweed mixture and prepare for application. Warm this mixture slightly in the hot towel cabbie.

3 Review client health history to ensure that the client is still a candidate for this treatment.

4 Tell the client what to expect during the treatment.

5 Ask the client to get on the table into a supine position just below the top sheet or towel while you step outside the room. He or she will be laying on the sheet of plastic face up.

6 Pre-treat the client by cleansing and toning the skin, one area at a time.

7 Perform any pre-treatment exfoliation procedures before applying the seaweed.

Procedure

8

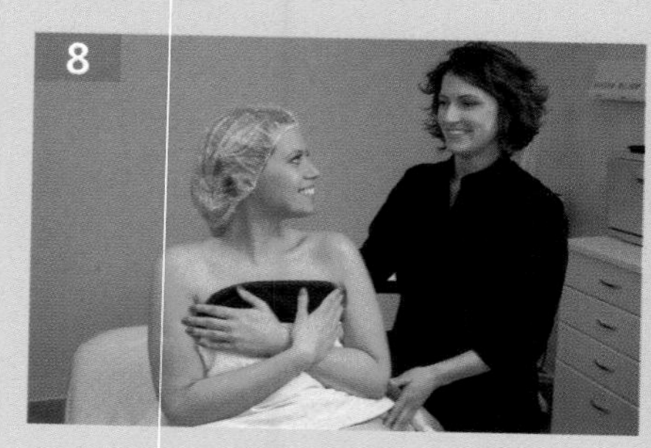

Assist client into a sitting position.

8 If the client is female, instruct her to cross her arms (to hold the modesty towel into place), and assist her into a seated position.

9

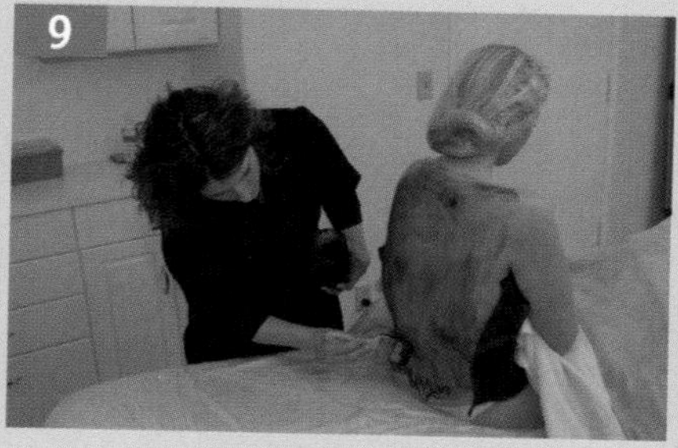

Apply the seaweed mixture to the back and shoulders.

9 Apply the seaweed mixture with your gloved hands or an oversized brush to the back and shoulders. Next help the client back to the supine position.

9a

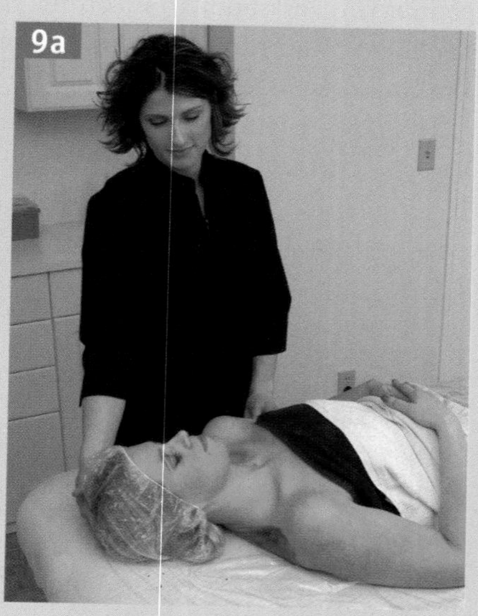

Help the client back to the supine position.

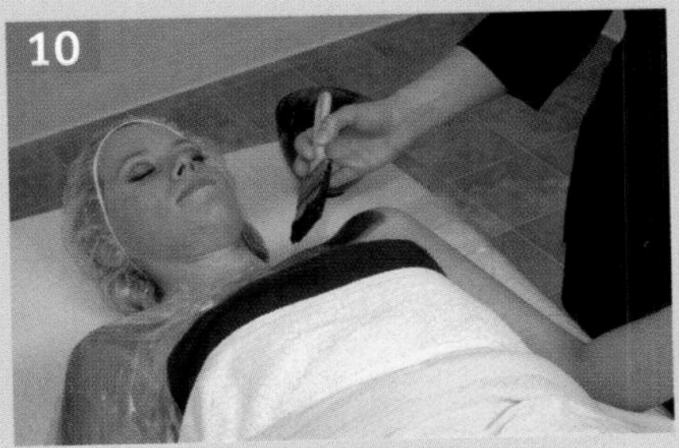
Apply mixture to the chest and arms.

10 Apply the mixture to the chest and arms. The stomach is optional.

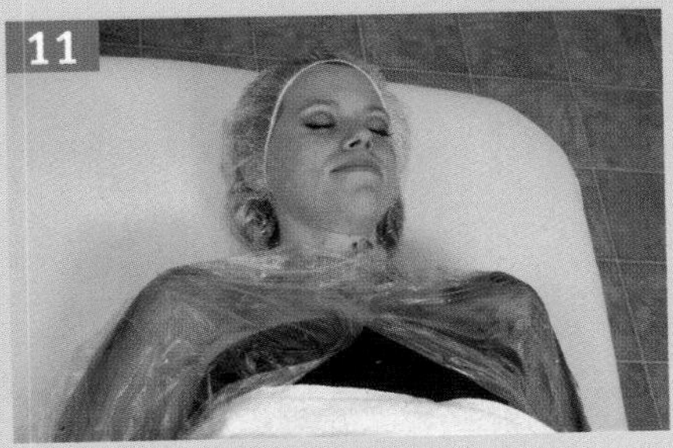
Wrap the client's upper body with plastic wrap.

11 Wrap the client's upper body with plastic wrap. Reposition the towel.

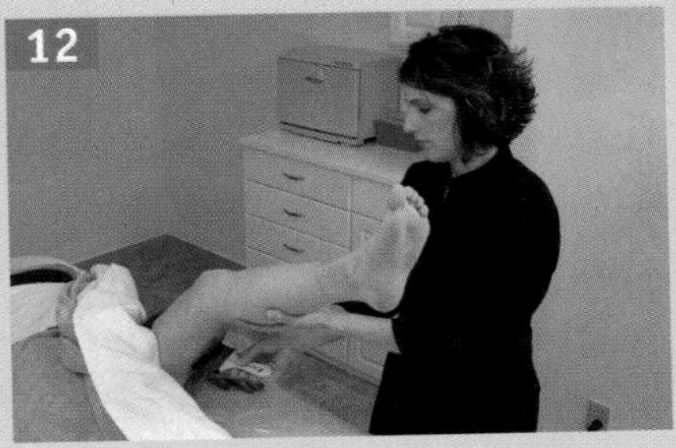
Apply the mixture to the legs and buttock area.

12 Apply the mixture to the legs and buttocks starting with the nearest leg. This is accomplished by gently raising the knees and applying the mixture to the backs of the legs and the buttocks.

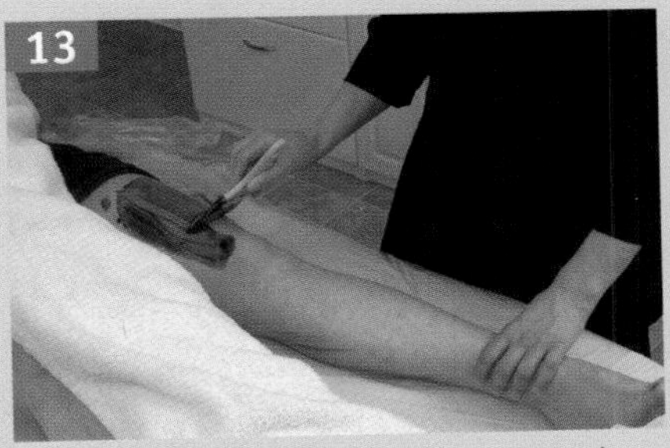
Apply the mixture to the front of the leg.

13 Slide the leg into a flat position and apply the mixture to the front of the leg.

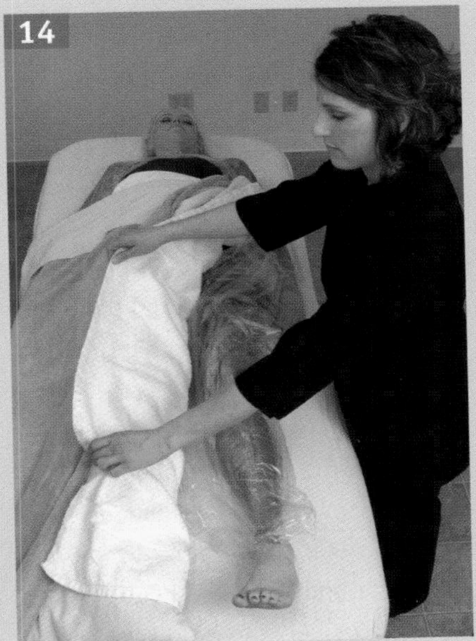
Pull plastic drape across the leg.

14 Pull the plastic drape across the leg over the mud, and reposition the towel.

15 Repeat this on the other leg.

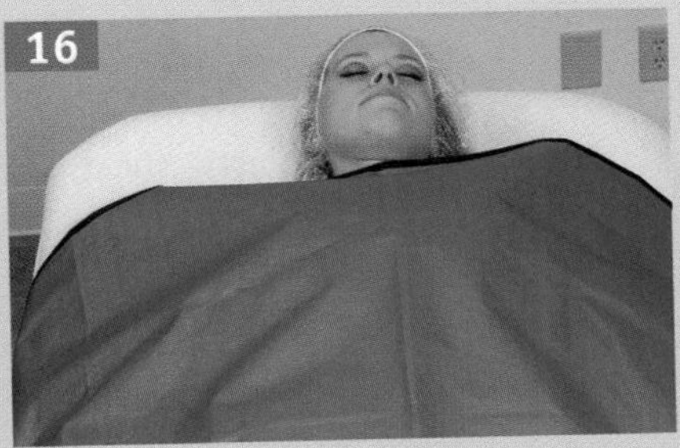
Cover the client with a blanket.

16 Cover the client with a thermal space blanket over the towel to ensure he or she stays warm.

17 Next fold up the layers or blankets onto the client. Use a towel around the neck to prevent heat loss. Process for the desired time, which is usually 25 minutes.

continues on next page

PROCEDURE 21–2, CONT. APPLYING AND REMOVING SEAWEED WRAP

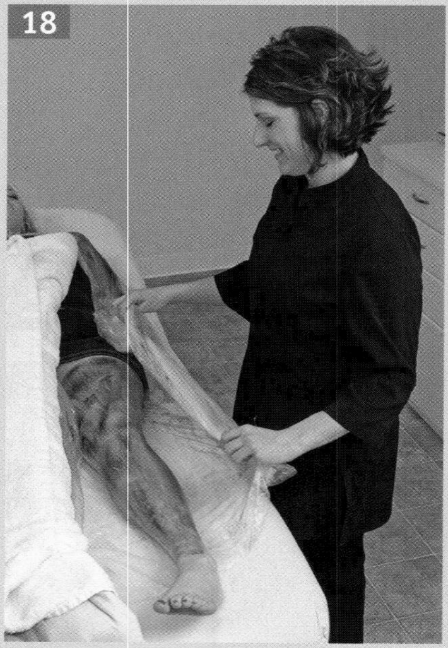

Fold away the plastic sheet and blankets.

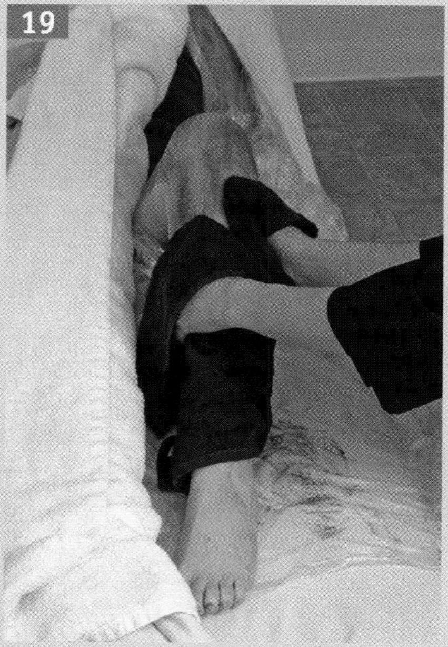

Remove all product from the front of the nearest leg.

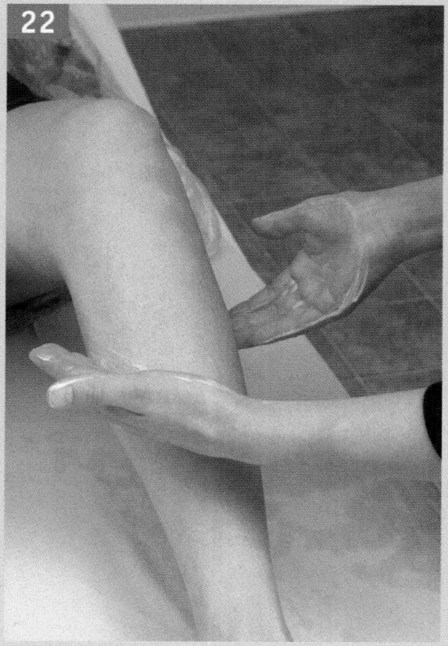

Apply body lotion or massage cream to leg.

18 Fold away the plastic sheet and blankets, one area at a time to ensure modesty. Remove product thoroughly with warm moist towels, tucking the plastic out of the way and re-covering the client with a clean bath towel. Start with the legs.

19 Starting with the nearest leg, remove all product from the front of the leg. Raise the knee to allow complete removal of product from the back of the leg. Shift the plastic out of the way and re-cover the client with a clean towel.

20 Repeat this process with the opposite leg. To remove the plastic from under the client, shift it as far as possible to the left side and have the client elevate his or her hips slightly to assist you. Slide the plastic completely from under the client's lower body, ensure that all product has been removed, and re-cover the client.

21 As an alternative, give the client a robe and assist him or her to the shower.

22 Apply body lotion or massage cream to the leg nearest you.

23 Apply the lotion to the opposite leg.

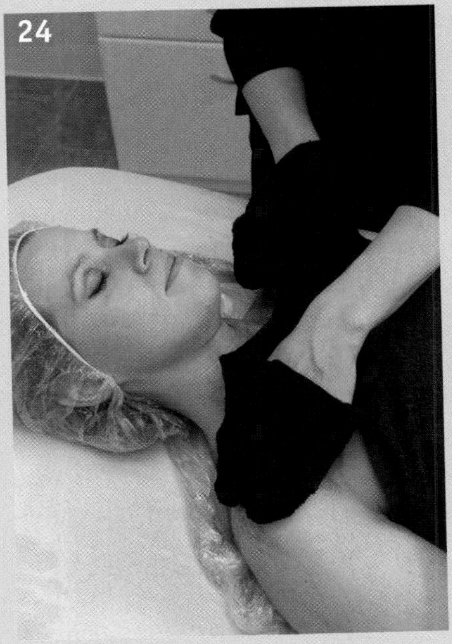

Move to client's upper body and remove mask.

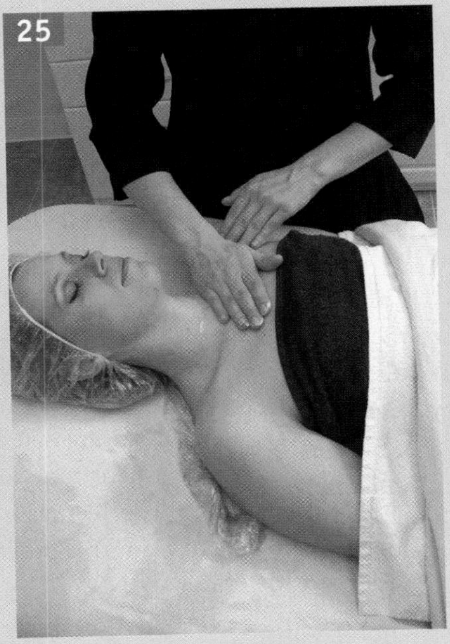

Apply lotion to the client's chest and arms.

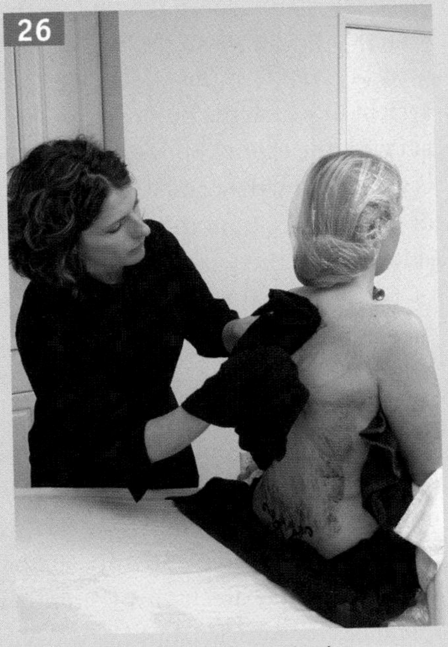

Remove mask from client's back.

24 Now move to the client's upper body and remove the mask, shifting the plastic away from the cleaned areas.

25 Apply lotion to the client's chest and arms. The stomach is optional.

26 Assist the client to a sitting position and remove the mask from his or her back.

27 Remove the last of the plastic.

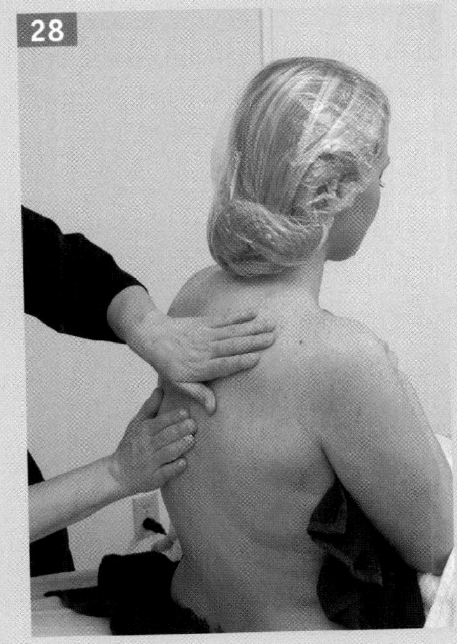

Apply lotion.

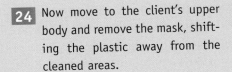

28 Apply lotion to the client's back. The client should now be in a seated position, coming back to reality slowly. The treatment is complete. Alternatively, you can use the same application and removal techniques as in Procedure 21-1.

Post-procedure

29 Offer the client water for rehydration.

30 Inform the client of any post-treatment instructions.

Clean-up and Disinfection

31 Follow clean-up and disinfection procedures in accordance with OSHA or state guidelines.

32 Disinfect implements according to OSHA or state regulations.

Herbal Wraps

There are several variations in basic wrapping techniques. These include **herb wraps,** which are herb-soaked linen sheets or elastic wraps resembling Ace® bandages that are wrapped tightly around the body in a mummy style. The goal of wrapping the client is to create a self-contained system in which the products applied are allowed to interact with the client's body. The beneficial effect of the wrap is achieved by the combination of heat and the properties of the herbs or from the ingredients applied to the client's skin prior to the wrap.

Each herb has a specific targeted effect. The herbs can increase circulation, provide soothing properties and nourishment to the skin, or may be **diaphoretic,** increasing perspiration. The sheets or bandages are usually soaked in an herbal brew and heated in a **moist heat unit** for approximately 20 minutes at 165 degrees. Sometimes this unit is mistakenly referred to as a **hydrocollator,** but the two are not the same. A hydrocollator heats special moist heat packs that are used by chiropractors and massage therapists for muscle pain. These devices are not designed to hold sheets (Figure 21–15) as they have an exposed heating coil in the bottom. The moist heat unit has a solid interior designed to hold water and soak the sheets. There is usually a drain outside at the back or bottom to facilitate emptying the unit. Be sure this drain is closed before adding water to the unit.

The herbs are usually provided in bulk form. Transfer a small amount of these herbal blends to a muslin bag filled about three-fourths full. The muslin pouch can be refilled during the day with fresh herbs. You can add more water to the heating unit. Start each day with a new batch; if that's not possible, do this at least every other day. You can store the mixture overnight in the refrigerator. It is a good idea to have several bags of the herbs available for your clients to purchase for home use.

When retrieving the linens or wraps, protect your hands from the heat by using rubber gloves. Use simple wood clamps when wringing the heavy wet muslin sheets out of the heating units and steaming herbal solution.

After applying the herbal wrap, cover the person with a blanket and apply a cold compress to the forehead. The treatment typically processes for approximately 30 minutes. Some spas use infrared heating lamps to keep clients warm. Remember that an herbal wrap is a heated treatment. As such, it is contraindicated for anyone who has open wounds or sores, is pregnant, has hypertension, or suffers from circulatory disorders, heart conditions, decreased feelings of sensation, or diabetes. This treatment may also not be appropriate for clients who tend to feel claustrophobic. Not every client is a candidate for this process.

Preparation for a Herbal Body Wrap Treatment

Fill the heating unit nearly three-quarters full with water to allow for submersion of herbs and wrap sheets. After the water reaches 165°F, completely submerge the muslin pouch filled with water-soluble herbs following manufacturer's directions. Allow the herbal mix to brew for approximately for 20 to 30 minutes. After the herbs have brewed completely, you have an herbal tea bath for the sheets. Submerse two 100% linen wrap sheets in the tea, allowing them to soak for 20 minutes. Linen is the preferred material due to its ability to maintain heat longer. While the sheets are soaking, prepare the treatment table with a wool or thick blanket followed by a thermal

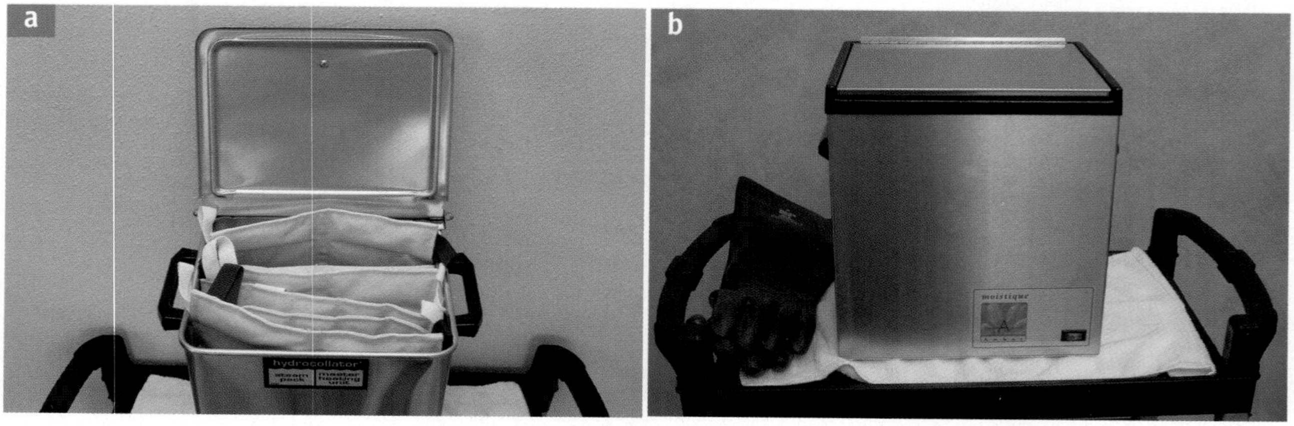

Figure 21–15 a) Hydrocollator and b) Moist heat unit.

blanket or plastic sheet to protect any underlying linens or blankets. Some technicians like to get the linen sheets hot in the moist heat unit and then transfer them to a hot towel cabinet to keep them warm before the client enters the room.

Client safety is an issue when dealing with hot sheets. Heat-sensitive clients may burn on the backs of thighs or buttocks if not properly monitored. Never leave this client alone, and if he or she complains of the temperature being too uncomfortable, remove the linens immediately.

Practice your wrapping technique as this is the most important step in the treatment. The temperature of the sheets is critical, because you want to induce the client to perspire (think sauna). To ensure that your client receives the full benefits of this treatment, instruct him or her to avoid showering immediately after the wrap; the herbs continue to work for several hours. Also, stress the importance of rest and replenishing any water loss that has occurred during this treatment. Remind the client to drink plenty of water to continue the detoxification process.

PROCEDURE 21–3 HERBAL BODY WRAP

MATERIALS AND IMPLEMENTS

- Moist heat unit
- Hot towel cabinet (optional)
- Thermal protective gloves
- Linen sheets (2)
- Long-handled metal tongs to handle herbal pouch and hot linens
- Spa treatment lounge setup with linens
- Towels and bath sheets
- Warm steam towels for product removal or, alternatively, sponges
- Thermal blanket
- Insulating blanket (wool is preferred)
- Herbs in muslin pouch or herbal ball
- Dry body brush
- Water and or tea for client

Preparation

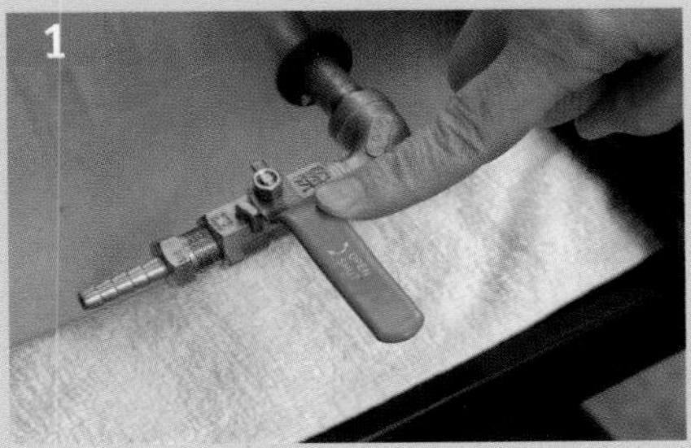

Before filling, make sure the drain valve is closed.

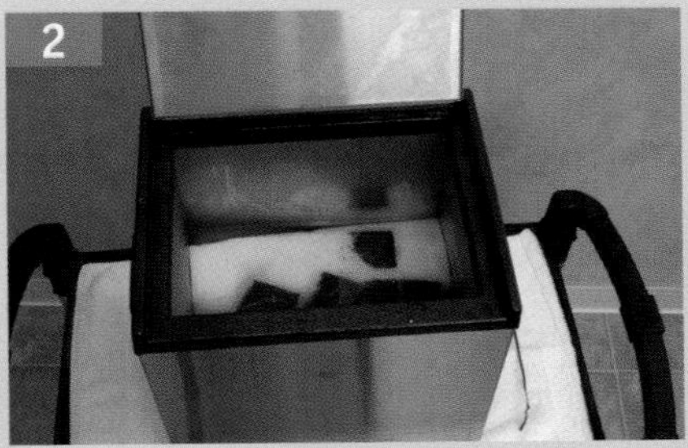

Place herbs in pouch in moist heat unit.

1 Prepare the moist heat unit following manufacturer's directions. The suggested temperature range is 150°F to 185°F.

Note: Before the unit is filled, make sure the drain valve is closed.

2 Place herbs in the pouch in the moist heat unit to brew, submerging them with the tongs. These need to process at least 30 minutes.

3 Fold the linens inward from each side lengthwise first, then crosswise so that it is folded in the pattern in which you will unfold it.

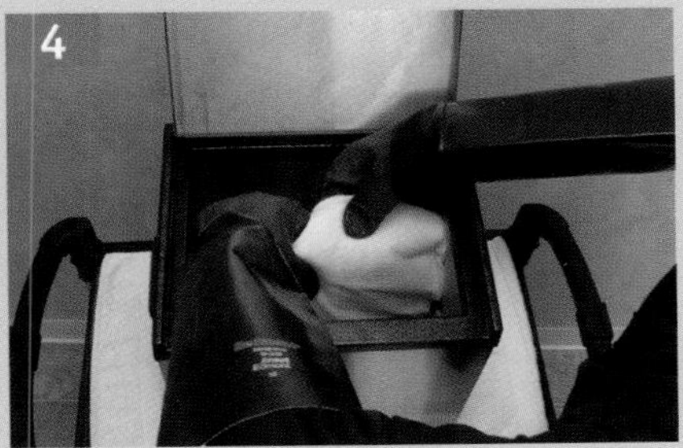

Place sheets in unit with thermal protective gloves.

4 Put on thermal protection gloves and place the sheets in the moist heat unit. Re-check the temperature per the manufacturer's guidelines.

continues on next page

PROCEDURE 21–3, CONT. HERBAL BODY WRAP

5 Set up the treatment room in standard spa treatment manner, from the treatment bed outward:

a. First: water protective cover
b. Wool blanket
c. Metallic spa sheet
d. Body pack film (optional)
e. Large bath towel (for dry brushing)
f. Spa towel across the head of the lounge

Optional: If working alone, you may find the linens difficult to handle, so prepare by putting on gloves. Remove the sheet from moist heat unit with tongs, wring it out quickly and thoroughly without unfolding it all the way, and place it in the hot towel cabinet to maintain temperature.

6 Review client health history to ensure that the client is still a candidate for this treatment.

7 Let the client know what to expect during the treatment, and determine his or her heat tolerance level.

8 Some technicians offer the client warm herbal tea to raise core body temperature. Alternatively, a client can take a shower or sit in the sauna.

9 Instruct the client to get onto the treatment table on the large bath towel, facedown, after you step outside the room. Client may opt to change into a swimsuit or disposable undergarments at this time.

Procedure

10

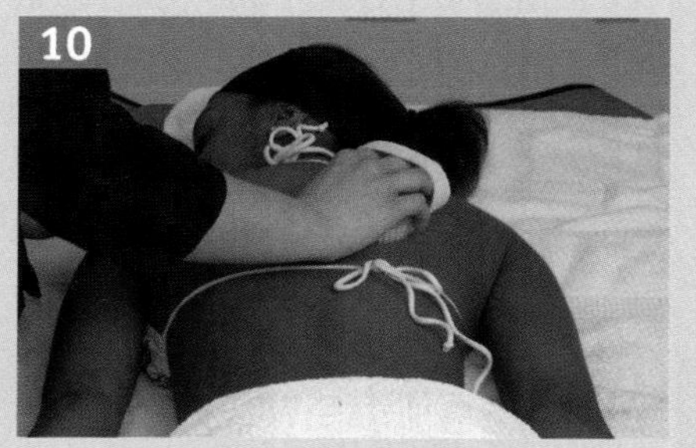

Begin with dry brushing.

10 Begin the treatment with a light massage, using effleurage movements or dry brushing the area to be treated. Dry brushing helps remove dead skin cells and stimulates the lymphatic system. Turn client and dry brush the front of the body.

11 Assist the client back up from the bed, keeping him or her draped in a large bath sheet if nude.

12

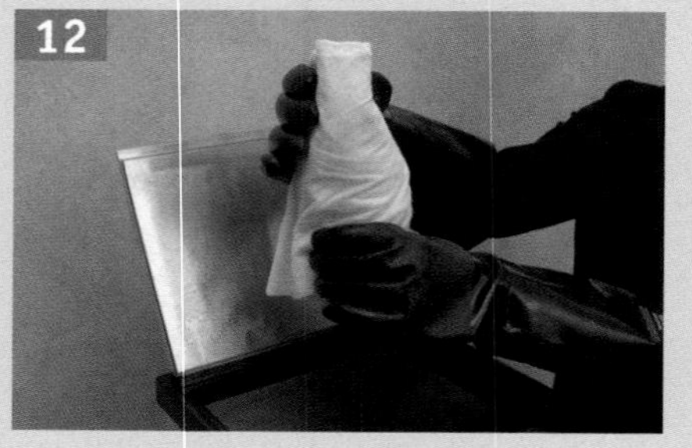

Remove and wring out one of the soaked linen sheets.

12 Remove the sheet from the hot towel cabinet. Alternatively if working directly from the moist heat unit remove one of the soaked linen sheets (wear proper hand protection to avoid burns) and wring it out thoroughly. Place the hot linen sheet on the bed, creating a long rectangle, which allows you to fold the sides around the client. Double-check the temperature to ensure it is not so hot as to burn the client's skin on prolonged contact. Ask the client to let you know if it feels too hot and you will get him or her off the sheet immediately.

12a

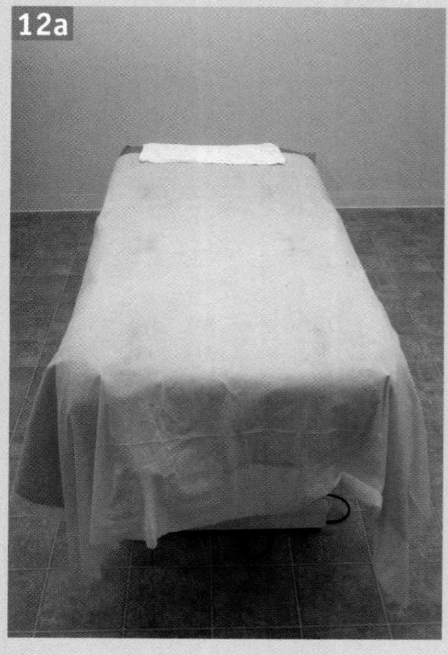

Place hot linen sheet on the bed.

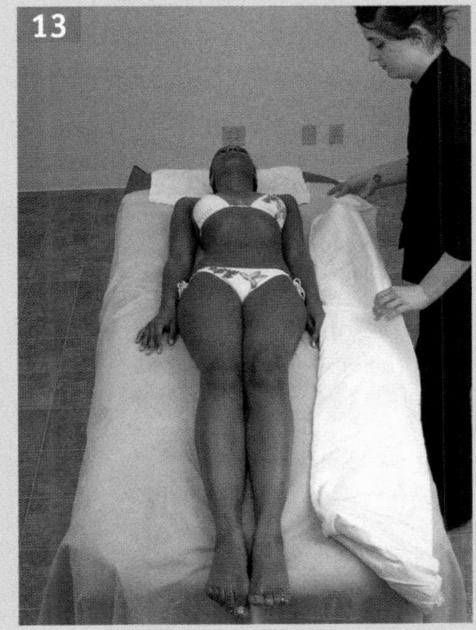
13

Assist the client back onto the bed.

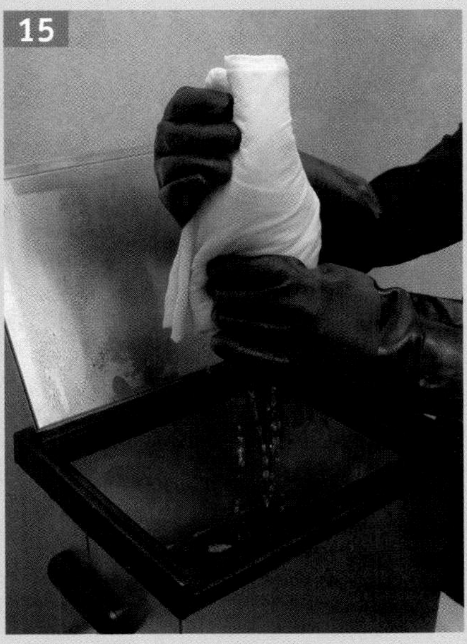
15

Remove the second linen and wring out thoroughly.

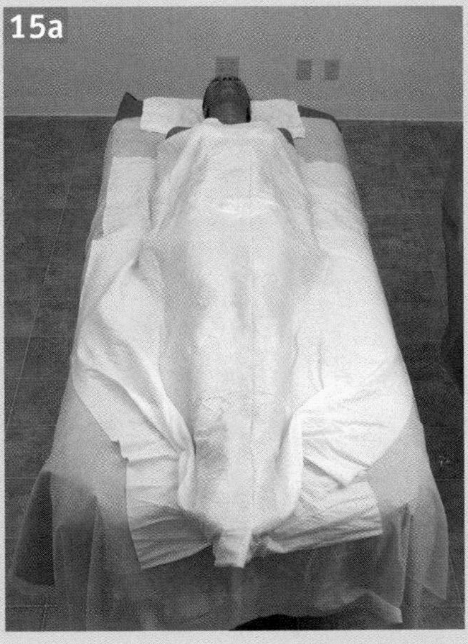
15a

Place the sheet on top of the client.

13 Assist the client back onto the bed lying faceup on the sheet.

14 Quickly wrap the linen sheet around the client's entire body. (You can also layer the sheet.)

15 Wearing thermal gloves, remove the second linen from the unit and wring it out thoroughly.

Quickly place it on top of the client so that the sheet is doubled, allowing more heat conservation.

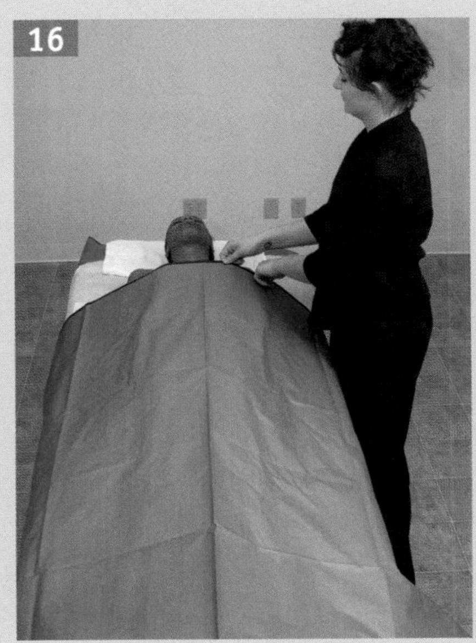
16

Wrap the thermal blanket over the herbal wrap sheet.

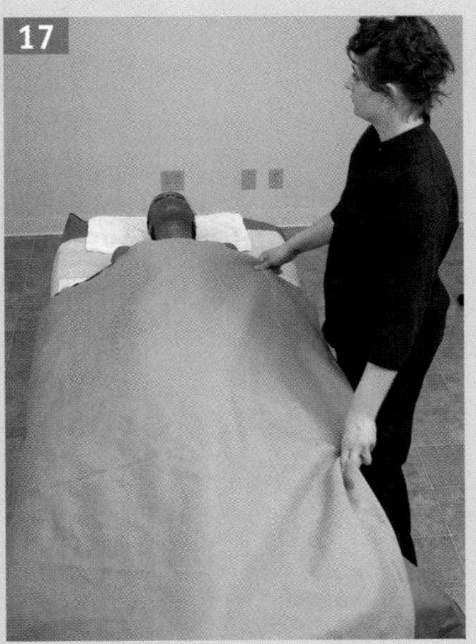
17

Wrap insulating blanket over the thermal blanket.

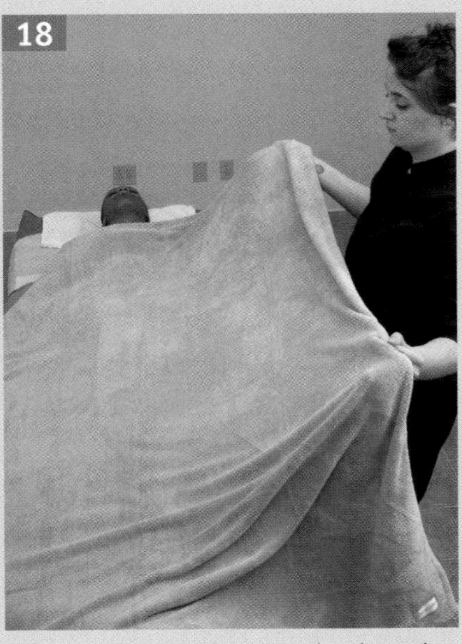
18

Wrap the wool blanket over the thermal blanket.

16 Wrap the thermal blanket over the herbal wrap sheet.

17 Wrap the insulating blanket over the thermal blanket.

18 Wrap the wool blanket over the thermal blanket.

continues on next page

PROCEDURE 21–3, CONT. HERBAL BODY WRAP

19a
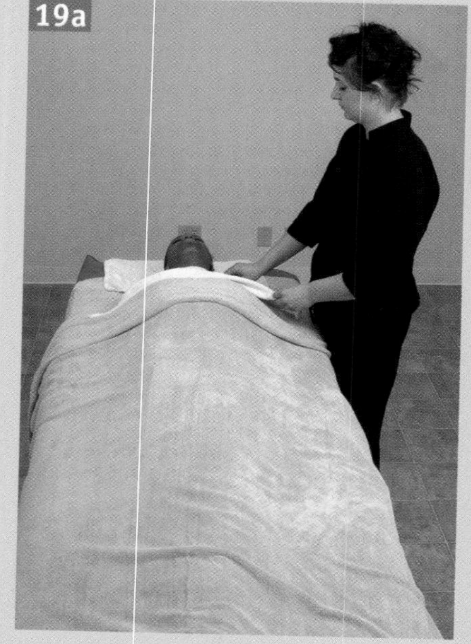
Use a towel around the neck area.

19 Add a second wool blanket, if needed, over the client to keep warm.

a. Use a towel around the neck to prevent heat loss.

b. Optional: Place a second wool blanket on top for additional heat retention.

c. Optional: Place a bolster under the client's knees.

20
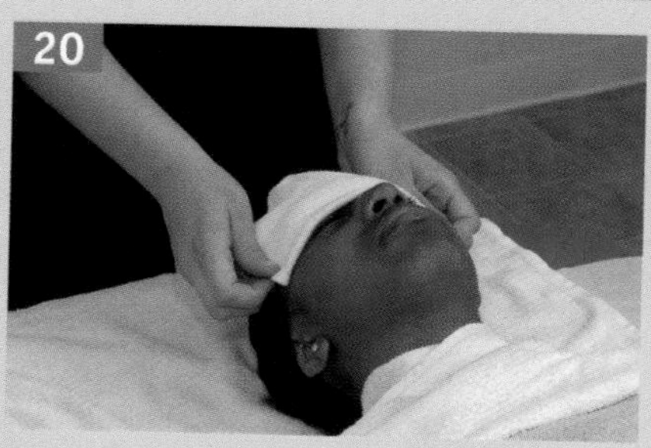
Apply a cool washcloth.

20 Apply a cool, folded washcloth to the client's forehead and across the eyes. For additional comfort, you can place a pillow under his or her head. If client gets too warm, open the blanket around the neck.

21 Leave the client wrapped for 20 to 30 minutes. During this time, perform a scalp massage or play soothing music.

22
 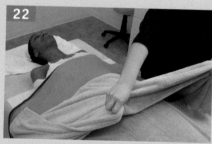
Remove the layers slowly.

22 After the wrap has processed, remove the layers slowly, allowing the client to get acclimated to

23
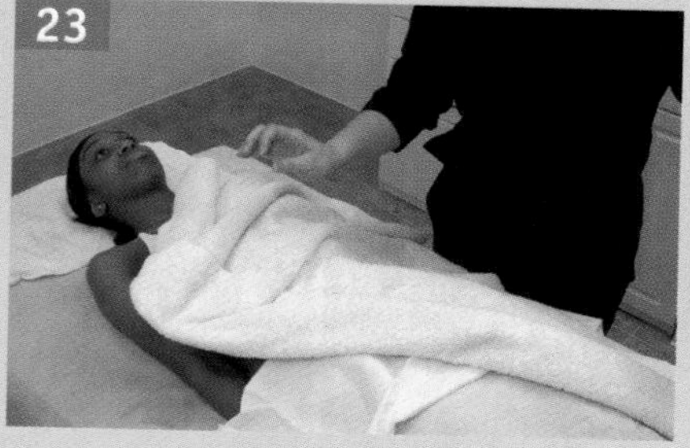
Cover client with dry towel.

the cooler temperature of the room.

23 Immediately cover the client with a dry towel to prevent chilling.

24
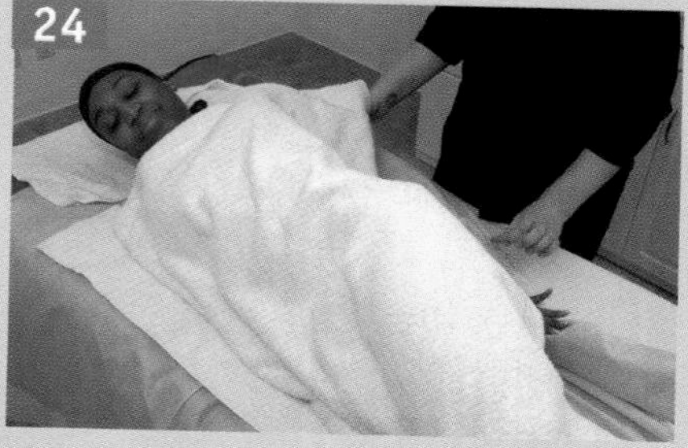
Slide the linen sheet out from underneath the client.

24 Have the client roll to one side and slide the linen sheet from underneath him or her. Repeat by rolling the client in the other direction and removing the sheet.

25 As this is a detoxifying treatment, no lotions should be applied.

26
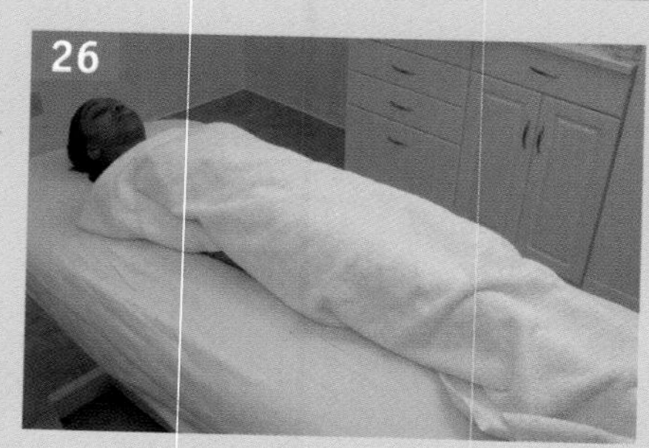
Have client lie down and rest.

26 Allow the client to lie back down and rest, if desired.

Post-procedure

27 Offer the client water to rehydrate.

28 Advise the client to avoid strenuous exercise, tanning beds, direct sun, and caffeinated beverages following the treatment.

29 Inform the client of any additional manufacturer post-treatment instructions.

Clean-up and Disinfection

30 Follow OSHA or state guidelines for clean-up and disinfection of the treatment room and linens.

31 Disinfect any implements following OSHA or state guidelines.

32 Clean and disinfect the moist heat unit following the manufacturer's directions.

Popular Herbals

Today many clients ask for all-natural or herbal body baths, treatments, and facials (Table 21–3). As an esthetician, it is important that you familiarize yourself with herbs and essential oils and what they do (Figure 21–16).

Table 21–3 Ingredients for an Herbal Scrub

INGREDIENTS	BENEFIT AND FUNCTION
Liquid soap base	Cleanses
Finely ground oat powder	Soothes
Honey	Moisturizes; antibacterial
Almond meal	Moisturizes
Walnut leaf powder	Skin cell regeneration; weakened cell reconstitution
Apricot kernel oil	Nutritious
Vitamin E oil	Antioxidant

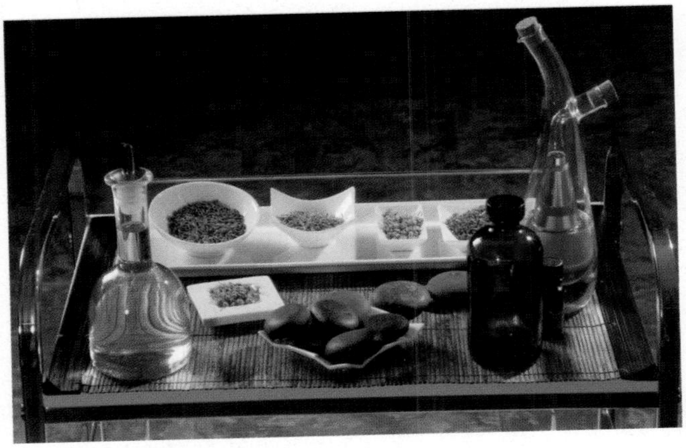

Figure 21–16 Herbs.

One of the common uses for herbs is the herbal bath. Herbal baths and medicinal bathing (also referred to as **thalassotherapy** or **hydrotherapy**), was traditionally utilized as a cosmetic, hygienic, and medicinal treatment. Herbal baths were employed in the treatment of skin conditions, including acne, dermatitis, eczema, psoriasis, and scalp itching, flaking, and dandruff. Herbal bath teas combine benefits of herbal aromatherapy and direct application of herbal nutrients to the skin. They are used as a body bath, footbath, herbal wrap, and as aromatherapy herbal pillows.

Herbal scrubs are fairly easy to perform, and the results are easily repeatable. Start off with a soap base and mix ingredients into the soap, one at a time, until you have achieved a paste. Massage this into the skin, working up a creamy lather. Rinse off, using a warm moist towel to remove any leftover material. Add a light moisturizer, if needed, or proceed with your next treatment.

The herbs in an herbal wrap typically consist of detoxifying, toning, stimulating, or relaxing and soothing herbs (Table 21–4). Detoxifying herbs may include eucalyptus, clove, rosemary, and ginger root. Soothing and relaxing herbs may include bergamot, cedar, chamomile, jasmine, patchouli, marjoram, sage, lavender, comfrey, and burdock. Body wraps differ from manufacturer to manufacturer, as well as in result desired.

CAUTION!

Be aware of any contraindications and your client's health history before using herbs in your therapies. For example, rosemary is contraindicative to individuals with high blood pressure, and clove and allspice can be very skin sensitizing. Use herbs sparingly.

Essential Oils and Wraps

In the context of spa treatments, aromatherapy is defined as the use of essential oils during facials, massages, and body treatments. These services incorporate essential oils at different times during the treatment for various therapeutic benefits (Figures 21–17 and 21–18 and Table 21–5).

The most common method involves massaging the diluted essential oils onto the body. The essential oil is

Table 21–4 Herbs Used in Wraps

HERB	FORM	BENEFIT
Allspice	Berry	Effective with arthritis and sore muscles; mild anesthetic
Basil	Leaf	Stimulates
Burdock	Root	Relieves bruises and inflammation
Clove	Stems	Astringent properties
Comfrey	Leaf	Soothes
Eucalyptus	Leaf	Increases blood circulation
Ginger	Root	Increases circulation; detoxifying agent
Lavender	Flower	Soothes
Rosemary	Leaf	Astringent; tones; stimulates
Sage	Leaf	Muscle relaxant

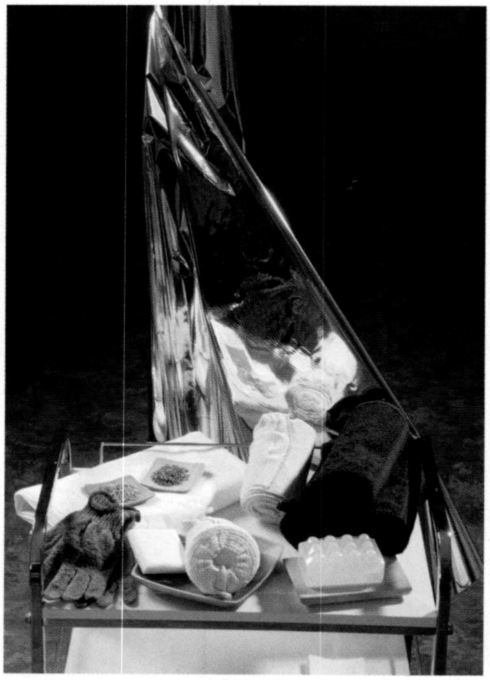

Figure 21–17 Wrap materials.

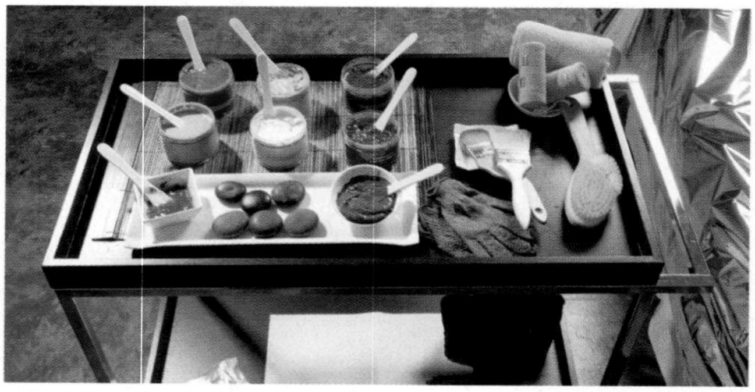

Figure 21–18 Supplies needed for wraps.

always mixed with carrier oil and is never applied directly to the body. Application of diluted oils should be done after the wrap due to fact that this could increase sensitivity or the client could have a toxic overload.

Cellophane, Space Blankets, or Foil Wrapping Agents

A foil or **cellophane body wrap** is designed to aid the detoxification process by locking in heat, moisture, vitamins, and minerals. It is designed to work with the body's own natural heat. The benefit of using these items is that in most cases they are disposable. Once you begin to work with algae, seaweed, and some masks, you will realize they stain the linens. Foil or cellophane wrap agents can form a protective barrier between the solutions used in your treatment and your linens.

Table 21–5 Supplies Needed for Wraps and Masks

ITEM	PURPOSE
Treatment table	According to service
Disposable undergarments	For client or use modesty towels
Treatment gown	For client modesty, depending on treatment
Headband or hair wrap	To protect the client's hair
Clean bandages, plastic, cellophane, metallic spa sheet or space blanket	Depends on treatment
Tape measure	To measure the client before and after treatment, if performing a slimming body wrap
Bowls (plastic)	To mix products as needed
Spatulas/brushes	To apply treatment products
Water	Used to mix with powder ingredients and masks; also need a glass of water for the client readily available
Clays, masks, herbs, essential oils, marine algae, or seaweed	Treatment products
Thermal blankets	To maintain heat (if required)
Client record card	To assess client and record details of treatment
Shower facility	To cleanse the skin before treatment and remove treatment products following a treatment
Exfoliating gloves	To break up masks for removal
Hot, steamed towels	To remove product if no shower is available

Blanket Wraps

Blanket wraps are used in place of the elastic body wrap. They involve the application of a blanket after a treatment to maintain heat or to cool the body. A typical application of a blanket wrap may include a mud bath followed by a shower, a soak in a mineral bath, or relaxation time in a steam room (Figure 21–19). This is followed by a wrap with a large cotton blanket that envelops the client like a cocoon for quiet and relaxation. The blanket wrap may be followed with a massage. This series truly demonstrates a full body spa experience.

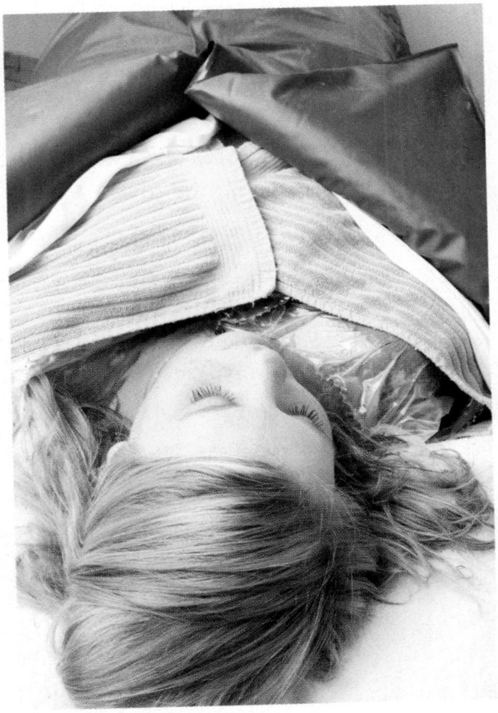

Figure 21–19 Sea mud full body wrap.

Dry Blanket Wraps or Cool Moist Blanket Wraps

You can use a dry blanket wrap after the client's core body temperature has increased in heated water or in the body treatment. It begins with a first-layer wrapping in a light cotton blanket, followed by a heavier wool one. This accelerates the release of toxins from the body. It is always recommended that the client drink plenty of water afterward to help rehydrate his or her system.

In the instances of cool, moist blanket wraps, the goal is to cool the client. In the case of treating sensitized or sunburned skin, you may apply an aloe vera mixture to the first blanket in which the client is wrapped and then follow it with another to prevent evaporation. Cool, moist blanket wraps also promote a soothing and comforting outcome.

Kneipp Body Wraps

The **Kneipp body wraps** were developed by a Bavarian monk, Father Sebastian Kneipp, who believed that disease could be cured by using water to eliminate waste from the body and that the cornerstone of health was through lifestyle, health education, and self-responsibility. Kneipp developed more than 100 different hydrotherapy treatments using water in solid, liquid, and vapor forms. His treatments included washings, wraps, packs, compresses, steam, and baths.

A Kneipp wrap envelops a body part with wet and dry cloths that are either hot or cold. Effects are achieved through temperature, length of application, and additives. Increased circulation promotes the removal of metabolic wastes and increases the oxygen and nutrient supply to the skin, resulting in a healthy glow.

Soothing Leg Treatment

For the following procedure (Figure 21–20), you will need a bottle of mineral water, preferably bottled at the source of a hot or thermal spring. The water will be used to rinse the skin in place of toner or regular water. This will help remineralize the skin and prevent stripping of the acid mantle usually caused by chlorine and processing by products in normal tap water.

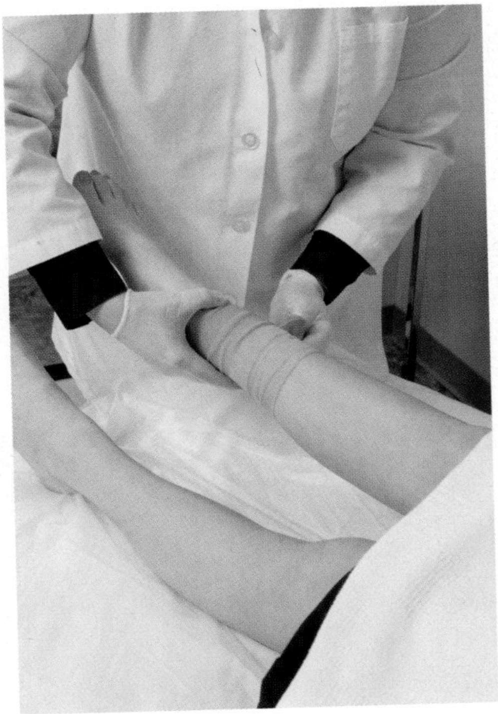

Figure 21–20 Leg wrap.

PROCEDURE 21–4 SOOTHING LEG TREATMENT

MATERIALS AND IMPLEMENTS

- Facial lounge with spa setup of linens and towels
- Section of protective plastic about 3 feet wide and 4 feet long
- Section of protective plastic about 6 feet wide and 4 feet long
- Fango or other mud
- Mineral water
- Cotton bandages or cloths
- Exfoliating granules
- Basin of hot water
- Ampoule appropriate for skin treatment
- Moisturizing cream appropriate for skin treatment
- Thermal blanket
- Decanting cups for supplies
- Mask brush
- Gloves (optional)
- Pressotherapy equipment (optional)

Preparation

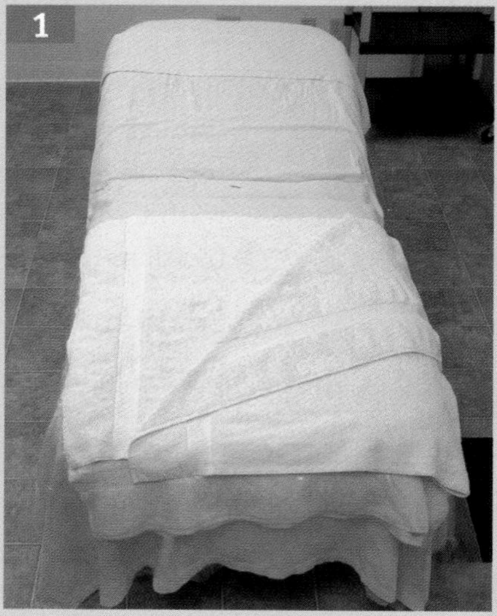

Prepare treatment table.

1 Prepare the treatment table with bottom linens and blankets.

2 Place the large plastic drape on the lower half of the bed. Place a towel over this to make handling easier.

3 Place the small plastic covering on top of this towel.

4 Place the top sheet or towel on top of the plastic covering.

5 Prepare the mixture of mineral water, fango mud, and exfoliating granules in a bowl. Keep in mind the client's skin type when choosing the level of exfoliation.

6 Review client health history to ensure that the client is still a candidate for this treatment.

7 Tell the client what to expect during the treatment.

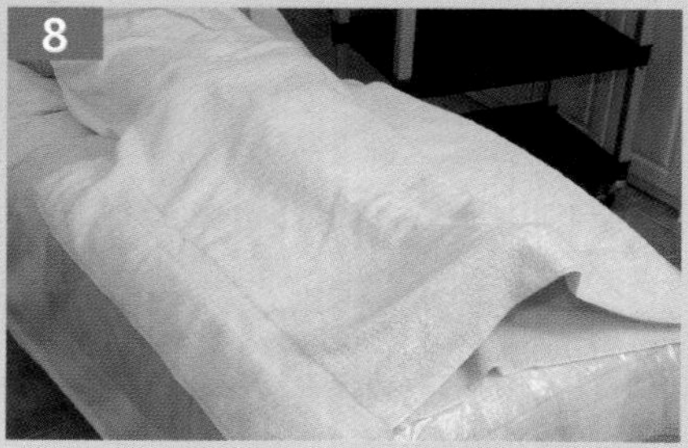

Instruct client to get onto the treatment table just below the top sheet.

8 Instruct the client to get onto the treatment table just below the top sheet or towel while you wait outside the room.

Procedure

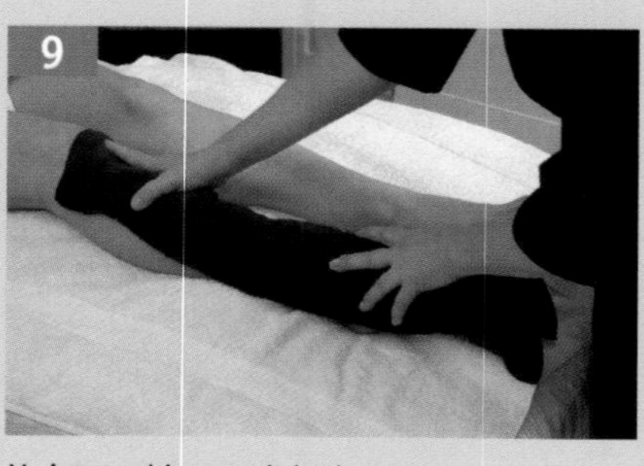

Moisten skin on right leg.

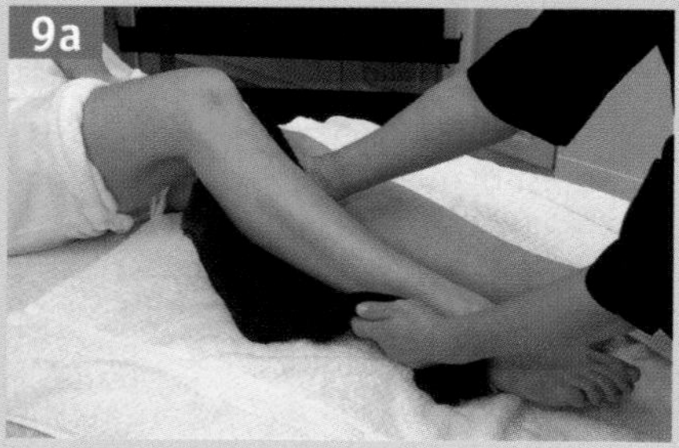

Moisten back side of the thigh area.

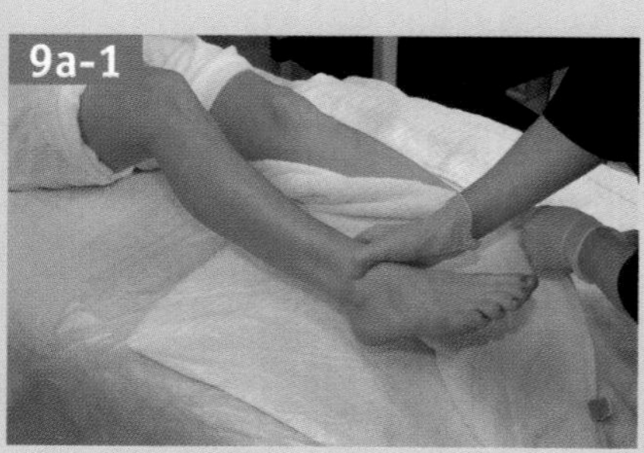

Place client's legs on the plastic.

9 Starting with right leg, moisten the skin by wiping the leg with a hot, wet towel. Have the client bend the knee to facilitate getting to the back of the thigh. Remove the towel and place client's legs on the plastic.

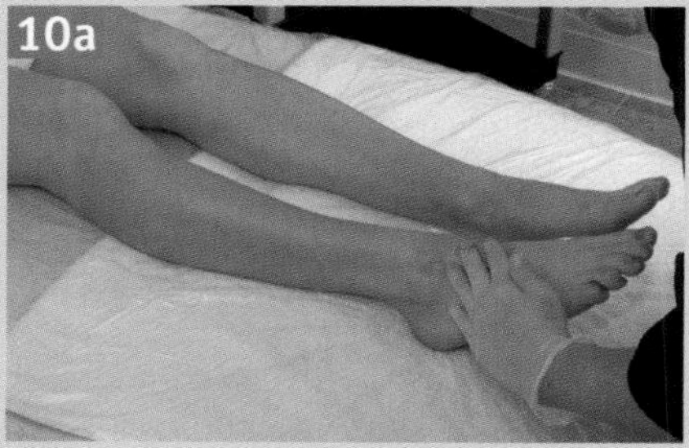

Start at the feet and work up the leg in circular motions.

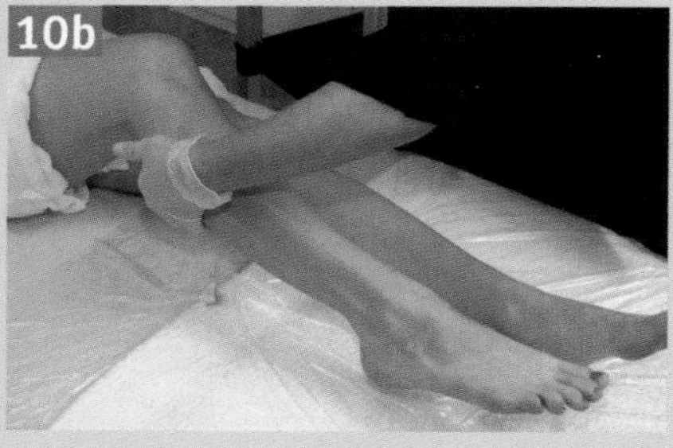

Apply the mixture to the front and back of leg.

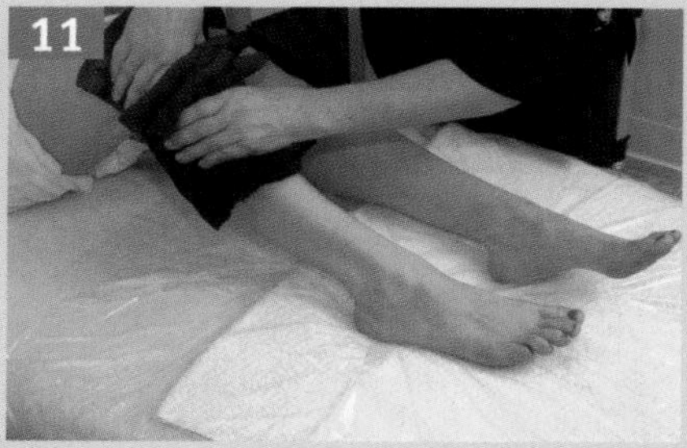

Remove the product.

10 Now on the moist skin, begin applying a mixture of thermal or mineral water, fango mud, and exfoliating granules.

a. Start at the feet and work up the leg, using upward, gentle circular motions with your hands. Be careful to avoid any scratched or wounded areas.

b. Gently raise the right knee. Apply the mixture to the front and back of leg.

11 Using the same steps as above, remove the product thoroughly with warm, moist towels that have been soaked in mineral water and warmed in towel cabinet.

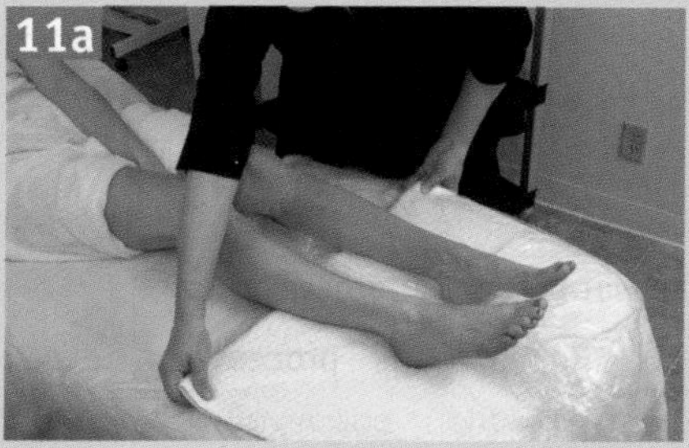

Slide plastic drape toward other leg.

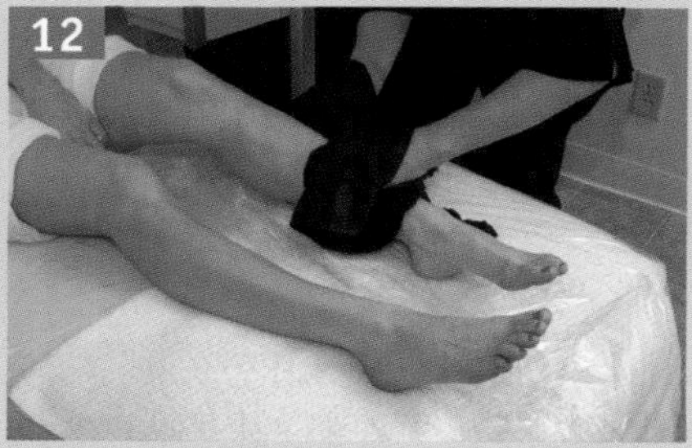

Repeat steps on left leg.

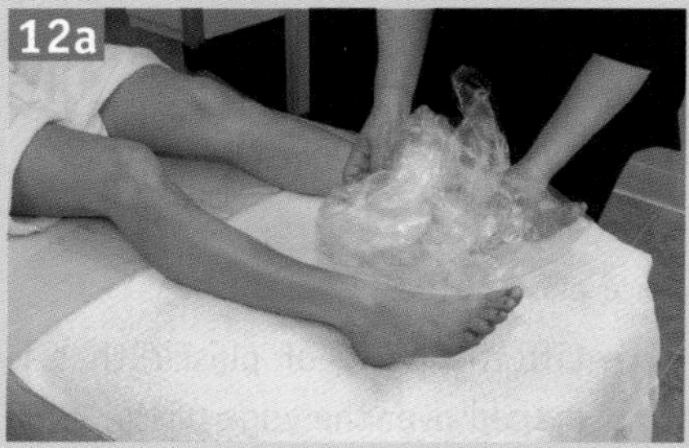

Slide the plastic drape from under the client and remove.

a. Slide the plastic drape that is under the client's leg toward the other leg (the center of his or her body).

b. Re-drape the client.

12 Repeat this process for the left leg. As you remove product from this leg, slide the plastic drape from under the client and remove.

The client is now laying on the towel on top of the second sheet of plastic.

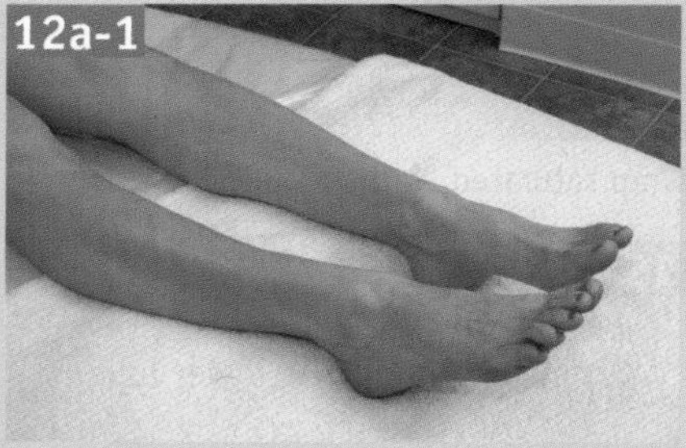

Client should be on the towel on top of the second sheet of plastic.

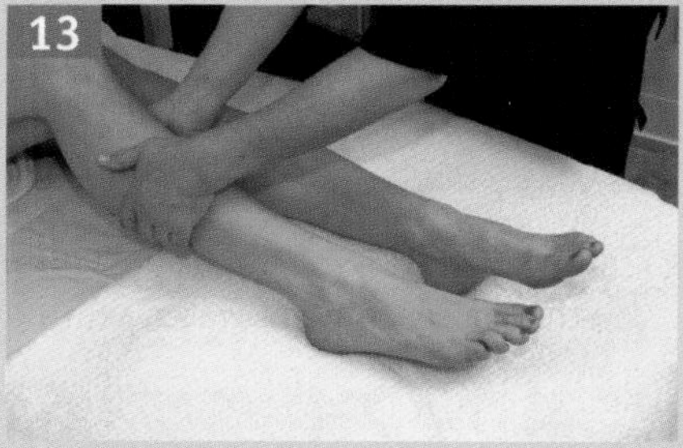

Apply mixture to front and back of the right leg.

13 Starting with right leg and using the same process as previously described, apply a mixture of ampoule and cream to the front and back of the leg.

continues on next page

HYDROTHERAPY AND OTHER SPECIALTY TREATMENTS

The Vichy Shower

The Vichy shower is thought to have originated in Vichy France, where the hot mineral springs have made the area one of the foremost locations for spas in Europe. This treatment can be incorporated into a diversity of body treatments (Figure 21–21). A key benefit for the client is that they stay relaxed on the table rather than having to get up and go to the shower. Many clients love the cascading sensation of the water.

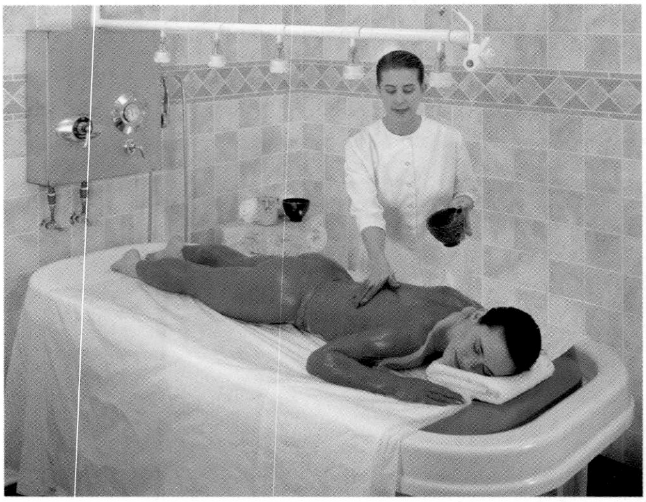

Figure 21–21 Vichy shower table being used for a body treatment.

The first step for a shower treatment is to empty the water pipes of the water that has been standing and has become cold and adjust the water temperature. The client must not be under the showerhead when you first turn it on or when you adjust the temperature, and the temperature must not exceed 104°F. Once you have achieved the optimal temperature, briefly close the valve while positioning the client on the table. Once the client is comfortable and lying on the table, open the valve and adjust the angle and volume of the heads as desired.

The second step is to adjust the intensity to the desired pressure. Pressures range from a fine mist to a jet and can be adjusted by twisting the head valves and using the optional handheld wand. After the treatment, drain all water from the heads by opening and closing the shower head valves until the water is absent.

Scotch Hose

A **Scotch hose** is a hose that projects water to stimulate the client from 10 to 12 feet away. This is a projection treatment as opposed to a shower treatment. Therapists are expertly trained to massage the client in specific precise patterns as opposed to an overall shower coverage. When operating the Scotch hose, remember to hold the hose when turning on the water and never let go of the nozzle when the water is flowing. You will remove the hose from the nozzle holder, turn on the water, and initially direct it toward the floor and drain until you have achieved an optimal temperature, which never exceeds 104°F. Please note that increasing or decreasing pressure will also affect the temperature. After using the hose to deliver an invigorating massage, empty the water from the hose and return the hose to the nozzle holder.

Baths

While baths may be used as herbal treatments, they also have other uses (Figure 21–22). Historically, the earliest recorded use of baths is attributed to the Romans. Some baths were located in upscale private residences but the public baths were popular gathering places for social interaction, dining, and relaxation.

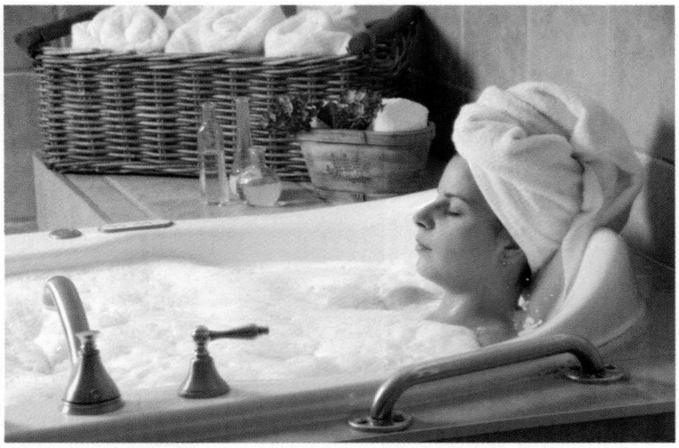

Figure 21–22 Baths have a significant value in stress reduction.

Following the example of the Romans, some spas offer communal pools of varying hot and cold temperature where clients may soak at their leisure. Resort spas may incorporate cultural bathing rituals and re-create the ambiance specific to those traditions. Japanese baths, Swedish bath houses, and mineral pool baths from local springs are all examples of the rites of the bath.

Private treatment room baths may be intended for soaking before or after another treatment or they may incorporate jetted systems of air or water. Essential oils may be added to the tub or rose petals floated on the water for beauty and ambiance. Some jetted tubs are equipped with a wand that the trained hydrotherapist uses for a water massage procedure. Tubs range from very basic claw-foot retro units to highly sophisticated computerized systems with programmed treatments that vary water pressure patterns along the body. While different bath protocols call for different water temperatures, client comfort is paramount. If clients do not enjoy a treatment, they will probably not repeat it.

While ambiance is important, so is safety. When purchasing a tub, look for a design that allows a client to enter and exit the tub safely.

It is imperative to properly disinfect the unit between clients; the labor involved is one reason these units are often not used to capacity. Always follow state and CDC guidelines for disinfection and sterilization, as well as manufacturer recommendations for cleaning the tub and using any disinfectants.

Raindrop Therapy

Raindrop therapy is a specialized massage with essential oils performed by trained massage therapists. Raindrop therapy originated almost two decades ago, a result of collaborative research between Dr. D. Gary Young and a Lakota medicine man. The therapy integrates a specialized massage technique/stroke with massage and essential oils to bring the body into structural and electrical alignment. Raindrop therapy is based on the theory that many types of scoliosis (a physical finding in which curvature of the spine is present) and spinal misalignments are caused by viruses or bacteria that lie dormant along the spine. These pathogens create inflammation, which, in turn, controls and disfigures the spinal column. Over the years this treatment has been found to be beneficial for its role in relaxing and detoxifying clients and in general wellness enhancement.

In raindrop therapy, specified oils are sequentially dispensed like little drops of rain six inches above the back and massaged along the vertebrae. The oils continue to work in the body for five to seven days following a treatment, with continued realignment and detoxification taking place during this time. The key to using the blends of oils is patience. Once the frequencies begin to balance in these areas, a structural alignment can occur. This treatment is relaxing, rebalancing, and beneficial to all clients who enjoy essential oil massage. Other effective uses of essential oils are adding a scent to your linens or towels, dispersing the aroma into the air during treatments, or performing a scalp massage with aromatic oils (Figure 21–23).

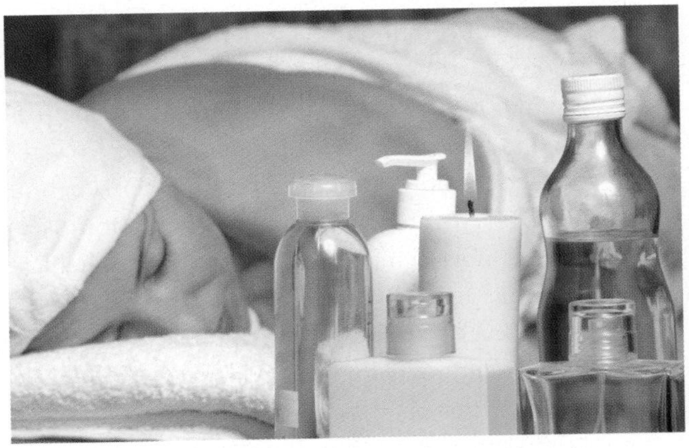

Figure 21–23 Aromatherapy is an important attribute of spa treatments.

Music Therapy

Modern science is confirming the ancient wisdom that music is medicine for the body, mind, and spirit. Sound, like light, travels in waves through the air and is measured in frequencies and intensities. Sound frequency refers to pitch—the high or low quality of sounds—and is measured in hertz (Hz), the number of cycles per second at which the wave vibrates. The lower the pitch, the slower the vibration; the higher the pitch, the faster the vibration. The research of Dr. Alfred Tomatis has established the healing and creative powers of sound and music.

> ***Here's a Tip***
>
> Given the power of music, estheticians need to be aware of what music they play in spas and salons.

Music's therapeutic effects include the following:

- Brain waves slow down and equalize. Certain baroque and New Age music can shift the consciousness from excited beta waves to resting state alpha waves.
- Mozart or Baroque help focus conscious awareness and increase mental organization.

- Gregorian chants and New Age music deepen and slow the breathing, which calms the mind.
- Heartbeat, pulse rate, and blood pressure are lowered with easy listening and softer music.
- Stress hormones in the blood decline significantly when a person listens to relaxing, soft music.
- The Mozart effect claims certain types of music, as well as singing and chanting, can short-term improve performance of certain types of mental tasks.
- Vibroacoustic therapy, developed by Norwegian Olave Skille, is a musical bath, wherein the client is immersed in a specific range of sounds either in water or on a bed, resulting in reduced muscle tension and improved body movement and coordination. The technique is now being used for a variety of medical conditions. Esthetically, it assists relaxation.
- Endorphin levels can increase with music, inducing a natural high and reducing pain.
- Perception of time changes with specific musical selections. Classical and Baroque music provokes orderly behavior, whereas highly romantic or New Age music softens stressful situations and seems to make time stand still.
- Productivity increases with the type of music one listens to. Classical music has been shown to increase work accuracy by 21.3%, whereas popular music only demonstrated an improvement of 2.4%.
- Memory has been enhanced using music and Dr. Georgi Lozanov's methodology.
- Music can create a sense of well-being and safety.

When working in a spa, you must consider many issues related to treatments: client confidentiality, privacy, health screening, indications and contraindications, and client preparation and comfort are all important factors. There is an unlimited number of spa body treatments available to you today to offer to your clients. First look at the space and equipment available. Investigate your market and decide which treatments best fit your clientele. Today's full-service spa offers a wide array of body treatments and hydrotherapy services, including body wraps and masks, Vichy showers, and hydrotherapy tubs.

REVIEW QUESTIONS

1. What are some table selection considerations for body treatments?
2. Discuss client security issues.
3. Why is it important to discuss how you handle privacy with your client?
4. Explain the benefits of one type of spa treatment.
5. What is the most popular spa treatment and why?
6. What are some differences in setup between a facial treatment and a body treatment?
7. Why should you never leave a client unattended during a treatment?
8. Discuss the pros and cons of bath treatments.
9. What are three benefits of a body treatment?
10. What are some benefits of a bath ritual?
11. Describe raindrop therapy.
12. Discuss the impact of music in a treatment.
13. Which type of music helps calm the mind?
14. Which type of music helps reduce stress?

CHAPTER GLOSSARY

blanket wraps: the application of a blanket after a treatment to maintain heat or to cool the body.

body mask: a body treatment involving the application of an exfoliating, hydrating, purification or detoxification mask to the entire body. Masks may include those with clay, cream, gel, or seaweed bases.

cellophane body wrap: a wrap that uses a plastic material to aid in the penetration of the product through means of producing or increasing perspiration.

diaphoretic: describes the acts of producing or increasing perspiration.

elastic wraps: bandages that can be rolled around a client and have an elastic composition allowing a tight and secure wrap.

herb wraps: body wrap treatment that includes the soaking of the wrap in an herbal tea blend prior to application.

hydrocollators: dry heat units that heat thermal packs to an optimal temperature. Commonly used in massage therapy, chiropactic or physical therapy practices.

hydrotherapy: spa treatments that use water.

Kneipp body wraps: wraps that envelop a body part with wet and dry cloths that are either hot or cold. Effects are achieved through temperature, length of application, and additives.

moist heat unit: units designed to hold water and to head linen wraps to an optimal temperature. Commonly herbal blends are added to the water.

Scotch hose: hose similar to a fire hose used in water therapy.

seaweed wraps: wraps that include application of a seaweed mask followed by a thermal blanket to seal in heat.

thalassotherapy: therapeutic use of sea water.

Vichy shower: overhead shower with adjustable water pressure used in body treatments.

wet room: a room lined with tile or other water impervious material and drains to service water treatments such as a Vichy shower.

CHAPTER 22

ALTERNATIVE THERAPIES

CHAPTER OUTLINE

- THE HISTORY OF ALTERNATIVE MEDICINE
- ENERGY BASICS
- ENERGY MANAGEMENT
- THE CHAKRA SYSTEM
- REIKI HANDS-ON HEALING
- ENERGY MEDICINES
- CRYSTALS AND GEMSTONES
- INTRODUCING ENERGY-BALANCING TREATMENTS TO CLIENTS

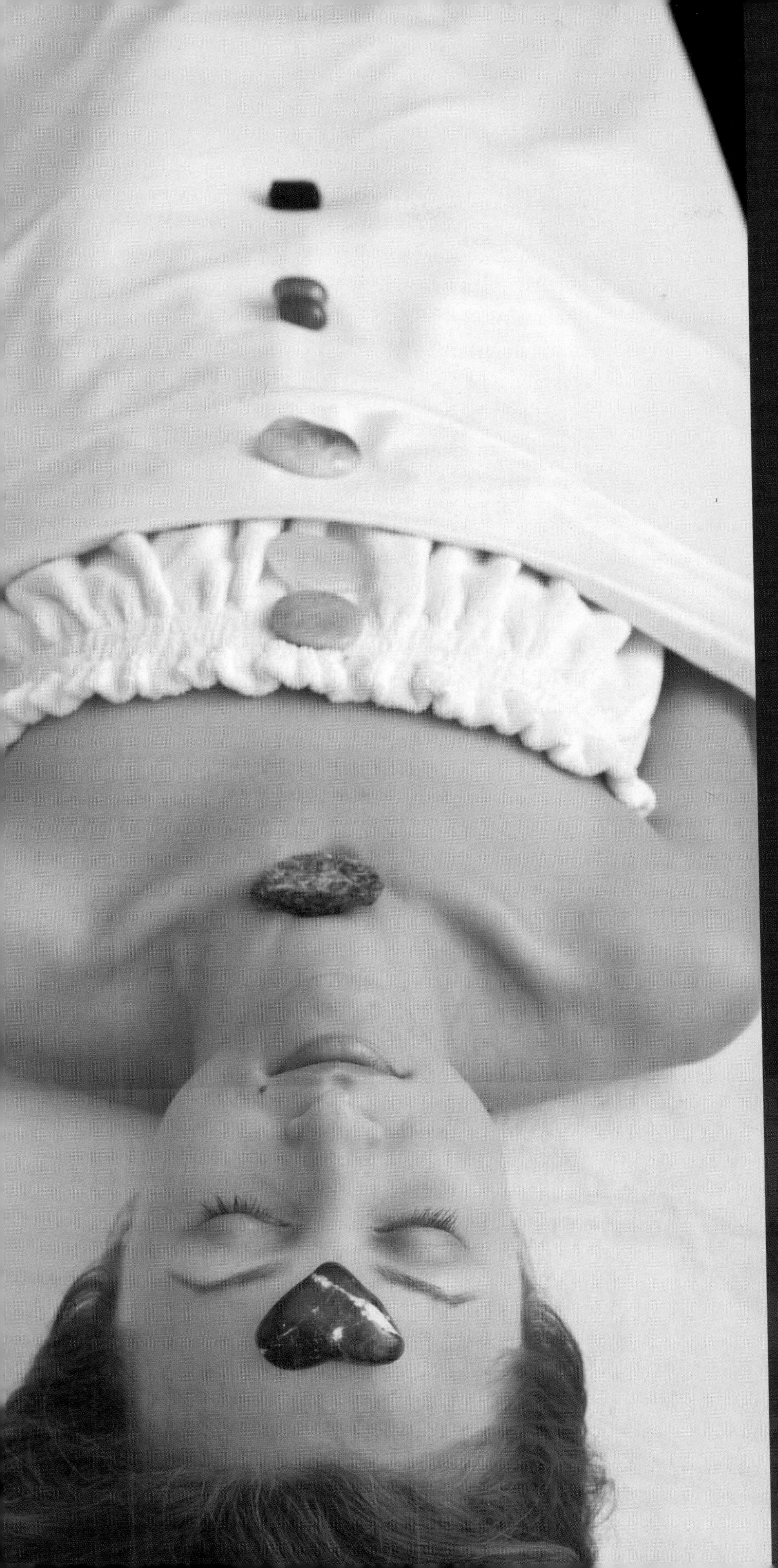

LEARNING OBJECTIVES

When you complete this chapter, you should be able to:

- Understand and perform various healing modalities.
- Explain how alternative therapies benefit daily life.
- Select alternative healing products for home care to sell from your facility.
- Select your healing stone collection.
- Know placement for hands-on treatments and gemstones.

KEY TERMS

Page numbers indicate where in the chapter the term is used.

balance 603
Chakras 608
complementary 615
crystals 614
emotional body 606
energy management 605
gemstones 613
Leaky Aura Syndrome 604
mental body 605
mental chatter 606
Reiki 608
Reiki attunement 612
spirit/energy body 607

True beauty comes from being balanced in body, mind, and spirit. When in **balance,** you represent your personal best qualities. When you are stressed or out of balance, the flip side of these qualities shows up. There really is no good or bad or right or wrong. Only you acting out of a balanced state or a out-of-balance state. To reveal your inner beauty, it is essential that you clear away stress, mental chatter, and negative energy to reveal your true self. You then automatically radiate your true essence, becoming authentic both inside and out.

You are unique and individual with innate talents that no one else can do quite like you do. When you focus on doing what you do best, there is no competition. You inspire others just by being you. The best way to attract positive, healthy clients who are happy to pay your fees is to be the best *you* possible. This chapter reveals ways to de-stress, quiet the negative self-talk in your mind, and calm your emotions so you can feel at peace and confident in your work. When you are able to find balance for yourself, you become the example that others want to follow.

Estheticians can now provide products and treatments using a variety of alternative healing techniques that encourage clients to schedule appointments on a weekly basis. When you focus on balancing the whole person, you help to heal emotional, mental, and physical aspects as well. These treatments help to reduce stress and anxiety by quieting mental chatter and calming the emotions, so you and your clients feel more at peace and centered and experience more intuitive insights. The difference is rejuvenation versus relaxation.

THE HISTORY OF ALTERNATIVE MEDICINE

The use of hands-on healing, plant medicines, and gemstones is not new. What we now call complementary and alternative medicine (CAM) was once the only medicine. For thousands of years, indigenous peoples have used and still use Mother Nature's bounty as a part of daily life. They believe that there is no separation between self and the environment. The spirit of man, nature, and the universe are one and the same. If someone is out of balance, nature can fill the void to restore balance. Therefore, what we do to nature, we do to ourselves, and vice versa.

With the inception of the industrial age, man came to view himself as separate from nature. Science became the only acceptable practice; leaving traditional methods of medicine and healing to be called primitive. Slowly, people started to separate from their receptive, intuitive selves to validate the logical, linear aspects of the mind.

Famous physicist Albert Einstein recognized this separation as creating a prison, writing: "A human being is part of the whole, called by us 'universe,' a part limited in time and space. He experiences himself, his thoughts and feelings as separate from the rest, a kind of optical delusion of his own consciousness." He believed that the only way to free ourselves from this prison was by "widening our circle of compassion to embrace all living creatures, the whole of nature and its beauty." (http://www.quoteworld.org).

Today, there is a resurgence of traditional practices focusing on the wholeness of nature as people feel the need to return to more natural roots. As an esthetician, you are a prime candidate to incorporate these services since you already provide hands-on treatments. Understanding how energy works and taking specific steps to enhance your techniques, you can set yourself apart from others using some of the CAM therapies offered in this chapter.

ENERGY BASICS

Energy is the basis for everything and is found in humans, animals, nature, and objects. Without energy you do not have vitality and life force. Within this energy field is a vibration or frequency that includes specific characteristics innate to that energy. Think of a tiger's instinct to hunt, a bird's instinct to fly, and a human's instinct to crawl and then walk. How does each species know to do these things? It is innate within the energy blueprint of the spirit.

Each person is born vibrant, whole, and full of his or her own spirit energy. Think of babies and small children at play. Ever notice how they radiate? They are full of their own energy and they beam. All of life is an adventure and they are full of spirit in their actions. You get pleasure watching them as they are so free and delightful to be around.

> **? Did You Know**
>
> *Spirit, energy body,* or *essence* are interchangeable words to describe the life force energy of all living things. Use the word or words that are most comfortable to you and your beliefs.

As you grow up, you become programmed and, little by little, you leave your energy behind. You fall and hurt yourself and leave a little energy there, your parents scold you and you leave more energy there, you get teased by others, and on and on. Life's experiences affect your spirit. By the time you reach adulthood, the energy body that was once whole and complete now looks like Swiss cheese. This is an analogy, of course, but you can understand these effects as they relate to feeling exhausted and out of touch with what matters most to you.

Your spirit has two parts, an inner face and an outer face. The inner face is the subtle energy body called the *Chakra system*. The outer face is the spirit energy that comes from within and exudes beyond the body called the *aura*. This unified energy field contributes to the health of the physical, mental, and emotional bodies.

Your aura is an energy bubble that surrounds you approximately 1 to 12 inches from your body. This bubble is semipermeable and moves with you when you move. As you approach other people, you bump up against their energy bubble. When this happens, you experience their energy and they experience yours. Some energy will resonate with yours and some may repel you.

When you are full of your own energy, the only energy that can penetrate is conscious spirit energy collected by the Chakras. When you have "energy gaps" from many years of leaving bits and pieces of your energy behind, you leave yourself open to absorbing other energies indiscriminately. Remember the analogy of Swiss cheese? This is called **Leaky Aura Syndrome**. The result is feeling exhausted, feeling other people's pain, sadness, anxiety and other unwanted energies.

As you consciously focus on filling your "energy gaps," you remove the holes where other energies might leak in. You feel protected and are able to perform treatments without the fear of absorbing unwanted energy. Most people try to gain more energy by focusing on the physical body alone. Although this may help, your attention would be better spent on rejuvenating the energy body. Following are some methods for balancing each aspect of the entire person.

FYI

Kirlian cameras, invented by a Russian couple, Semyon and Valentina Kirlian, in the 1930s, are used to photograph the colors of the aura so that people without psychic vision are able to see the energy of the Chakras made visible. Figure 22–1a was taken before any energy work had taken place. Figure 22–1b was taken minutes after the subject received energy balancing.

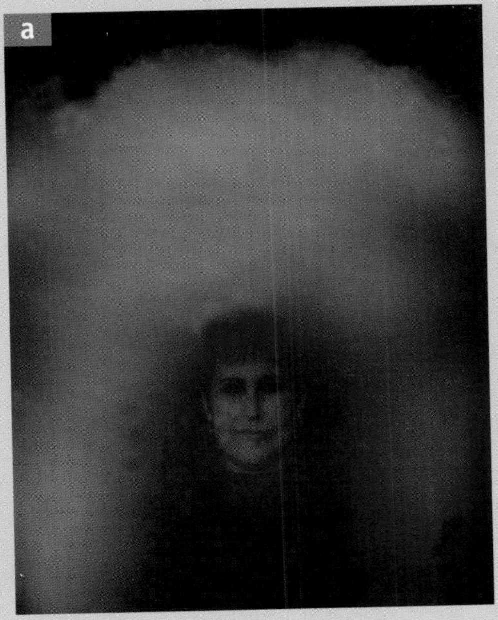

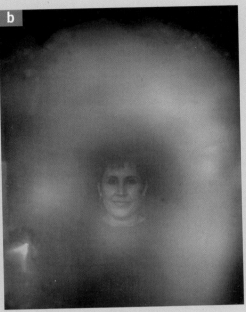

Figure 22–1a Aura picture before.

Figure 22–1b Aura picture after.

ENERGY MANAGEMENT

The phrase "balancing body, mind, and spirit" has been used for years in the context of health and wellness. While many people refer to it, there has been no simple way to understand and discuss the topic with clients. Balancing body, mind, and spirit really covers four areas: the physical, mental, emotional, and spirit bodies. Each has its own intelligence, characteristic qualities, and best methods for reaching balance. **Energy management** is a multisensory system that you can incorporate into your practice to help your clients reach and maintain balance in each of these areas (Figure 22–2).

The Four Bodies

The physical body is a body you are familiar with. It has sensory intelligence connected with the sensory nervous system. You can see, feel, hear, taste, and touch. Your sensory nature is connected to nature's rhythm and is part of your energy blueprint (Table 22–1).

? Did You Know

The same things that create free radicals also throw you off balance energetically:

- **UV Radiation**
- **Stress**
- **Alcohol**
- **Tobacco**
- **Processed foods and sugar**
- **Drugs, prescription and otherwise**

Performing treatments on yourself daily or even weekly helps you to maintain balance.

The **mental body** is your computer brain and the information that has been programmed into it through childhood and life experiences. Your brain processes information received, providing your social outlook on life and reactions to daily events; this is called *cognitive*

Energy Management Chart

Service/Product Provided		Physical Body	Mental Body	Emotional Body	Spiritual/ Energy Body
Reiki	霊気	✓	✓	✓	✓
Massage	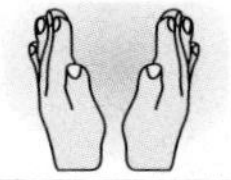	✓	some effect	some effect	some effect
Exercise/Diet	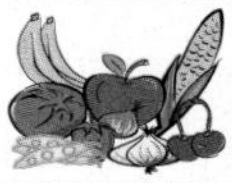	✓	some effect	some effect	some effect
Herbology/ Supplements	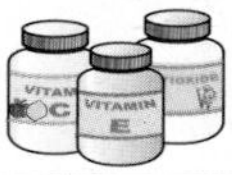	✓	✓	✓	some effect
Aromatherapy	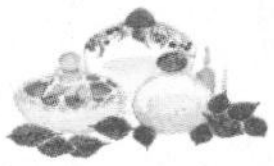	some effect	✓	✓	some effect
Music/Visualizations	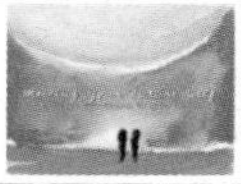	some effect	✓	✓	✓
Flower Essences	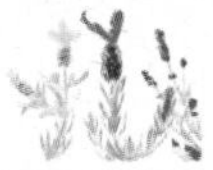	some effect	✓	✓	✓

Figure 22–2 Energy management chart.

Table 22–1 The Four Intelligences of the Physical, Mental, Emotional, and Spirit Bodies

THE FOUR INTELLIGENCES OF THE PHYSICAL, MENTAL, EMOTIONAL, AND SPIRIT BODIES		
Physical Body	Sensory Intelligence	The five senses are connected to the body's central and peripheral nervous systems. Basic intuitive instincts, such as "fight or flight" and "gut feelings" are controlled here.
Mental Body	Cognitive Intelligence	*Cognitive* refers to the rational, concrete mind and each individual's ability to gather and assess information. This information is stored in memory and becomes the individual's programmed belief system and perception on life.
Emotional Body	Feeling Intelligence	This includes a person's receptive, sub-conscious nature, which allows feelings of empathy. It is the window to the multidimensional aspects of Intuitive Intelligence in which we experience feelings of resonance at the fourth, or heart, Chakra.
Spirit/Energy Body	Intuitive Intelligence	Intuition provides the ability to connect to the collective unconscious—beyond time and space. This is where a-ha! moments and intuitive insights come from.

intelligence. With enough data, you are preconditioned to respond to a multitude of occurrences. Someone who is highly programmed is always self-conscious. He or she takes everything personally and is constantly seeking approval. **Mental chatter** is another result of programming run amok.

The **emotional body** is your innate feeling intelligence. It includes knowing your creative talents and self-worth with the ability to tell the difference between who you *are* and who others *want* you to be. Your values come from within, not from others or what you own. Your feeling intelligence is part of your inherent nature

> **Did You Know**
>
> Psychology was derived from the Greek word *psyche,* meaning "breath," a synonym for the soul. The Greeks believed that the soul, or "psyche," was responsible for one's behavior. In its original context, psychology was the study of the soul, self, and mind.

and provides access to heartfelt resonance. When something resonates in the heart, you know instinctively that it is true. You are drawn to it because it "feels" right to you. When you do not stay true to your innate values and feelings you may suffer from disorders such as depression or anxiety or even physical disease.

Your **spirit,** essence or **energy body,** is one and the same. It is your intuitive intelligence. Your spirit connects you to a sense of "knowing" that is not cognitive. It provides your life force energy and innate talents and gives you a passion for life. It radiates from within and surrounds you in your aura. When your spirit is healthy you are healthy. You make the world a better place just by being you. It is that simple. Your thoughts, actions, and consistent patterns either fill or deplete your energy. Someone with a healthy spirit has a twinkle in his or her eyes. That person's essence radiates at first glance. They have a certain presence that is appealing to be around. When someone's spirit is depleted, you see an emptiness or dullness in the eyes. He or she is not present in spirit and may even appear to be running on auto-pilot, as in the saying, "the lights are on, but nobody's home." Because the spirit is not visible to the naked eye, it frequently is ignored. Not feeding your spirit can lead to depression, anxiety, and physical disease.

Keeping the Four Bodies in Balance

Physical: To keep your physical body healthy and in balance, you need to feel safe and secure in your body and environment, exercise, eat the right foods, get proper rest and sleep, and take supplements and antioxidants for nutritional support. Reiki, hands-on healing therapy, reduces stress and balances the physical body on all levels.

Mental and Emotional: Balancing the mental and emotional bodies is similar. While exercise and diet have a positive effect on the physical body, there are items from nature that specifically target issues related to the mental and emotional bodies such as improving mental clarity and focus, quieting negative self-talk, and calming emotional stress and anxiety. Reiki, essential oils, herbs and herbal elixirs, flower essences, gemstones, and products infused with any of these energies work to balance these two bodies. Music and guided visualizations also help to balance these areas if they are uplifting to listen to.

Spirit: How do you revive a depleted spirit? It takes like to heal like. To balance the spirit you need spirit energy, such as Reiki universal life force energy, flower essences which contain plant spirit, gemstones with nature's spirit, and products infused with any of these spirit energies. Music and guided visualizations also help to heal the spirit if the vibration of the music is calibrated with spirit energy. Another way to feed the spirit is doing work, hobbies, and play that you love to do. You have innate gifts and talents that you do well regardless of training. When you utilize these talents, you feed your spirit. The pleasure of doing what you enjoy brings you vitality and feeds all of your intelligences.

USING ESSENTIAL OILS AND HERBS FOR BALANCE

Aromatherapy is an effective way to bring balance to the emotional and the mental bodies. Smell is the most powerful sense because it connects directly to the brain. Essential oils from plants and flowers contain volatile oils that are considered to be the plant's hormones. These hormones have chemical components that react with the hormone centers in the human brain, triggering some sort of physiological change. Depending on the essential oil compounds and their properties, clients who have aromatherapy treatments may experience feeling stimulated, balanced, relaxed, improved health, and more. Following are some essential oils that you can use to encourage balance in the mental and emotional bodies:

- Rosemary, peppermint, and coriander seed: Enhance mental clarity and focus
- Lavender, Roman chamomile, Melissa, clary sage, neroli: Calm the emotions
- Ylang ylang, St. John's wort, pettigrain, bergamot, lemon verbena: Lift the spirits

Herbs are plant materials that are taken internally rather than inhaled. You may choose from capsules, tablets, teas, and herbal elixirs, which are also called *herbal tinctures*. They work more on the physical body since they are ingested through the digestive tract and are assimilated through the body. The following herbs may be used to help balance the mental and emotional bodies.

- Ginkgo biloba, gotu kola, rosemary, peppermint: Enhance mental clarity and memory recall
- Scullcap, lemon balm, chamomile: Calm the emotions
- St. John's wort, oatstraw, lemon balm: Lift the spirits

Another excellent method for soothing, reenergizing and re-balancing is conscious breathing in a mini-meditation. When you are feeling stressed or stuck, deep breathing and Reiki offer a quick fix that can be done anywhere or any time, eyes open or closed. Place one or both hands on your second and fourth Chakras. Expand your abdomen as you take a deep, deep breath that fills your lungs, and hold it for two to three seconds. Release your breath through the mouth completely before you inhale again.

Think of what you would like more of and breathe in that quality. Release unwanted energies with each exhale. Try some of the qualities listed here:

- Breathe in Acceptance and breathe out Judgments.
- Breathe in Confidence and breathe out Doubt.
- Breathe in Gratitude and breathe out Resentment.
- Breathe in Abundance and breathe out Limitations.
- Breathe in Peacefulness and breathe out Anxiety.
- Breathe in Love and breathe out Anger.
- Breathe in Awareness and breathe out Fear.

Make up your own affirmations and focus on what you want to create more of in your life.

THE CHAKRA SYSTEM

There are seven major energy centers within the subtle energy body, called **Chakras,** that circulate life force energy throughout the body (Figure 22–3). The Chakras are like the organs of your spirit. In the physical body, if your organs are healthy and functioning at their optimal level, you have physical health. When the Chakras are balanced and operating at their optimal level, you have energetic health. The energy body feeds the physical body and the physical body feeds the energy body. One system supports the other.

Dating back nearly 2,600 years, the word *Chakra* comes from the Sanskrit word meaning "wheel of light." Aligned in the center of the body near the spinal column, each Chakra represents a different aspect of your essence and personality and is associated with a color, sense, sound, endocrine gland, and organs. They collect universal spirit energy and distribute it throughout the body. The energy of the Chakras radiates from within and surrounds you in your aura. The colors of the aura represent the health of both the physical and spirit bodies.

Everything starts on an energy level. Being consistently out of balance energetically can affect the health of the associated organs as well as mental, emotional, and spiritual health. Take a look at Table 22–2 for a brief description of the Chakras, their associated color, sense, note, organ(s), and endocrine gland.

The Chakra system represents many aspects of your life and personal growth. Chakras one through three are foundation Chakras and relate to the physical, material world—who you are, your perception of life, how others view you, and how you represent yourself. These Chakras also have to do with programming and conditioning—what you learned from your family and social environment while growing up. Living through social programming, you can only react to circumstances. You speak and see only what you believe to be possible—what is referred to as "operating on autopilot."

Spiritual development is connected with Chakras four through seven as they represent you on a conscious level. Operating through the upper four Chakras, you have use of all of your intelligences—feeling, intuitive, sensory and cognitive. You have connection to your heart, voice, vision, and intuitive insight to create your life rather than react to it. You receive information from a higher source, have clear vision of the big picture, and know how you fit into the picture. You are able to speak clearly about your vision from the heart. When you come from this place, you feel at peace and comfortable in your own skin and environment. Feeling comfortable in your body, you connect to a sense of purpose and have passion for life. By offering services to balance the Chakras you are assisting clients to reconnect to their whole self—body, mind, and spirit. Anything with spirit energy will work to balance the Chakra system. Review Table 22–2 for information on each Chakra.

REIKI HANDS-ON HEALING

Reiki, pronounced *ray'-key*, is a healing and balancing energy transmitted through the palms of the hands that lifts your spirits and allows you to come into balance. Beyond relaxation, Reiki calms the emotions and quiets the mind, leaving you with a sense of inner peace and knowing. It is one of the few healing arts that works to balance the entire person—the physical, mental, emotional, and spiritual aspects of each individual.

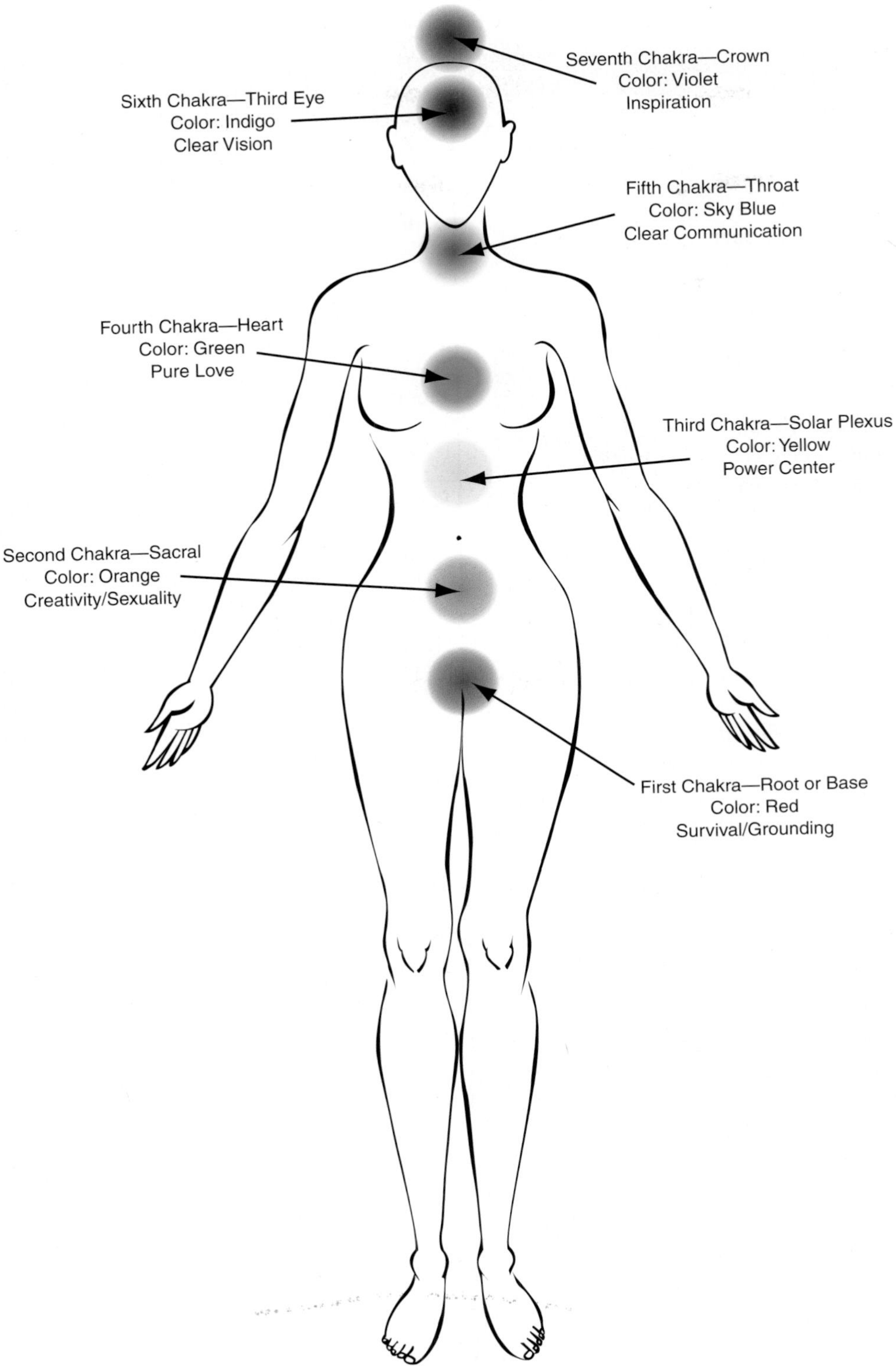

Figure 22–3 Chakra Chart.

Rei means "universal, the spirit energy that surrounds and permeates everything," and *ki* means "life force energy, your personal spirit energy that comes from within." Combine these two energies and you have a very powerful balancing and healing potential. By learning a simple series of hand positions covering the Chakra system, you can add value to your services and facials. Although Reiki does not include massage manipulations, you can intersperse Reiki hand positions into your current facial massage and procedure.

Table 22–2 Chakra Descriptions

CHAKRA	COLOR	GLANDS/ORGANS	
Seventh—Crown: intuitive intelligence The seventh Chakra is your personal connection to universal energy. This Chakra connects you to innate knowing, allowing insights and intuitive intelligence to come through. When you are open at this Chakra you have understanding of universal wisdom and a sense of union to all. Blocking the seventh Chakra can lead to lack of connection, feeling empty, despair, or depressed.	**Violet** Inspirational, Wise, Illuminating	**Element** Cosmic Energy **Sense** 7th Sense	**Glands/Organs** Pineal, CNS, Cerebral Cortex, Right Eye **Note** B
Sixth—Third Eye: holistic mind, visionary The sixth Chakra is your center for clear vision. It allows you to see the big picture and where you fit into the big picture. This Chakra is considered the holistic mind, allowing you to develop the systems to realize your vision. Out of balance you lack vision related to life purpose and your future self.	**Indigo** Intuitive, Spiritual, Respectful	**Element** Light **Sense** ESP	**Glands/Organs** Pituitary, CNS, Cerebellum, Left Eye, Nose & Ears **Note** A
Fifth—Throat: individuality, sense of purpose The fifth Chakra is the center for clear communication and expression through words, both written and verbal. When in balance the fifth Chakra allows you to speak clearly about your vision. You have the freedom to express your voice without limitations. Out of balance your voice is either stifled or too imposing.	**Blue** Cooling, Calming, Meditative	**Element** Ether **Sense** Hearing	**Glands/Organs** Thyroid, Para-Thyroid, Throat, Hypothalamus, Mouth **Note** G
Fourth—Heart: emotional connection to the rhythm of nature The fourth Chakra is located at the heart and is considered to be the pulse of life and attunement to nature's cycles. This Chakra is responsible for unconditional love. Acceptance and inner identity begins here. Your spirit speaks to you at the heart providing you with resonance to feel what is authentic to you. In balance you have compassion and understand the inter-relatedness of all life. Out of balance you are disconnected from your true self.	**Green** Balancing, Harmonizing, New Growth **Pink** Loving, Gentle, Caring	**Element** Air **Sense** Touch	**Glands/Organs** Thymus, Lymph glands, Heart, Circulatory & Immune Systems, Lungs, Arms & Hands **Note** F
Third—Solar Plexus: concrete mind The third Chakra is your center of power and personal will. This Chakra relates to the logical/linear mind and can become out of balance by a strong ego where the focus is on imposing your will on others. This Chakra relates to your learned, programmed mind and how you think you are supposed to be, look, and behave. When in balance you have vitality, a positive self-image, and a balanced sense of self. Out of balance you move into ego, imposing your beliefs and will on others.	**Yellow** Energizing, Revitalizing, Uplifting	**Element** Fire **Sense** Sight	**Glands/Organs** Pancreas, Gall Bladder, Liver, Stomach, PNS, Muscles, Diaphragm **Note** E

Table 22-2 *continued*

CHAKRA	COLOR	GLANDS/ORGANS	
Second—Sacral: below the navel, female energy	**Orange**	**Element**	**Gland/Organs**
The second Chakra is an emotional center for creativity and sensuality. This Chakra allows you to connect with others through feelings, desire, and sensation. Women's reproductive organs are located here to help bring balance to the male energy of the first Chakra. In balance you are receptive, connected to your true nature and intuition. Out of balance you might be denying your instinctive, emotional self, too needy or dominated by emotions.	Creative, Sensual, Fiery	Water	Ovaries, Female Reproductive organs, Spleen, Skin, Kidneys
		Sense	**Note**
		Taste	D
First—Root: base of the spine, male energy	**Red**	**Element**	**Gland/Organs**
The first Chakra is the foundation for the rest of the Chakra system. Being the most physical, it represents the connection between your body and mother earth. It governs the basics such as shelter, food, clothing, feeling secure in your body and surroundings. Since the male reproductive organs are located in the first Chakra the energy is more male and connected to basic survival instincts. In balance you are grounded and secure in your body and environment. Out of balance you might be in survival mode, overly aggressive, or not grounded in your actions.	Stimulating, Powerful, Hot	Earth	Adrenals, Colon, Lymph & Skeletal Systems, Male Reproductive organs
		Sense	**Note**
		Smell	C

The Origin of Reiki

Reiki was developed in the late nineteenth to early twentieth centuries by Dr. Mikao Usui, a Japanese sensai—meaning teacher—from Kyoto, Japan. When his students inquired about performing healing treatments with the hands, he is said to have started a quest to rediscover this ancient practice. His travels and research led him to recover the keys to activate and direct universal life force energy in sacred Tibetan writings. From these sources and years of implementation, he perfected the form of Reiki practiced today.

The practice of "laying on of hands" has been written about in sacred texts throughout history as a means to bless or invoke healing. All tribal cultures and major religions practiced some form of this healing. Up until the French Revolution, the kings and queens of France and England used a method of healing touch called "the Divine Touch." This tradition was gradually lost as the scientific method became the norm. Now, with a resurgence of traditional wellness practices, the benefits of hands-on healing are becoming more and more widespread within the beauty industry.

The Benefits of Reiki

Everyone has healing energy in their hands. What is the first thing you do when you have a cut or wound? You instinctively put your hands on it. This eases the pain and starts the healing process. Reiki elevates your current healing ability to new levels, providing wellness and balance from within. It is a simple and safe way to help yourself and others. Following is a list of benefits it offers to the body, mind, and spirit:

- Reiki lifts the spirits and brings balance to all aspects of the body, mind, and spirit.
- Reiki reduces stress and anxiety by quieting mental chatter and calming the emotions so you feel peaceful and centered and rejuvenated.
- Reiki flows out through the hands, so you do not receive other people's negative backwash.
- It is safe to use any time on any body. You can use it on yourself, others, plants, pets, and products.
- Reiki works to heal the cause of imbalance and eliminate it.
- It may be combined with other therapeutic and healing techniques.

- It does not conflict with medical procedures or medication. It may be used to relieve pain and speed up the healing process.
- Is not a religion and does not conflict with religious beliefs.
- Used regularly, Reiki helps to lessen the affects of daily stressors and protect you from absorbing unwanted energies.
- Once you are attuned to Reiki, you are attuned for life (see below).

The Three Levels of Reiki

Reiki involves three levels, or degrees, of energy activation called *attunements*. Each degree promotes an expanded consciousness and amplifies the universal healing energy beyond the previous level. **Reiki attunements** are performed by a Reiki master teacher to open and connect a student to universal healing energy on all levels of the physical, mental, emotional, and spirit bodies. Each attunement provides a clearing of someone's current energy in order to raise his or her vibration to the next level.

First Degree or Level 1 allows for hands-on healing. This includes first-level energy attunements and instructions on how to perform hands-on treatments on yourself and others. With regular use of Level 1, unhealthy habits and practices that do not resonate with your new energy level may naturally move out of your life. It is recommended to wait at least two weeks before receiving your second-level attunements.

Second Degree or Level 2 allows for distance healing. This level amplifies the Reiki 1 healing energy to a higher degree. This training enables you to provide full-body treatments from a distance. You learn to clear emotional and mental energy as well as physical spaces. Second-degree Reiki has a profound effect on your overall well-being, bringing more balance to the emotional self and body/mind connection. It is recommended to practice consistently on yourself and wait six months to a year before going to Reiki Master level.

Third Degree or Reiki Master allows you to activate others. This level promotes an expanded consciousness and amplifies the universal healing energy beyond the previous level. Master level is for those who have a calling to work on a broader scale of healing and teaching. At Level 3 you are able to attune others to Reiki levels 1, 2, and 3.

Once you receive your attunements, the more you practice on yourself the better you will feel and the easier it will be to share your experience and sell this service. Practicing three to four times a week will help you to maintain balance daily. When you take time to heal yourself first, you become the example others want to follow.

Occasionally you will find that someone does not respond to your treatment. This is fine; you are only the facilitator and are not responsible for their healing. You provide the opportunity, and clients either respond to the energy or do not.

Choosing a Reiki Master Teacher

If you are interested in offering Reiki healing to clients, you must have proper Reiki training by a certified Reiki master teacher. Because energy work is very intimate, select a teacher who makes you feel comfortable. This person will be your mentor, and you want to feel safe going to them when you have questions. Once attuned, you will be energetically connected to this person for life. Money should not be the key factor in choosing your teacher. More important is the teacher's character and experience in teaching Reiki. Following are some important questions to ask:

- Is your Reiki master a good example of his or her work, both inside and out?
- Does he or she practice Reiki regularly on himself or herself?
- How much teaching has this person done?
- Does he or she specialize in teaching a certain target market?
- How long did this teacher take for their progression to Reiki master?

Remember that it takes at least two weeks between attunements to acclimate to your new energy level. It is preferable to find a teacher who has followed and teaches by these guidelines as well. Although weekend courses have become available in the recent past, to attune people in two or three of the levels without waiting in between, this is contrary to Dr Usui's teachings.

Beware of teachers who claim their Reiki is "better" or the "authentic" Reiki. Dr. Usui was the original source for Reiki training. When you are accessing universal life force energy, you cannot improve on this energy—there is no "better." Someone who is trying to convince you that his or her way is better is coming from linear, left-brain programming and not the original Usui teachings.

ENERGY MEDICINES

Energy medicines are a category of products that feed the spirit and fill in your "energy gaps." They contain "spirit energy" from nature and universal life force energy. As you work to fill the spirit, you automatically address emotional and mental conflicts as well. Caught early, energy medicine can help to improve the health of the physical body. You can play an important role in your client's wellness by using and providing products in this category to sell as part of a home-care regimen.

Bach Flower Remedies

In the mid-1930s, Dr. Edward Bach left a successful medical practice in London to develop a new system of medicine that was derived from nature. In his work in London, he had observed patients with consistent emotional states corresponding to certain conditions of ill health. As a result, he grew dissatisfied with the medical practices of his time, which focused on treating the symptoms rather than the cause of a disease. His philosophy was this: "Take no notice of the disease, think only of the outlook on life of the one in distress."

He developed 38 formulas he called flower essences. Not to be confused with essential oils, flower essences are considered to be the vibration, or "spirit," of a plant. Flowers are picked at their peak of growth and placed in water to capture the essence of the plant. Alcohol is added to preserve the shelf life of the solution.

Each plant has its own healing characteristics and issues it helps to resolve. Flower essences help to resolve mental and emotional issues on an energy level by helping to fill in the "energy gaps" in a depleted spirit. You infuse the plant spirit with yours by taking a few drops orally under your tongue, placing it on the pulse points, or spraying it in a mist.

Although there are many flower essences to choose from, it is best to start with the original formulas developed by Dr. Bach; they are also the easiest to find. Packaged in little tincture bottles with droppers, they are easy to use and carry with you. Please note that it may take more than one bottle to completely resolve an issue energetically.

Following are the top seven Bach Flower Essences and Rescue Remedies:

1. White Chestnut clears mental chatter.
2. Walnut helps you to set boundaries and provides protection from outside sources.
3. Larch improves self-esteem and confidence.
4. Rock Water helps you let go of unattainable standards you set for yourself and others.
5. Vervain finds middle ground for those who tend to go to extremes.
6. Holly heals emotional wounds so you can accept and love yourself.
7. Rescue Remedy essence and cream combines five flowers and is beneficial for any imbalance or stressful situation.

Gem Elixirs

You can purchase gem elixirs or make them by placing one or more of the stones of your choice in clean water. Let them sit overnight and then use the infusion as part of a beverage or spray mist.

Energy Infusions

Energy infusions are products that have been attuned energetically with universal healing energy. Reiki is ideal for infusions because you can attune products in addition to people. At the Master level, you can attune cosmetics, skin care products, aromatherapy products, and herbal remedies. Gem elixirs and energy infusions help to balance the mental, emotional, and spirit bodies.

CRYSTALS AND GEMSTONES

Selecting Stones

Gemstones are considered to be any rock, crystal, or stone used for jewelry and adornment. Ancient cultures believed their beauty instilled them with magical powers. Used as talismans they helped to protect, enhance, uplift, and strengthen an individual. The Egyptians held ceremonies for crystal gazing, called *scrying,* to induce altered states of mind in order to receive messages from spirit and see into the future. Edgar Cayce, the sleeping prophet of the 1930s, spoke of a huge cylindrical crystal as the power source for the lost continent of Atlantis, giving its citizens incredible powers.

The mystery and attraction of gemstones is still present today and can be used as a means to enhance the

? Did You Know

A talisman is an object, stone, or piece of jewelry believed to provide the wearer with magical powers.

well-being of clients. Colorful stones and clear quartz contain spirit energy that helps to balance the human spirit. Each stone has a vibrational pattern based on its color and composition. Using them in treatments provides added value to your clients. You may place them over the Chakras, infuse their energy in water to drink, use as a spray mist, or just hold them and admire them in your hands.

If you choose to incorporate this type of treatment into your menu of services, the first thing to do is select your healing stone collection. Polished stones are the easiest to use and clean. **Crystals** work well if you consider the size and shape. If they are too large, they become heavy; if they are too delicate, they are difficult to maintain. Use larger crystals for decoration and smaller ones to place either on your client or around them on the facial bed. Recommended stones are: black tourmaline, red jasper, carnelian, citrine crystal, citrine polished, aventurine, rose quartz, apatite, sodalite, fluorite (Figure 22–5).

Review your Chakra chart (see Table 22–2) and include at least one stone for each Chakra color. Remember that the fourth Chakra represents two colors, pink and green. Attend a gem and mineral show, or locate a lapidary, New Age, or herbal bookstore that carries an assortment of crystals and polished stones. Choose stones that resonate with you. Some will seem to call out to you at first glance. These are perfect to add to your collection. Table 22–3 lists popular healing stones by color in four basic categories.

If you decide to keep two collections, one personal and one professional, separate the two, using your personal collection only for yourself. Store your client collection where you have easy access to them during treatments. Clear the energy of your new collection by using one of the cleansing methods discussed later in this chapter. You will maintain the integrity of their energy by cleaning them after each use with clients.

Getting to Know Your Stones

Once you have selected your stones, it is time to get familiar with them on an intuitive level. Collect your stones and a small memo pad and pen and find a quiet place, preferably outside in a quiet place, to sit with your collection. Select one of your stones and write the name of this stone on the first page of your pad. Open your left hand (the receiving hand) with palm up, and place this stone on your palm. Focus on the color, shape, and feel of the stone for a moment. Breathe in the color and imagine yourself as a part of the stone. Remaining silent, close your eyes and your hand with the stone, and notice any insights or sensory information you receive. Write any thoughts that come to mind. Do not worry if it makes sense or not, just write. Designate a page or two for each stone. It may take a few days or even weeks to receive and record your information. Take as long as needed until you feel your list is complete.

If you find that you draw a blank with this technique, that is okay. It may take some time and practice to strengthen your intuitive abilities. Until then, use the guidelines provided in this chapter to perform your treatments.

Sanitizing and Clearing Your Stones

There are different methods you can use to clear your healing stones so that they are sanitary and free of other people's energy. It is important to do this after each use with clients.

Table 22–3 Popular Healing Stones

1. WARM STONES STIMULATING/ ASSERTIVE	2. MUTED STONES BALANCING/ RECEPTIVE	3. COOL STONES CALMING/ INTUITIVE	4. CLEANSING STONES CLEARING/ GROUNDING PROTECTIVE
red, orange, yellow	clear, green, pink	blue, turquoise, indigo, violet, purple	brown, black, white, gray
red jasper picture jasper orange calcite carnelian citrine amber tiger's eye	clear quartz aventurine jade malachite rose quartz rhodochrosite strawberry quartz	apatite turquoise chrysocolla sodalite lapis lazuli purple fluorite amethyst	black tourmaline mahogany obsidian hematite selenite (WS; water-soluble) snowflake obsidian onyx, labradorite

1. Sanitize your stones by washing them with soap and water and then placing them in a disinfecting solution. Clear the energy by placing the stone under running water for 30 to 60 seconds.
2. If you are attuned to second- or third-degree Reiki, you may also clear your stones by using the Reiki symbols you learn at these levels.
3. If your stones are water-soluble or water-sensitive (WS), you can use one of the following methods:
   - Pour a mound of dry sea salt into a bowl or plate and place your stones in the middle of the mound. Let them sit overnight to clear the energy.
   - Place your stones in the bottom of a Tibetan singing bowl, and run the wooden handle around the rim for 30 seconds.

Color's Role in Healing

Color plays a major role in our lives. Each color has its own frequency or vibration that can help us to get energized, stimulated, or relaxed or to even lift our spirits. The seven colors of the rainbow are associated with the seven colors of the Chakras. If a Chakra is out of balance, you can use color to restore balance. Techniques used range from gemstones, colored light, pictures, and even water infused with color.

Look at the color wheel in Figure 22–4. Warm colors, including red, orange, and yellow, are the most stimulating and energizing. Blues and purples are cool and considered to be the most calming and enlightening. The closer to red the color is, the more stimulating it will be. The closer to blue, the more calming it will be. Yellow is energizing and helps to lift the spirits, while green, the color in the middle of the rainbow, represents balance and is considered to be the most healing.

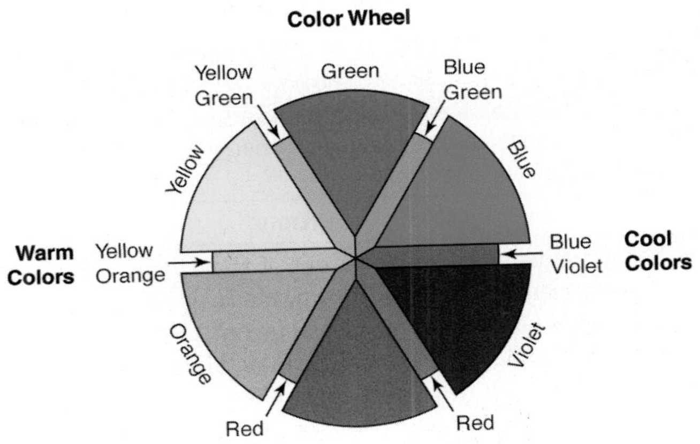

Figure 22–4 Color wheel.

Each color has an intensity range, meaning how bright or soft the color appears. The intensity of bright colors will generate more energy than soft colors. Adding white to any color (called a *tint*) will soften the effects of that color. Adding black (called a *shade*) will deepen the meaning. For example, aventurine is a soft, light green in color. It encourages balance and equilibrium while softening the protective shell around the heart. Malachite, with its deep and rich green color, encourages depth of emotion and feeling.

Colors opposite each other on the color wheel are called **complementary** because of their extreme contrast. Mixing two complementary colors balances the energy. Placing a complementary color on one's Chakra will help to balance overactive energy that is present. Understanding these color associations will help you to make the best choices for your clients.

Clear quartz represents all of the colors of the rainbow. Try this experiment. Select a quartz crystal and place it on a solid white background. Shine a bright light into the crystal. As you move the light around, you will see small rainbows appear in the inclusions of the stone. Because of this, clear quartz is like the wild card of stones. It will work on any Chakra for anyone. When in doubt, it is always safe to use both the polished and crystal versions of this stone.

As with any treatment, there are some contraindications to using color. Some stones tend to be more reactive than others. For example, red stones such as red jasper may cause overstimulation and a physical reaction such as twitching. If your client is already somewhat bold and aggressive, red will accentuate this behavior. Replace red at the first Chakra with a light blue stone for its calming effects or the complementary color of green to balance the excessive energy. Another example is amethyst; its spiritual intensity has also been known to cause reactions. If your client already likes and uses this stone, consider it safe to use in his or her treatment. If you are not sure, a good alternative is fluorite with purple and green, because it strengthens the connection between the spirit and heart. Trust your intuition and don't be afraid to experiment until you find the right blend of colors and stones for your clients (Table 22–4).

The Laying of Gemstones

Now that your stones are clear and you understand the importance of color, you can make selections for a treatment. Think of the outcome you want for your client,

Table 22–4 Healing Stones Chart

CATEGORY 1 – WARM	GEMSTONE QUALITIES – STIMULATING, ENERGIZING, ASSERTIVE
Red, Orange, Yellow	Use these stones to stimulate and energize your client.
Red Jasper	**Client Conditions**
Picture Jasper Orange Calcite Citrine Amber Tiger's Eye	• First Chakra – Lacking confidence, not grounded or asserting themselves, in survival mode, not feeling safe in their body or environment. Red. • Second Chakra – Feeling blocked, lack of creativity and passion, out of touch with emotions, feeling unloved. Orange. • Third Chakra – Lacking a sense of self, caught up in the mind, negative self-talk, or convinced that their way is the only way. Yellow.
CATEGORY 2 – MUTED	**GEMSTONE QUALITIES – BALANCING, RECEPTIVE, RESTORATIVE**
Clear, Green, Pink	Use these stones to restore balance and healing ability.
Clear Quartz	**Client Conditions**
Aventurine Jade Malachite Rose Quartz Rhodochrosite Strawberry Quartz	• Fourth Chakra – Lack of compassion, disconnected from nature's rhythm, no resonance in work, play, or relationships. Soft – medium green. • Feeling unlovable, harsh on self and others, lacking in self-care. Pink. • On auto-pilot, going through the motions. Deep green.
CATEGORY 3 – COOL	**GEMSTONE QUALITIES – CALMING, INSIGHTFUL, RECEPTIVE**
Blue, Indigo, Violet	Use these stones for clear vision and speaking your voice.
Apatite	**Client Conditions**
Turquoise Blue Lace Agate Sodalite Lapis Lazuli Fluorite Amethyst	• Fifth Chakra – Feeling anxious, stressed, irritable, angry, overly expressive or aggressive. Soft – medium blue. • Sixth Chakra – Lack of focus, vision and life purpose. Has tunnel vision. Doesn't see the possibilities available to them in life. Indigo and deep blue. • Seventh Chakra – Lack of direction, feeling empty, depressed, in despair about life. Violet, purple.
CATEGORY 4 – CLEANSING	**GEMSTONE QUALITIES – CLEARING, GROUNDING, PROTECTING**
Black, Brown, White, Gray	Use these stones to clear negative energy and ground your client in present time.
Black Tourmaline	**Client Conditions**
Mahogany Obsidian Snowflake Obsidian Hematite Onyx Selenite Labradorite	• Not grounded – seems to be out of their body. Full of chaotic, negative energy. Brown, black. • Daydreams – full of great ideas but not able to ground them and bring them to reality. Gray, black, and white. • Don't know how to protect themselves from other people's energy. They have a tendency to be overly sensitive and absorb energy like a sponge from people and environments. Black, brown, gray and white.

and then use the guidelines listed in Table 22–3 and the Healing Stone Table 22–4 to help you select the right blend of stones.

In a simple layout, you will use one gemstone per Chakra in the associated Chakra color. If there is an overabundance of energy in a particular area, you will want to address that area by calming it down with light blue or its complementary color. You may then place the appropriate Chakra-colored stone on top of this stone.

If a client complains about having a lot of stress, find out where he or she is feeling it most. Is it in the chest, head, or stomach? Place a light blue stone such as blue lace agate on this area. If the client is angry or aggressive, use this stone at the first chakra to calm. Does the client have too much negative self-talk? Then, use the stone on the third and sixth chakras. Wherever there is an overabundance of unwanted energy, light blue will infuse peaceful energy there.

If your client is sluggish and wants to perk up, stay away from blue and use red or orange. Maybe he or she is feeling insecure and unsure. If so, use a yellow stone like citrine at the third chakra to boost confidence and self-esteem. Following is a list of popular stones that are beneficial to each chakra.

Black tourmaline, first Chakra: This is a very powerful healing stone that everyone can use to protect, ground, and clear negative energy. Place this stone on the first Chakra or have the client hold it in the left hand during a treatment (Figure 22–5).

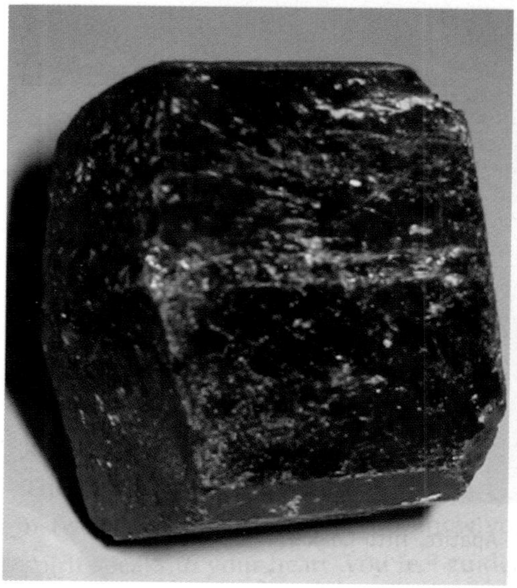

Figure 22–5 Black tourmaline, first Chakra.

Red jasper, first Chakra: The red jasper stone connects you to Mother Earth. It helps to ground energy and provide respect for self, others, and surroundings, and it clears the blood and stimulates life force energy through the physical body. Use this stone when you are not sure of yourself or the next step to take (Figure 22–6).

Carnelian, second Chakra: This stone inspires sensuality and receptivity. It lifts the emotions and sparks desire and imagination to create from an intuitive level. Carnelian helps to enhance self-confidence and assertiveness. Use it to own and accept the feminine aspects of power needed to balance the male and female energies within each person (Figure 22–7).

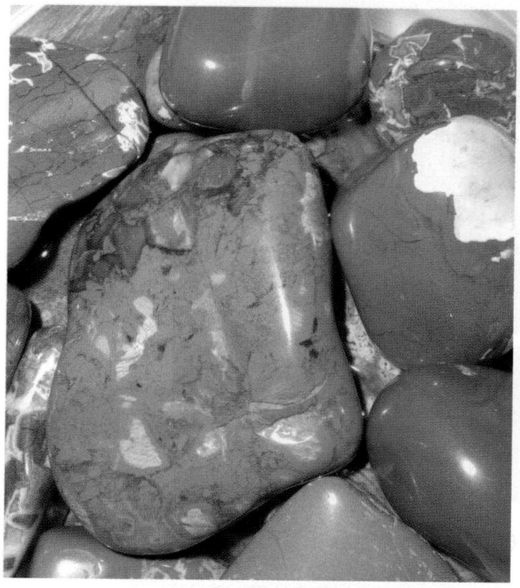

Figure 22–6 Red jasper, first Chakra.

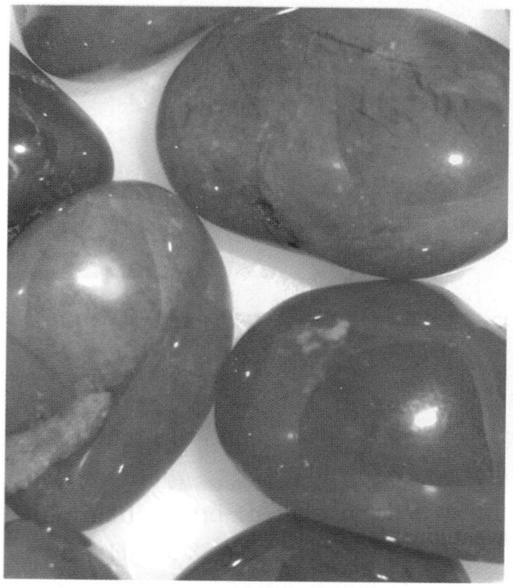

Figure 22–7 Carnelian, second Chakra.

efits that are spiritual and illuminating, allowing higher knowing. The beauty is deep within. Ideal for soul

you will know how to treat each client based on their concerns.

Citrine, third Chakra: Citrine contains the energy of the sun in a stone. It helps you get in touch with per-

Rose quartz, fourth Chakra: This stone opens your heart to love and nurture yourself. When

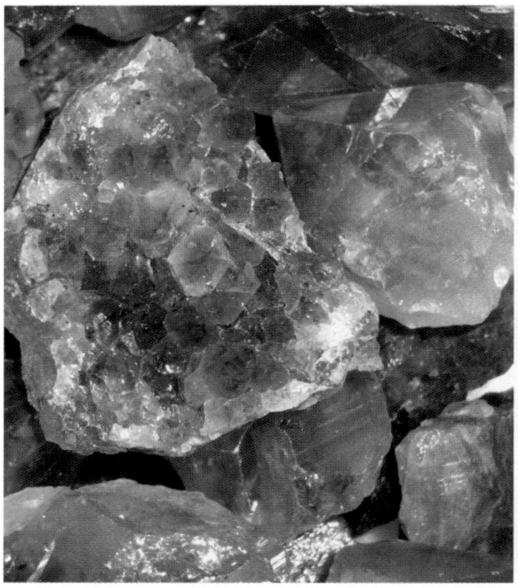

Figure 22–15 Amethyst, seventh Chakra.

INTRODUCING ENERGY-BALANCING TREATMENTS TO CLIENTS

Energy-balancing treatment is a future direction of esthetics as we work toward de-stressing the client. They can be incorporated in a simple manner or, as with other esthetic areas, studied in depth. They address common issues related to a hectic lifestyle, such as stress, anxiety, excessive mental chatter, and more. Clients are seeking simple and healthy ways to achieve peace of mind and feel more grounded and connected. Mini-treatments provide a safe haven and a weekly service you can sell to clients. Or, by adding these components to a current facial, you add perceived value to that facial.

Speak about the benefits with clients rather than specifics. As your clients experience these new services, they will most likely ask more questions. At that time you can go into more of the details that you learned earlier in this chapter. A good statement to start with would be, "The new Energy-balancing, multisensory treatments I offer help to reduce stress and anxiety by quieting mental chatter and calming the emotions, so you will feel peaceful and centered and experience more a-ha! moments. The difference is rejuvenation versus relaxation." Following is a list of other benefits:

- Beyond relaxation, you feel a sense of well-being and inner peace.
- Day-to-day problems that normally bother you will not have the same charge.
- You feel more centered and grounded and able to focus on what matters most to you.

Here are some tips for making it easy for clients to choose these services.

- Let them know that the results last longer when they receive three consecutive treatments.
- Provide a monthly package deal offering three treatments within that time period.
- Include home-care products to sell with your package, and let them know that these products will help them to maintain balance between visits with you.
- Include small indulgences with each treatment that they can take home with them, such as healing stones, aroma sachets with herbs, or essential oils.

PROCEDURE 22-1 30-MINUTE REJUVENATION PROCEDURE

IMPLEMENTS AND MATERIALS

- Massage table or facial lounge
- Towels and linens
- Essential oil selection
- Healing stone collection
- Mood music or guided visualization

Preparation

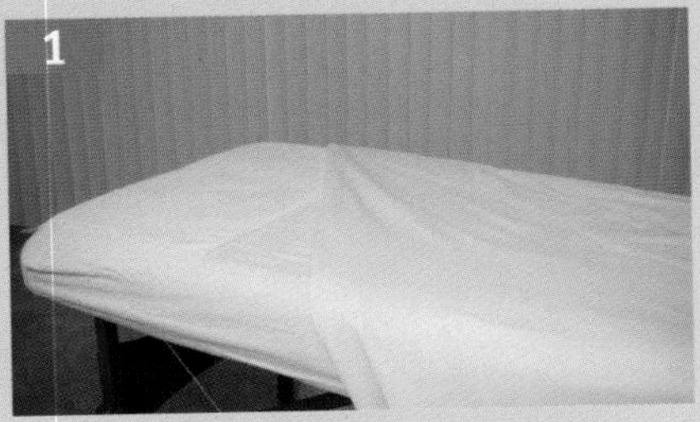

Drape massage table.

1 Drape the massage table or facial bed with one sheet.

2 Use a hand towel under the head.

3 Set out the aromatherapy selection with one or two calming and one or two invigorating oils.

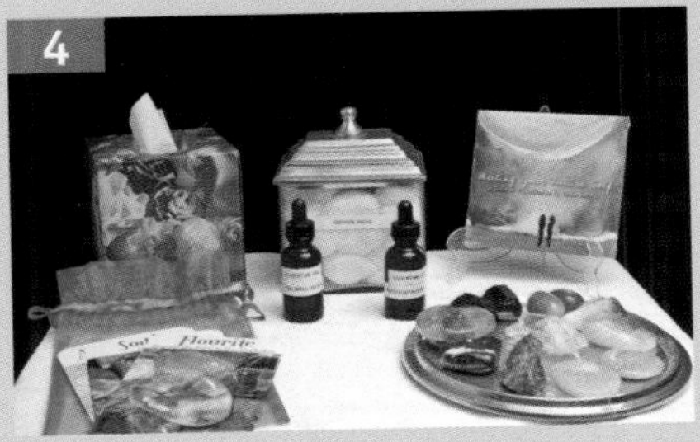

Set out stones.

4 Set out the healing stone collection, including black tourmaline, carnelian, citrine, aventurine, rose quartz, apatite, sodalite, and fluorite.

5 Have your client select their choice of mood music or guided visualization.

This procedure is modified from a full-facial treatment and will not include removing makeup or wrapping the hair. The goal is to offer a half-hour session combining Reiki and healing stones to rejuvenate the energy body.

6 Instruct the client to remove jewelry and clothing on his or her upper body. Provide a drape.

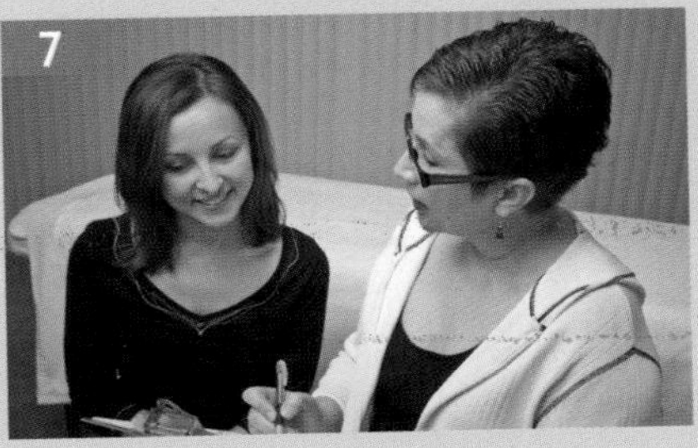

Consult with client before treatment.

7 To show a difference before and after the treatment, ask these questions when the client first arrives and then again at the end of the treatment, before the client gets off the facial bed.

On a scale of 1 to 10 (10 being the highest), how would you rate your:

- Stress level?
- Level of mental chatter?
- Emotional/anxiety level?

Procedure

8 Make the client comfortable on the facial bed. Wrap him or her with the sheet and place a blanket over the torso, legs, and feet, if needed. When he or she is comfortable, dim the lights and turn on the mood music.

9 Put one or two drops of a calming essential oil on a cotton ball and have your client take three to four deep breaths while breathing in this scent.

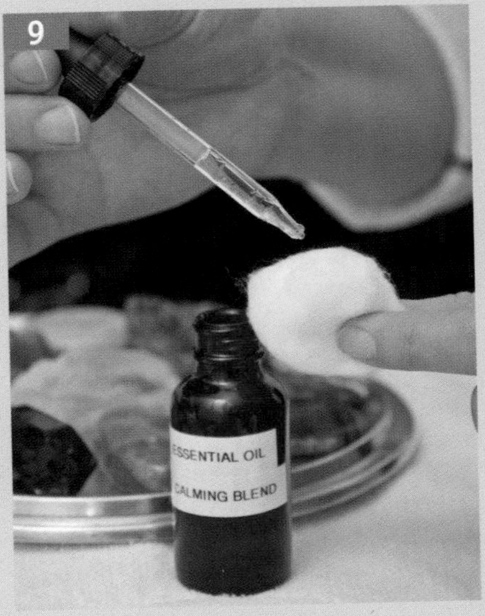

Put calming oil on cotton ball.

continues on next page

PROCEDURE 22-1, CONT. 30-MINUTE REJUVENATION PROCEDURE

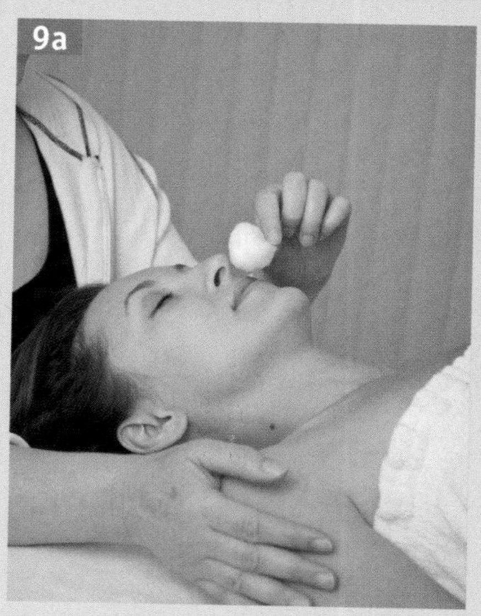

Have client breathe in scent.

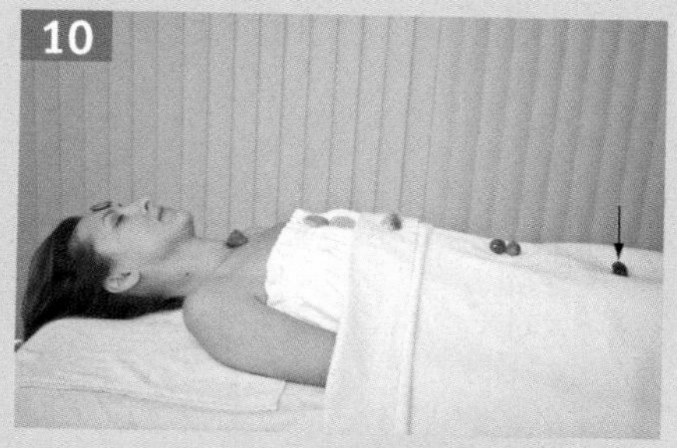

Place the healing stones on the appropriate chakras.

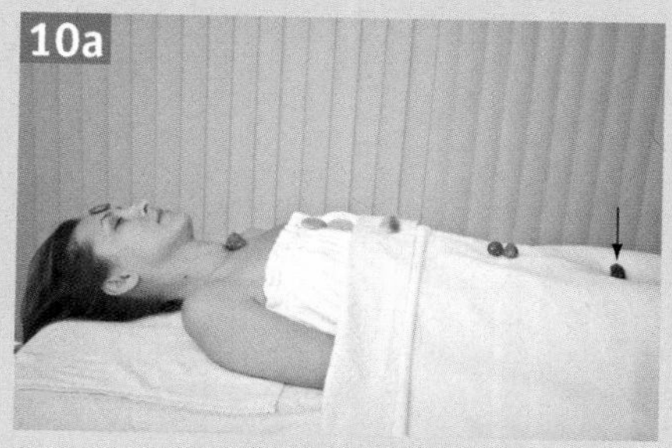

First chakra: black tourmaline.

10 Place the healing stones on the appropriate Chakras, starting with the first. Use larger smooth and flat stones when possible so they do not roll off of the client. Let your client know where you will be placing the stones.

- First Chakra, black tourmaline, on top of the sheet at the pubic area.

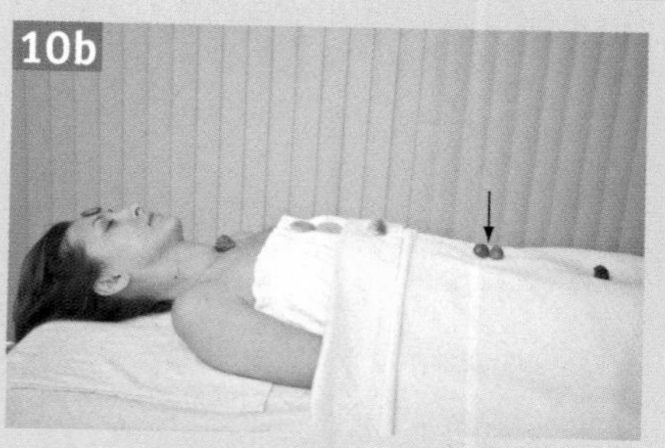

Second chakra: carnelian.

- Second Chakra, carnelian, 1 to 2 inches below the belly button.

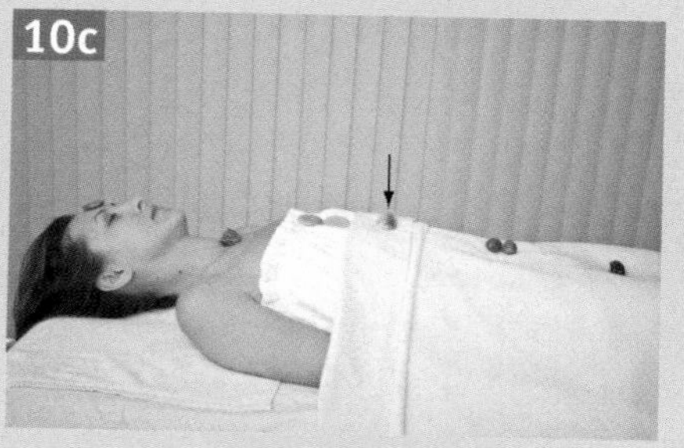

Third chakra: citrine.

- Third Chakra, citrine, at the opening of the rib cage under the sternum.

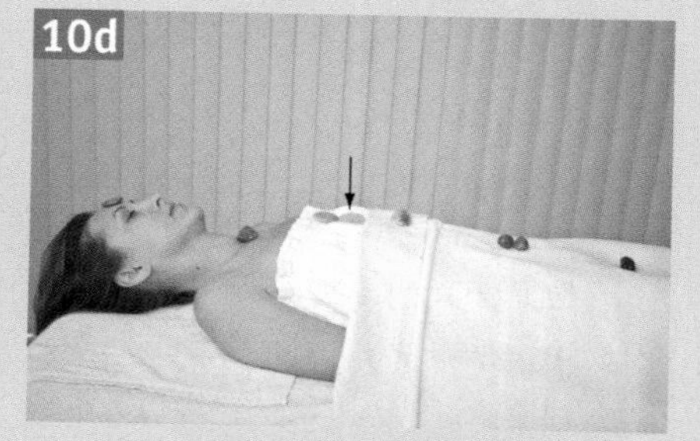

Fourth chakra: aventurine and rose quartz.

- Fourth Chakra, aventurine and rose quartz, at the heart area .

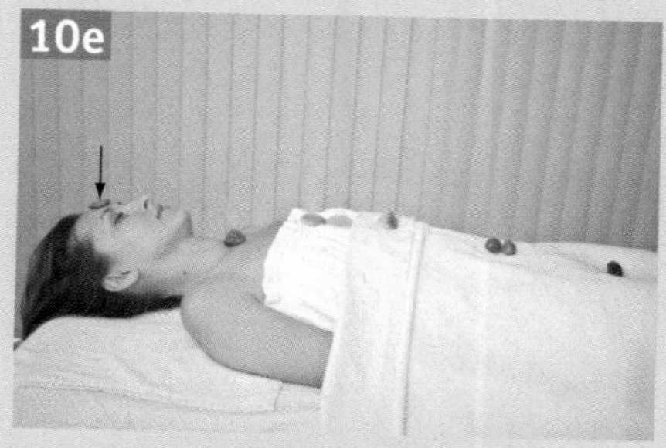

Fifth chakra: apatite or clear quartz.

- Fifth Chakra, apatite or clear quartz, in the hollow of the throat.

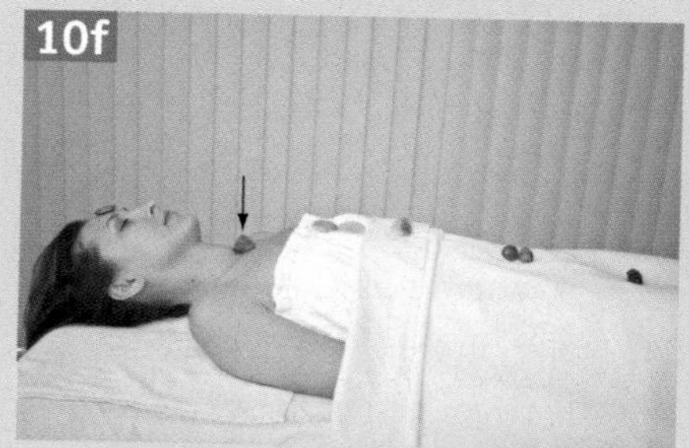

Sixth chakra: sodalite.

- Sixth Chakra, sodalite, on the third eye.
- Seventh Chakra, fluorite or amethyst, touching the top of the head or under the towel and head if the stone is flat and small enough.

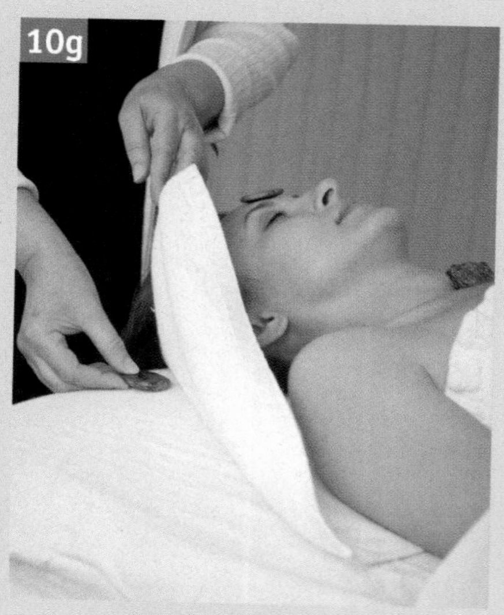

Seventh chakra: fluorite or amethyst.

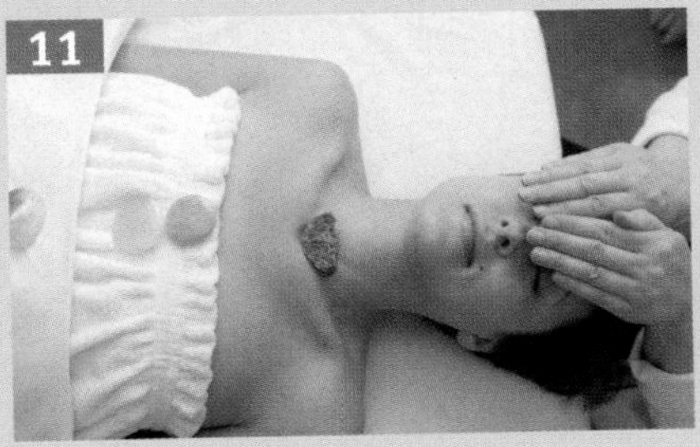

Rest palms lightly on the forehead.

11 Place your hands in the first Reiki position over the eyes, covering the sixth Chakra. Rest your palms lightly on the forehead, with hands and fingers cupping—but not touching—the eyes and upper face. Hold for 2 to 3 minutes. Be careful not to put too much pressure on the healing stone that is located on the center of the forehead.

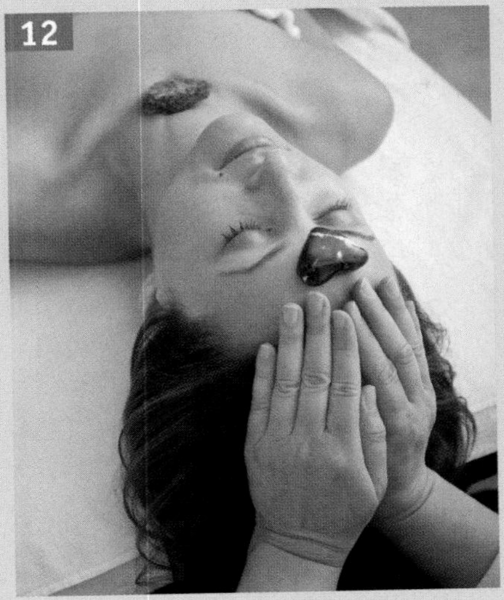

Holds hands side-by-side with fingers. pointing up.

12 Move your hands to the second Reiki position at the top of the head, covering the seventh Chakra. Hold hands side-by-side with fingers pointing up, cupping the top of the head for 2 to 3 minutes.

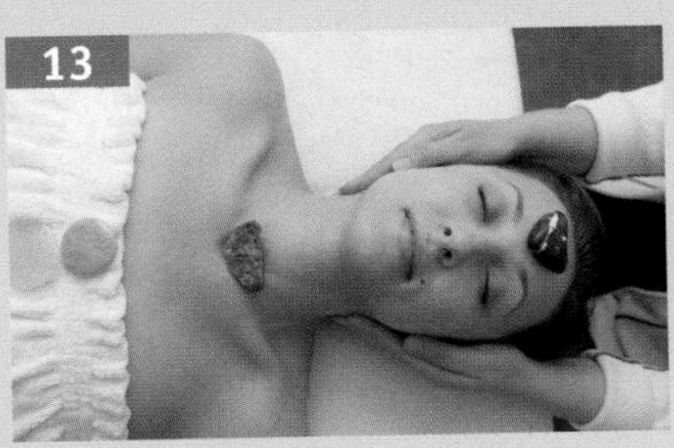

Cup hands completely over the ears.

13 Slowly separate your hands to the third Reiki position, covering the ears. Cup hands completely over the ears for 2 to 3 minutes.

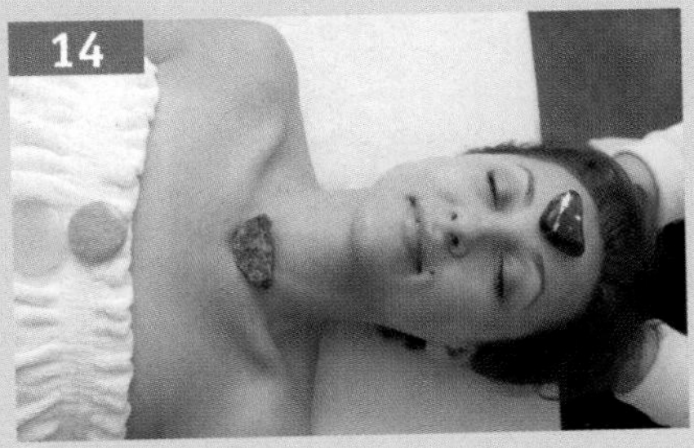

Cradle the head.

14 Gently move both hands to the fourth Reiki position under the head. Cradle the head in your hands. With your fingers, apply pressure below the occipital ridge and pull up. Hold for 2 to 3 minutes. Be careful not to disturb stones on the head and neck areas when moving your hands to this position.

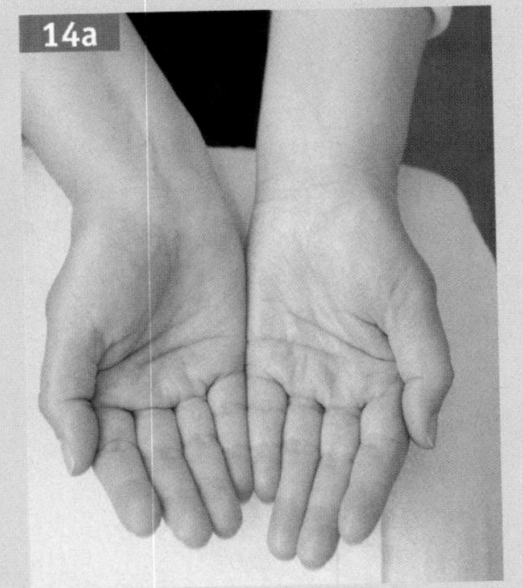

Hand position for cradling.

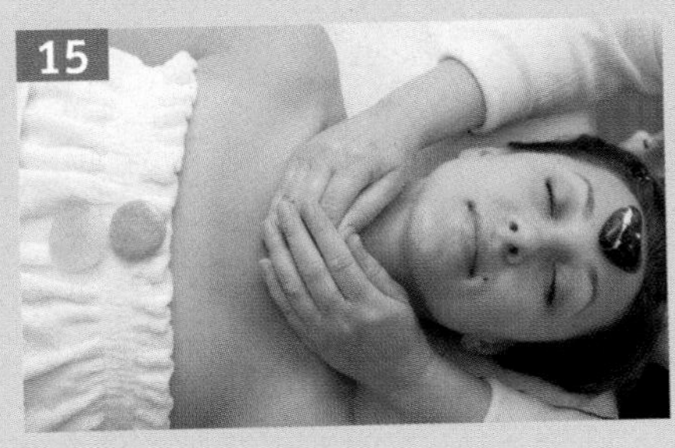

Cover throat area.

15 Slowly separate the hands and move into the fifth Reiki position, covering the throat area. Be careful not to hold this area too tightly as some clients experience claustrophobia related to the neck. Hold this position for 2 to 3 minutes.

continues on next page

PROCEDURE 22–1, CONT. 30-MINUTE REJUVENATION PROCEDURE

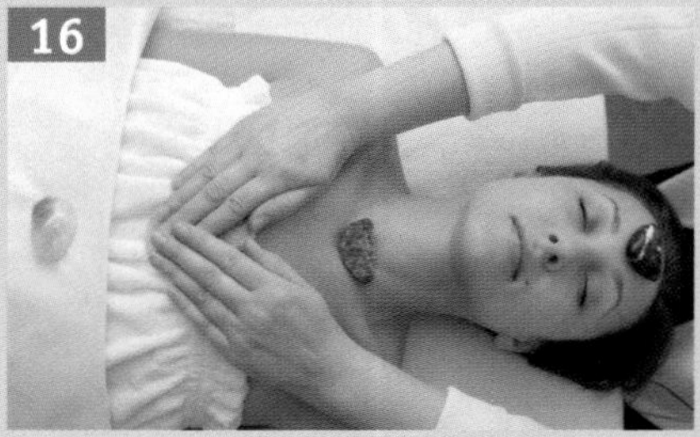

Hold hands over the heart chakra.

16 Move your hands into a V-formation on the décolleté to the sixth Reiki position, over the heart. Hold both hands over the heart Chakra for 2 to 3 minutes.

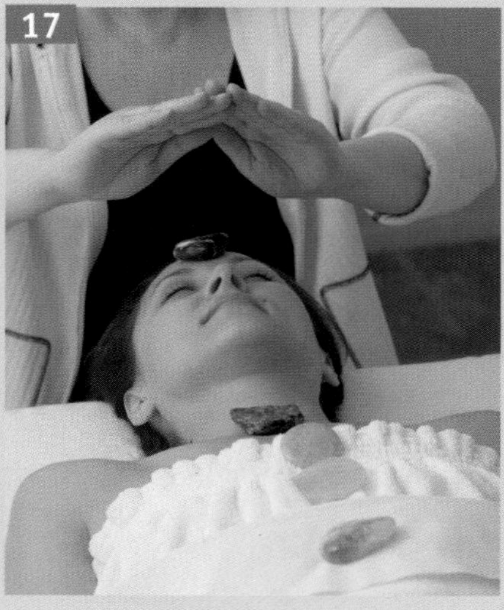

Keep hands together.

17 Keeping your hands together, slowly move them off your client. Keep them together until they are in front of you again.

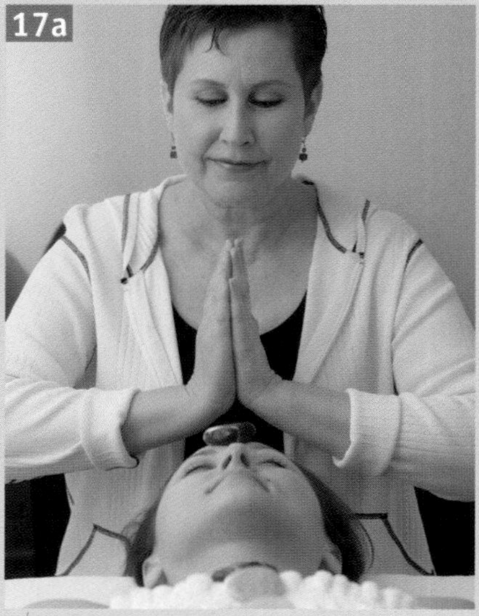

End session.

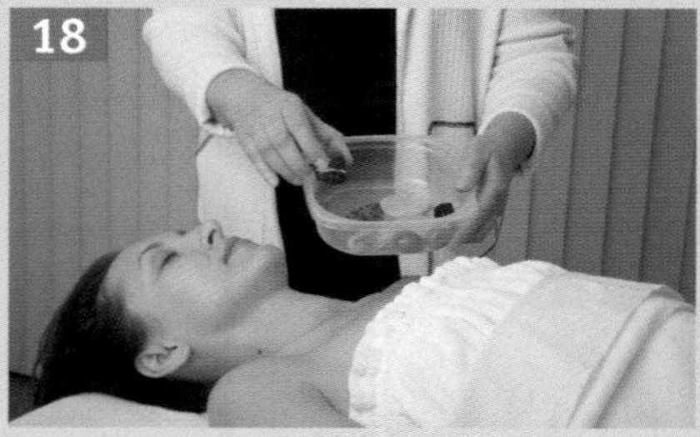

Remove the stones.

18 Remove the stones, one by one, and place them in a container to be sanitized.

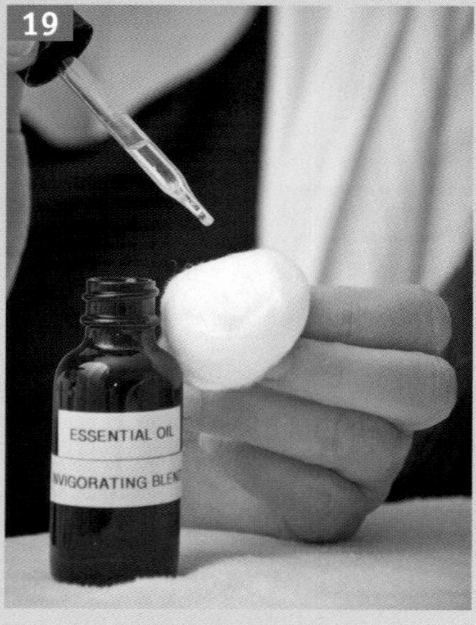

Prepare essential oil.

19 Use one of the invigorating essential oils on a cotton ball to help stimulate your client and gently wake him or her up.

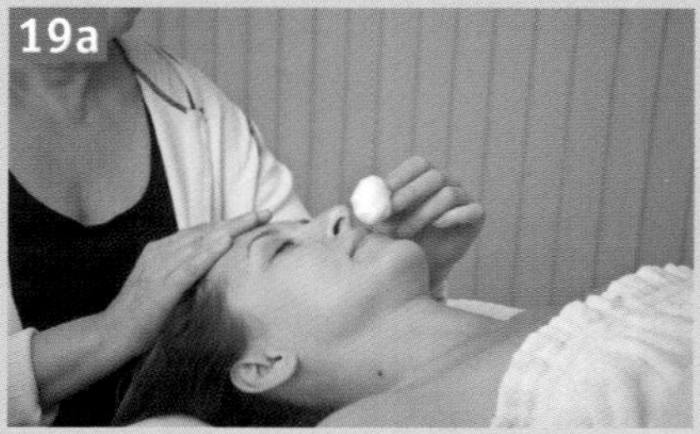

Gently wake up client.

Post-procedure

When the client is somewhat alert, ask him or her how he or she feels and then ask the same three questions you asked before. Compare the difference in responses.

Clean-up and Disinfection

20 Follow state and regulatory guides for cleaning and disinfecting the treatment room, linens, and implements.

21 Clean stones with hot soapy water and strong disinfectants.

Remember that like attracts like and spirit energy heals the spirit. When you take time to heal yourself first, you become the example others want to follow. You will attract positive, healthy clients to you who want your unique services. Use the tools in this chapter to create your signature services and products.

You have all the answers within you—there is no need to change. Just peel away the layers and expose the wonderful and unique essence that is you!

REVIEW QUESTIONS

1. What is balance?
2. What are the benefits of offering alternative therapies in your practice?
3. Name the four components of energy management.
4. Name three methods to balance the mental and emotional bodies.
5. How does aromatherapy affect your mood?
6. How would you describe Reiki to clients?
7. What significance does color play when selecting healing stones for your treatment?
8. How does energy affect you on a daily basis?
9. What are flower essences and how do they work?
10. How would you promote this service to a client?

CHAPTER GLOSSARY

balance: quieting mental chatter, calming the emotions and reviving the spirit, resulting in a sense of inner peace, feeling grounded, more aware, connected and intuitive.

Chakra: one of seven main energy centers of the body. They are found situated at the base of the spine, at the navel, the solar plexus, the heart, throat, the midde of the forehead and the crown of the head. Chakras are major marma points or mahamarmas. Litterally Chakra means "energy wheel."

complementary: completing or making whole. Complementary and alternative medicine (CAM)

CHAPTER GLOSSARY

balances Western medicine by introducing Nature to help bring balance to all aspects of a person before disease can take hold.

crystals: multi-faceted gemstones with 6 sides culminating at a point called a termination. The 6 sides are said to be Chakras 1–3 and 5–7 with the point representing the Heart or fourth Chakra. There are many crystal varieties. Clear quartz crystals embody the full spectrum of light and are made of silica which is an element also found in the human body. Crystals amplify energy, good or bad. This is why it is important to clear your energy and that of your stones regularly.

emotional body: feeling intelligence includes a peron's receptive, subconscious nature, allowing feelings of empathy and resonance.

energy management: a methodology to balance all aspects of body, mind, and spirit that includes the practice of assessing one's energy and providing ways to renew and restore balance.

gemstones: gemstones are considered to be any rock, crystal, or stone used for jewelry and adornment.

Leaky Aura Syndrome: a condition where the aura has developed "energy gaps" from years of leaving bits and pieces of energy behind. This leaves one open to absorbing other energies indiscriminately, resulting in feeling exhausted.

mental body: cognitive intelligence refers to the rational, concrete, learned knowledge. This information is stored in memory and becomes the programmed belief system and perception on life.

mental chatter: Constant self-talk in the mind, especially negative or judgmental thoughts that keep you occupied on trivial issues.

Reiki: universal life force energy transmitted through the palms of the hands that helps to lift the spirits and provide balance to the whole self, body, mind and spirit.

Reiki attunement: performed by a Reiki master teacher to open and connect to universal healing energy on all levels of the physical, mental, emotional, and spirit bodies. The attunement provides a clearing of someone's current energy in order to raise his or her vibration to the next level.

spirit/energy body: also known as spirit or essence, is the life force energy coming from within and radiating beyond the body. The inner face of the Chakras combined with the outer face of the Aura.

CHAPTER 23

AYURVEDA THEORY AND TREATMENTS

CHAPTER OUTLINE

- WHAT ARE AYURVEDIC TREATMENTS?
- WHAT MAKES A SPA TREATMENT AYURVEDIC?
- FIVE VEDIC PRINCIPLES TO APPLY TO TREATMENTS
- THE DOSHAS
- VATA BODY-MIND CHARACTERISTICS
- PITTA BODY-MIND CHARACTERISTICS
- KAPHA BODY-MIND CHARACTERISTICS
- AYURVEDIC TREATMENTS

LEARNING OBJECTIVES

After completing this chapter, you should be able to:

- Discuss what Ayurveda means, where it comes from, how old it is, and the types of treatments it includes.
- Name the unique qualities of Ayurvedic treatments.
- Describe how the five elements form the three doshas.
- Discuss the positive qualities of each of the doshas as they relate to clients.
- Name lifestyle choices and habits that disrupt the doshas and cause problems.
- Describe how customizing treatments can help balance the doshas.
- Name the benefits of ayurvedic treatments.
- Define the types of ayurvedic services that are offered.

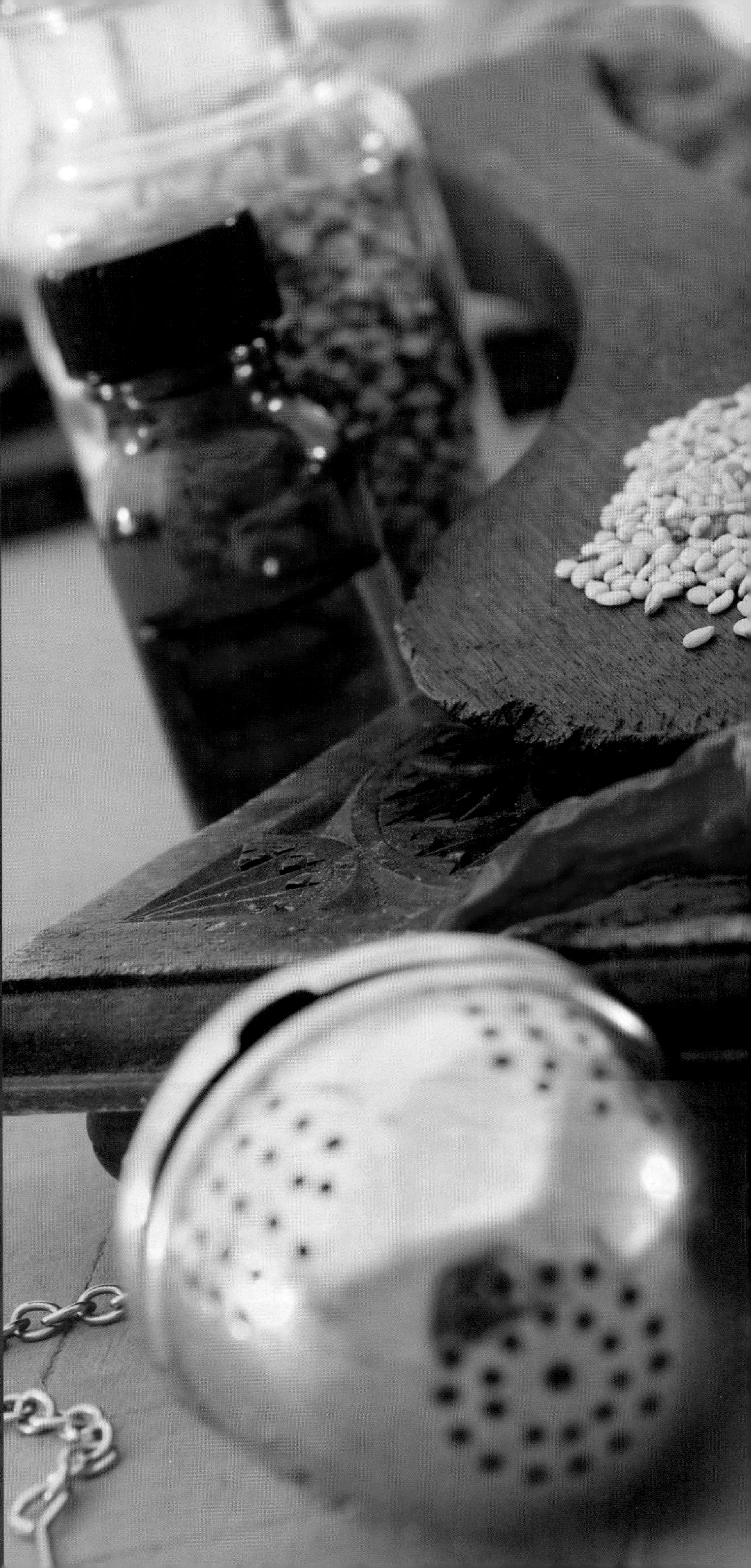

KEY TERMS

Page numbers indicate where in the chapter the term is used.

Ayurveda 629	**marma 639**	**Vata dosha 631**
doshas 631	**panchamahabhutas 631**	**Vedas 630**
Kapha dosha 632	**Pitta dosha 632**	**vikruti 632**
kansa vataki 655	**prakruti 632**	

Ayurveda is an ancient healing art that originated in India along the banks of the Indus River system (Figure 23–1). It is thought to be the oldest, most complete body of information available to us that provides a map for each person to find his or her path toward individual natural beauty and personal wellness. The word *Ayurveda,* pronounced "are-you-vay-da," means "the science of life," a study of longevity, or simply knowing about how to live, be well, and manifest one's own natural beauty.

Ayurveda is still practiced all over India today and, with increased interest from foreign travelers, it is experiencing a huge worldwide revival. Once thought of as a passing trend, Ayurveda is now a well-established modality in the spa and beauty industry, where the profound depth of its simple treatments are loved and appreciated by clients who seek a more holistic approach to skin and body care.

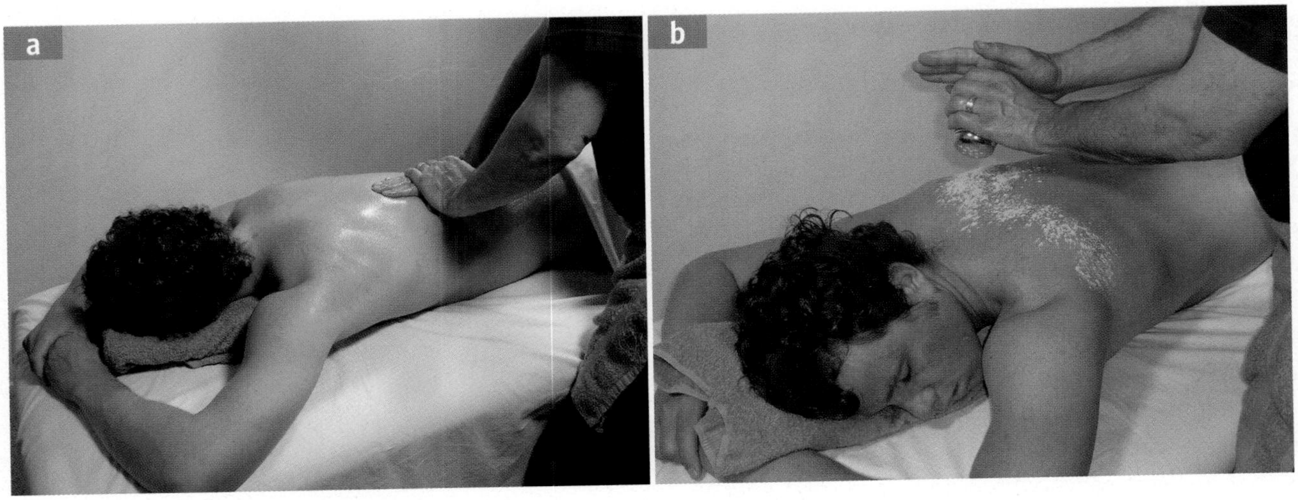

Figure 23–1 An ayurvedic treatment.

WHAT ARE AYURVEDIC TREATMENTS?

Ayurveda is sometimes called the "mother of all healing" because the treatments demonstrate the finest qualities of a mother—love and respect for each and every client, gentleness, understanding, and unconditional support. It is the source of many types of body care used today, including: foot reflexology, polarity therapy, full-body oil massage, deep tissue massage, kinesiology, physiotherapy, aromatherapy, and hydrotherapy (Figure 23–1). It also gave birth to modern medical treatments such as nutrition, herbal supplementation, homeopathy, acupuncture, psychiatry, and surgery, including cosmetic surgery.

Ayurveda provides care and wisdom from every available source, including more esoteric studies such as astrology; mantra, or healing through prayer and chanting; color therapy; music or sound therapy; gem therapy and the use of stones; and alchemical preparations.

WHAT MAKES A SPA TREATMENT AYURVEDIC?

Ayurvedic services have been practiced in India for the last few thousand years. Such treatments include a great variety of skin care and massage techniques, most of which use herbal oils, steams, wraps, and herbal exfoliates and masks.

Ayurvedic treatments should embrace a set of principles that are outlined in the **Vedas,** the ancient writing of the rishis who were Indian mystics that first recorded Ayurveda and are the root text for all ayurvedic studies. These principles may sound a little esoteric but their application is completely practical. The result is a depth and richness to treatments that is the unique quality and heart of Ayurveda.

FIVE VEDIC PRINCIPLES TO APPLY TO TREATMENTS

Ayurveda looks at spa treatments as a dance of subtle energy exchange between the client, the therapist, and the environment rather than simply a sequence of physical hands-on techniques, which means every sensation experienced is potentially healing or harmful. The client is genuinely honored both as a unique individual and as the embodiment of both mind and spirit. Their perfections are celebrated and challenges addressed using products that are pure, and natural and carry vital energy. Let's now look at each of the five principles in detail.

Principle and Application No. 1

On the most basic level, the human body is energy and light. These pure vibrations are responsive to all other outer vibrations, including emotion. This explains why every sensation a client experiences during a treatment affects how he or she looks and feels. This is called the six-sense approach (Figure 23–2):

- **Sound:** the voice of the receptionist or answer machine, how much we talk, what we say, the music we play, noises that comes from inside or from outside the room
- **Sight:** the design of the spa, the color scheme, staff uniforms, the furnishings, the arrangement of the rooms, product package design, the cleanliness and organization of treatment areas, anything that the client sees during a visit
- **Smell:** all smells, pleasing as well as distracting, intentional or accidental, such as aromatherapy, flowers, spa products, cleaning agents, pools or showers, and even other local businesses
- **Touch:** the first hug or handshake; the type of therapeutic touch, be it light or deep, slow or fast, vigorous or gentle, straight or circular; the feel of sheets, robes, blankets, oil, water, or any feeling or sensation that comes from contact with the skin
- **Taste:** the memory a client carries from anything that has touched the tongue, even a lick of a chocolate face mask; other tastes are types of drinks and snacks served to clients, hot or cold, juice or great coffee, before or after treatment or at any time a client visits the spa

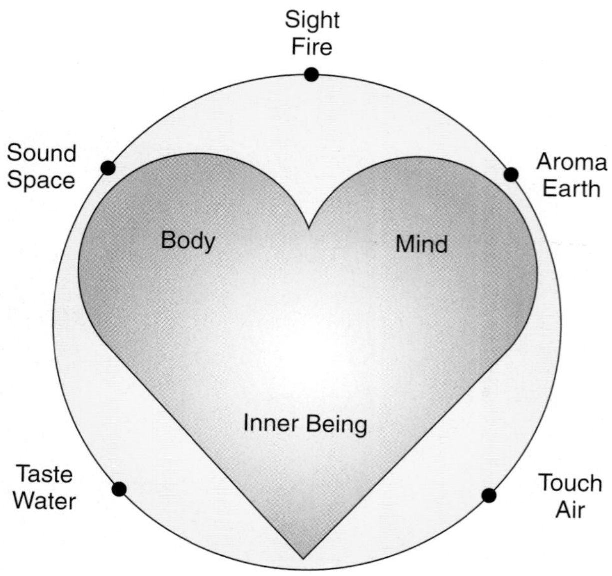

Figure 23–2 The six senses.

- **Heart Feeling:** how you and all staff members connect with clients in a personal, yet professionally genuine, manner; in many ways the most important "sense" of all and the one that builds a loyal and devoted clientele

Principle and Application No. 2

Human beings are an intricately integrated system of physical, mental, and spiritual energy. Rather than look at just a client's problem, such as wrinkles, acne, or puffy eyes, Ayurveda looks at the whole person, how his or her life works, and what his or her world is like. Using kind eyes and an open heart, notice details of the client's physical being: height; weight; body frame; facial structure; and the condition of skin, hair, and nails. Pay attention to the client's body language; his or her voice and what he or she talks about; mood; feeling; stresses; and joys. Be interested to know about the client's work and home life, how well he or she sleeps, and what makes him or her tick. Use this to craft a spa experience that not only pleasantly serves but moves the client in a positive direction.

Principle and Application No. 3

The way a person looks, thinks, behaves, and feels is the result of a combination of subtle energies, or five great elements, also called **panchamahabhutas,** that came together the second that person is conceived. These elements have qualities that are of fire, water, earth, wind, and space, and they dance together in the body as partners called the *three universal natures,* or **doshas.** Learning the characteristics of each dosha helps us better understand challenges a client faces as a natural manifestation of the forces at work in his or her being. It helps us not judge and guides us toward personalized solutions and customized treatments for clients.

Principle and Application No. 4

Each client has natural perfections and inherent challenges. Though we each have a unique blend of subtle energies making us who we are, there is not a best blend. The journey toward beauty and balance is a very personal one, and each person can only be his or her personal best.

The job of the ayurvedic esthetician is to accentuate the client's positive qualities and work with him or her to help bring resolution to difficulties or problems, realizing that each person is as unique as the journey he or she chooses.

Principle and Application No. 5

Ayurvedic beauty and personal-care products should be gently cleansing or provide needed nutrients that are digestible to the skin. They must cause no harm to the body and have no side effects. Ayurvedic specialists believe all products should be made of ingredients that would be safe to eat. They should be organically grown and fresh so as to not only cleanse or nourish but also to provide refreshing life force to the skin. Ingredients may include organic, cold-pressed oils, dried herbs, powdered grains, flower petals, or dried fruit rind and naturally occurring minerals. Specialty manufacturers offer products formulated to meet ayurvedic principles.

If each of these principles can be fully embraced the whole spa experience will be individually customized with the result that the client will feel cared for to perfection and have a deeply balancing and memorable experience.

THE DOSHAS

These principles are important, but the one that provides the main framework for customizing treatments and making them so memorable is the third principle, which introduces the idea that each client is unique and should be treated individually. Each client is the manifestation of subtle energy, a blend of the three doshas, called their *constitutional mind-body type.*

Dosha is a Sanskrit word, the meaning of which is similar to the Greek idea of body humor. A dosha is sometimes described as an invisible force that is responsible for all of the physiological and psychological processes in the body-mind system. Doshas cannot be measured by science or perceived by the ordinary senses; they are vibrational modes in subatomic matter. We experience them in the rhythms of nature, the motion of the planets, and the complexity of DNA. According to Ayurveda, the amount of each dosha a person has determines not only the way the person looks but also how that person thinks, speaks, acts, and feels. Doshas are not fixed in quantity or location and do have the natural tendency to change, move, and become unbalanced.

Vata, which means "to move or enthuse," combines qualities that are like space and wind. It is the most subtle, least tangible, and yet most powerful of all the doshas, as it alone can travel around the body without assistance. The **Vata dosha** is responsible for all movement in the body—both voluntary, such as walking, involuntary, such as the heart beating—and, on a subtle level, even for the movement of thoughts through the mind. The more Vata one has, the more that person moves about naturally.

Pitta, which means "to heat or burn," hopefully combines the qualities of the fire and water elements. Like steam that is made when fire and water combine, the **Pitta dosha** is forceful and hot. It is responsible for all transformations in the body, such as the transformation of food to cell nutrients or transformations in the mind of information to personal understanding. It works with all of the biochemical messengers in the body and is tightly linked to the hormonal and endocrine systems. The Pitta dosha is responsible for all metabolic processes, such as digestion; the more Pitta one has, the warmer the skin.

Kapha, which means "to embrace or keep together," combines qualities that are like earth and water. Just like dust and rain mixed together make clay, Kapha dosha is responsible for the body's form and all lubrication in the system such as the moisture in our mouth and sinuses, the fluid in our joints, and the fat around our organs. The **Kapha dosha** is responsible for physical form and lubrication; the more Kapha one has, the more substantial and strong the person's body will be.

Each person has a unique combination of the Vata, Pitta, and Kapha doshas, or subtle energetic qualities (Figure 23–3). The individual combination is called the **prakruti.** The doshas exist, move, and change in the body and may or may not be in perfect balance. When a person's doshas change, they are called the **vikruti.** When a person's prakruti does not match his or her vikruti, the doshas are considered out of balance. Imbalance usually occurs when any one or more of the doshas accumulate in the body, most often due to poor digestion, lack of exercise, or entrenched mental habits. That is when any type of physical, mental, emotional, or spiritual problem may arise. For example, Kapha dosha, which is in charge of giving form to the body in balance, gives the skin perfect hydration and firmness, whereas extra Kapha dosha manifests as more form than needed, namely swelling or cellulite.

Prakruti Is Your Personal Blueprint

Prakruti means "the first creation" and is determined at conception. In modern terms we can think of it as somewhat like DNA structure, chains of potential qualities and predispositions. Our prakruti does not change throughout our life; it is our norm, our baseline, for our personal wellness and beauty.

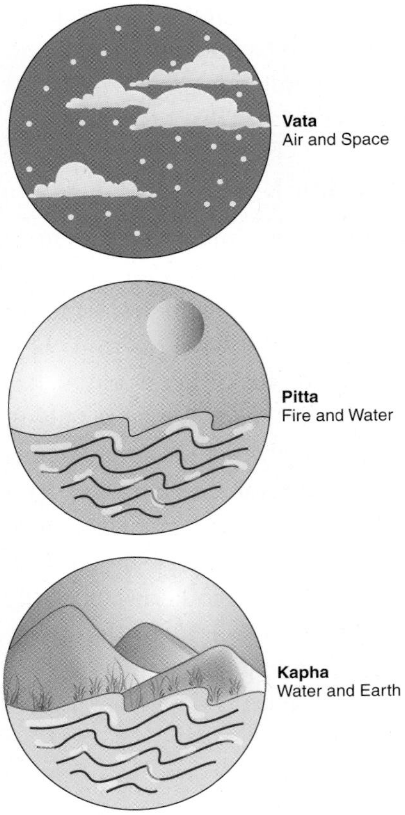

Figure 23–3 Symbols for the three doshas, top to bottom: Vata, combining space and air qualities, Pitta, combining fire and water qualities and Kapha, combining earth and water qualities.

Vikruti Is Your Present State of Subtle Energy

Vikruti is the balance of doshas at any given time. Our dosha balance can change with every thought, action, sense stimulation, and environmental condition. This is why the teachings of Ayurveda have always included prenatal care, lifestyle choices, and environmental considerations. Vikruti is often the imbalance of the doshas that is understood to be the root cause of all health and beauty issues.

The Qualities of the Five Elements

Just as the doshas, elements in the body can change in force or quantity, being in or out of balance. Of the five elements, space and earth change the least. The other three elements, air like the wind, fire like daily temperatures, and water like the amount of mist and rain, change all the time. You will notice this with the change in weather and, as you get older, you will notice how much the climate affects how you feel inside. But these elements are moving inside the body all the time too. Seasonal changes demand that the body be flexible enough to strike a balance so you are always juggling with your lifestyle choices to keep the body's own subtle intelligence flowing steady, offering you a chance to shine.

Following is a list of each element with two common qualities of that element. For each quality we have listed how this quality would be noticed in your client.

- **Space**
  Cold: someone whose skin is cold to the touch or has cold hands and feet
  Open: an open-minded client, the first to try new things
- **Air**
  Active: the fidgety, talkative client who has a hard time settling down
  Inspirational: the staff member whose presence feels like a breath of fresh air
- **Fire**
  Heat: the client whose skin flares up easily or who complains about a room being stuffy
  Upward-moving: someone with tremendous drive and ambition
- **Water**
  Cool: a client with soft, moist skin
  Lubricating: someone who is able to move smoothly around difficulties
- **Earth**
  Solid: a client with firm skin that ages well
  Stable: the regular client who loves traditional and time-proven treatments and practices

If the elements are in balance, the result is beauty and health. If one element is allowed to accumulate, then problems will eventually manifest. Following is a list of conditions caused by out-of-balance elements:

- Extra earth: cellulite
- Extra water: puffiness or edema
- Extra fire: redness or inflammation
- Extra air: dryness or flaking
- Extra space: osteoporosis

Dosha Overview

Table 23–1 is an example of forms used in spas or clinics to determine a client's ayurvedic skin type. It is important for a client to fill out a form like this one on a "how I feel today/now" basis, rather than "normally" or "usually," so that you can see what may need rebalancing. The client does have to choose just one quality from each group of three choices across the page. They should check everything they think represents their qualities, then add up the totals in each vertical column.

In this introduction to Ayurveda we will focus on the positive aspects of each dosha. Many attributes may seem to overlap from dosha to dosha, so this chapter will focus on the more unique ones.

VATA BODY-MIND CHARACTERISTICS

The Vata client's elemental qualities are space and air. This client's traditional attributes are defined by the words *dry, cold, light, irregular, mobile, subtle,* and *rough*. Generally, this client is slender, small, and light-boned with light musculature. His or her movements are quick and light, possibly jerky. This client talks a lot, mostly about experiences, travels, dreams, feelings, and sensations. The hands are cool with long fingers and drier, thinner nails. His or her facial features are smaller and may be irregular, and the hair tends to be wiry and drier. He or she has eyes that are bright and lively, darting, interested, and enquiring and often have dark irises. This client has fine, even lips. The skin tends to be thin, with fine pores, and slightly dry. He or she rarely breaks out and does not blush or tan easily. The ideal Vata personality is energetic, enthusiastic, open-minded, centered, creative, and artistic. He or she is great at multitasking, is a great mediator, communicates well, and is even-tempered, pleasantly objective, inspirational, multitalented, free-spirited, understanding, knowledgeable, and flexible.

What Unbalances the Vata Dosha?

It is very common for clients to have their Vata dosha out of balance. Most aspects of modern living unbalance Vata energy, whether these things affect body, mind, or spirit. A few of the physical triggers include lack of rest, lack of supportive touch, poor dietary habits, air travel, overexercise, and childbirth, as well as living in cold weather, working in smoggy or noisy environments, or recovering from surgery. Mental triggers include fears of change, too much rushing, and feeling a lack of support.

Balancing the Vata Dosha

When the Vata dosha is unbalanced, it is very often the simple and obvious things that somehow are forgotten. Suggest that your client get regular rest, keep warm, eat balanced meals at regular times, and to take some time for himself or herself—perhaps for quiet time, a hot bath, or a massage.

Table 23–1 Ayurvedic Skin and Body/Mind Assessment Sheet

MY SKIN . . .		
is dry, especially when I travel, in winter, or in windy weather.	is sensitive. Soaps and cosmetics easily give me itchiness or a rash.	is prone to congestion.
is fine. I can easily feel my bone structure.	is medium thickness. I can feel muscles when I touch my face.	is thicker. I feel full flesh when I touch my face.
is cold and rough or flaky.	is warm and soft to the touch.	is cool and moist to touch.
tans deeply and easily. I love the sun.	burns easily and gets freckles. Heat can make me irritable.	tans slowly. Heat makes me feel clammy quickly.
enjoys oils and rich creams.	prefers light lotions or gels.	hates heavy or oily cosmetic preparations.
has fine lines, especially around my eyes.	has visible blood vessels, especially on my nose and cheeks.	pores are enlarged, especially on my nose and chin.
on my lips cracks easily.	on my lips is prone to bleed or get sores.	on my lips gets sticky.
looks gray and lifeless when I'm stressed or tired.	looks sallow or flushed when I'm stressed or tired.	looks pale or puffy when I'm stressed or tired.
rarely has breakouts.	is prone to inflamed and yellow breakouts.	is prone to blackheads, whiteheads, or deep cysts.
Vata score:	**Pitta score:**	**Kapha score:**
I . . .		
am slim and fine-boned.	have a medium, athletic build.	am heavy-boned and have a curvaceous figure.
have lively, darting eyes.	have intense magnetizing eyes.	have a calm, soft gaze.
talk a lot.	ask a lot of precise questions.	say little, but think deeply.
have a poor memory.	remember dates and figures easily.	am slower to learn but have a great memory.
am prone to worry and mood swings.	am prone to angry outbursts.	am prone to depression.
hate cold.	get irritable in heat, especially humid heat.	prefer the shade.
am energized by heat and sunshine.	thrive in nature.	enjoy medium heat with breeze.
spend easily at sales.	like to buy top-of-the-line items.	save money easily.
easily overextend myself.	work hard and play hard.	am prone to lethargy or getting in a rut.
am often late to appointments.	am always early or on time.	prefer regular time schedules.
carry hand lotion and lip balm.	wear sunglasses often.	carry a large purse.
like to touch, feel, and hold things.	am aware of color and design.	am sensitive to smell.
love to travel.	need to be in charge.	prefer to be left alone.
am creative and sensitive.	am intelligent and courageous.	am strong-willed and caring.
often forget to eat meals.	love tasty foods.	eat comfort foods.
have dry, coarse hair.	have silky, straight hair.	have thick, heavy hair.
sleep poorly.	have colorful dreams.	sleep easily.
like fine, soft fabrics.	like elegant, expensive jewelry.	like homey accessories.
behave like a rabbit.	behave like a fox.	behave like a turtle.
shop for fun, especially for shoes.	enjoy reading and movies, especially documentaries.	have no problem relaxing at home.
Vata Total:	**Pitta Total:**	**Kapha Total:**

Treatment Tips for Balancing the Vata Dosha

Following are some points for treating the client with an out-of-balance Vata dosha. The key words for a Vata-balancing treatment are *warm, calm,* and *nourish.*

Temperature

Keep temperature warm and consistent, whether in the treatment room, around the spa, or for product. Warm your hands before you touch a client and warn a client if a product has to be cold to be therapeutic.

Talk

When the Vata is high, conversation can get fast and dizzy. Aim for as little talk as possible, as this client desperately needs peace. Give him or her permission to have a quiet rest. Keep your advice brief and grounded. You may need to repeat advice often for for the client to remember it.

Touch

Be gentle and consistent with touch but not too light or it tickles. Circular movements, especially clockwise circles, are very calming.

Techniques

You can suggest any treatment that uses oil and warmth. That may include a heated table, a warm oil massage, a body wrap or steam, or a nourishing facial with a warm mask. Warmth on the belly is particularly calming. Give your client a hot water bottle or hot pack to hold during any facial and offer another hot pack for the feet.

Snack

Serve hot or room temperature drinks and cooked snacks that taste sweet or salty, such as cookies or crackers.

Other

You may need to set boundaries on your time. When the Vata is out of balance, it is easy to get caught up in a whirlwind of enthusiasm or confusion and have time fly by. Keep grounded and keep your eye on the clock so you have time to work at a reasonable pace.

PITTA BODY-MIND CHARACTERISTICS

The Pitta client's elemental qualities are fire and water. The words defining his or her traditional attributes are *hot, oily, light, regular, intense, fluid,* and *sharp.* This client is of medium build, well-balanced, and athletic with good posture. His or her movements are commanding, self-assured, direct, and self-contained. The speech is precise, well-informed with good vocabulary, very clear, and assertive. The hands are warm to the touch with a strong handshake. His or her nails are even, almond-shaped, and pink in color. The client's features are classical and well balanced, while the hair is lighter with fine, straighter texture. His or her eyes are sharp, bright, twinkling, and engaging. The lips even have good color. His or her skin is of average thickness, with peaches-and-cream or coppery tones, oilier in the T zone, and warm to the touch, and he or she blushes easily.

The ideal Pitta personality is one who is passionate, powerful, and charismatic and who accomplishes a lot. This person is warm, compassionate, discriminating, visual, ethical, flexible, joyful, sensual, unconventional, vital, patient, nurturing, loyal, disciplined, practical, a clear communicator and a planner. He or she loves a challenge and sets high standards.

This client is self-assured, punctual, results-oriented, and appreciative of organization and cleanliness. He or she needs to feel at least a little in control; this person loves written information and will buy the top-of-the-line products because he or she is conscious of appearances. He or she likes clean, refreshing services.

What Unbalances the Pitta Dosha?

The Pitta dosha increases when the weather is hot and humid, when one is working under tight time schedules, when passion or anger is high, and when subject to auto fumes or spending too much time in front of computer screens. Common triggers for a Pitta imbalance include working too intensely; eating spicy foods; overeating red meat, salt, or shellfish; experiencing a lack of water; drinking too much coffee or alcohol (especially spirits); smoking; or generally anything of great intensity physically, emotionally, or mentally.

Balancing the Pitta Dosha

The keys to keeping the Pitta dosha in balance are physical and mental relaxation. These clients need to try to go with the flow and experience more humor in their lives. Since Pitta refers to heat, they need to physically and mentally cool down. Fresh air and a cool environment are positive steps toward balancing the fire.

Treatment Tips for Balancing the Pitta Dosha

Following are some points for treating the client with an out-of-balance Pitta dosha. The key words for a Pitta-balancing treatment are *cool, soothe,* and *relax.*

Temperature

Keep the treatment room fresh by opening a window if you can, or use a fan or ion generator. If a treatment demands high temperatures or the weather is very hot, offer ways of taking the edge off the heat, such as a sip of cool water, a cool washcloth on the forehead, a small face fan, a cool spray of rosewater, a cooling footbath, or cool marble stones.

Talk

These can be your most demanding clients, as they tend to ask a lot of challenging questions or try to help you plan your life. Be polite but firm and never bluff if you don't know the answer. Offer to check, find them a book, or offer a brochure for more information. Try to focus them on feeling body sensations rather than thinking so they can relax and simply enjoy the experience.

Touch

Your touch must be precise, firm, and well-trained and have a logic or reason. Pitta will make skin tissue feel tight and stressed; your touch should "fluff up" the tissue and encourage a smile.

Techniques

Cool, wet treatments such as cool compresses, mud masks, and seaweed wraps work well. Cool but light eye pads or eye pillows help take a lot of tension out of the face as heat tends to build up around the eyes.

Snack

Cool, fresh fruits and vegetables with juices or excellent-quality water are your best choice. It can be very simple but should be presented in ways that are visually appealing. Presentation is a close second to great taste.

Other

Punctuality, cleanliness, tidiness, and professionalism are key. If you run more than five minutes late and are untidy or disorganized, you will quickly lose points with these clients.

KAPHA BODY-MIND CHARACTERISTICS

The key elements of a Kapha are earth and water. This client's traditional attributes are defined as *dense, ample, cool, oily, stable, thick, smooth,* and *dull.* He or she has a strong build with square or rounded shapes and is heavy-boned and well proportioned. The movements are graceful, rolling, gentle, soft, and grounded. The client is soft-spoken and quiet; this person may use few words but speaks from the heart. The hands are strong, cool, and square with strong, even, square nails. Generally, this person has larger, even, full features with thick, heavy, plentiful hair. The eyes are large, moist, and tranquil with a mouth that tends to be large with full lips and even teeth. The skin is thick with great tone and slightly oily. It is well hydrated, strong, and ages well.

An ideal Kapha personality is one that is stable, grounded, confident, consistent, and responsible. This person is independent, loves routine, and is sincere, flexible, accepting, joyful, sensual, vital, patient, nurturing, generous, loving, loyal, honest, and reliable.

What Unbalances the Kapha Dosha?

Lack of movement is the key to Kapha imbalance. Lack of exercise, too much sitting, or sleeping or eating just before bed are all triggers. Too much beer or heavy comfort foods add to the feeling of dullness. Depression, lack of emotional support, or feeling stuck are also contributors.

Balancing the Kapha Dosha

Think movement and lightness to help balance this dosha. Regular exercise, light breakfasts, and light dinners are all helpful. Light, warm, or dry foods, lots of vegetables, and not too much water are beneficial. Involvement is another form of movement and any form of social involvement may be helpful.

Treatment Tips for Balancing Kapha Dosha

Following are some points for treating the client with an out-of-balance Kapha dosha. The key words for a Kapha-balancing treatment are *freshen, comfort,* and *gently stimulate.*

Temperature

Keep the temperature in the treatment room comfortable, not too hot or too cold.

Talk

You may need to inspire, question, or make the conversation for the client. Don't expect verbal praise. This client will show gratitude with a tip or referral or maybe with a gift card. Keep him or her from falling into a deep sleep so he or she can enjoy all of the aromas and touch techniques.

Touch

Your touch should be deeper, kindly, and with good focus. Gentle strokes as for lymph drainage are stimulating while still luxurious and comfortable.

Techniques

Give this client deep cleansing facials, lymphatic massage, sauna, wraps, and traditional beauty services, such as a manicure and pedicure.

Snack

Offer snacks that are pretty and taste spicy or sweet.

Other

Remember that this client is not used to getting attention or being remembered. He or she is moved by small gifts.

AYURVEDIC TREATMENTS

Ayurvedic Skin Care

The Philosophy

The understanding in ayurvedic skin care is that the more a person nurtures and treasures himself or herself in positive ways, the more radiant that person becomes physically and expressively, regardless of shape or proportion. In Ayurveda outer beauty includes not only what is visually perceived in the qualities of the skin, hair, and body contours; it also includes grace in posture and movement and the subtle quality of freshness and vitality and magnetizing brightness of being. This beauty is understood to be the product of overall good health and not simply a cosmetic event. The emphasis is on self-knowledge and the development of habits that help beauty blossom at any age.

Inner beauty relates to inner qualities of being, which includes emotional and mental states. As with physical outer beauty, inner beauty is molded by diet and lifestyle choices but is also developed by mind training. The secret aspect of beauty refers to the energy, insight, and inspiration it takes to make the personal choices and develop the personal habits it takes to achieve outer and inner beauty. This takes time, patience, and a willingness to be open and learn from experience.

These three aspects have been described as being like a scale, with outer beauty on one side, inner beauty on the other, and secret beauty in the middle holding the balance. Ayurvedic beauty is the path toward this balance.

The Products

Ayurvedic cosmetics have been used for the last 3,000 years, and in all that time they have shown nothing but positive results. The products were derived from plants, herbs, essential oils or extracts, pure vegetable oils, pure water, **ghee** (clarified butter), honey, pure milk, and whole fruits and vegetables. Traditionally they were made fresh at home along with foods and medicines.

Ayurveda teaches that the skin is a major organ of absorption and that the attributes of topically applied products can pass into skin to be absorbed through the fine capillaries directly into the bloodstream, where they provide raw materials that build healthy skin. It has been calculated that essential oils applied topically are 60% to 75% more medicinally powerful than herbs that are ingested, so Ayurveda teaches that if you cannot eat it safely, do not put it on your skin.

Ayurveda also teaches that all things that have life carry "intelligence" that is a vibratory energy that has the ability to organize and bring balance to life. There are Ayurvedic products that are simple organic-base oils, essential oil blends and simple powdered herbs and clays, but there are also sophisticated formulations that use traditional Ayurvedic herbs in creams or lotions.

The Treatments

There is no typical "ayurvedic" facial, just as there is no typical "American" facial. There are many different sequences and all types of products, from totally traditional to more Western-style products using Indian herbs. Many use the same basic procedures as in the West—cleanse, steam, moisturize, and so on—but the order varies considerably. Ideas common to both include the importance of the whole treatment environment, the caring attitude of the therapist, hygienic procedures for equipment, correct selection of products, and a regular home-care routine.

The goal of an ayurvedic facial is to create a deep sense of peace in the mind as well as the body and to bring balance to the subtle energies of the body, causing a healthy radiance in the face. The products used bring balance to a client's particular ayurvedic skin type. Products labeled Vata, Pitta, or Kapha are balancing for those dosha skin types. The treatment environment, quality of touch, and treatment procedures are customized to match the client's dosha type. Marma points are a vital part of the massage portion of the facial. The basic needs are to cleanse, nourish, and moisturize.

There are many herbs used in ayurvedic skin care to cleanse and nourish the skin, as well as more common ingredients, such as ground almonds, citrus fruit peel, milk, honey, and sugar (Table 23–2). This list includes some herbs that are not well known in the West, but their inclusion here gives you an idea of the number used and the range of actions for each. Oils and essential oil blends are also used to rejuvenate the skin and sometimes replace moisturizing creams in a treatment.

Table 23–2 Herbs

AMALAKI	RUDRAKSHA
Rasayana for Pitta	Healing for the skin, the blood, and circulation
Promotes tissue regeneration	Has spiritual properties
Increases blood cell count	Has emotional properties
Is high in vitamin C	**TRIFALA**
Antioxidant	Skin toner and rejuvenative
ASHWAGANDA	Antioxidant
Nurturing and clarifying mentally	**TULSI (HOLY BASIL)**
Rejuvenates and heals	Clears the aura
Adaptagenic (calms nervous system)	Supports the immune system
Enhances radiance	Antifungal
BRAHMI (GOTA KOLA)	**TUMERIC**
Enhances circulation	Antimicrobial, antioxidant, healing agent
MAHASUDADARSHAN	Moisturizes
Purifies blood	**SHATAVARI**
Antimicrobial	Has anticancer properties
Cleanses blemishes	Environmental protectant
MANJISTHA	Healing soothing, anti-inflammatory
Purifies blood	Softens the skin
Clears lymphatics	Has strong radiance properties
Enhances immune function	**VACHA (CALAMUS)**
Enhances circulation	Revitalizes nerves
Enhances skin quality	Breaks up congestion in the subtle channels
Enhances skin vitality	Is a traditional ingredient in wrinkle formulas
NEEM	Has strong radiance properties
Purifies and detoxifies blood	Revitalizes the body's life force
Has antiviral, antifungal, and antibacterial properties	
Astringent	
Moisturizes	

The herbs and oils can be blended to target particular dosha needs for balance. Following are descriptions of blends targeting particular doshas.

Vata blends should be sweet, warming, grounding, calming, nourishing, hydrating, toning, warming, focusing, clarifying, energy giving, and emotionally balancing.

> ### *Here's a Tip*
>
> Ayurvedic skin care is more than a matter of using exotic Indian herbs and oils. In its purest form it is about helping each client better understand his or her body-mind type and how to best bring balance in his or her own life.

Base oils may include jojoba, avocado, rosehip seed, and sesame. Essential oils may include carrot seed, clary sage, frankincense, rose, rosewood, rose geranium, rose, palmarose, neroli and vanilla. Herbs may include shatavari, ashwagandha, basil, bala, vacha, ginger, and nutmeg.

Pitta blends should be fresh, clean, freeing, cooling, calming, and soothing and should increase patience, sensitivity, and self-love. Base oils may include jojoba, coconut, apricot, olive, shea nut, meadow foam seed, ghee, and sunflower oils. Essential oils may include bergamot, calendula, blue chamomile, fennel, frankincense, immortelle, jasmine, lavender, neroli, rose, sandalwood, spearmint, vertiver, and ylang ylang. Herbs may include neem, shatavari, amalaki, licorice, fennel, cardamon, bringraj and manjista.

Kapha blends should be warming, rich but light, luxurious, comforting, clearing and gently stimulating, energizing, uplifting, and inspiring. Base oils may include jojoba, safflower, sesame, apricot, and grape seed. Essential oils may include bergamot, cinnamon, coriander, clary sage, ginger, juniper berry, lavender, lemongrass, myrrh, neem, nutmeg, orange, patcholi, rosemary, sage, and thyme.

Essential oils for all skin types (tridoshic) include rose, jasmine, lavender, sandalwood, frankincense, melissa, and fennel.

Magical Marmas

The word **marma** is most commonly translated as "vital," "hidden," or "secret energy points," but *marma* also refers to the channels that connect these energy points as well as the energy that runs in these channels. Marmas on the face measure about the width of half a finger. Marmas can also be called *varma*. *Varma* means "a tender spot," so if you are not certain about a location, feel around gently until you locate a more sensitive spot. That will be the marma point.

The marmas are connected by **nadis**, subtle energy channels, 72,000 of which converge at the navel. The nadis carry information, energy, and light, which is why when we work with marmas many clients report feeling more able to focus and more vital and even look brighter and shine more. The fact that there are so many connections at the navel is one reason why a tummy warmer is so comforting and balancing. Using marmas helps balance the doshas through their very close connection with the lymphatic systems, circulation of blood, and nerve impulses as well as the hormonal system.

Marma points work closely with the lymphatic system, and some are identical to points known as *lymphatic gates* in Western tradition or *shiatsu points* in oriental traditions. Though acupuncture sites are the same as marma points, the energy network on which marma points communicate and connect are not the same as the acupuncture meridians. Marmas are connected to the Chakras, and the seven Chakras are themselves considered major marmas.

Marmas are described as the places on the skin where energy and matter come together or where the mind communicates with the body. The sites in your body pick up how you are feeling and what you are thinking, communicating this message to your skin and, eventually, to all of the systems in your body. This explains why your skin glows when you are happy or in love, looks taut when you are stressed, and lacks tone when you feel sad.

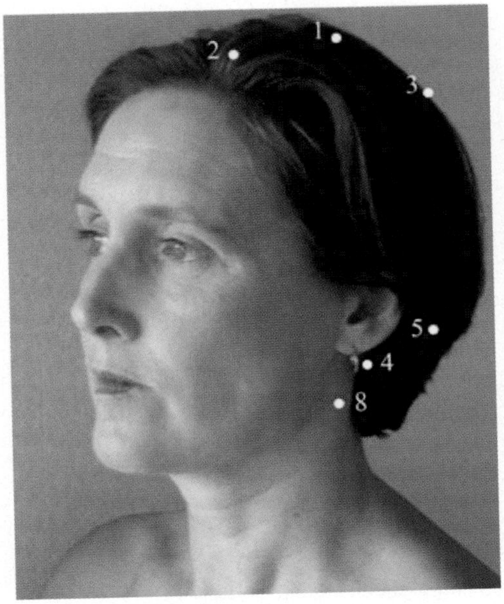

Figure 23–4 Marma points on the scalp and neck (side view).

There are 107 major marmas used in full body therapeutic sequences, 37 of which are on the head and neck and chest (Figure 23–4). More than a third of the major energy points are touched during a facial, which is why they are so pleasurable and enhance the feeling of well-being (Figure 23–5).

FOCUS ON: *Marmas*

Along with the 107 major marmas, there are 84,000 minor marma points all over the body; some sources refer to the skin itself as the 108th marma. Marma points can be thought of as an intelligence network that keeps the body in touch with itself and its needs. It is useful to think of them as eyes that are looking around their particular location and ears listening to subconscious thoughts. If they are closed or not fully functional, the body does not get the communication it needs.

Marma points are damaged or closed by physical traumas, such as accidents or injuries. It is not unusual for a client to report feeling emotionally altered after an accident or to be uncomfortable even after bones and tendons have healed. According to ayurvedic understanding, this is because the marmas have been traumatized and are not fully functioning and the needs of the tissues are not fully seen or heard. Physical trauma can and often does occur at birth, which is why infant massage is practiced even in the poorest villages in India.

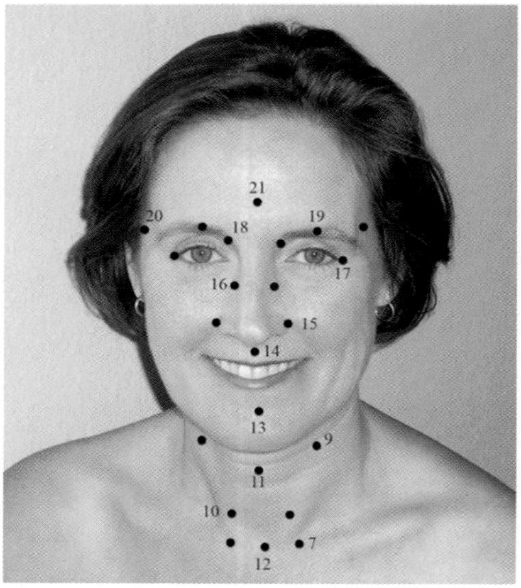

Figure 23–5 Marma points on the face.

Marmas can be closed by stress. The phrases "being out of touch with myself" or feeling "closed down" are exactly what we experience when mental tension has closed the marma network. Diet and lifestyle can be contributors. Touch of all kinds is vital for a healthy life so hold, hug, and love your clients and those you love. It is good for their marmas.

The main way to open marmas is gentle touch. It might be a touch with the hand over an area where the marma is, gentle finger pressure, massaging in small circles over the marma point, or touch with a variety of tools such as warm stones. Marmas are also opened by exercise, especially with hatha yoga postures, aroma therapy, light therapy, and chanting or singing.

Marmas help the skin care for itself. They are the network that communicates the skin's needs to the body, which meets those needs (Figure 23–5 and Table 23–3). But marmas do not work just with the physical body; they work with the mind and affect the deepest part of your being.

When marmas are open and healthy, there is good communication and the needs of the skin are well met. The skin is well nourished, hydrated, and cleansed and so will age slowly and look vibrant. Open marmas helps the mind to be open, relaxed, and inclined to make healthy choices. On the innermost level when marmas are open, you feel basically good and inspired. You have an inner sense of peace and contentment that shows in a gentle radiance.

When the marmas are closed, the skin and supporting tissues are not getting their needs met and the skin manifests a range of problems, such as too dry, very oily, congested, infected, or swollen. The posture degenerates, pain and tension gather in the body, and premature aging sets in. Intuition is impaired. There is depression, less sense of purpose, or poor memory. If you ever hear clients say "I just have no idea how to cope anymore," they are experiencing closed or semi-closed marmas. It could be that your therapeutic, loving touch may be all that is needed for them to reconnect and find ways to help themselves.

Following is a basic marma point massage. Through advanced studies, you can learn to customize this massage for each specific dosha and to employ more intricate techniques. Marma massage is always performed with the client reclining on a facial lounge or massage bed. It may be a specialty stand-alone treatment prior to a Shirodhara or in conjunction with another ayurvedic therapy.

CAUTION!

This is a basic procedure. Pressure and protocols vary slightly with the dosha type being treated. You should seek supplemental training to master this technique.

Opening Sequence

This short sequence is taught by Dr. Vasant Lad as a wonderful way to start any ayurvedic treatment, making the client feel completely comfortable and relaxed. It can be used before any treatment in which you need the client to feel quickly relaxed.

Table 23–3 Benefits of Balancing Facial Marma

BENEFITS OF BALANCING FACIAL MARMA	
1. MURDHNI or ADHIPATI	Calms the mind, kindles deeper understanding, fosters contentment, heightens perception and assists with spinal alignment
2. BRAHMA RANDRA	Helps insomnia, elevates mood, eases headaches, and balances body weight
3. SHIVA RANDRA	Helps lower blood pressure, relieves dizziness, and improves memory and sense of alertness
4. KARNAMULA	Helps relieve jaw tension, eases ear congestion, and states of anxiety or mental tension

Table 23–3 *continued*

5. KRIKATIKA	Helps relieve tension in the neck and back and improve posture
6. SIMANTA	Feels nurturing and helps rest and relaxation
7. AKSHAKA	Helps to balance the liver (right) and spleen (left), which helps dispel anger and boost energy
8. MANYAMULA	Improves circulation to the face and stimulates lymph
9. SIRA MATRIKA	Helps to improve facial circulation and voice
10. SIRAMANTHA	Helps to improve the voice and ease throat and neck pain
11. KANTHA	Helps to improve thyroid function and the ability to express feelings and regulate mood
12. KATHANADI	Helps to clear the voice and upper respiratory congestion
13. HANU	Helps to improve circulation to the face and connect with inner feelings
14. OSHTA	Helps to ease dizziness and fainting, improve mental clarity, and sexual desire
15. KAPOLA NASA	Helps clear sinuses, strengthen lungs, and cope with stress
16. URDHVA GANDU	Helps to clear the sinuses and brighten the eyes
17. APANGA	Helps relieve eye strain and puffiness or inflammation
18. ASHRU ANTARA	Helps to ease eye strain and headaches
19. BHRUH and ASHRU MADHYA	Relieves stress, benefits eyes, and eases headaches
20. SHANKHA	Improves memory and helps with feeling more connected and calm
21. AJNA or STHAPANI	Helps relieve tension and bring peace and harmony to the mind

PROCEDURE 23–1 OPENING SEQUENCE MASSAGE

IMPLEMENTS AND MATERIALS

- Facial lounge with standard linen and towel setup
- Appropriate products for facial treatment to be performed
- Appropriate supplies for treatment to be performed
- No special supplies are needed for these manipulations.

Preparation

1 Prepare facial lounge and towels.

2 Gather supplies and products as necessary.

Procedure

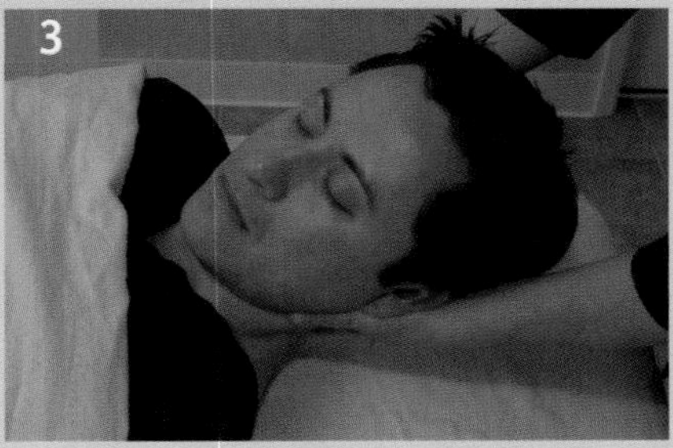

Release tension in the neck.

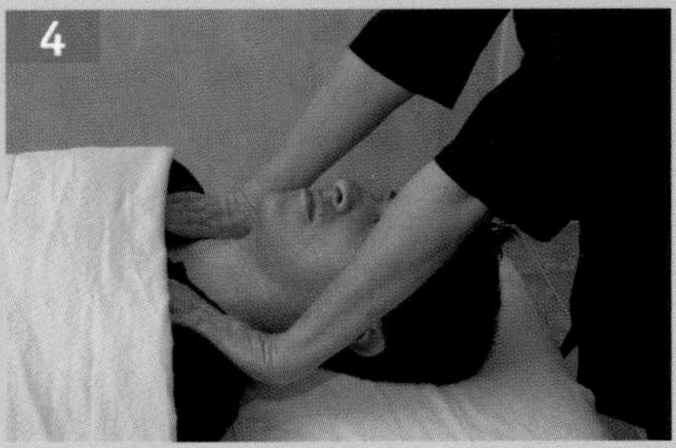

Press on the shoulders.

3 Cradle the head, resting your fingertips along the occipital line at the back of the head, with thumbs either closing or resting in front of the ear. Raise the head slowly and gently until there is a complete stretch in the back of the neck. Hold for a moment. Lower the head very slowly. Repeat twice more.

4 Keep your elbows straight, rest your hands on the shoulders, and lean forward. Release the pressure, take in a big, deep breath with your client, let the breath out, and lean on the shoulders again. Repeat twice more.

continues on next page

PROCEDURE 23–1, CONT. OPENING SEQUENCE MASSAGE

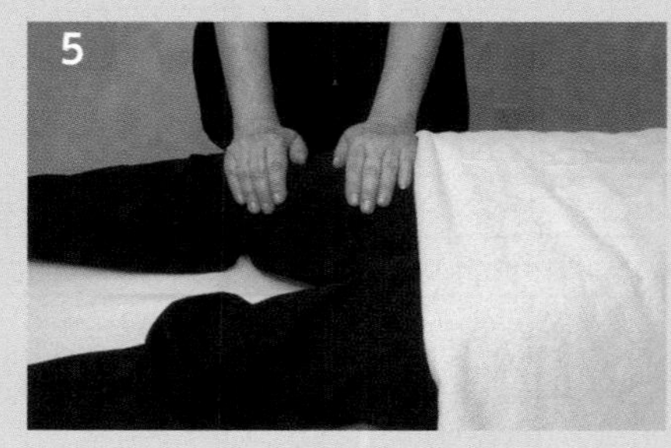
Touch the knees.

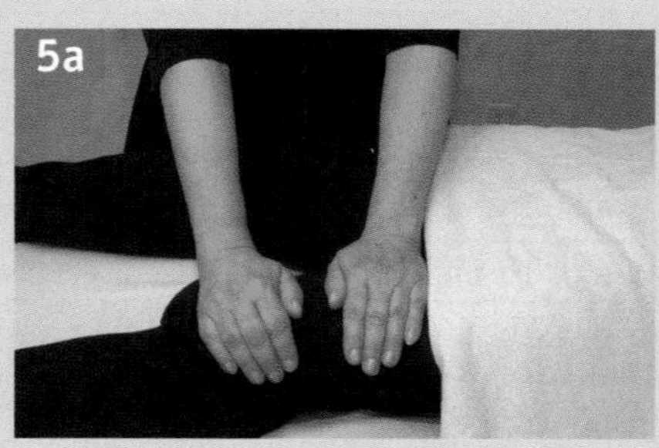
Rotate the knee cap.

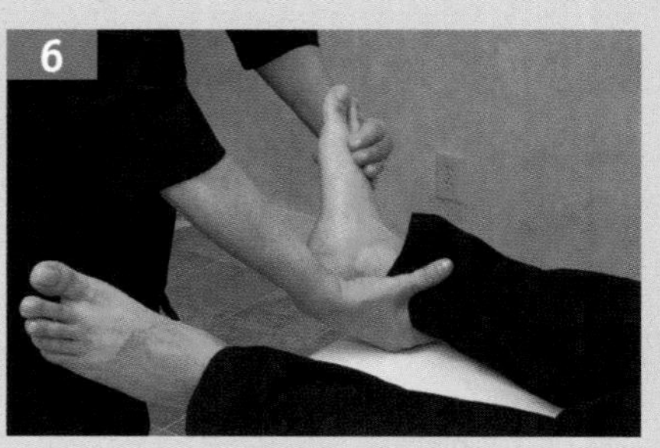
Rotate the ankles.

5 Move to the side of the client and move the covers so that you can touch the knees. Start with the right knee. Rest the left hand on the right thigh and then rotate the kneecap five times counter clockwise and then five times clockwise. Reach over and repeat on the other knee.

6 Move to the foot of the bed. Rotate the ankles, slowly, through a full range of motion: right foot first, three times counter-clockwise, three times clockwise. Repeat on the left foot.

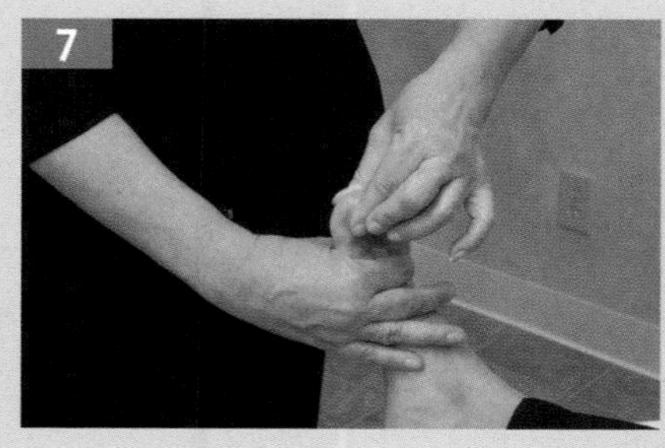
Gently pull the toes.

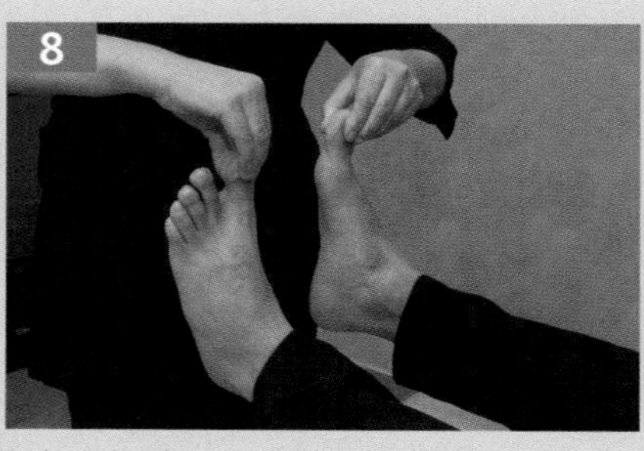
Relax the feet.

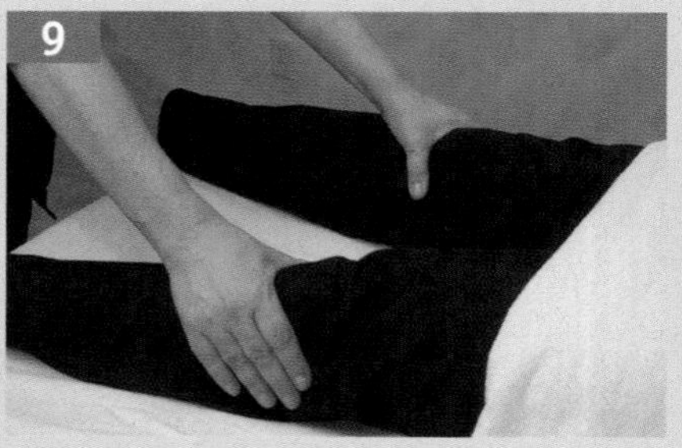
Hold at the knees.

7 Start with one foot, grasp the big toe and stretch, then rotate. Repeat with the other foot.

8 Lift the feet with both big toes, stretch, and gently jiggle the ankles. Repeat with each pair of toes, ending with baby toes.

9 Hold both legs at the knees, with your thumb resting in the hollow at the bend of the knee. Hold this position for a few moments.

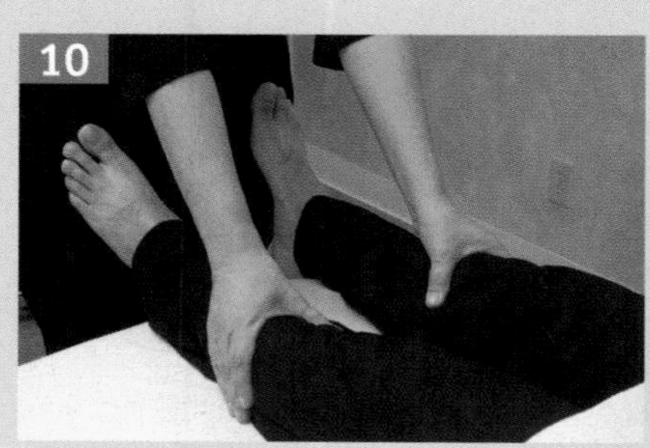
Hold the calf muscle.

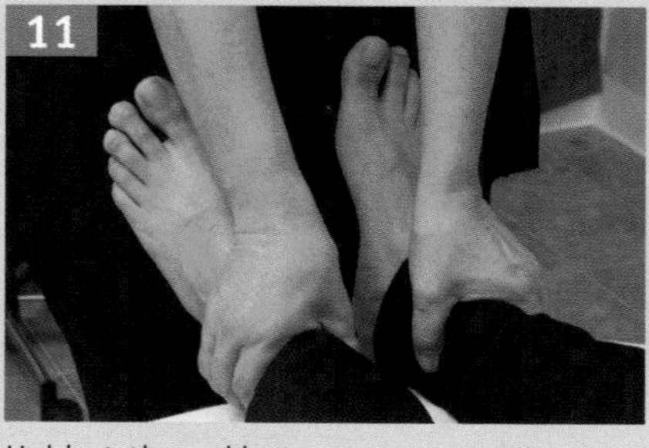
Hold at the ankles.

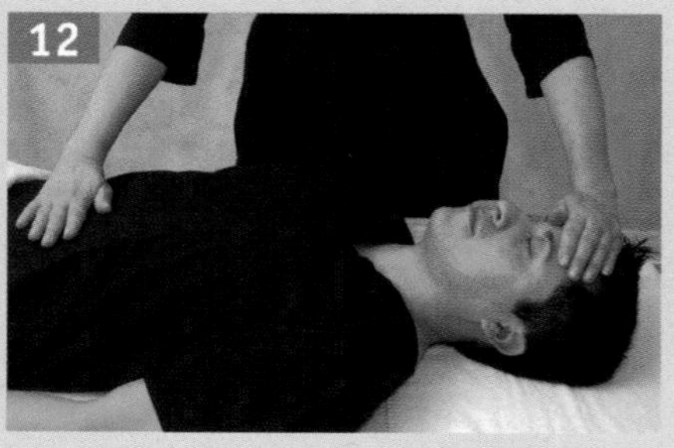
Place one hand on the client's abdomen and one on the forehead.

10 Hold the top of the calf muscle as in step 9.

11 Hold at the ankles, thumbs resting one inch below the medial maleolus.

12 Move to the side of the bed and place one hand on the client's abdomen and one on the forehead. Hold for a few moments.

Post-procedure

Now you may move into any other procedure desired.

Clean-up and Disinfection

13 Perform standard clean-up and disinfection procedures following state guidelines.

14 Prepare the room for the next client.

PROCEDURE 23–2 BASIC MARMA POINT MASSAGE

IMPLEMENTS AND MATERIALS

- Standard facial lounge setup with linens and towels
- Disposable sponges, gauze squares, or warm towels
- Ayurvedic massage oil blend, 5 to 10 drops
- Sun protection moisturizer (appropriate for client's skin type)

Preparation

1 Prepare treatment lounge.

2 Gather supplies and products.

3 Warm the oil in a massage oil heater or other warming device. This makes the treatment more luxurious and allows for quicker penetration into the skin.

4 Review the client's history with him or her and assure the appropriateness of procedure. Then select the appropriate ayurvedic massage blend based on the client's dosha.

Procedure

You may find it more comfortable to do the massage with one hand while the other hand stabilizes and retains contact with the client in a supportive manner.

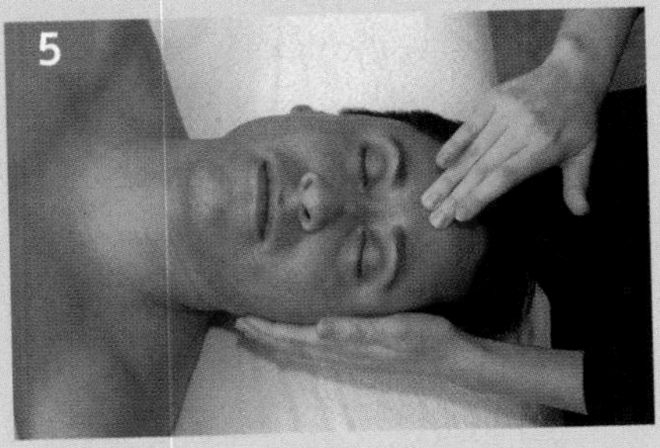

Position 1.

5 Position 1, on the midline of the head, **11** finger widths above the eyebrows. Using your thumb, middle finger, or fourth finger, perform 15 to 30 gentle clockwise circles.

6 Position 2, on the midline of the head, 8 finger widths above the eyebrows. Using your thumb, middle finger, or fourth finger, perform 15 to 30 gentle clockwise circles.

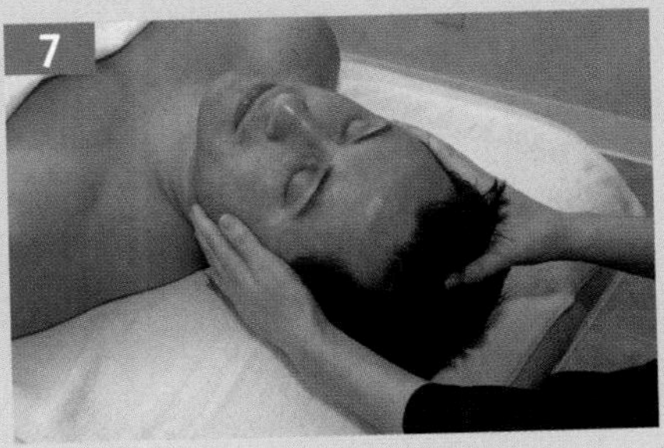

Position 3.

7 Position 3, on the midline of the head, 15 widths above the eyebrows. Lift and stabilize the head with one hand while massaging with the other. Using your thumb, middle finger, or fourth finger, perform 15 to 30 gentle clockwise circles.

8 Position 4. For this zone, do first behind the left ear, and then roll head gently to the other side and repeat on right ear. Using your thumb, middle finger, or fourth finger, perform 15 to 30 gentle clockwise circles.

continues on next page

PROCEDURE 23-2, CONT. BASIC MARMA POINT MASSAGE

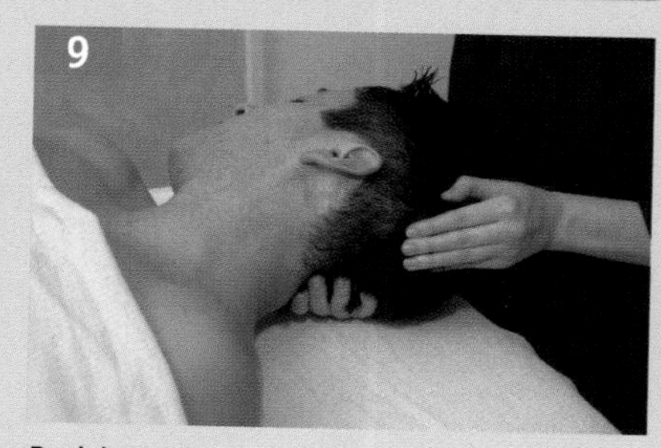

Position 5.

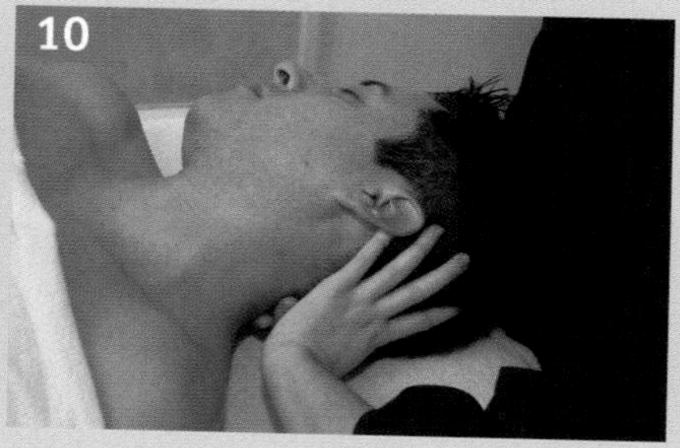

Position 6.

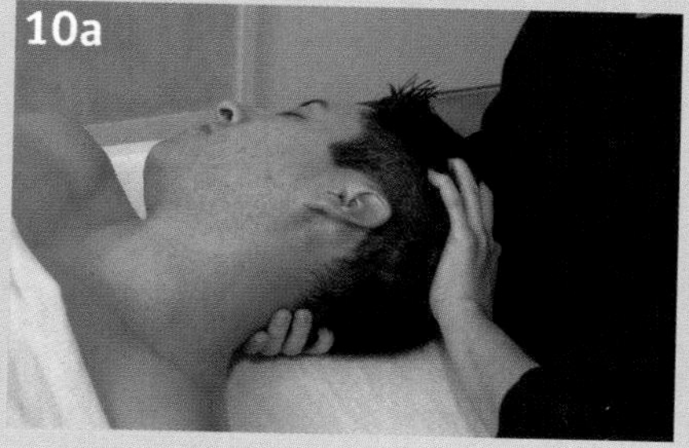

Lift and stabilize the head.

9 Position 5. Place hands on both sides of the head at the top of the spine. Support the head with one hand and massage with the other, rotating your hands as needed to completely massage both sides of the head. Work deeply enough to manipulate the skin and muscles of the scalp. Use all of your fingertips to move over the scalp, using sufficient pressure to gently move the scalp over the skull and systematically work over entire scalp.

10 Position 6, all of the joints in the skull. Use all of your fingertips to encourage the scalp to move over the skull, systematically working over the entire scalp. Lift and stabilize the head with one hand while massaging with the other.

11 Position 7, on the top of the collarbone where it joins the breast bone. Press and release down toward the waist. Repeat 3 times.

12 Position 8, the side of the neck, 4 finger widths below the earlobe. Apply gentle lymph drainage in a press-release pattern, repeating 3 times.

13 Position 9, either side of the upper windpipe. Apply gentle lymph drainage in press-release, pattern repeating 3 times.

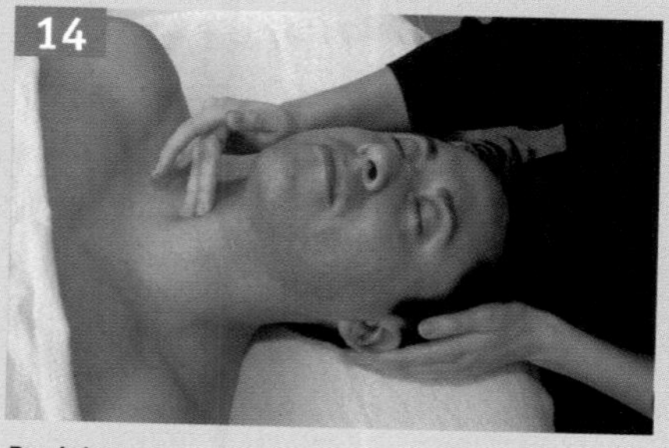

Position 10.

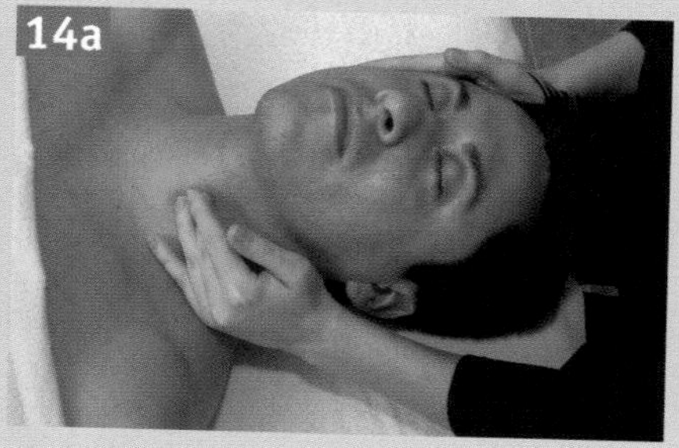

Position 10.

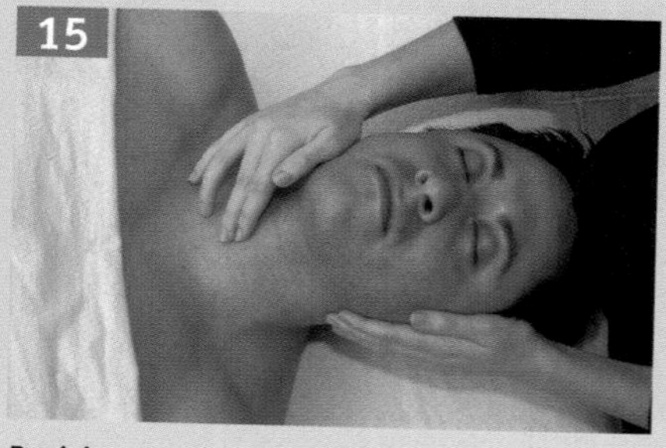

Position 11.

14 Position 10, either side of the lower windpipe. Apply gentle lymph drainage in a press-release pattern, repeating 3 times.

15 Position 11, mid-neck or around the Adam's apple. Apply gentle clockwise circular massage, repeating 3 times.

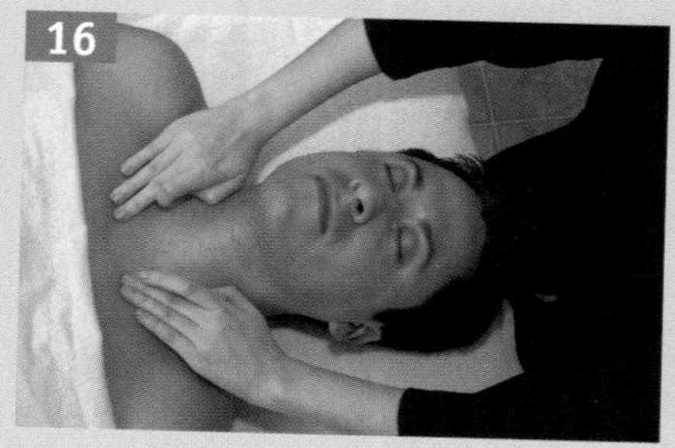

Position 12.

16 Position 12, slightly behind the top of the breastbone. Apply gentle lymph drainage. Press and release gently toward the waist. Repeat three times.

17 Position 13, in the middle of the chin. Press and release gently 10 times.

18 Position 14, in the middle of the upper lip. Press and release gently 10 times.

19 Position 15, where each nostril joins the face. Press and release gently 10 times.

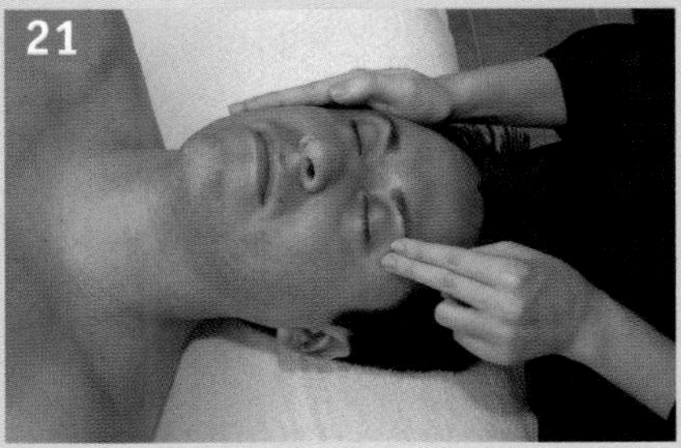
Position 17.

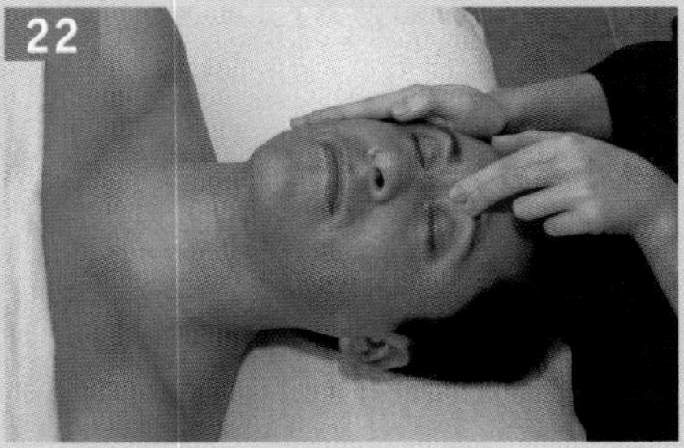
Position 18.

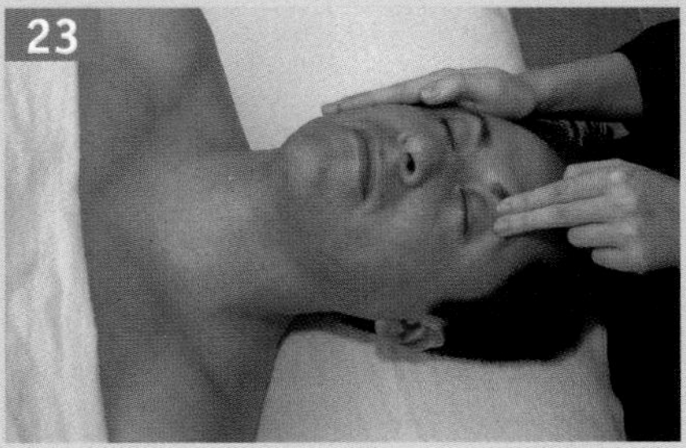
Position 19.

20 Position 16, halfway up the nose on either side. Press and release gently 10 times.

21 Position 17, in the outer corner of each eye. Press away from the eye toward the boney orbit. Press and release gently 10 times.

22 Position 18, below the inner corners of the eyebrows on the upper boney orbit. Gently press away from the eye toward the top of the head. Press and release gently 10 times.

23 Position 19, in the middle of the eyebrows. Press and release gently 10 times.

24 Position 20, in the hollows of both temples. Gently rub with 10 small circles.

25 Position 21, in the middle of the forehead on the midline 2 finger-widths above the eyebrows. Gently rub single finger in clockwise spiral, starting very tiny and slowly expanding to cover the entire middle of the forehead.

26 Decant appropriate ayurvedic oil into palms of your hands but do not rub hands together.

27 Position 22. Cradle the client's face along the jawline and ask him or her to inhale the aromatic essence of the oil.

28 Position 23. Stroke under the chin. Wrap your fingers under the client's chin with fingers interlaced, and using alternating hands pull outward toward the ear lobes, following the soft tissue on the underside of the jaw and using moderately firm pressure. Repeat 5 strokes with each hand.

29 Position 24. Chin to temple glide. Using 2 fingers of each hand, trace along the jawline from the center of the chin to the temple, and perform 5 circles on the temporal region.

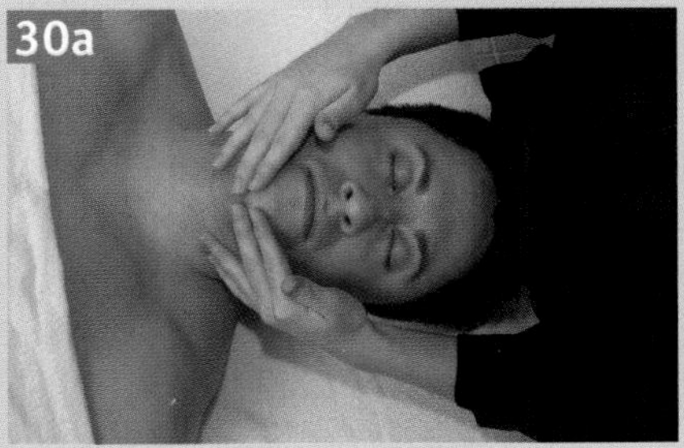
Position 25: Center of the mentalis.

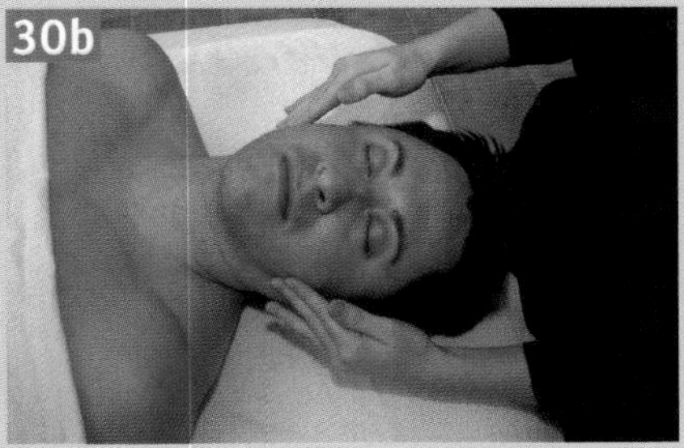
Position 25: Slide up over the chin to a point on jawline.

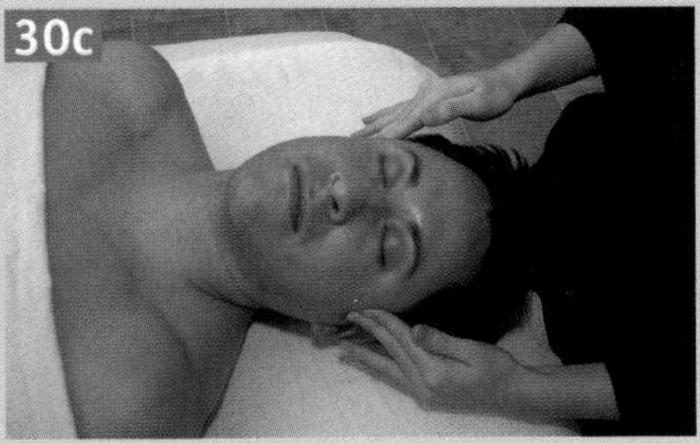
Position 25: Slide to a point on the jawline in line with the masseter muscle.

30 Position 25. Chin to temple release using 2 fingers from each hand simultaneously.

a. Perform 3 press release patterns on the center of the mentalis.
b. Slide up over the chin to a point on the jawline below the outer corners of the mouth and perform 5 circles.
c. Slide to a point on the jawline in line with the masseter muscle, and do 3 press/release patterns.

continues on next page

PROCEDURE 23-2, CONT. BASIC MARMA POINT MASSAGE

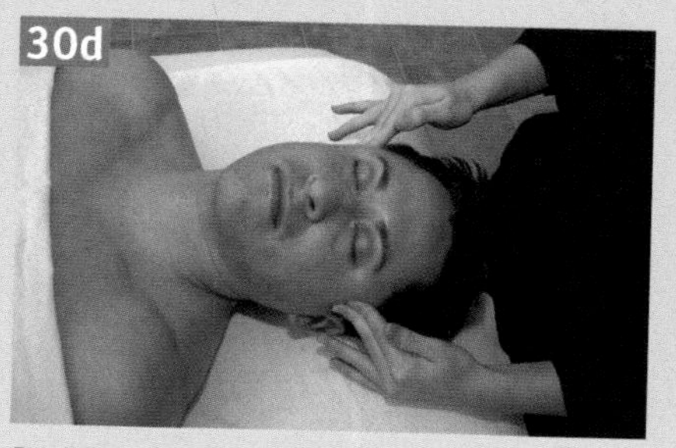

Position 25: Travel to temple.

d. Travel to the temple and perform 5 circles in temporal regions.

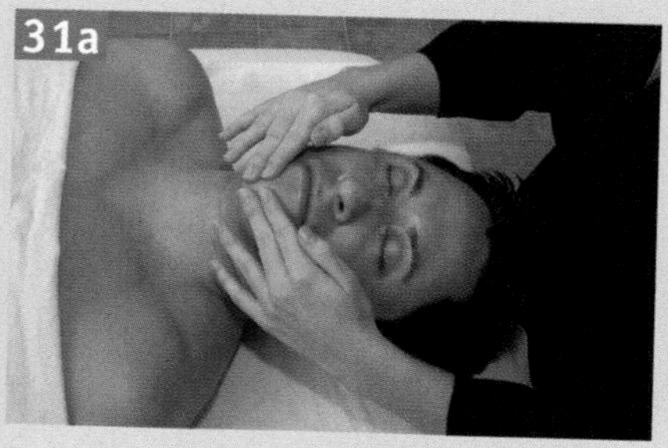

Position 26: Center of the mentalis.

31 Position 26. Up the face movement using 2 fingers from each hand simultaneously.

a. Perform 3 press-release patterns on the center of the mentalis.

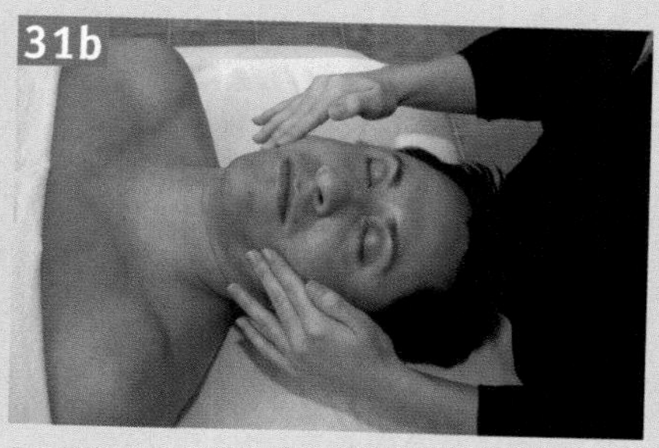

Position 26: Glide to the corners of the mouth.

b. Glide to the corners of the mouth and perform 5 small circles.

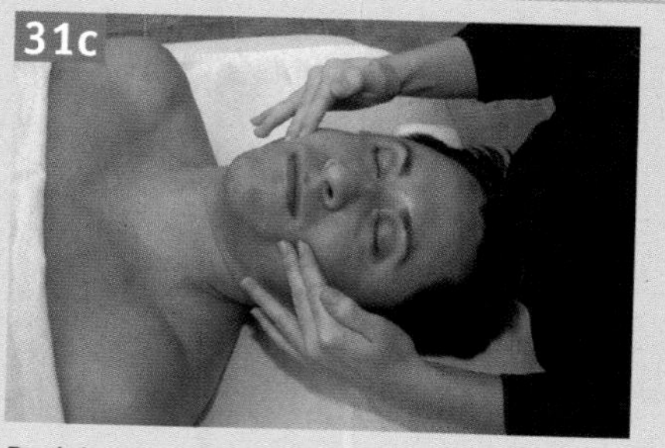

Position 26: Glide to the underside of the masseter.

c. Glide to the underside of the masseter and perform 3 press-release patterns.

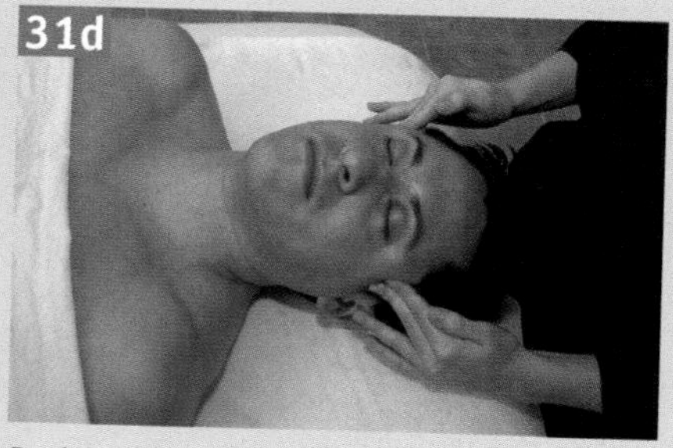

Position 26: Glide to the temples.

d. Glide to the temples and perform 5 circles.

32 Position 27. Center of lip to mastoid (both hands simultaneously).

a. Starting at center of upper lip using one finger from each hand, perform 3 press-release patterns.
b. Slide to either side of the upper lip at the outer corners of the mouth and perform 5 small circles.
c. Slide to the front of the masseter muscle and press and release firmly 3 times.
d. Slide toward the ear and then up and over the ear to the mastoid process.
e. Perform 5 circles on the mastoid process.

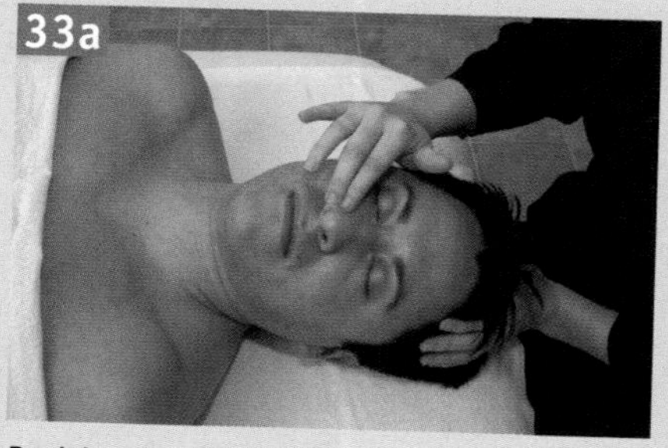

Position 28: Flare of the right nostril.

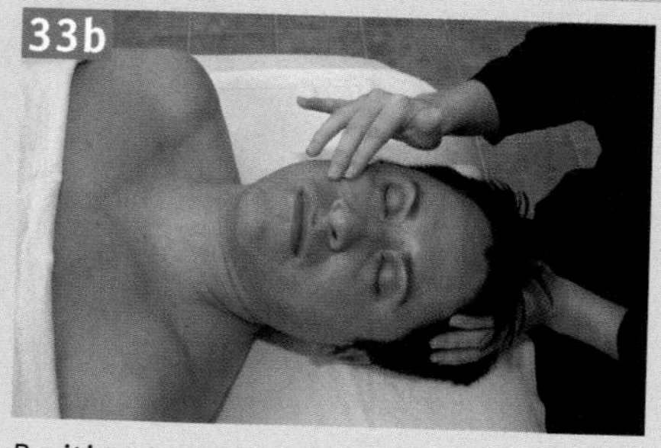

Position 28: Stroke across the cheek bone to the ear.

33 Position 28, nose to mastoid. This is done one side of the face at a time. The hand not being used for massage is resting on the top of the client's head.

a. At the flare of the right nostril, perform 3 press-release patterns.
b. Stroke under the cheekbone to the ear, and then slide up and over to the mastoid process.

33c

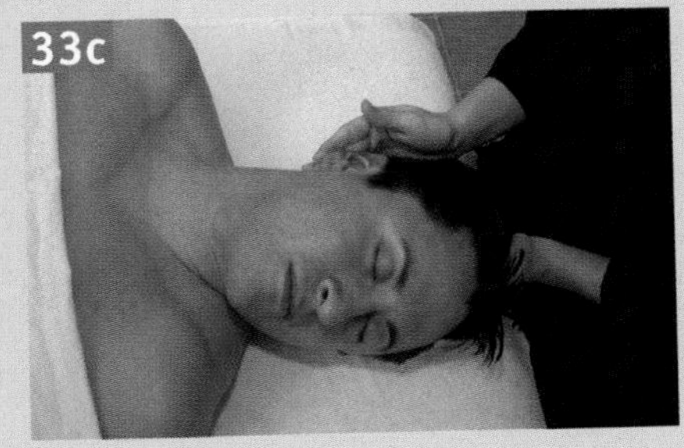

Position 28: Perform 5 circles on the mastoid process.

c. Perform 5 circles on the mastoid process.

d. Repeat on the left side of the face.

34a

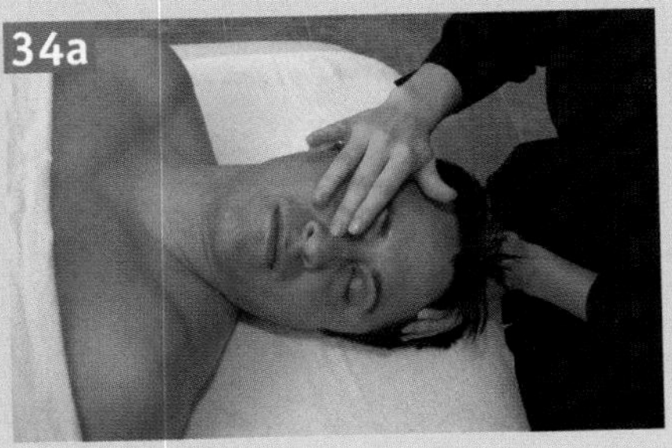

Position 29: Mid-nose to mastoid.

34 Position 29. Mid-nose to mastoid. This is performed on both sides of the face simultaneously.

a. Starting at the point about halfway up the nose where the cartilage meets the cheek, perform 3 press-release patterns.

34b

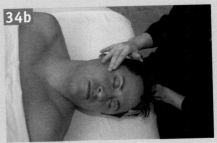

Position 29: Slide across cheek to the ear, up and over the ear to the mastoid process.

b. Slide across cheek to the ear, up and over the ear to the mastoid process.

34c

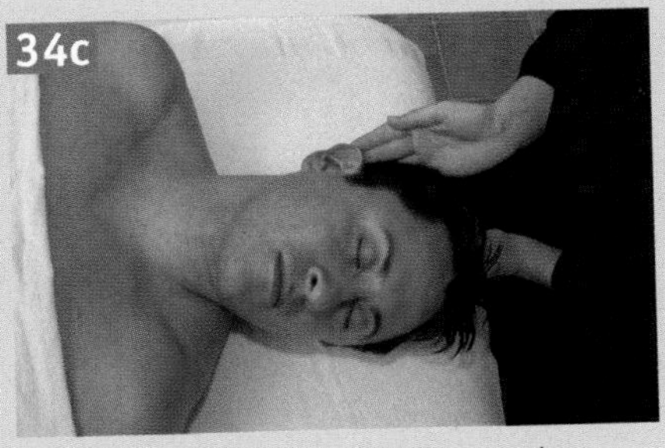

Position 29: Perform 5 circles on the mastoid process.

c. Perform 5 circles on the mastoid process.

35 Position 30, under eyes. Perform one eye at a time with the other hand resting on the client's head for stability and security. All pressure in this area should be on the lower ridge of the orbital bone toward the toes of the client, not into the eye socket area.

a. Starting at the inner corner of the eye socket, perform 3 press-release patterns.

b. Glide about a quarter of the way across the eye and repeat.

c. Glide about half of the way across the eye, and repeat.

d. Glide about three-quarters of the way across the eye and repeat.

e. Glide to outer corner of the eye, and "jiggle" the tissue gently but firmly.

36 Position 31, nose to brow. This is done with both hands at the same time until you are working above the eyes.

a. Starting at the tip of the nose, glide up the nose to just below the inner corner of the eyebrow. Allow your left hand to travel up and cover the left side of the client's head.

b. At the inner corner of the eye, perform 3 press-release patterns.

c. Glide a quarter of the way along the brow bone and repeat.

d. Glide half of the way along the brow bone and repeat.

e. Glide three-quarters of the way along the brow bone and repeat.

f. Glide to the end of the brow bone and repeat.

37 Position 32, brow pinch. This is done with the thumbs and index fingers of both hands at the same time.

a. Starting at the inner corners of the brow, gently but firmly pinch and release.

b. Shift 1 finger width toward the outer brow and repeat.

c. Repeat this pattern across the brow, ending at the outer corners.

continues on next page

PROCEDURE 23–2, CONT. BASIC MARMA POINT MASSAGE

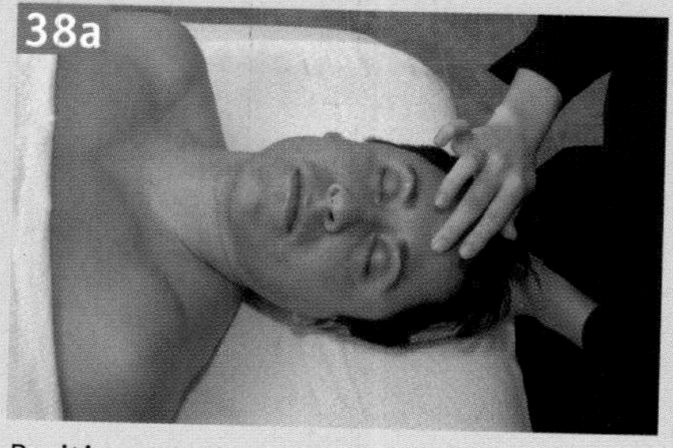

Position 33: Nose-forehead spiral.

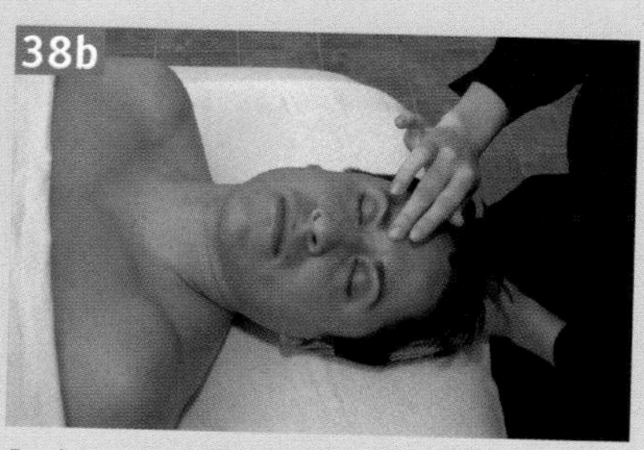

Position 33: Start with a tiny circle and slowly enlarging the movement, trace a spiral that grows to encompass the entire forehead.

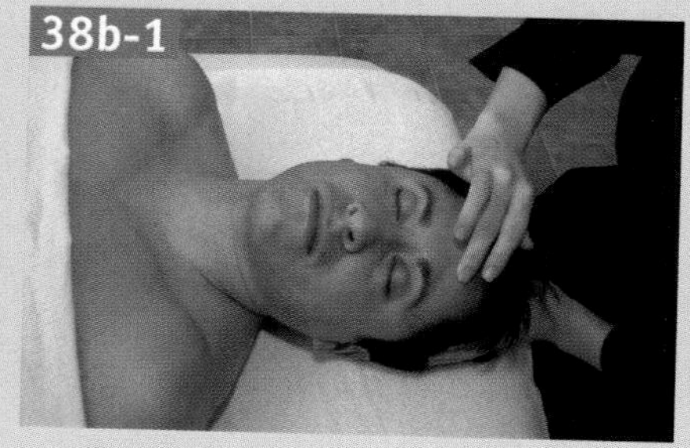

Position 33: Start with a tiny circle and, slowly enlarging the movement, trace a spiral that grows to encompass the entire forehead.

38 Position 33, nose-forehead spiral

a. Place one hand on top of the client's head. Using 2 fingers of the free hand, slide up from the tip of the nose to the forehead, just above and between the brows.

b. Starting with a tiny circle and slowly enlarging, trace a spiral that grows to encompass the entire forehead.

39 Position 34, zigzags. This movement is a bit stimulating to slowly rouse the client.

a. Glide back to the center point just above the brows. Still using just one hand, place multiple fingers in a row perpendicular to the brow across forehead.

b. Trace zigzags across the forehead to one temple and then back across the forehead to other temple.

40 Position 35. Next offer a more vigorous massage of the scalp and ears using pads of fingers or full hands, as best fits the client's head and your hand size.

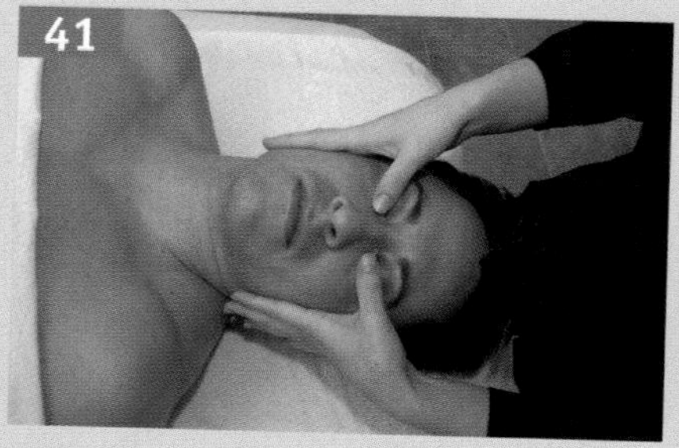

Position 36

41 Position 36. Now rest the thumbs on the closed eyelids of the client and close the ears with the middle fingers. Hold position for a minute.

42 Position 37. Remove any excess massage oil with a warm moist towel, wet disposable sponges, or cotton pads.

43 Position 38. Complete with appropriate SPF product or move into additional facial steps as desired.

Post-procedure

44 Gently rouse the client and offer him or her water or an appropriate beverage for their dosha.

45 As this is very relaxing, advise the client to get up carefully. Make sure the client is alert.

46 Answer any questions the client may have about the massage and any anticipated results.

47 Encourage the client to drink water for the next few hours to continue the internal cleansing process. Also, make the client aware that since this can be a detoxifying treatment, they may experience some side effects (possibly headache or mild nausea, or no symptoms at all).

Clean-up and Disinfection

48 Clean the treatment room and work area following OSHA and state guidelines.

49 Disinfect all linens and supplies and throw away any disposable items.

50 Prepare the room for the next client.

Shirodhara Treatment

Shirodhara (she-row-dar-ra) literally means to play a threadlike stream of oil on the head (Figure 23–6). It is offered as a 30-minute add-on after other relaxing treatments to deeply relax and refresh the client. Sometimes oils are used that are beneficial to the hair and scalp; in fact this treatment was introduced to the spa industry as a warm oil scalp treatment. Now a variety of oils and sometimes herbal buttermilks are being used, which takes the benefits far beyond soft hair.

For a Shirodhara treatment, the client lies on the back with the head slightly tilted back while you pour a warm oil or cool buttermilk over the middle of the forehead for 10 to 20 minutes. This stimulates the marma, or vital energy point, on the middle of the forehead, sending a message to the brain to release serotonin. This is sometimes called the *pleasure response,* as the body is easily able to enjoy the experience of letting go and relaxing deeply. On a more subtle level, energies around the spine are freed, which helps calm and clear the mind. In Tibetan Ayurveda, Shirodhara is called "psycho-spiritual" massage. It is a process that demands a mindful attitude on the part of the therapist. If you create a safe and "sacred" space, the client will have an experience that will help him or her become more in touch with his or her innermost being.

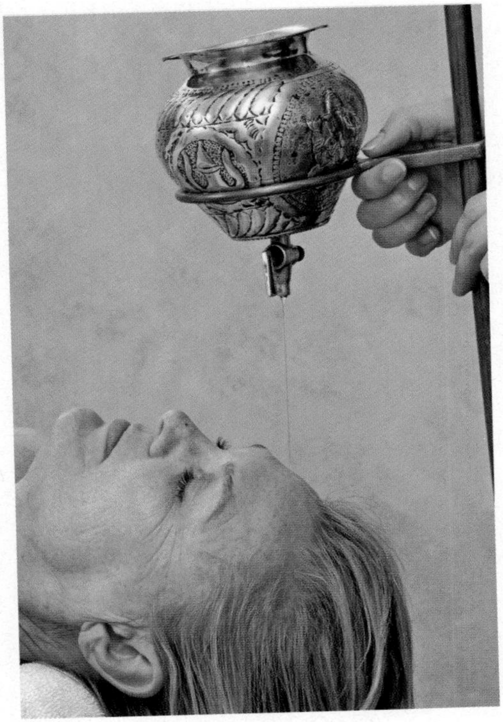

Figure 23–6 Shirodhara treatment.

Shirodhara has similar benefits to a great night's sleep. It promotes deep relaxation while gently energizing the body. It also helps with stress headaches, alleviation of insomnia, and improving the quality of your sleep. It improves mental clarity and decision-making abilities, strengthens meditative states, and even assists in substance abuse recovery.

FOCUS ON: *Shirodhara Contraindications*

Do not perform Shirodhara on clients who have the following conditions:

- **Late-term pregnancy (Client will be on her back for a prolonged time, causing discomfort.)**
- **Neck pain or whiplash injury**
- **Very low blood pressure (Shirodhara lowers blood pressure.)**
- **Intoxicated or under the influence of recreational drugs**
- **Epilepsy**
- **Brain tumors**
- **Cuts or rashes on the scalp**
- **An aversion to flowing oil**
- **Currently receiving cranial-sacral therapy**
- **In a hurry to leave (The client needs to relax and be grounded before driving.)**

Environmental Considerations

Follow these steps to ensure the best treatment environment possible for your client.

- The treatment room must be quiet, with as little foot traffic as possible moving past the door. As clients become sound-sensitive even small noises can feel surprisingly irritating.
- You must be able to sit still while the oil is pouring.
- The room should have lighting and sound systems that are independent from the rest of the facility.
- Ideally the room should be near a shower or a quiet hair-washing area; alternatively the client will return home and wash his or her hair.
- A silent aromatherapy diffuser is a wonderful addition.
- Candles help make a special atmosphere, if allowed by law.

- Music should be calming instrumentals that are not suggestive of a particular place or scene.
- Possible add-ons include application of oil to the abdomen and a cool compress on the eyes.
- Hot stones on the feet are helpful, as are tension-relief products on the neck and shoulders.

Shirodhara Pre-Treatment Information

Before you take the client to the treatment room, check the client's medical history for contraindications, and then explain the treatment and have your client read over and sign a Shirodhara Information and Advice sheet. This form should include a description such as the following:

The Shirodhara treatment can evoke an extremely deep relaxing state and have a profound effect on the psyche. It is not uncommon for some to experience dreamlike states, lights, colors, and/or strong emotions. Others simply experience lightness, clarity, and a sense of open awareness that is both freeing and somewhat magical. Experiences like these can often leave us feeling more open but also a little more vulnerable. For this reason, we strongly recommend that after your Shirodhara treatment, you neither drive, return directly to work, or go into any circumstance that you deem to be stressful. Allow at least 30 minutes after your treatment to dress slowly and be our guest for tea and a snack. Then return to a place that is quiet and supportive for a few hours.

PROCEDURE 23-3 SHIRODHARA TREATMENT

IMPLEMENTS AND MATERIALS

- Massage table
- Shirodhara equipment (bowl, stand, dispenser)
- Oil warming equipment
- 2 sheets and 1 blanket
- 1 head support pillow
- 1¼ pints refined sesame oil
- Hand towel
- Plastic spa sheet
- Facial tissue
- Paper towel
- Candles (optional)
- Music and music player

Preparation

1 Evaluate the client to assure that treatment is appropriate. Use the quesionnaire in Table 23–1 to determine the client's dosha. More Pitta clients seem to appreciate slightly cooler oil or a moving stream; more Vata clients prefer a wider stream and warmer oil; and Kapha clients are easily satisfied.

2 Prepare the treatment room, using the plastic spa sheet to protect the lounge and draping it over the end of the table so that it falls into the catch basin; the oil will flow from the hair down the plastic into the bowl.

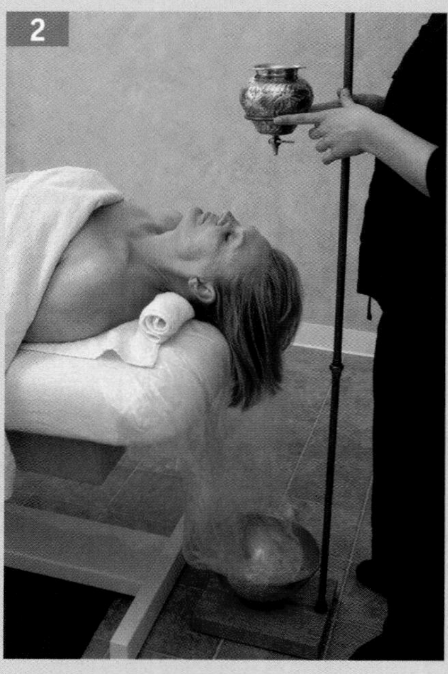

Prepare treatment room.

3 Gather and prepare the supplies you will need.

4 Gather the products you will need for the treatment.

5 Set the treatment oil to warm in the hot towel cabinet or a massage oil warmer. (It is better

to have it too hot than too cold, although not so hot as to burn.)

6 Have extra room-temperature oil available to adjust the heat of the oil, as needed. Oil should be above body temperature and feel warm to the inner wrist or hand.

7 Prepare for the client and wash your hands.

Procedure

The treatment is performed in a very simple sequence:

8 Commence with your opening movements as desired.

9 Optional: Perform Marma Point Massage.

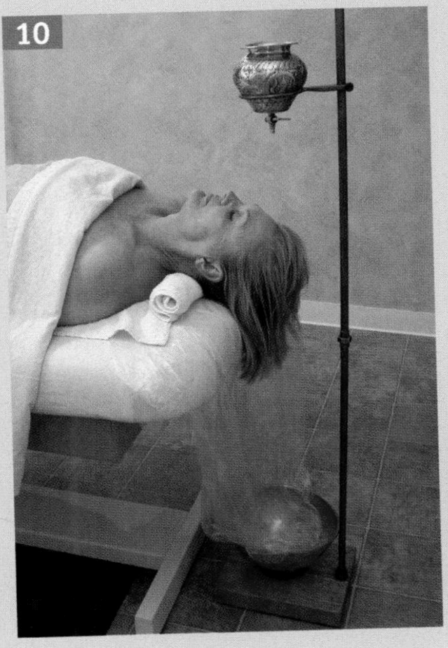

Position the client.

10 Position the client so the head is slightly over the end of the massage table and you can see a gentle slope to the forehead. Use a pillow or small, rolled-up towel for extra neck comfort, if needed. As they move, make sure the spa plastic sheeting is underneath the client's head so as to protect your linens and guide the flowing oil onto the side of the bowl. Allowing oil to flowl onto the side of the bowl is quieter and less disturbing than having it drip into the bowl.

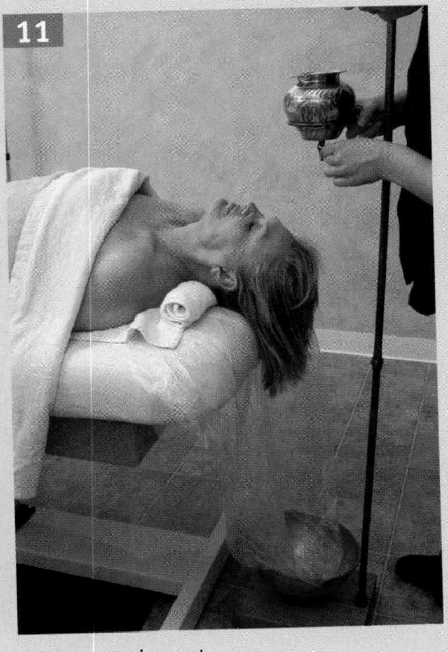

Arrange equipment.

11 Position the Shirodhara equipment so the top of the oil stream is about 4 inches above the client's forehead. Arrange the bowl that is for catching the oil on the floor, allowing the spa plastic sheeting to drape into the bowl.

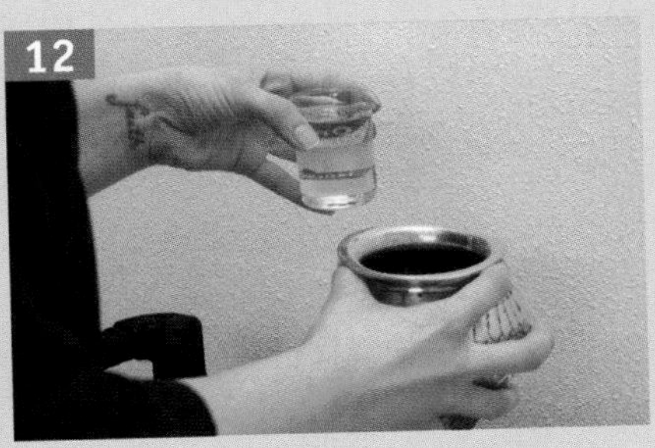

Double-check the temperature of the oil.

12 Double-check the temperature of the oil before filling the Shirodhara vessel. Add room-temperature oil as needed to achieve proper temperature. The oil should be no more than 2–3 degrees above body temperature which is pleasantly warm on the hand.

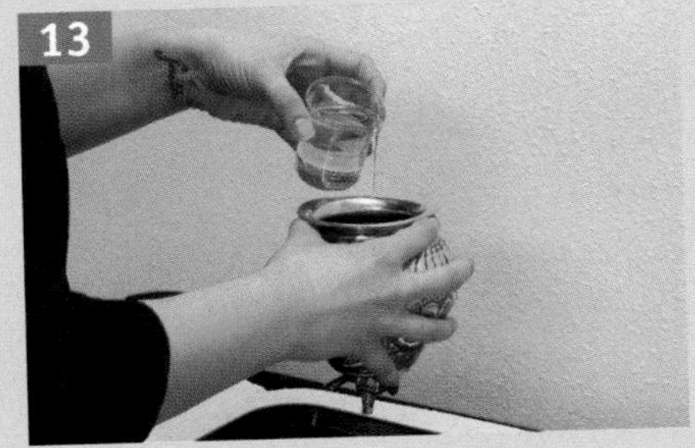

Fill vessel with the warmed oil.

13 Remove the Shirodhara vessel from its stand and fill it with the warmed oil; then replace the vessel in the stand. (Do not fill while vessel is positioned over client's head.) Check settings so oil flow is appropriate for the client.

continues on next page

PROCEDURE 23-3, CONT. SHIRODHARA TREATMENT

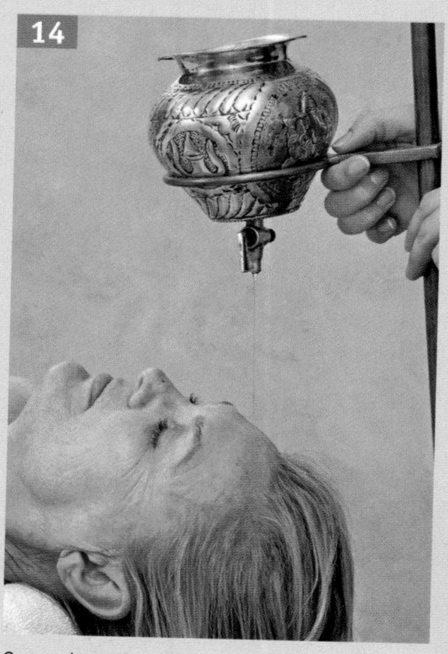
Open the valve.

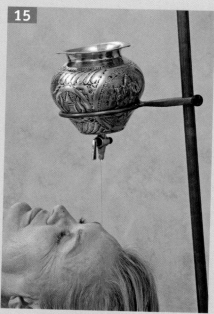
Check temperature of the oil.

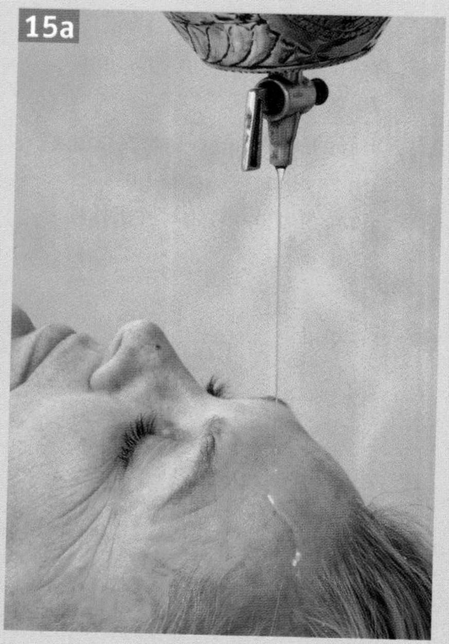
Gently play the oil slightly from side to side.

14 Open the valve so that oil begins to flow into the hair; then introduce the stream of oil to the middle of the forehead, with a focus on the third eye position.

15 Check that the temperature of the oil is comfortable to your client. With practice you will be able to gently play the oil slightly from side to side while maintaining a steady stream.

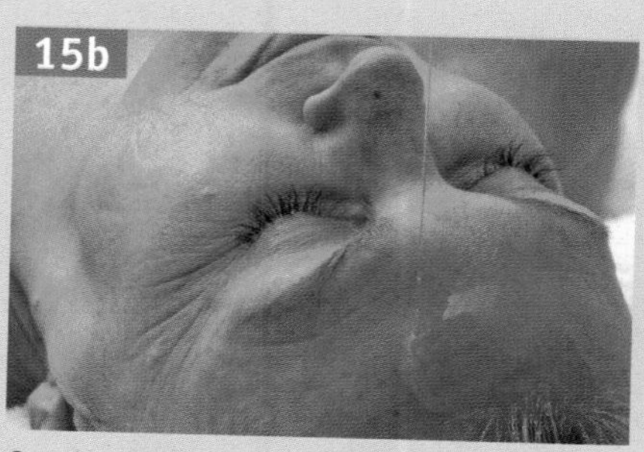
Gently play the oil slightly from side to side.

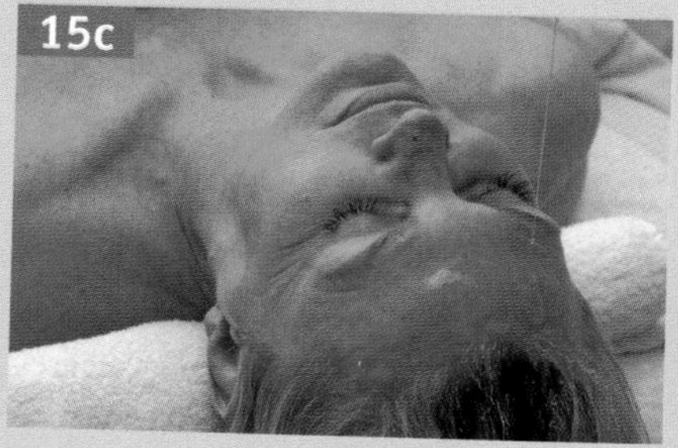
Gently play the oil slightly from side to side.

CAUTION!

Never leave the room while the oil is playing, perform any other treatments while the oil is playing, or give Shirodhara while your client is in a steam tent, herbal linen wrap, or other detox treatment. If your client should become upset, ask if he or she is all right but do not get into conversation. Offer to stop the oil and let the client know you can start it again at any time.

16

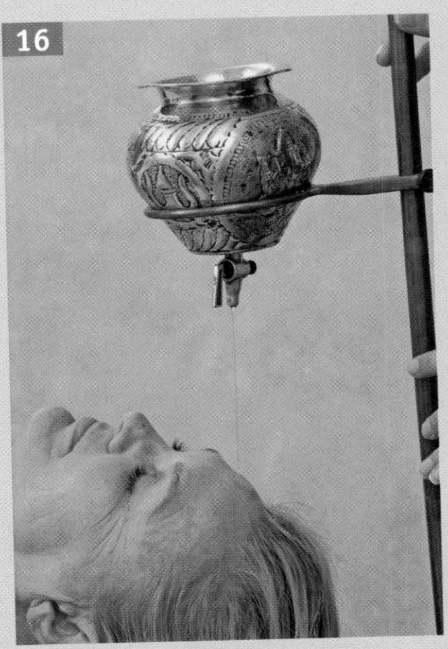

Guide the stream back over the hairline.

17

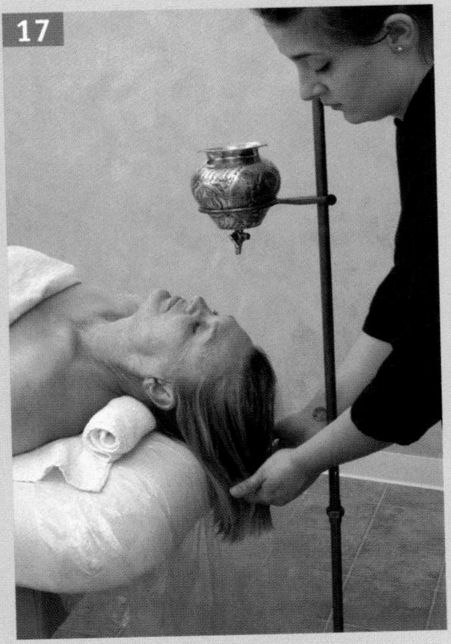

Gently squeeze excess oil from the hair.

17a

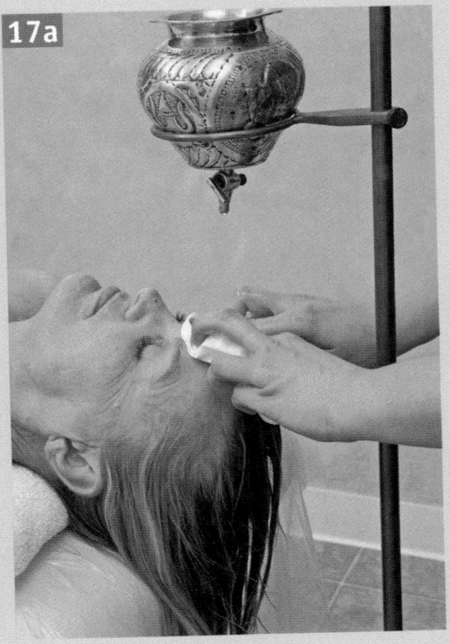

Blot the forehead.

16 Watch the oil level carefully. When the oil is down to the last quarter-inch, guide the stream back over the hairline and into the hair and then turn off the tap. Turn it off before it reaches the point where it wants to drip, as this would be very uncomfortable for the client.

17 Work your hands through or around the client's hair, depending on its length, gently squeezing excess oil from the hair while lightly massaging the scalp. Blot the forehead with a folded tissue to wipe off any excess oil. Use a towel or paper towel to wipe oil out of the hair and loosely wrap it in a hand towel.

17a-1

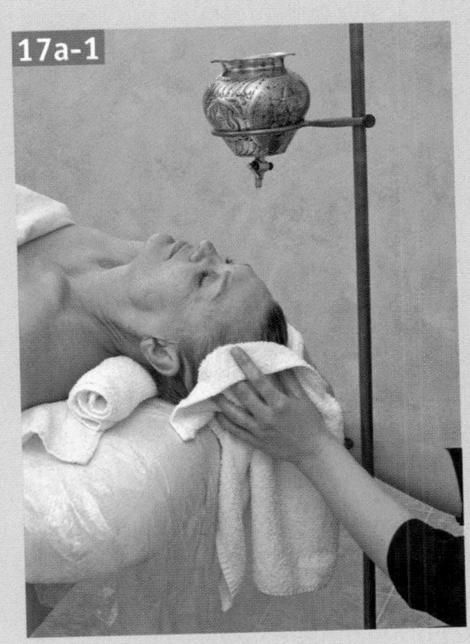

Wipe and loosely wrap hair in a hand towel.

18

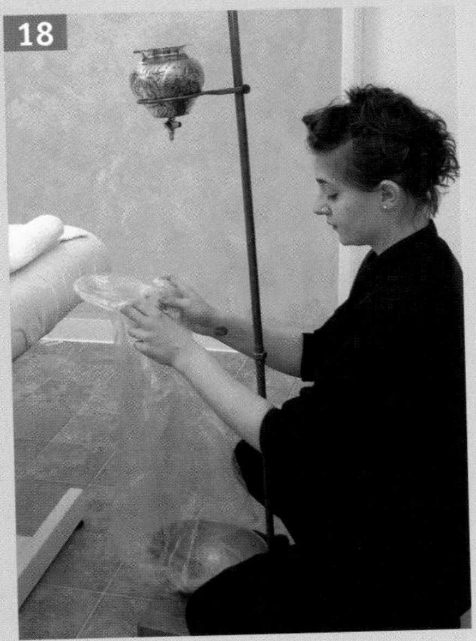

Drop the spa plastic into the catching bowl.

18 Drop the spa plastic into the catching bowl as well as the oil vessel and remove.

continues on next page

PROCEDURE 23-3, CONT. SHIRODHARA TREATMENT

18a

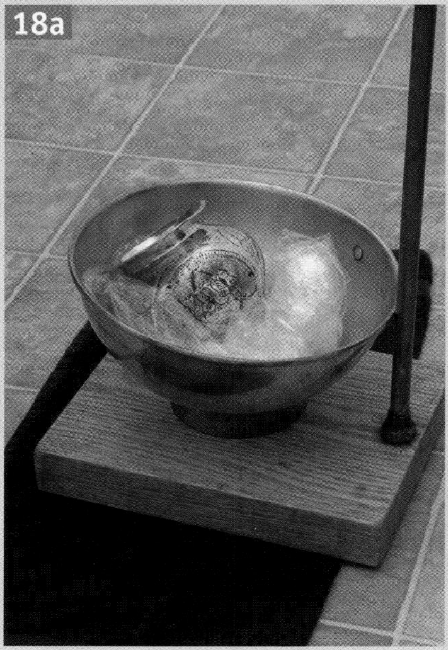

Remove equipment.

19 Some clients do not like to move and prefer to rest for about 5 minutes. Alternatively, others ask for a brief scalp and ear massage. Have the client ease down the table just enough so that his or her neck and head are supported for the massage.

20 Hold the covered head for a moment and then move to the foot of the bed and gently hold the client's ankles.

21 Let the client rest for 5 minutes.

Post-procedure

22 Take the client to the shower if it is available. If none is available, provide a plastic cap to cover the client's hair and protect clothing until he or she can return home.

Here's a Tip

To more easily remove the oil from the hair, advise your client to add shampoo to the hair before introducing any water. The shampoo breaks down the oil. The client should lather and then add water and rinse, repeating if needed.

23 Offer a drink and a snack before he or she leaves.

24 Shirodhara should always be the last treatment in any series. The only reason to give further work after Shirodhara would to help a client feel more grounded: taking time on the closing sequence, adding a short hand massage, and encouraging the client to relax until he or she is fully alert before departing. Your high-drive clients are most at risk as they may not be in touch with their slightly altered mental state.

Clean-up and Disinfection

25 Drain all the *unused* oil out of the vessel back into product container. Wash vessel with hot soapy water.

26 Drain the *used* oil into a bottle for submission to your local recycling center and wash the large collecting bowl in hot soapy water.

27 Dispose of the plastic spa sheet.

28 Follow state regulations for standard clean-up and disinfection.

Other Ayurvedic Treatments

Ayurveda has had thousands of years to develop a world of unique treatments. These are the most common ayurvedic treatments being offered in spas today:

Ayurvedic Mud: In this treatment, a thin layer of clay and herbs is applied from the elbows to the fingertips and knees to the tips of the toes. The clay cleanses while the herbs reenergize the body. This is very refreshing and rejuvenating for the whole body.

Ayurvedic Face Rejuvenation Sequence: This is a unique and comprehensive touch technique for the face, scalp, neck, shoulders, and upper chest using strokes and secret, vital point (marma) massage. These points have been used traditionally to bring balance to both body and mind.

REGULATORY AGENCY ALERT

Be advised laws that vary from state to state and the lines between skin care and massage are sometimes blurred, especially in full-body skin care. If in doubt about the legality of a treatment, check with your local regulating board.

Ayurvedic Facial: This facial uses simple oil blends and natural herbal compounds in a sequence of cleansing, marma massage, steam or compress, mask, and moisturizing that brings balance to the client's dosha.

Garshana: This is a dry, gentle exfoliation for the face or body using raw silk gloves. Treatments for the face are performed after makeup removal. For the body, one or two therapists use the garshan silk gloves in a dry exfoliation before a body treatment. Garshan (rubbing) stimulates flow and circulation in the tissues and leaves the body silky and enlivened.

Kansa Vataki: In this treatment, the client's feet are coated in aromatic ghee (clarified butter) and then rubbed with a small bowl made of three metals. Traditionally used to help eye problems, this treatment is marvelously relaxing and wonderful for easing tension around the eyes and helping to normalize skin tones. It is currently used as an add-on service for pedicures and facials.

Marma Point Face Rejuvenation: Warm aromatic oils are caressed into the face using points and strokes that enliven energy channels in the face. This creates a youthful glow and enlivened state of consciousness, happiness, and peace.

Nadi Swedena: Steam is applied to the back, neck, or any other joints that need a little extra loving care or relief from the pain of tension. The gentle herbal steam of Nadi Swedana is an excellent way to move beneficial oils and herbs deeper into the skin. It is very pleasurable and relaxing and makes it easier for the body to let go without deep-pressure massage techniques.

Swedana: This term applies to any therapy that induces sweating, such as facial steams, herbal compresses, or herbal linen wraps. These treatments provide deep cleansing to the skin and must be followed by a good shower.

Tibetan Eye Rejuvenation: In this treatment, an aromatic oil is applied to the feet, followed by warm heat delivered by textured terra-cotta stones and a cooling eye pillow or compress applied to the eyes. The oil and heat draw stress and tension away from the face, particularly from around the eyes, leaving them moist and clear.

This chapter has aimed to give an overview of basic ayurvedic theory and provide some details about some specific treatments. It should be viewed as a brief introduction to a vast body of information that has been treasured by humanity for the last 6,000 years. Though originally from a distant land and an ancient wisdom Ayurveda has a tremendous amount of insight to offer us all in modern times. It both deepens a therapist's understanding of their client and the client's experience of their treatment. Brought to us by mystics and explained in terms of subtle energy, Ayurveda is both practical and offers very tangible results. So please do not hesitate to try these techniques, offer these questionnaires, and make use of this information.

REVIEW QUESTIONS

1. Where did Ayurveda come from and how old is it?
2. What are some modern practices that have emerged from Ayurveda?
3. Name one principle that makes a treatment ayurvedic and give an example of the application of that principle.
4. What are the senses that are included in the six-sense approach? Give one example of each in a spa/skin care setting.
5. List the three doshas and list the two elements that form each dosha.
6. List the five elements for each dosha and give one general quality and one problem that you would see in skin if there was too much of that element.
7. Describe a Vata skin in balance.

REVIEW QUESTIONS

8. List Pitta skin attributes.
9. Describe a client with Kapha skin type.
10. List three personality traits for each dosha type and one way you adjust your marketing skills to engage that type of client.
11. Give a definition of a marma point and list three that help relaxation.
12. List one ayurvedic herb and its use in skin care.
13. What are the three steps essential in ayurvedic skin care?
14. What is a Shirodhara treatment? List two reasons for giving this treatment and two precautions.
15. Define two additional ayurvedic treatments.

CHAPTER GLOSSARY

Ayurveda: the world's oldest and most complete system of holistic healing. Literally means the study of life or science of longevity.

dosha: one of the three subtle energies that determine metabolism and intelligence of the body-mind system. The three doshas are vata, pitta and kapha. Literally means "impurity" or that which can become unbalanced.

Kapha dosha: the dosha that gives structure to the body, lubricates tissues, provides strength, and supports immune function. This dosha has qualities that are like earth and water.

kansa vataki: foot massage using a small bowl made from three metals.

marma: sensitive points on the body where there are greater concentrations of the body's life force. There are 108 marma points used therapeutically but thousands of minor marmas. Literally means vital, hidden or secret energy points.

panchamahabhutas: the five great elements: space, air, fire, water and earth.

Pitta dosha: the dosha that is responsible for all metabolic functions and transformations. This dosha has qualities that are like fire and water.

prakruti: individual or natal constitution. Literary means ones "nature."

Vata dosha: the dosha that is responsible for all movement in the body, voluntary and involuntary. This dosha has qualities that are like air and space.

Vedas: a collection of root texts of ayurvedic knowledge. Literally means "pure knowledge" or the principles of creations.

vikruti: imbalance of doshas.

ADDITIONAL TERMS

The following terms are included as a reference as they are all common ayurvedic terms clients or coworkers might use or ask about.

agni: the universal organizing principle of conversion such as the power to digest food or understand experiences.

ama: body toxins from undigested food that causes illness.

ashram: place for spiritual development.

aura: a subtle energy fields that surrounds the body that is visible or can be felt by some people. Aura colors have been photographed using Kirlian photography.

Chakra: one of seven main energy centers of the body. They are found situated at the base of the spine, at the navel, the solar plexus, the heart, throat, the middle of the forehead and the crown of the head. Chakras are major marma points or mahamarmas. Literally means "energy wheel."

dhatus: the seven tissues of the body, plasma, blood, muscle, fat, bones, bone marrow, reproductive organs.

ghee: clarified butter used for massage or for cooking.

gunas: qualities or attributes given to substances or people such as light, dry or cold. There are twenty fundamental gunas in ayurveda.

guru: spiritual teacher. Literally means one that removes the darkness of ignorance.

karma: one's future being determined by present or past actions. Literally means "action."

kundalini: primal energy that is awakened by special spiritual practices.

lepas: cleansing pastes or poultices for the skin.

malas: body wastes.

mandala: geometric shaped images used for meditation.

mantra: one or more syllables sung or chanted to help bring balance to the mind-body system. The most commonly known and used mantra is OM pronounced AUM.

nabhi: navel.

nadi: subtle energy channel. Ayurvedic name for pulse.

ojas: the pure essence of the body that is the power behind immune function and is what gives the body a healthy glow.

prana: life giving force or vital force.

pranayam: breath control exercises that should be done only with a qualified teacher.

rajasic: energetic, aggeressive.

Sanskrit: the language in which the roots of Ayurveda were written. It is sometimes called the language of creation.

samadi: state of pure joy.

sattvic: gentle, calm, nourishing.

shirobhyanga: head massage.

shirodhara: a fine warm stream of oil or cool stream of buttermilk is poured over the forehead to deeply calm the nervous system. Shirodhara causes the release of serotonin, which deeply relaxes the body, melting tensions. It alleviates discomfort in the head, neck, and shoulder area, as well as engenders profound feelings of pleasure, inner balance, mental clarity, and radiance to the completion.

sidhi: psychic power.

six sense approach: the belief that the health and balance of the body of the body/mind system is influenced by the perceptions of all the senses: sight, smell, taste, touch, hearing, and the intuitive sense felt with the heart. Simply put, we are always influenced by the environment in which we find ourselves.

snana: bathing.

snehana: oil massage to lubricate the body.

soma: nectar.

srota: channels in the body that carry food, blood, air or energy.

sundar: beauty.

tamasic: heavy, dull, and destructive.

tej: healthy glow or radiant beauty.

triphala: commonly used herb for cleansing and toning the digestive tract.

ubtan: a blend of flour and powdered herbs used dry oviha paste to remove oil after message.

vaidya: ayurvedic physician.

yantra: geometric symbol that represents a primal sound or syllable.

yoga: exercise that involves postures and breathing techniques. Literally means "union with the divine."

PART 6

MEDICAL

Chapter 24 Working in a Medical Setting
Chapter 25 Medical Terminology
Chapter 26 Medical Intervention
Chapter 27 Plastic Surgery Procedures
Chapter 28 The Esthetician's Role in Pre- and Post-Medical Treatments

CHAPTER OUTLINE

- MEDICAL AESTHETICS
- HOW ESTHETICIANS WORK WITH PHYSICIANS
- SCOPE OF PRACTICE
- THE MEDICAL AESTHETIC PRACTICE
- TRAINING AND EDUCATION
- INTERFACING WITH MEDICAL PROFESSIONALS

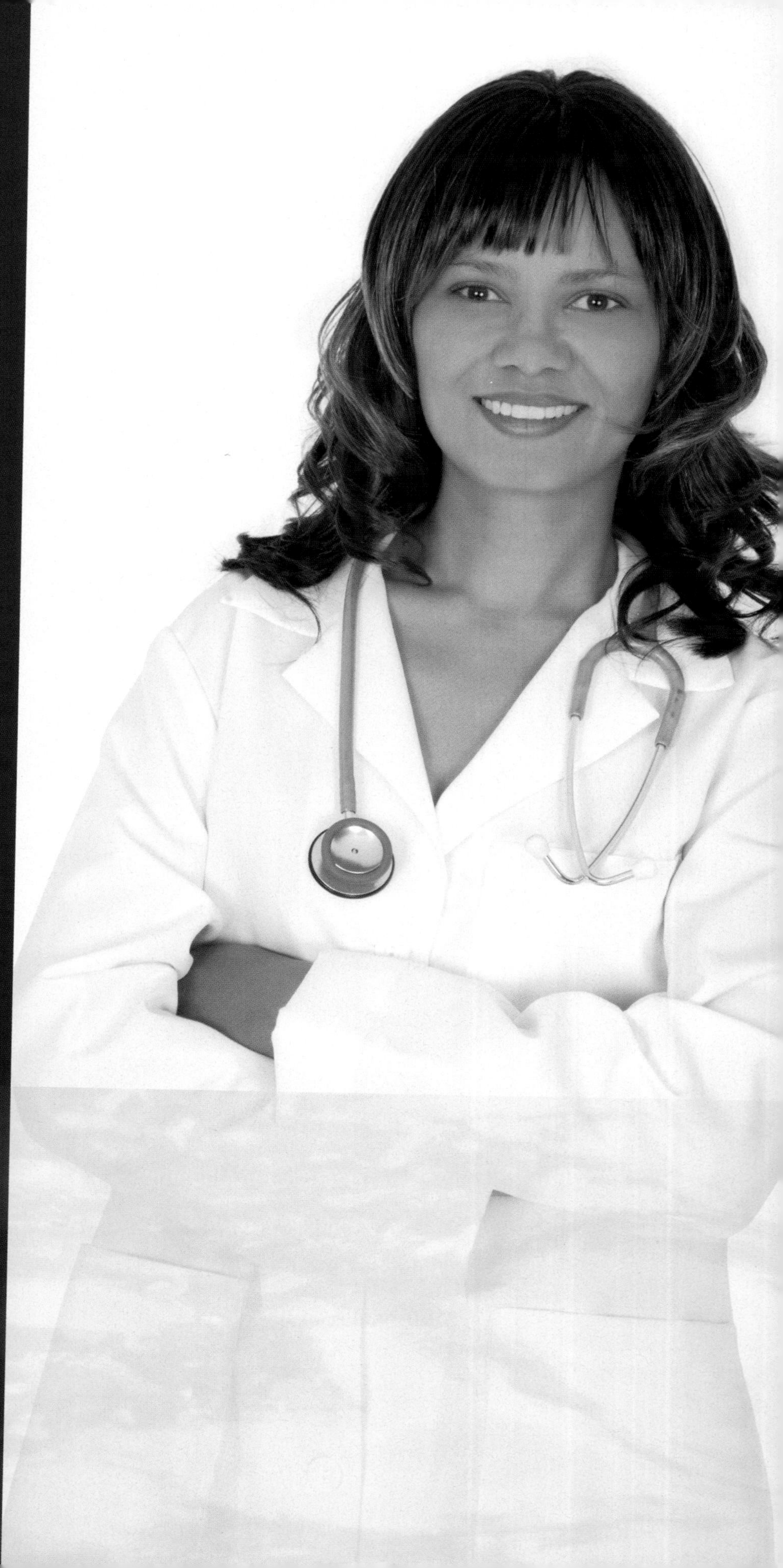

LEARNING OBJECTIVES

After completing this chapter, you should be able to:

- Explain how estheticians work with physicians.
- Name the key personnel in a medical aesthetic setting.
- Discuss common misconceptions in the field of medical aesthetics.
- Explain what the term *scope of practice* means for estheticians.
- List the various types of medical aesthetic practices.
- Name the various procedures performed in a medical practice.
- Discuss the difference in training and education for physicians and estheticians.
- Consider best practices for interfacing with medical professionals.
- Explain the scientific method.
- Discuss the role of HIPAA in the medical aesthetics practice.
- Explore legalities in the medical aesthetic environment.
- Discuss best practices for coping with office politics in a medical environment.

CHAPTER 24

WORKING IN A MEDICAL SETTING

KEY TERMS

Page numbers indicate where in the chapter the term is used.

anecdotal evidence 669
board certified 665
control group 668
cosmetic dermatology 665
cosmetic plastic surgeon 665
dermatological surgeon 665
dermatologist 665
hypothesis 668
medical spa 665
medi-spa 665
placebo 668
reconstructive surgeon 665
scientific method 668
scope of practice 664

Over the past several decades the role of the esthetician has expanded to include a broader range of skin care services in a variety of health, beauty and wellness, facilities, such as skin care clinics, medical spas, and wellness centers. While each facility has its own specific requirements, many are now integrating modern techniques with centuries old beauty traditions to create a holistic program of skin care that embraces mind, body, and spirit. This comprehensive approach to aesthetic procedures has strengthened the connection between health and beauty professionals and has created a growing acceptance of the role of the esthetician in a medical setting. It has also raised the bar for estheticians who must be prepared to increase their skills and improve their business knowledge to meet the demands of this growing trend.

MEDICAL AESTHETICS

The current interest in medical aesthetics originates from many new developments, including scientific advancements in products, equipment, and techniques. The introduction of noninvasive procedures, such as microdermabrasion and collagen and botox injections, along with a greater acceptance of more invasive procedures, such as cosmetic surgery, are now encouraging many individuals to experiment beyond traditional comfort zones.

This adventurous new spirit is largely attributed to baby boomers (those born between 1946 and 1964), a generation unwilling to surrender a youthful appearance as they enter middle age. In search of more results-oriented treatments, baby boomers have played a significant role in the acceptance of modern medical aesthetic procedures. Coupled with one of the greatest disposable incomes in history, this affluent generation has helped turn the business of treating appearances into a multi-billion-dollar industry that continues to have an enormous economic and cultural impact on our society.

HOW ESTHETICIANS WORK WITH PHYSICIANS

The natural link between health and beauty has created a marvelous synergy between estheticians and physicians that has grown from a simple referral system to an entirely new business model. Estheticians, long interested in enhancing the treatments they performed in the salon, have been instrumental in promoting the efficacy of more-advanced medical procedures. As estheticians began referring to physicians, it became apparent that the treatments and services they provided, such as facials, pre- and and postoperative skin care, and makeup application, complemented the work of physicians in a way that added real value to medical practices. Physicians soon realized that not only are the treatments estheticians performed skilled and reliable, estheticians are also able to play a supportive role in client consultation and education, a situation that ultimately enhances the overall benefit to the patient.

Common Misconceptions

The skilled esthetician has become an integral part of the medical aesthetic practice; however, it is important for those working in this relatively new frontier to note that the credentialing status of the esthetician has not changed. This can be confusing to the esthetician who is taught to understand that his or her role has expanded. While there is little doubt that advanced technology and a growing acceptance of the esthetician in a medical practice has significantly altered the esthetician's role, when it comes to credentials the esthetician's title has not changed.

Esthetician Credentials

Training and education requirements for estheticians in the United States continue to vary by state, with the number of hours required for licensing ranging anywhere from 260 to 1,500 hours of training and the majority falling somewhere around the 600-hour mark.

The current state of esthetic licensing requirements is a controversial one that has many calling for increased education, more progressive regulations, and national standards. The two-tier licensing structure is a popular concept that segregates esthetic training and licensing into two separate modules: A 600-Hour Basic and 600-Hour Advanced or Master Esthetician program has gained the support of a large number of estheticians and educators. However, to date this model actually exists as law in only two states, Utah and Virginia, although it should be noted that others have expressed an interest in following suit.

Unfortunately, changing laws is often a long and tedious process that can take years, a situation that has estheticians and industry leaders frustrated and has prompted many estheticians to take the initiative for increasing their own education by entering one of a growing number of advanced esthetic training programs. This is a great testimony to the esthetician's dedication to education, but it has no legal significance; for example, it has not resulted in either a "medical esthetician" or "paramedical esthetician" license, terms that are commonly used to denote the esthetician's role in a medical environment but have no legal value.

In search of qualifying credentials that acknowledge their contribution to a more results-oriented and scientific approach to skin care, some estheticians have chosen to use the title "Clinical Esthetician." These estheticians often have private practices and may work primarily with physicians on a referral basis, but, again, this title is not officially recognized by esthetic licensing boards.

Esthetician License in the Medical Practice

If you wish to practice in a medical or clinical setting, you should also be aware that some states have apprenticeship requirements which can interfere with the esthetician's ability to operate under their own esthetic license in a medical practice. For example, if you are working in a state that requires estheticians to serve an apprenticeship under another fully licensed esthetician or cosmetologist for a specific time period before becoming fully licensed to operate on your own, it will be important to question your state board as to how you will fulfill this requirement if there is no such qualified person on staff.

But even if your state does not require an apprenticeship you should question your state board on the point of recognizing your esthetician license in a medical office, as this raises serious legal and liability questions. For example, if the licensing board that regulates estheticians does not sanction certain procedures the esthetician is asked to perform in the medical practice, how is the esthetician protected from liability? In many cases the esthetician working in a medical aesthetic practice is asked to choose between assuming the role of an esthetician or that of a medical assistant. These issues are currently the topic of much debate around the country. If you have strong feelings about such topics, there are many ways to voice your opinion. You can start by taking an active role in trade associations and organizations that promote, define, and advocate for the role of the esthetician in the medical practice. This is a great opportunity to learn more about the history of the field of esthetics and to become involved in the legislative issues that will ultimately affect *your* future.

SCOPE OF PRACTICE

When you complete the required number of hours of esthetic training in your state, you are eligible to take the licensing exam offered by the state board of registration responsible for regulating estheticians in your state. If you pass, you will be awarded an esthetician license.

Depending on the regulations in your state, your new license will allow you to perform certain esthetic procedures. These are set forth by the licensing board that regulates estheticians in your state; this is typically the Board of Cosmetology. Look closely at these regulations. These are the laws that define your **scope of practice,** or what types of treatments and services you can perform under your esthetician license. These regulations may also indicate limitations or restrictions on your scope of practice.

Hopefully, you have reviewed the laws governing estheticians in your state as part of your current training program. If you did not receive a copy of these regulations from the school or university you attend, you can request a copy from your state board. While state laws for estheticians vary, all are a matter of public information. If you are concerned or have a question that is not clearly defined in the state regulations you received, always check with your state licensing board. Many states post their statutory requirements and other pertinent information on the Internet.

CAUTION!

Remember that performing treatments or services beyond the scope of your license can have serious legal consequences. When in doubt about a service, treatment, or procedure seek appropriate counsel from the State Board of Registration for Estheticians in your state. As an added precaution, check with your insurance agent to make sure you are fully protected against liability for all of the work that falls under your job description.

Physicians and nurses must also be licensed. Licensing for these medical personnel is regulated by the State Board of Registration for Medicine and the State Board of Registration of Nursing, respectively. Each board has its own set of rules and regulations, which are used to define their licensing requirements and scope of practice.

When you accept a position as an esthetician in a medical practice, you must be conscious of the limits of your license as well as the roles and responsibilities of your colleagues. With so many new advancements in today's medical aesthetic practice, one of the concerns for estheticians entering the medical environment is that the boundaries may become blurred. Estheticians are reminded that should they be asked to perform duties that are outside the scope of their training, certification, and expertise there can be legal consequences. If you are caught between the requirements of your job description and the scope of your license, it is important to seek the advice of qualified professionals. As a general rule, when in doubt, don't.

THE MEDICAL AESTHETIC PRACTICE

Dermatology and plastic, or cosmetic, surgery are among the most common medical specialties associated with medical aesthetics. Estheticians have a long history of mutually respectful working relationships with physicians in these practices. However, today this more traditional model of medical aesthetics is changing with many other physicians, such as general internists, obstetricians, gynecologists, ophthalmologists, and cosmetic dentists, entering the beauty business. This is yet another topic that is raising many questions within the medical field.

There are several reasons for the broadened interest in medical aesthetics. Significant advances in technology, the financial constraints of managed care, and a genuine interest in some specialties to take a more holistic approach to health, beauty, and wellness are just a few of the reasons other medical professionals have become interested in medical aesthetics. It is also no secret that the field of esthetics has grown into a multi-billion-dollar industry that many recognize as a tremendous financial opportunity.

Dermatology

Dermatologists are physicians who specialize in diseases of the skin, hair, and nails. As such they are and have been a natural source of referrals for those working in the beauty field, such as estheticians and hairdressers.

Due to the previously mentioned technological advancements and other cultural and psychological factors, the field of dermatology has expanded its role in recent years to place greater emphasis on appearance-related skin conditions, or what is commonly referred to as **cosmetic dermatology.** Dermatologists who specialize in cosmetic dermatology treat appearance-related skin conditions, such as wrinkles, scars, hyperpigmentation, and hyperplasia. They also treat skin cancers, skin diseases, and other dermatology problems.

Another growing subspecialty of dermatology is dermatological surgery. **Dermatological surgeons** are dermatologists who also perform plastic or cosmetic surgery. This title may also be used to refer to those dermatologists who use lasers to perform advanced dermatological procedures, such as laser skin resurfacing.

Plastic Surgery

Plastic surgeons are physicians who specialize in performing surgery for cosmetic or reconstructive purposes. **Cosmetic plastic surgeons** are generally associated with elective surgical procedures, or those that are not medically necessary but desired for appearance-related concerns, such as blepharoplasty, rhytidectomy, abdominoplasty (eyelid, face, and tummy lifts), breast augmentation or reduction, and liposuction.

Conversely, **reconstructive surgeons** are generally associated with surgical procedures that are medically necessary and are used to correct abnormalities associated with birth defects, such as cleft lips; accidents; injury-related and other physical deformities; and the removal of life-threatening diseases, such as skin cancer lesions.

General plastic surgeons, facial plastic surgeons, and ophthalmic surgeons are other surgeons who are commonly associated with cosmetic and reconstructive surgery. Estheticians referring to or interested in working in these types of surgical practices should look for physicians who are **board certified,** a title reserved for those physicians who have taken and passed the exam required for board certification in their respective specialties.

The Medi-Spa

The **medical spa,** or **"medi-spa"** as the name is often coined, is a relatively new business model that has shown steady progress in recent years. Medical spas offer a wide range of medical aesthetic procedures and traditional spa services that may be incorporated within a physician's private practice, a clinic, a laser or wellness center, or hospital setting.

There are many variations of the medical spa in development that may offer any number of esthetic treatments and wellness and medical procedures, such as facials, massage, botox and collagen injections, laser treatments, chemical peels, and acupuncture. These services are typically performed by a staff of medical personnel and complementary health and beauty service providers, such as physicians, nurses, estheticians, electrologists, nutritionists, massage therapists, acupuncturists, and naturopathic doctors.

If you wish to practice in a medical spa, you should be aware that laws governing the medical spa and or medical aesthetic practice vary from state to state. Because most of the laws governing medical spas are new, they have raised considerable debate among professionals, trade associations and professional organizations, educators, and legislators within each field and have prompted a long list of questions that must be answered before any official prototype or national standard can be established.

FYI

The National Coalition of Estheticians, Manufacturers, Distributors, and Associations defines a medical spa as a facility that, during all hours of business, shall operate under the on-site supervision of a licensed health-care professional operating within his or her scope of practice, with a staff that operates within their scope of practice as defined by their individual licensing board if licensure is required. The facility may offer traditional, complementary, and alternative health practices and treatments in a spa-like setting.

TRAINING AND EDUCATION

As the medical aesthetic model of skin care unfolds, training and education have taken center stage. This has created yet another area of controversy that calls for a better understanding of how each practitioner is educated.

Those entering esthetician training programs often come from diverse backgrounds and education levels. Some enter esthetics school right out of high school while others may be transitioning from careers in which they have years of experience and perhaps a college degree. Esthetician programs have also become a popular choice for other licensed professionals, such as electrologists, massage therapists, and nurses.

Because esthetics draws such a varied population, there are typically huge differences in training and education, which the esthetic instructor must endeavor to cross. The unevenness in educational background can pose concerns for students as well, but if you find yourself in these circumstances, consider yourself fortunate. Learning in a diverse environment generally provides a much broader perspective and greater experience working with a variety of people that can ultimately prove extremely beneficial in the workplace.

Esthetic Education Model

Although college-level courses for estheticians do exist, the majority of esthetic programs are offered as a clock-hour curriculum. This means that the student must attend classes for a set number of hours each week. For those enrolled in full-time programs, this is usually 30 to 40 clock-hours of class and/or practical hands-on training time per week. However, due to variations in state regulations the length of clock-hour programs for estheticians differs. For example, if you attend an esthetics course in a state that mandates 300 hours of training to become eligible to take the licensing exam, and the set number of clock hours per week is 30 hours, it will take you 10 weeks to graduate. In comparison, if the licensing board in your state requires 1,200 hours of training with a maximum number of hours of 30 hours per week, you will attend school for approximately 40 weeks or 9 months.

Some states may have additional requirements for estheticians, such as an apprenticeship. Under these circumstances estheticians might be obligated to fulfill a certain number of hours or even years working under the supervision of some other licensed individual.

Medical Education Model

Those in the medical field are educated according to an academic model that comprises college-level courses. College courses are based on a credit-hour system, whereby a certain number of credits are awarded to each course. Full-time students are generally enrolled in a specified number of required courses, which are offered over a set time period, such as a semester. To graduate, the student must fulfill the required number of course credits for his or her program or curriculum.

In an academic model, upon graduation the student receives a degree, such as a bachelor or baccalaureate degree, which typically requires four years of education. Advanced degrees require additional schooling beyond the bachelor's degree. For example, a master's degree usually requires an additional two years of education while a doctoral degree typically requires four additional years of education. Variations in the number or years of training can be expected based on whether a student is full time or part time.

In this model a physician is among the most educated professionals in the academic environment, with a compulsory requirement of eight years of education beyond the high school diploma. This typically includes four years of undergraduate college-level courses to fulfill the requirements of a baccalaureate degree plus four years of medical school, at the end of which he or she is awarded a Doctor of Medicine degree (MD). In addition to an academic program, doctors are generally required to undergo a year of internship followed by two to four years of residency in their field of specialty, after which they are eligible to take an exam to become board certified. As you can see, this is a lengthy and arduous commitment to education that goes far beyond the criteria established for most other professions.

Nurse Training

The nurse is a key player in the medical aesthetic practice and is someone who works closely with the physician to provide medical care. While each medical practice has its own hierarchy, in some medical aesthetic practices the nurse may be your immediate supervisor. The esthetician working under the supervision of a nurse should be aware of the nurse's training requirements.

There are several nursing programs that result in licensing. Each requires a different level of education. These programs are typically based on the academic model of education. The Registered Nurse, or RN, requires the most education, traditionally a four-year college-level curriculum; upon graduation the nurse is awarded a BS or Bachelor of Science degree. The Licensed Practical Nurse (LPN) generally requires two years of training, which results in an AAS or Associate of Arts & Science degree. Of course, the nurse may continue to study beyond these requirements to earn a master's degree. Other certificate programs for nurses, such as vocational nursing programs, are also available. Those who graduate from certificate or hospital-based programs are awarded a diploma or certificate of graduation as opposed to a college degree.

INTERFACING WITH MEDICAL PROFESSIONALS

It is critical for estheticians who choose to work in a medical aesthetic practice to have a healthy respect for the education and training of their colleagues. This is not meant to imply that each person in a work environment should be any less valued or respected than another. Ideally all professionals should respect what each person brings to the table. Still it must be understood that there are significant differences in what each staff member is qualified to do. In addition, estheticians working in a medical practice need to have a complete understanding of the standards and requirements imposed upon all personnel working in a medical practice.

First and foremost, those working in a medical environment must operate in strict accordance with Occupational Safety and Health Administration (OSHA) standards and the Health Insurance Portability and Accountability Act (HIPAA). These government-imposed regulations place enormous value on patient safety and confidentiality. In addition, health-care providers must contend with ethical and liability issues that may not exist in the salon environment. It is imperative that you understand and respect these guidelines. An inability to follow set protocol or a careless remark can have serious legal consequences in a medical setting.

? Did You Know

The United States government has enacted federal privacy standards to protect patients' medical records and health information. These laws must be followed in all medical settings, including skin care clinics and medical spas.

The Department of Health and Human Services (HHS) developed the Health Insurance Portability and Accountability Act (HIPAA), to serve as protection to individuals with regard to obtaining information about their health in a medical setting. HIPAA legislation also states that all communication that takes place in a medical setting must be kept confidential. This means that clients or patients visiting a medical spa or clinical skin care setting can file formal complaints about practitioners engaging in a breach of confidentiality. Estheticians working in these medical settings should be aware that they can be held liable for sharing information with others about clients or patients and should be extremely careful not to talk about clients or patients with other estheticians or with other clients or patients. For more information visit http://www.hhs.gov.

The Scientific Method

Another very important consideration in the medical environment involves how medical professionals solve problems. All medical protocols are based on the **scientific method** (Table 24–1), a philosophy of reasoning that is based on first generating and then testing a **hypothesis.** This method has been used by scientists as far back as the seventeenth-century astronomer Galileo and is the basis for all scientific investigation and discovery. Medical professionals rely on the scientific method to evaluate drugs, procedures, and equipment before use on the general public and to develop theories that can be applied with as much accuracy as possible to predict patient outcomes.

Research methodology plays a significant role in testing hypotheses and drawing a conclusion that can be applied with confidence. To limit the number of variables in an experiment, scientists typically assemble two groups: the experiment group and a control group. The experimental group is given the factor—say, a new medication or product—being tested. Another group, called the **control group,** is not given that factor—or, in this case, the medication or product. This group is given a **placebo,** something that appears similar but is not the same substance as what is given to the experimental group. Scientists then carefully observe and record the results of each group, measuring the differences and calculating what is referred to as *statistical significance,* or enough of a difference to warrant the conclusion. If the results meet appropriate standards for significance, scientists then publish the results of the study, which become standard practice until some new discovery is made. This is certainly an oversimplification of what often takes years to measure accurately in medicine; however, it is meant to give you some idea of the enormous task involved in testing the scientific method.

While the scientific method is readily accepted in medicine, it is not commonly associated with cosmetics, where the ubiquitous "miracle in a jar" is often perceived as targeting the consumer's emotions without a great deal of factual information to back up the promised results. This can be a source of frustration between medical and esthetic professionals, who have different standards when it comes to drugs, products, and treatments. Physicians, accustomed to the scientific process in which it can take years of experimentation before a drug meets the standard for patient use, may have little patience for cosmetic claims which generally require less research. This is primarily due to the fact that cosmetics are focused on appearances rather than medicinal use.

Table 24–1 The Scientific Method

THE SCIENTIFIC METHOD IS A FIVE-STEP PROCESS THAT INVOLVES:
1. ***Observation*** or study of the issue in question.
2. Research and raising a ***question*** about what has been observed.
3. Formulation of a ***hypothesis*** or an educated guess to explain your observation.
4. ***Experimentation*** to prove or disprove your hypothesis.
5. ***A conclusion*** or explanation that documents the result of your experimentation.

? Did You Know

The U.S. Food and Drug Administration (FDA) is a federal government agency responsible for ensuring the safety of all consumer products, namely food, drugs, and cosmetics. But did you know that while all drugs are subject to mandatory approval before they are marketed, the FDA only controls cosmetics from a *disapproving* basis?

Essentially what this means is that the FDA only regulates the cosmetic industry when it disapproves of a claim or product; it does not "approve" cosmetics; and it only takes steps when a harmful or "bad" cosmetic is brought to its attention. When this happens, the FDA conducts an investigation. If the cosmetic is found to be unsafe, or that its manufacturer is making untrue claims or drug claims about it, the FDA will move to warn the company or remove the product from the market.

Furthermore, the FDA does not require cosmetic manufacturers to list their products or formulas with the FDA. This is done on a voluntary basis only. It should be noted, though, that the Federal Packaging and Labeling Act instated by the FDA in 1977 does require cosmetic manufacturers to list all of the ingredients used in their products. A more complete comparison of drugs and cosmetics is outlined in the Food, Drug and Cosmetic Act of 1938, which is available from the FDA.

However, as more advanced cosmetic treatments and products make their way onto retail shelves and into the treatment rooms of salons and spas, the basic principles of the scientific method along with its associated clinical trials are becoming equally important to the field of esthetics. Today many manufacturers support product development with research that substantiates the claims of product ingredients and measure product efficacy with case studies that document the improvement in the subject's appearances. While many of these studies are primarily based on **anecdotal evidence** rather than scientific evidence—which means that the results are based on observation and theory rather than scientific experimentation—they are nevertheless meaningful.

Terminology

A thorough understanding of medical terminology is another critical factor for the esthetician who wishes to integrate seamlessly into the medical aesthetic practice. Whether the esthetician is working in a medical spa, hospital, or private physician's practice, he or she will be expected to understand and use the correct clinical terminology. He or she will also be expected to interpret medical language using the appropriate lay terms for patient understanding. A failure to interpret language correctly can have serious consequences for both staff and patients.

Medical Record Keeping

The correct use of medical terminology is especially important when it comes to medical chart writing. The notes on charts may be shared with a number of other professionals, such as other physicians, lawyers, and insurance agents. The esthetician working in a medical office is expected to be knowledgeable in whatever method of chart writing is used in that practice, incorporating the appropriate abbreviations for documentation. For clinical purposes, the esthetician must also become accustomed to framing his or her language in the most objective terms possible, steering clear of judgmental phrases that could be misinterpreted in reports. The SOAP method of charting is a protocol that is often interjected for this purpose. The term SOAP is an acronym for Subjective Objective Assessment Plan, a systematic approach of chart writing that reduces medical record keeping to the *subjective*, or patient's, description of the problem; an *objective* description of what is actually observed; an *assessment*, or evaluation or diagnosis of the problem; and the *plan* for treatment. To become proficient in these methods, the esthetician may need additional education or training.

Office Culture

Culturally, the medical aesthetic environment is significantly different than any other salon or spa business environment to which the esthetician may be accustomed. One of the most important things to remember is that those seeking treatment in a medical setting are first and foremost, *patients*, not clients. This simple definition of those seeking services in a medical aesthetic practice dramatically alters the role of every professional working in this setting.

While some medical offices have a more relaxed attitude when it comes to patient and staff relations, it is very important for those working in a medical office to maintain an appropriate level of professionalism. Be courteous and congenial, but remember that you are not there to make friends with patients, and unlike the salon or spa where a certain amount of fraternization may be overlooked, crossing professional boundaries is not likely to be tolerated in the medical setting. Confidentiality and patient safety must be a top priority at all times.

Human Resource Management

Organizational hierarchy exists in any office; however, unlike larger corporations where there may be several managers who share responsibilities across departments, or a salon environment in which employees may be encouraged to think independently and share in the decision-making process, the medical practice often adheres to a strict top-down human resource methodology whereby all direction comes directly from the doctor, who maintains complete control over all facets of operation. Such a situation may prove intolerable to you if you prefer autonomy or are used to making decisions on your own. At the other extreme, you could find yourself in a medical setting that has very little structure and a management team that has no desire to educate staff. If you are someone who needs a great deal of direction, this will not be the right situation for you.

Nepotism

Not unlike other small businesses, the medical aesthetic practice may operate as a family-owned business. This can have both positive and negative effects.

In a family-run business, key positions are often delegated to close family members, such as a spouse, sibling, child, or some other relative. If you have ever worked for a family-owned and operated business, you can appreciate the close-knit camaraderie that can exist in this type of atmosphere. This frequently flavors the decision-making process and can significantly alter the personality of the entire organization.

On the negative side, family-managed businesses may be prone to an unfair evaluation of the staff that results in favoritism toward family members. The best advice anyone can give to those working in such a situation is to act in a professional manner at all times. Be friendly and courteous, but at the same time be mindful of protocol and personalities. If the situation is one in which you feel you are constantly at odds, it is in your best interest to find another position.

On a positive note, there are many family-run operations spearheaded by very forward-thinking and unbiased individuals who have a healthy respect for what each member of the team brings to the success of an operation. Under these circumstances management can be instrumental in exerting considerable influence over the primary decision maker, a situation that can bode well for all parties.

As you consider the various medical aesthetic employment options, remember that there are pros and cons in every work situation. You may not like all of your coworkers and there may be room for administrative improvement in the best of work conditions. If you can learn not to take things personally, show up every day with a good attitude, communicate professionally, and leave with the feeling that you have performed to the best of your capabilities, you are bound to be successful. Remember, a confident and helpful attitude is a welcome addition to any office environment.

REVIEW QUESTIONS

1. Provide a brief history of the evolution of the esthetician in a medical setting.
2. What significance do the terms *medical esthetician, paramedical esthetician*, and *clinical esthetician* have? What impact do these terms have on the credibility of the esthetician working in a medical setting? Explain your reasoning.
3. Define the phrase *scope of practice*. Team up with a classmate to research the scope of practice for estheticians working in a medical setting as defined by the laws in your state.
4. What is a medical spa? Describe the esthetic services typically found in this setting. How do other types of medical aesthetic practices compare to this environment? Support your discussion with research.
5. Name the various service providers that might be found in the medical setting. Follow up with research on two to three medical spas in your area. What types of service providers did you find in these medical spas? Would you say these are typical or atypical? Why or why not? Discuss your findings with your classmates.
6. What is a dermatologist? Discuss the difference between a dermatologist, cosmetic dermatologist, and a dermatological surgeon.
7. What is a plastic surgeon? Describe the primary difference between a cosmetic plastic surgeon and a reconstructive plastic surgeon.
8. What are the educational requirements for estheticians? for physicians? for nurses?
9. Compare and contrast the clock-hour model of education to the credit-hour or academic model of education. What impact do these two education models have on the way estheticians and medical professionals work together?

10. Team up with several classmates to create a list of best practices for working with medical professionals. How does this list compare to those of your classmates?
11. Define the scientific method. How would an esthetician apply this to his or her work in the medical setting?
12. Supply the FDA definition for drugs and cosmetics. How does this affect the way cosmetics and drugs are advertised?
13. How does the FDA regulate the cosmetic industry? Do you approve or disapprove of the current laws regulating cosmetics? Defend your argument.
14. How does HIPAA affect the role of the esthetician working in a medical setting?
15. What is meant by *office politics*? What is meant by *nepotism*? Would you enjoy working in a family-owned business? Why or why not?

CHAPTER GLOSSARY

anecdotal evidence: based on observation and theory rather than scientific experimentation.

board certified: title reserved for those physicians who have taken and passed the exam required for board certification in their respective specialties.

control group: the group in an experiment that is not given the factor, medication, or product in question.

cosmetic dermatology: a subspeciality of dermatology that treats appearance-related skin conditions, such as wrinkles, scars, hyperpigmentation, and hyperplasia.

cosmetic plastic surgeon: physicians who specialize in elective surgical procedures, or those that are not medically necessary but are desired for appearance related concerns, such as blepharoplasty, rhytidectomy, abdominoplasty (eyelid, face, and tummy lifts), breast augmentation or reduction, and liposuction.

dermatological surgeon: a dermatologist who performs plastic or cosmetic surgery; may also refer to those dermatologists who use lasers to perform advanced dermatological procedures, such as laser skin resurfacing.

dermatologist: a physician who specializes in and treats diseases of the skin, hair, and nails.

hypothesis: an educated guess that is based on an observation or study of an issue in question.

medical spa: a medical facility that offers medical aesthetic procedures and traditional spa or esthetic services in a spa-like setting.

medi-spa: a term used interchangeably with medical spa.

placebo: in research methodology, a substance that appears to be similar but is not the same substance as, what is given to the experimental group.

reconstructive surgeon: a physician who specializes in surgical procedures that are medically necessary and are used to correct abnormalities associated with birth defects, accidents, injuries, and other physical deformities, and the removal of life-threatening diseases such as skin cancer lesions.

scientific method: a philosophy of reasoning that is based on first generating and then testing a hypothesis.

scope of practice: refers to the type of treatments and services one can perform under license.

CHAPTER 25

MEDICAL TERMINOLOGY

CHAPTER OUTLINE

- HOW MEDICAL TERMINOLOGY WORKS
- THE HISTORY OF MEDICAL TERMINOLOGY
- THE BASICS OF MEDICAL TERMINOLOGY
- ROOT WORDS
- PREFIXES
- SUFFIXES
- PRONUNCIATION

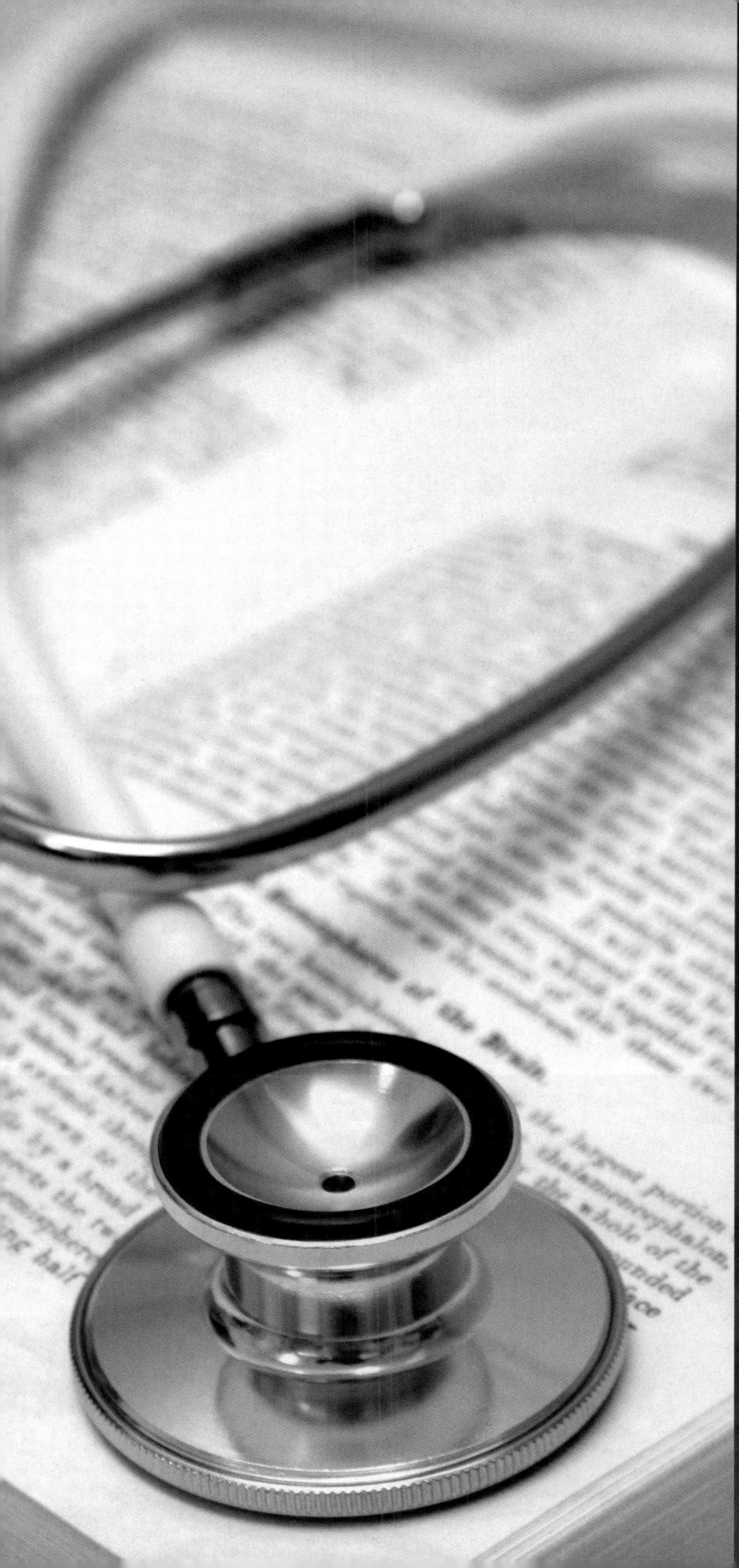

LEARNING OBJECTIVES

When you complete this chapter, you should be able to:

- Discuss and define medical terminology.
- Explain the history and origin of medical terminology.
- Instruct on how to conduct a word analysis.
- Describe the use of plurals.
- Define root words.
- Describe the use of prefixes.
- Describe the use of suffixes.
- Explain pronunciation.

KEY TERMS

Page numbers indicate where in the chapter the term is used.

adjective 683
combining form 676
combining vowel 676
diminutive 683
modifies 676
noun 683
plural 683
prefixes 675
pronunciation 685
root words 675
suffixes 675
word analysis 676

Just as teachers, auto mechanics, and computer engineers use words specific to their profession, so do medical personnel. As an esthetician, you probably will not be using the word *megabyte* unless you are referring to someone that has a rather large mouth. If you were a computer analyst, you would use the word. Likewise, a virus will have a different meaning to you than it will to a computer analyst. The vocabulary you will be using is referred to as *medical terminology*.

HOW MEDICAL TERMINOLOGY WORKS

As medical science grew and improved upon itself, as new functions were understood and processes discovered, the medical community adopted a language of its own. This language, or vernacular, was needed in order to help physicians and other allied health professionals keep straight the prolific amount of vocabulary involved in medicine. By knowing the meaning of Greek or Latin **root words**, or base parts of words, a user can understand the meaning of words that include those roots. The use of **suffixes** (word parts added to the ends of words) and **prefixes** (word parts added in front of words) gives further clarity. For example, take the word *nephrology*. The root *nephr* means "pertaining to the kidneys," and the suffix *-ology* means "the study of something." Therefore, *nephrology* is the study of the kidneys (Figure 25–1).

Medical terminology includes the use of personal names as well. Usually, this occurs in the context of a treatment or disorder that is named after the person who first studied or discovered it. For example, Dercum's disease is named for Francis X. Dercum, an American neurologist.

By knowing the basics of medical terminology, you will be able to decipher the meaning of a word even if you haven't heard it before. For example, if you are a specialist in medical skin care, you may run across the word *dermatitis*. While you may know that this word has something to do with skin that itches or has a rash, your knowledge of medical terminology would help you ascertain that this word's exact meaning of dermatitis is "skin inflammation."

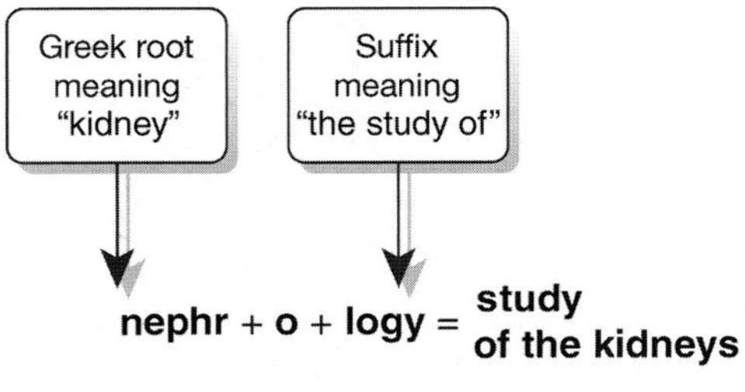

Figure 25–1 Diagrammatic breakdown of the word *nephrology*.

THE HISTORY OF MEDICAL TERMINOLOGY

When early physicians were first working to identify anatomical structures, abnormalities, and functions, doctors were scattered across a wide geographic area and communication was slow and unreliable. Imagine trying to keep track of the same item in several different languages. With so many words being added to the lexicon, it became necessary to set in place a formalized, structured methodology for the naming process. These early doctors needed to implement a system that imposed consistency and prevented their colleagues from naming things in multiple ways. Thus, the current system of medical terminology was born. Understanding how this system has evolved over the centuries will help you make sense of unfamiliar terms you encounter in your work.

Egyptian, Greek, and Roman Influences

Some of the earliest medical writings were made by an Egyptian named Imhotep, now universally thought to be the "father of medicine." Some 2,200 years went by before the "father of modern medicine," the Greek Hippocrates, was born. Hippocrates recognized the need for a universal language of medicine. To make order of the terminology used during that time, Hippocrates referred to the texts left behind by Imhotep. The knowledge that Imhotep passed on to his Greek protégés was fine-tuned and adopted by the Romans. At the time, most Greek and Roman medical terms were based in mythology, legend, and physical description. Since most of these myths and legends were meant to explain the unexplainable, the remnants of these words left in medical terminology are often amusing. For example, in Homer's *The Odyssey,* drinking from the River Lethe leads to fatigue and sluggishness, or *lethargy.* Legends have also made permanent marks in the medical lexicon. The terms *atlas, Achilles' heel,* and *cancer* all have origins in legends of the day.

The Middle Ages and Renaissance Period

People of the Middle Ages relied on clinical description when coining medical terms, even though those descriptions were often medically and politically incorrect. For example, during this period a person with a foot deformity was said to have a *clubfoot.* This disorder was so named because of the sound that person made when walking on medieval castle floors.

During the Renaissance, maritime advancements in ship building and cartography allowed more extensive travel. This perpetuated a similar intercontinental influence in medical terminology as physicians traveled between countries. Cross-cultural hybrids of words began to appear, such as *orthopedics,* which comes from the Latin *ortho* ("straight") and the Greek *paedic* ("child").

Contemporary Times

In modern times the medical community has put forth an organized effort to renovate prior mistakes and inaccuracies in nomenclature. Organizations and individuals have and are constantly seeking out misnomers and other errors in the medical terminology. Often, several names for one item are retired and one name becomes the universally accepted name in accordance with the goals of medicine. Today's colleges and medical schools offer extensive classes in medical terminology and students are encouraged to use this vocabulary when talking to peers.

THE BASICS OF MEDICAL TERMINOLOGY

Now that you have read the background of medical terminology, you are ready to begin the process of learning about the words themselves and some of the basics and exceptions that make medical terminology so complex. As a patient, or student, you may have heard and understood words that are easily recognizable. For example, most people know what *arthritis, tonsils,* and *kidneys* are. But you may not know what a *phlebotomist* or what *laparoscopy* is.

Word Analysis

Medical terminology is much like a puzzle. By using **word analysis** and dissecting a word, you can isolate the different word parts and unlock the puzzle. Once you can isolate the different word parts and define them, you can use this knowledge to define many other related words.

When decoding a medical term, begin at the end of the word, or the suffix, and then go back to the beginning. For example, one word with which many people are familiar is *mammography.* The suffix of the word is -*graphy,* which means "to record." The root word is *mamm,* which refers to the breasts. Therefore, *mammography* is a recording of—or an image of—the breast.

To find a suffix, isolate the different parts of the word. Look for an "o" in the middle of the word or another **combining vowel.** The root word and the combining vowel together are called the **combining form.** Again, let's use the word *mammography:*

mamm / o	/graphy
Combining Form	Suffix

ophthalmoscope:

ophthalm / o / scope

pathology:

path / o / logy

leukocyte:

leuk / o / cyte

amniocentesis:

amnio / o / centesis

Sometimes a medical term has more than one root word. Since the combining vowel connects the root word to the suffix, you will most often find a corresponding number of combining forms in a particular word. Table 25–1 provides some examples.

In many cases, there is a prefix before the combining form. A prefix **modifies** the root word, usually quantifying or qualifying it. For example, *poly* means "many," and *intra* means "within."

intravenous	intra / ven / ous
polyneuropathy	poly / neur / o / pathy

Table 25–2 shows some terms and how they break apart.

Table 25–1 Root Word Examples

TERM	FIRST COMBINING FORM	SECOND COMBINING FORM	SUFFIX
Gastroenterology	Gastro	Entero	-logy
Otolaryngologist	Oto	Laryngo	-logist
Electroencephalography	Electro	Encephalo	-graphy

Table 25–2 Examples of Combining Vowels and Suffixes

	PREFIX	ROOT WORD	CONNECTOR VOWEL	SUFFIX
ophthalmoscope		ophthalm	o	-scope
pathology		path	o	-logy
leukocyte		leuk	o	-cyte
amniocentesis		amni	o	-centesis
intravenous	intra	ven		-ous
polyneuropathy	poly	neur	o	-pathy

Note that not all words shown in the two tables are structured in the exact same format. For example, the word *intravenous* has no combining vowel. When the suffix begins with a vowel, as is the case with *-ous,* the combining vowel is dropped.

Plurals

As you know, the plural form of many words in the English language is often difficult to ascertain. In some instances, the words are completely different (mouse/mice) or they are the same as the singular form (deer/deer). A similar challenge exists in medical terminology. Some might argue that the use of proper plurals can be one of the more challenging aspects of medical terminology. The problem is so pervasive that even many of physicians experience difficulty with them.

In reality, plurals generally follow some basic rules. If you learn these rules, you will be prepared to tackle any challenges that arise. Table 25–3 provides some of the more common rules of forming plurals.

Table 25–3 Basic Rules of Thumb for Forming Medical Plurals

IF THE SINGULAR ENDING IS:	SINGULAR EXAMPLE:	THE PLURAL RULE IS:	PLURAL FORM:
is	Diagnosis	Drop the *is* and add *es*.	Diagnoses
um	Ileum	Drop the *um* and add *a*.	Ilea
us	Alveolus	Drop the *us* and add *i*.	Alveoli
a	Vertebra	Drop the *a* and add *ae*.	Vertebrae
ix	Appendix	Drop the *ix* and add *ices*.	Appendices
ex	Cortex	Drop the *ex* and add *ices*.	Cortices
ax	Thorax	Drop the *x* and add *ces*.	Thoraces
ma	Sarcoma	Retain the *ma* and add *ta*.	Sarcomata
on	spermatozoon	Drop the *on* and add *a*.	Spermatozoa
nx	Larynx	Drop the *x* and add *ges*.	Larynges
y	Deformity	Drop the *y* and add *ies*.	Deformities
yx	Calyx	Drop the *yx* and add *yces*.	Calyces
en	Foramen	Drop the *en* and add *ina*.	Foramina

The 10 Common Exceptions to Basic Plural Rules:

1. Sometimes the proper plural of a word ending in *is* is formed by dropping the *is* and adding *ides*. For example, *epididymis* becomes *epididymides*.
2. Sometimes the proper plural of a word ending in *us* is formed by dropping the *us* and adding *era* or *ora*. For example, *viscus* becomes *viscera; corpus* becomes *corpora*.
3. Some words ending in *ix* or *ax* have more than one acceptable plural form. For example, the plural of *appendix* can be either *appendices* or *appendixes*; however, the most common plural form is the *ices* ending.
4. The proper plural for certain words ending in *ion* can be formed simply by adding an *s*. For example, *chorion* becomes *chorions*.
5. The plural form of the term *vas* is *vasa*.
6. The plural form of *pons* is *pontes*.
7. The plural form of the dual-meaning word *os* is *ora* when referring to mouths and *ossa* when referring to bones.
8. The plural form of *femur* is *femora*.
9. The plural form of *cornu* is *cornua*.
10. The plural form of *paries* is *parietes*.

? Did You Know

Prefixes and suffixes change or modify a word's meaning. For example, the word *famous* means "well or widely known." With the prefix *in-*, the word becomes *infamous*, which means "having an exceedingly bad reputation."

ROOT WORDS

The root is the most basic component of a word, and it is the basis for which the meaning of a word is constructed. Often, roots can stand alone, as is the case with *graph, cycl(e), pyr(e), crypt,* and *term*. Most roots in medical terminology, however, do need other components. For example, the roots *gastr, carcin,* and *lapar* need to be combined with prefixes, suffixes, or even other roots. Refer to Table 25–4 for examples.

All words have a root. The root of a word will give you the clues you need to reveal the word's meaning. For example, the root of *becoming* is *come*. Since you know what *come* means, you have the first clue you need to encode the meaning of the whole word. As another example, take the word *misogynist*. If you dissect this word using word analysis, it looks like this:

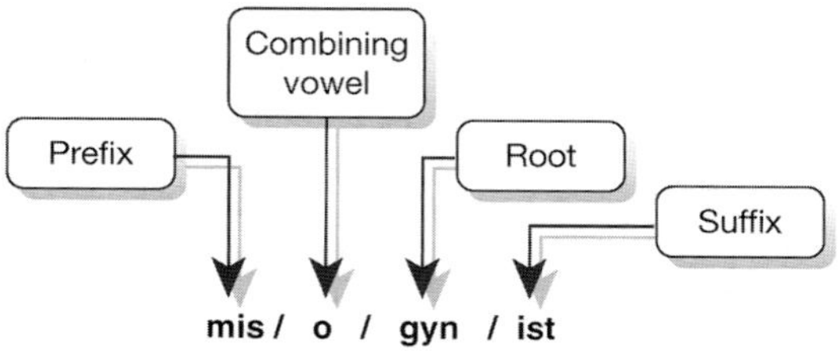

It is one thing to be able to dissect the word and another to be able to name the individual parts. It is something else entirely to know what those individual parts mean:

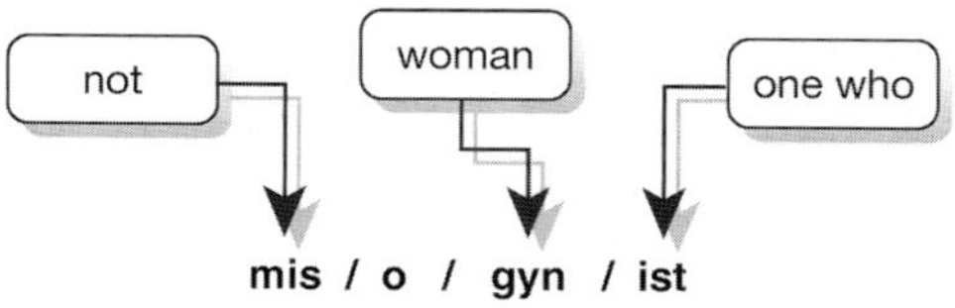

Words with the same root have related meanings. For example:

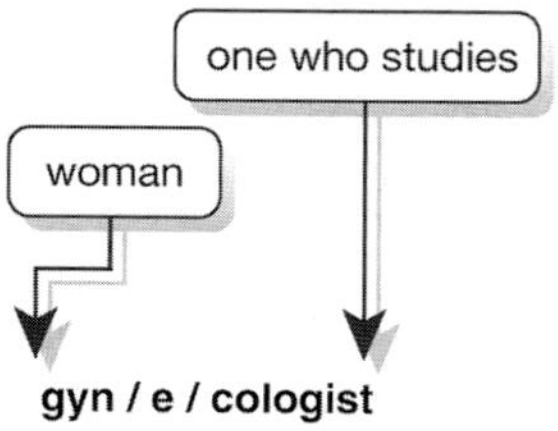

A word can contain more than one root. For example, *matrilineal* contains the roots *matri* (mother) and *lineal* (line). *Matrilineal,* therefore, means "determining descent through the female line."

Table 25–4 Examples of Root Words

ROOT	WORD	DEFINITION
Gastr	Gastritis	Inflammation of the stomach
Carcin	Carcinogen	To produce cancer
Lapar	Laparotomy	Abdominal surgery

COMMON ROOT WORDS USED IN MEDICAL TERMINOLOGY

GREEK ROOTS:

ACANTH: thorn
ACR: extremity
ACTIN: ray
ADEN: gland
AER: gas or air
ALG: pain
ALL: different
ANCON: elbow
ANDR: male
ANGI: vessel
ANTH: flower
ARTHR: joint; speech
ANTHROP: human being
ANTR: cavity
AUT: self
AUX: to increase
BA: to walk
BALL, BOL: to throw or to place
BI: life
BLAST: seed or bud
BLEPHAR: eyelid
BOL, BOUL: will
BRACY: short
BRADY: slow
BROM: foul scent; bromine
BRONCH(I): airway
CARCIN: cancer
CARDI: pertaining to the heart
CARP: wrist
CAU: to burn
CELE: hernia or swelling
CENTE: to puncture
CEPAHAL: head
CHEIL, CHIL: lip
CHIR: hand
CHOL: bile
CHORD: cord
CHROM, CHROMAT: color
CHRON: time
CLAS: break
CLY: to wash or to rinse
COCC: berrylike
COL: colon
COLL(A): glue
CONDYL: knob
CRANI: cranium
CRINE: to secrete
CRY, CRYM: cold
CRYPT: hidden
CYCL: circle
CYE: to be pregnant
CYST: bladder; cyst
CYT: cell
DACTYL: finger or digit
DEM: people
DERM, DERMAT: skin
DESM: ligaments
DIDYM: twin or testicle
DROM: course
DYN, DYNAM: power
EC, EK, OIC, OIK: house
ECH: to repeat
EDE: to swell
EO: dawn or red
ERG: to work
ERYTHR: red
ESTHE, AESTHE: to feel
GALA, GALACT: milk
GAM: union
GE: earth
GER, GERONT: old age
GLAUC: silver or gray
GLOT: tongue
GLYC: sugar
GNO: to know or have knowledge
GON: to produce
GONI: angle
HELI: sun
HEM, HEMAT: blood
HEPAT, HEPAR: liver
HETER: different
HIST, HISTI: tissue
HOD, OD: road or path
HYAL: glass
HYDR: fluid
HYGR: moisture
HYSTER: uterus
IS: same
ISCH: to suppress
ISCHI: hip
KER, KERAT: horny tissue
KINE: motion
LAL: to talk
LAPAR: abdomen
LARYNG: larynx
LECITH: yolk
LEI: smooth
LEP: to seize
LEPT: delicate
LEX: to read
LIP: fat
LOG: word
LYMPH: pertaining to the lymphs
MACR: large
MAST, MAZ: breast
MEGA: large
MEL: limbs
MELAN: dark
MEN: moon; menstruation
MENING: membrane
MER: part
MES: middle
MICR: small
MIS: hate
MIT: thread
MNE: to remember
MORPH: to form or to change
MY, MYO, MYOS: muscle
MYEL: spinal cord
MYX: mucus
NARC: stupor
NE: new

COMMON ROOT WORDS USED IN MEDICAL TERMINOLOGY, CONT.

NECR: dead tissue
NEPHYR: kidney
NEUR: nerve, nervous system
NOS: disease
ODONT: tooth
ODYN: pain
OLIG: few
ONC, ONCUS: tumor
OO: egg
OP, OPT: eye
OPTHALM: pertaining to the eye
ORCH: testicle
ORTH: straight
OSM: sense of smell
OST: bone
OT: ear
OX, OXY: sharp; oxygen
PAG: united
PALI: return
PAN: all
PATH: disease or feeling
PED, PAED: child
PEN: deficiency
PEP, PEPT: to digest
PETR: rock
PHA: to speak
PHAG: to eat
PHAN: to appear
PHLAC(T): to protect
PHLEB: vein
PHON: sound
PHOR, PHER: to bear; to go
PHOT: light
PHRAG: to contain within
PHRAS: to speak
PHREN: mind
PHY: to grow
PHYLL: leaf
PHYTE: plant or growth
PLAS(T): to form or mold
PLATY(S): broad
PLEG: paralysis
PLEUR: side
PLEX: stroke
PLO: fold
PNEA: breathing
PNEUM: air
POD, PUS: foot
POIKIL: irregular
POLY: many
POR: passageway
PRESBY: old
PROCT: anus or rectum
PSUED: false or fake
PSYCH: mind
PTO: to fall
PY: pus
PYL: gateway
PYR, PYRE: heat or fire
RHIN, RHINE: nose
SARC: flesh
SCHIZ, SCHIS: to split
SCLER: hardened
SCOP: to view
SEP: to rot
SOM, SOMAT: body
SPA: to jerk
SPHYGM: pulse
STA: to stand
STAPHYL: bunches
STEN: narrow
STERN: chest
STIG: mark or point
STOL, STAL, STLE: to send; contract
STOM, STOMAT: mouth or opening
SYRING: tube
TACHY: fast
TAX: to arrange
TELE: completion
THE: to put
THEL: nipple
THERM: heat
THORAC: chest
THROM: clot
TON: tension
TOP: to place
TOX: poison
TRACHEL: neck
TRICH: hair
TROP, TREP: to turn or to respond accordingly
TROPH: development
UR, URE: having to do with urine or urination
XEN: stranger
XER: dry
ZYM: to ferment

LATIN ROOTS:

AC(U): point
ACT, AG: to act
ADIP: fat
AL: winged
ALB: white
ALVEOL: cavity
AMBUL: to walk
ANNUL: ring
APIC: tip
AQU: water
ARC(U): arched
ARE: space
ARTICUL: joint
ATRI: room
AUD: to hear
AUR: ear
AX: axis
BARB: beard
BI, BIN: two
BILI: bile
BUCC: cheek
BULL: blister
CAL: to be warm
CALC: calcium
CALCAR: spur

COMMON ROOT WORDS USED IN MEDICAL TERMINOLOGY, CONT.

CALL: hardened skin
CAN: glowing
CAP, CAPT, CEPT: to receive
CAPILL: hair
CAPS: box
CENT: one hundred
CEREBR: brain
CERN, CRET, CRE: to separate or to secrete
CERVIC: neck
CESS: to yield
CID: to fall
CING: to bind
CIPIT: head
CIS: to cut
CLAV (1): club
CLAV (2): key
CLIV: slope
CLUS, CLOS: to close
COLL: neck
CORD: heart
CORN: horny
CORP, CORPUS: body
CORT: the outermost layer
CRE, CRESC, CRET: to grow
CUB: to lay down
CURR, CURS: to go
CUSPID: point
CUSS: to shake
CUT: skin
DEC, DECIM: ten
DENT: tooth
DEXTR: to the right side
DIGIT: toes and fingers
DOL: to feel pain
DORM(IT): to sleep
DORS: back
DUC, DUCT: to lead
DUR: hard
EGO: I
ERR: wander or to deviate
FA: to speak
FACI: surface
FACT, FIC: to make
FASCI: band
FEBR: fever
FER: to carry or produce
FERR: iron
FIBR: fiber
FIBUL: clasp
FIL: thread
FISS: to separate
FLAGELL: whip
FLAV: yellow
FLEX: to bend
FLU, FLUX: to flow
FOLL: bag
FRAC, FRAG: to break or to bend
FRUCT: fruit
FUN: cord
FUNG: fungus
FURC: fork
FUS: to pour
FUSC: dark
GEMIN: paired
GEN(U): Bknee
GEST: to carry
GINGIV: gums
GLAB(R): smooth
GRAV: heavy
GREG: to flock
GUST: to taste
HAL, HALIT: to breath
HER, HES: to stick
HIAT: to remain open
I, IT: to go
ILE: ileum
INGUIN: groin
INSUL: island
JACUL: to dart
JECT: to throw
JUNCT, JUG: to join
LAB: to fall
LABI: lip
LACRIM: tear
LACT: milk
LAMELL: a thin plate
LAT: to carry
LATER: side
LENT: lens
LEV (1): to the right side
LEV (2): lightweight
LIEN: spleen
LIG: to bind
LINE: line
LOB: lobe or ear
LUC: light
LUM: light
LUMB: loin
LUN: moon
MACUL: spot
MAGN: large
MAL: cheek
MAL(E): bad
MALLE: hammer
MAMM: breast
MAN(U): hand
MATR, MATERN: mother
MEAT: to pass
MEDI: middle
MENT (1): chin
MENT (2): mind
MIL(L): one thousand
MOLL: soft
MORT: death
MOT: to move
MUC: mucus
MULT: many
MUR: wall
NAR: nostril
NAS: nose
NERV: nerve

COMMON ROOT WORDS USED IN MEDICAL TERMINOLOGY, CONT.

NEV: birthmark
NIGR: black
NOCT: night
NOM: name
NON, NOVEM: nine
NUC: nut
NUTRI, NUTRIT: to nourish
OCT, OCTAV: eight
OCUL: pertaining to the eye
ORB: circular
OS, OR: mouth
OSS: bone
OV: egg
PALAT: palate
PALP: to touch
PAR: to produce
PAT: to open
PATI: to suffer
PECTOR: breast
PED: foot
PEL(L), PULS: to beat
PELL: skin
PET, PETIT: to seek
PIL: hair
PLANT: sole of the foot
PLEX: to interweave
PLIC(IT): to fold
PLUR: more
POSIT: to put
POT: sense of power
PRIM: first
PRON: face down
PROXIM: near
PRUR: to itch
PULMO(N): lung
PUNCT: point
PUR: pus
QUADRU: four
QUART: four
QUINQUE: five
QUINT: five
RADI: radius or ray
REG, RECT: to make straight
REN: kidney
RET: net
RIG: stiff
RIM: crack
ROS: to eat away at
ROT: round
RUB: red
RUG: wrinkle
RUPT: to break
SALI, SILI, SULT: to jump
SANGUI: blood
SCRIB, SCRIPT: to write
SEB: grease
SEC, SECT, SEG: to cut
SECOND, SECUND: second
SEMI: half
SEMIN: seed
SEN: old
SEP, SEPT (1): to separate
SEP, SEPT (2): seven
SESQUI: one and a half
SEXT: six
SICC: dry
SOL: sun
SOLV, SOLUT: dissolve
SOMN: sleep
SON: sound
SORB, SORPT: to draw inward
SPIC: cone
SPIN: thorn
SPIR: to breath
SQUAM: scale
STA: to stand
STRAT: layer
STRI: striated
STRING, STRICT: to draw tight
STRU, STRUCT: to build
TACT: to touch
TEN, TENT: to hold
TEND, TENS: to stretch
TERMIN: ending
TERTI, TER, TERN: three
TRACT: to drag
TRI: third
TRUS: to push
TUBER: to swell
TUM: to swell
TUSS: cough
UN: one
UNGU: nail
VAGIN: sheath
VAL: strength
VARI: varied
VARIC: swollen
VAS: vessel
VEN: vein
VENT: belly
VERT, VERS: to turn:
VESIC: blister
VISCER: entrails
VIT: life
VITR: glass
VULS: to tear

PREFIXES

Knowing the Greek and Latin roots of a word's prefix can also help you determine the meaning of words. As mentioned earlier, prefixes modify the root words by either qualifying or quantifying them. Quantity can be indicated with the prefix *poly-,* which designates a general number, or a prefix that points to a specific number, such as *tri-*. Quantity can also be designated as a negation, as in words with the prefixes *in-* or *im-,* meaning "without."

Prefixes can qualify a root in terms of time or direction. *Ante,* for instance, means *before,* and if we connect it with *mortem* we end up with *antemortem,* or "prior to death."

FOCUS ON: *Decoding Words*

Pneumonoultramicroscopicsilicovolcanokoniosis. Yes, this is an actual word coined in the 1930s to be the longest word in the dictionary. What does it mean? It is a medical condition where there is damage to the lungs caused by inhaling silica dust from a volcano. Medical terminology is filled with words that seem incomprehensible. By "dissecting" these words into discrete units, you can understand even the most complex terms.

SUFFIXES

Just as prefixes appear in front of words, suffixes appear at the end of words. Like a prefix, a suffix also modify a word's meaning. Unlike a prefix, a suffix helps make the word an adjective, a verb, or a noun. For example, the root word *gen(e)* means "to produce." *Gene,* a form of this root, is a noun. However, the word *genetic* is an adjective. Knowing the meaning of a suffix is just as important as knowing the root word and the prefix in discerning the meaning of a medical term.

Table 25–5 Adjective Endings

ADJECTIVE ENDINGS	EXAMPLE
-ac	Cardiac Heart
-al	Skeletal Skeleton
-ary	Salivary Saliva
-ic	Pelvic Pelvis
-ical	Surgical Surgery
-ous	Venous Vein
-tic	Paralytic Paralysis
-ar	Muscular Muscles

When dissecting a term for interpretation, start at the suffix, if the word has one. If there is a suffix, the process of unlocking the word's meaning begins with the clues given by the suffix. As mentioned above, the most important clue the suffix provides is the whole word's part of speech.

Knowing the Greek and Latin origin of a word's suffix can help us determine the meaning. Suffixes modify root words by indicating whether a word is a **noun,** an **adjective,** a **plural,** or a **diminutive** (Tables 25–5, 25–6, and 25–7).

Table 25–6 Noun Endings

NOUN ENDINGS	MEANING	EXAMPLE
-iac	Indicates person afflicted with certain diseases or conditions	Hemophiliac
-ia	An unhealthy state	Anesthesia
-is	Forms the noun from the root	Cutis Skin
-ism	Condition, state of being	Alcholism Alcohol
-ist	One who specializes	Radiologist
-itis	Inflammation	Arthritis
-logy	Study of	Biology
-plasty	Form or fix	Rhinoplasty
-oma	Tumor or mass	Carcinoma
-scopy	Process of visual examination	Laproscopy
-y	Condition, process	Neuropathy Nervous system Disease
-gen	To be produced	Pathogen

Table 25–7 Diminutive Endings

DIMINUTIVE ENDING	MEANING	EXAMPLE
-ole	Small, little, minute	Artiole Artery
-icle	Small, little, minute	Particle Piece
-ule	Small, little, minute	Veinule Vein

COMMON PREFIXES USED IN MEDICAL TERMINOLOGY

GREEK PREFIXES:

A-, AN-: not or without
AMPHI-, AMPHO-: both
ANA-: up or again
ANTI-: opposite
APO-: away
CATA-: down or against
DYS-: bad or difficult
EC-, EX-: outward or outside
EN-, EM-, EL-: inward
ENDO-, ENTO-: within
EPI-: upon
ES-, EIS-: into or inward
EU-: normal
EXO-, ECTO-: external
HYPER-: more
HYPO-: less
META-: change or transfer
PARA-: beside or associated with
PERI-: around or nearby
PRO-: before
PROS-: toward or in addition to
SYM-: with or together

LATIN PREFIXES:

A-, AB-, ABS-: from
AD-, AC-, AG-, AL-: near, to or toward
AMBI-, AMBO-: both
ANTE-: before
CIRCUM-: around
COM-, CON-, CO-: with
CONTR-: opposite
DI-, DIS-, DIF-: apart
E-, EX-, EF-: out or complete
IM-, IN-: into
INFRA-: below
INTER-: between or among
INTRA-, INTRO-: within
JUXTA-: on the side of or close to
OB-, OF-, OP-, OC-: toward or completely
PER-: through or wrongly
POST-: after or behind
PRE-: before
PRO-: forward or in front
RE-, RED-: again
RETRO-: backward or back
SE-: away
SUB-, SUC-, SUF-, SUP-: under or somewhat
SUPER- SUPRA-: above
TRANS-, TRAN-, TRA-: across
ULTRA-: beyond

COMMON SUFFIXES USED IN MEDICAL TERMINOLOGY

GREEK SUFFIXES:

-AL: pertaining to or like
-AN: pertaining to
-ARY: placement for
-ATE: to make
-ECTOMY: removal of
-EMIA: condition affecting the blood
-GENOUS, -GENIC: producing
-IA, -Y: state of
-IASIS: diseased condition
-IC, -TIC: pertaining to or like
-ICIAN: one who specializes in
-ICS, -TICS: the study of
-ID, -IDA, -IDEA: related to
-IN, -INE: chemical derivative of
-ISK, -ISCUS: little
-ISM, -ISMUS: condition of
-IST, -AST: one who
-ITIS: inflammation of
-IUM: part of, lining for, or in the area of
-IUM, -ION: little
-IZE: to make or to treat
-LOGY: the study of
-LYSIS: dissolution by
-MA, -ME, -M: the consequences or results of
-MANIA: madness or insanity about
-METER: measure
-METRY: study of measure
-NOMY: study of
-ODE, -OID: in the shape of
-OMA: tumor resulting from or contained within
-OSIS: characterized as being diseased
-OUS: full of or pertaining to
-PATHY: disease of
-PHILIC, -PHILOUS: loving
-PHOBIA: fear of
-PLASTY: formation of
-RRHEA: abnormal flow
-SCOPE, -SCOPY: to see
-SIS, -SIA, -SY, -SE: process by which
-STOMY: surgical opening of
-T, -TE: one who, or that which
-TER: means for placement of
-THERAPY: remedy for or by
-TOMY: surgery on or by
-URIA: condition affecting urine
-US: member of or person

COMMON SUFFIXES USED IN MEDICAL TERMINOLOGY, CONT.

LATIN SUFFIXES:

-ABLE, -IBLE: able to

-ACEOUS: belonging to or resembling

-ACIOUS: inclination toward

-AL, -IAL, -EAL, -UAL: pertaining to

-AN, -ANE: pertaining to

-ANCE, -ANCY: state of being, quality of being

-ANT, -IANT: to be

-AR: pertaining to

-ARY: pertaining to

-ATE, -ITE: characterized by having

-BUL, -BULA, -BLE, -BULUM: resulting from, act of, or placement of

-CRUM: means of or resulting from

-CULE, -CLE: small

-CULUM: resulting from or act of

-EL, -ELLE: small

-ELLUS, -ELLA, -ELLUM: small

-ENCE, -ENCY: state of being, quality of being

-ENT, -IENT: to be

-ESCE: to begin or to be somewhat

-ETTE, -ET: small

-FORM: having the shape of

-FY, -FIC: to make or to cause

-IA: state of being or act of doing

-IC, -TIC: pertaining to

-ID: inclination toward

-IGATE, -EGATE: to drive

-IL: small

-ILE, -IL: pertaining to

-ILE: able to

-ILLUS, -ILLA, -ILLUM: small

-IN: pertaining to

-ION: act of or resulting from

-ITIOUS: characterized by

-ITUDE: state of or able to

-ITY, -ETY, -TY: state of being or quality of

-IVE: inclination toward

-LENT: full of or predisposed to

-MEN, -MIN: resulting from or act of

-MENT, -MENTUM: resulting from or act of

-OR: one who, or that which

-OR: state of being or resulting from

-ORY: inclination toward

-ORY: placement for

-OSE: full of

-OUS, -IOUS, -EOUS: full of

-TRUM: means of or resulting from

-ULE, -OLE, -LE: small

-ULOUS: inclination toward

-ULUS, -ULA, -ULUM, -OLA: small

-UNCLE: small

-UNCULUS: small

-UOUS: inclination toward

-URE: act of or resulting from

-US: act of or resulting from

-Y: state of being or act of doing

PRONUNCIATION

Pronunciation is a fundamental, yet key, concept for anyone in the medical fields. Regardless of the vast wealth of knowledge a person may have in his or her brain, it is difficult to view the person as credible unless he or she can properly pronounce words in the vernacular. In medical terminology, many words are long and complicated and rather easy to mispronounce, so it is important to learn the proper pronunciation of each.

Developing accurate pronunciations skills takes both patience and diligence. There are some general points to remember. For example, some words have silent letters; they are paired with other letters, and the combination has one sound. See Table 25–8 for some examples.

Table 25–8 Silent Letters

LETTER COMBINATION	SOUND	EXAMPLE	PRONUNCIATION
Pt	t	pterygoid	ter' î-gold
Ps	s	psorias	sor-i'ah-sis
Pn	n	pneometer	ne-om'it-er
Gn	n	gnathitis	na-thît'is
Mn	n	mnemonic	ne-mon'ik

Another rule concerns prefixes. If a prefix ending in a vowel comes before the combinations *pt, gn,* or *pn,* then the first letter is pronounced:

hemoptysis he-mop´tî-sis
prognathism prog´nah-tizm
polypnea pol"ip-ne'ah
dysgnathia dis-na'the-ah

The third rule involves combinations of the vowels oe and ae (English spelling), which are pronounced as the long *e* sound. When preceded with the letter *c* (as in *ce, cae,* or *coe*), these combinations are pronounced like the word *see; ge, gae,* and *goe* are pronounced as if they begin with the letter *j*: *jee.*

haema he'mah
rugae roo `je
coelum se`lom
septicaemia sep"tî-se'me-ah
caecum se'kum

Another rule involves the pronunciations of words that include combinations of the letters *ph, rh, ch, x,* and *dys* (Table 25–9):

Practicing in the company of medical professionals can be daunting. However, estheticians who know the fundamentals of medical terminology will develop a working rapport with those professionals. Understanding parts of speech and their uses in English, the standard medical language, will help you learn and become adept at mastering medical terminology.

Table 25–9 Letter-specific Pronunciations

LETTER COMBINATION	SOUND	WORD	PRONUNCIATION
Ph	f	phrenoplegia	fren"o-ple'je-ah
Rh	r	rhytidosis	rit"î-do'sis
Ch	k	cochlea	kok'le-ah
x	z	xanthic	zan'thik
dys	dis	dysphagia	dis-fa'je-ah

REVIEW QUESTIONS

1. Explain some of the early medical discoveries made by the Egyptians, the Greeks, and the Romans.
2. What is medical terminology? Why is it necessary?
3. What are root words, suffixes, and prefixes?
4. How should you dissect a word to decipher its meaning?
5. What is a combining vowel?
6. What is a combining form?
7. What is the plural of *vertebra*? What is the plural of *diagnosis*?
8. What do the letter combinations *gn, pt,* and *ps* all have in common in medical terminology?
9. Separate the following words into their combining forms:

   interarticular ______________________

   quinquepartite ______________________

prescription ______________________
calcepenia ______________________
annulus ______________________
biped ______________________
purulent ______________________

10. Define the words above.

interarticular ______________________
quinquepartite ______________________
prescription ______________________
calcepenia ______________________
annulus ______________________
biped ______________________
purulent ______________________

CHAPTER GLOSSARY

adjective: part of speech used to describe a noun.

combining form: resulting combination of a root word, a combining vowel, a prefix, a suffix, or any combination.

combining vowel: vowel used to combine root words with suffixes and prefixes.

diminutive: suffix that is added to a word to note smallness or being smaller than something else.

modifies: to qualify or limit the meaning of a word.

noun: part of speech that is used to name a person, place, thing, quality, or action. It is usually the subject or object of the action in a sentence.

plural: form of a word meant to indicate that there is more than one.

prefixes: parts of Greek or Latin words used at the beginning of a word to alter or modify its meaning.

pronunciation: process of accurately speaking a word as it is meant to be spoken.

root words: parts of Latin or Greek words that serve as the basis for medical terminology.

suffixes: parts of Greek or Latin words used at the end of a word to alter or modify its meaning.

word analysis: process by which the different parts of the words are dissected and interpreted to determine the meaning of the original word.

CHAPTER 26

MEDICAL INTERVENTION

CHAPTER OUTLINE

- MEDICAL INTERVENTION DEFINED
- AN INTRODUCTION TO BOTOX
- AN INTRODUCTION TO DERMAL FILLERS
- AN INTRODUCTION TO SCLEROTHERAPY
- AN INTRODUCTION TO MEDICAL PEELS

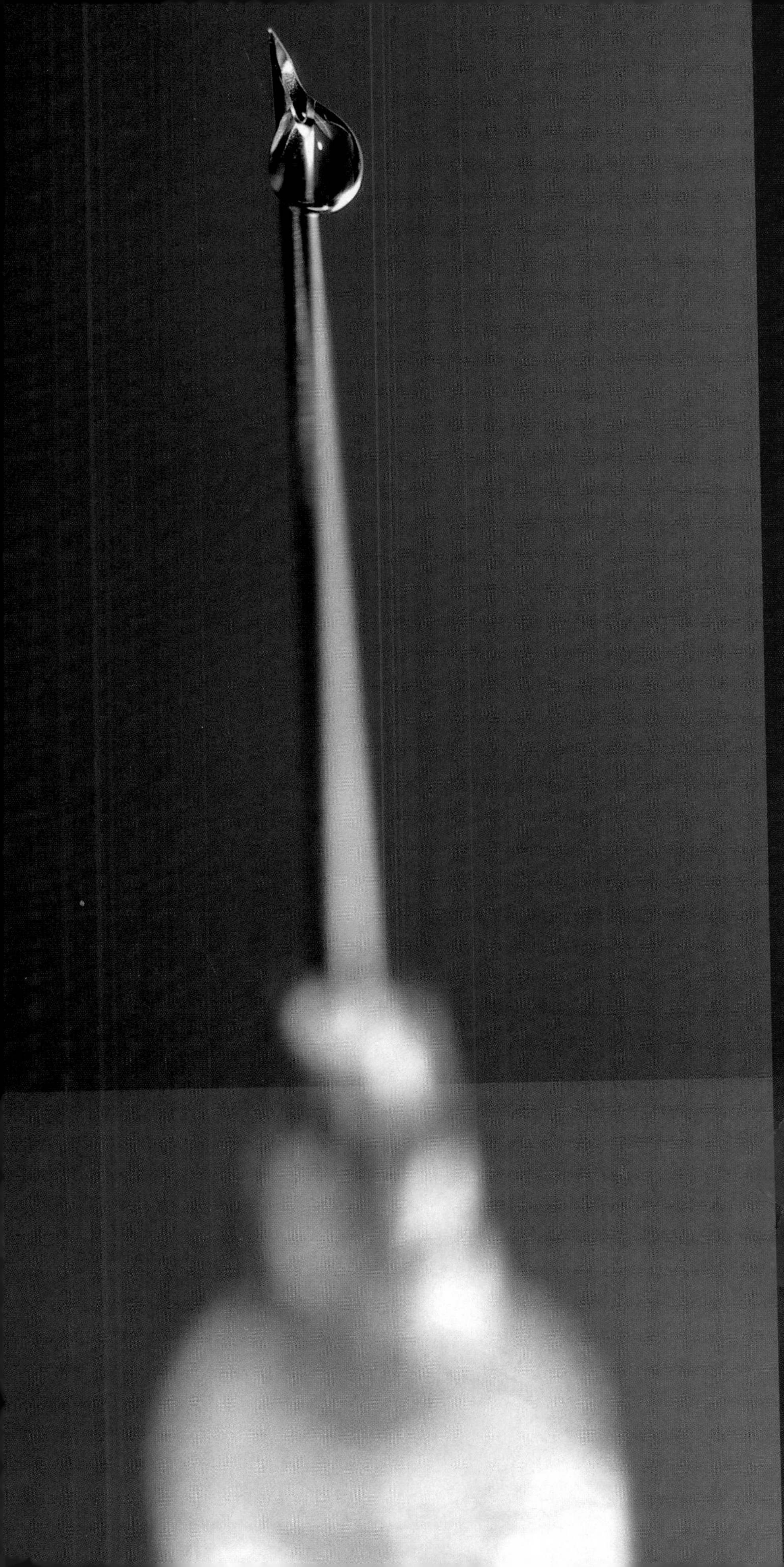

LEARNING OBJECTIVES

After completing this chapter, you should be able to:

- Introduce and define *medical intervention*.
- Explain what Botox is and how to use it in an esthetic environment.
- Explain what dermal fillers are and how to use them in an esthetic environment.
- Define the common types of dermal fillers used.
- Explain what sclerotherapy is and how to use it in an esthetic environment.
- Discuss medical peels, how they differ from esthetic peels, and how they are used.

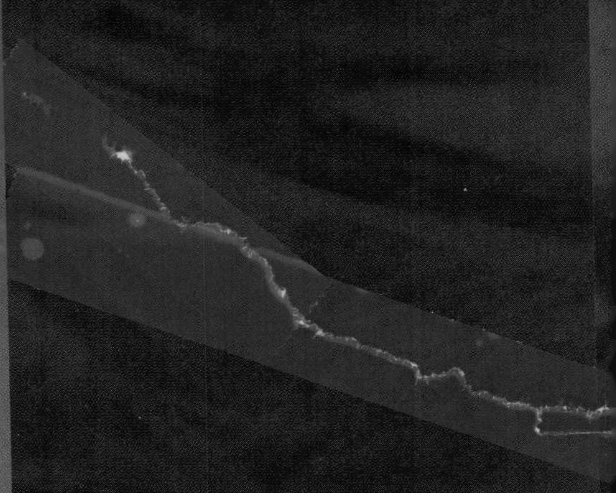

KEY TERMS

Page numbers indicate where in the chapter the term is used.

autologous 698
avian 697
blepharospasm 693
blood-brain barrier 695
botulinum toxin 693
bovine collagen 697
cautery 705
cervical dystonia 693
cleaving 697
complications 701
dynamic movement 693
dyschromias 704
glabella 692
hyaluronic acid 700
nasolabial lines 692
necrosis 700
Non-animal Stabilized Hyaluronic Acid (NASHA) 701
nonimmunogenic 697
platysmal bands 694
ptosis 693
punctate keratitis 696
sclerotherapy 691
strabismus 693
tinnitus 705
varicose veins 702

Facial beauty creates attention and has an impact on a person's status in society. While standards of facial beauty differ from country to country and culture to culture, there are basics that define beauty. Those basics include symmetry, balance, proportion, and harmony (Figure 26–1). Lines, wrinkles, and sagging skin were once considered an irreversible consequence of the aging process. Past generations grudgingly accepted wrinkles and crow's feet as their right of passage into the golden years. Some wore their lines proudly as a testament to their survival of war, depression, and oppression. Today, the opposite is true. As more baby boomers have moved into their 60s, they have been responsible for the creation of the multibillion-dollar industry called nonsurgical aesthetics. Wanting to sustain a youthful appearance, consumers have forced the development of products and services to meet their needs. This has led to the use of Botox®, injectable fillers, and medical peels. In addition, **sclerotherapy**—treatment for the elimination of small blood vessels, enlarged veins, and dilated capillaries—has become exponentially more popular. What is the esthetician's role in this movement?

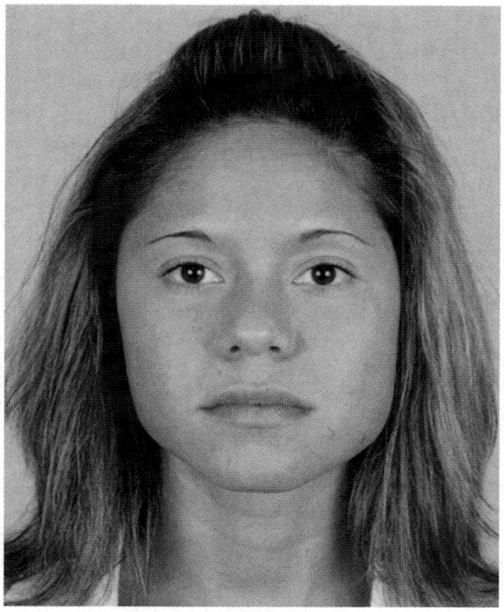

Figure 26–1 A youthful face.

MEDICAL INTERVENTION DEFINED

There are two sides to the field of esthetics: the esthetic side and the medical side. The esthetic side deals primarily with procedures with which you have become accustomed: microdermabrasion, facial toning, esthetic peels, and the like. For certain clients, though, the fight against the effects of aging requires the use of more aggressive approaches. These clients want services that include injectable products such as Botox, dermal fillers, and injection vein therapy. While you can suggest these services to clients, these products are categorized as medical intervention and are performed by highly trained medical personnel.

The Esthetician's Role

In most states, trained medical professionals, such as doctors or nurses, are the only individuals qualified to perform these procedures. This means that not all facilities offer these services. However, you, the esthetician, who has a rapport with your clients, will often be the one to suggest the options, answer the questions that inevitably ensue, and ease the client's concerns about these procedures. In fact, you may be the first to discuss with a client the benefits of injection dermal therapy, sclerotherapy, and advanced peeling techniques. Thus, you need to be thoroughly familiar with these procedures.

New products come onto the market regularly, so you must be vigilant about updating information you give to clients and checking its accuracy. You can best accomplish this by reading all available materials and having regular discussions with the physician or nurse injector in the clinic where you work or to whom you may refer clients. Regular discussions benefit everyone involved—the client, the esthetician, the doctor, and the injector—by ensuring that everyone is imparting the same information to the client.

If you do not work within the medical setting, it is important to establish a relationship with a local medical professional to whom you feel comfortable referring clients. This is a positive two-way street, because the more information they share with you, the more valuable an asset you will be in referring clients to them. It is to them, or their staff, you will turn to gain more information about procedures and products discussed in this chapter.

General Information Estheticians Can Give Clients

There is some general information that you can share with a client without consequences. This includes information about types of products, durability of products, and what to expect in post-care.

General Information about Dermal Fillers

There are several general points about dermal fillers that you can share with your clients, including the different types of fillers, the durability of products, the best indications for dermal fillers, anesthesia for the treatment, and post-care.

Products and FDA Approval Status

You should always be able to name the products your clinic carries, which products are preferred, and why. Knowing which pharmaceuticals are approved by the U.S. Food and Drug Administration (FDA) and which are not is also an important component of your knowledge base. While many physicians obtain unapproved dermal fillers from other countries, it is important to understand why drug products are approved and others are not. This is not necessarily printed knowledge but more "sophisticated gossip" that will find its way into the medical office. While you would not typically share this information with a client, you may be asked about a particular prescripton product, and it is nice to know, usually from a company sales representative, a pharmaceutical's status with the FDA.

Product Durability

The most common question that an esthetician hears from clients concerns product durability. A procedure is expensive and may be uncomfortable and time-consuming (sometimes requiring two to three appointments to achieve the desired result). For these reasons, most clients want to know how long the product lasts. The answer to this question depends on several variables, including the type of material used, the placement, the depth of the placement, and whether this is the primary or secondary injection session.

The first variable in a dermal filler procedure, the type of material used, has almost everything to do with how long the procedure's effects last. That is to say, certain products have a longer durability than others; for example, the effects of hyaluronic acid last longer than those of bovine collagen. As you educate the client about product choices, begin with the concept that certain products inherently last longer.

The second variable that affects durability is the location of placement, or the indication. Some areas of the face absorb the product more quickly than others. For example, the lips absorb more quickly than acne scars on the lateral aspects of the face, and the **nasolabial lines,** which run from the nose to the mouth, absorb more quickly than a **glabella,** area between the brows, that is treated with a dermal filler and then paralyzed with Botox (Figure 26–2). In other words, movement or friction plays into the durability of a product.

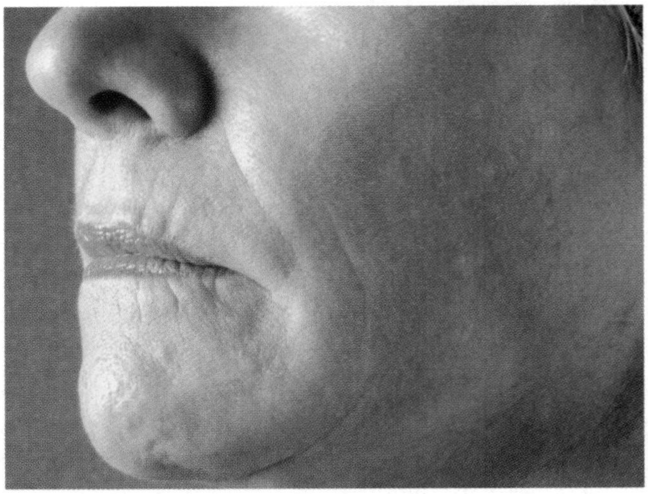

Figure 26–2 Nasolabial lines.

The depth of placement is also an important factor. If a product is placed more deeply than is recommended, it will absorb more quickly. The clearest example of this concept is the placement of Restylane Fine Line® or Zyderm I® into the mid-papillary dermis. Both are intended to be placed in the upper epidermis. The limited correction that is provided by the wrong placement will last only weeks compared to the durability of the proper placement, which should last months.

Finally, an important and little-recognized component of durability is the number of previous treatments. It is well known that the *original* result that is achieved with dermal fillers lasts only four to eight months, but the material will reside in the tissues for more than a year. When a client has another treatment six months *after* the original treatment, the correction is easier and the original product provides a foundation on which to lay new product, making the result easier to achieve and longer lasting.

While Botox's variables are not as significant as those of the dermal fillers, you should still be aware of the key points necessary to educate the Botox client. When discussing Botox with the client, be aware of the indications for the procedure, the durability of Botox, potential discomfort, and treatment consequences, such as bruising or complications such as eyelid **ptosis,** or drooping eyelids.

The indications for Botox include frown lines, forehead lines, crow's feet, upper and lower lip lines, and chin pebbling. There are, of course, nuances to these treatment indications, such as skin laxity, volume of lines and wrinkles, and anticipated appearance. Whether or not the injector can give the client the result he or she seeks should be left for discussion with the injector. Do not promise something that you cannot control and do not know to be true.

Clients frequently ask about the durability of Botox. While timeframes vary, a good response to this question is three to five months. As with dermal fillers, durability depends on the area treated, the length of time since the last treatment, and the desires of the client. Clients who request full paralysis will have less durability, because once the muscle begins to move the client is back in the office, usually about three months after the procedure. If, on the other hand, the client is willing to have some movement or partial paralysis of the muscle, he or she might be happy for as long as five months. Botox can be uncomfortable for some people, but typically clients tolerate the procedure well and are out of the office in 15 minutes. Bruising can be a frequent treatment consequence with Botox, especially around the eyes. Counseling the client to discontinue aspirin or other products that may contribute to bruising two days prior to treatment can be helpful. However, the client should check with his or her primary physician to consider the advisability prior to discontinuation of any medications. If the client is bruised, it can take as long as two weeks for the area to resolve, especially around the eyes.

Finally, the most feared complication is that of eyelid ptosis, in which the eyelid is paralyzed and unable to open fully. This complication is related to glabellar treatment, *not crow's feet*. The nerves and muscles that control the eyelids are above the arch of the brow. If the injector is not careful about the placement of the treatment near the eyebrow, eyelid ptosis can occur.

FOCUS ON: *Dispensing Advice*

As an esthetician, you can provide basic, helpful information to a client seeking dermal filler or Botox treatment. However, estheticians should never dispense medical advice. Be careful about the advice you give and how you recommend treatments. You do not want the client to misunderstand you as making endorsements for particular products.

AN INTRODUCTION TO BOTOX

Botox Cosmetic, the product name for **botulinum toxin,** is the answer to some of the most common complaints of aging. According to some, it is the greatest advancement in recent cosmetic medicine. It can erase fine lines and wrinkles and improve facial contour, and it addresses eye shape in a matter of days without the need for surgery. In short, Botox can stave off what most clients fear the most: going under the knife to effect a younger appearance.

Botox Cosmetic has been used for many situations since the early 1970s. Originally, Botox was used to treat conditions such as **blepharospasm, strabismus, cervical dystonia,** and cerebral palsy. Today, it is most recognized, and FDA approved, for the treatment of lines and wrinkles associated with **dynamic movement,** a term that describes muscle movement below the skin, which creates lines in the skin itself, such as in frowning.

Botox is a refined version of the bacteria that causes the illness known as botulism. For most people considering the use of Botox, this is of particular concern. However, following a refining process, Botox is safe for human consumption in the clinical doses in which it is used. This makes all the difference. Botox has become the tool that doctors and nurses turn to every day for the treatment of wrinkling associated with glabellar frown lines, vertical forehead lines, crow's feet, upper lip lines, lower lip lines, corners of the mouth, and **platysmal bands,** wrinkling around the neck, to name a few.

The American Society of Plastic Surgeons, one of several societies that keep statistics on cosmetic plastic surgery, reports that Botox is the number one nonsurgical procedure for both men and women. More than 2 million women and more than 250,000 men had Botox treatments in 2003. With the growing acceptance and marketing penetration, there is no doubt that Botox continues to experience significant market growth with each passing year. Other nonsurgical procedures—such as chemical peels, microdermabrasion, or even dermal fillers—do not come close to these numbers. So what makes Botox so appealing to the public and estheticians alike?

Indications for Botox

Glabellar frown lines are the most commonly treated indication for Botox Cosmetic. When evaluating a patient for treatment, look for several key points, including the lines of the glabella (Figure 26–3). Are they singular or multiple? Does the area pull in just one spot or in multiple areas? How far do the lines extend vertically? and How deep are the lines and how heavy is the glabellar region over the eyes?

Forehead lines are the horizontal lines that are created when the brow is lifted. Treating the forehead can be one of the more challenging indications because the depth of the lines may be an indication of potential brow laxity. Complete relaxation can be responsible for brow ptosis, especially in the hands of the inexperienced injector. When evaluating the brow for treatments, look for several key indicators: brow heaviness or droopiness, lid heaviness, glabellar involvement, and depth of lines (Figure 26–4a and b).

Crow's feet are those pesky little lines around the eyes (Figure 26–5a and b). They can begin in the early 20s and deepen as years go on. The lines are created by the contraction

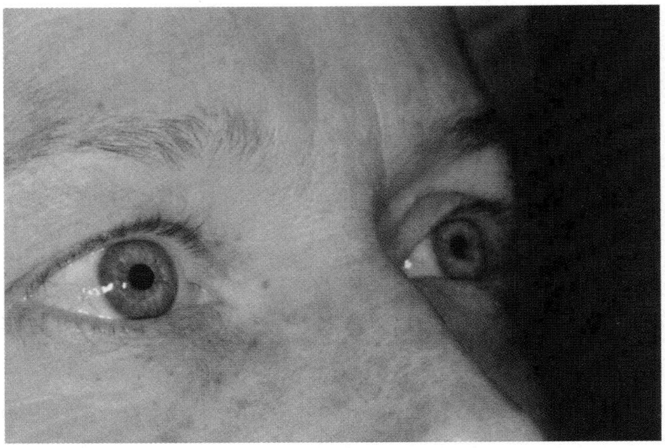

Figure 26–3 An appropriate client for glabellar Botox.

Indications for Botox

Indications for Botox
Upper third of the face (frontalis, corrugator supercilli/procerus, orbicularis oculi muscle)
Middle third of the face (levator labii superiosis alaequenasi, nasalis)
Following cosmetic surgery
Abnormal muscle hypertrophy
In combination with other rejuvenating procedures (dermal fillers/soft tissue resurfacing)
Facial nerve disorders
Breast augmentation
Parotid gland fistula
Headaches

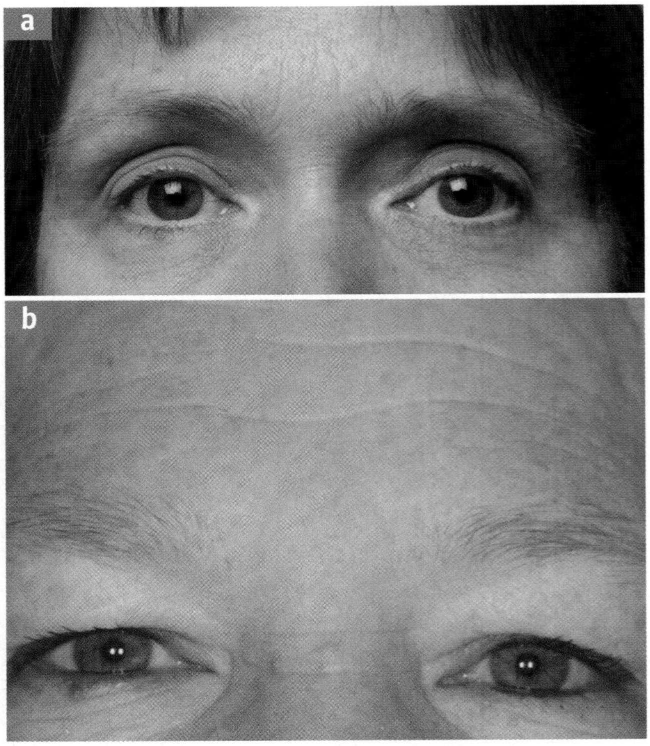

Figure 26–4 a) An appropriate candidate for forehead Botox; b) An inappropriate candidate for forehead Botox.

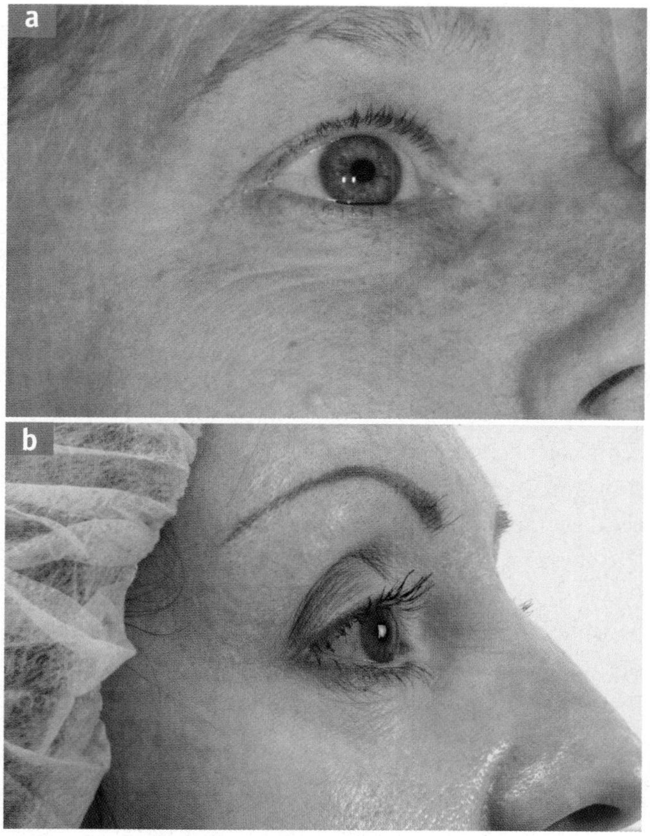

Figure 26–5 a) An appropriate candidate for crow's feet Botox; b) An inappropriate candidate for crow's feet Botox.

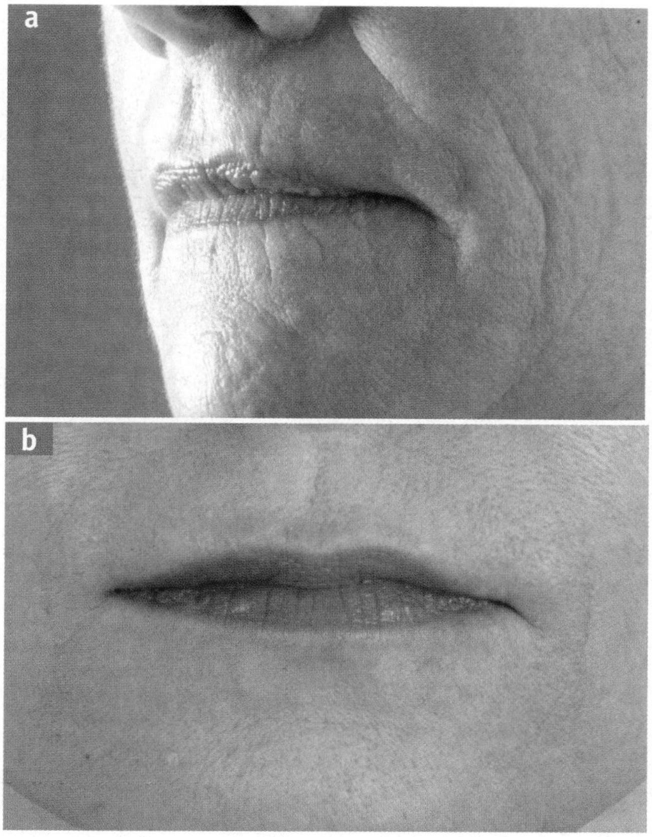

Figure 26–6 a) An appropriate candidate for vertical lip line Botox; b) An inappropriate candidate for vertical lip line Botox.

of the orbicularis oculi. When evaluating the lines around the eyes, look for the following indicators: depth of line, muscle activity, skin laxity under the eye, and visible blood vessels.

Marionette lines are those lines that extend from the corners of the mouth down toward the jawline. These lines are often associated with skin laxity in the upper face and often cannot be treated with Botox alone. However, Botox will assist the muscles in lifting up the corners of the mouth to improve the appearance. When evaluating this area, look for the amount of skin laxity, the degree of shadowing, and the amount of downturn in the corners of the mouth.

Vertical lip lines or smoker's lines plague most women by the time they are in their 50s. Lipstick seeps into these lines, allowing color to progress through the line. Moreover, they create a puckered look around the mouth. When evaluating this area for treatment, look for the intensity of the movement, the depth of the line, the length of the line, and the appearance of the line in a relaxed state (Figure 26–6a and b).

Many times the neck can give away a person's age. Treatment of the neck bands with Botox is an increasingly popular treatment that avoids surgery and improves the appearance of the neck almost overnight. When considering a client for treatment, evaluate the neck for vertical bands that are apparent in the resting position (Figure 26–7a and b). These bands may or may not be accompanied by horizontal rings, which are also appropriate for treatment.

Complications and Side Effects of Botox

Botox does not cross the **blood-brain barrier,** the mechanism in the brain capillaries that is selectively permeable. This unique feature keeps Botox at the site it is injected. Therefore, any side effects we discuss are limited to those effects at the muscle site. For example, poor placement of Botox in glabella treatment may cause eyelid ptosis. The side effects of Botox include eyelid ptosis, brow ptosis, overtreatment, or asymmetry after injection. The other, less common side effects include headaches, flu-like symptoms, and nausea.

There are more serious yet uncommon adverse reactions associated with the use of Botox in the treatment

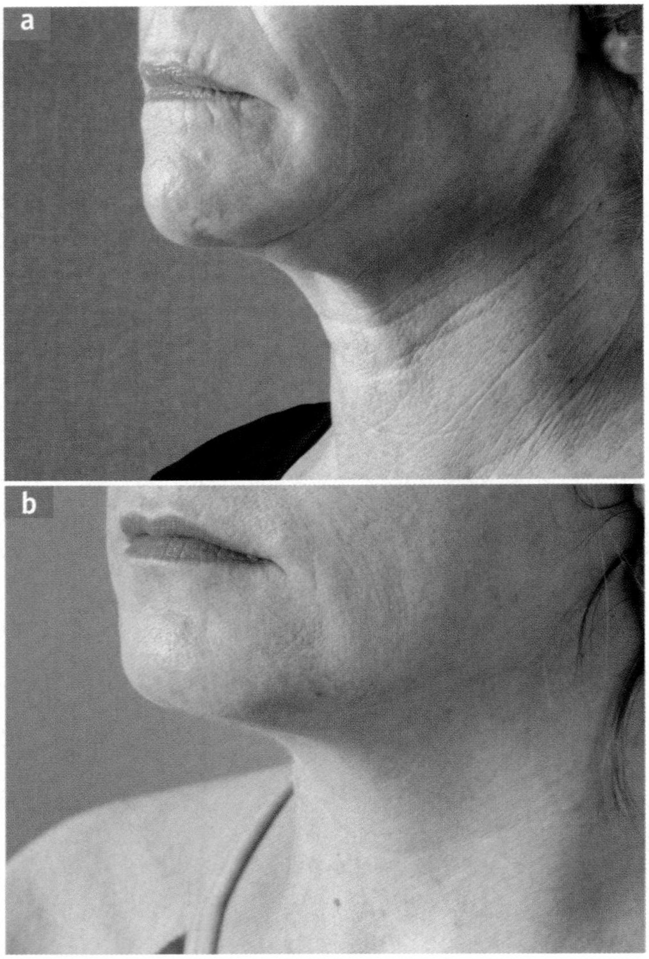

Figure 26–7 a) Appropriate candidate for neck ring and platysma band Botox; b) An inappropriate candidate for neck ring and platysma band Botox.

of cervical dystonia and blepharospasm. According to Allergan, the manufacturer of Botox, "The most frequently reported adverse reactions in clients with cervical dystonia are dysphagia (19%), upper respiratory infection (12%), neck pain (11%), and headache (11%)." The other more serious adverse events are associated with the treatment of blepharospasm and include ptosis (20.8%), superficial **punctate keratitis** (6.3%), and eye dryness (6.3%)."

Some clients experience another side effect of Botox: Their bodies develop protein antibodies, which neutralizes the Botox and renders it useless. This event is rare but it does occur. According to Allergan, about 1% to 2% of the Botox population will develop blocking antibodies. There are several hypotheses about the development of blocking antibodies, including frequency of treatment and the number of units used at each session. In these cases, you will need to help the client consider another treatment. However, those few people whose bodies resist Botox are not disqualified from treatment with other botulinum toxins, such as Myobloc®. In addition, the client may be treated with a dermal filler.

AN INTRODUCTION TO DERMAL FILLERS

With the general trend toward living longer, healthier lives, it is only natural that people want to look as good as they can for as many extra years as possible. However, as we get older and collagen production begins to decrease, the signs of aging become more and more pronounced. The face begins to sag, muscular activity shows in the form of wrinkles and lines, and sun damage becomes apparent. As the skin ages, it becomes lax and decreases in volume. This causes the facial asymmetry and proportion—markers for youth and beauty—to become less noticeable. While plastic surgery remains an option for many, some people consider it too extreme, too expensive, or too invasive. For these people, the perfect solution to reduce the signs of aging is the use of dermal fillers (Figure 26–8).

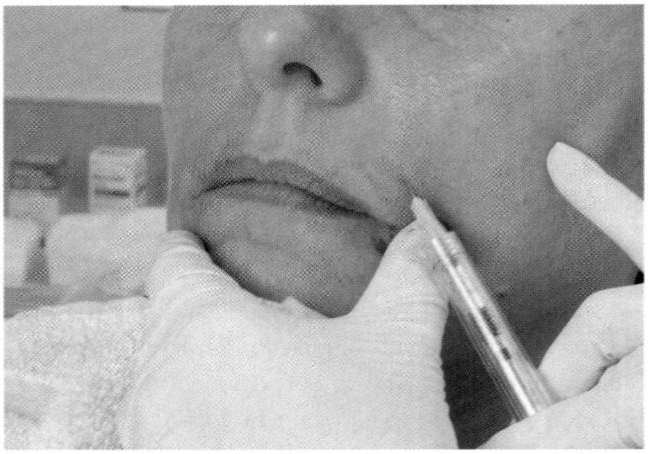

Figure 26–8 Client receiving a dermal filling treatment.

A perfect injectable material should have several qualities: It should be easy to place and forgiving in placement; it should be hypoallergenic, and it should have few, if any, risks, such as infections, bleeding, scarring, tissue reactions, and product migration. It should also be reasonably priced, durable with reproducible results, relatively painless to inject, and approved for use in the country in which you live. It is also important that the product be easy to wear, and produce minimal bruising, swelling, or irritation. While these requests seem reasonable, the perfect dermal filler simply does not exist, and with good reason. While some of the requirements are easy to solve, other issues, such as reproducible results, treatment consequences, or risks, are not as controllable, because the process of dermal filling is technique sensitive. That means that the result that is achieved with one injector may or may not be duplicated with another injector. In fact, duplicating the result from treatment to treatment with the same injector can be challenging.

Dermal fillers can be made of natural and synthetic materials. The natural products include bovine collagen (derived from cowhide), autologous collagen (derived from human sources), NASHA (Non-Animal Stabilized Hyaluronic Acid), **avian** hyaluronic acid (derived from birds), and calcium hydroxylapatite. The most common synthetic material is liquid silicone. All of these products improve the volume loss, correct facial asymmetries and proportions, smooth lines, and fill wrinkles. Each product has its advantages and will provide a better result in certain conditions, indications, or certain skin types.

Bovine Collagen

Bovine collagen is the product that began the craze known today as *dermal filling*. The original collagen was discovered in the 1970s and approved for use in 1981. It is a heterologous dermal filler, meaning that it is derived from a species other than humans. As the name implies, it is derived from cows—specifically, the hide. To harvest the product, the cowhides are broken down into their base elements, which include collagen. The collagen is then purified with elements that make it **nonimmunogenic,** meaning it won't produce an immunologic response. This will make it as neutral as possible for use as an injectable product. That said, allergies are possible, so skin testing prior to treatment is necessary.

In skin testing, a small amount of collagen is placed on the forearm (Figure 26–9). The waiting time for allergy analysis is 29 days, and treatment must not occur before that time. Many injectors feel is important to do two skin tests, since it is reported that at least 2% of the injected population will become allergic to the product once it is injected in the face. It is thought these allergies show up on the second exposure simply due to the additional allergen (bovine collagen) that is presented to the body (Figure 26–10).

Nevertheless, bovine collagen allergies are about 3% to 5% of the population, despite **cleaving** during the production process. A consequence of the cleaving of the collagen is that it renders it unstable. To this effect, the collagen breaks down rather quickly. As a general rule, bovine collagen lasts between 6 and 12 weeks. Indications for bovine collagen use include the treatment of lines and wrinkles (Figure 26–11), acne scars, lip augmentation (Figure 26–12), glabellar correction (Figure 26–13), and crow's feet (Figure 26–14).

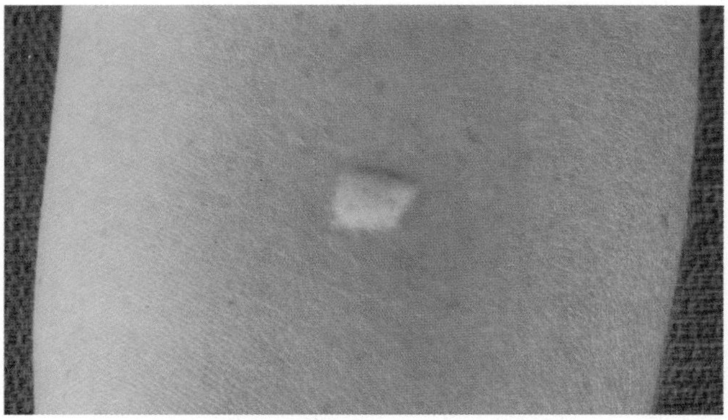

Figure 26–9 Skin test immediately after implantation.

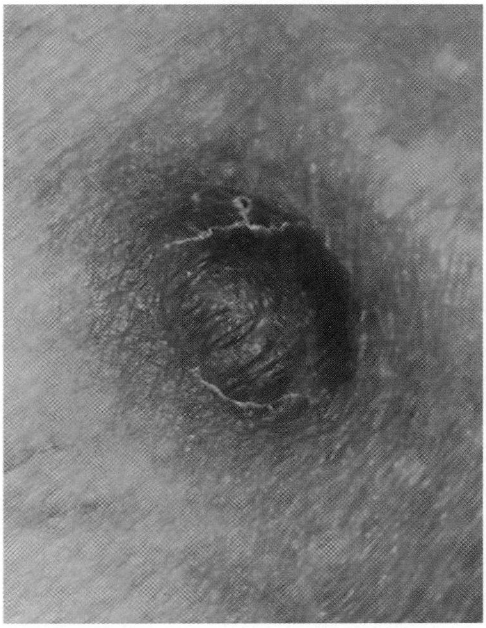

Figure 26–10 A positive collagen skin test.

Contraindications for bovine collagen treatments include an allergy to the product, a history of anaphylactic reactions of any sort, autoimmune diseases, those individuals undergoing desensitizing to beef products, pregnancy, and lactation.

There are three brand names for bovine collagen; Zyderm I®, Zyderm II®, and Zyplast® (Figure 26–15). Each product has a different weight of collagen and a

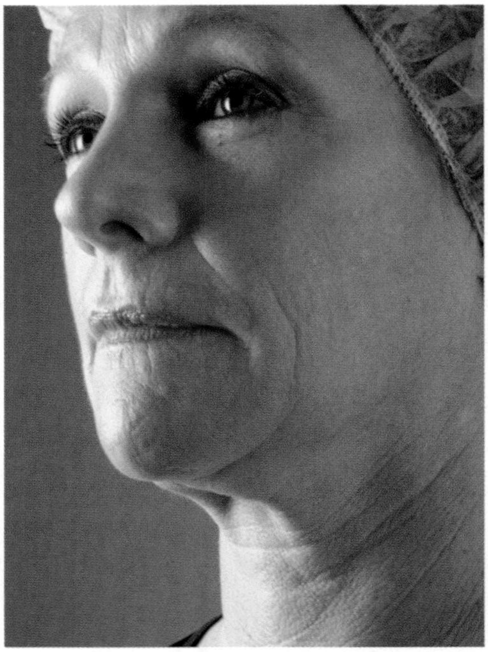

Figure 26–11 A candidate for line dermal filler.

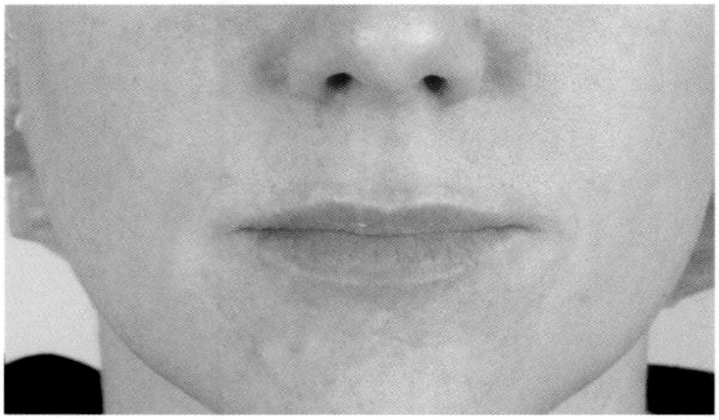

Figure 26–12 A candidate for lip augmentation.

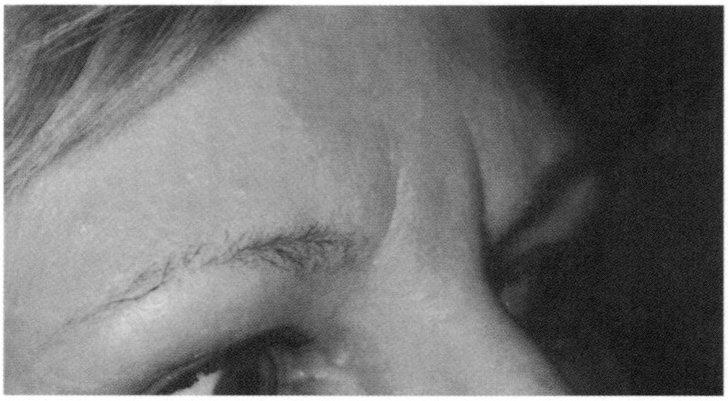

Figure 26–13 A candidate for glabella line correction.

specific purpose and indication (Figure 26–16a and b). All three types of bovine collagen must be refrigerated

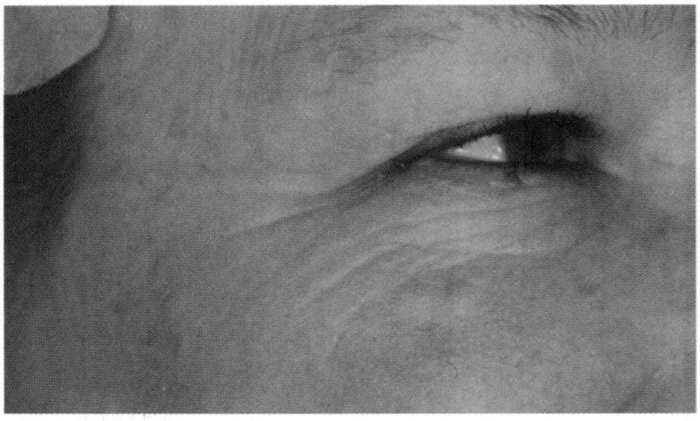

Figure 26–14 A candidate for crow's feet correction.

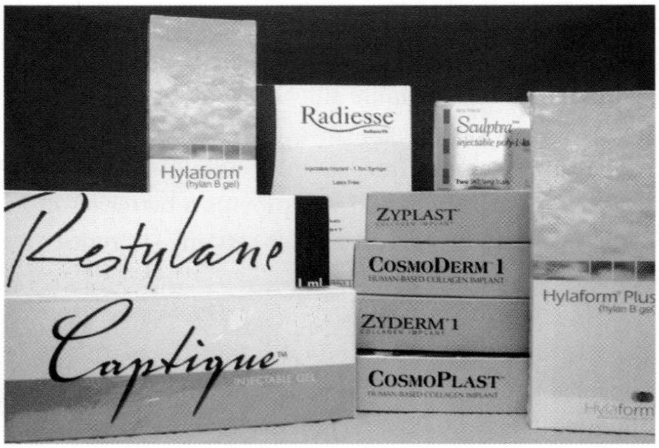

Figure 26–15 Dermal filler brands.

and should not be left out of the refrigerator overnight. All bovine are made by INAMED (formerly McGhan Medical Corporation), as are autologous collagen products, Cosmoderm® and Cosmoplast®.

Human Collagen

Human collagen is called **autologous,** meaning that it is derived from the same species in which it is used. The evolution of human collagen began as a result of the many allergies and short durability associated with bovine collagen. The need for a collagen-based dermal filler from human origins became increasingly apparent (Figures 26–17a and b and 26–18a and b). The most significant benefit of using autologous collagen is that it does not cause allergic reactions and as such does not require skin testing. That said, on rare occasions this substance has been known to cause hypersensitivities. These hypersensitivities have been traced to washes used to prepare the autologous collagen. Human collagen with trade names of Dermologen® and Cymetra® was originally derived from cadavers. While this seemed a good idea at the time

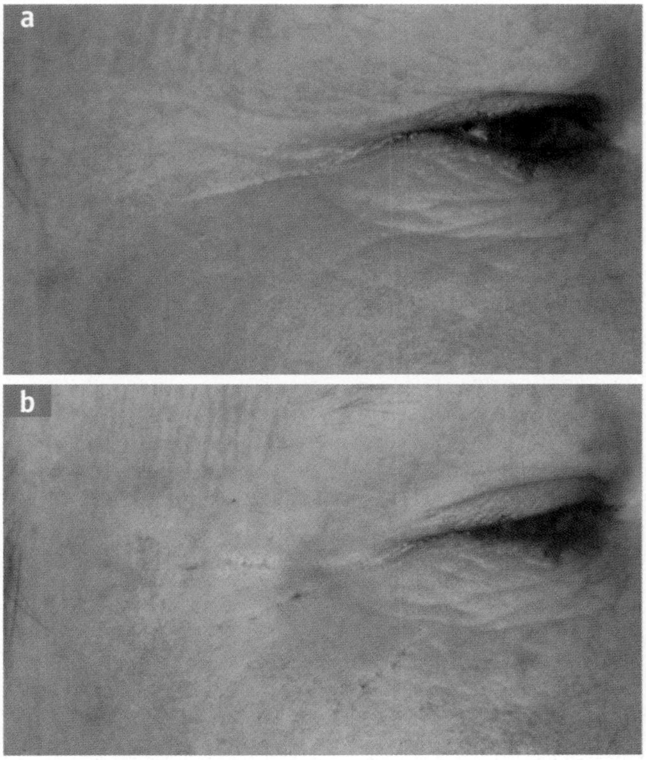

Figure 26–16 a) Before filler injected into the crow's feet and b) after.

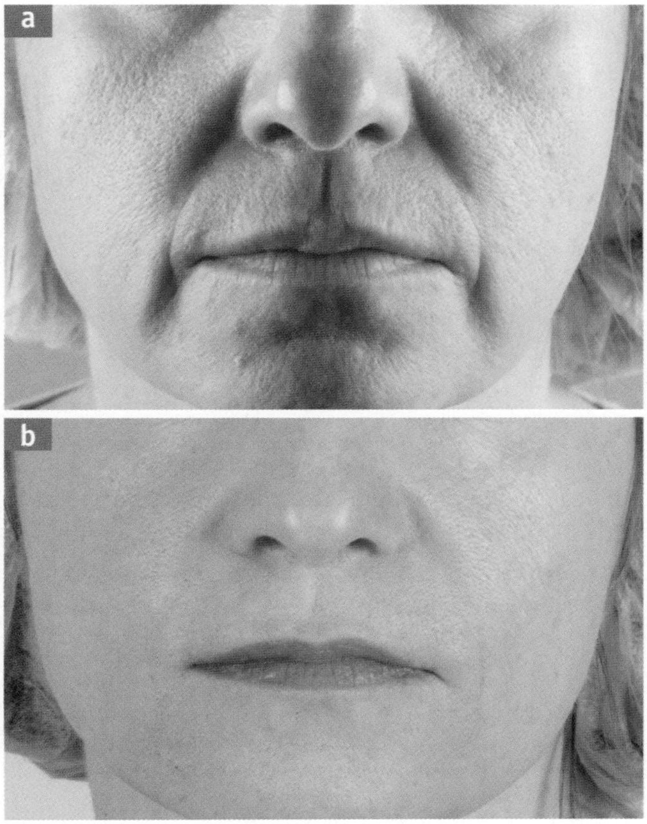

Figure 26–17 a) Before treatment of nasolabial folds and b) after.

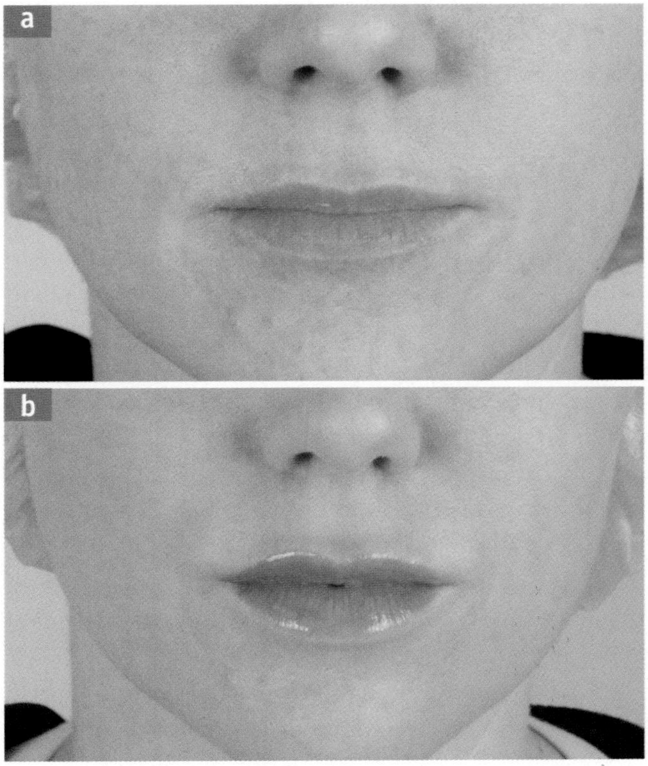

Figure 26–18 a) Before treatment of lip augmentation and b) after.

(cadaver cartilage is used routinely in some surgical procedures), the proliferation of AIDS and hepatitis C caused clients concern, and the popularity of this product waned.

Due to the difficulty of harvesting product and the potential for complications in the multistaged process for production, transportation, and delivery, the need for a more reliable form of autologous collagen still persisted. The result was two products, Cosmoderm® and Cosmoplast® (Figure 26–19). These products are manufactured from human collagen in a perfected laboratory setting.

Cosmoderm

Cosmoderm is 6.5% human dermal collagen by weight. It is suspended in a sodium chloride solution (normal saline) with lidocaine. It is injected into the shallow reticular dermis to treat deeper rhytides in the glabellar region, nasolabial folds, marionette lines, and oral commissures. It can also be used to treat acne scarring. Cosmoderm behaves much like Zyderm II and is used in similar applications.

Cosmoplast

Cosmoplast is less likely to degrade than either Cosmoderm or Zyderm II. It is 3.5% human collagen mixed with a

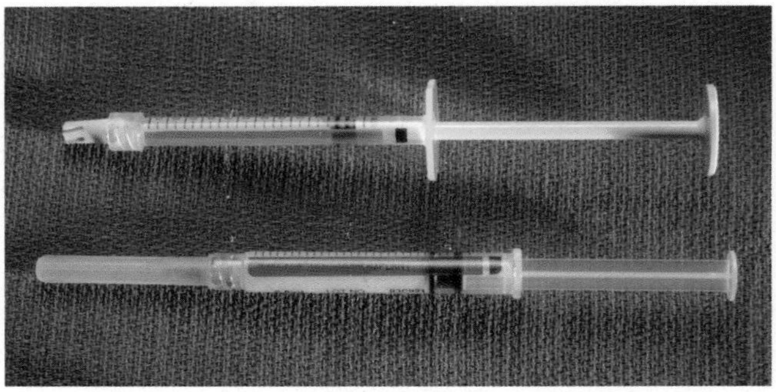

Figure 26–19 Dermal fillers in syringes.

compound, which creates a network that is more structurally sound, similar to the process used for Zyplast. Because it is more viscous, it is injected into the deep reticular dermis. It is used to treat coarser rhytides around the mouth and nasolabial regions. Cosmoplast should not be used in the glabellar region due to a risk of localized tissue **necrosis.** Like Zyplast, Cosmoplast has the ability to project the tissues better than Cosmoderm and therefore should be used in areas that require advanced projection, such as lips.

Hyaluronic Acid

Even as human bioengineered collagen seemed to address the issues of potential allergy risks, medical professionals and injection specialists still sought a dermal filler that could safely and effectively replace the volume of the skin and repair the defects caused over time. This research led to one of the most popular nonsurgical tools available today, **hyaluronic acid.**

Hyaluronic acid is a naturally occurring polysaccharide (sugar) found in every part of the body, and it is the main component of mammalian connective tissues. About 50% of hyaluronic acid found within the human body is housed in the skin. It is also plentiful in the fluid of the eyes as well as in joints, where it operates as a lubricant and a shock absorber. Hyaluronic acid's chemical makeup enables it to hold up to a thousand times its weight in water, making it a necessary component of the skin's natural moisturizing functions. For this reason, it is a highly desired addition to moisturizers and cosmetics. As an injectable product, it brings many of the necessary characteristics of the perfect dermal filler to the table, so it is quickly becoming the most widely used and preferred dermal filler on the market.

Also called *hylans,* the most common hyaluronic acid injectables we will examine are Hylaform®, Captique®, and Restylane®. While there are many others, these are FDA approved and are therefore more meaningful for those of us in the United States (Table 26–1). We will study the differences between the hylan materials using the differentiators of concentration, cross-linking, and source.

Table 26–1 Hylans Used as Dermal Fillers

NAME OF PRODUCT	FDA APPROVED	MANUFACTURER
Hylaform®	Yes	Inamed
Hylaform® Plus	Yes	Inamed
Captique®	Yes	Inamed
Restylane®	Yes	Q-Med
Restylane FINE LINE™ *hyaluronic acid*	No	Q-Med
Restylane PERLANE™ *hyaluronic acid*	No	Q-Med
Juvederm®	No	LEA Derm
Macrolane®	No	Q-Med
Dermalive®	No	Dermatech
DermaDeep®	No	Dermatech
Matridur®	No	Medical Aesthetic Supplies, Ltd.
Matridex®	No	Medical Aesthetic Supplies, Ltd.
Achal (1% sodium of hyaluronic acid)	No	Tedec Meiji Farma
Hylan Rofilan® Gel	No	Rofil Medical International
Viscontour®	No	Aventis Dermatology

FDA, U.S. Food and Drug Administration.

Other available hylans, such as Juvederm® and Perlane®, do not yet have FDA approval. In addition, be aware that there are several products that are composed of hyaluronic acid in combination with other products. These products include Hyacell®, a hyaluronic product that contains zinc, selenium, vanadium, and embryonic extracts; Dermalive® and DermaDeep®, which are acrylic hydrogel surrounded by hyaluronic acid; and Achal, which is a sodium of hyaluronic acid—so in the truest sense, is it not a hyaluronic acid.

Hylaform Gel

Hylaform Gel is described as an animal-based hyaluronic acid. The hyaluronic acid is "derived from rooster combs and other domestic fowl," but, while animal-based, it is significantly more stable than bovine collagen and has greater durability. Hylaform is also cross-linked with diveinyl sulfone. This cross-linking process helps to increase the stability of the hyaluronic acid and increase the durability of the product in the tissues. Hylaform is used widely as a filler for scars, diminishment of rhytides, and lip augmentation.

Those who are familiar with both bovine collagen and Hylaform report that it injects more smoothly, without risk of clumping. In studies, Hylaform showed a durability, or showed the best results, up to approximately five months after injection. After that time the product began to diminish and the correction faded. Initial treatment responses included the usual bruising, swelling, and erythema. Persistent erythema appeared in less than 2% of the tested population and resolved without long-term treatment. While Hylaform is derived from animal products, because hyaluronic acid is the same in all species, skin testing is not required.

Restylane

The FDA approved Restylane for soft tissue augmentation in 2003. It is one of the newest and most highly regarded of the dermal fillers on the market today. Restylane is a synthetic hyaluronic acid, meaning that it is man-made. It is synthesized from cultures of streptococcus equi. The product is then cross-linked with epoxides to stabilize it. Since this product does not use an animal source, it has been called **Non-animal Stabilized Hyaluronic Acid**, or **NASHA.** Because the product is non-animal in nature, it is believed that the human body recognizes the hyaluronic acid to the same degree it recognizes naturally occurring hyaluronic acid. In a clinical study with 158 Caucasian clients, it was noted that after eight months of treatment, 78% of the clients continued to have marked improvement in the treated areas. This may speak to the degradation process, which is termed *isovolemic,* or attracting water as it degrades. As with Hylaform, in studies, Restylane treatments had treatment responses of erythema, swelling, and bruising. It was noted in one Restylane study that persistent erythema in the first week after injection could be in response to exercise, sun exposure, and menstruation. It is believed this is related to the water-collecting properties of hyaluronic acid.

Restylane is popular for treatment to the nasolabial folds, lip augmentation, oral commissures, and marionette lines and to augment the result of Botox in the glabella. Recently Restylane has become a popular choice for improving the jawline and replacing volume in the face as well as treating the tear troughs under the eyes.

Complications and Side Effects of Dermal Fillers

Side effects and complications are unexpected yet known possibilities of a given treatment. They occur randomly and no one can predict which client will experience them. It is important to know how to handle these situations, both before they might happen and after they do.

Dermal Filler Side Effects

A side effect is not the result of a mistake, but side effects do happen. Effective management of side effects depends on the steps you take both prior to and at the earliest stages of recognition that a side effect has occurred. Familiarize yourself with the dermal filler process and become comfortable with the possible consequences associated with the treatment. Prepare your client by informing him or her of these side effects, and have the client sign off on a consent form. If the client is aware of the possibility of side effects, he or she will be much less likely to become upset or dissatisfied should they occur.

If side effects do occur, a client will seek your reassurance that the treatment consequences are normal and expected. He or she may also want input about how long it will take for the result to become apparent and for the bruising, swelling, and erythema to dissipate. Your response should be helpful and reassuring, but appropriate. Do not extend yourself outside your area of expertise. Your demeanor and your mastery of the knowledge will create trust between you and the client.

Dermal Filler Complications

Similarly, while the possibility of a **complication** is real, the likelihood is rare and can be minimized by taking proactive steps during the consultation, treatment, and determination that a complication has occurred. Overall, your job is to support the client, but it is in your best interest to avoid speaking poorly of the physician or injector. If you venture an opinion that does not support the situation or is not fully knowledgeable, it can be damaging for all parties involved. Your support and understanding can improve the client's attitude and can help to create productive communication between injector and client.

Communication is the key to successful damage control. First, it is of great importance that you inform the client of the risks and the client has signed a consent form prior to the procedure. Second, know the processes that ought to be in place in the event of a complication. Know whom to ask for help in your place of employment, or, if you are an independent technician, refer the client

FYI

Never give medical advice. If you think a client has a possible problem or needs more detailed information, recommend that he or she seek proper medical attention.

back to the attending physician. Never attempt to correct a medical condition on your own. Being compassionate and sympathetic to the client's feelings at this time is the most important thing you can do.

Combining Botox and Dermal Fillers

Upper lip lines can be a bit tricky to treat. Those that are deeper require a thicker material buried in the reticular dermis layered with a lighter material to solve the fine lines that remain (Figure 26–20). One unfortunate problem is that the upper lip can be easily overcorrected, making it appear fat or unnaturally large. While the lines may be gone, the client now has an altered facial shape with an unruly-sized upper lip—which is a rather large price to pay. Therefore, when consulting with the client about the treatment, explain that the treatment will not make the lip lines go away. In fact, a 50% improvement is likely, which should be considered a superior result. On the initial visit, the injector corrects no more than 50%. When the dermal filling is complete, the injector adds six to eight units of Botox around the upper and lower lips (Figure 26–21). This is spaced evenly to provide a symmetrical aesthetic result. This technique provides a weakening to the orbicularis oris without a paralysis, which, of course, is not the goal. The dermal filler will hold for approximately four to six months (depending on the product used); the Botox will hold for two to three months. The client should return in a month for additional dermal filling to top off the result and ensure the best results.

Crow's feet are often solved with the use of Botox alone; however, those clients with significant volume loss are not completely satisfied with Botox alone. These clients usually have very lax, sun-damaged skin. Additional treatment with a dermal filler in the deeper crow's feet provides a superior result with a durability that will make the client happy. Caution the client that the thin nature of the skin surrounding the eyelids will make lumping and bumping more obvious. The skin may also be transparent enough to show the dermal filler. Therefore, the injector must take care in volume and placement.

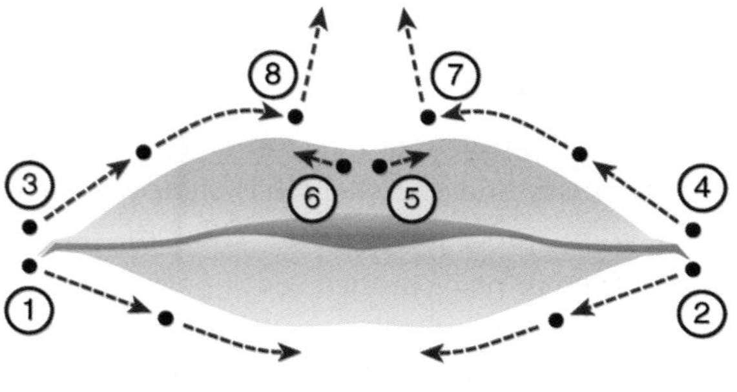

Figure 26–20 Placement of the dermal filler for the upper lip.

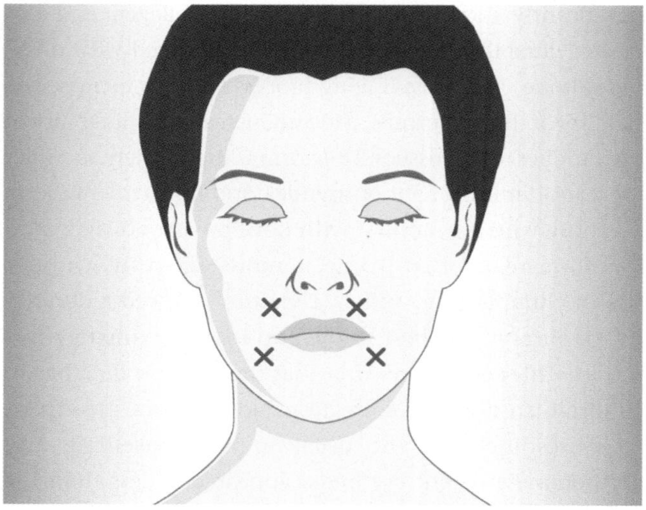

Figure 26–21 Placement of the Botox after dermal filling.

Before the introduction of Botox, glabella treatment with a dermal filler was the treatment of choice. However, there are many times that a glabella will simply not respond completely without the use of a dermal filler. Carefully filling the lines of the glabella and augmenting the treatment with Botox will provide an improved result for those clients with years of glabellar motion (Figure 26–22a and b).

AN INTRODUCTION TO SCLEROTHERAPY

Dilated blood vessels, also known as **varicose veins**, are a problem for many people. They appear as red, blue, or purple veins through the skin's surface, most often on the lower extremities (Figure 26–23). As we age, these can also be found on the hands. These are a result of the failure of valves within the veins. Most often varicose veins—and especially spider veins—are relatively harmless, even if they are unsightly.

Causes of Problem Veins

There have been many studies into the root causes of varicose veins. The results have been as varied as they have been inconclusive. However, there are several generalities

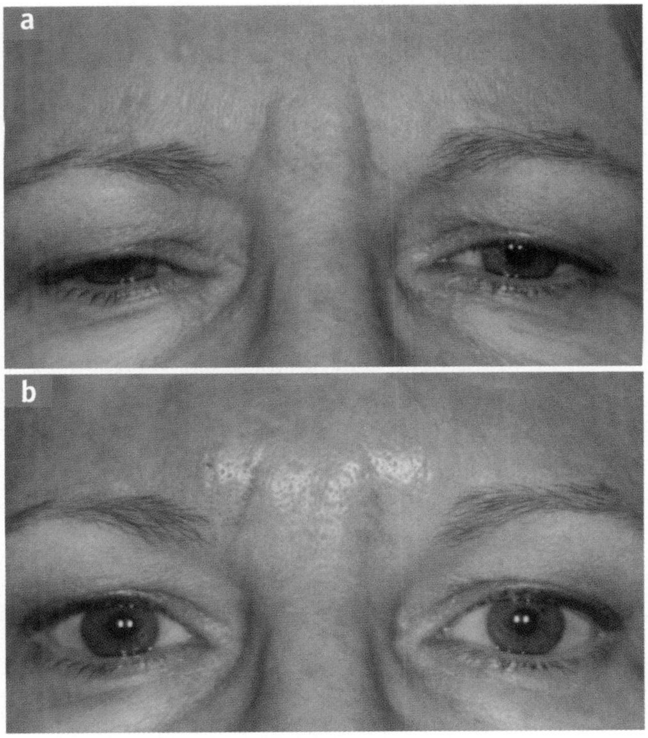

Figure 26–22 a) Client before the addition of Hylaform and after treatment with Botox and b) Client after the addition of Hylaform and Botox.

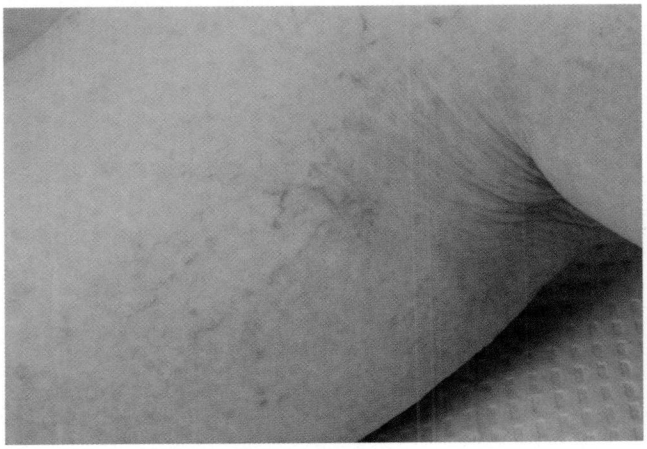

Figure 26–23 Varicose veins.

that most people will agree increase certain people's chances of having varicose veins.

The first of these is gender. Most studies have found that women are about twice as likely to have varicose veins than men. This may be linked to women's high-heeled shoes, leg crossing, or hormonal changes resulting from menstruation or pregnancy.

Geography is the second major consideration. A host of studies have concluded that varicose veins are significantly less common in non-Western countries. This may be due in part to longer periods of time spent standing or more sedentary lifestyles. While there are no conclusive results about why geography is a factor, the more stressful, fast-paced lifestyle of many countries in the West may have a lot to do with it.

The next reason is almost universally understood to be true. Age has a lot to do with the appearance of varicose veins. The longer the veins have been pumping blood, the more likely they are to fail. Natural wear and tear, especially in the light of other variables, increases the likelihood of varicose veins.

Another factor is weight. Physiologically, it makes sense that the more weight a person carries, the more likely the venous return system will be compromised. Obese people, particularly women, have a greater instance of intense varicosities; however, studies have not made a direct link.

The final variable that might cause an individual to have varicose veins is genetics. While this may increase the likelihood, like weight, there is no conclusive evidence.

Vein Therapy

Vein therapy, more commonly known as *sclerotherapy*, might be familiar to you, because you are already developing those small spider veins on your legs (Figure 26–24). But the disease is more complicated than a few spider veins. Some women have pain and larger vessels associated with the disease. Because this disease is so common (more than 50% of women have this problem in some form), you should know about varicose veins and the options for treatment.

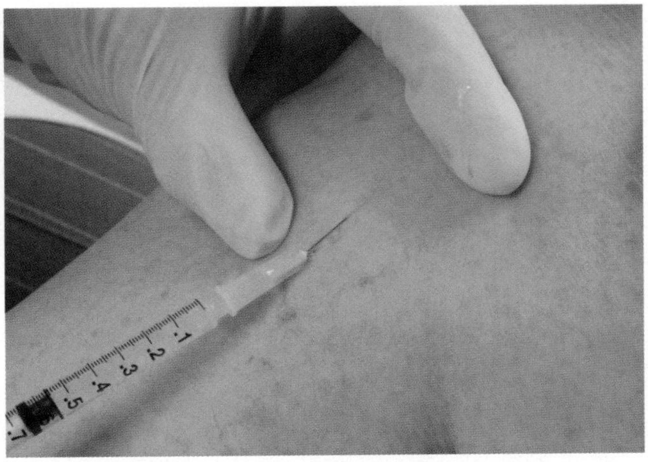

Figure 26–24 Sclerotherapy of spider veins.

The Esthetician's Role in Sclerotherapy

The esthetician's role in vein therapy will most likely be limited to answering client questions about the possibilities for treatment and the treatment process itself. The answers to these questions should be general and accurate but should not constitute medical advice.

A client's most common question about vein therapy is "Can this leg/vein be treated?" The treatment is, of course, like all treatments: It is based on indications and contraindications. Therefore, there are certain people who will be disqualified from treatment: Clients with HIV, AIDS, diabetes, bloodborne diseases, circulatory problems, anticoagulation therapy, and heart disease may not be candidates for the treatment. Additionally, veins that are varicosed from the groin to the knee or all the way to the ankle may warrant a surgical procedure rather than injection therapy. However, the large majority of women with spider veins can be treated successfully with injection sclerotherapy. Recommend that your clients find a reputable and experienced physician or nurse injector to provide the treatment. Being able to refer clients to practitioners for certain conditions makes you a valuable and trusted asset to the client; therefore, it is a good idea to keep a list of practitioners you trust. It would also be helpful for you to prepare the client in simple terms about the commitments of sclerotherapy. This preparation will help him or her to be a more qualified candidate for the physician. Client preparation includes post-care (information you can obtain from the referring physician) but generally includes wearing support stockings, avoiding the sun for several weeks, and adjusting the exercise program to avoid bumping the treated area.

The second question that the client will ask is "Does it hurt?" This question is a bit trickier to answer, because the pain factor is directly related to the solution that is used to treat the blood vessel. Be aware of the different solutions that are available and be able to educate clients about the pain factor during treatment. The general answer, however, is that the treatment can sometimes be uncomfortable, but it is not terribly painful.

Finally, people often want to know what you have had done. If you have had the treatment, whether it is sclerotherapy, Botox, or dermal fillers, you bring safety and authority to the situation. However, your experience may not be the experience that the client will have, so be careful in describing your treatment or post-treatment course as if it is the standard. If you use your experience, be sure you state it as such: This is how it was for me or this is what happened to me. This way you do not create an uncomfortable situation if the client's situation is not exactly the same.

> **Here's a Tip**
>
> If you have had procedures done and you share that information with your clients, be sure to add that results may vary from client to client. Then they will not expect their results to match yours.

AN INTRODUCTION TO MEDICAL PEELS

Chemical peels, which appeal to young and old alike, are treatments using agents that peel layer(s) of skin, refining the skin and allowing newer and healthier skin to present itself. Chemical peels are the preferred treatment for many signs of aging, including variations in skin color, called **dyschromias** and fine lines. A peel can be an individual procedure or a single step in a multifaceted treatment. There are a number of different types of peels and different peel depths. Generally the results of a peel can be flaky skin, redness, and edema, and there is a heightened risk of scarring. Some deeper peels can cause serious injury. Medical peels offer heightened levels of success, but also the greatest potential for consequences, because the acids used by physicians are more intense in action than the peels used by estheticians.

> **FYI**
>
> There are four levels of peeling: very superficial, superficial, moderate, and deep.

> **Here's a Tip**
>
> Chemical peeling is basically an accelerated exfoliation induced by a chemical agent. Superficial peeling agents cause increased slough of the stratum corneum, and deeper peels cause necrosis and inflammation in the epidermis, papillary dermis, or reticular dermis.

> **REGULATORY AGENCY ALERT**
>
> Know your state guidelines on the usage of chemical peels. There is a wide variation of regulation from state to state.

Types of Peeling Agents

There are many different types of peeling agents. Among the most familiar are glycolic acid, Jessner solution, salicylic acid, trichloroacetic (TCA), and phenol. Each has a specific purpose and each has advantages and disadvantages as a peeling agent. Additionally, each is technique-sensitive, meaning that the end result depends on the knowledge and skill of the technician using it. The more experienced the technician, the better he or she is at the process of the treatment and thus the end result for the client.

Glycolic and Lactic Acids

Glycolic or lactic acid as peeling agents, come in three basic strengths (although the percentages can be varied): 30%, 50%, and 70%. For medical use usually the solution is a pH of 2 or less and higher percentages are used. Glycolic or lactic acids are indicated for photodamage presenting as dyschromia, fine lines, and rough textures. They are also used for acne treatments.

These peels are light (though they can be deeper under certain circumstances), safe, nontoxic, and generally have very few complications. Since the rise in popularity of microdermabrasion, glycolic or lactic peels have become less popular. This is unfortunate because these peels have a specific and useful place in treating skin superficially, even though they have very specific follow-up care procedures.

Jessner Peel

Jessner peel solution is a combination of three different acids—14% salicylic, 14% resorcinol, and 14% lactic—in an ethanol base. There are often attempts to increase the percentages of the salicylic acid in this solution to increase its efficacy in treating acne, but any increase in the salicylic acid will lead to clumping and debris in the solution. Therefore, it is best to stick with what is known as 14%/14%/14% to avoid the peel solution separating. Jessner solution provides a superficial peel, focusing on exfoliating and digestion of the debris associated with acne. Jessner solution is also frequently used in combination with other acids, usually TCA, to potentate the result.

Salicylic Acid (Beta) Peel

Salicylic acid is an beta hydroxyl acid found in willow bark, though it is manufactured chemically from sodium phenolate. The salicylic acid, or "beta peel," comes in strengths from 12.5% to 30%. This peel is most effective for the treatment of acne and should be directed accordingly.

> **★ REGULATORY AGENCY ALERT**
>
> When using Jessner's solution, make sure that the solution matches what is allowed by your state and is suitable for your client. Failure to do so could result in a lawsuit.

Salicylic acid is also found in some medical offices as a 50% paste and is used for the treatment of sun damage on the extremities. This is a very specialized peeling process and should be left to the physician for two reasons: the use of an unfamiliar peeling paste and the potential for salicylate toxicity. While it is unlikely that you will be faced with salicylate toxicity, it is still important to understand the symptoms: headache, dizziness, vomiting, and **tinnitus** (ringing in the ears). Avoid the possibility by limiting the area to be treated at one time: Do the face, the arms, or the back, but never multiple areas unless directed to do so by your supervising medical professional.

Trichloroacetic Acid

Trichloroacetic acid, or TCA, is a common peeling agent in the medical spa. It comes in a variety of strengths, usually increasing incrementally by 5% points, for example, 10%, 15%, 20%, 25%, and so on. It has many benefits, including that it is nontoxic, stable, easy to use, and able to create a variety of results (Figures 26–25 and 26–26). The most commonly recognized TCA peel is the Obagi Blue Peel, which usually utilizes 30% TCA. TCA penetrates to the papillary dermis or the upper reticular dermis when a full frost is achieved (Figure 26–27). The frost is the result of the chemical (TCA) coagulating the protein in the skin. When the chemical is applied to the skin, it acts as a **cautery** in coagulating the protein. Overall, TCA is an easy-to-use, predictable, medium-depth peel in the hands of a properly trained professional.

Designer Peels

The definition for designer peel may seem to be whatever the spa is marketing. In reality, the term *designer peel* has a specific definition and indication. Designer peels are a combination of multiple solutions, usually herbal and homeopathic substances, such as azelaic acid, lactic acid, mulberry root,

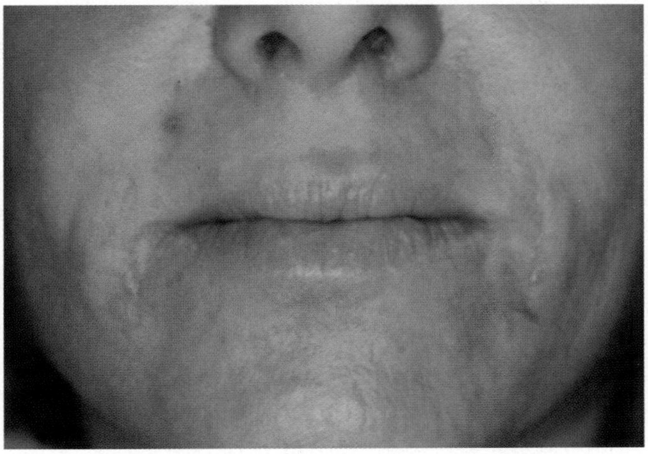

Figure 26–25 Client before a TCA Peel.

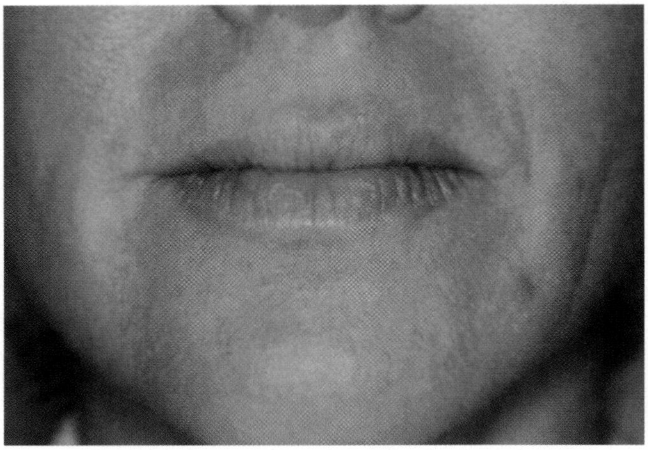

Figure 26–26 Client healed after a TCA peel.

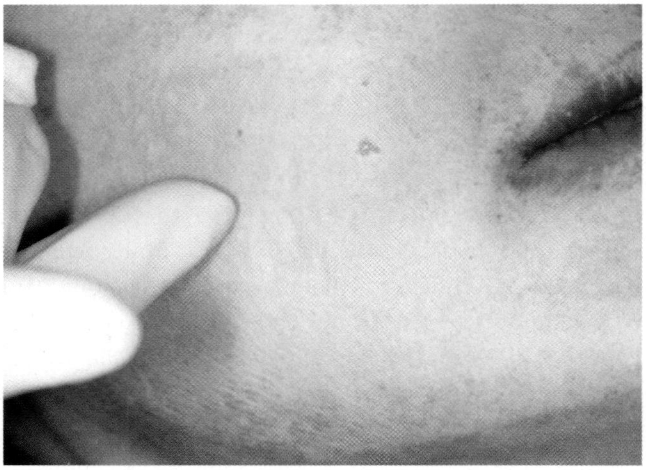

Figure 26–27 TCA frost.

bearberry, echinacea, and gotu kola, azelea, lavender, licorice or kojic acid. these peels are often used in conjunction with microdermabrasion treatments. These ingredients alone will have minimal efficacy alone; the result is often therapeutic. If this is the goal of your client, then their use is warranted. For more aggressive treatments, they are best used in conjunction with stronger peeling agents, like AHAs.

Other Solutions

Other peeling solutions that are important to note include phenol or pyruvic acid. The most commonly used deep-peeling agent is the Baker-Gordon, or B.G., solution. This is a combination of phenol, Septisol, and croton oil. This combination results in a 45% to 55% concentration of phenol. This peel penetrates to the reticular dermis, and, as with TCA, coagulates with the proteins in the skin and gives a frost. The Baker-Gordon phenol peel is used for deeper lines and aged skin. It always (except in a rare case) leaves the skin with too little pigment, a condition known as hypopigmentation.

Pyruvic acid, a keto-acid, is less often used, and there is less documented evidence on its importance as a peeling agent. Ask for clinical evidence supporting its use and performance before incorporating it into your program (Table 26–2).

Benefits of Medical Peels

Every day, human skin undergoes the normal process of sloughing older dead skin cells. In their place, newer cells have traveled up through the layers of skin. Chemical peels accelerate this process in three different manners. First, resurfacing the stratum corneum stimulates epidermal growth. This makes the epidermis thicken. Second, chemical peels cause necrosis, or destruction of damaged skin. Ideally, the damaged or dyschromatic skin will be replaced with healthier, normalized tissue by means of the skin's wound healing processes. Deeper peels induce the production of new collagen and ground substance within the dermis. This occurs as an inflammatory response to wounding deeper basal layer and papillary dermis tissue.

Contraindications for peels include sunburns, open lesions (such as a cold sore), a rash of any kind, or an infection on the face.

Table 26–2 Peeling Agents

TREATMENT	THESE TREATMENTS:	THESE TREATMENTS DO NOT:
Trichloracetic Acid Peels	• Flatten scarring • Reduce rhytides • Correct photodamage • Improve hyperpigmentation	• Reduce pore size • Eradicate all rhytides • Remove telangiectasia • Remove deep scarring
Jessner's Solution and Glycolic and Lactic Acid Peels	• Reduce rhytides • Correct photodamage • Improve hyperpigmentation	• Reduce pore size • Eradicate all rhytides • Remove telangiectasia • Remove deep scarring

Contraindications, Complications, and Side Effects of Medical Peels

Contraindications for medical peels are usually quite obvious but warrant discussion. Among the contraindications for peeling are excessive telangiectasia, infections, rashes, open lesions, and sunburns. Also, a client who has just had a facelift or eyelid lift is not a candidate for skin peeling. Finally, the client who has been on Accutane in the last year is not a candidate for facial peeling.

Common side effects include redness, burning, and itching. These side effects are usually short-lived and bearable. Downtime will depend on the peel depth.

Peel complications are more severe, and often to the detriment to the client. Chemical peel complications can range from minor irritations to permanent scarring. In very rare cases, chemical peel complications can be life-threatening. The strength of chemicals used increases the risk of chemical peel complications; the phenol chemical peels, for instance, have a very high risk of serious chemical peel complications, due to the strong acids involved. Clients who undergo a peel treatment ought to be concerned about severe burns, infection, scarring, and allergic reaction.

As an esthetician, there is only so much you can do to manage the effects of aging and other skin conditions on your clients. Sometimes, medical resources need to be incorporated. Aside from deeply invasive procedures, medical intervention involving injectable therapies, such as Botox; dermal fillers; peels; or sclerotherapy may be beneficial to meet a client's goals. While a qualified medical professional must perform these procedures, it will be you that recommends, counsels, and often arranges a procedure for a client. Thus, knowing the subtle nuances of these procedures as well as their indications will not only make you more qualified to talk about these medical interventions, but it will help you gain the client's trust and respect, which you can only acquire by acting in a client's best interest.

REVIEW QUESTIONS

1. Explain what medical intervention is. How is it different from the treatments that are normally performed in a spa setting?
2. What reasons might a client consider medical interventions that are beyond normal esthetic treatments?
3. Are estheticians qualified to perform these procedures? If not, who is?
4. Why is it important for an esthetician to be familiar with medical intervention treatments?
5. What are some of the common questions a client might have about medical intervention procedures? How would you answer these questions?
6. What is Botox indicated for?
7. How long will Botox last? What considerations will affect the durability?
8. What are the possible complications and side effects of Botox?
9. What are dermal fillers and what are they used for?
10. What is the durability of Bovine collagen?
11. Identify the different types of dermal fillers. What would determine if one might be better for a particular client than another?

REVIEW QUESTIONS

12. What are some of the side effects of dermal fillers? Why is allergy testing necessary?
13. Why might someone consider combining Botox and dermal fillers?
14. What is sclerotherapy?
15. What are the four levels of peel depth?
16. How do chemical peels make the skin appear younger and fresher?
17. What are the main peel agents? What are their peel depths?
18. What are peels contraindicated for?

CHAPTER GLOSSARY

autologous: derived from the same species of which it is implanted.

avian: pertaining to birds.

blepharospasm: spastic movement of the orbicularis oculis; usually a result of frequent and prolonged eye strain.

blood-brain barrier: mechanism that alters the permeability of brain capillaries, so that some substances, such as certain drugs, are prevented from entering brain tissue, while other substances are allowed to enter freely.

botulinum toxin: bacterium from which Botox is derived.

bovine collagen: heterologous collagen which is derived from the skin of cows.

cautery: an agent or instrument used to destroy abnormal tissue by burning.

cervical dystonia: prolonged, repetitive muscle contractions that may cause twisting or jerking movements of the of the neck.

cleaving: to split a complex molecule into a simpler molecule.

complications: any unwanted and unexpected consequences of performing a treatment.

dynamic movement: movement caused by active movement of muscles and nerve impulses.

dyschromias: abnormal display of facial hyperpigmentation due to solar damage.

glabella: the point above the nose between the eyes, often subject to dynamic movement.

hyaluronic acid: a glycosaminoglycan that has no protein component that can hold up to 400 times its own weight in water. A hydrating fluid found in the skin; hydrophilic agent with water-binding properties. Also known as *sodium hygluronat.*

nasolabial lines: dynamic wrinkles that connect the nose to the mouth.

necrosis: cell or tissue death.

NASHA: Non-animal Stabilized Hyaluronic Acid.

nonimmunogenic: unlikely to cause a hypersensitive or antigenic reaction.

platysmal bands: bands aroung the neck which are a result of dynamic movement of the neck and jaw.

ptosis: drooping of the eyelids.

punctate keratitis: calluses resulting from prolonged and frequent exposure to friction.

sclerotherapy: injection into a vein of a chemical irritant that causes fibrosis and, later, elimination of the lumen, to treat varicose veins, hemorrhoids, or esophageal varices.

strabismus: eye disorder in which the optic axes in either eye can not focus on the same object.

tinnitus: ringing in the cars.

varicose veins: condition characterized by incompetent valves in the veins, most commonly in the legs.

CHAPTER 27

PLASTIC SURGERY PROCEDURES

CHAPTER OUTLINE

- FACE-LIFT (RHYTIDECTOMY)
- FOREHEAD-LIFT (BROW-LIFT)
- EYE LIFT (BLEPHAROPLASTY)
- NOSE JOB (RHINOPLASTY)
- FACIAL IMPLANTS
- BREAST IMPLANTS (AUGMENTATION MAMMAPLASTY)
- BREAST-LIFT (MASTOPEXY)
- BREAST REDUCTION (REDUCTION MAMMAPLASTY)
- BREAST RECONSTRUCTION
- TUMMY TUCK (ABDOMINOPLASTY)
- LIPOSUCTION (SUCTION-ASSISTED LIPOPLASTY)

LEARNING OBJECTIVES

After completing this chapter, you should be able to:

- Demonstrate a basic working knowledge of common plastic surgery procedures.
- Explain procedures to clients and answer basic questions about those procedures.
- Interact with medical professionals and understand client needs about those procedures.

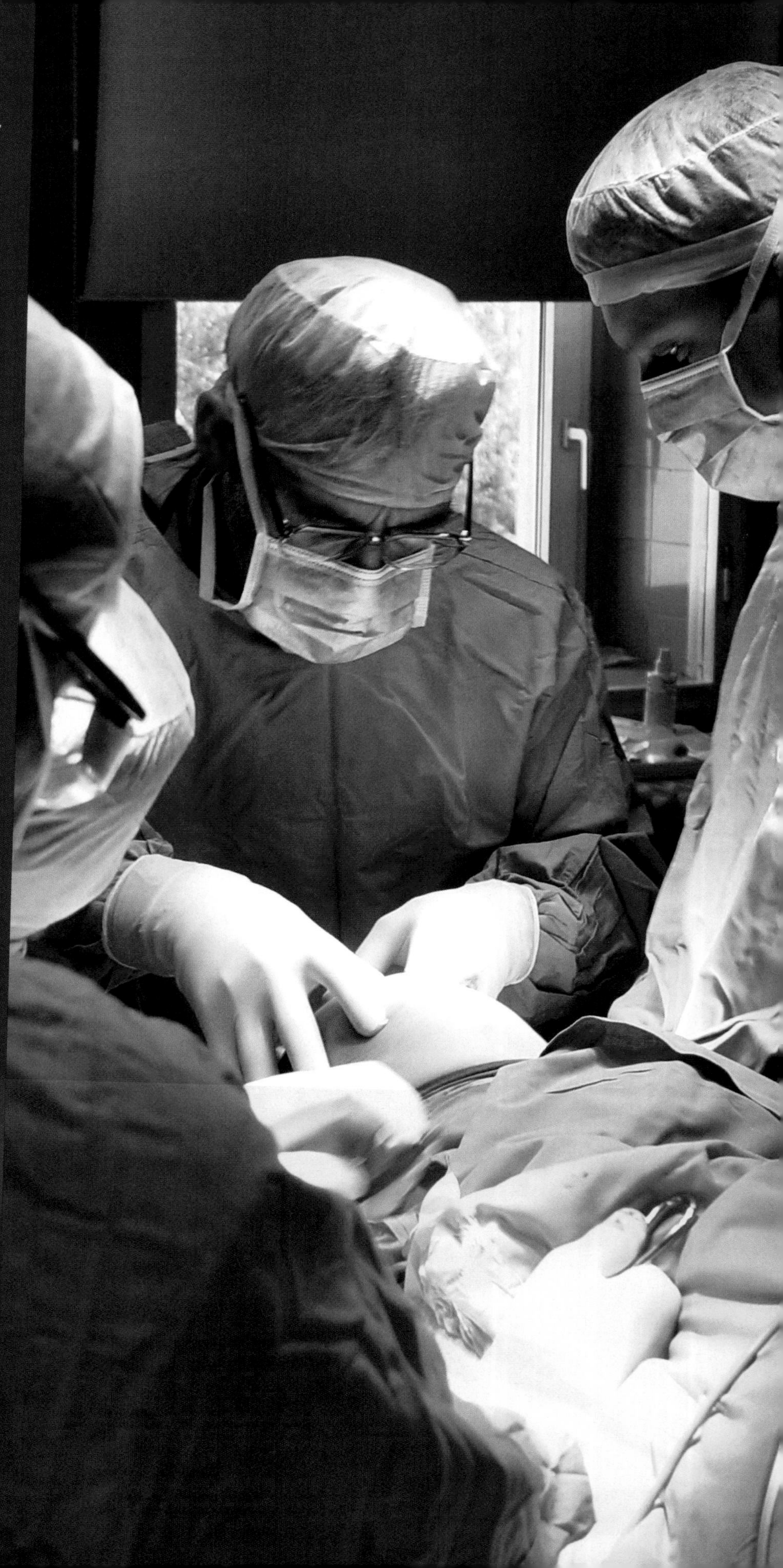

KEY TERMS

Page numbers indicate where in the chapter the term is used.

abdominoplasty 727
areolas 723
bariatric surgery 727
blepharoplasty 713
breast implants 725
circumareolar 722
classic forehead-lift 714
closed rhinoplasty 718
conjunctiva 716
deviated nasal septum 717
dorsum 719
electrocautery 716
endonasal 718
endoscopic 714
fascia 727
Graves' disease 716
inframammary crease 722
liposuction 728
mammaplasty 720
mastectomy 724
mastopexy 722
mentoplasty 718
nasal turbinates 717
nasolabial folds 712
open rhinoplasty 718
pendulous breasts 723
periorbital fat 716
photophobia 717
reconstructive rhinoplasty 717
rhinoplasty 717
rhytidectomy 712
striae distensae 727
submental 712
superficial musculoaponeurotic system (SMAS) 713
synthetic 718
thread lift 713

With more than 78 million "baby boomers" in the United States and more than 10,000 people per day turning 50, it is no surprise that more cosmetic plastic surgery procedures are being performed. This generation and their successors are living longer; have, overall, a higher disposable income than other generations; and, possibly because of their lifelong exposure to beauty as depicted in television and movies, are less tolerant of the signs of aging. Consequently, they seek qualified professionals to help them look and feel younger. Often an esthetician is their first contact in this search. While it is not an esthetician's role to convince or dissuade any client about a surgical procedure, it is important to be familiar with the alternatives available to a client and the most common surgical methods of intervention.

FOCUS ON: *Anesthesia*

Physicians have a variety of anesthetic techniques to choose from for any particular procedure. Patients whose surgery is done under local anesthesia with intravenous (IV) sedation will be awake but relaxed. Although they may not feel any pain, these patients may feel some tugging and occasional discomfort. Patients who have surgery while under general anesthesia will sleep during their procedures. The patient's health, the extent of the procedure, and physician and client preferences dictate the method used.

FACE-LIFT (RHYTIDECTOMY)

One of the most popular and satisfying cosmetic surgical procedures today is the face-lift. The medical term for a face-lift is **rhytidectomy**; it is derived from the Latin words *rhytid* (wrinkle) and *ectomy* (to remove). Although the incisions for a face-lift extend up into the hairline, the procedure does virtually nothing to the upper part of the face. Thus, a face-lift is often combined with a forehead-lift, eyelid surgery, and/or facial liposuction. Concurrent with a face-lift, "skin resurfacing" can be used to fine-tune the facial skin (e.g., a chemical peel, dermabrasion, or laser resurfacing). Rhytidectomy and skin resurfacing complement each other, but one is not a substitute for the other. Resurfacing best treats superficial lines and wrinkles, pigmentation, and irregularities.

Indications

Rhytidectomy is the most effective in eliminating loose skin and deep wrinkles in the lower third of the face and neck areas; it can give definition to the jawline (jowls) and remedy **nasolabial folds**, the creases or lines that run from the corner of the nose to the corner of the mouth. It can also eliminate vertical "cords" in the neck that are caused by prominent medial borders of the platysma muscle. Fatty neck tissue can also be remedied during a face-lift with liposuction or sharp resection of the **submental** fat pad. Submental is the area within the triangular margins of the mandible where the double chin resides, below the mentalis. Most face-lifts are done on patients in their 40s to 60s, but a physician may take on an 80-year-old patient for a face-lift if the physician determines that the patient is healthy and a suitable candidate for the surgery.

Mechanism of Action and Target Tissues

Rhytidectomy smoothes loose facial and neck skin by removing excess fat, removing excess skin, and/or tightening underlying muscles. There are basically three face-lift techniques, and sometimes a physician will use a combination of the three, which are based on the depth of the dissection plane. The dissection planes are superficial, medium, and deep. The remaining skin flap is then re-draped over the underlying support structure and secured with complex suturing.

Pre-Procedure Considerations

Because the rhytidectomy incision may extend into the scalp, patients with very short hair may be advised to grow their hair to cover the resulting incision in the scalp while it heals. Optimal healing is enhanced with proper preoperative and postoperative skin care. *It is mandatory that a patient stop smoking for at least one to two weeks before surgery* because smoking inhibits blood flow to the skin and may delay the healing process or even cause loss of skin.

FYI

Most, if not all, cosmetic plastic surgeons require the patient to quit smoking prior to surgery because of the predictable problems it creates during the healing process. The worst-case scenario is necrosis, or death of skin tissue. This can result in infection, delayed healing, and scarring.

Regardless of the type of anesthesia used, or where the surgery is performed, patients should arrange for someone to drive them home after surgery and for someone to stay with them to help them with their daily activities for one to two days. It is not unusual for patients to stay in a recovery facility for up to several nights after the operation.

Procedure Techniques

Although many face-lifts are performed under local anesthesia with intravenous sedation, some surgeons prefer general anesthesia. The final choice depends on the patient's wish, the extent of the surgery, ancillary procedures, and/or the surgeon's preference. Rhytidectomy is a major operative procedure that physicians can perform in an outpatient surgical center or an office-based facility; some physicians prefer to do the procedures in a hospital, where their patients have a brief stay afterward.

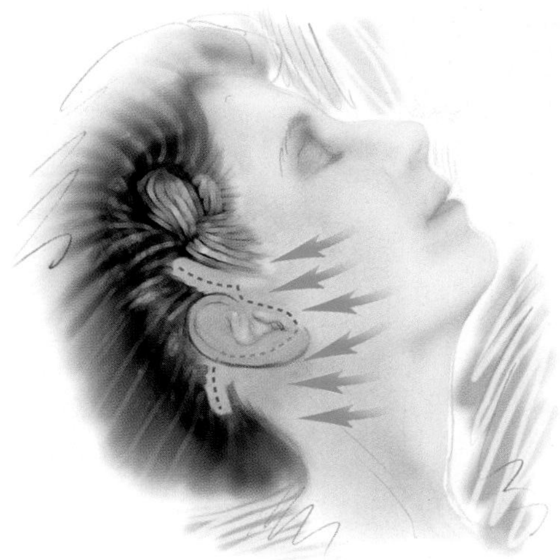

Figure 27–1 Repositioning skin for face-lift.

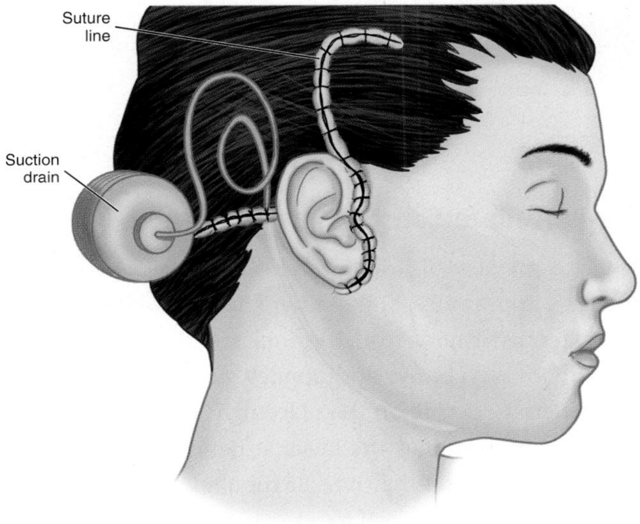

Figure 27–2 Sutured wound.

There are several rhytidectomy techniques, which depend on the depth of the dissection plane: 1) the "classic" plane that only involves a skin flap (superficial plane); 2) the **superficial musculoaponeurotic system** (mid-plane), or **SMAS;** this is the layer of tissue that covers the deeper structures in the cheek area and is in continuity with the platysma; 3) the subperiosteal face-lift (deep plane); and 4) a combination of these techniques (Figures 27–1 and 27–2).

Thread Lift

The "thread" face-lift procedure, also known as a **thread lift,** is a simple, minimally invasive, FDA-approved procedure using the innovative placement of subcutaneous sutures. The sutures are made of clear polypropylene material with tiny, evenly spaced barbs or cogs. These "threads" are placed in the subcutaneous layer (through small incisions) and arranged in an umbrella-like fashion with sufficient tension to gently suspend or lift the sagging tissues. The placement and number of sutures varies from patient to patient.

These "threads" are best used for subtle repositioning of saggy cheeks, jowls, or eyebrows in individuals with good elasticity of the skin (Figure 27–3a and b). The body surrounds each "thread" with collagen. The thread lift does not replace a traditional face-lift because it cannot fully correct skin that sags too much; thus it is not as effective for a neck-lift.

This procedure is performed under local anesthesia. If done by a properly trained and experienced physician, this procedure is quick, effective, and safe. Surgery time is usually under one hour, but it varies, depending on the area treated and the number of threads used. In most cases, there is minimal discomfort with some slight bruising and swelling. Ice compresses are recommended for the first 48 hours. Patients can usually return to work or normal activities in a few days. The length of time the results last depends on the age of the patient, the degree of sagging, and the number of threads used. Additional threads may be added with time, as needed.

FOREHEAD-LIFT (BROW-LIFT)

A forehead-lift (brow-lift) is a cosmetic or functional surgical procedure that targets the upper third of the face (i.e., forehead and eyebrows). It does absolutely nothing for the middle or lower face. Further, it is important to understand that the texture of the skin is not altered by a forehead-lift. Thus, it is not uncommon for patients to have concomitant skin resurfacing (peels/dermabrasion/laser), face-lift, and/or blepharoplasty to improve the overall texture of the skin as well as to give the face a more youthful appearance. A forehead-lift procedure is usually done in patients who are between the ages 40 of 65.

Indications

A forehead-lift is used to smooth wrinkles (*rhytids*), soften deep frown lines and furrows between the eyes, and/or to elevate the brow for a more pleasing and restful look. A patient who is having a forehead-lift may also have eyelid surgery (**blepharoplasty**) at the same time, especially if he or she has significant overhang of the

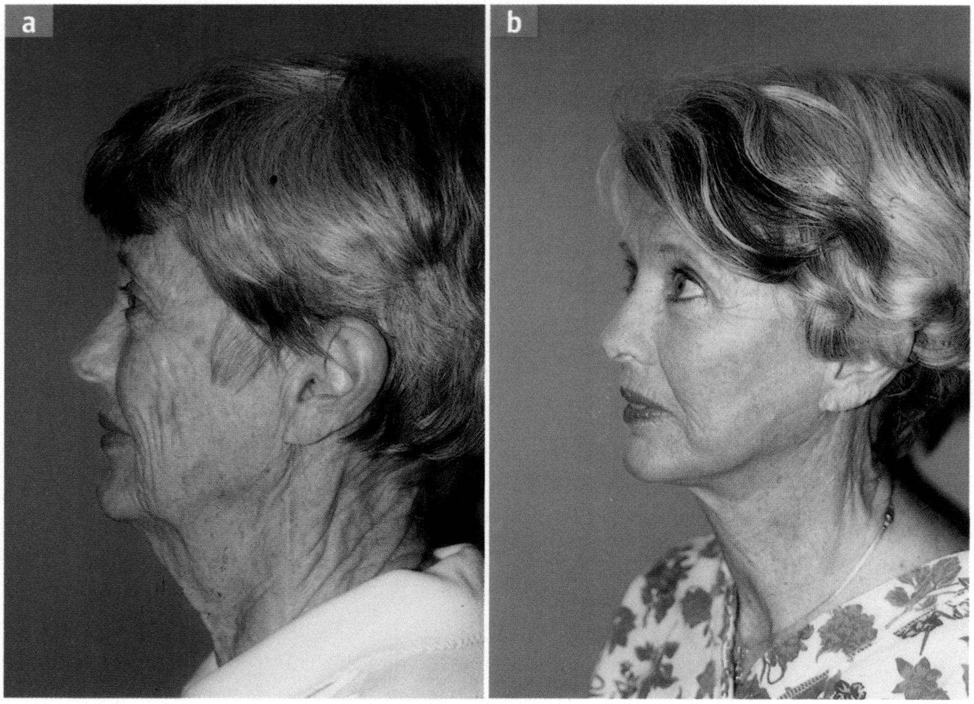

Figure 27–3 Before and after face-lift.

upper eyelids. Sometimes patients who believe they need upper-eyelid surgery find that a forehead-lift better meets their needs (i.e., severely drooping eyebrows can impair the superior field of vision).

Patients who are bald or who have a receding hairline may still be good candidates for a forehead-lift. The surgeon simply alters the incision location or performs a more conservative operation.

Mechanism of Action and Target Tissues

There are two main surgical techniques for a forehead-lift: the **classic forehead-lift** ("open technique") and the **endoscopic** or minimal incision forehead-lift. The main difference between these two techniques is the placement, number, and size of the incision(s). Both techniques involve the manipulation and excision of muscles and skin that cause wrinkles, deep frown lines, furrowing, and/or droopy eyebrows. Using the classic technique, the surgeon usually hides the incision just behind the hairline, extending from ear to ear. With the endoscopic method, the surgeon uses a viewing instrument (endoscope) to look for locations to make multiple small incisions. Both techniques yield similar results (Figure 27–4a and b), but the endoscopic technique typically has quicker recovery.

Pre-Procedure Considerations

To get a preview of how a forehead-lift might change a patient's appearance, the cosmetic surgeon places his or her extended thumbs on the upper and outer edges of the patient's eyebrows and applies gentle, upward pressure. Then, to decide on the placement of the incision(s), the surgeon examines the facial structure, the condition of the skin, and the hairline. If the patient's hair is very short, he or she may wish to let it grow out before surgery to hide the resulting scar(s).

Procedure Techniques

Although most forehead-lifts are performed under local anesthesia and intravenous sedation, some surgeons prefer general anesthesia. Both the classic forehead-lift and the endoscopic forehead-lift are usually performed in a surgeon's office-based facility or an outpatient surgery center. However, these procedures are occasionally done in the hospital.

Both the classic and endoscopic techniques require the same preparation: The patient's hair is tied back and trimmed behind the hairline where the incisions will be made. For most patients undergoing the classic technique, a coronal incision follows a headphone-like pattern, slightly behind the natural hairline, starting just above

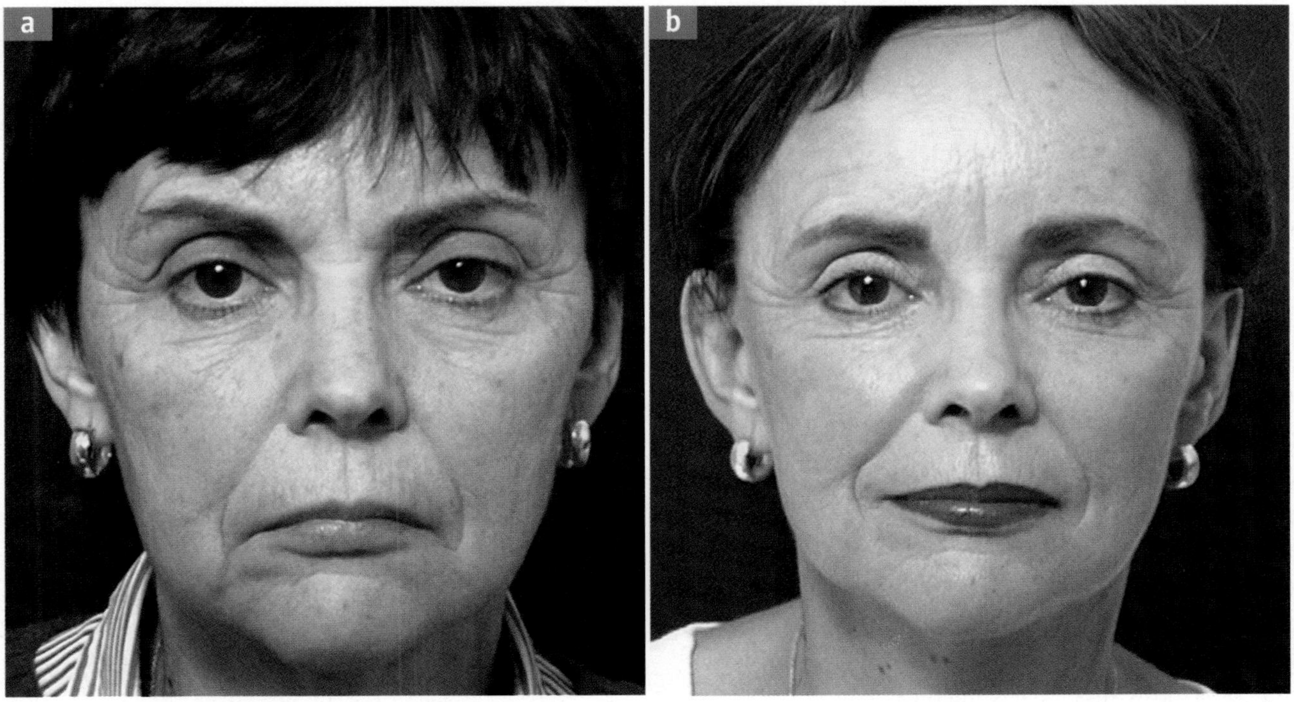

Figure 27–4 Before and after forehead-lift.

ear level and running across the top of the forehead and down to just above the opposite ear (Figure 27–5). If the patient has a high forehead, the mid-portion of the incision is made directly at the hairline to avoid further rising of the forehead. This incision, which has the advantage of lowering the hairline, generally heals favorably. The disadvantage could be noticeable scarring.

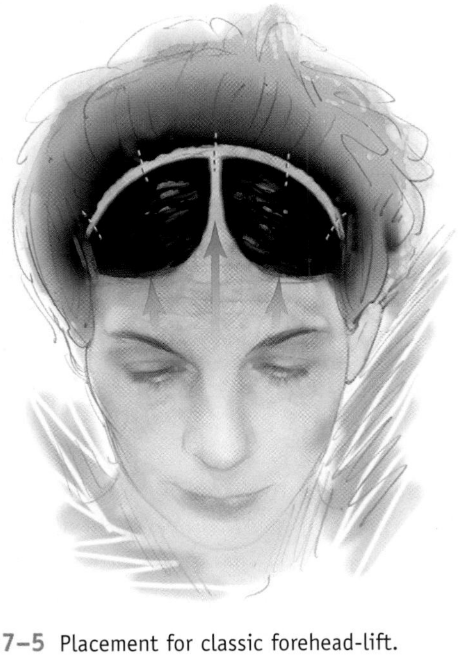

Figure 27–5 Placement for classic forehead-lift.

Conversely, if the hairline is very low, the surgeon can raise it by placing the incision near the top of the head. Patients with bald or thinning hair may opt for a midscalp incision so the resulting scar follows the natural junction of two bones in the skull and is less conspicuous; however, it may still show.

Forehead-lift procedures take between one to two hours to perform. Most patients go home the same day, and they need transportation to and from surgery and assistance with daily activities for several days after the surgery.

EYE LIFT (BLEPHAROPLASTY)

Patients with baggy upper eyelids and bulging lower eyelids may opt to have an eye lift, or blepharoplasty, done. In 2003, the American Society of Aesthetic Plastic Surgeons reported more than 260,000 blepharoplasty procedures, making a blepharoplasty the most-often-performed procedure of all cosmetic surgeries. It can be done alone or in conjunction with a face-lift, brow-lift, or other cosmetic procedure.

Indications

The best candidates for a cosmetic blepharoplasty are usually men and women with redundant skin in the upper eyelids and/or baggy lower eyelids. This can be caused by any number of factors, including genetics, aging, lifestyle issues, or sun damage.

Blepharoplasty cannot alter dark circles, fine lines, or wrinkles around the eyes, nor can it change sagging eyebrows. Instead, a lift in the temple region elevates eyebrow overhang.

Mechanism of Action and Target Tissues

During this procedure, the surgeon excises redundant eyelid skin. If needed, he or she will also excise a strip of orbicularis oculi muscle along with the upper eyelid skin. If bulging exists, some **periorbital fat** is also excised.

Pre-Procedure Considerations

Typically, a physician will take a history and perform a physical examination on a patient to evaluate that patient's general health. The physician is likely to do a visual field test, an assessment of tear production, and an assessment of the patient's eyelids to determine the tissues that need to be addressed and whether any additional procedures are appropriate (such as laser resurfacing or a brow-lift). A few medical conditions make blepharoplasty more risky, including thyroid problems, such as hypothyroidism and **Graves' disease,** a form of hyperthyroidism, and a lack of sufficient tears.

Procedure Techniques

A blepharoplasty may be performed in a surgeon's office-based facility, an outpatient surgery center, or in a hospital. Patients usually receive local anesthesia with intravenous sedation or a systemic anesthesia, which makes him or her feel drowsy and relaxed. General anesthesia may also be used. After receiving anesthesia, the patient is prepped and draped in a sterile fashion.

For both upper and lower eyelid blepharoplasty, the surgeon places the incisions on, adjacent to, or parallel to the patient's natural lines and creases around the eyes. The incision may be extended to the crow's feet lines on the outer corners of the eye to minimize appearance of the resulting scars (Figure 27–6). In the upper eyelids, the surgeon excises a long, elliptical island of skin, with or without muscle. Through this incision, the surgeon removes excess fat (Figure 27–7). In the lower lids, the skin flap is dissected and, if needed, excess periorbital fat, the fat pockets above and below the eye, is excised (Figure 27-8). After hemostasis is attained with **electrocautery,** the technique of using an electrical device to cut and seal blood vessels to control bleeding, the surgeon trims excess skin and muscle, sutures with fine nonabsorbable sutures, and covers the sutures with steri-strips.

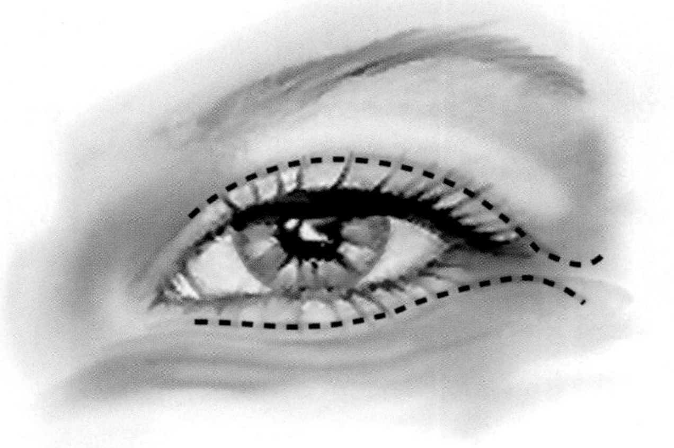

Figure 27–6 External incision for upper and lower blepharoplasty.

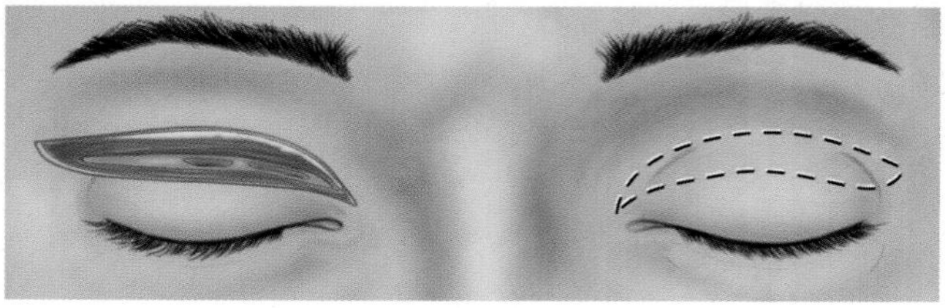

Figure 27–7 Upper eyelid excision.

In situations in which there are bulging pockets of fat beneath the lower eyelids but no skin redundancy, the surgeon may perform a transconjunctival blepharoplasty, (one that extends across the **conjunctiva,** the mucus membrane that lines the eyelids), making the incision inside the conjunctiva, or lower eyelid, leaving no visible external scar (Figure 27–8a and b). This is usually performed on younger patients with thicker, more elastic skin. The periorbital fat is excised and the conjunctiva can be closed with a special suturing technique.

Together, upper and lower blepharoplasty usually takes 45 minutes to 2 hours, depending on the extent of the surgery. If done separately, each procedure will take less time. If there are excess wrinkles below the eyes, the patient can have a laser resurfacing done at the same time.

Post-Surgical Concerns

Dressings and Wound Care

Typically, the eyes are not bandaged after surgery. Rather, the surgeon may lubricate the eyelids with ointment and place ice compresses over the eyes while the patient reclines. As the anesthesia wears off, the eyelids may feel tight and sore. If this occurs, the patient should respond

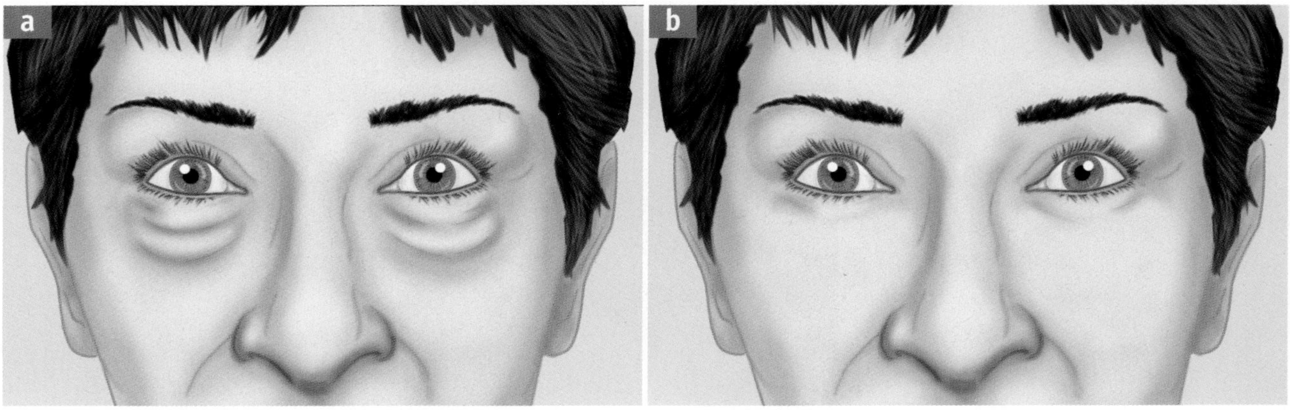

Figure 27–8 Before and after removal of under-eye bags.

well to over-the-counter pain medications. If the pain is severe, the surgeon must be notified immediately. Patients may also experience excessive tearing and light sensitivity (**photophobia**) for several weeks after surgery. Many surgeons recommend the use of eye drops for patients who experience dryness, burning, or itching.

Sutures

The upper and lower wounds are closed with nonabsorbable sutures. If the incision for the transconjunctival approach is closed with fine absorbable sutures, they can be left in place. In fact, absorbable sutures are usually left in place, while permanent sutures are removed two to five days after surgery.

Bathing and Hair Care

By the third or fourth postoperative day, most patients are able to shower and gently wash the face and hair with mild soap or shampoo. They should not rub their eyes for several weeks after surgery. Patients should not have hair coloring or other chemical services until the surgical wound is completely healed.

NOSE JOB (RHINOPLASTY)

One of the most common aesthetic procedures is rhinoplasty, commonly known as a nose job. It is a very delicate operation requiring specialized training and experience. Most rhinoplasty procedures are performed for cosmetic reasons; these procedures are called cosmetic rhinoplasty. When a rhinoplasty is done to relieve nasal airway obstruction, it is called **reconstructive rhinoplasty,** which can be done alone or in conjunction with a cosmetic rhinoplasty, if warranted. A **deviated nasal septum,** a condition in which the middle wall inside the nose deviates into the airway passages, and/or enlarged **nasal turbinates,** areas of bone and mucosa projecting from the walls of the nasal cavity, can contribute to nasal airway obstruction; these conditions are repaired (reconstructive rhinoplasty) with a septoplasty and/or turbinectomy, respectively. Although complex procedures may require a short hospital stay, most patients return home the same day.

Indications

The goal of a cosmetic rhinoplasty is to create harmony between the nose and other facial features. **Rhinoplasty** can reduce or increase the size of the nose, change the shape of the tip, change the shape of the bridge, narrow the span of the nostrils, or change the angle between the nose and the upper lip. Rhinoplasty is often performed with chin and/or cheek implants.

Although there is no upper age limit for cosmetic nasal surgery, most surgeons prefer to delay operating on younger patients until they have completed their growth spurts, which is usually in the mid-teens for girls and the mid- to late teens for boys.

Mechanism of Action and Target Tissues

Through strategically placed incisions, the surgeon exposes the main structural support (nasal bones, septum, and alar cartilages) for the nose. He or she then fractures, sculpts, and trims to attain the desired size and shape. Upon completion, the surgeon re-drapes the skin and mucosa and closes with key sutures (Figure 27–9a and b).

Pre-Procedure Considerations

Factors that can influence the procedure and results include the structure of the nasal bones, the support cartilage at the tip of the nose, the shape of the septum, the shape of the face, the thickness of the skin, and

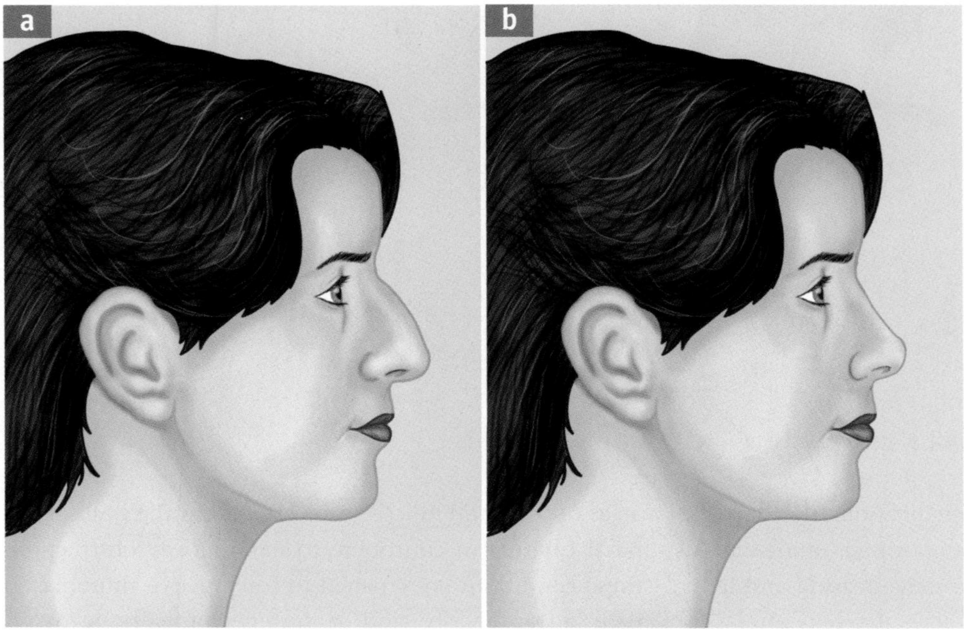

Figure 27–9 Before and after rhinoplasty to remove hump on nose.

even the patient's age and race. Menstruation may affect intraoperative and postoperative bleeding.

Procedure Techniques

Depending on the extent of the procedure and the patient's and/or surgeon's preference, rhinoplasty can be performed under local or general anesthesia. There are two surgical techniques: the **endonasal,** inside the nose, approach, commonly known as a **closed rhinoplasty,** or surgery in which incisions are inside the nose and do not leave an external scar, and the **open rhinoplasty,** or surgery in which there is an incision between the nostrils which can leave a faint scar. Through strategically placed incisions, both techniques allow access to the nose's framework of bone and cartilage. The majority of the incisions in either closed or open rhinoplasties are within the nasal cavity to avoid visible scarring.

The framework is exposed and sculpted to create the desired shape; for example, the nasal hump and septal cartilage may be trimmed to reduce the profile of the nose and/or to elevate the tip of the nose (Figure 27–10). In some cases, the surgeon fractures, or saws, a **synthetic** or manufactured implant or cartilage from another part of the nasal bones—where they meet the cheeks and bridge of the nose—and then compresses the loose nasal bones to form a new shape. Total surgery time depends on the surgeon's experience and the type, difficulty, and scope of the procedure(s) performed.

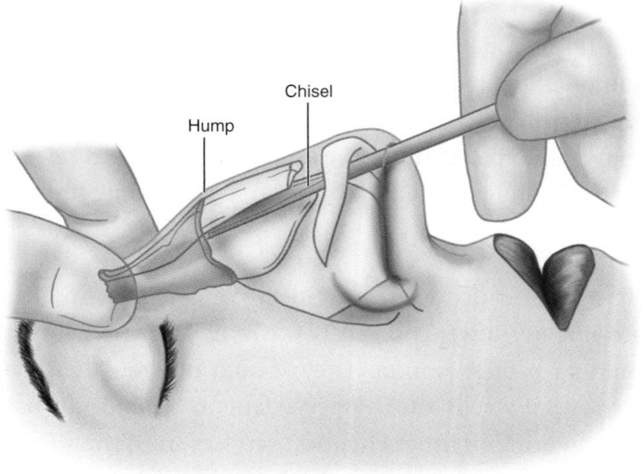

Figure 27–10 Removing hump from nose.

FACIAL IMPLANTS

Facial implants are designed for augmentation, reconstruction, or rejuvenation of the face. They have been used for more than 20 years to improve and/or enhance facial contours and provide harmony and balance to the face.

Indications

A weak or receding chin makes the nose look larger than it is and makes fleshy necks look more pronounced. Because aging can cause a loss of chin projection, adding a chin implant (**mentoplasty**) at the time of a face-lift or a rhinoplasty can improve the neck contour, profile, and jawline. Cheek implants correct flatness in the mid-face by increasing the projection of the cheekbones, which serves to rejuvenate the mid-face region. Nasal implants are used to better define or add projection to the **dorsum** (the top profile) of the nose. Facial implants are often combined with other facial cosmetic procedures such as a rhinoplasty, face-lift, and/or submental liposuction.

Mechanism of Action and Target Tissues

Facial implants come in a variety of synthetic, solid, and semisolid materials, sizes, and styles for the chin, cheek, nose, and jaw. Small synthetic implants are inserted between soft tissue and bone over the desired area. After healing, the skin drapes smoothly over the implants, conforming to the bone, and the implants are usually undetectable. By virtue of its physical properties, the desired area is augmented (i.e., high cheekbones and/or a better-defined chin, which is especially apparent in the profile). The results are essentially permanent.

Pre-Procedure Considerations

Patients with gum or dental problems may not be candidates for intraoral placement of facial implants. As with other facial surgeries, smoking will inhibit blood flow to the skin and will delay healing of the incisions.

Procedure Techniques

Facial implant surgery may be done with either local anesthesia combined with a sedative or with general anesthesia. Surgery usually takes place in an office-based facility, a freestanding surgical center, or a hospital outpatient facility. The procedure follows a similar pattern for all facial areas.

Chin

An incision is made either externally in the natural crease line just under the chin or internally, inside the mouth, where gum and lower lip meet. The surgeon creates a pocket between the bone and soft tissue, inserts the implant, and sutures the incision. During the procedure, the surgeon selects the proper size and shape implant for the patient. Insertion of a chin implant may take anywhere from 30 minutes to 1 hour (Figure 27–11).

Nose

The dorsum of the nose can be enhanced with synthetic implants placed as a sole procedure or in conjunction with a cosmetic or reconstructive rhinoplasty. The implants may be inserted through the incisions made for those procedures.

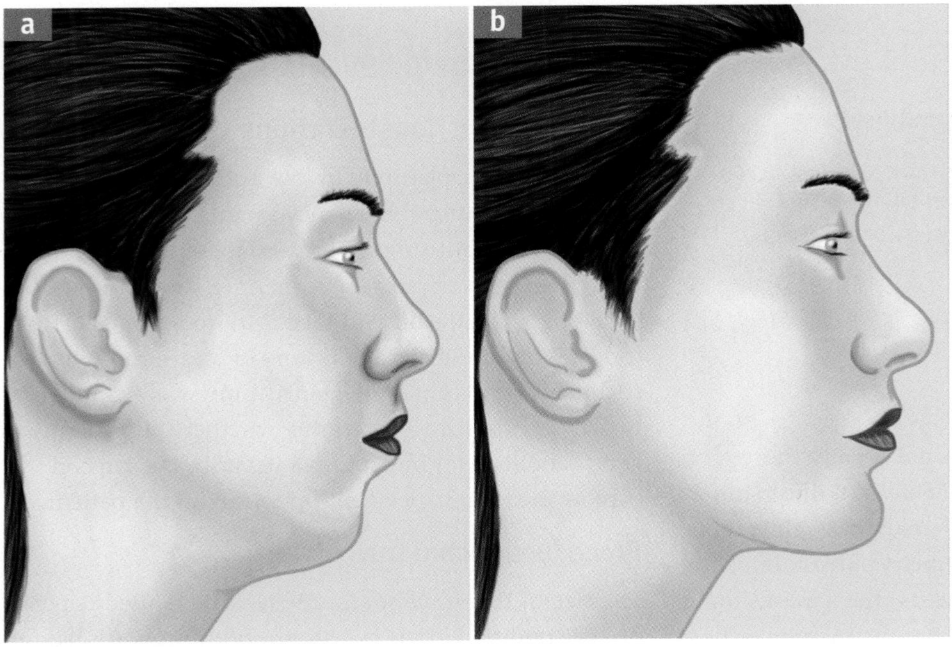

Figure 27–11 Weak chin, before and after implant.

BREAST IMPLANTS (AUGMENTATION MAMMAPLASTY)

Augmentation **mammaplasty** is the insertion of synthetic implants in a woman's breasts to enhance the size and shape of her bust. Because gravity, pregnancy, and the effects of aging eventually alter the size and shape of virtually every woman's breasts, it is not surprising that breast implant surgery is one of the most common cosmetic procedures sought by women in the United States (Figure 27–12).

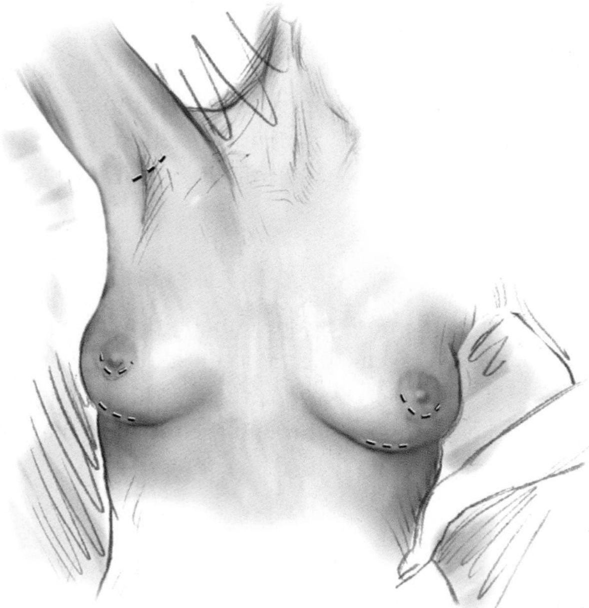

Figure 27–12 Possible incision sites.

> **FYI**
>
> There is no evidence that breast implants affect a woman's fertility, future pregnancies, or ability to nurse.

Indications

Women who seek breast implants are usually those who wish to enlarge and/or reshape their breast(s) due to inherited small breast size, weight loss, childbirth, aging, tubular breast(s), and/or breast asymmetry. Breast implants can also be used to reconstruct breasts after a mastectomy for breast cancer. (See the Breast Reconstruction section later in this chapter.)

Mechanism of Action and Target Tissues

During this procedure, the surgeon positions a synthetic breast implant either behind the breast tissue only or behind the pectoralis muscle and breast tissue to increase projection and breast size while achieving the most natural appearance possible. The incision placement and positioning of the breast implant (relative to the pectoralis muscle) depends on the patient's anatomy and the surgeon's recommendation and/or preference.

There are a variety of implant designs, all of which have advantages and disadvantages. New choices become available all the time, so the client should discuss this thoroughly with the physician.

> **? Did You Know**
>
> In 1992, because of safety concerns, the U.S. Food and Drug Administration (FDA) restricted the use of silicone gel-filled implants to women willing to participate in long-term studies with specific indications for surgery. These implants have now been approved for use.

> **FYI**
>
> If the breasts are sagging, a patient might consider a breast-lift (mastopexy) in conjunction with the augmentation.

Pre-Procedure Considerations

Patients who are planning to lose a significant amount of weight or planning a pregnancy might consider postponing breast implant surgery, because these events can alter breast size in an unpredictable manner. At the initial consultation, the surgeon will take a thorough medical history and inquire about any history of breast cancer and/or results of previous mammograms. A physical examination is then performed to determine whether the patient is a good candidate for breast implants. If so, the surgeon will explore breast enhancement options with the patient.

Procedure Techniques

The size of the implant and the technique used depends on the condition of the breasts, the body proportions, and the patient's expectations. Other options include incision

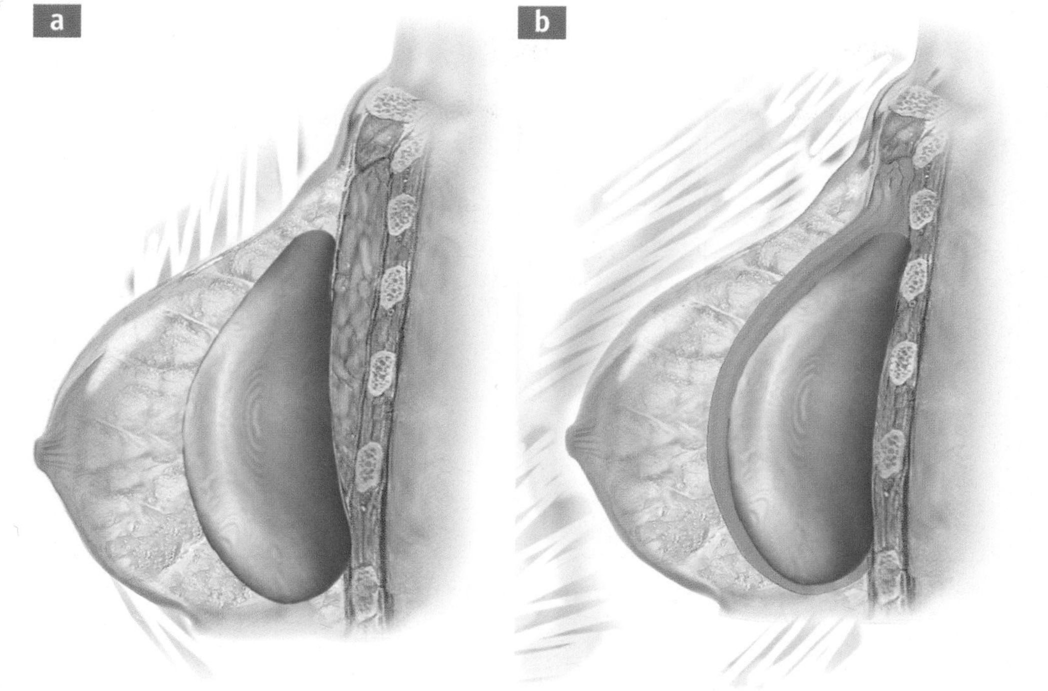

Figure 27–13 Subglandular and submuscular implant.

placement, size and type of implant, and whether the implants will be placed beneath the pectoralis muscle or between the pectoralis muscle and the breast gland (Figure 27–13).

Mammograms and Breast Implants

Although usually not necessary, it is not unreasonable to obtain a mammogram before breast implant surgery. It may pick up early breast cancer and/or serve as a baseline mammogram to compare with future studies. In some instances, the surgeon may recommend another mammographic examination some months after surgery.

Women in the appropriate age group should continue routine mammograms after breast augmentation. Some women with a high risk for breast cancer may require additional breast diagnostics such as ultrasound or an MRI. However, the presence of breast implants makes it technically more difficult to take and read mammograms and could delay or hinder the early detection of breast cancer. As such, the technician should use special techniques to optimize the interpretation of the mammogram.

While you as an esthetician will probably not have to deal with postoperative complications for breast augmentation, reduction, or restoration, it is important that you communicate with surgeons regarding what may occur for your clients who have had these procedures. Follow the physician's counsel for how to handle these cases. Discuss complications that may occur, including infection, necrosis, capsular contraction, and scarring.

FOCUS ON: *Breast Radiography and Implants*

Although there is no scientific evidence that breast implants cause breast cancer, they may change the way mammography is done to detect cancer. Technicians should be experienced in the special techniques required to obtain a reliable X ray of a breast with an implant.

FYI

After breast augmentation, patients will still be able to perform breast self-examination.

BREAST-LIFT (MASTOPEXY)

With age, breast skin loses its elasticity, and factors such as pregnancy, nursing, and gravity often cause the breasts to sag. In addition, some women may also have stretch marks and loss of volume in their breasts due to weight

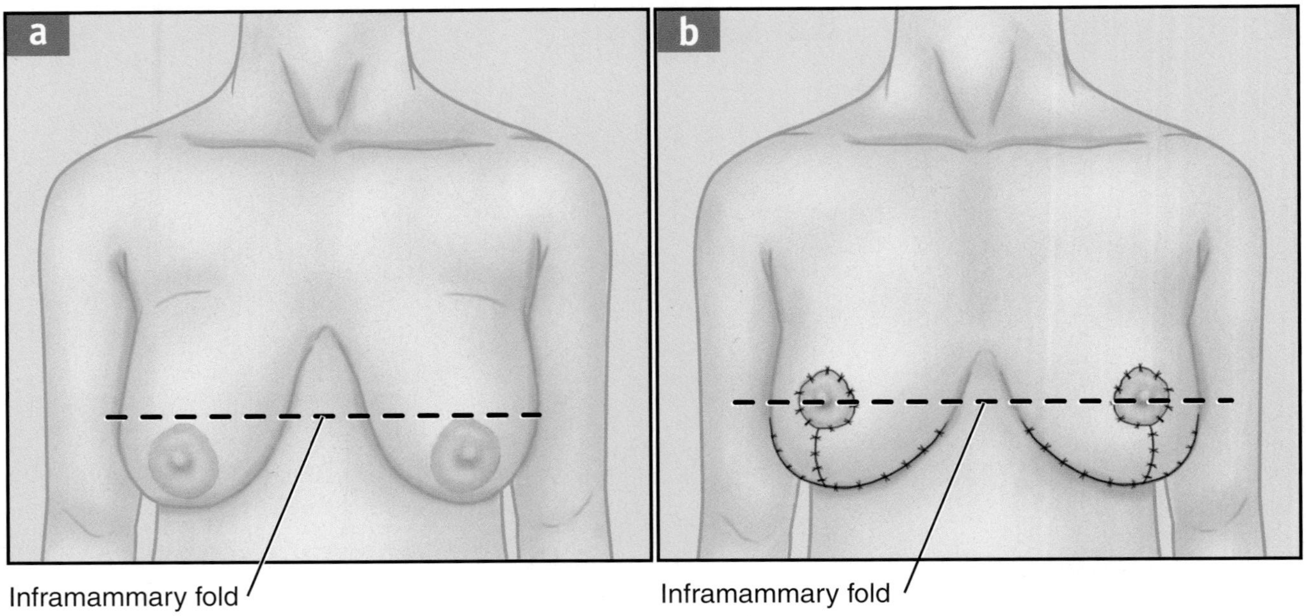

Figure 27–14 Ptosis of the breast and mastopexy.

fluctuations and natural breast atrophy. This droopiness of the breasts, or ptosis, results because the skin envelope is much larger than the volume of breast tissue. This can be remedied through a breast-lift (**mastopexy**), a surgical procedure designed to make the breasts perkier, fuller, and more youthful looking.

Indications

If a patient's nipples are below the level of the **inframammary crease,** the area below the armpit, when standing (Figure 27–14), she is a candidate for a breast-lift. Although breasts of any size may be lifted, the best results are usually achieved in women with small, sagging breasts. Because of the greater weight, women with large breasts will most likely have shorter lasting effect of any breast-lift surgery. Mastopexy does nothing in the way of increasing the breast volume. Thus, if a patient wants larger breasts, breast implants can be inserted at the time of the breast-lift.

The best candidates for mastopexy, as for all cosmetic procedures, are healthy, emotionally stable women with realistic expectations.

Mechanism of Action and Target Tissues

Because the main cause of droopy breasts is skin laxity and/or atrophy of the breasts, the goal of a breast-lift is essentially a tailoring (reduction) of the skin envelope such that it drapes over the available breast tissue to create a perkier and fuller breast—with a more natural placement of the nipple/areolar complex and overall contour.

Breast-lift procedures can be done using different incision patterns to place the resulting scar in such a manner as to camouflage it within creases or boundaries of sharp color demarcations (e.g., the dark areola). These patterns include a **circumareolar** incision one that follows around the areola, a vertical incision (connecting the circumareolar incision to the inframammary incision), and a horizontal incision beneath the breast—much like the incisions for a breast reduction. In some instances, it may be possible to avoid the horizontal incision beneath the breast.

After the cosmetic surgeon removes excess breast skin, he or she shifts the nipple/areolar complex to a more youthful position on the resulting breast mound. The nipple/areolar complex remains attached to underlying mounds of breast tissue. This usually allows for the preservation of sensation and the ability to breast-feed.

FYI

Although breast-lift surgery does not increase the risk of developing breast cancer, it may be a good idea for some patients—depending on age and family history—to obtain a baseline mammogram before surgery and again several months after surgery. This will assist a physician who reads that patient's future mammograms looking for any changes in breast tissue; he or she will be able to rule out any changes that took place during the surgery. After a breast-lift, patients will still be able to self-examine the breasts.

Pre-Procedure Considerations

Before a breast-lift, a surgeon examines and measures a patient's breasts while the patient is sitting or standing. The surgeon considers the size and shape of the patient's breasts, the size of the **areolas,** or nipples, and the extent of sagging before selecting the best surgical approach. The goal is to optimize the results while leaving the least noticeable scars possible.

Although mastopexy usually does not interfere with breast-feeding, pregnancy is likely to stretch the breasts again and offset the results of the breast-lift procedure. Thus, patients planning to have children should postpone a mastopexy.

Patients should make arrangements ahead of time for someone to drive them to and from their procedure and to assist them with their daily activities during the recovery period.

Procedure Techniques

A breast-lift surgery can be performed using local or general anesthesia. For cost containment and convenience, a surgeon usually performs a breast-lift on an outpatient basis in the surgeon's office-based surgical suite, an outpatient surgery center, or a hospital.

There are two types of breast-lift procedures: the full lift and the modified lift. Mastopexy usually takes 1½ to 3½ hours, and the length of the procedure varies according to the surgeon's experience and technique. If the patient is having a breast implant inserted along with the breast-lift, the surgeon will place the implant in a pocket directly under the breast tissue, or deeper, under the pectoralis muscle of the chest wall. Regardless of the technique, the surgeon repositions the nipple/areolar complex to the approximate level of the inframammary crease—as viewed from an upright, lateral profile. Then, the surgeon closes the incisions with interrupted (buried) subcuticular sutures and running or interrupted (superficial) nonabsorbable sutures. This is the most common procedure for breast-lift; it involves an anchor-shaped incision following the natural contour of the breast (Figure 27–15).

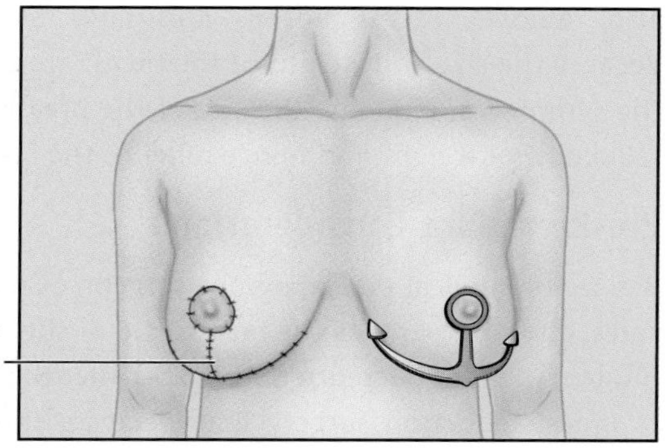

Figure 27–15 Anchor-shape suture line.

BREAST REDUCTION (REDUCTION MAMMAPLASTY)

Women with large, heavy-hanging breasts, **pendulous breasts,** often experience an assortment of troublesome symptoms, including, but not limited to, back and neck pain, skin irritation, physical deformities, and breathing problems. Breast reduction, technically known as reduction mammaplasty, is a surgical procedure to create smaller, better-shaped, and proportional breasts. Breast reduction surgery has among the highest patient satisfaction rates of any cosmetic and reconstructive surgical procedure.

Indications

Women from their teens into their 80s can have breast reduction surgery. In general, it is usually wise to wait until at least age 20 to make sure the breasts have stopped growing.

Breast reduction surgery is usually not done for appearance alone; it is done to reduce the size of pendulous breasts, relieving medical problems and symptoms caused by their weight. These symptoms include the following:

- Back and neck pain
- Bad posture and deformities of the skeleton
- Breathing problems
- Pain from sports or vigorous activity
- Chronic back, upper neck, and shoulder pain
- Skin rash under the breasts
- Deep, painful grooves in the shoulders from the pressure of a bra strap
- Restricted levels of activity
- Self-esteem problems, particularly in adolescent girls
- Difficulty wearing or fitting into certain bras and clothing

FYI

Women whose breasts are sagging but not too large might receive more benefit from a breast-lift, also known as mastopexy.

Mechanism of Action and Target Tissues

Breast reduction surgery is a tailoring/sculpting surgical procedure that reduces the size of large, pendulous breasts to make them less weighty. Unlike mastopexy, where only the skin is removed, breast reduction surgery also removes excess fibrous and fatty breast tissue. Because the size and weight of the breast are the cause of the symptoms, reducing the size of the breasts results in reduction of weight and hence relief of the symptoms.

Pre-Procedure Considerations

Before the surgical procedure, the surgeon examines, measures, and photographs the breasts. He or she will use the photographs for reference during and after the procedure.

Breast reduction surgery may decrease the ability to breast-feed. Therefore, a woman wishing to do so should probably delay the procedure until she is done having children. Further, the overall appearance of the breasts may change after having a baby.

Before surgery, patients should make arrangements for someone to drive them to and from their procedure and to assist them with their daily activities during the recovery period.

Procedure Techniques

Breast reduction is most often performed under general anesthesia, causing the patient to sleep during the procedure. There are several surgical techniques available for breast reduction surgery, but the most common one involves an anchor-shaped incision that goes around the areola, down from the areolar incision to an inframammary crease incision (Figure 27–16).

Most breast reduction surgeries are performed on an outpatient basis, and patients are usually allowed to go home within hours of the operation. However, if an extremely large amount of breast tissue is to be removed, the surgeon may require the patient to stay overnight in the hospital for monitoring.

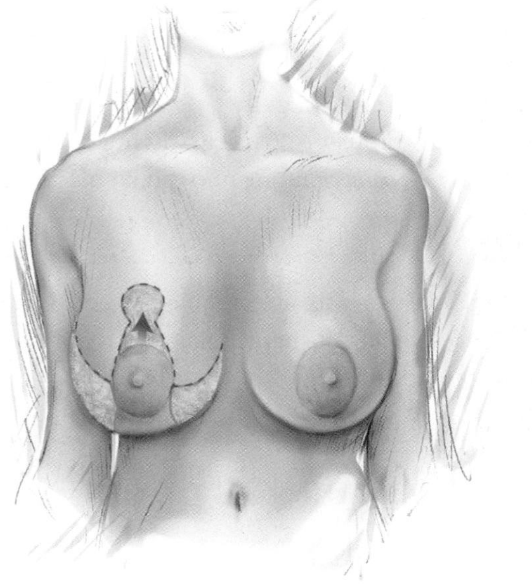

Figure 27–16 One type of incision used for reduction and mastopexy.

BREAST RECONSTRUCTION

Breast reconstruction procedures are very popular and rewarding options for breast cancer patients and have been welcomed by thousands of women around the world. About 75% of all breast cancer patients opt to have reconstructive work done on the involved breast and sometimes also on the other to regain better symmetry. While it is not yet possible to create an exact replica of the human breast, the goal of plastic surgeons is to create a breast mound to approximate the form, feel, and appearance of a natural breast.

Indications

Breast reconstruction is available to most women after a mastectomy. The best candidates are women whose cancer, as far as can be determined, seems to have been eliminated by **mastectomy** (Figure 27–17). The timing of the surgery is based on the individual client's medical situation and her team of medical doctors. For some it is done immediately and for others it is delayed. Either way, satisfactory results can be achieved.

Mechanism of Action and Target Issues

Using local or distant tissue (with or without an implant), the surgeon creates a breast mound in an attempt to give symmetry to the woman's post-mastectomy chest wall.

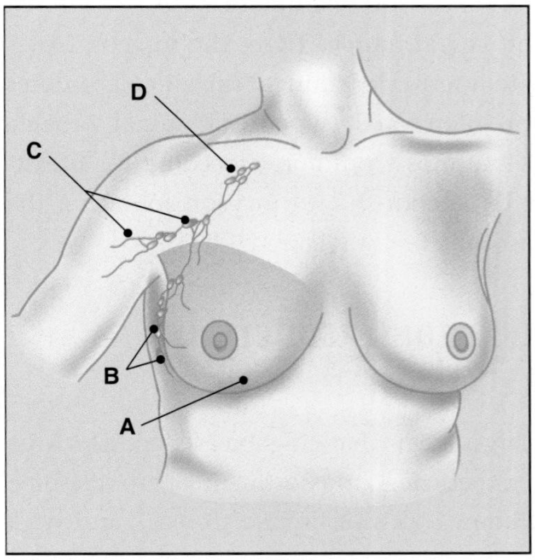

Figure 27–17 Simple mastectomy.

> **FYI**
>
> Breast reconstruction has no known effect on the recurrence of disease in the breast. If the cancer does recur, breast reconstruction will not generally interfere with subsequent chemotherapy or radiation treatments.

Pre-Procedure Considerations

In the initial stage of breast reconstruction, creation of the breast mound is almost always performed using general anesthesia, allowing the patient to sleep pain-free throughout the procedure. If follow-up procedures are required, they may be done under a general or local, depending on the surgeon's preference and other factors.

Procedure Techniques

Breast reconstruction is not a simple procedure, and depending on the surgical option used, it usually involves more than one operation. The woman and her surgeon have many options to consider. The final choice depends on the woman's age, needs, anatomy, tissue, health, physical limitations, and surgeon's ability and experience. The initial stage is usually performed immediately after the mastectomy, under the same anesthesia.

Patients must conform to the physician's guidelines for pre- and post-procedure care. Most require the patient to quit smoking, as the incidence of breast tissue necrosis in smokers is very high. As previously mentioned, smoking can result not only in poor healing but also, possibly, infection or tissue necrosis and sloughing.

Surgical Options

Local Tissue with Implants

Mastectomy patients who have adequate surrounding tissue to cover an implant will not require the use of an expander before receiving an implant. For these women, the surgeon proceeds with inserting an implant, usually under the pectoralis muscle. Essentially, **breast implants** give projection beneath local tissue or under the repositioned flaps that are not bulky enough to give the necessary projection.

Skin Expansion

This technique combines skin expansion and subsequent insertion of an implant (Figure 27–18a and b). A balloon connected to a thin flexible tube is inserted between the skin and pectoralis muscle or between the pectoralis muscle and ribs. At the other end of the tube is a tiny port-valve that is also buried beneath the skin.

Beginning sometime after surgery, the surgeon periodically injects saline solution into the valve to gradually distend the expander. After weeks to months, when the overlying tissue is sufficiently stretched, the expander may be removed and replaced with a permanent implant. However, some expanders are designed to remain as the final implant.

Distant or Flap Reconstruction

A more complex approach to breast reconstruction involves creation and transfer of a tissue flap containing

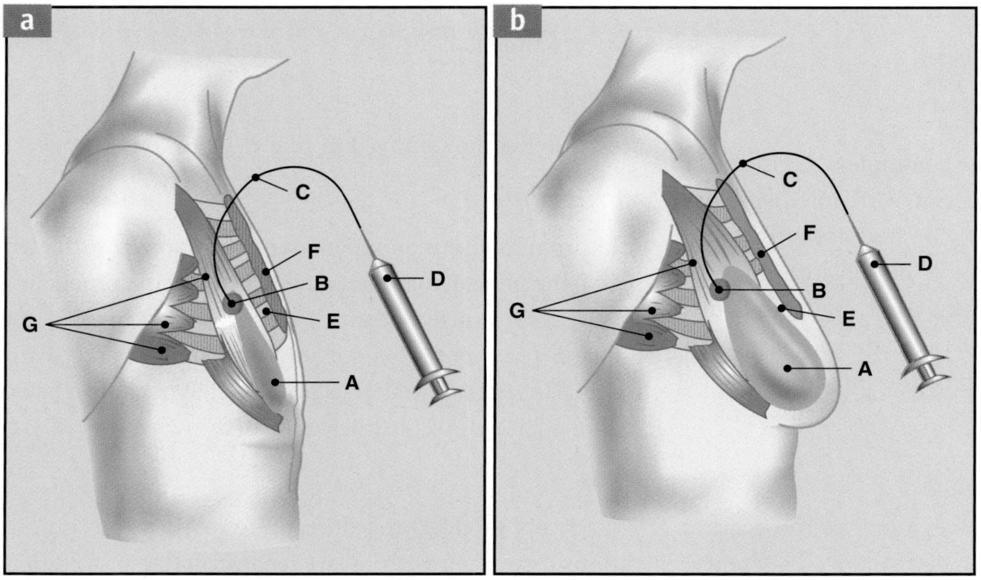

Figure 27–18 Tissue expander non-inflated and inflated.

skin with fat and/or underlining muscle, which is taken from other parts of the body, such as the back, buttocks, or abdomen. In the latter case, the patient may receive the added benefit of an improved abdominal contour through a tummy tuck.

Musculocutaneous Flap

In this type of flap surgery, the tissue remains attached to its original site via its blood supply. These flaps consist of skin, fat, and muscle. With its vascular leash intact, it is tunneled beneath adjacent skin and placed in the mastectomy site, creating a pocket for an implant or, if there is adequate tissue beneath the island of skin, creating the breast mound itself, without the need for an implant (Figure 27–19). This is also called the transverse rectus abdominis myocutaneous or (TRAM) flap.

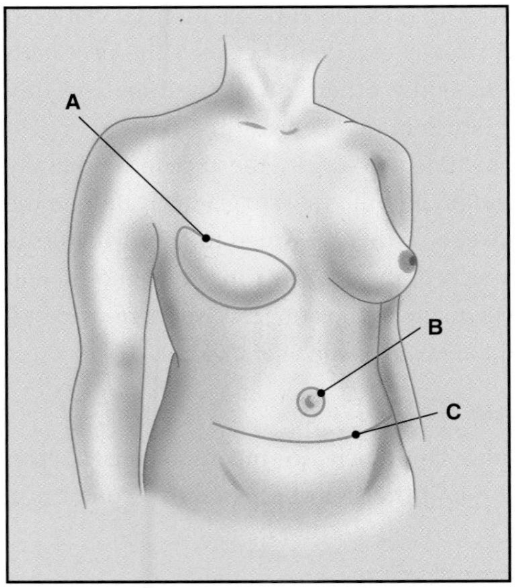

Figure 27–19 Tram flap incision lines.

Free Flap

This flap technique is the most complex, requiring a plastic surgeon who is experienced with microvascular surgery. The surgeon removes the desired donor flap and severs its vascular leash. Common donor areas include the abdomen, thighs, or buttocks. After meticulous dissection the flap is transplanted to and, the vascular leash is, reconnected to blood vessels in the proximity of the mastectomy site.

Follow-up Procedures

Most breast reconstruction involves a series of procedures that occur over time. Based on the woman's preference, it may be necessary to enlarge, reduce, or lift the natural breast to match the reconstructed breast and optimize the final result. The initial reconstructive operation is usually the most complex.

The nipple and areola are reconstructed and/or tattooed in a subsequent procedure. There are numerous options based on the individual client and the physician's preference. A physician will refer patients to a permanent color technician based on the physician's experience with that person, feedback from clients, and results of the technician's past work.

Postoperative Considerations

Post-Procedure Skin and Tissue Changes

Usually, a reconstructed breast will not exhibit the same contour as the pre-mastectomy breast, nor will it match the opposite breast. It will probably feel firmer and look rounder or flatter than the opposite, natural breast.

FYI

It is not yet possible to restore normal sensation to the reconstructed breast or to the nipple/areolar complex; however, in time, some feeling may return.

Postoperative Activity

Many reconstruction options require a surgical drain to remove excess fluids from surgical sites. The drains are removed within one to two weeks after surgery. As a general rule, the patient is advised to avoid overhead lifting, strenuous sports, and sexual activity for three to six weeks following surgery. If implants are used without flaps and reconstruction is done apart from the mastectomy, the recovery time may be less.

Sutures

Most stitches are removed in one week to ten days.

Mammograms

Aside from routine mammograms on the non-reconstructed breast, the surgeon may recommend periodic mammograms on the reconstructed breast. If reconstruction involves an implant, patients should seek out a radiology center with technicians experienced in techniques that obtain a reliable mammogram on reconstructed breasts.

Risks

As with any surgical procedure, there are risks and complications associated with breast reconstructive procedures.

Although relatively uncommon, some patients experience bleeding, fluid collection, infection, and excessive scar tissue. For risks associated with breast implants, review the section of this chapter on breast implants.

Scarring

There will be scars at both the tissue donor site and at the reconstructed breast, and recovery will take longer than with an implant.

TUMMY TUCK (ABDOMINOPLASTY)

Abdominoplasty, more commonly known as a "tummy tuck," is a major surgical procedure that produces a smoother, firmer, flatter abdomen and a thinner waist. With some techniques, it even tightens the pubis and lifts the anterior thighs. An abdominoplasty can remove **striae distensae** ("stretch marks") between the umbilicus and the pubic area; those remaining are tightened, making them less noticeable.

> **FYI**
>
> A tummy tuck is not a weight-loss procedure or substitute for exercise or a healthy diet.

Indications

The best candidates for abdominoplasty are men or women who are in relatively good shape but are bothered by redundant lower abdominal skin, excess fat, and/or weakened abdominal muscles that are unresponsive to diet or exercise. The surgery is particularly helpful to women who, through multiple pregnancies, have stretched their abdominal muscles and skin beyond the point where they can return to normal by dieting or exercising. Women who are planning a pregnancy should postpone an abdominoplasty. Abdominoplasty is becoming an even more popular operation with the increase in patients who have had massive weight loss after **bariatric surgery** (gastric bypass) for morbid obesity. If the abdominal wall musculature/ **fascia** are firm and flat with minimal skin laxity, simple liposuction may be all that is required.

Mechanism of Action and Target Tissues

The tummy tuck is basically a tailoring procedure to recontour the abdomen and hips. The surgeon excises excess skin and repositions the remaining skin over the umbilicus. If the abdominal wall (muscular layers) bulges out, the surgeon tightens it at the vertical midline.

Pre-Procedure Considerations

Before the surgical procedure, the surgeon performs a complete health history. In addition, because several factors contribute to the overall final result of a tummy tuck, the surgeon performs a physical examination to evaluate weight, skin elasticity, muscle tone, overall fat distribution, nutrition, and the extent of procedure needed. In general, patients who start out in top physical condition with strong abdominal muscles will recover from abdominoplasty much faster.

Smokers should quit smoking at least two weeks before surgery and not resume for at least two weeks after surgery. Patients should avoid overexposure to the sun before surgery, especially to the abdomen, and they should avoid a radical diet, as both can inhibit the body's ability to heal.

Procedure Techniques

Either general anesthesia or regional/local anesthesia with intravenous sedation is used in abdominoplasty. Many surgeons perform "tummy tucks" in an outpatient surgical center or an office-based facility; others prefer a hospital, where patients have a brief stay. The patient's underlying health status plays a role in the decision about where the surgery is performed.

There are several different abdominoplasty techniques. The surgeon chooses a procedure based on the extent of the laxity of the patient's abdominal/fascial wall, the redundancy of the skin, the elasticity of the skin, and the amount of fat. Several incisions can be used in this operation; they are placed in such a way that they are covered with most underwear and some bathing suit bottoms. For a better body contour, liposuction of the surrounding area can be done in conjunction with the abdominoplasty.

Miniabdominoplasty

If the problem is localized between the pubic hairline and the umbilicus, a surgeon may do a partial abdominoplasty. In this procedure, the surgeon makes an incision just above the pubic hairline that extends laterally in the direction of the anterior superior iliac spine. If there is laxity in the muscle wall/fascia, this may be tightened with permanent, nonabsorbable sutures. The surgeon dissects the cutaneous flap (skin and underlying subcutaneous fat) from the underlying fascia of the abdominal muscle—from the pubic hairline up to the umbilicus.

After dissecting it from the underlying muscle/fascia, the surgeon stretches the cutaneous flap down to the incision line over the pubic hairline; he or she then excises the excess cutaneous flap and sutures it into its new position. The length of the incision is determined by how much skin needs to be excised.

With partial abdominoplasty, the incision is much shorter and the umbilicus may not require surgical manipulation—unless, as the skin is tightened and stitched, the resulting tension pulls the umbilicus into an unnatural shape. If this occurs, the surgeon makes a "buttonhole" in the centerline of the cutaneous flap to receive the umbilicus without distortion caused by the tension on the flap. Thus, it is possible to have a partial abdominoplasty without a scar around the umbilicus. Partial abdominoplasty may take one to two hours.

Full Abdominoplasty

The most common procedure is a full abdominoplasty. The incision is the same as in the partial abdominoplasty but may extend further laterally onto the hips. Moreover, the dissection of the cutaneous flap is more extensive. If the surgeon dissects it from the underlying muscular/fascia beyond the umbilicus and up to the ribs (Figure 27–20), he or she makes another incision around the umbilicus to free it from the cutaneous flap. If there is a laxity of the abdominal muscle/fascia, the surgeon tightens it along the vertical midline with nonabsorbable sutures—from just above the pubic hairline up to the mid-portion of the rib cage, creating a stronger, more contoured abdominal wall and a smaller waist (Figure 27–21).

LIPOSUCTION (SUCTION-ASSISTED LIPOPLASTY)

Liposuction is the most commonly performed cosmetic procedure in the United States. It is also known as *liposculpture, lipoplasty*, and *suction-assisted lipectomy (SAL)*.

Indications

Liposuction is a surgical procedure primarily used for the removal of stubborn areas of fat that do not respond to diet or exercise. Such areas include the abdomen, hips, buttocks, thighs, knees, upper arms, cheeks, jowls, submental area (double chin), and breast tissue in men.

Whether to do a simple liposuction procedure and/or an accompanying "lift" procedure depends on the amount of excess skin versus the amount of excess fat. Although age is not a major consideration, older patients

> **? Did You Know**
>
> *Cellulite* is a medical term used to describe an uneven, dimpled, "cottage cheese" texture to the skin overlying fat; it commonly appears on the buttocks, thighs, and/or hips. It is not responsive to liposuction because it is too superficial.

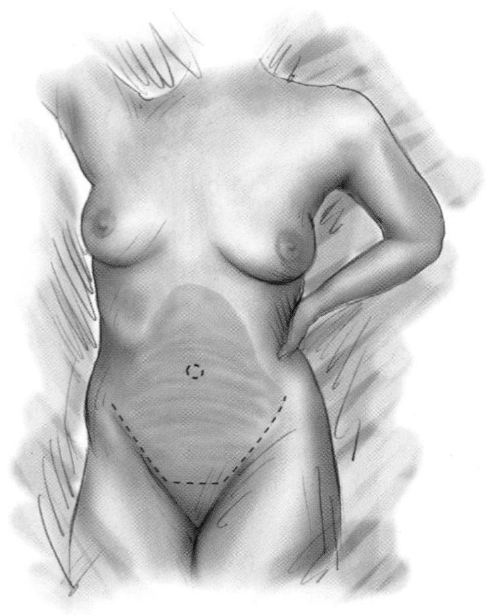

Figure 27–20 Extent of incision.

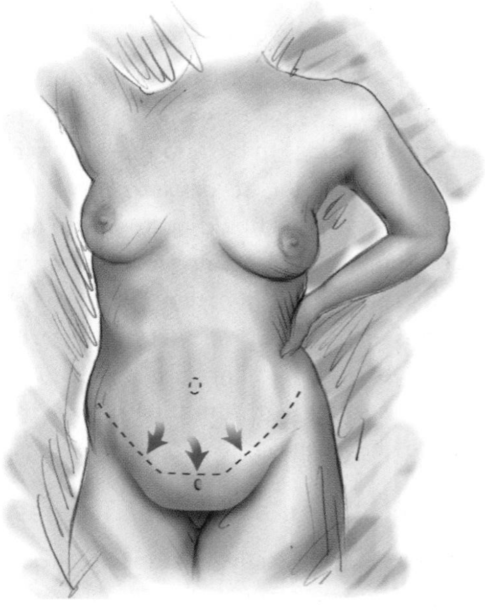

Figure 27–21 Excess skin repositioned.

may have diminished skin elasticity and may not achieve the same results as a younger patient with tighter skin. Liposuction does not cure cellulite, or "dimpled" skin.

Mechanism of Action and Target Tissues

There are several liposuction techniques; they share a common principle of suction via a handheld cannula that is inserted through a tiny stab wound incision (approximately 1.5 cm) in the skin. The cannula is connected to a suction machine via a flexible tube. For small areas, special cannulas are connected directly to a large hand-held syringe that generates suction. The hand-held cannulas have a blunt tip and holes along its shaft. Depending on the techniques, the fat is suctioned directly, or ultrasound waves break the walls of the fat cells, and the resulting fluid is suctioned through the cannula. The skin, muscles, nerves, and blood vessels are left intact. There is an artistic component to the surgeon's ability to create the desired contour by manipulating the cannula to remove the appropriate amount of fat.

Pre-Procedure Considerations

Patients considering this procedure should avoid medications that affect blood coagulation.

Procedure Techniques

Liposuction may be performed in an office-based surgical facility, in an outpatient surgery center, or in a hospital. In general, patients having small volume (<1.5 liter) liposuction usually return home the same day. For large volume (>1.5 liter) liposuction, an overnight stay for observation may be required to monitor blood pressure and fluid balance. Liposuction generally takes between one to four hours, depending on the particular area, size of the area, type of anesthesia, and the technique used.

After a sterile preparation and draping with sterile barriers, the surgeon makes a small "buttonhole" incision near the area where fat is to be removed; for example, for *submental* liposuction, the tiny stab incisions are placed behind the ear and one is placed just beneath the chin; for liposuction of the arms, a tiny incision is made near the elbow and/or in the armpit crease. The surgeon manipulates the cannula under the skin to contour the desired result (Figure 27–22).

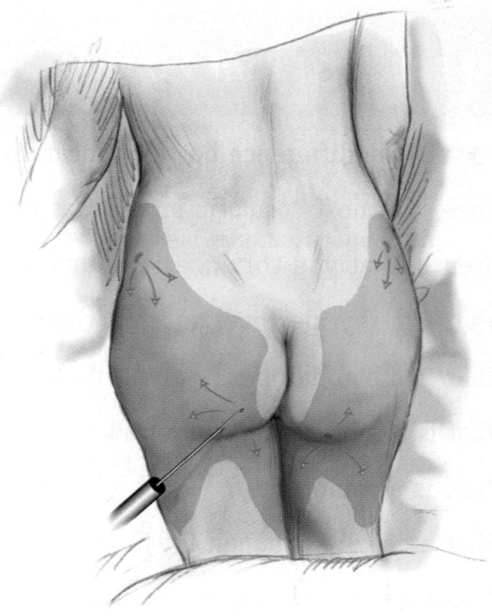

Figure 27–22 Common areas of liposuction.

In the early days of liposuction, no fluid was injected into the target area ("dry technique"). Today, suction-assisted lipectomy (SAL) is commonly done using the wet technique or without ultrasound-assisted liposuction (UAL). The surgeon's choice of technique is determined by a combination of factors, including the precise area to be treated, the amount of fat to be removed, and the surgeon's training, experience, and preference.

> **FYI**
>
> *Body contouring* refers to the group of aesthetic procedures used to change the body contour. It includes abdominoplasty or tummy tuck, brachioplasty, liposuction, thigh buttock-lift, reduction mammaplasty, and mastopexy (breast-lift).

The better the esthetician understands common surgical procedures, the better they will be able to answer questions that clients may ask when considering cosmetic surgery. We will also be better prepared to support clients who have these procedures done and to respect the healing processes involved. Estheticians working in a medical office may be an integral part of client education and pre- and postoperative care which we shall further discuss.

CHAPTER 28

THE ESTHETICIAN'S ROLE IN PRE- AND POST-MEDICAL TREATMENTS

CHAPTER OUTLINE

- PRE-MEDICAL OR LASER INTERVENTION PROCEDURES
- PRE-SURGICAL HOME CARE
- POST-PROCEDURE GUIDELINES
- WHEN TO REFER BACK TO THE PHYSICIAN

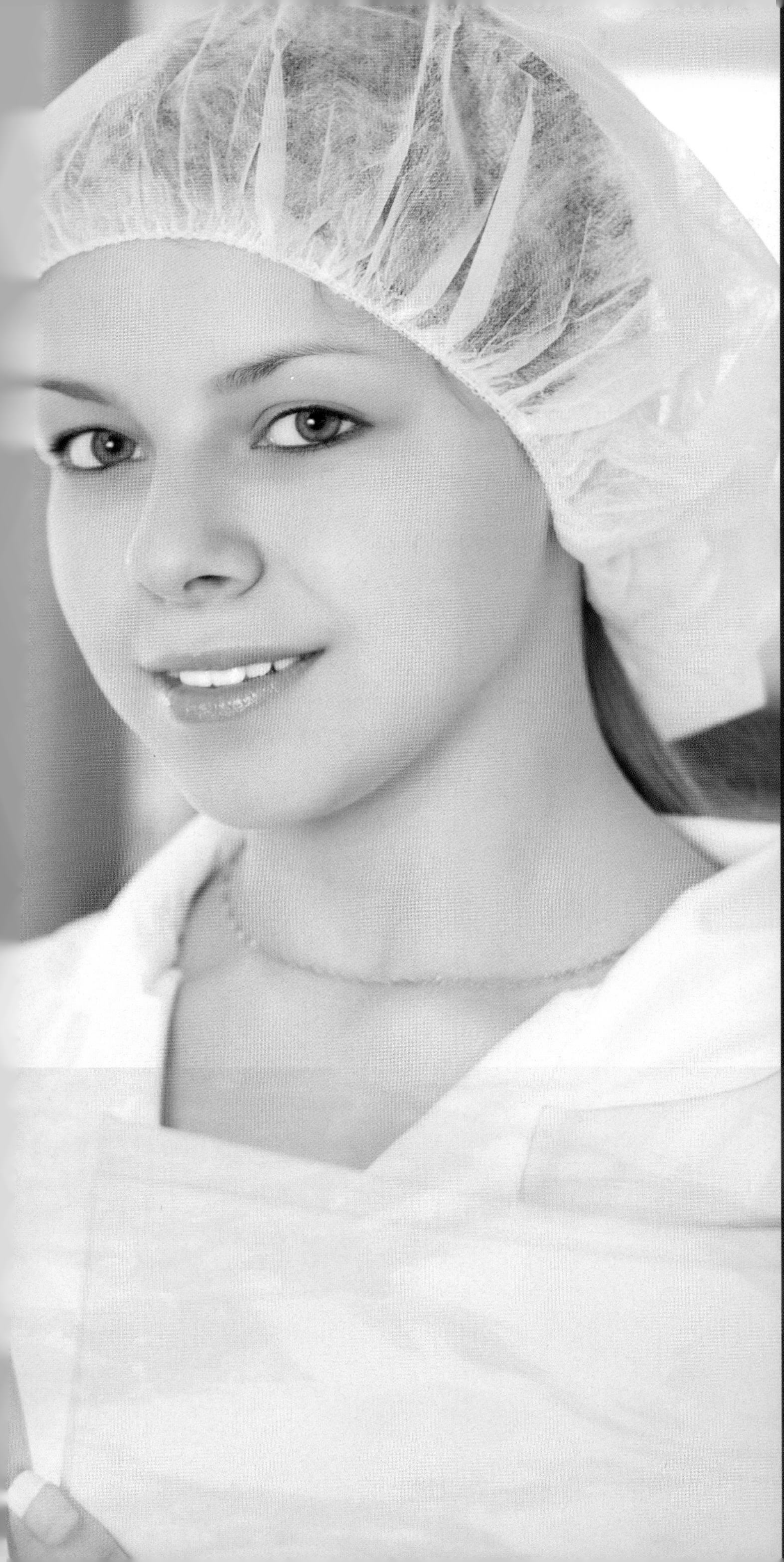

LEARNING OBJECTIVES

After completing this chapter, you should be able to:

- Name pre-procedures estheticians can perform to enhance surgical procedures and ablative laser procedures.
- Discuss home care products used before surgery.
- List post-medical procedure esthetic protocols.
- Discuss home care products used post-surgery.
- Decide when to refer the client back to the physician for care.

KEY TERMS

Page numbers indicate where in the chapter the term is used.

ablative 736
allergic reaction 743
Aquaphor® 739
Arnica montana 741
chin/neck bra 743
collagen remodeling 735
collagen shrinkage 735
facial bra 741
Famvir® (famciclovir) 739
hydroquinone 738
laser resurfacing 735
liposuction 742
reepithelialization 739
Valtrex® (valacyclovir hydrochloride) 739
Zithromax Z Pak® (azithromycin) 739

Many clients choose ablative laser procedures performed by a physician, including **laser resurfacing**, laser peels, and laser fractional resurfacing. Laser procedures result in biological and physiological reactions to the skin with immediate erythema, edema, crusting, and/or scabbing. Other results include **collagen shrinkage**, (the breakdown of collagen fibers when exposed to heat), **collogen remodeling**, (the rebuilding and strengthening of fibers during the healing process) and, ultimately, the improvement of skin tone and texture.

Under the direction of the physician, you can play a major role in a client's care, both before and after a medical procedure, ultimately improving the client's skin with your services and knowledge of home care products. For a client to obtain the best results from any surgical intervention or ablative laser procedure, his or her skin needs to be in the best possible condition before the procedure is performed. The better the condition of the skin, the better the results from a medical intervention. After a procedure, you can help clients adhere to medical intervention guidelines to minimize the risk of infection and maximize the client's outcome.

During this time, you can also offer assistance in product selection for home care products, using your knowledge of these products to steer a client to what will work best for him or her, and minimizing skin reactions for the most sensitive clients. Above all, you need to know when to move forward and when to refer the client back to his or her doctor for counseling or medical assistance.

FYI

When speaking with medical professionals regarding a person under their care, it is most appropriate to use the term *patient* to identify that person. When speaking about a person who is not under a physician's care but instead comes to your place of business for esthetic services, that person is a *client*.

PRE-MEDICAL OR LASER INTERVENTION PROCEDURES

Before a client undergoes a medical or ablative laser procedure, you can provide treatments and advice that will help the client get the most from that investment. These pre-medical and/or laser treatments give you the opportunity to counsel the client on the importance of post-procedure skin care and long-term skin maintenance.

FYI

An ablative procedure, such as a resurfacing procedure, is one that disrupts the epidermis and/or dermis.

Eight weeks before a client has any surgery or ablative procedure, you can begin a treatment plan for the client that will change and adapt to his or her needs. The client's skin type, level of photoaging, and physician protocol will determine the plan that you follow. You may use one type of treatment or a combination of treatment protocols, depending on the client's skin assessment and what you feel may be the best treatment plan to achieve your goals for his or her skin.

In-medical office or clinic treatments include classical cleansing facials, superficial chemical peels, microdermabrasion, ultrasonic, microcurrent facial toning, or enzyme peels. Be sure to conduct a thorough consultation with the client before starting any treatments (Figure 28–1). You can include additional protocols based on the physician's guidelines. For example, manual lymph drainage can be very beneficial to stimulate circulation, remove wastes, and minimize swelling. In-clinic treatments should be done weekly or as protocols for the specific service are recommended (Figure 28–2). As this client may be nervous or apprehensive about his or her upcoming procedure and may have a difficult time concentrating on detailed information, make sure to send the client home with written information. Reassure him or her that it is normal to be anxious, nervous, or worried and recommend conveying these concerns to the doctor.

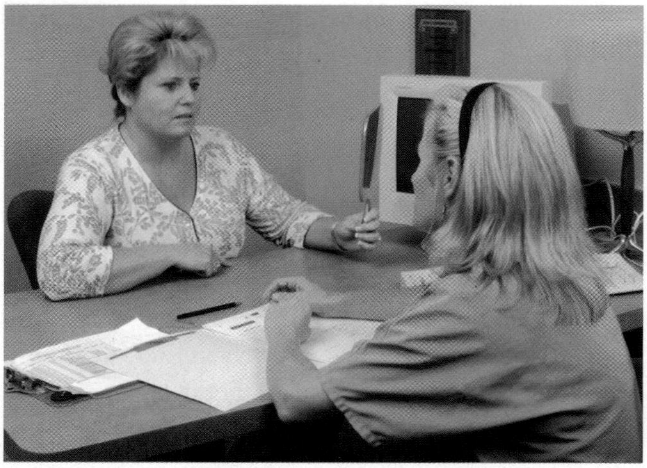

Figure 28–1 Esthetician counseling client.

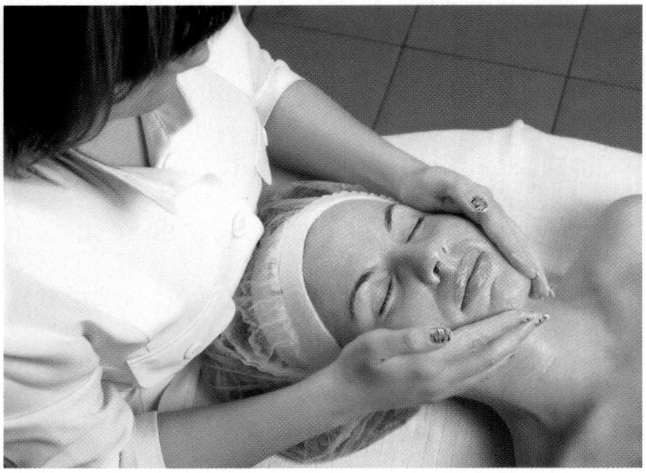

Figure 28–2 Client enjoying a facial pre-treatment.

Superficial Chemical Peels

These peels include AHA, BHA, retinoic acid, or Jessner's; select a peel starting with the lowest concentration and gradually increase in strength as the client tolerates. These treatments help to stimulate the home care program by exfoliating the upper layers of the epidermis and serve as an additional skin-lightening measure. Make sure the client stops using home care AHAs, retinoic acid, or scrubs two to three days before and for three to five days after a peel, depending on its strength. Follow manufacturer's guidelines and avoid being too aggressive, which may result in traumatizing the skin. This is your time to use your experience, education, and critical thinking skills to improve the client's skin; with your help, his or her skin can become progressively better in tone and texture and the client will not have to deal with possible side effects or complications of any procedure.

REGULATORY AGENCY ALERT

If you are not working under a physician's supervision, use only those acids that are within your scope of practice. Know your state regulations on this point.

Microdermabrasion

Microdermabrasion is an alternative to chemical peels, especially on strong, oily, thick skin that has had extreme sun exposure. Make certain that the client stops using AHAs, BHAs, scrubs, or retinols two to three days prior to and two to three days following a microdermabrasion treatment. Whether you use a crystal or non-crystal device machine, use power and pressure settings appropriate for the skin and follow your manufacturer's guidelines for the number of passes to be made. Do not irritate the skin more than is necessary.

CAUTION!

On clients with sensitive or irritated skin, such as those who have rosacea or those with extensive couperosity.

FOCUS ON: *Preparing for Microdermabrasion*

Make sure the client stops using AHA, BHA, scrubs, or retinoic acid 2 to 3 days prior to and following a microdermabrasion treatment.

Enzyme Peels

Enzymes such as papain, bromelin, trypsine, or blends of these dissolve keratin, thereby softening and aiding in the hydration of the skin. Papaya is the gentlest of these and is often used on very sensitive skin. Follow manufacturer guidelines for product selection based on skin type. Some of these formulas are more aggressive than others so it is important to know your product and the skin type for which it is most effective.

Ultrasonic

The gentle hydrating as well as exfoliating benefits of this treatment make it particularly suited to pre-surgical treatments. For thin, more delicate skin, ultrasonic treatments are less irritating and aggressive than microdermabrasion. Once the cavitation (peeling) step is completed, sonophoresis is an excellent choice to penetrate serums or skin-brightening agents. If your device incorporates micro-amp, then this heightens the service by working for skin homeostasis. Depending on the enzymes that you use and the type of ultrasonic device that you have, the option of performing an enzyme exfoliation first and then incorporating ultrasonic sonophoresis becomes an alternative. Or you can perform microdermabrasion and then incorporate the sonophoresis and microcurrent aspects of the ultrasonic. Iontophoresis may also be used in place of sonophoresis. Appropriate integration of modalities can enhance options for client treatment.

Microcurrent Facial Toning

The muscle strengthening aspects of this treatment can be intermixed with other treatments to help condition and tone the skin prior to surgical or laser intervention (Figure 28–3). Follow manufacturer guidelines for frequency and information on how to incorporate this treatment with others. The toning achieved can work well to enhance surgical procedures because the facial infrastructure is in better condition. For long-term enhancement of surgical lifting, once the client is healed after surgery, you can resume toning treatments. Keep in mind that initially you will need to see the client at least twice weekly, and after that you can follow manufacturer's guidelines for maintenance.

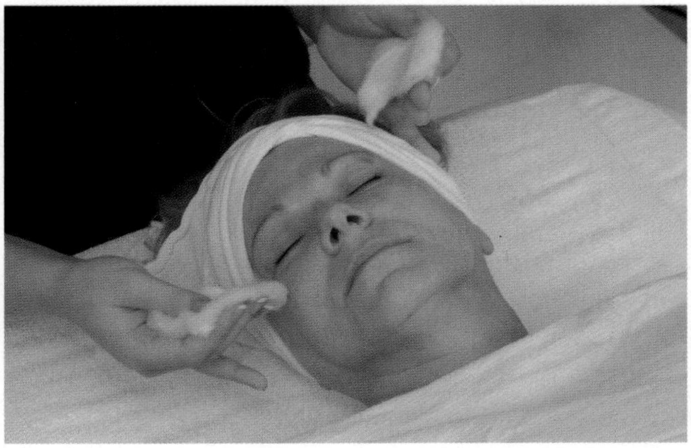

Figure 28–3 Client enjoying pre-treatment facial toning.

Lymph Drainage

Lymph drainage is used both pre- and postoperatively to stimulate the movement of fluid in the connective tissues, therefore reducing inflammation and increasing relaxation. In addition to draining lymphatic fluids from the area, the treatment emulates a wave-like sensation, which soothes muscle tension and the nervous system and creates a deep relaxation not present in other types of massage or treatments. For facial surgical procedures, ask the physician for guidelines about incorporating manual lymph drainage. Often this is done two weeks before the procedure as part of another treatment or as a biweekly stand-alone treatment. These treatments should be spaced two to three days apart. In most cases, lymph drainage speeds recovery time for post-surgery trauma by reducing edema and increasing healing tissue synthesis.

? Did You Know

Manual lymph drainage gives the client a deep relaxation not offered by other types of massage.

3 Days Pre-op

The last pre-surgical treatment should be a soothing, hydrating facial treatment using cool steam, high-frequency, light-to-little standard massage, lymphatic drainage massage, and sunscreen. At this point, the client's skin is conditioned and ready for their scheduled procedure. You do not want the skin to be overly sensitive on the day of surgery. This is an opportunity to be encouraging, comforting, and supportive to what may be a very nervous client. He or she may enjoy (and need) a soothing hand or foot treatment to aid relaxation.

PRE-SURGICAL HOME CARE

Many times the doctor may have a kit of products for the client to use before surgery or a laser procedure. The client usually starts using the products in this kit about eight weeks in advance. Regimes for both preoperative surgery and pre-laser treatments are similar; the key difference is the addition of **hydroquinone,** a skin lightening agent, for some laser treatments.

Pre-Laser Home Care

Pre-laser products focus more intensively on exfoliation. Advise the client when to discontinue the use of acids as to not compromise the pre-surgical treatments that are to be performed in-clinic.

Pre-laser home care kits include:
- **AHAs and or BHAs for exfoliation**
- **Hydroquinone or other skin-lightening agents**
- **Hydrating moisturizer with amino acids**
- **Tretinoin/retinoic acid, vitamin A derivatives**
- **Environmental protection/sunscreen containing an SPF of at least 30 and physical as well as chemical sunscreens**

Following are typical routines for using the home care products in a pre-laser skin care kit:

A.M.
1. Cleanser
2. Lightener (avoid eye area)
3. Moisturizer
4. Sunscreen

P.M.
1. Cleanser
2. Lightener (avoid eye area)
3. Retinoic acid
4. Moisturizer

Preoperative Home Care

As with laser-resurfacing or other cosmetic procedure, the client will tolerate the post-surgical phase much better if his or her skin is in optimum condition. If the client is having a combination of procedures—such as a face-lift and laser resurfacing—you need to combine both treatment plans. Depending on skin type and classification, clients need to use, at a minimum, products designed to exfoliate, hydrate, condition, and protect.

Pre-surgery home care kits include:
- **Cleansers: AHA, BHA, or enzymes for exfoliation; chamomile or allantoin for soothing**
- **Exfoliators: AHA, BHA, vitamin A derivatives, enzymes**
- **Hydrators/moisturizers: amino acids, hyaluronic acid, bioflavinoids, green tea, vitamins C and E**
- **Eye cream: amino acids; peptides; vitamins A, E, C; arnica; sodium hyaluronate**
- **Sunscreen: UVA and UVB protection with an SPF of at least 30**

Following are typical routines for using the home care products in a pre-surgical skin care kit:

A.M.
1. Cleanser
2. Exfoliant
3. Hydrator/moisturizer (may combine exfoliants in this step)
4. Sunscreen

P.M.
1. Cleanser
2. Exfoliator
3. Hydrator/moisturizer

POST-PROCEDURE GUIDELINES

Post procedure in-clinic protocols vary slightly between post-laser and post-surgery clients. It is very important that you do not perform any treatments without the physician's approval. Resume routine facials only when the client has been released from the physician's care.

CAUTION!

Perform post-procedure treatments only with a physician's consent.

After CO_2/Erbium Nd:YAG Laser Resurfacing

Each physician's home care guidelines vary for patients who have had laser resurfacing procedures (Figure 28–4). Physicians provide their patients with kits for home use and dictate the use and application of those home care products based on research and preferences. It is important that clients adhere to the guidelines. General post-laser guidelines include:

- Days one to five after the procedure: The physician will initially apply a specialized dressing (for example, Silon®, Flexan®, or Spenco Second Skin®) to promote wound healing. The doctor then uses petroleum or a water-based ointment, **Aquaphor®**, on unaffected areas, such as lips, and around the eye area. If the dressing falls off at home, the patient may need to have it replaced and should call the physician. The patient should continue taking prescribed antibiotics, such as, **Zithromax Z Pak®** a broad spectrum antibiotic, or Keflex®, and an antiviral medication, such as **Famvir®** or **Valtrex®**, as directed.

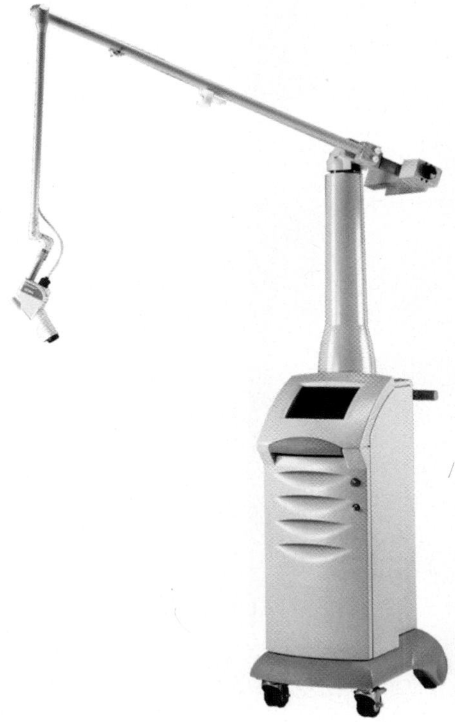

Figure 28–4 CO_2 laser. Courtesy of Lumenis® Ltd.

CAUTION!

The client's skin is extremely delicate and needs to be treated very gently after laser resurfacing procedures.

Applying ice packs or a bag of frozen peas on the site is instrumental in reducing post-resurfacing swelling and discomfort. **Reepithelialization**, the regrowth of the skin occurs anywhere from three to four days and up to seven to fourteen days. The patient's skin can easily be traumatized during this process. Your role is one of hand-holder and support during this time.

- Days five to ten after the procedure: Once the physician removes the dressing, the patient should begin to apply solution soaks (usually 1 teaspoon vinegar to 1 cup of water) every two to three hours as the physician indicates. This is followed by an application of petroleum or water-based ointment, Aquaphor. Keep the skin well lubricated. The skin *must not* dry out! During this period of reepithelialization, clients have a tendency to bruise easily and skin may even peel (Figure 28–5a and b). Any sign of a edema, oozing, rash, pimples, eruptions, and/or fever needs to be reported to a physician immediately, as these may be signs of an infection.
- Days 10 to 30 after the procedure: Your client should continue with home care products using dense hydrating moisturizers, and peptide creams. Erythema or intense redness can remain up to two to three months after laser treatments. This is the time to incorporate mineral powder makeup as camouflage therapy. The use of protective sunscreen is mandatory with an SPF of at least 30 to prevent hyperpigmentation or other side effects.
- One month post-laser: The physician may direct your client to have a light AHA or enzyme exfoliation, which most patients can tolerate. Often the skin is still peeling and this product may further the healing. All treatments for three to six months should focus on

CAUTION!

Do not use microdermabrasion or glycolic, salicylic, lactic, or other acid or exfoliating technique on a post-laser client until the physician gives approval.

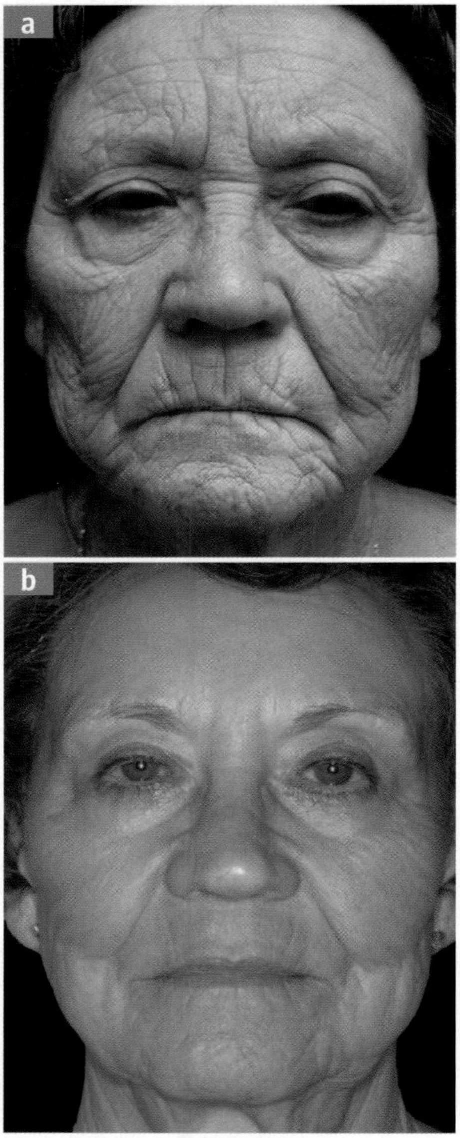

Figure 28–5 Client pre- and post-CO_2 laser. Courtesy of Lumenis® Ltd.

hydrating and soothing. Avoid using warm steam on a post-laser client.

Post-Surgical Procedures

Post-procedure guidelines depend on the procedure being performed. Many times multiple procedures are performed simultaneously or consecutively. This will dictate what home and in-clinic care will be recommended. The safest guide is to follow physician's directions and to ask questions if standard protocols seem to be contraindicated for your specific client. Never perform services unless or until approved by the physician. For example, the physician may approve camouflage makeup but not facial services. It is best to get releases for services in writing.

FOCUS ON: *Doctor's Orders*

Every client and every procedure are different. Always follow the doctor's guidelines and recommendations for post-surgical procedures.

Rhytidectomy or Face-lift

Face-lift (Figure 28–6a and b) or forehead-lift postoperative guidelines call for rest and adherence to physician's directions. Following are more specific guidelines that a physician might give a patient:

- One week after surgery: The patient should rest at home and take Tylenol or prescriptive narcotics for pain. He or she can use ice packs intermittently to reduce

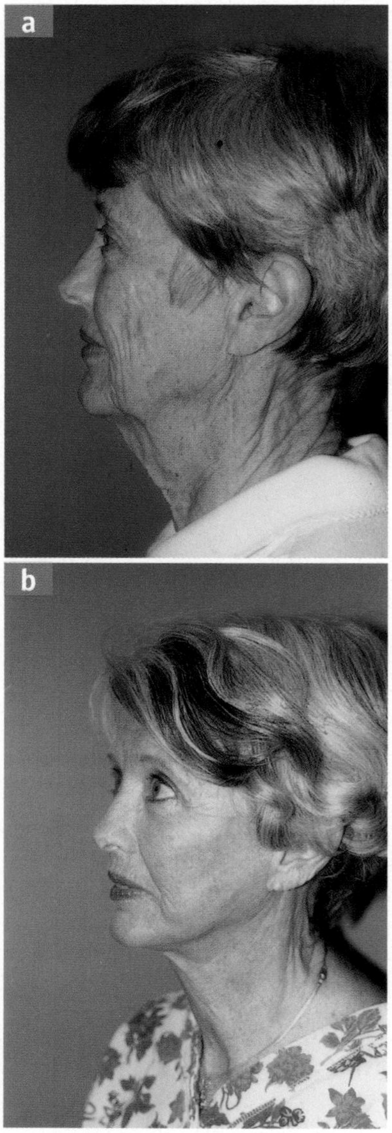

Figure 28–6 Client pre- and post-face-lift.

post-surgical swelling. The patient should keep jaw movement at a minimum by taking liquid meals through a straw. The patient can cleanse using a warm, soft cloth on all unbandaged areas as well as a light, hydrating moisturizer. The physician will see the patient two to three days after surgery. If drains have been used, the physician will remove them and replace bandages with a **facial bra** to enhance healing of newly placed skin, muscles, and nerves (Figure 28–7). Some physicians incorporate the use of **Arnica montana,** a natural herbal remedy taken three to five days before and up to two weeks following surgical procedures to reduce the amount and duration of bruising.

- Days 8 to 15 after surgery: The patient should follow a gentle cleansing regimen, avoiding all suture and staple sites. He or she should cleanse these sites with a hydrogen peroxide and water solution followed with an antibiotic ointment. The patient can apply moisturizer and sunscreen with a minimum SPF of at least 30 daily, avoiding all suture and staple sites. During this time, the patient will see medical professionals (the doctor or nurse) for removal of sutures and staples. The physician may direct you, the esthetician, to perform manual lymph drainage to reduce swelling and camouflage with mineral powder foundation to hide skin discolorations.
- Two weeks after surgery: The client should continue home care and can apply camouflage makeup. He or she may be advised to apply a scar-management product to reduce inflammation and prevent formation of keloid scaring.

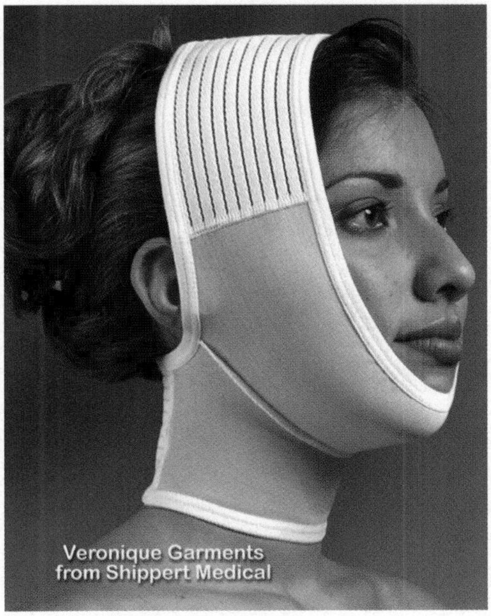

Figure 28–7 A facial bra.

CAUTION!

Advise your client to avoid touching or applying a substance to any suture or staple sites following surgery.

Silicone scar tapes and liquid preparations are also used for scar management. You may continue manual lymph drainage twice weekly and may apply a soothing, non-drying, hydrating facial mask. Clients often need some exfoliation, and gentle forms of enzymes are the product of choice. Avoid use of hot steam or hot towels as the skin will be more sensitive. If the client experiences any stinging, remove the enzyme and apply cool, wet towels. Avoid chemical peels, microdermabrasion, heat/steam, or any stimulating treatments at this point.

- Three weeks or more after surgery: Most clients can return to their pre-surgery home care regimen. They can now use AHAs, BHAs, antioxidants, hydrating moisturizers and sunscreens. In the clinic, many clients will still feel some numbness located near or at incision sites. You can apply manual lymph drainage as a part of a routine facial treatment to facilitate healing. The client should continue scheduling in-office follow-up appointments with the physician over the next six months to evaluate skin tightening, wound healing, and the client's final outcome.

Blepharoplasty

Blepharoplasty procedures, or eye lifts, heal quickly compared to other procedures, although the client may have some issues with dry eyes and/or bruising (Figure 28–8a–d).

- Days one to seven after surgery: The patient should rest and apply prescribed eye drops or ointment as indicated by the physician. He or she can use ice packs intermittently to reduce post-surgical swelling and apply topical antibiotic at the suture site if directed by the physician. The patient can take Tylenol or other prescriptive medication for pain as directed. The nurse or physician will remove sutures in 5 to 10 days. The physician may suggest that the patient take Arnica montana, a homeopathic remedy two to three days before and up to two weeks after any surgical procedure to reduce the amount and duration of bruising. If a laser procedure was also performed on the lower lids, the physician will remove bandages or dressings at day five if they have not fallen off. The physician will tell the patient to apply post-laser soaks and then to keep the area well lubricated with petroleum or a water-based ointment, such as Aquaphor.

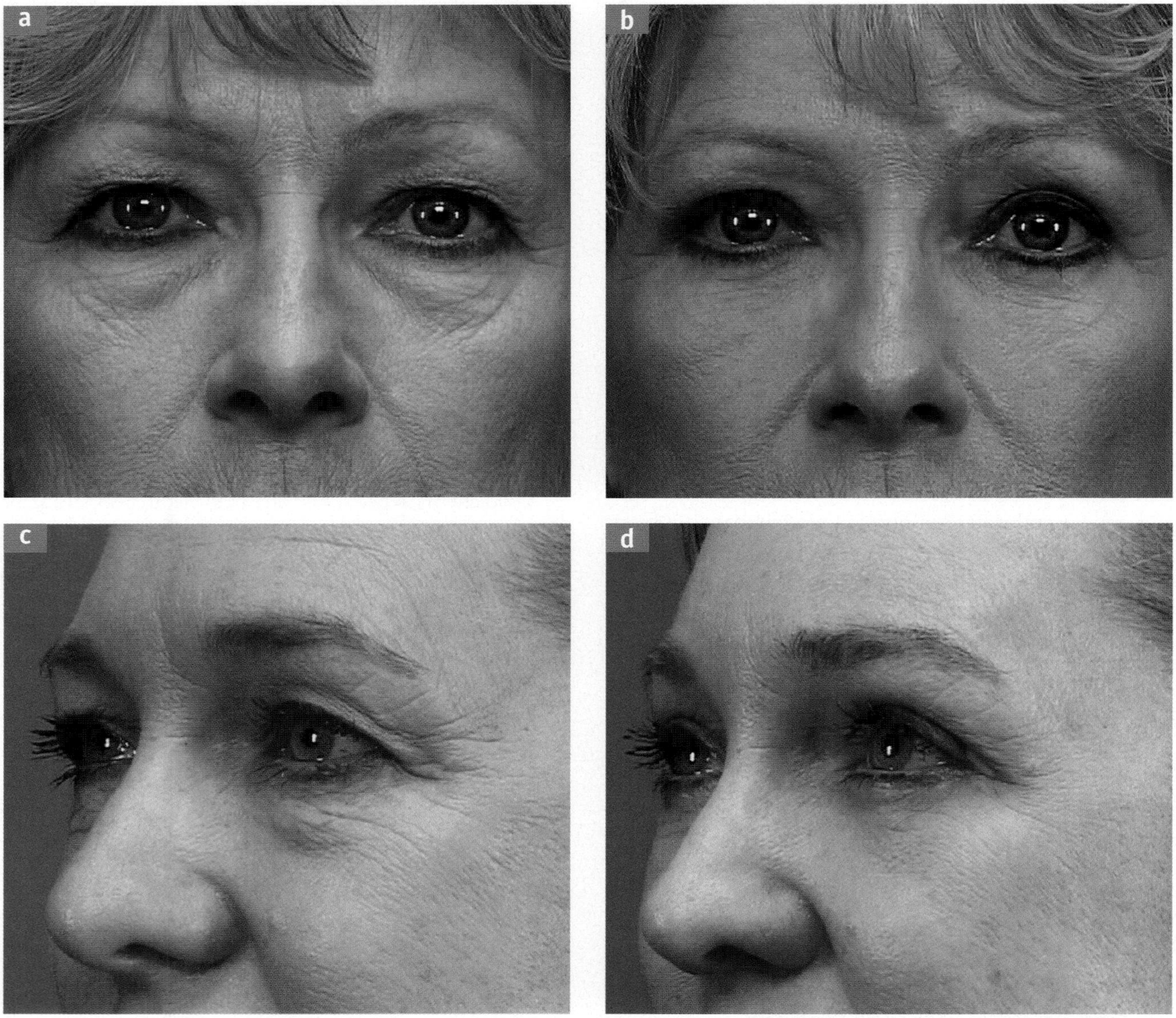

Figure 28–8 Client pre- and post-blepharoplasty.

- Days 7 to 12 after surgery: If the patient also had laser surgery, he or she will be instructed to follow the protocol for using the laser kit items (hydrocortisone, squalene, or peptide cream and sunscreen). If indicated by the physician, light camouflage mineral-based makeup may be applied. An in-office follow-up visit is generally scheduled with the physician.
- Two to three weeks after surgery: At this point the client may return to using hydrating eye cream as before surgery and continue camouflage makeup. As long as the client did not have a laser procedure, you may employ manual lymph drainage and then apply a hydrating/soothing eye mask as a complement to a routine facial treatment.
- Two to six months after surgery: The client should see his or her physician at intermittent follow-up appointments during these months so that the doctor can evaluate suture lines and the final appearance of the upper and /or lower lids.

Jowl/Neck/Chin Liposuction

Clients undergoing **liposuction** experience quick healing with a short recovery period (Figure 28–9). Bruising and swelling are the most common side effects.

- One to three days after surgery: The patient should rest at home to reduce any swelling or edema from the procedure. He or she must wear a **chin/neck bra**,

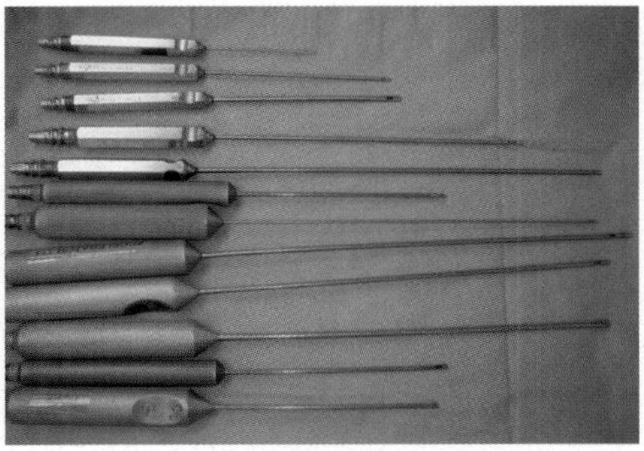

Figure 28–9 Liposuction cannula and machine.

a supportive device that must be worn continuously for the first 48 to 72 hours to enhance healing of the skin and reduce bleeding. Tylenol or prescriptive narcotics may be taken for pain as ordered by the physician. The client should make an appointment with the physician two to three days after surgery. If suitable, the client can take Arnica montana four to five days before and up to two weeks after any surgical procedure to reduce the amount and duration of bruising.

- Day four to four weeks after surgery: The client should follow a gentle cleansing regimen as the wound heals, cleaning these sites with a solution of water and gentle soap followed with an antibiotic ointment. He or she can apply moisturizer, avoiding suture and staple sites. The client should wear a facial bra as much as possible at home and at bed time. The physician may ask a client to perform mild massage to the neck area to reduce any lumps or skin texture irregularities after liposuction. Or the physician may ask you to perform manual lymph drainage to reduce post-procedure swelling. If ordered by the physician, you can apply light camouflage mineral-based makeup to reduce the discoloration from the post-procedure bruising.
- Four weeks and more after surgery: Most clients can return to their normal home care regimen. They can now use AHAs, BHAs, antioxidants, hydrating moisturizers, and sunscreens. Clients may still feel some numbness located near or at incision sites. The client should see his or her physician at intermittent follow-up appointments during these months so that the doctor can to evaluate the overall tightening of the neck and jaw line.

WHEN TO REFER BACK TO THE PHYSICIAN

You need to be able to recognize signs of a wound that is not healing properly. Any time a client exhibits unexpected redness, skin eruptions, edema, or oozing—with or without a fever—you should immediately refer that client to his or her physician for evaluation. Also, patients can have contact dermatitis, a response to topical agents or an **allergic reaction,** an acquired response to environemtal substances such as topical skin preparations, tape, or ointments. If any of these indicators are present, do not perform any procedures without a physician's approval. The most critical time for infection is the first few days after surgery or resurfacing, and the patient should be under direct physician care at that point. However, delayed complications can occur, and you need to be vigilant to protect your client's health.

As with all procedures, strict adherence to pre- and post-operative protocols defines the eventual outcome. You, the esthetician, become the client educator, coach, and liaison with the physician and thus have a great opportunity to enhance the effectiveness of surgical and laser procedures. You can give your client the much-needed support before, during, and after a procedure. The cycle continues as the patient again becomes the client and resumes routine visits for education, products, and treatments.

REVIEW QUESTIONS

1. What types of laser procedures are ablative?
2. Collagen shrinkage occurs at the end of which procedures?
3. What drug might be recommended to reduce hyperpigmentation?
4. What are two common antiviral medications that physicians may order preoperatively?

REVIEW QUESTIONS

5. When does reepithelialization occur after laser resurfacing?
6. Esthetician care post-face-lift includes which measures?
7. How long should the chin/face bra be worn after liposuction?
8. What is a common procedure performed after surgery to reduce swelling and edema?
9. When should the esthetician refer the client back to a physician?

CHAPTER GLOSSARY

ablative: in surgical uses it refers to the ability to surgically cut or remove using a laser.

allergic reaction: an abnormal reaction and hypersensitivity to topical or oral substances that are ordinarily harmless. Signs and symptoms include hives, swelling, rash, and skin eruptions and can progress to respiratory distress.

Aquaphor®: a water-soluble, bland emollient ointment.

Arnica montana: mountain plant (also known as *leopard's bane*) found in the Alps; a homeopathic herb known for speeding the post-operative recovery process, reducing uncomfortable swelling and bruising, and, often, post-operative pain.

chin/neck bra: a supportive device worn after surgery of the chin or neck area.

collagen remodeling: an increase of new collagen deposits within the dermis caused by thermal heating from a laser system.

collagen shrinkage: thermal heating from a laser system can break down the collagen bonds and structures leading to shrinkage and contraction of the dermis by 20% to 30%.

facial bra: protective bandage worn around one's chin and neck after face lifts and liposuction procedures.

Famvir® (famciclovir): antiviral medication that can stop or shorten a recurrent herpes simplex outbreak.

hydroquinone: a topical medication that is used for bleaching or reducing excessive melanin lesions in the epidermis.

laser resurfacing: a laser procedure utilizing the CO_2 or Erbium laser that involves vaporization of the epidermis and/or dermis for facial rejuvenation; used to smooth wrinkles or lighten acne scars and stimulate growth of new collagen.

liposuction: a surgical procedure used for the removal of stubborn areas of fat.

reepithelialization: the formation of new epidermis and dermis over an area of injury. The epithelial cells from the wound margin and the philosebaceous units migrating to repair damage.

Valtrex® (valacyclovir hydrochloride): antiviral medication that can stop or shorten a recurrent outbreak of herpes simplex.

Zithromax Z Pak® (azithromycin): wide-spectrum antibiotic that is derived from erythromycin. It is highly effective against Staphylococcus aureus, bacteria frequently living on the skin or in the nose of a healthy person, which can cause a wide range of skin infections.

PART 7

BUSINESS SKILLS

Chapter 29 Financial Business Skills
Chapter 30 Marketing

CHAPTER OUTLINE

- CALCULATING BUSINESS RISK
- THE BUSINESS PLAN
- FINANCIAL PLANNING
- PROTECTING BUSINESS ASSETS
- EMPLOYEE COMPENSATION
- UNDERSTANDING THE IRS

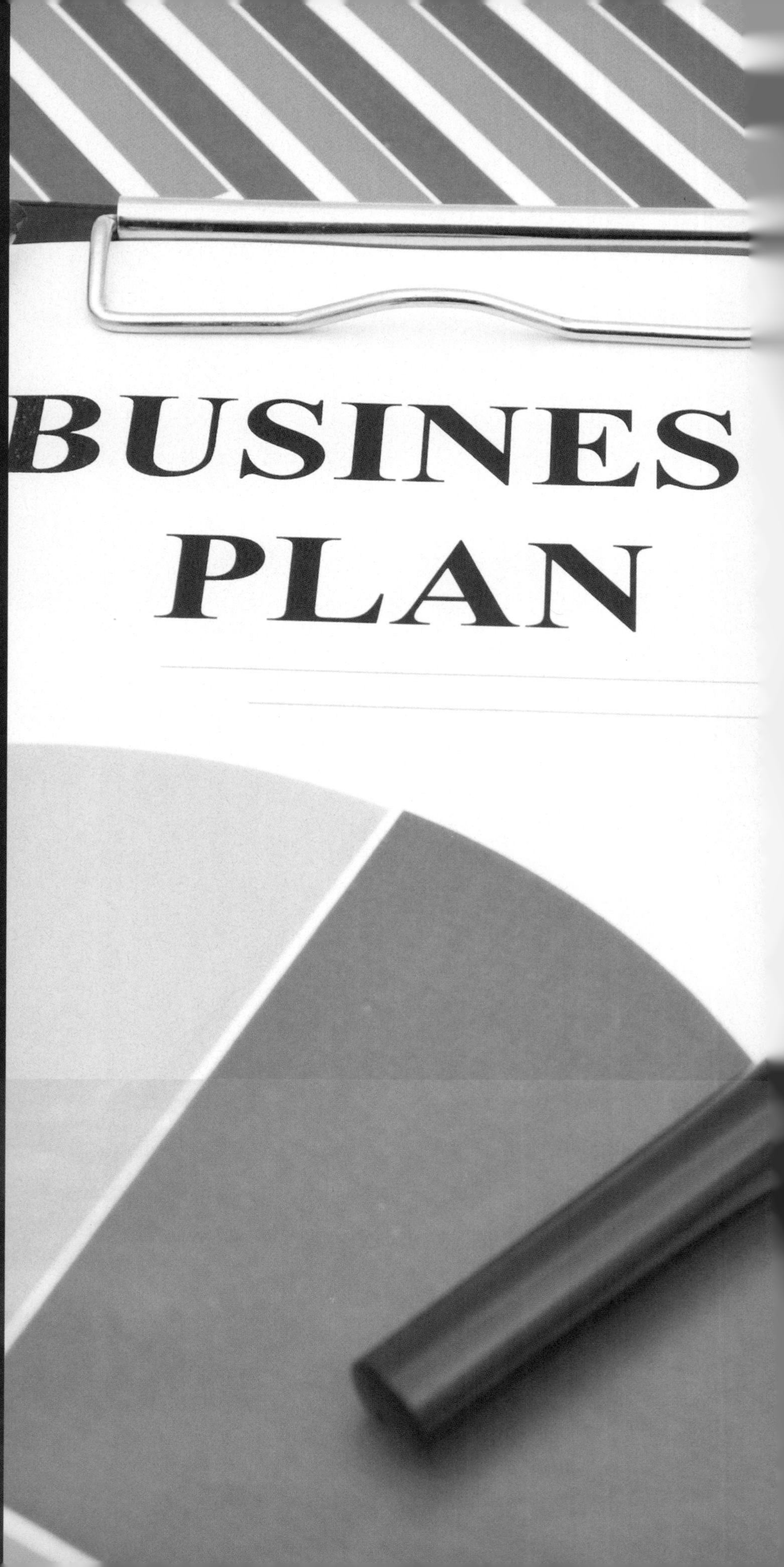

CHAPTER 29

FINANCIAL BUSINESS SKILLS

LEARNING OBJECTIVES

After completing this chapter, you should be able to:

- Discuss the risks involved in business ownership.
- Explain the importance of drafting a business plan.
- Describe several methods that can be used to finance a business.
- List the main financial tools used to track business.
- Explain why insurance is important to the small business owner.
- List the primary methods of compensation used in the skin care industry.
- Explain the importance of understanding IRS guidelines.

KEY TERMS

Page numbers indicate where in the chapter the term is used.

assets 752
balance sheet 752
break-even analysis 752
business plan 749
capital 751
cash flow statement 752
costs of goods sold 752
Employer Identification Number (EIN) 756
Federal Unemployment Tax 758
generally accepted accounting principles (GAAP) 752
gross profit 752
income statement 752
independent contractor 755
Individual Tax Identification Number (ITIN) 756
insurance 754
liabilities 752
net profit 752
owner's equity 752
promissory note 751
resale tax 761
risk 749
risk management 753
self-employment tax 759
Social Security Number 756
venture capitalists 751

Are you someone who has always dreamed of owning your own business? Perhaps you chose a career in esthetics with just that idea in mind. If so, you are not alone. Many enter the field of esthetics with the goal of one day opening their own business. Skin care is an exciting industry that is emotionally gratifying and financially rewarding. It is also one that has become fiercely competitive.

In the last two decades the business of skin care has expanded into a variety of new business models that include salons, spas, fitness facilities, medical aesthetic practices, and wellness centers. There are countless variations on these themes, but to compete in this new environment one thing is absolutely certain: You need excellent business and financial management skills.

CALCULATING BUSINESS RISK

When you think about taking risks, you probably think of outrageously dangerous behaviors, like sky diving, gambling, or car racing. But the truth is there is risk involved in just about everything you do. **Risk** refers to the chance of incurring some type of harm, damage, or loss. Fortunately, this does not prevent most of us from engaging in everyday tasks, such as walking the dog or driving to work. However, the ability to take risks has new meaning when you invest heart, soul, and finances to start your own business.

When it comes to starting a business, risk involves very careful consideration of one's ability to put forth their time, energy, and money with no guarantee of the return. If you have an entrepreneurial spirit, these risks may come naturally to you, but you should not take them lightly. It would be foolish to move forward without carefully weighing the many pros and cons of owning and operating a business.

Before you decide to open your own business, take the time to examine industry trends, analyze the competition, and study economic conditions. Developing strong critical thinking skills before becoming a salon or spa owner will better prepare you to make the many business decisions that you will face down the road.

THE BUSINESS PLAN

Prospective business owners use a basic tool called a **business plan** to help them develop a plan of action and hopefully avoid many of the risk factors and stumbling blocks associated with business failure, including a lack of sufficient capital or managerial experience. A good business plan maps out a complete strategy for how a business will operate. It should include several important categories: an executive summary, a marketing plan, a strategic design and development plan, an operations plan, and, most importantly, a solid financial plan.

Here's a Tip

If you think a business plan is unnecessary, think again. Poor planning is one of the top reasons for business failure.

If you have a strong business background, tackling the outline presented in Figure 29–1 may come easy, but not all estheticians enter the field with the knowledge required to write a business plan. Do not be discouraged; even those with business experience may have the need to gather additional support. Fortunately, there are numerous resources available to the small business owner. Search the Internet or visit your local library and you will find entire texts, journals, and software programs devoted exclusively to the subject of business planning. These tools are helpful for those who wish to tackle this project themselves, but a word of caution: Even if you consider yourself someone who is capable of writing a business plan, it is wise to employ professional help in areas where you lack actual experience.

The expert advice of a small business consultant, accountant, or marketing specialist can be invaluable in developing a plan of action that will virtually walk you through each process step by step. While hiring outside help comes at a cost, the knowledge gained at the beginning of your entrepreneurial journey is generally well worth the initial investment and is likely to save you a great deal of time and money in the long run.

Executive Summary

This section of your business plan should provide the reader with a complete overview of your entire strategy.

Here's a Tip

When developing a business plan, it is important to address each category in detail. Each of the main components in the business plan outline should answer *who, what, where, when,* and *how* you will carry out each facet of your plan. As you begin this task, remember to keep your audience in mind. This is particularly important when it comes to finances, especially if you intend to use your business plan to make a case for borrowing money.

I. Executive Summary
  - **a.** Name, nature, and location of your business
  - **b.** The business structure you will use to operate your business—for example, a Sole Proprietorship, Partnership, Corporation, or Limited Liability Company
  - **c.** A summary of all of the main categories of your plan

II. Marketing Strategy
  - **a.** Current economic conditions
  - **b.** Target market
  - **c.** A competitive analysis
  - **d.** Unique selling proposition
  - **e.** The methods you will use to promote your business, such as advertising, publicity, public relations, direct marketing, sales promotions, and personal selling

III. Strategic Design and Development
  - **a.** The physical layout of your facility
  - **b.** The four Ps: Product, Price, Promotion, and Place
  - **c.** A strategic value assessment
  - **d.** The suppliers and vendors you intend to use
  - **e.** Pricing and sales strategy for services and retail products
  - **f.** An analysis of your strengths, weaknesses, opportunities, and threats [SWOT Analysis]

IV. Operations
  - **a.** The day-to-day operational strategies you will use to conduct business in terms of the financial management, technological tools, and personnel you will employ
  - **b.** Key personnel and their roles
  - **c.** Policies and procedures for staff
  - **d.** Client policies
  - **e.** Methods of employee compensation
  - **f.** Salary levels and the rationale for each amount
  - **g.** Employee training and education
  - **h.** Resources for maintaining and protecting your business, such as a business attorney, accountant, insurance agent, human resource manager, and marketing or public relations manager

V. Financial Information
  - **a.** Initial start-up costs
  - **b.** Estimate of expenses for the first 3 years of operation
  - **c.** Balance sheet stating the initial assets, liabilities, and net worth of your business
  - **d.** A break-even analysis for retail products and services
  - **e.** 1- to 3-year projections, including financial statements for each year (balance sheets and income and cash flow statements)
  - **f.** Sources of capital, including personal funds and business loans
  - **g.** Use of all sources of capital
  - **h.** Plan for repaying all loans

VI. Conclusion

Figure 29–1 Business plan outline.

Be sure to identify the name and location of your business and provide enough information about your background to give the reader confidence that you can carry out your plan.

Marketing Plan

Chapter 30 of this text includes information on marketing strategies you can use for your business. Your marketing plan should take into account all of these marketing strategies and should clearly identify all of the methods you will use to develop brand recognition and promote business, such as advertising, public relations, publicity, sales promotions, direct marketing, and personal selling skills.

Strategic Design and Development Plan

Your strategic design should include a detailed account of the Four Ps: Product, Price, Promotion, and Place. (See Chapter 30 for a full discussion of the Four Ps.) A complete description of your facility and the products and services you will offer, along with realistic goals and objectives, is the key to executing an action-oriented plan. Think of strategic design as the nuts and bolts of your business plan. This is the step that will catapult you into action.

Operations Plan

The development of concrete administrative and organizational procedures, such as which accounting method your business will operate under; the technology that will be used to perform bookkeeping, track sales, and schedule appointments; and the name of the person who will be responsible for managing your skin care business are the heart of operations. Policies and procedures as they relate to two of the most important aspects of business operations, personnel and clients, are critical to this phase of development.

Financial Plan

Without a doubt, a solid financial management strategy is the single most important factor in any business plan; it is critical to those seeking additional funds to start their business. Many new business owners require help with this section, but any advisor is only as good as the information the business owner provides. Be prepared to provide your financial advisor with a detailed account of all of the expenses associated with start-up and maintenance, including the cost of products, equipment, supplies, furnishings, and so on.

Conclusion

Many business plans incorporate an ending or conclusion to summarize the business owner's goals. While this may seem redundant, it often helps both the writer and reader to clarify questions and identify information that may be missing or confusing.

FINANCIAL PLANNING

The first question any prospective business must answer is "Where will I get the money to start this business?" There are three primary sources for raising **capital**, or the amount of money you need to invest in your business. These include 1) your own savings, 2) loans, and 3) investors. Unless you are independently wealthy, chances are you will have a limited amount of funds to invest in your own business; however, you should expect to use those funds. While you may view this as a considerable handicap, consider that most lenders take the attitude that if you are not willing to take a risk on yourself, why should you expect others to do the same?

There are a variety of loans available to small business owners. These come with varying degrees of responsibility and finance charges, or interest rates that must be paid back on a regularly scheduled basis. To obtain such money, you need to qualify as a good risk. This generally includes an assessment of your personal financial rating, or credit score. If you decide to borrow money, you will also need to think about a plan for paying it back. Falling behind on loan payments can place your business in serious financial jeopardy.

Money contributed by outside investors or private individuals, such as **venture capitalists** and small business investment companies, generally comes in the form of an exchange or return on their investment, which in this case means a portion of your income. While this can be very appealing to the new business owner, keep in mind that venture capitalists generally want to exert some control over the way you conduct your business.

There may be other "angels" in your life, such as friends and family who are willing to invest in your business. If you decide to borrow from family members and friends, be sure to draft a **promissory note**, a legal document that clearly defines the terms of your loan agreement. There are other government-sponsored and private agencies that exist to help women and minorities start their own businesses. If you qualify, this is a viable path for additional resources.

FYI

The Small Business Administration (SBA) is an independent federal agency set up to help small business owners. The SBA is a valuable resource for those seeking financial and or business management advice, with links to a wealth of professional resources, such as the Service Core of Retired Executives (SCORE), Small Business Development Centers (SBDC), and the Small Business Training Network (SBTN), a virtual campus that provides online business courses to prospective entrepreneurs and small business owners. The SBA also plays an active role in helping both new and already existing small businesses raise capital, acting primarily as a guarantor for loans from private investors and other institutions. To learn more about qualifying for a loan from the SBA, visit its Web site at http://www.sba.gov.

Financial Tools

Once you have acquired the money needed to finance your business, you need to keep careful track of it. There are several tools designed to help you manage finances that your accountant can put in place for you. These include the balance sheet, income statement, and cash flow statement, all of which should be set up in accordance with **generally accepted accounting principles (GAAP),** or the standard procedures established by the accounting profession (Figure 29–2).

Technology

Because of the computer, managing day-to-day operations is no longer the tedious task it was in the past. Using computer software to perform ordinary bookkeeping and accounting tasks, such as tallying daily sales totals, generating profit and loss statements, tracking cash flow, paying bills, and calculating payroll is now commonplace.

In addition to basic bookkeeping and accounting tasks, many salons and spas are now using computer software to maintain employee schedules, perform sales transactions, manage payroll, and control inventory. With many convenient and affordable third-party vendors readily available, some skin care businesses are also using software to schedule client appointments and sell gift certificates and products online.

The Balance Sheet

The **balance sheet** provides a snapshot or overview of your business at a given point in time and is measured in terms of assets and liabilities. **Assets** are anything your business owns. **Liabilities** are the debt or monies your business owes to creditors. The balance sheet also shows the **owner's equity**, or what the owner's interest is in the assets of the company after all of the business' liabilities have been deducted; this is typically referred to as the *net worth of a business*. All of this information will help you to gain a clear picture of the overall health of your business.

The Income Statement

The **income statement,** also referred to as a profit and loss statement, takes a longer view of your financial picture. This statement reflects your revenues, or the total amount of money your business takes in from the sale of products and services, reported as your **gross profit** minus the **costs of goods sold**, or what it costs you to provide the products that you sell. To determine the real income or **net profit** of a business, you must subtract all of the expenses associated with operating your business.

The Cash Flow Statement

The **cash flow statement** provides a clear picture of how much money is flowing in and out of the business on a regular basis. Cash flow is usually calculated over the course of a year and is assessed in terms of its positive and negative value. Those businesses that are able to maintain a positive cash flow will have enough cash on hand to cover expenses. On the other hand, owners of businesses with a negative cash flow will have to borrow money to meet expenses. Continually borrowing money to meet expenses places the small business at risk. Naturally, most businesses strive to maintain a positive cash flow.

Break-Even Analysis

How many cleansers, toners, facials, and body treatments will you need to sell to cover all of the expenses associated with operating your business? This information is determined by the **break-even analysis**, or the point at which all costs are covered and your business begins to earn a profit.

Calculating the break-even point is a complex process when it comes to skin care, as this figure must be calculated separately for services and retail products. This can be a lengthy and arduous task and is best performed with the expert assistance of an accountant. You may be tempted to forego performing a break-even

ASSETS	LIABILITIES & OWNER(S) EQUITY
CURRENT ASSETS	CURRENT LIABILITIES
Cash $________	Accounts Payable $________
Accounts Receivable $________	Short-Term Notes Payable $________
Inventory $________	Other $________
Prepaid Rent $________	
Total Current Assets $________	Total Current Liabilities $________
FIXED ASSETS	LONG-TERM LIABILITIES OR DEBT
Fixtures $________	Notes Payable $________
Equipment $________	Bank Loans $________
Land $________	Other Loans $________
Buildings $________	
Total Fixed Assets $________	Total Long-Term Liabilities $________
TOTAL ASSETS $________	TOTAL LIABILITIES $________
	Owner's Equity or Net Worth $________
	Retained Earnings $________
	Total Equity or Net Worth $________
	TOTAL LIABILITIES & NET WORTH $________

Figure 29–2 A balance sheet.

analysis; however, this is not a good idea. Understanding how many products and services you need to sell on a weekly, monthly, and quarterly basis to break even is an important business function that can help you to meet expenses and set goals to create even greater profit.

PROTECTING BUSINESS ASSETS

Wearing a seatbelt, exercising, and avoiding toxic substances are things people do to decrease the possibility of injury. These are day-to-day **risk management** practices. The same philosophy applies to businesses.

Most small business owners are cautious and do everything they can to prevent injury to their employees and customers, but they are well aware that accidents do happen. The first rule of prevention in any risk management program is strict adherence to local, state, and federal guidelines regarding disinfection and public and occupational safety. Remember that operators of skin care businesses are expected to follow Occupational Safety and Health Administration (OSHA) guidelines. It is also imperative that every service provider operating under a license in your salon or spa adheres to his or her scope of practice.

To avoid the risk of injury to customers, smart business owners take the time to train and supervise their employees, using carefully drafted protocols and procedures for virtually every facet of operation. This should include periodic safety checks of the entire facility to ensure public safety. For example, replacing a worn rug or faulty piece of equipment can help to avert an accident. Implementing a crisis management program is another important measure a business owner can take to help safeguard his or her business in the event of disaster.

CAUTION!

As an insured business owner, it is your responsibility to make sure that every service provider working in your place of business is licensed by the appropriate state licensing board. Take extra precautions to see that each service provider practices within the scope of his or her license and be sure to list every service provider on your insurance policy before allowing him or her to perform any procedure in the salon or spa.

Insurance

It would be impossible for the majority of businesses to cover the expense of re-building should some unforeseen disaster occur. Here is where the transfer of risk to a third party, through insurance policies, comes into play. **Insurance** is the best protection against business casualties or the loss of something that the small business owner cannot afford to be without.

? Did You Know

Insurance is regulated by state law. Certain types of business insurance, such as workers' compensation, are required by law in all states. Contact the Office of the Insurance Commissioner for specific insurance guidelines and the laws in your state.

There are several basic types of insurance, including property or casualty, liability, malpractice, life, health and disability insurance, and workers' compensation. An insurance agent may recommend that you purchase other types of insurance, such as business interruption, as well. Make sure you are dealing with a reputable and qualified agent; he or she will help you purchase the policies that are required by law and that best fit your needs.

Recently, the insurance industry has become concerned with covering the use of new technologies in spas and skin care salons. Because state laws are often vague when it comes to the use of advanced equipment and procedures, some insurance companies are now requiring skin care business owners to provide proof of adequate training before purchasing insurance for certain advanced skin care or hair removal equipment and procedures. Make sure you are covered for all of the procedures performed by your business and for all of the equipment you and your employees use. If you have any questions, ask your agent.

If you are going into business for the first time, you should investigate personal liability insurance. Learning more about the best way to protect yourself and your family from unforeseeable events, such as personal injury and loss, can give you the peace of mind that comes from knowing you have done all you can to maintain your interests. Seek the expert advice of a competent business attorney and reputable insurance agent.

EMPLOYEE COMPENSATION

It is well known that the skin care business is labor intensive, which is an important consideration in any financial planning. What many new business owners do not realize, though, is that *how* they pay service providers is just as important as *how much* they pay them. As you develop a strategy for compensating your employees, keep in mind that while payroll is generally your biggest expense, you also need to think about the way you pay your employees, and most importantly your service providers, which will have a direct impact on the profitability of your business.

Skin care businesses vary in how they compensate service providers, utilizing both salary, or fixed wages, such as an hourly rate, and commission-based pay structures, or some variation of these methods. Currently there is much discussion in the industry about the benefits of each method. Whichever method of compensation you decide to use, consider that payroll is a very complex and highly charged subject for both the employer, who is taking a huge risk with the hope of gaining a profit, and the employee, who wants to be valued for what he or she contributes to your business.

On this point, the best advice for anyone starting his or her own skin care business is to study the options, talk to business owners who are using the various systems, attend the many seminars and workshops available through trade organizations and industry conferences on this topic, read whatever research is available, and then decide. This is not a topic to be taken lightly.

Independent Contractors

The use of independent contractors has become standard practice in many spas and salons. However, this method can present complications that may not be in the best interest of salon owners, particularly those who wish to build a team-based business. If you decide to engage service providers in this manner, you should be aware that the terms of your relationship must adhere to strict IRS guidelines.

? Did You Know

Tips are generally accepted in most spas and salons. But did you know that tips must be reported as income? The IRS offers salon and spa owners several options for reporting tip income. Discuss these strategies with your accountant, and look for more information in the IRS Publication 3144, *Tips on Tips: A Guide to Tip Income Reporting.*

According to the IRS, an **independent contractor** is someone who sets his or her own fees, controls his or her own hours, has his or her own business card, and pays his or her own taxes. Independent contractors can conduct business pretty much however they choose within legal parameters, controlling the means and methods by which they accomplish their work and are free to work for other businesses. Estheticians who elect to work as independent contractors should be aware that they are responsible for adhering to all laws set forth by their licensing board and any, local, state, and federal rules and regulations that apply to small business owners in their trade.

Business owners that engage service providers as independent contractors will want to establish a legal contract that outlines in detail the exact terms of the agreement between the two parties. Be warned, however: Do not hire a service provider as an independent contractor and then have the person work as an employee at your business. Some businesses owners do this to avoid paying mandatory insurance and taxes, such as Social Security tax, Medicare, workers' compensation, federal and state income taxes, and liability insurance. If you do this, you will be placing your business in serious jeopardy.

CAUTION!

Worker status is an important factor in determining tax obligations and one that the IRS takes very seriously. Any business owner who hires an independent contractor must abide by the legal definition of the term as outlined by IRS requirements. If you need help determining employee versus independent contractor status, see IRS Form SS-8, "Determination of Worker Status for Purposes of Federal Employment Taxes and Income Tax Withholding."

The IRS uses three general categories to determine independent contractor status: behavioral control, financial control, and the relationship between the two parties. Explanations of these criteria, along with a complete description of what constitutes an employee, can be found in several IRS documents for employers, including IRS Publication 15, Circular E, *Employer's Tax Guide,* and IRS Publication 15-A, *Employer's Supplemental Tax Guide,* and are succinctly outlined in IRS Publication 1779, an easy to read brochure which can be accessed online. IRS Form SS-8, "Determination of Worker Status for Purposes of Federal Employment Taxes and Income Tax Withholding" is available for those who require additional help making the distinction between employee and independent contractor. For more information visit the IRS Web site at http://www.irs.gov.

Look at all of these documents closely before deciding to hire service providers as independent contractors. If your arrangement with a service provider does not fit the government's definition of independent contractor, you as the business owner will be considered the employer and will be charged for back payment of the employee's taxes that should have been deducted originally, along with heavy penalties or fines.

? Did You Know

An esthetician who meets the lawful IRS definition of an independent contractor is considered self-employed and is responsible for paying all of his or her own federal and state income taxes plus an additional self-employment tax. He or she may also be responsible for making periodic estimated income tax payments to cover tax liabilities. Failure to do so could result in tax penalties.

UNDERSTANDING THE IRS

"In this world nothing can be said to be certain, except death and taxes."

Benjamin Franklin

Benjamin Franklin was a wise man; however, he is not likely to have anticipated the complexity that prevails in today's tax laws. Although technology appears to have made it a lot easier for individuals to prepare and file their own income tax returns, it has not eliminated the need for a small business owner to retain the professional expertise of a qualified business and/or tax attorney, certified public accountant, and skilled bookkeeper. The advice of qualified professionals in matters of the IRS can be invaluable when it comes to avoiding tax consequences.

Tax Identification Numbers

The IRS uses two important numbers to identify taxpayers: the Social Security number (SSN) and the Employer Identification Number (EIN).

Your **Social Security Number** is your individual taxpayer number. If you do not have a social security number already, you can apply for one at the nearest Social Security office in your area. You may also request an application, or SS-5 Form, by phone or fax or download this form from the Social Security Web site at http://www.socialsecurity.gov.

The **Employer Identification Number (EIN)** is used to identify businesses that maintain employees. However, some banks require an EIN for any business entity, including a sole proprietorship that has no employees. To obtain an EIN, you must fill out Form SS-4 (Figure 29–3). You can obtain one from the IRS via phone or fax, or you can download the form from the IRS Web site at http://www.irs.gov.

If you are a non-resident or resident alien working in the United States, the IRS will issue you an **ITIN**, or an **Individual Tax Identification Number** to process your tax obligation to the U.S. government.

Employee Tax Status

As a spa or salon owner you are responsible for correctly reporting and classifying the tax status of anyone who works for you. If you hire employees, you are required to keep several important forms on file and distribute them to your employees: Form W-2, Form W-4, and Form I-9.

Form W-4

As an employer, you will need to supply each employee with Form W-4, the "Employee's Withholding Allowance Certificate" (Figure 29–4 on page 758), which an employee uses to specify marital status and number of dependents. Information on this form determines how much tax will be withheld from the employee's paycheck.

Form W-2

If you have employees, you are required to file a Form W-2, "Wage and Tax Statement" (Figure 29–5 on page 759), for each one. This form summarizes the employee's wages for a specified calendar year and is used by the employee to determine his or her tax obligations to the state and federal government on his or her individual tax return. The IRS Web site supplies specific instructions for filling out and filing this form.

Form I-9

By law, employers must verify that their employees are eligible to work in the United States. You must use Form I-9 (Figure 29–6 on page 760) for this purpose; this form is available from the Immigration and Naturalization Service (INS).

Form 1099

The independent contractor is responsible for calculating his or her own deductions and filing his or her own tax returns; however, salon and spa owners who hire independent contractors must provide the contractor with a statement of earnings for the tax year. You must fill out Form 1099 for anyone to whom you paid more than $600 annually; on the form, you report the gross amount you paid the contractor.

Filing Tax Returns

As a salon or spa owner, you will be responsible for filing tax returns for your business. This requires careful record keeping that includes a detailed account of all of your business income and expenses.

Tax returns are filed according to a specified time period, which is defined as either a fiscal or calendar year. This is determined by the accounting method under which your business operates. Service businesses generally follow a calendar year; however, there are certain exceptions. Your tax accountant can help you to determine the correct protocol for your situation.

Those who use the calendar year are generally required to file state and federal tax returns on or before April 15

Form **SS-4** (Rev. July 2007) Department of the Treasury Internal Revenue Service

Application for Employer Identification Number

(For use by employers, corporations, partnerships, trusts, estates, churches, government agencies, Indian tribal entities, certain individuals, and others.)

▶ See separate instructions for each line. ▶ Keep a copy for your records.

OMB No. 1545-0003

EIN

Type or print clearly.

1 Legal name of entity (or individual) for whom the EIN is being requested

2 Trade name of business (if different from name on line 1) | 3 Executor, administrator, trustee, "care of" name

4a Mailing address (room, apt., suite no. and street, or P.O. box) | 5a Street address (if different) (Do not enter a P.O. box.)

4b City, state, and ZIP code (if foreign, see instructions) | 5b City, state, and ZIP code (if foreign, see instructions)

6 County and state where principal business is located

7a Name of principal officer, general partner, grantor, owner, or trustor | 7b SSN, ITIN, or EIN

8a Is this application for a limited liability company (LLC) (or a foreign equivalent)? . . . . ☐ Yes ☐ No | 8b If 8a is "Yes," enter the number of LLC members . . . . ▶

8c If 8a is "Yes," was the LLC organized in the United States? . . . . ☐ Yes ☐ No

9a **Type of entity** (check only one box). **Caution.** If 8a is "Yes," see the instructions for the correct box to check.

☐ Sole proprietor (SSN) ______
☐ Partnership
☐ Corporation (enter form number to be filed) ▶______
☐ Personal service corporation
☐ Church or church-controlled organization
☐ Other nonprofit organization (specify) ▶______
☐ Other (specify) ▶
☐ Estate (SSN of decedent) ______
☐ Plan administrator (TIN) ______
☐ Trust (TIN of grantor) ______
☐ National Guard ☐ State/local government
☐ Farmers' cooperative ☐ Federal government/military
☐ REMIC ☐ Indian tribal governments/enterprises
Group Exemption Number (GEN) if any ▶

9b If a corporation, name the state or foreign country (if applicable) where incorporated | State | Foreign country

10 **Reason for applying** (check only one box)
☐ Started new business (specify type) ▶ ______
☐ Hired employees (Check the box and see line 13.)
☐ Compliance with IRS withholding regulations
☐ Other (specify) ▶
☐ Banking purpose (specify purpose) ▶______
☐ Changed type of organization (specify new type) ▶______
☐ Purchased going business
☐ Created a trust (specify type) ▶______
☐ Created a pension plan (specify type) ▶______

Figure 29–3 Employer Identification Number (EIN).

of every year unless this date falls on a Saturday, Sunday, or legal holiday. This information is highly publicized. For those operating on a fiscal year basis or those who file as a corporation, the filing date varies and again, should be reviewed with your tax accountant to determine your individual status.

Business Taxes

As a small business owner, you should familiarize yourself with your tax obligations. However, unless you are a tax accountant or a business attorney, keeping up on the tax codes can be overwhelming. Your best asset in this arena is a qualified and trusted tax accountant who stays abreast of changing tax laws and requirements and can advise you on your own tax obligations. In addition, the IRS publishes a complete guide for small business owners, entitled Publication 334, *Tax Guide for Small Businesses*. This publication is free and available online or by mail. The IRS Web site also hosts online classroom lessons that can help you better understand the various tax requirements.

Income Tax

Your income tax obligations and the forms you must file will vary based on the business entity or structure under which you form your company. For example, you can choose to operate your business as a sole proprietor, partnership, corporation, S corporation, or limited liability company. Your business attorney and tax accountant will help you to determine the best entity and appropriate forms for your business needs.

Payroll Tax Deductions

There are several important deductions you should be aware of when calculating employee payroll taxes.

Personal Allowances Worksheet (Keep for your records.)

A Enter "1" for **yourself** if no one else can claim you as a dependent . . . . A ______

B Enter "1" if:
- You are single and have only one job; or
- You are married, have only one job, and your spouse does not work; or
- Your wages from a second job or your spouse's wages (or the total of both) are $1,500 or less. . . B ______

C Enter "1" for your **spouse.** But, you may choose to enter "-0-" if you are married and have either a working spouse or more than one job. (Entering "-0-" may help you avoid having too little tax withheld.) . . . . C ______

D Enter number of **dependents** (other than your spouse or yourself) you will claim on your tax return . . . . . . D ______

E Enter "1" if you will file as **head of household** on your tax return (see conditions under **Head of household** above) . E ______

F Enter "1" if you have at least $1,500 of **child or dependent care expenses** for which you plan to claim a credit . . F ______

(**Note.** Do **not** include child support payments. See Pub. 503, Child and Dependent Care Expenses, for details.)

G **Child Tax Credit** (including additional child tax credit). See Pub. 972, Child Tax Credit, for more information.
- If your total income will be less than $58,000 ($86,000 if married), enter "2" for each eligible child.
- If your total income will be between $58,000 and $84,000 ($86,000 and $119,000 if married), enter "1" for each eligible child plus "1" **additional** if you have 4 or more eligible children. G ______

H Add lines A through G and enter total here. (**Note.** This may be different from the number of exemptions you claim on your tax return.) ▶ H ______

For accuracy, complete all worksheets that apply.
- If you plan to **itemize or claim adjustments to income** and want to reduce your withholding, see the **Deductions and Adjustments Worksheet** on page 2.
- If you have **more than one job** or are **married and you and your spouse both work** and the combined earnings from all jobs exceed $40,000 ($25,000 if married), see the **Two-Earners/Multiple Jobs Worksheet** on page 2 to avoid having too little tax withheld.
- If **neither** of the above situations applies, **stop here** and enter the number from line H on line 5 of Form W-4 below.

--- **Cut here and give Form W-4 to your employer. Keep the top part for your records.** ---

Form **W-4** | **Employee's Withholding Allowance Certificate** | OMB No. 1545-0074 **2008**

Department of the Treasury Internal Revenue Service

▶ **Whether you are entitled to claim a certain number of allowances or exemption from withholding is subject to review by the IRS. Your employer may be required to send a copy of this form to the IRS.**

1 Type or print your first name and middle initial.	Last name	2 Your social security number
Home address (number and street or rural route)	3 ☐ Single ☐ Married ☐ Married, but withhold at higher Single rate. **Note.** If married, but legally separated, or spouse is a nonresident alien, check the "Single" box.	
City or town, state, and ZIP code	4 **If your last name differs from that shown on your social security card, check here. You must call 1-800-772-1213 for a replacement card.** ▶ ☐	

5 Total number of allowances you are claiming (from line **H** above **or** from the applicable worksheet on page 2) | 5 |

6 Additional amount, if any, you want withheld from each paycheck . . . . | 6 | $

7 I claim exemption from withholding for 2008, and I certify that I meet **both** of the following conditions for exemption.
- Last year I had a right to a refund of **all** federal income tax withheld because I had **no** tax liability **and**
- This year I expect a refund of **all** federal income tax withheld because I expect to have **no** tax liability.

If you meet both conditions, write "Exempt" here . . . . ▶ | 7 |

Under penalties of perjury, I declare that I have examined this certificate and to the best of my knowledge and belief, it is true, correct, and complete.

Employee's signature
(Form is not valid unless you sign it.) ▶ **Date** ▶

8 Employer's name and address (Employer: Complete lines 8 and 10 only if sending to the IRS.)	9 Office code (optional)	10 Employer identification number (EIN)

For Privacy Act and Paperwork Reduction Act Notice, see page 2. Cat. No. 10220Q Form **W-4** (2008)

Figure 29–4 Form W-4, Employee's Withholding Allowance Certificate.

These include federal income tax, Social Security, and Medicare taxes. The government provides tax charts to help you showing the withholding amounts for each of these taxes. Your accountant or payroll service provider will use these to determine the specific amounts to withdraw from each employee's paycheck. These figures are determined by the employee's individual tax status as indicated on Form W-4. As an employer, you are required to match employee contributions to Social Security and Medicare.

Form 941 is used to report the amount of federal, Social Security, and Medicare taxes withheld and paid for by each employee and the employer's matching deductions for Social Security and Medicare. This form is filed on a quarterly basis.

Federal Unemployment Tax

Employers are responsible for paying another very important tax, the **Federal Unemployment Tax.** This

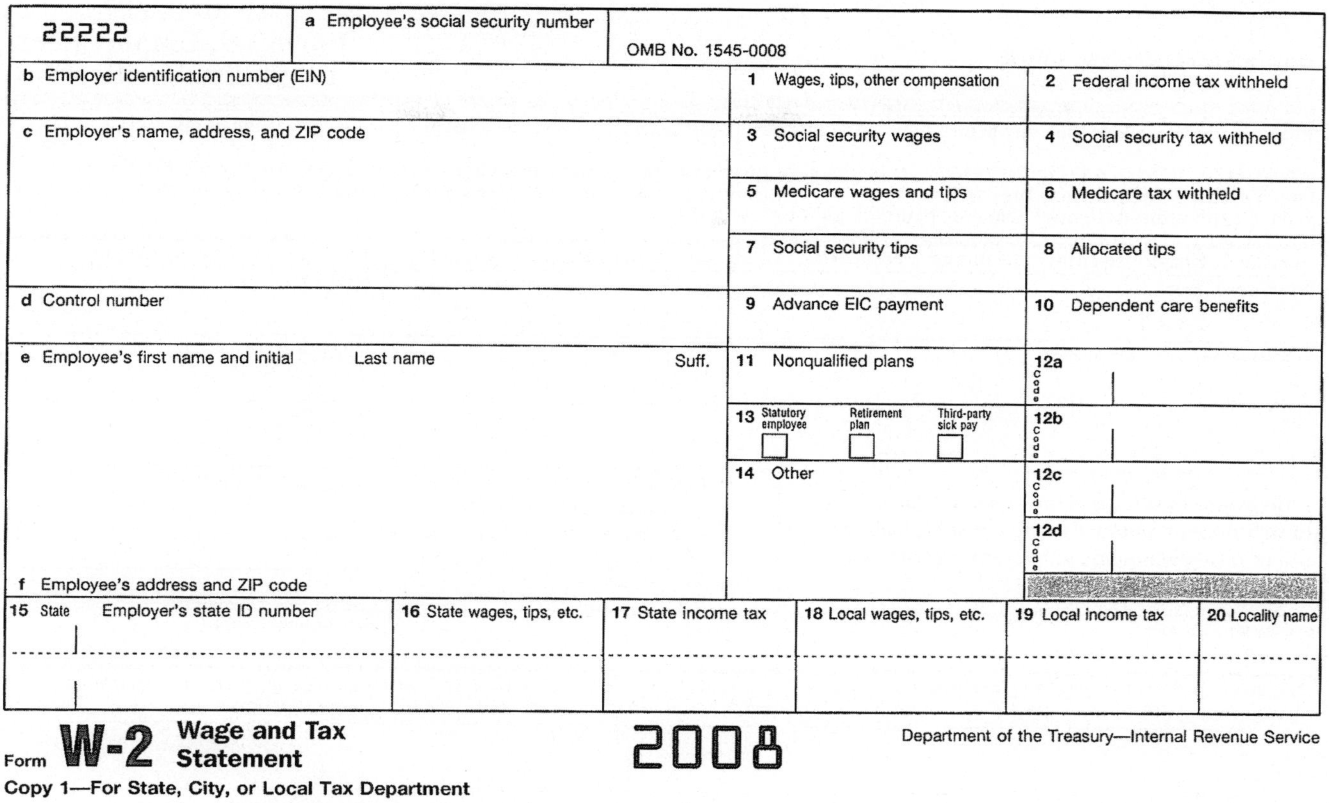

	a Employee's social security number			
22222		OMB No. 1545-0008		
b Employer identification number (EIN)		1 Wages, tips, other compensation	2 Federal income tax withheld	
c Employer's name, address, and ZIP code		3 Social security wages	4 Social security tax withheld	
		5 Medicare wages and tips	6 Medicare tax withheld	
		7 Social security tips	8 Allocated tips	
d Control number		9 Advance EIC payment	10 Dependent care benefits	
e Employee's first name and initial Last name Suff.		11 Nonqualified plans	12a Code	
		13 Statutory employee ☐ Retirement plan ☐ Third-party sick pay ☐	12b Code	
		14 Other	12c Code	
			12d Code	
f Employee's address and ZIP code				

15 State Employer's state ID number	16 State wages, tips, etc.	17 State income tax	18 Local wages, tips, etc.	19 Local income tax	20 Locality name

Form **W-2** Wage and Tax Statement   **2008**   Department of the Treasury—Internal Revenue Service

Copy 1—For State, City, or Local Tax Department

Figure 29–5 Form W-2, Wage and Tax Statement.

is a joint program between state and federal governments that is used to cover employees who lose their jobs and file for unemployment assistance. However, employees are not required to make a contribution to the Federal Unemployment Tax, so there is no payroll deduction associated with this tax. These taxes are the sole responsibility of the employer. Form 940, which is filed annually, is used to report the employer's payment. Specific guidelines associated with filing this tax are available from the IRS. There are also several online training programs for those interested in learning more about how this tax is calculated.

State Income Tax

The Federation of Tax Administrators provides a direct online link to each state's Department of Revenue. Information regarding tax obligations for businesses is also available directly from each state's Department of Revenue. You should review this material with a qualified tax accountant who is familiar with the law as it applies to your individual business and who can walk you through the requirements in your state.

Self-Employment Tax

Independent contractors, sole proprietors, partnerships, and limited liability companies are all required to pay a **self-employment tax.** Payment of this tax makes you eligible to receive retirement benefits, disability benefits, survivor benefits, and hospital insurance or Medicare in much the same way as an employee would. It should be noted that a failure to report or an underreporting of income can result in lower Social Security benefits upon retirement.

Other Deductions

As an employer, you may decide to offer employees other benefits, such as health insurance or a retirement plan. These are excellent benefits for employees that also provide you, the employer, with appealing tax deductions. If you offer these benefits, you will need to track the amounts as well.

Estimated Tax Payments

Self-employed individuals who expect to owe taxes to the government are required to make estimated tax payments

OMB No. 1615-0047; Expires 06/30/08

Department of Homeland Security
U.S. Citizenship and Immigration Services

Form I-9, Employment Eligibility Verification

Please read instructions carefully before completing this form. The instructions must be available during completion of this form.

ANTI-DISCRIMINATION NOTICE: It is illegal to discriminate against work eligible individuals. Employers CANNOT specify which document(s) they will accept from an employee. The refusal to hire an individual because the documents have a future expiration date may also constitute illegal discrimination.

Section 1. Employee Information and Verification. To be completed and signed by employee at the time employment begins.

Print Name: Last | First | Middle Initial | Maiden Name

Address *(Street Name and Number)* | Apt. # | Date of Birth *(month/day/year)*

City | State | Zip Code | Social Security #

I am aware that federal law provides for imprisonment and/or fines for false statements or use of false documents in connection with the completion of this form.

I attest, under penalty of perjury, that I am (check one of the following):
- ☐ A citizen or national of the United States
- ☐ A lawful permanent resident (Alien #) A ______
- ☐ An alien authorized to work until ______
  (Alien # or Admission #) ______

Employee's Signature | Date *(month/day/year)*

Preparer and/or Translator Certification. *(To be completed and signed if Section 1 is prepared by a person other than the employee.) I attest, under penalty of perjury, that I have assisted in the completion of this form and that to the best of my knowledge the information is true and correct.*

Preparer's/Translator's Signature | Print Name

Address *(Street Name and Number, City, State, Zip Code)* | Date *(month/day/year)*

Section 2. Employer Review and Verification. To be completed and signed by employer. Examine one document from List A OR examine one document from List B and one from List C, as listed on the reverse of this form, and record the title, number and expiration date, if any, of the document(s).

List A		OR	List B	AND	List C
Document title:	______		______		______
Issuing authority:	______		______		______
Document #:	______		______		______
Expiration Date *(if any)*:	______		______		______
Document #:	______				
Expiration Date *(if any)*:	______				

CERTIFICATION - I attest, under penalty of perjury, that I have examined the document(s) presented by the above-named employee, that the above-listed document(s) appear to be genuine and to relate to the employee named, that the employee began employment on *(month/day/year)* ______ **and that to the best of my knowledge the employee is eligible to work in the United States. (State employment agencies may omit the date the employee began employment.)**

Signature of Employer or Authorized Representative | Print Name | Title

Business or Organization Name and Address *(Street Name and Number, City, State, Zip Code)* | Date *(month/day/year)*

Section 3. Updating and Reverification. To be completed and signed by employer.

A. New Name *(if applicable)* | B. Date of Rehire *(month/day/year) (if applicable)*

C. If employee's previous grant of work authorization has expired, provide the information below for the document that establishes current employment eligibility.

Document Title: ______ Document #: ______ Expiration Date (if any): ______

I attest, under penalty of perjury, that to the best of my knowledge, this employee is eligible to work in the United States, and if the employee presented document(s), the document(s) I have examined appear to be genuine and to relate to the individual.

Signature of Employer or Authorized Representative | Date *(month/day/year)*

Form I-9 (Rev. 06/05/07) N

Figure 29–6 Form I-9, Employment Eligibility Verification four times per year. Form 1040-ES is used to report federal estimated tax payments and Form 1-ES is used to report state estimated tax payments for this purpose. These quarterly tax payments are due on April 15, June 15, September 15, and January 15 of each tax year.

Sales Tax

Those selling retail products in the salon or spa must also be aware of **resale tax** obligations. Sales tax laws vary from state to state, but in general if you sell retail products you are required to pay an additional sales tax on each product you sell. This typically requires a permit or resale certificate. For more information about retail sales and how to apply for a permit, contact the Office of the Secretary of State in your state.

Deferred Income Tax

Deferred income tax is an important factor in the sale of gift certificates which salon owners may issue for either a cash value or goods and services. There are tax obligations associated with each. Deferred income can be very confusing to the small business owner, who may be unprepared for the huge tax obligations that can prevail if he or she does not track the sale and redemption of gift certificate sales carefully. Establishing a method for handling cash revenues until a gift certificate is redeemed is a critical part of the process. If you do not understand your tax obligations concerning gift certificates or have trouble setting up a system of accountability, seek the advice of a qualified business or tax attorney and tax accountant who are familiar with the laws in your state.

Tax Penalties

Whether you decide to work as an independent contractor or own your own spa or salon, you will assume all of the benefits and responsibilities associated with being your own boss. This includes penalties for late filing, late payments, and/or errors in reporting taxes. Remember that ignorance is no defense in terms of following the law. A failure to comply with legal business obligations or, worse, to intentionally attempt to defraud the federal government of revenue, can result in significant tax penalties and may have other serious legal consequences, including fines and/or imprisonment.

Financial planning is a complex business matter that cannot be covered fully in one chapter; however, if you are interested in becoming a spa or salon owner, you should have general knowledge of the many financial business management obligations associated with owning a business. Remember that there is no substitute for expert legal and accounting advice. When it comes to developing a solid financial plan, seek the support of trusted and qualified professionals in these matters.

REVIEW QUESTIONS

1. Define business risk. How might a new spa or salon owner calculate the risks involved in business ownership?
2. What is the primary importance of a business plan?
3. Explain the importance of the balance sheet, income statement, and cash flow statement to the salon owner.
4. What is a break-even analysis? How can calculating a break-even analysis help the salon owner?
5. Why does the small business owner need insurance?
6. How might the use of advanced skin care equipment in the salon impact the salon owner when it comes to purchasing insurance? Team up with a classmate to research insurance laws in your state.

REVIEW QUESTIONS

7. Describe each of the main methods of compensation used in the skin care business. Defend your argument for the one that most appeals to you as a business owner. How might this method compare to others, from an employee's perspective?
8. What is an independent contractor? Discuss the pros and cons associated with hiring service providers as independent contractors. Team up with a classmate to research the IRS guidelines for this type of employment.
9. What is Federal Unemployment Tax? Why is this tax necessary?
10. What is self-employment tax? How might this impact a small business owner's cash flow?
11. Describe the various types of payroll taxes. Which form is used to determine an employee's withholding allowance?
12. Discuss the tax repercussions associated with the collection of money from gift certificates.

CHAPTER GLOSSARY

assets: anything your business owns.

balance sheet: provides a financial overview of a business at a given point in time in terms of its assets and liabilities.

break-even analysis: the point at which all costs are covered and your business begins to earn a profit.

business plan: a strategy for understanding key elements in developing business; also serves as a guide to making informed business decisions.

capital: the amount of money invested in a business.

cash flow statement: indicates how much money is flowing in and out of a business on a regular basis.

costs of goods sold: what it costs to provide the products and services that you sell.

Employer Identification Number (EIN): the number used to identify businesses that maintain employees.

Federal Unemployment Tax: a joint program between state and federal government that is used to cover employees who lose their jobs and file for unemployment assistance.

generally accepted accounting principles, (GAAP): the standard procedures established by the accounting profession.

gross profit: the total amount of money a business takes in from the sale of products and/or services.

income statement: a profit and loss statement.

independent contractor: a non-employee service provider in accordance with IRS guidelines who is able to control the means and methods by which they accomplish their work (and is responsible for adhering to all laws set forth by their licensing board and any local, state, and federal rules and regulations that apply to small business owners in their trade).

Individual Tax Identification Number (ITIN): the number issued by the IRS to a non-resident or resident alien working in the United States to process their tax obligation to the United States government.

insurance: provides protection against business casualties; or the transfer of risk to a third party, as in the form of an insurance policy.

liabilities: the amount of debt or money your business owes to creditors.

net profit: the real income of a business after all of the expenses associated with operation are subtracted.

owner's equity: the owner's interest in the assets of the company after all of the business' liabilities have been deducted.

promissory note: a legal document that defines the terms of a loan agreement between two parties.

resale tax: a tax imposed upon those who sell retail products.

risk: the chance of incurring some type of harm, damage, or loss.

risk management: the methods used to safeguard your business against loss or damage.

self-employment tax: a tax imposed upon those who are self-employed, which allows them to receive retirement benefits, disability benefits, survivor benefits, and hospital insurance or Medicare, in much the same way an employee would.

Social Security Number: the number used to identify an individual taxpayer.

venture capitalist(s): a private individual (or group of individuals) who invest in businesses with the goal of gaining a return on their investment or profit.

CHAPTER 30

MARKETING

CHAPTER OUTLINE

- THE DEFINITION OF MARKETING
- CUSTOMER VALUE
- STRATEGIC VALUE
- CUSTOMER RELATIONSHIP MANAGEMENT
- THE PROMOTION MIX
- THE MARKETING PLAN
- THE BROCHURE, OR MENU OF SERVICES
- THE INTERNET
- THE USE OF TECHNOLOGY
- MARKETING RESPONSIBLY

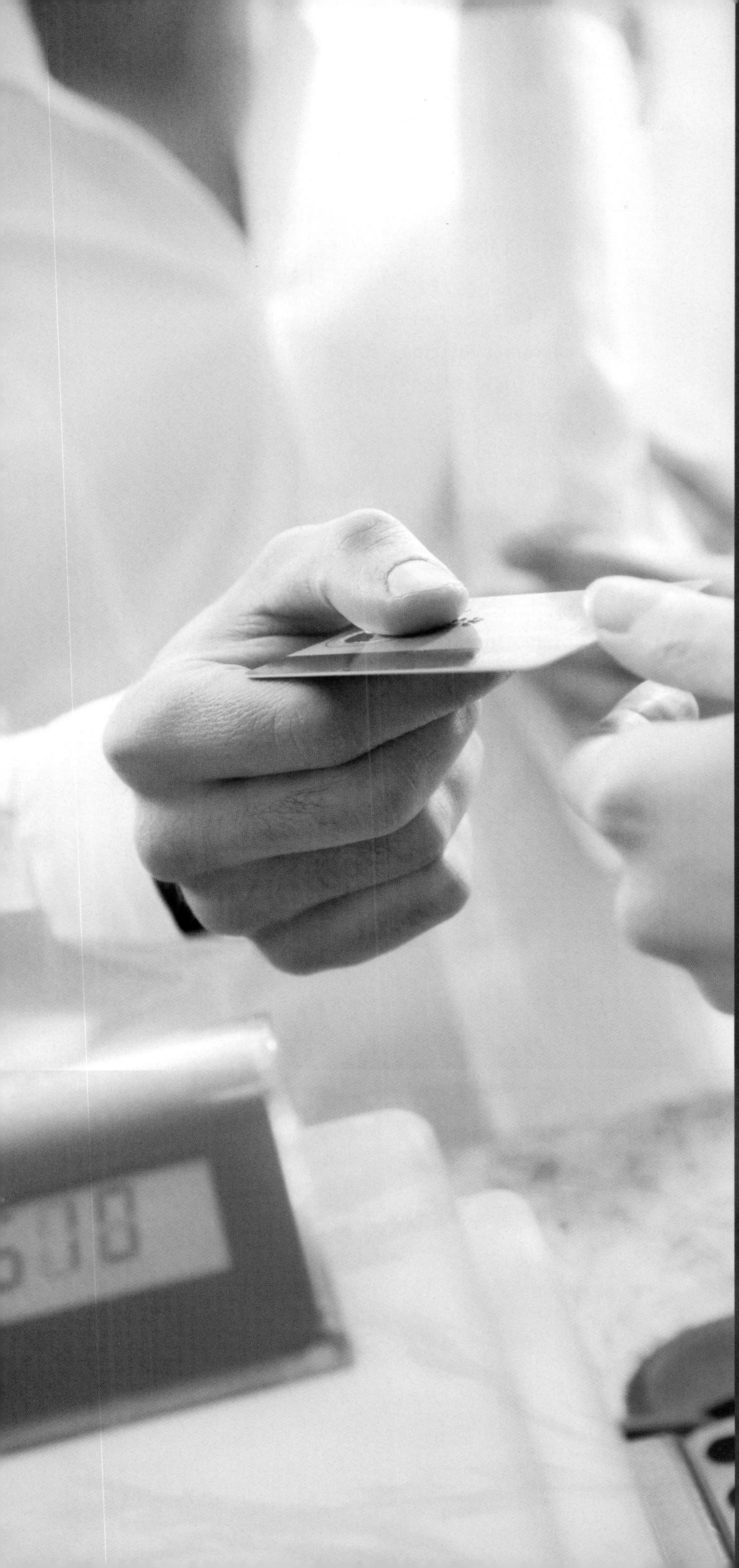

LEARNING OBJECTIVES

After completing this chapter, you should be able to:

- Explain the basic principles of marketing.
- Explain the role of demographics in creating customer value.
- Discuss the various methods of marketing communications.
- List the six main methods of marketing promotion.
- Explain the value of developing a complete marketing plan.
- Discuss several cost-effective ways to market a salon.
- Discuss the use of technology in the salon.
- List those government agencies responsible for overseeing marketing.

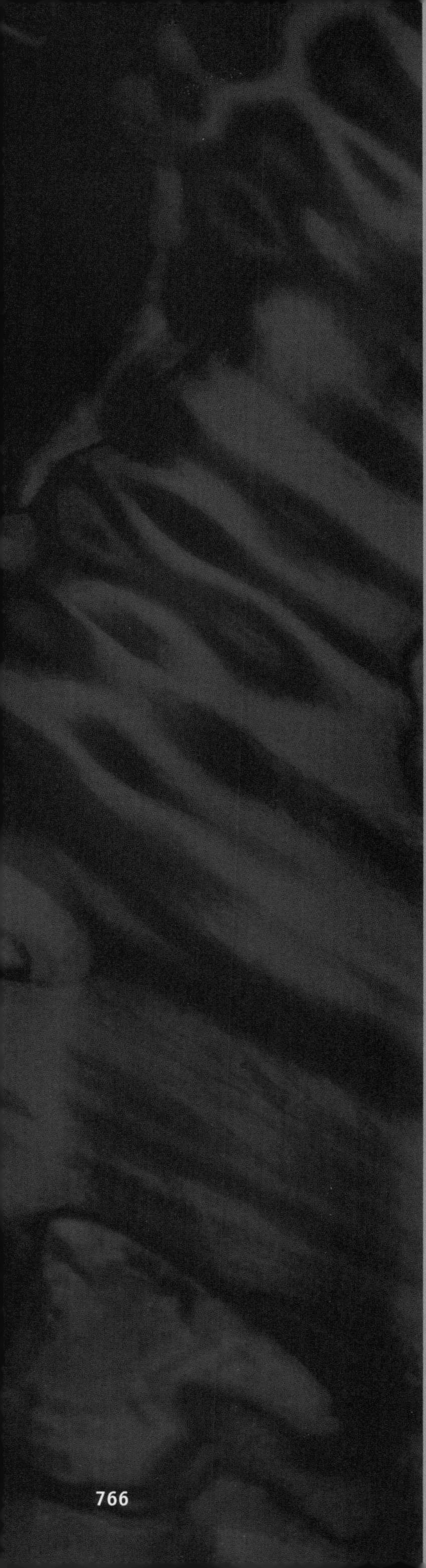

KEY TERMS

Page numbers indicate where in the chapter the term is used.

advertising 771
brochure, or menu of services 774
customer relationship management 770
direct marketing 772
Internet 775
marketing 767
marketing plan 774
personal selling 773
place 768
price 768
product 767
promotion 768
promotion mix 771
publicity 772
public relations 772
sales promotion 773

One of the most important elements in any business plan is marketing—and for good reason. Marketing is what drives business. In today's highly competitive skin care industry, it can also mean the difference between a business with an average financial return and one that is phenomenally successful. There are many resources available for business owners with limited marketing experience. However, it is wise for the new business owner to have a general understanding of the entire marketing process before embarking on a plan or hiring a consultant (Figure 30–1).

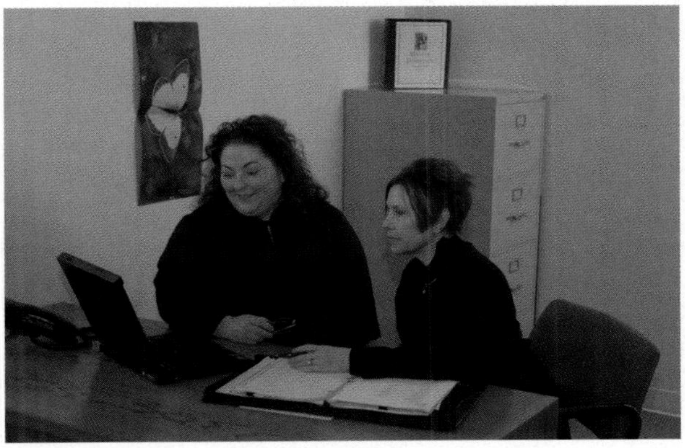

Figure 30–1 Marketing drives business.

THE DEFINITION OF MARKETING

Mention the word *marketing* and most people immediately think of advertising. However, advertising is just one aspect of **marketing**, which in fact, covers a much broader business strategy for how ideas, goods, and services are bought and sold or exchanged.

The Marketing Mix

All marketing begins with what are commonly referred to as the *Four Ps:* product, price, promotion, and place. These factors, also referred to as the *marketing mix,* outline a complete business strategy that can be adjusted as needed over time.

FOCUS ON: *Marketing*

Marketing is a broad business strategy that is based on developing a mutually beneficial exchange between a buyer and a seller. In the skin care business, clients, or buyers, have certain needs or wants. Skin care business owners, or sellers, aim to satisfy those needs and wants with their products and services. In the process of marketing, something of value is exchanged between the two, so that, ideally, each is better off after the exchange. A complete marketing strategy that embraces this philosophy and focuses on the benefit to the consumer is the first step in developing a thoughtful marketing plan.

Product

The term **product** refers to more than the ingredients used to conduct services or the jars displayed on your retail shelves. In marketing, this term refers to your complete business concept and includes both tangible and intangible characteristics, such as the items you sell, menu of services, philosophy, and logo that will ultimately be associated with your business.

The business of skin care typically involves products and services and the equipment used to perform those services. The types of products and services you select for use in your skin care practice will have a significant impact on your overall concept. For example, products and treatments that are results-oriented versus relaxation-oriented will make a definite statement about your business—but they are not the sum total of your product.

When it comes to providing skin care services, the service provider is a vital part of building the product concept. A capable staff is essential to operations and especially important in building client confidence. Give this aspect of your marketing plan a great deal of attention. Hiring qualified staff at the onset is critical to gaining repeat business and maintaining a successful operation over time.

Image is another significant factor that helps business owners to establish what is referred to as *brand recognition*. Today's skin care businesses are housed in any number of facilities, including beauty salons, separate skin care salons, spas, and medical aesthetic facilities. Before you can develop a solid marketing plan, you must decide on the main focus of your business and establish a brand name that embodies the image you wish to project. There are other aspects of branding, such as a good public relations program, which will help you to develop a positive public image. This is all part of developing your "product."

Price

The **price** or monetary value applied to goods and services sold varies according to the type and size of the facility. But all pricing should be calculated according to the cost associated with providing that service or product. For example, the cost of a service includes both the direct costs associated with performing that service, such as, labor, time, and materials, and the indirect costs, such as rent and utilities.

Your pricing strategy should also take into account the demand for your product or service. Take a good look at the number of skin care businesses in the area and what they charge. Will you undercut or charge more than those prices? That will depend on your spa concept, but do not overlook your target market. Given the number of salons and people in the area, how many clients can you expect to visit your skin care facility each year? Study carefully customers' ability to pay along with the demand for services. This information will play a significant role in your pricing strategy and your profitability.

Promotion

Most people equate marketing with the **promotion** aspect or the strategies used to persuade others to purchase products and services. These generally involve several methods of communication, including personal selling, advertising, public relations, direct marketing, sales promotions, and publicity. Business owners generally use a combination of these strategies to bring attention to their product and services, but the key to using them successfully is consistency. A carefully planned promotional strategy that is implemented on a regular schedule will help you to make the most of your marketing dollars.

Place

Place refers to the distribution channel or method for delivering goods and services to clients. While many of the retail products you sell may go through several channels of distribution—for example, from a manufacturer to a wholesaler to a distributor to you—in a service-based business it is hard to separate place from the service provider. In this case, determining the key points of value as they relate to your location, convenience, accessibility, and customer service are extremely important (Figure 30–2).

PRODUCT	Your complete business concept, including the products and services that you sell, your philosophy, and service providers
PRICE	The monetary value applied to the goods and services you sell
PROMOTION	The communication methods you use to persuade customers to purchase your products and services
PLACE	The distribution channel or method for delivering your goods and services to clients.

Figure 30–2 The four Ps form the basis of a strategic marketing plan.

CUSTOMER VALUE

In our media-driven culture, marketing is often credited with persuading consumers to buy a host of things they may not necessarily need or want. While there is no doubt that marketing methods can be persuasive, it is important to remember that when it comes to skin care, consumers have many choices. More importantly, today's educated skin care consumer is unlikely to fall for clever marketing and advertising campaigns that do not provide something of value.

One of the most important factors in understanding the marketing process is recognizing that it serves both buyers and sellers. Consumers (buyers) have needs or wants. Business owners (sellers) aim to satisfy those needs and wants with their products and services. In the process of marketing, something of value is exchanged between the two so that ideally each is better off after the exchange. When looked at from this perspective, you can see that ultimately there must be a benefit to the consumer.

> **Here's a Tip**
>
> Clients today are extremely knowledgeable about esthetic services and are looking for value for their purchase. This does not necessarily translate to a discount or sale; however, it is important to remember that whether a client's goal is skin improvement or relaxation, he or she is an educated consumer and expects results.

Studying the demographics of your customer base is an important part of evaluating how best to meet customers' needs. Demographics, or the study and analysis of the characteristics of a particular group of people, including age, sex, income, education level, and spending habits, is a major component of market research. Gathering information on these variables is a great place to begin looking at the best products and services for your market. This strategy is particularly important to those targeting a specific market, such as a high-income clientele. Salon owners can also use such information to make important decisions about the pricing of products and services their salons offer.

> **Activity**
>
> Gathering demographic information is an important part of the marketing process. Begin by investigating the demographic resources available to you in your community. Start with your local town hall. What information can you find there? How is it categorized? What other local resources are available? Do these add any substantial value? What other state or national resources may be helpful? How will you incorporate this information into your marketing plan?

In addition to outside demographic studies, many salons implement internal strategies to collect information. For example, they may use an independent survey to determine what magazines or newspapers their clients read, what television shows they watch, or what radio stations they listen to. This type of data gives a salon owner a great deal of information about clients' lifestyle and values (Figure 30–3). It can also help the salon owner to select media that will support their advertising goals.

Salon owners also spend a considerable amount of time analyzing clients' spending habits. A solid understanding of the type of skin care products and services his or her clients use and how much they typically spend on these products and services is an important part of building a successful sales program that meets client's needs and satisfies business objectives.

STRATEGIC VALUE

Although marketing seems like a fairly straightforward practice, it nevertheless requires a thoughtful analysis of the exchange process. Smart business owners invest a great deal of time identifying the benefits and features of the products and services they sell as well as how the consumer benefits from using each. These are important considerations in positioning and pricing products and services on the market or creating what is called *strategic value*.

> **Activity**
>
> Select a product or service in your facility and identify its benefits and features. How will you communicate these benefits to your client? List several creative methods for delivering information to clients about the product or service you have selected. Be sure to include a personal selling dialogue that carefully explains the main features and benefits of the product or service.

Learning as much as possible about clients' intangible preferences is an equally important piece of the puzzle. For example, do consumers want quality skin care at an affordable price, or would they be willing to pay above-average prices to receive treatments that are considered elite or status-oriented? Another point that is generally important to the consumer is whether or not a service is easily accessible or convenient. The amount of time required to obtain a service may also have a significant impact on whether or not the client ultimately decides to make a purchase. Knowing just what is important to the population with which you are working will help you to target the right points to achieve success.

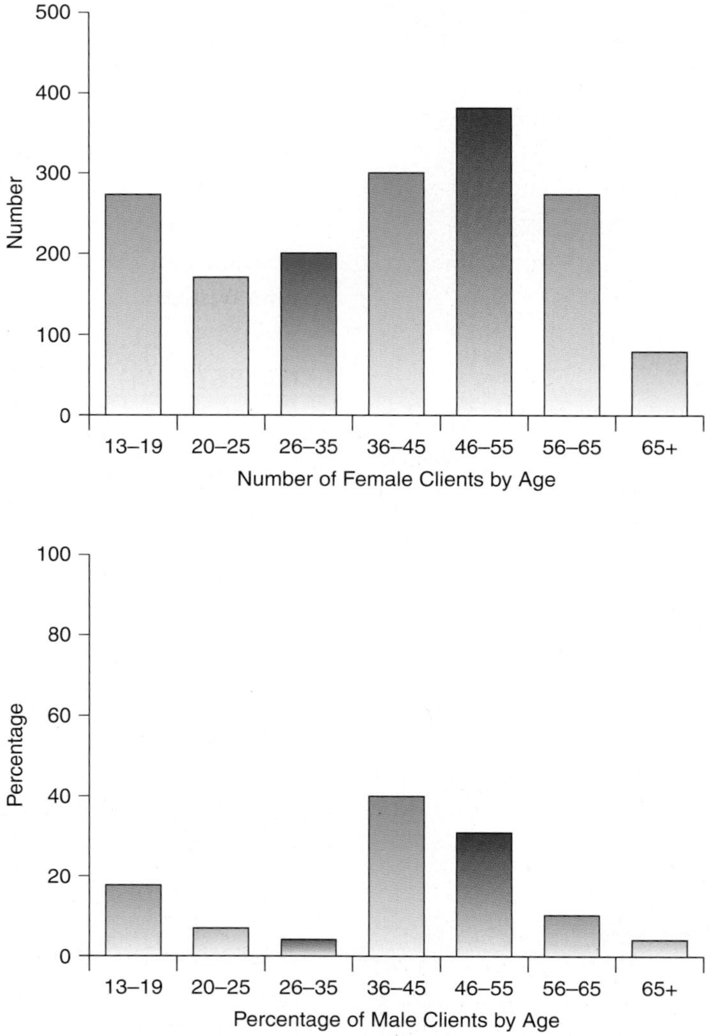

Figure 30–3 An analysis of the type of services and products clients desire will help you to better meet their needs.

CUSTOMER RELATIONSHIP MANAGEMENT

Today's consumer-centric marketing orientation has made managing customer relations, or **customer relationship management,** the primary focus of all marketing efforts. This concept is especially important to new salon (skin care) owners who should understand that customers are the most valuable asset in any business.

Another critical factor in the current marketing environment is quality control. Many businesses make a great first impression but fall short of the client's expectations during repeat visits. The quality of products and services and the manner in which *every* member of a staff treats clients *each and every time* they visit the salon or spa is an important part of marketing (Figure 30–4).

A total quality management program that takes a critical look at all aspects of operations can help you develop

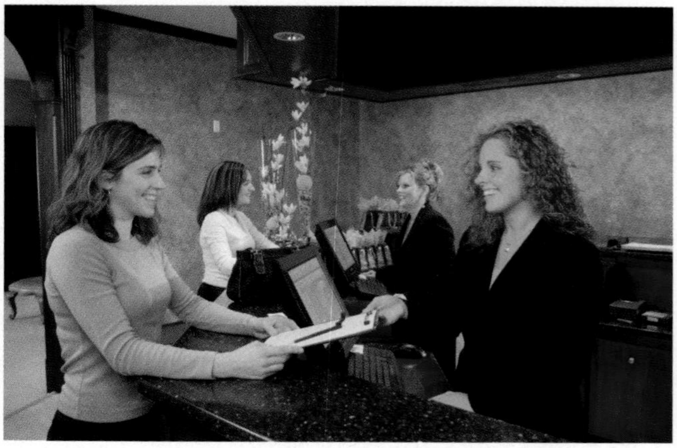

Figure 30–4 All staff must be equally invested in developing positive customer relations.

Here's a Tip

Ongoing evaluation of your skin care methods and continued efforts on the part of all staff to provide clients with a quality experience will help you to increase customer satisfaction and maintain a competitive business edge.

strong long-term personal relationships with customers and can also keep staff members from becoming complacent. By focusing on the needs of the customer and continually striving to understand, improve, and create new methods for meeting these needs, you can alleviate some of the challenges associated with maintaining a competitive business edge.

THE PROMOTION MIX

Once you have a thorough understanding of your client base and the value that you provide, you can begin to think about how you will market your business. There are several methods of promotion that you can use, including advertising, public relations, publicity, direct marketing, personal selling, and sales promotions. These are generally referred to as the **promotion mix.**

As you decide on the best ways to promote your business, remember that all marketing relies on good communication and think in terms of *who* you will direct your product or service to (or the target market); *what* message you want to convey about the product or service; *how* you will communicate that message; and *where* you will deliver it.

Advertising

While the term *advertising* is often used loosely to refer to any method of promotion, in marketing, the term **advertising** refers to promotional efforts that are paid for and intended to increase business. Some of the more popular methods of paid advertising used by skin care businesses include classifieds, newspapers, magazines, radio or television, and direct mail.

- *Classified ads* typically comprise text only and are arranged under subheadings that categorize the product or service being offered. For example, a salon may be listed under the subheading of "Beauty" or "Skin Care" in the local telephone directory. Newspapers and magazines may also incorporate classified sections that similarly identify "Beauty" sections. Generally speaking, these are less expensive ways to advertise.
- *Newspapers*, another cost-effective method of advertising, provide salons with an excellent opportunity to reach a huge volume of consumers. Depending on the size and distribution of the paper, some newspapers will include the cost of creative services in the price of the ad. Most newspapers also offer special rates based on how many days or weeks you run the ad.
- *Magazines* tend to charge higher prices for ads than newspapers do, but they are a good way to reach a specific target market. However, salon owners should understand what that market is before signing a contract: The readership of a particular magazine may be too narrow a population for the business owner's needs. Still, magazine advertising can be very helpful in building name recognition and defining a salon's image (Figure 30–5).
- *Radio* and *television ads* are generally more expensive and require continuity to be effective. While both provide an excellent opportunity to reach large numbers of potential clients, advertising on major radio and television stations can be cost-prohibitive for the small salon or spa. Local community or cable networks are a good alternative and may offer salons and spas more affordable options.
- *Direct mail* is a good way to reach valued customers and target potential clients. Maintaining an up-to-date database with current client information is the key to successful and cost-effective direct-mail efforts. Salons can also purchase mailing lists from marketing agents

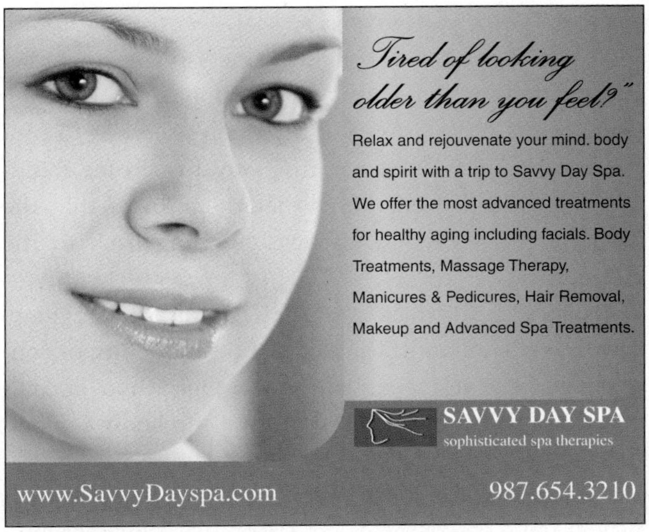

Figure 30–5 A display ad.

or create lists using information accessed freely from public service agencies, such as the local chamber of commerce. Customizing databases to access a specific target market is a good way for salons to reach those clients who might value particular services.

Public Relations

This widely accepted marketing strategy has taken center stage in the marketing arena in recent years and is perhaps the most involved method of promotion available to small business owners. While a small business owner can easily accomplish some of the methods used to generate good public relations, such as developing good community and interpersonal relations, most methods are best performed by public relations professionals who understand how to implement this complex marketing strategy.

Public relations strategies focus on generating positive publicity for a business. To accomplish this, goal marketing specialists use several methods of promotion, such as advertorials, press releases, and media kits to target those in a position of influence, such as magazine editors and broadcast and print journalists. They also encourage business owners to perform good works and plan events to raise community awareness. These tasks involve a considerable amount of research, networking, and time. They also require excellent communication skills that can take years to develop.

Publicity

There are many ways to garner **publicity**, or free media attention. A business owner can get a salon's name in the news free of charge through any number of focused efforts, such as a press release, a public speaking appearance, or participation in a special event. Community service is a good way for small business owners to attract media attention and gain favorable publicity. Attending civic events or volunteering the salon's services to promote worthy causes is a caring way to become familiar with local citizens and to let them know that the owner is interested in giving something back to the community.

Offering to do makeup for the local theater group, speaking to community groups and organizations, or conducting a class on proper skin care for high school or adult education programs are just a few ways to boost a salon's public image and may have the added bonus of encouraging people to patronize the salon. An owner might want to extend the scope of his or her charity work by contributing to those causes he or she feels most passionate about.

Here's a Tip

In spite of hard work, many business owners feel awkward about bringing attention to their charity and community service work, awards, and other accolades. From a publicity viewpoint, however, it is important that they take credit for their efforts. Nothing can compare to the publicity derived from being recognized as a respected member of the business community dedicated to doing good works.

For example, an owner may decide to donate a certain percentage of the salon's profits to breast cancer research during a specified time period. Although this type of work is time-consuming, many find great satisfaction in knowing they are helping to make a difference.

Direct Marketing

Direct marketing refers to any direct attempt to reach the consumer. This very popular method of marketing typically includes the distribution of coupons, postcards, sales letters, and newsletters directly to the consumer (Figure 30–6). While many small business owners are wary of the cost expenditure involved in this method of promotion, it should be noted that there are outlets for delivering these options cost-effectively. The real challenge lies in creating a direct mail piece that prompts the consumer to respond.

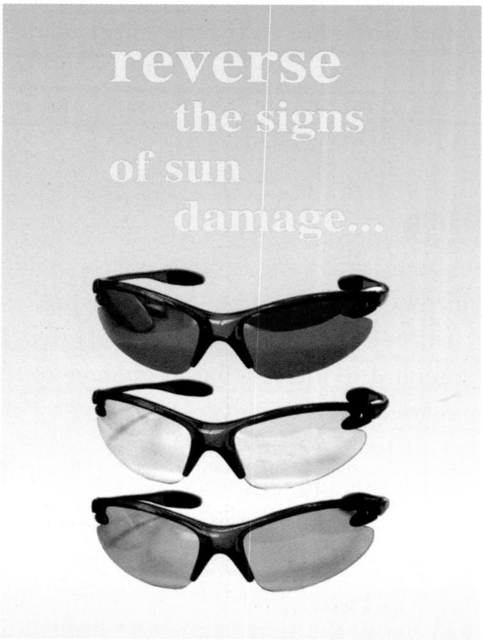

Figure 30–6 A direct mail postcard or e-newsletter is a great way to bring your message to a targeted population.

A successful direct marketing campaign is based on two important factors: the offer and the target audience. Creating an offer that has value to the consumer is critical to the success of any direct mail promotion, but any offer is only as good as the mailing list it is directed toward. Understanding whether or not the target market will respond favorably to an offer is key to getting the results you want.

If you decide to use this method of promotion, be conscious of the excessive use of certain techniques, such as telemarketing and electronic mail, that have prompted many recipients to put their names on nationally sponsored "Do Not Call lists" and install spam filters on their computers. Be sure to set appropriate limits so as not to annoy recipients. Overuse of these techniques can ultimately have a negative impact on your business.

Personal Selling

Personal selling involves a one-to-one exchange with the consumer and is one of the most cost-effective marketing strategies available to skin care business owners. Skin care professionals have the tremendous advantage of being able to work closely with clients, a situation that places them in the enviable position of being able to sell directly to clients on a regular basis. But this added benefit does not automatically guarantee success.

Personal selling requires excellent communication skills, which are not always an integral part of a service provider's training. To make this technique work it is important for skin care owners to train staff members on a number of fronts, including:

- Using excellent interpersonal communication skills to find out what clients want and need in terms of skin care.
- Viewing sales as a professional responsibility and an important part of their job description.
- Using their knowledge of the client and their communication skills to conduct one-on-one sales meetings with clients that ultimately help clients to resolve their skin care concerns.
- Developing techniques for overcoming sales resistance that allow the esthetician to maintain professional credibility (Figure 30–7).

Sales Promotions

Airlines offer frequent flyer programs, restaurants are famous for early bird specials, cosmetic companies give away free gifts with purchases of greater value, and department stores have one-day sales events. The list of sales promotions is endless, but the goal is always the same. All **sales promotions** are aimed at drawing attention to products and services with the goal of increasing the volume of business.

There are many creative ways to bring attention to the various salon treatments and products that you sell. For example, you can offer referral or reward programs, conduct retail product sales, promote seasonal services and packages, or offer special coupons to new or repeat customers. Remember, though, that any sales promotion should focus on the value to the consumer. For example, if you offer clients frequent customer or membership programs, be sure to state the value they will receive for purchasing a series in advance (Figure 30–8). Will that

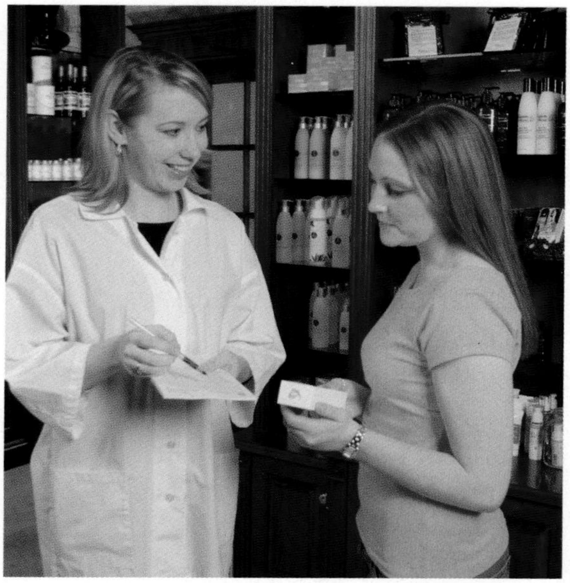

Figure 30–7 Good communication skills are critical to developing strong retail sales.

FOCUS ON: *Sales Training for Staff Members*

Excellent interpersonal communication skills are essential in the skin care business. Estheticians must be comfortable talking with clients and making recommendations for services or products that will improve the client's skin and help him or her to reach their goals. Clients expect recommendations and see this as an esthetician's professional responsibility. Developing a conscientious and ethical sales program should be a significant part of any business owner's marketing plan.

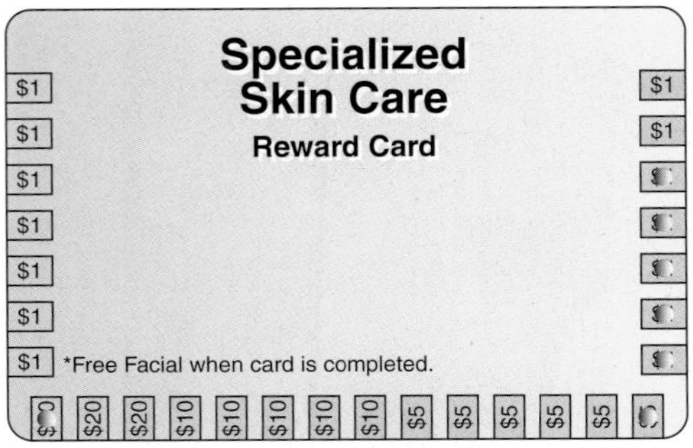

Figure 30–8 Series savers are a great way to encourage repeat business.

value be a financial reward, such as a discount, or will clients gain an additional service free of charge?

THE MARKETING PLAN

A good **marketing plan** states a business owner's goals and objectives as well as the strategies he or she will use for achieving those goals. This document should define a target market and state the owner's unique selling proposition, or how this business will be better than or different from the competition, along with a thorough description of the methods that the owner will use to attract business—for example, the promotion mix.

> **FYI**
>
> Your own marketing plan should provide a detailed account of all of the marketing methods and tools you will use to achieve your goals, including:
>
> - **Advertising**
> - **Public relations**
> - **Publicity**
> - **Sales promotions**
> - **Direct marketing**
> - **Personal selling**
> - **The Internet**

Establishing Goals

Smart business owners understand the value of implementing a marketing plan according to set goals and objectives. There are five primary objectives to consider in marketing skin care, and they are especially important in building sales promotions:

1. Create an ongoing interest in standard offerings.
2. Encourage repeat business.
3. Fill in slow periods.
4. Promote new products and services.
5. Increase retail sales.

Building a program that incorporates these goals and plans for marketing efforts on a weekly, monthly, and quarterly basis will help a business owner stay on track and increase business.

The Marketing Budget

Opinions differ on just how much money should be spent on marketing and advertising per year. Some salons set a fixed percentage of the annual budget based on projected revenues. Others choose to let market conditions and direct results dictate how they spend their advertising dollars. While there is no set standard, consider that an owner of a new business can expect to spend more money for marketing and advertising initially. Marketing expenses may level off once brand recognition is firmly established. However, this does not mean an owner can stop spending money on marketing. Marketing is a dynamic and ongoing process.

The most important thing for any small business owner to remember is that marketing is critical to maintaining a successful business. Marketing should not be thought of as something that is done if there is money leftover or something that can be discontinued once a business is up and running. Successful marketing campaigns require careful planning and an ongoing financial commitment.

Another important factor in budgeting is recognizing that marketing and advertising stimulate business and offer the largest benefit when business is slow. Therefore, when sales are sluggish, it may not be in a salon's best interest to cut back on advertising.

Whether the salon owner chooses a percentage-based model or calculates their budget according to market conditions and direct results, all decisions should be based on sound professional judgment. A good marketing program is often not about how much money is spent, but rather how well it is spent.

THE BROCHURE, OR MENU OF SERVICES

The **brochure**, or **menu of services**, is a key presentation piece and one of the more expensive printed marketing materials in which a salon will invest. The primary purpose of a brochure is informational: It should include everything clients need to know about the salon's or spa's treatments and services. However, the brochure should be designed with the target market in mind and, most importantly, reflect the basic image and philosophy of the salon. Whether a brochure is simple or elaborate, or whether it includes information on several straightforward or more fanciful treatments, will have a great deal to do with the type of salon and its clientele. For example, a brochure for a small skin care clinic focused on providing moderately priced treatments will look different than a brochure for a larger, full-service facility that caters to a high-end clientele.

This does not mean that a simple brochure with a limited number of treatment options cannot be attractive or enticing. There are many ways to be creative when developing a brochure (Figure 30–9). Using themes and incorporating special logo or design features can enhance the overall presentation.

As important as an attractive presentation is the text inside. The brochure must be clear, well written, organized, and legible. Dividing services into appropriate sections, such as face and body treatments, can make it easier for the client to access information. The writing must be free of grammar and spelling errors, and the salon's phone number, address, and Web site address should all be correct, easy to find, and readable. A professional consultant can be instrumental in writing the brochure, scrutinizing the details, and supervising printing, ultimately bringing all of these components together into a user-friendly brochure that encourages clients to pick up the phone.

Most salons today also include their policies in the brochure. This is a good way to provide clients with important information, such as how the salon handles cancellations and late arrivals, what methods of payment they accept, or any special comfort or safety considerations (for example, their policy on children visiting the salon or on cell phone use). The hours of operation and directions to the salon are other helpful features that address frequently asked questions. Some salons avoid including price information in the brochure in case prices change; that would necessitate reprinting the entire brochure. Clients often appreciate the inclusion of pricing information, though, because it allows them to zero in on the cost of services. Including all of this information in a separate price index can help limit confusion and avoid problems.

THE INTERNET

The **Internet** is a complex communications system that is capable of linking multiple computers worldwide. This sophisticated network has become an incredible resource for reaching millions of people and one that any business owner should include in a marketing program and budget. Developing a Web site is an involved process that goes beyond the scope of this text, but it is important to note that developing a Web site requires more than acquiring a URL, or Web address, and pasting the business's brochure on the Internet.

The primary goal of any Web site is to entice people to call or visit a salon. Simply posting a menu in its entirety is not the best use of a site. A good Web site makes consumers aware of the salon's offerings and what they can expect when they visit it. It may also identify frequently asked questions that will help consumers to better

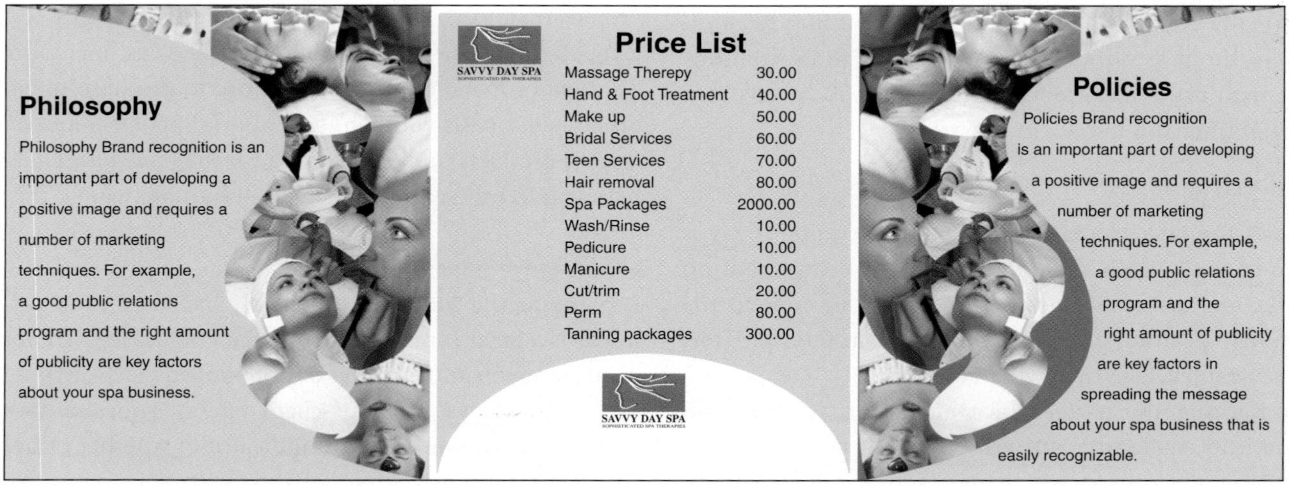
Philosophy
Philosophy Brand recognition is an important part of developing a positive image and requires a number of marketing techniques. For example, a good public relations program and the right amount of publicity are key factors about your spa business.
SAVVY DAY SPA
Price List
Massage Therepy 30.00
Hand & Foot Treatment 40.00
Make up 50.00
Bridal Services 60.00
Teen Services 70.00
Hair removal 80.00
Spa Packages 2000.00
Wash/Rinse 10.00
Pedicure 10.00
Manicure 10.00
Cut/trim 20.00
Perm 80.00
Tanning packages 300.00
SAVVY DAY SPA
Policies
Policies Brand recognition is an important part of developing a positive image and requires a number of marketing techniques. For example, a good public relations program and the right amount of publicity are key factors in spreading the message about your spa business that is easily recognizable.

Figure 30–9 A brochure or menu of services should reflect the basic image and philosophy of the salon.

> **Here's a Tip**
>
> The Internet can help you reach many potential clients, but developing a Web site can be an involved and complex process. Before you undertake such a project, do additional research and seek professional assistance to make it a rewarding rather than frustrating experience.

understand the benefits and features of a particular product or service. This is a great way to demonstrate expertise and get people to ask more questions. Using the Internet to sell gift certificates or deliver special announcements, such as information on upcoming events, a newsletter, or sales promotions via e-mail is another excellent cost-effective way to promote business.

There are many inexpensive options available for those looking to develop a Web site, including software programs, templates, and any number of Web development services and consultants. If you decide you would like to create a site for your business, be selective about your options and take time to develop your strategy. Make sure that all of the information that appears on the site is correct and truthful. Remember that millions of people will have instantaneous access to information about your business.

THE USE OF TECHNOLOGY

The world of technology has made it a lot easier to market a business. With salon software programs that can schedule appointments, sell gift certificates and retail products, track sales, and creates marketing promotions, it is really a matter of taking the time to utilize technology in the most productive way. And as those comfortable with using technology will tell you, it can save you a lot of time and money in the process.

Analyzing Sales Promotions

One of the best uses of technology in the salon today is sales analysis. With thousands of dollars being spent on marketing and retail sales, salon owners are now in the fortunate position of being able to look at their progress on several levels at the push of a button.

Analyzing the performance of sales promotions on a monthly, quarterly, and yearly basis is a great way to get a handle on market swings, address slow periods, and develop marketing programs. All of these factors can ultimately help you improve your marketing efforts. Most software programs have the capability of printing graphic reports, which make evaluating the numbers even easier. However, finding out exactly what is working and what is not takes a bit more investigation.

Tracking Sales, Client Information, and Employee Performance

Product and service sales are the primary revenue stream of any skin care business. There are several ways to evaluate how well your business is performing in these two critical areas. The first involves analyzing the overall performance of individual products and services (Figure 30–10). The second involves studying individual client profiles. The third requires an in-depth look at individual employee performance.

Products and Services

Tracking the performance of each product and service you sell will tell you a lot about what is popular with clients and what is not. It may also point to a need to increase marketing efforts. For example, there is little doubt that gift certificate sales are likely to be higher at holidays, or that product sales will increase during sales promotions, but what about the sale of series and spa packages on an everyday basis? Are these valuable revenue-generating treatments being overlooked on a day-to-day basis? Encouraging clients to purchase face or body treatments bundled in series savings or value-added packages is a great way to boost repeat business.

If you have recently introduced a new product, track the methods used to market that product. Are you able to correlate an increase or lack of sales to a particular promotional campaign or, on the other hand, a lack of a campaign? Taking a look at all facets of sales, including the type of marketing efforts you use to promote them, on a regular basis will help you to promote or eliminate certain products and services, a task that can ultimately help you to use your marketing dollars more wisely.

Customer Profiles

Looking at the individual spending habits of each customer is a great way to find out what clients need and or want from you and whether or not you are meeting those needs. An analysis of your client referral and retention rate will provide an excellent indicator of whether or not your clients are ultimately satisfied with your salon and services. These numbers are extremely useful in helping

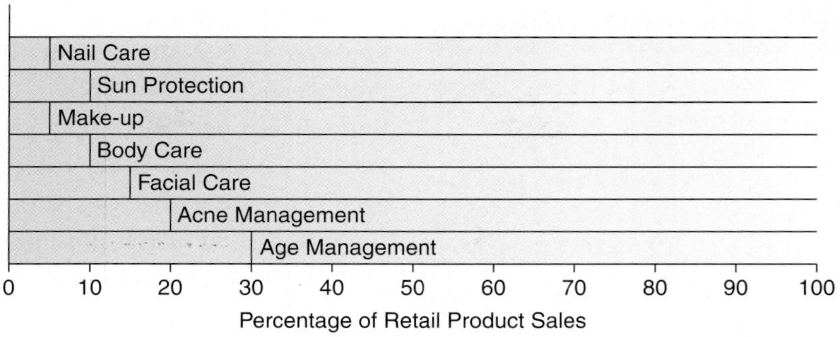

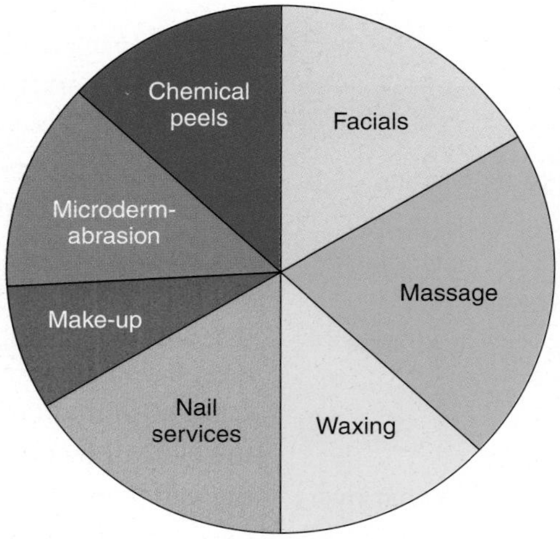

Figure 30–10 Tracking your efforts will help you to determine the most productive methods for marketing your skin care salon.

you address these critical issues with your staff and service providers as well.

Employee Performance

Because personal selling is such an integral part of any salon marketing program, one of the most important areas of concern for business owners when measuring sales and marketing efforts is employee performance. Technology is invaluable in this area and can assist the salon owner in taking an unbiased and detailed look at each individual's performance.

Whether you are calculating the individual's ability to bring in new business or measure individual sales performance, technology can easily track how many services or products each individual has sold on a daily, weekly, or monthly basis. Some software programs also have a built-in calculator for determining commission rates.

Sales analysis tools can be a great help in setting individual goals as well. Some salons implement special bonuses or incentives, such as education vouchers, days off, or special commission rates to boost new product sales or motivate employees to increase sales.

Using the Computer as a Marketing Tool

Your computer is an excellent resource for automatically prompting the implementation of everyday promotional items, such as referral cards, reminder notices, birthday and thank-you cards, which are important tools of the trade that keep business flowing. Marketing software programs are also invaluable when it comes to printing mailing labels, creating gift cards, and delivering newsletters and other direct marketing promotions via the Internet, but your personal computer should not be used to create important business collateral such as brochures and business cards. These materials are best created by skilled professionals.

MARKETING RESPONSIBLY

Marketing has the important and sometimes dubious distinction of influencing consumer purchasing decisions. However, there are laws and agencies in place to make sure businesses conduct their marketing efforts responsibly.

Here's a Tip

Technology can help you to implement a number of automatic business builders, such as

- **Referral bonuses**
- **Reminder notices**
- **Loyalty programs**
- **Gifts cards**
- **Series savers**
- **Membership certificates**

REGULATORY AGENCY ALERT

It is important for business owners to be familiar with the rules and regulations of the Food and Drug Administration (FDA), the Federal Trade Commission (FTC), the Consumer Product Safety Commission (CPSC), and Better Business Bureau, as well as state and local regulatory agencies.

There are several U.S. government agencies that oversee marketing practices. The Federal Trade Commission (FTC) is the primary agency responsible for regulating all business conduct, overseeing such important business functions as patent and trademark laws and pricing. The Food and Drug Administration (FDA) is responsible for governing the packaging and labeling of all food, drugs, and cosmetics. This organization publishes several booklets and pamphlets for the cosmetic industry, which you can find easily on the Internet. The Consumer Product Safety Commission (CPSC) is responsible for filing claims against companies that produce unsafe or defective products. Other local government and private agencies such as the U.S. Attorney General's office and the Council of Better Business Bureaus also serve as watchdogs to protect the consumer.

If you are thinking about becoming a business owner, it is wise to learn the laws and basic rules set forth by these agencies. All salon owners should make every effort to avoid using deceptive or fraudulent techniques when it comes to marketing any product or service sold in their salon or spa. Service providers must be equally diligent when representing products and services and refrain from making any claim that they do not know to be true.

Marketing is a broad-based business strategy that requires extensive research and planning that goes beyond the scope of this text. It is also what drives business. If you are interested in opening your own skin care salon it is important to develop a solid understanding of the basic principles of marketing and to be familiar with the various methods available for promoting your business. Studying the demographics of your target market is an integral part of the overall process. However, when it comes to developing a complete marketing program and marketing materials, it is wise to seek the support of qualified marketing professionals who can help you to assess the feasibility of your plan and develop the right image and strategies for your business from the start.

REVIEW QUESTIONS

1. Define the term *marketing*.
2. What are the four Ps used in creating a marketing strategy for a skin care salon?
3. Explain the six marketing strategies identified in the promotion mix.
4. Why are demographics important to marketing?
5. What role does customer value play in product selection?
6. Explain the concept of features and benefits in marketing.
7. List several methods used to advertise.
8. What are sales promotions?

9. What is a unique selling proposition (USP)?
10. How can technology be used to create cost-effective marketing strategies in the salon?
11. What government agencies are responsible for overseeing marketing practices and what role does each have?

CHAPTER GLOSSARY

advertising: refers to promotional efforts that are paid for and directly intended to increase business.

brochure, or menu of services: a key marketing presentation piece that lists the treatments and services that are available at your salon.

customer relationship management: the management of customer relations.

direct marketing: a marketing strategy that refers to any direct attempt to reach the consumer.

Internet: a complex communications system that is capable of linking multiple computers worldwide.

marketing: a business strategy for how ideas, goods and services are bought, sold or exchanged.

marketing plan: states your marketing goals and objectives and the strategies that you will use to achieve those goals.

personal selling: a marketing strategy that involves a one to one exchange or dialogue with the consumer.

place: refers to the distribution channel or method for delivering your goods and services to clients.

price: the monetary value applied to goods and services sold.

product: in marketing this term refers to your complete business concept and includes both the tangible and intangible characteristics associated with your marketing strategy.

promotion: the marketing methods used to persuade others to purchase your products and services.

promotion mix: the communication methods used to promote business in marketing. These include advertising, public relations, publicity, direct marketing, personal selling, and sales promotion.

publicity: a marketing strategy used to gain free media attention.

public relations: a marketing strategy that is used to generate positive publicity about your business.

sales promotion: a marketing strategy aimed at drawing attention to your products and services with the goal of increasing the volume of business.

REFERENCES AND RESOURCES

CHAPTER 2

OSHA- http://www.osha.gov/

CDC- http://www.cdc.gov/

1. Health Educators Inc. (2001). *Education for the Modification Industry.* Cleveland OH: Health Educators Inc.

CHAPTER 3

1. Pugliese, P. T. M.D. (1999). *Advanced Professional Skin Care.* Bernville, PA: APSC Publishing

CHAPTER 4

1. Lees, Mark. (2007). *Mark Lees Skin Care, Beyond the Basics: Third Edition.* Clifton Park, NY: Thomson/Delmar Learning Publishers

CHAPTER 5

1. Hill, Pamela R.N. (2006). *Milady's Aesthetician Series: Botox, Dermal Fillers, and Sclerotherapy.* Clifton Park, NY: Thomson/Delmar Learning Publishers

CHAPTER 6

1. Hill, Pamela R.N. (2006). *Milady's Aesthetician Series: Botox, Dermal Fillers, and Sclerotherapy.* Clifton Park, NY: Thomson/Delmar Learning Publishers

CHAPTER 7

1. Lees, Mark. (2007). *Skin Care Beyond the Basics: Third Edition.* Clifton Park, NY: Thomson/Delmar Learning Publishers
2. Harrison, J. (2008). *Aromatherapy: Therapeutic Use of Essential Oils for Esthetics.* Clifton Park, NY: Milady/Cengage Learning Inc.
3. Harrison, Jimm. Phytotherapy Institute for Healthy Aging and Holistic Beauty.

CHAPTER 8

1. Aesthetic Dermatology News. (2008, May/June), 30.
2. Alam, M., Dover, J., and Arndt, K. (2007, June). Use of cutaneous lasers and light sources: Appropriate training and delegation. *Skin Therapy Lett., 12(5),* 5–9.
3. Allen, C.J. (2008, January/February). Societies issue consumer alerts. *Aesthetic Dermatology News, Vol. 3 (1),* pp. 1–16.
4. American Society for Dermatologic Surgery. (2006). Keeping patients safe: A guide to combating the practice of medicine by unqualified, unsupervised individuals [Online]. Available: http://www.ASDS.net.
5. ANSIZ 136.3.2005. American National Standard Institute for Safe Use of Lasers in Health Care Facilities. Orlando: Laser Institute of America.
6. Arndt, K., Dover, J.S., and Anderson, R.R. (2006, Dec). The state of non-traditional acne treatments (Supplement). *Skin & Aging, 14(12).*
7. Bellew, S.G., Lee, C.,Weiss, M.A., and Weiss, R.A. (2005). Improvement of atrophic acne scars with a1, 320nm Nd: YAGlaser: Retrospective study. *Dermatol Surg., 31(9),* 1218–1221.
8. Biesman, B.S., Baker, S.S., Carruthers, J., Silva, H.L., and Holloman, E.L. (2006). Monopolar radiofrequency treatment of human eye lids: A prospective, multicenter, efficacy trial. *Lasers in SurgMed, 38(10),* 890–898.

9. Brahmavar, S., and Hetzel, F. (2001). Medical lasers: Quality control, safety standards, and regulations, [Online]. Available: http://www.aapm.org.

10. Cosmetic Laser Solutions Medical Spa. (n.d.). Gentle YAG for skin tightening in Boston [Online]. Available: http://www.bostonhealthandbeauty.com

11. Courtesy information of Thermage™

12. Courtesy information of Rockwell Laser Industries

13. Courtesy information of Dusa Pharmaceuticals

14. Courtesy information from Lumenis® LTD.

15. Dennis, V., Crowgey, S., and Grimes, B. (1996). *Laser series*. Unpublished manuscript.

16. Dennis, V., Crowgey, S., and Grimes, B. (1996). Laser series. Unpublished manuscript.

17. Dover, J., Lim, H., Rigel, D., and Weiss, R. (EDs). (2004). *Photoaging*. NewYork: Marcel Decker, Inc.

18. Dwyer, Melody. DO. Boise, Idaho.

19. Elman, M., and Lebzelter, J. (2004). Light therapy in the treatment of acne vulgaris. *Dermatol Surg., 30(2),* 139–146.

20. FDA classification system [Online]. Available: http://www.qrasupport.com. http://www.fda.gov.

21. Fisher, G.H., Jacobson, L.G., Bernstein, L.J., Kim, K.H., and Geronemus, R.G. (2006). Non ablative radiofrequency treatment of facial laxity. *Dermatolog Surg., 31(s3),* 1237–1241.

22. Gerson, Joel; D'Angelo, Janet; Lotz, Shelley. (2004). *Milady's Standard Fundamentals for Estheticians, ninth edition,* Clifton Park, NY: Delmar Learning

23. Goldberg, D.J., Rohrer, T., Dover, J., and Alam, M. (2005). *Lasers and Lights: Vascular, pigmentation, scars, medical applications, v.1.* Philadelphia: Mosby Elsevier Health Science.

24. Goldberg, D.J., Rohrer, T., Dover, J., and Alam, M. (2005). *Lasers and Lights: Rejuvenation, Resurfacing, Hair Removal, Treatment of Ethnic Skin.* Vol. 2. Philadelphia: Mosby Elsevier Health Science.

25. Goldman, M. (ED). (2006). *Cutaneous and Cosmetic Laser Surgery.* Philadelphia: PA: Mosby Elsevier Health Science.

26. Goldman, M.P., Mauricio, M., and Rao, J. (2004) Intravascular 1320nm laser closure of the great saphenous vein: A 6 to 12 month follow-up study. *DermatolSurg, 30(11),* 1380–1385.

27. Goldberg, D.J., and Russell, B.A. (2006, Jun). Combination blue (415nm) and red (633nm) LED phototherapy in the treatment of mild to severe acne vulgaris. *J Cosmet Laser Ther., 8(2),* 71–75.

28. Hansen, I. (2007, Jan/Feb). Fractional resurfacing. *Medesthetics,* 28–35.

29. Hansen, I. (2007, Mar/Apr). Light-based acne treatments. *Medesthetics,* 24–30.

30. Hill, P. (2007). *Advanced Face and Body.* Clifton Park: Cengage Learning

31. Idaho Board of Medicine.Intense pulsed light and/or laser devices [Online]. Available: http://www.bom.state.id.us.

32. JGM Associates, Inc. (1993). *Therapeutic Applications of Advanced Laser Products,* 1, Tutorials. Burlingham, MA

33. Kaufmann, J. (2007, May 1). Alexandrite laser may be tool of choice for hair removal. (White paper) *Dermatology Times.*

34. Kauvar, A. (2007) Photodynamic Therapy. New and Future applications of PDT. (Conference program). Dallas: American Society of Laser Surgery and Medicine.

35. Kronemyer, B. (2005, Jan/Feb). Gentlewaves obtains the first FDA approval for LED-based wrinkle treatment. *Aesthetics Buyers Guide,* 228–229.

36. Kronemyer, B. (2007, May/June). Skin tightening, devices evolve to meet patient demand. *Aesthetics Buyers Guide,* 33–52.

37. Kronemyer, B. (2007, Jan/Feb). Smart lipo cleared as first laser lipolysis. *Aesthetics Buyers Guide,* 22–24.

38. Lowe, N.J., Luftman, D. and Sawcer, D. (1994). Q-switched ruby laser. Further observations on treatment of professional tattoos. *J Dermatol Surg Oncol., 20(5),* 307–311.

39. Mariwalla, K., and Rohrer, T. (2005). Use of lasers and light-based therapies for treatment of acne vulgaris. *Lasers in Surg and Med, 37(5),* 333–342.

40. Medical Insight, Inc. *Aesthetic Buyers Guide* [Online]. Available: http://www.miinews.com

41. Medical Insights, Inc. (2007, June). Home use devices (Executive summary).

42. Merkel, Williams, M.D. Grand Junction, Colorado.

43. Moretti, M. (ed.) *The Aesthetic Guide, The Aesthetic Buyers Guide, Vol. 11(1)* (pp. 888–120).

44. Moretti, M. (2007). Body shaping and skin tightening drive global aesthetic industry to $ 15 billion by 2011 (Market study from *Medical Insight, Inc.*) [Online]. Available: http://www.surgicenteronline.com.

45. Moretti, M.(Ed.). (2005). Clinical round table (supplement). European Aesthetics Buyers Guide, 18–22. Available: http://www.eurobg.com

46. Olympic Dermatology and Laser Clinic (online) Available: http://www.olympicdermatology.com.

47. Rao, J., and Goldman, M.P. (2006). Prospective, comparative evaluation of three laser systems used individually and in combination for axillary hair removal. *Dermatol Surg., 31(12),* 1671–1677.

48. Resinisch, L. (1996). Laser physics and tissue interactions. *Otolaryngologic Clinics of North America, 29(6),* 893–913

49. Rockwell, J. and Chamberlain, J. (2000). *RLI: Medical users guide for laser safety.* Cincinnati: Rockwell Laser Industries.

50. Rokhsar, C., Lee, S., and Fitzpatrick, R. (2005, September). Review of photo rejuvenation: devices, cosmeceuticals, or both? *Dermatol Surg, 31(9),* 1166–1178.

51. Sadick, N.S. (2005). Combination radiofrequency and light energies: electro-optical synergy technology in esthetic medicine. *DermatolSurg., 31(s3),* 1211–1217.

52. Sadick, N., Rotund, A., Wanner, M., and Manstein, D. (2007). Technology for fat-related disorders workshop (Conference program). Dallas: American Society of Laser Medicine and Surgery.

53. Shamban, A.T. (n.d.). Photopneumatic (PPx) pore-cleansing acne treatment: A break through treatment option for non-responders to acne therapies [Online]. Available: http://www.aesthera.com

54. Smalley, P.J. Technology Concepts International.

55. Trost, D., Zacherl, A., and Smith, M.F.W. (1992). Surgical laser properties and their tissue interaction. In F.W Mansfield and J.T. McElveen (Eds.) *Neurological Surgery of the Ear,* (pp. 131–161). Philadelphia: Mosby Elsevier Health Science.

56. U.S. Department of Labor, Occupational Safety & Health Administration. (1991). STD01-05-001-PUB8-1.7 Guidelines for laser safety and hazard assessment [Online]. Available: http://www.osha.gov.

57. U.S. Department of Labor, Occupational Safety & Health Administration. Blood borne pathogens standards-29CFR1910.1030 [Online]. Available: http://www.osha.gov.

58. Vandruff, C. (ED.). (2008, March/April). *Aesthetic Trends and Technology, Vol.7(7)* (pp. 33–69).

59. Weaver, S.M. and Sagaral, E.C. (2003). Treatment of Pseudofolliculitis barbae using the long-pulse Nd: YAG laser on skin types V and VI. *Dermatol Surg., 29(12),* 1187–1191.

60. Weiss, R.A., McDaniel, D.H., Geronemus, R.G., Weiss, M.A., Beasley, K.L., Munavalli, G.M., and Bellew, S.G. (2006). Clinical experience with light-emitting diode (LED) photomodulation. *Dermatol Surg., 31(s3),* 1199–1205.

61. Yaghmai, D., Garden, J.M., Bakus, A.D., Spenceri, E.A., Hruza, G.J., and Kilmer, S.L. (2004). Hair removal using a combination radiofrequency and intense pulsed light source. *J Cosmet Laser The, 6, 201–2*

CHAPTER 10

1. Arroyave, E. M.D. (2006). *Understanding Cosmetics Procedures: Surgical and Nonsurgical.* Clifton Park, NY: Thomson/ Delmar Learning Publishers

2. Hill, Pamela R.N. (2006) *Milady's Aesthetician Series: Peels and Peeling Agents.* Clifton Park, NY: Thomson/Delmar Learning Publishers

3. Lee, Mark. (2007) *Skin Care Beyond the Basics: Third Edition.* Clifton Park, NY: Thomson/Delmar Learning Publishers

CHAPTER 11

1. Hill, Pamela. (2006). *Milady's Aesthetician Series: Microdermabrasion.* Clifton Park, NY: Thomson/Delmar Learning Publishers.

2. Pugliese, P.T. M.D. (2005). *Advanced Professional Skin Care: Medical Edition.* Bernville, PA: The Topical Agent LLC

CHAPTER 12

1. Lee, Mark. (2007). *Mark Lees Skin Care, Beyond the Basics: Third Edition.* Clifton Park, NY: Thomson/Delmar Learning Publishers

CHAPTER 13

1. Erasmus, Udo. (2002). *How Bad Are Cooking Oils?* www.udoerasmus.com/articles/udo/hbaco_pv.htm
2. Harrison, J. (2008). *Aromatherapy: Therapeutic Use of Essential Oils for Esthetics.* Clifton Park, NY: Milady/Cengage Learning Inc.
3. Harrison, Jimm. Phytotheraphy Institute for Healthy Aging and Holistic Beauty.
4. Lindgren, Frank T.; Nichols, Alex V.; Freeman, Norman K.; Wills, Robert D. *Potential Contamination in the Analysis of Metyl Esters of Fatty Acids by Gas-Liquid Chromatography;* UC Berkeley.

CHAPTER 14

1. Lees, Mark. (2007). *Skin Care Beyond the Basics: Third Edition.* Clifton Park, NY: Thomson/Delmar Learning Publishers

CHAPTER 15

1. http://www.nlm.nih.gov
2. http://www.rxlist.com
3. http://www.drugs.com
4. Michalun, N. (2001). *Milady's Skin Care and Cosmetic Ingredients Dictionary,* Thomson/Delmar Learning
5. Spratto, G.R., Woods, A.L. (2005). *2005 PDR Nurse's Drug Handbook,* Thomson/Delmar Learning
6. http://www.fda.gov
7. Deglin, JH and Vallerand, AH Davis's (2007). *Davis's Drug Guide for Nurses.* F.A. Davis, Philadelphia, PA.
8. http://www.emedicine.com/PED/topic581.htm
9. http://www.diabetes.org/type-1-diabetes.jsp
10. Roth-Skidmore, Linda (1999). *1999 Nursing Drug Reference,* Mosby St. Louis, Missouri

CHAPTER 16

1. Lees, Mark. (2007). *Skin Care Beyond the Basics: Third Edition.* Clifton Park, NY: Cengage Learning.

CHAPTER 17

1. French-Moody, R. (2004). *Milady's Guide to Lymph Drainage Massage.* Clifton Park, NY: Thomson/Delmar Learning Publishers

CHAPTER 18

1. ANSIZ 136.3.2005. American National Standard Institute for Safe Use of Lasers in Health Care Facilities. Orlando: Laser Institute of America.
2. Aesthetic Buyers Guide [Online]. Available: http://www.miinews.com
3. Bickmore, H. (2004) Milady's Hair Removal techniques. Clifton Park, N.Y: Milady. Medical Insight, Inc.
4. Bitter, P.H. (2000) Noninvasive rejuvenation of photo damaged skin using serial, full face intense pulsed light treatments. *Dermatol Surg. 26(9),* 835–843.
5. Courtesy information from Marcel Besse, Light Biosciences and Omnilux medical Photo Therapeutic LTD.
6. Courtesy of Lumenis® LTD.
7. Courtesy information of Light Bioscience Product
8. Courtesy information of Thermage™

9. Courtesy information of Dusa Pharmaceuticals
10. Dover, Jeffery; Lim, Henry; Rigel, Darrell; Weiss, Robert. (2004). *Photoaging,* New York, NY: Marcel Decker, Inc.
11. Gerson, Joel; D'Angelo, Janet; Lotz, Shelley. (2004). *Milady's Standard Fundamentals for Estheticians, ninth edition,* Clifton Park, NY: Delmar Learning.
12. Goldberg, D.J., Rohrer, T., Dover, J., and Alam, M. (2005). *Lasers and Lights: Vascular, pigmentation, scars, medical applications,* Vol 1. Philadelphia: Mosby Elsevier Health Science.
13. Goldberg, D.J., Rohrer, T., Dover, J., and Alam, M. (2005). *Lasers and Lights: Rejuvenation, Resurfacing, Hair Removal, Treatment of Ethnic Skin, vol. 2.* Philadelphia: Mosby Elsevier Health Science.
14. Goldman, M. (ED). (2006). *Cutaneous and Cosmetic Laser Surgery,* Philadelphia: Mosby Elsevier Health Science.
15. Goldman, M.P., Weiss, R.A. and Weiss, M.A. (2005). Intense pulsed light as a nonablative approach to photoaging. *Dermatol Surg., 31(9),* 1179–1187.
16. Hill, P. (2007). *Advanced Face and Body.* Clifton Park: Cengage Learning.
17. Kauvar, A., ASLMS 2007 Photodynamc Therapy Presentation: New and future applications PDT.
18. Kauvar, A. (2007) Photodynamic Therapy. New and Future applications of PDT. (Conference program). Dallas: American Society of Laser Surgery and Medicine.
19. Moretti, M.(ed.) *The Aesthetic Guide, The Aesthetic Buyers Guide, Volume 11*(1) (pp. 88–120).
20. Nestor, M., Goldberg, D., Goldman, M., Weiss,R., and Rigel, D. (2000 March). Photorejuvenation-Nonablative skin rejuvenation using intense pulsed light. (White paper). *Skin and Aging.*
21. Nestor, M., Goldberg, D., Goldman, M., Weiss, R., and Rigel, D. (2003). New perspective on Photorejuvenation. Skin and Aging. II (5). [Online] Available: http://www.skinandaging.com.
22. Olympic Dermatology and Laser Clinic [Online] Available: http://www.olympicdermatology.com.
23. Rao, J., and Goldman, M.P.(2006). Prospective, comparative evaluation of three laser systems used individually and in combination for axillary hair removal. *Dermatol Surg., 31(12),* 1671–1677.
24. Rockwell, J. and Chamberlain, J. (2000). RLI: Medical users guide for laser safety. Cincinnati: Rockwell Laser Industries.
25. Ross, V. (2006). Laser versus Intense Pulsed Light: Competing Technologies in *Dermatology. Lasers in Surgery and Medicine: 38: 261–272.*
26. Smalley, P.J. Technology Concepts International.
27. Vandruff, C. (ED.). (2008, March/Aprl). Aesthetic Trends and Technology, Volume 7(7) (pp. 33–69).
28. Willem, A., Toorrontequi, J. et al. (2007) Hair stimulation following laser and intense pulsed photepilatoin: review of 543 cases and ways to manage it. *Lasers in Surgery and medicine: 39:297*–301.

CHAPTER 19

1. Hill, Pamela; Todd, Laura. (2008). *Milady's Aesthetician Series: Advanced Face and Body Treatments for the Spa.* Clifton Park, NY: Cengage Learning.
2. Bickmore, H.R. (2004). *Milady's Hair Removal Techniques: A Comprehensive Manual.* Clifton Park, NY: Thomson/Delmar Learning Publishers

CHAPTER 21

1. Hill, Pamela; Todd, Laura. (2008). *Milady's Aesthetician Series: Advanced Face and Body Treatments for the Spa.* Clifton Park, NY: Cengage Learning.
2. Alexcae Moren, S. (2005). *Spa and Salon Alchemy: The Ultimate Guide to Spa and Salon Ownership.* Clifton Park, NY: Thomson/Delmar Learning Publishers

CHAPTER 22

1. Alexcae Moren, S. (2005). *Spa and Salon Alchemy: The Ultimate Guide to Spa and Salon Ownership.* Clifton Park, NY: Thomson/Delmar Learning Publishers

CHAPTER 23

1. Sachs, M.; Sachs, R. (2007). *Ayurvedic Spa*. Twin Lakes, WI: Lotus Press

CHAPTER 24

1. D'Angelo, Janet et al. (2003). *Milady's Standard Comprehensive Training for Estheticians*. New York: Milady, an imprint of Delmar, a division of Thomson Learning, Inc.
2. D'Angelo, Janet. (2006). *Spa Business Strategies*, New York: Thomson/Delmar Learning
3. Dietz, Sallie. (2004). *The Clinical Esthetician: An Insider's Guide to Succeeding in a Medical Office*. New York: Thomson/Delmar Learning.
4. Gerson, Joel. *Milady's Standard Fundamentals for Estheticians*, 10E. New York: Thomson/Delmar Learning, 2007
5. Lees, Mark. *Skin Care Beyond the Basics:* Third Edition. New York: Thomson/Delmar Learning, 2007.

CHAPTER 25

1. Chabner, Davi-Ellen. (2005). *Medical Terminology: A Short Course,* 4th ed. Philadelphia: W.B. Saunders.
2. Hill, Pamela R.N. (2006). *Milady's Aesthetician Series Medical Terminology: A Handbook for the Skin Care Specialist.* Clifton Park, NY: Thomson/Delmar Learning Publishers
3. http://ec.hku.hk/mt/suffix3.htm
4. http://www.dummies.com/WileyCDA/DummiesArticle/id-1185.html
5. http://www.mtworld.com/tools_resources/medical_plurals.html

CHAPTER 26

1. Hill, Pamela R.N. (2006). *Milady's Aesthetician Series: Botox Dermal Fillers and Sclerotherapy.* Clifton Park, NY: Thomson/Delmar Learning Publishers
2. www.allergan.com

CHAPTER 27

1. Arroyave, E. M.D. (2006) *Understanding Cosmetics Procedures Surgical and Nonsurgical.* Clifton Park, NY: Thomson/Delmar Learning Publishers

CHAPTER 28

1. Deitz, S. (2004). *Milady's The Clinical Esthetician: An Insiders Guide to Success in a Medical office.* Clifton Park, NY: Thomson/Delmar Learning Publishers

CHAPTER 29

1. D'Angelo, Janet et al. (2003). *Milady's Standard Comprehensive Training for Estheticians.* New York: Milady, an imprint of Delmar, a division of Thomson Learning, Inc.
2. D'Angelo, Janet M. (2006). *Spa Business Strategies: A Plan for Success.* New York: Thomson/Delmar Learning.
3. Gambino, Henry. *Marketing & Advertising for the Salon.* New York: Thomson/Delmar Learning, 1996.
4. Gerson, Joel, *Milady's Standard Fundamentals for Estheticians.* 10 E New York: Delmar Learning, an imprint of Delmar, a division of Thomson Learning, Inc. 2007

CHAPTER 30

1. D'Angelo, Janet et al. (2003). *Milady's Standard Comprehensive Training for Estheticians.* New York: Milady, an imprint of Delmar, a division of Thomson Learning, Inc.
2. D'Angelo, Janet M. *Spa Business Strategies: A Plan for Success.* New York: Thomson/Delmar Learning, 2006.
3. Gambino, Henry. (1994). *Milady's Esthetician's Guide to Business Management,* New York: Milady Publishing Company
4. Gerson, Joel. *Milady's Standard Fundamentals for Estheticians.* 10 E New York: Delmar Learning, an imprint of Delmar, a division of Thomson Learning, Inc. 2007

Glossary

A

abdominoplasty: tummy tuck.

ablation: the removal of surface material from the body. Ablative devices refer to those that vaporize, cut, or remove all or part of the epidermis and/or dermis.

ablative: in cosmetic medical uses, a procedure in which there is a removal and heating of the epidermis and sometimes portions of the dermis by a CO2 and/or Erbium Nd:YAG laser. In surgical uses it refers to the ability to surgically cut or remove using a laser.

absolutes: an extraction method using a solvent (hexane) to extract the essence from the plant material.

absorption: attraction of energy particles, liquid, or gas to a particular chromophore or target in the skin. The uptake of one substance into another.

acetylcholine: enzyme found in various tissues and organs, associated with muscle movement.

acetylsalicylic acid (ASA): aspirin.

acidophilic normoblast: part of the blood cell line and formed from the polychromatic normoblast, this cell (8 to 10 microns diameter) loses its nucleus at this stage.

Acquired Immune Deficiency Syndrome (AIDS): disease caused by the HIV virus that breaks down the body's immune system.

actin: a protein in a muscle fiber that, together with myosin, is responsible for contraction and relaxation.

actin filaments: connected to the catenins, they help stabilize cell adherence.

actinic keratoses: pink, sometimes scaly, abnormal skin lesions that are regarded to be precancerous. These lesions develop as the result of sun damage and may present on the face, ears, neck, shoulders, arms, and most commonly on the hands.

active ingredient: ingredient in a drug that causes a change to the structure or function of the body.

active transport: a process that requires expenditure of ATP energy to move molecules across a cell membrane; also called facilitated transport.

acupuncture: the practice of inserting very fine needles through the skin to specific points to help relieve pain or cure disease. Origin: China.

acute: the rapid-onset, short-term initial stage of disease. Contrast with chronic.

acute coronary syndrome (ACS): general term used for any condition which causes chest pain resulting from limited blood flow to the heart.

adduction: side-to-side movement.

adductor group of muscles: smaller muscles that work to keep the legs together during most physical activity.

adenosine triphosphate (ATP): a multifunctional nucleotide that transports chemical energy within cells for metabolism and converts oxygen to carbon dioxide.

adherens junctions: provides strong mechanical attachments between adjacent cells.

adjective: part of speech used to describe a noun.

adrenal glands: endocrine glands, located just above the kidneys, that produce hormones needed by the nervous system to transport nerve impulses.

adrenaline: a hormone secreted by the adrenal glands during an emergency response, such as stress. Adrenaline elevates the heart rate, increases blood pressure, and triggers the release of cortisol.

adult acne: acne that develops in the 20s and above; often caused by hormone fluctuations, or external factors, such as comedogenic (pore-clogging) skin care products.

adulteration: the process of adding natural or synthetic compounds, or cheaper but similar oils, to "stretch" or alter the fragrance of an essential oil.

advertising: refers to promotional efforts that are paid for and directly intended to increase business.

aerosolized: ultramicroscopic particles suspended in the air or in a gas.

afferent: (L. ad, "to lead" + ferre, "to bear") Adjective meaning leading or bearing toward some organ, such as nerves conducting impulses toward the brain or blood vessels carrying blood toward an organ; contrast with efferent.

AGE Products: AGE stands for advanced glycation endproducts, which are particles created in glycation that cross-link with proteins and lipids, resulting in tissue damage.

agni: the universal organizing principle of conversion such as the power to digest food or understand experiences.

agranulocytes: nongranular white blood cells.

airbrush makeup: the process of applying makeup to the skin using an airbrush device.

airbrushes: small air operated tools that spray liquids such as makeup.

akt: a pathway used as an intermediate signal as part of the DNA signaling cascade.

ala: flaring cartilaginous expansion on the side of each nare.

albumin: a grouping of certain water-soluble proteins as those found in blood or egg whites; the most abundant blood plasma protein.

alkaloids: secondary metabolites found in plants. They are nitrogen-containing organic compounds such as caffeine, morphine, nicotine, and quinine, which are very physiologically active in the human body.

allantoin: an anti-inflammatory compound isolated from the herb comfrey; used in creams, hand lotion, hair lotion, aftershave, and other skin-soothing cosmetics for its ability to heal wounds, skin ulcers, and to stimulate the growth of healthy tissue.

allergic reaction: an abnormal reaction and hypersensitivity to topical or oral substances that are ordinarily harmless. Signs and symptoms include hives, swelling, rash, and skin eruptions and can progress to respiratory distress.

alpha d-tocopherol: an antioxidant nutrient and popular form of vitamin E used in skin care and health supplements, generally isolated from soy or wheat.

Alzheimer's disease: chronic, progressive neurological condition characterized by early onset of dementia.

ama: body toxins from undigested food that causes illness.

amino acids: organic acids that form the building blocks of proteins. There are 20 amino acids utilized within the human body. Nine of these are essential amino acids and must be supplied by the diet.

anabolism: part of the metabolic process wherein larger molecules are built up from smaller molecules.

analgesic: a pain-killing effect.

anaphylaxis: serious, hypersensitive allergic reaction characterized by respiratory distress, hypotension, edema, rash, and tachycardia. Immediate medical attention is necessary.

anastomosis: the connection point of different parts of a branching network.

anchoring system: ties the plaque to the cytoplasm through the cytoskeleton; located inside the cell behind the plasma membrane.

androgens: male hormones.

anecdotal evidence: based on observation and theory rather than scientific experimentation.

anemia: condition characterized by a deficiency in iron.

angina: chest pain resulting from a lack of oxygen to the heart.

ankylosing spondylitis: stiffening of the vertebrae in the spine, resulting in loss of movement.

antacid: any agent that neutralizes stomach acid.

antagonist: something that opposes the action of another.

antianginals: class of drugs used to prevent the onset of an anginal attack.

antianxiety drugs: any drug that prevents or limits the severity of the symptoms of an anxiety disorder.

antiasthmatics: any drug that prevents or limits the severity of the symptoms of an asthma attack.

antibacterial: 1.) Destroying or stopping the growth of bacteria. 2.) Agent that destroys or prevents the growth of bacteria.

antibiotic: any variety of natural or synthetic substances that inhibit growth of or destroy microorganisms. Used extensively in treatment of infectious diseases.

antibodies: components of the immune system that neutralize antigens.

anticholinergics: class of drugs used to limit spasms and cramping, particularly of the digestive and urinary tracts.

anticonvulsants: class of drugs used to prevent or limit the severity of spastic activity resulting from certain neurological conditions.

antidepressants: class of drugs used to prevent or limit the severity of the symptoms of depression.

antiemetics: class of drugs used to prevent or limit the severity of the symptoms of nausea and vomiting.

antigen: 1.) a modified type of serum globulin synthesized by lymphoid tissue in response to antigenic stimulus. 2.) any material that elicits an immune response.

antihistamines: class of drugs used to block the action of histamine.

antimicrobial: 1.) destructive to or preventing the development of microorganisms. 2.) agent that destroys or prevents the development of microorganisms.

antioxidants: substances that neutralize free radicals, thereby decelerating the aging process and leaving tissues and cells healthy and able to function properly.

antipsychotic: class of drugs used to prevent or limit the severity of the symptoms of psychosis.

antiretrovirals: class of drug which are used to treat retroviruses, viruses that use the infected individuals DNA to replicate.

antispasmodics: see anticonvulsants.

antithrombotics: class of drugs that are used to prevent platelet coagulation.

antiulcer drugs: class of drugs used to prevent or limit the severity of the symptoms of peptic ulcers.

aorta: arterial trunk that carries blood from the heart to be distributed by branch arteries through the body.

aortic semilunar valve: valves that prevent blood from flowing back into the heart.

apnea: temporary ceasing of normal breathing function, often during sleep.

apocrine glands: coiled structures attached to hair follicles found in the underarm and genital areas. They produce a thicker form of sweat and are responsible for producing the substance that, when in contact with bacteria, produces body odor.

aponeurosis: any of the deep and thick facia, resembling flattened tendons, that attach muscles to bones.

apoptosis: (Gr., apo, away from + ptosis, a falling) Genetically determined cell death; "programmed" cell death.

Aquaphor®: a water-soluble, bland emollient ointment.

aqueous extract: an herbal water infusion.

areola: the circular area of darker pigmentation surrounding the breast nipple.

Arnica Montana: mountain plant (also known as *leopard's bane*) found in the Alps; a homeopathic herb known for speeding the post-operative recovery process, reducing uncomfortable swelling and bruising, and, often, post-operative pain.

arrhythmia: heart condition characterized by irregular heartbeats. Arrhythmias can be harmless or potentially serious.

arterioles: smallest component of the arteries; connects with capillary beds.

asepsis: sterile; a condition free from germs and any form of life.

aseptic technique: the process of properly handling sterilized and disinfected equipment and implements to prevent contamination.

ashram: a place for spiritual development.

aspartate: four-carbon amino acid found, with malate, to be the first products of the C4.

assets: anything your business owns.

asthenia: weakness or lack of strength.

ataxia: defective muscle coordination.

atria: two upper chambers of the heart that receive blood (singular atrium).

atrial flutter: cardiac arrhythmia characterized by a rapid activity of the atrial muscles.

atrioventricular valves: valves that prevent blood from flowing back into the ventricles of the heart.

attenuation: the act of removing light energy from a beam before it exits a second medium; a method of blocking laser energy.

aura: a subtle energy field that surrounds the body that is visible or can be felt by some people. Aura colors have been photographed using Kirlian photography.

autoclave: apparatus for sterilization by steam pressure usually at 250° F. (121° C.) for a specified length of time.

autoimmune disorders: disorders or diseases in which the body produces disordered immunological response against itself. Normally the body's immune mechanisms are able to distinguish clearly between what is a normal substance and what is foreign. In autoimmune diseases this system becomes defective and produces antibodies against normal parts of the body to such an extent as to cause tissue injury.

autologous: derived from the same species of which it is implanted.

autonomic motor systems (autonomic nervous system, ANS): the system that controls involuntary functions of the circulatory, respiratory, endocrine, and digestive systems and controls the actions of involuntary muscles, such as the heart.

AV conduction: component of the cardiac electrical system.

avian: pertaining to birds.

Ayurveda: the world's oldest and most complete system of holistic healing. Literally Ayurveda means the study of life or the science of longevity.

B

B cell: a type of lymphocyte derived from bone marrow stem cells that matures into an immunologically competent cell (under the influence of the bursa of fabricius in the chicken, and the bone marrow in nonavian species); following interaction with antigen, it becomes a plasma cell, which synthesizes and secretes antibody molecules involved in humoral immunity. Also called B lymphocyte.

B lymphocyte: cell that manufactures antibodies involved in immunity.

back bubble: the bubbling of liquid and air into the holding bowl of the airbrush during the mixing and cleaning processes.

bacteria: one-celled microorganisms with both plant and animal characteristics; also known as microbes. Capable of surviving on living and nonliving matter. Bacteria may be either pathogenic or nonpathogenic.

balance: quieting mental chatter, calming the emotions and reviving the spirit, resulting in a sense of inner peace, feeling grounded, more aware, connected and intuitive.

balance sheet: provides a financial overview of a business at a given point in time in terms of its assets and liabilities.

balneotherapy: body water treatments that use mud or fango, Dead Sea salt, seaweed, enzymes, or peat baths. Many of these treatments originated in ancient Greek and Roman bathhouses. While water treatments were originally used primarily for medicinal purposes, they eventually evolved into relaxation treatments as well.

barbiturates: addictive central nervous system depressants.

bariatric surgery: gastric bypass surgery.

basalt: a common grey to black fine grained volcanic rock.

bases: alkaline substances; substances with a pH above 7.

basophil: white blood cell characterized by the presence of blue cytoplasmic granules that become stained by a basophilic dye.

basophilic normoblast: a blue colored cell formed from the division of the pronormoblast this cell (6 to 18 microns diameter) produces polychromatic normoblasts.

benzene ring structure (Aromatic ring): hydrocarbon containing 6 carbon atoms and 6 hydrogen atoms; is responsible for some of the most effective antibacterial and antimicrobial compounds found in essential oils.

benzodiazepines: group of drugs with a sedative effect; predominantly used to treat anxiety and sleep disorders.

bicuspid valve: heart valve located between the left atrium and ventricle that regulates blood backflow between the two chambers.

bioavailable: describes a substance's ability to be used as a performance ingredient by the skin.

biochemistry: the study of chemicals and chemical reactions in the body.

biologically inert: describes ingredients that will not cross-react with chemicals that occur naturally in the body.

bipolar radio-frequency (RF) energy: a current that flows on a path of least resistance between positive and negative electrodes that are placed at opposite ends of treatment forceps or device head. No dispersive electrode is needed.

blanket wraps: the application of a blanket after a treatment to maintain heat or to cool the body.

blastocoel: a fluid-filled or yolk-filled cavity surrounded by a blastoderm.

blastoderm: primary epithelium formed in early embryonic development of many arthropods when the nuclei migrate to the periphery and undergo superficial cleavage; usually encloses the central yolk mass.

blastula: (Gr., blastos, "germ" + L. ula, "dim") an early stage in the development of an embryo; it consists of a sphere of cells enclosing a fluid-filled cavity (blastocoel).

blepharoplasty: an eye lift; plastic surgery procedure that removes excessive skin and/or fat in the upper and/or lower eyelids.

blepharospasm: spastic movement of the orbicularis oculis; usually a result of frequent and prolonged eye strain.

bloodborne: described transmission thorough direct blood-to-blood contact, such as sharing needles or through blood transfusion.

bloodborne pathogens: pathogenic microorganisms present in human blood that can cause disease in humans. These pathogens include, but are not limited to, hepatitis B virus (HBV), hepatitis C virus (HCV), and the human immunodeficiency virus (HIV).

blood-brain barrier: mechanism that alters the permeability of brain capillaries, so that some substances, such as certain drugs, are prevented from entering brain tissue, while other substances are allowed to enter freely.

blood pressure: force exerted by circulation of blood on the walls of blood vessels.

board certified: a title reserved for those physicians who have taken and passed the exam required for board certification in their respective specialties.

body dysmorphic disorder (BDD): psychosocial disease that causes individuals to be inappropriately concerned, obsessed, or fixated with their appearance.

body mask: a body treatment involving the application of an exfoliating, hydrating, purification or detoxification mask to the entire body. Masks may include those with clay, cream, gel, or seaweed bases.

botulinum toxin: bacterium from which Botox is derived.

bovine collagen: heterologous collagen which is derived from the skin of cows.

brachii: bicep, or muscle of the upper arm; name literally means "two heads," because it originates from two heads attached to the scapula (collar bone) and the humerus.

brachialis: important muscle for the arm's ability to flex at the elbow.

break-even analysis: the point at which all costs are covered and your business begins to earn a profit.

breast implants: to increase the size of the breast(s) using synthetic material such as silicone or saline implants.

brochure, or menu of services: a key marketing presentation piece that lists the treatments and services that are available at your salon.

bronchodilators: group of drugs which are used to reverse acute bronchial constriction.

buffering: refers to adjusting the pH of a product to make it more acceptable to the skin.

business plan: a strategy for understanding key elements in developing business; also serves as a guide to making informed business decisions.

C

capital: the amount of money invested in a business.

carboxylic acid: organic compounds containing the carboxyl functional group, a carbon with a double-bonded oxygen and an alcohol group attached.

cardiac fibers: muscle cells in the heart.

cardiovascular system: system that controls the steady circulation of the blood through the body by means of the heart and blood vessels. Also known as the circulatory system.

carotenoids: terpenoid compounds with 40 carbon atoms (tetraterpenoids). Those that contain oxygen are called *xanthophylls*—such as lutien found in tomatoes; Those without oxygen, are subcategorized as *carotenes*— beta-carotene being the most popular of those. These deeply pigmented compounds have a wide range of powerful health-giving properties.

cash flow statement: indicates how much money is flowing in and out of a business on a regular basis.

catabolism: part of the metabolic process wherein larger molecules within cells are broken down into smaller molecules which are then used for energy or waste.

catalyst: something that triggers a change.

catechins: a crystalline flavinoid compound with antioxidant properties

catechol-O-methyltransferase inhibitors: agents that break down levodopa, allowing greater availability in the central nervous system.

catenin: a protein important in stabilizing cell adherence to avoid abnormal spread of cells.

cautery: an agent or instrument used to destroy abnormal tissue by burning.

cell cycle: the regular sequence of events in the life of a cell, during which the cell grows, prepares for division, duplicates its contents and divides to form two daughter cells.

cell-mediated immunity: a part of the immune system that does not involve antibodies and the function of which is carried out mainly by T-cells.

cell wall: the rigid outermost layer of the cells found in plants, some protests (type of single-cell organism), and most bacteria. Found in plants composed principally of cellulose. Not found in animal cells.

cellophane body wrap: a wrap that uses a plastic material to aid in the penetration of the product through means of producing or increasing perspiration.

cellular membrane: also called plasma membrane. A semipermeable lipid bi-layer common to all living things.

cellulitis: potentially serious infection of the skin that presents as a small, red area surrounding a skin injury; those at risk include the elderly and those with a compromised immune system.

central serous retinopathy: occular condition characterized by fluid leaking from the macula resulting in blurred vision.

ceramides: a lipid component of the intercellular cement within the stratum corneum layer.

cervical dystonia: prolonged, repetitive muscle contractions that may cause twisting or jerking movements of the neck.

Chakra: one of seven main energy centers of the body. They are found situated at the base of the spine, at the navel, the solar plexus, the heart, throat, the middle of the forehead and the crown of the head. Chakras are major marma points or mahamarmas. Literally chakra means "energy wheel."

chalazia: small, lumpy cysts in the eyelids.

chemical reactions: reactions between two elements or two compounds that result in chemical changes.

chin/neck bra: a support device worn after surgery of the chin or neck area.

cholesterol: a lipid component of the stratum corneum.

chondroitin sulfate: a proteoglycan found in the dermis.

chromophore: responsible for molecular color. Elements that laser light is attracted to; melanin, hemoglobin, or dye particles.

chronic: long-term or persistent disease. Contrast with *acute*.

chronic acid reflux disease: recurrent condition characterized by stomach acids slipping into the esophagus, resulting in a burning sensation in the chest.

chronic metabolic acidosis: condition characterized by abnormally low pH levels.

chronic stress: long-term stress that occurs when the body's fight or flight response doesn't shut off, which can lead to a wide variety of health problems.

circumareolar: refers to the circumference of the areola.

classic forehead lift: the lifting technique involving a cornal incision that follows a heaphone-like pattern, slightly behind the natural hairline.

cleavage: the early mitotic and cytoplasmic divisions of an embryo.

cleaving: to split a complex molecule into a simpler molecule.

clinical inflammation: inflammation that can be plainly seen with the naked eye or with the aid of a magnifying loop.

closed comedones: non-inflammatory follicle impactions that appear as small bumps just under the skin surface. Called closed comedones because the follicle opening is extremely small.

closed rhinoplasty: surgery of the nose involving internal incisions, which do not leave a visible scar.

clotting factors: specific proteins that act together in clotting; defects in specific protein changes result in clotting conditions such as hemophelia.

cluster of differentiation (CD): all cells are coated with antigenic substances; each of the more than 160 clusters has a different chemical molecule that coats the surface. Every T and B cell has about 105 molecules on its surface.

co-enzymes: a vitamin or hormone that assists in an enzyme's activity, or acts as a co-factor.

coherent light: parallel rays of light that travel spatially and temporally in phase with each other.

collagen remodeling: an increase of new collagen deposits within the dermis caused by thermal heating from a laser system.

collagen shrinkage: thermal heating from a laser system can break down the collagen bonds and structures leading to shrinkage and contraction of the dermis by 20% to 30%.

collagenase: self-destruct skin enzyme that destroys collagen.

collateral circulation: blood vessels that supply blood and nutrients to the body.

combining form: resulting combination of a root word, a combining vowel, a prefix, a suffix, or any combination.

combining vowel: vowel used to combine root words with suffixes and prefixes.

complement system: a complex series of enzymes in the blood that coats microbes with special molecules making them more susceptible to phagocytosis.

complementary: completing or making whole. Complementary and Alternative Medicine (CAM) balances Western medicine by introducing Nature to help bring balance to all aspects of a person before disease can take hold.

complications: any unwanted and unexpected consequences of performing a treatment.

conduction: the sharing or transfer of heat between objects.

conjuctiva: the mucous membrane that lines the eyelid.

conjunctivitis: inflammation of the mucous membranes of the eyes and eyelids.

connective tissue: fibrous tissue that binds together, protects, and supports the various parts of the body; examples are bone, cartilage and tendons.

connexins: transmembrane proteins that permit the flow of ions that cause contraction of the heart muscle and strong contraction of the uterus during labor.

contaminate: 1.) to soil, stain, or pollute or otherwise render impure. 2.) to render unfit for use through introduction of a substance that is harmful or injurious.

contaminated: the presence or reasonably anticipated presence of blood or other potentially infectious material (OPIM) on an item or surface.

control group: the group in an experiment that is not given the factor, medication or product in question.

corium: (L. *corium*, "leather") the deep layer of the skin; dermis.

corneocyte: another name for a stratum corneum cell.

cornified: (L. *corneus*, "horny") adjective referring to epithelial cells that have undergone conversion into nonliving, keratinized cells.

cornified envelope: a highly cross-linked layer of proteins found in the stratum corneum.

Corpus luteum: a temporary endocrine structure that develops from the ovarian follicle during the menstrual cycle; essential to establishing and maintaining pregnancy.

corpuscles of Ruffini: nerve endings in the subcutaneous tissue of the human finger that detect stretch of connective tissue and send slow continuous signals when stimulated, heat detectors; also known as organ of Ruffini.

Cortisol: a hormone that allows the body to address a threatening situation by releasing energy from fat cells for use in the muscles.

cosmetic dermatology: a subspecialty of dermatology that treats appearance-related skin conditions, such as wrinkles, scars, hyperpigmentation, and hyperplasia.

cosmetic plastic surgeon: physicians who specialize in elective surgical procedures, or those that are not medically necessary but are desired for appearance related concerns, such as blepharoplasty, rhytidectomy, abdominoplasty (eyelid, face, and tummy lifts), breast augmentation or reduction and liposuction.

costs of goods sold: what it costs to provide the products that you sell.

couperose: areas of small, red enlarged capillaries of the face and other areas of the body.

cross-linking: a process in which collagen and elastin fibrils in the dermis collapse, causing the support system for the skin to collapse.

cryogen: liquified gas that is cooled below room temperature to -150 degrees C.

cryotherapy: the dermatological removal of lesions by freezing, usually with liquid nitrogen.

crystals: multi-faceted gemstones with 6 sides culminating at a point called a termination. The 6 sides are said to be Chakras 1–3 and 5–7 with the point representing the Heart or 4th Chakra. There are many crystal varieties. Clear quartz crystals embody the full spectrum of light and are made of silica which is an element also found in the human body. Crystals amplify energy, good or bad. This is why it is important to clear your energy and that of your stones regularly.

Cushing syndrome: condition of the endocrine system characterized by a multitude of disorders.

cutaneous: pertaining to the skin (e.g., a skin infection).

customer relationship management: the management of customer relations.

cyanosis: bluish coloring of the skin resulting form reduced levels of hemoglobin in the blood.

cycle: repeating unit that makes up the pattern of biological rhythms.

cyclin: a protein important in the control of the cell division cycle and mitosis.

cyclin-dependent kinase (CdK): adds phosphate to a protein along with cyclins and is a major control switch for the cell cycle.

cytochromes: color-coded proteins that exist in the cytoplasm of a cell and are involved in the cellular transport system.

cytokine: (Gr., kytos, "hollow vessel" + kinein, "to move") molecule secreted by an activated or stimulated cell (for example, macrophages) that causes chemical immune responses in certain other cells.

cytokinin: a type of hormone that promotes growth by stimulating cell division.

cytoplasm: the watery fluid of the cell, including the protoplasm, containing food material necessary for growth, reproduction, and self-repair.

cytoskeleton: in the cytoplasm of eukaryotic cells, an internal framework of microtubules, microfilaments, and intermediate filaments that anchor, organize, and moves organelles and other structures.

cytotoxic (killer) T cell: (Gr., *kytos*, "hollow vessel") a special type of T cell activated during cell-mediated immune responses, that recognizes and destroys virus-infected cells.

D

daughter cell: a cell that results after a division of a stem cell. The original cell is called the mother cell/division.

decontaminate: the use of physical or chemical means to remove, inactivate, or destroy bloodborne pathogens on a surface or item to the point where they are no longer capable of transmitting infectious particles. The surface or item is rendered safe for handling, use, or disposal.

defatting agents: agents that remove fats and lipids, along with dirt, makeup and debris, from the surface of the skin.

deionization: a process that neutralizes ions in water to be used in the manufacture of skin care and cosmetics.

demodex folliculorum: a skin mite that has been associated with rosacea.

dendrite: tree-like branching of nerve fibers extending from a nerve cell; short nerve fibers that carry impulses toward the cell.

dendritic cell: cells that serve to fix and process cutaneous antigens; they contain large granules named Birbeck granules. Also known as Langerhans cells.

deoxygenated: formerly oxygen-rich blood routed back to the heart, via the veins, after its nutrient load has been distributed.

depression: 1.) patterns of fatigue, inability to concentrate, feelings of low self-worth, and possible thoughts of suicide. 2.) condition characterized by low mood, loss of interest, loss of energy, weight changes, changes in appetite, changes in sleep patterns, fatigue, inability to concentrate, feelings of low self-worth, and possible thoughts of suicide.

dermal scattering: how light scatters or spreads within the skin tissue.

dermatan sulfate: a glycosaminoglycans; a complex carbohydrate in the dermis.

dermatoheliosis: coined term describing damage to the skin caused by long-term sun-exposure.

dermatological surgeon: a dermatologist who performs plastic or cosmetic surgery; may also refer to those dermatologists who use lasers to perform advanced dermatological procedures, such as laser skin resurfacing.

dermatologist: a physician who specializes in and treats diseases of the skin, hair, and nails.

dermis: 1.) live layer of connective tissue below the epidermis 2.) contains the collagen and elastin fibers and acts as the main support structure of the skin.

desmocollins: projects proteins; is a calcium dependent, and extends from the plaques that interlock with identical proteins from the adjacent cell. A member of the desmosome family.

desmogleins: a member of the demosome family; projects cadherin proteins, is calcium binding and extends from the plaques that interlock with identical proteins from the adjacent cell.

desmoplakin: one of the two proteins that make up the plaques in the cell membrane.

desmosome: (Gr., desmos, "bond" + soma, "body") 1. structures that assist in holding cells together. 2. buttonlike plaque serving as an intercellular connection containing many complex proteins; can be affected by auto-immune disorders.

deviated nasal septum: a condition in which the middle wall (septum) inside the nose deviates into the airway passages; can cause problems with breathing through the nose.

dhatus: the seven tissues of the body, plasma, blood, muscle, fat, bones, bone marrow, reproductive organs.

diabetes: disease that results when the pancreas does not secrete enough insulin.

diaphoretic: describes the acts of producing or increasing perspiration.

diastole: part of the normal rhythm of the heart during which the heart chambers fill with blood.

dihydrotestosterone (DHT): a form of male hormone that stimulates the sebaceous glands to produce sebum.

dilution amount: the amount, usually defined as a percentage, that essential oils are diluted in a formula when added to a cream, oil or perfume blend.

diminutive: suffix that is added to a word to note smallness or being smaller than something else.

diplopia: a condition of seeing double.

direct marketing: a marketing strategy that refers to any direct attempt to reach the consumer.

disaccarides: two saccharides together; sugars made up of two simple sugars such as lactose and sucrose.

disinfection: the second-highest level of decontamination; nearly as effective as sterilization but does not kill bacterial spores; used on hard, nonporous surfaces.

dispersing electrode: "grounding pad" placed on the individual's thigh or area of large tissue mass that receives the radio-frequency energy and returns it back to the RF unit.

distillation: 1.) process that removes mineral and trace elements from the water. 2.) process used to extract essential oils from a plant using hot water, hot water and steam, or steam alone.

dl-tocopherol: synthetic form of vitamin E.

DNA synthesis: a complex process that reproduces the critical information in each cell for proper functioning and reproduction.

dorsum: the top profile of the nose.

dosha: one of the three subtle energies that determine metabolism and intelligence of the body-mind system. The three doshas are vata, pitta and kapha. Literally dosha means "impurity" or that which can become unbalanced.

dowager hump: a bump that forms along the spine due to slow bone loss over time.

drug: according to the FDA: "articles (other than food) intended to affect the structure or function of the body."

drug claim: to make a claim that a product affects the structure or function of the body.

dynamic movement: movement caused by active movement of muscles and nerve impulses.

dyschromia: abnormal display of facial hyperpigmentation due to solar damage.

dysmorphic: abnormally formed.

dyspepsia: a symptomatic condition characterized by abnormal or painful digestion.

dysphagia: difficulty swallowing.

dysphoria: feelings of depression, discomfort, or unhappiness with no known cause.

dysphonia: abnormal hearing.

dysplastic: abnormal growth; often used to describe cancerous lesions.

dystonia: abnormality characterized by prolonged, repetitive muscle contractions that may cause twisting or jerking movements of the body part affected.

E

ectoderm: (Gr., ektos, "outside" + derma, "skin") outer layer of cells of an early embryo (gastrula stage); one of the germ layers, also sometimes used to include tissues derived from the ectoderm.

efferent: (L. ex, "out" + ferre, "to bear") leading or conveying away from some organ, for example, nerve impulses conducted away from the brain, or blood conveyed away from an organ; contrasts with afferent.

elastase: self-destruct skin enzyme that destroys elastin.

elastic wraps: bandages that can be rolled around a client and have an elastic composition allowing a tight and secure wrap.

elaunin: elastin-type fiber found in the dermis believed to be an intermediate form of elastin.

electrocautery: an electrical device used to cut the skin or to seal blood vessels to control bleeding during surgery.

electrodessication: a device that emits low levels of radio-frequency and high-frequency current, which arcs onto the skin and dries or destroys a targeted superficial lesion.

electrolytes: ions required by cells to regulate the electric charge and flow of water molecules across the cell membrane.

electromagnetic spectrum of radiation (EMR): made from all forms of energy whose spectrum extends from long radio waves to ultrashort gamma waves.

embryo: (Gr., "full to bursting") the first stage of human life; starts with fertilization of a women's egg (ovum) by a male's sperm.

emotional body: feeling intelligence includes a person's receptive, subconscious nature, allowing feelings of empathy and resonance.

employer identification number: the number used to identify businesses that maintain employees.

emulsifier: a substance used in creams, lotions and other skin-and hair-care products that allows oil and water to mix without separating.

end-bulbs of Krause: thermoreceptors that detect cold, found in the skin, conjunctiva of the eye, mucus membranes of lips and tongue, the penis and clitoris, and the fingertips.

endocarditis: inflammation of the muscles lining the heart.

endocrine glands: 1.) ductless glands that release hormonal secretions directly into the bloodstream. 2.) a group of specialized glands that affect the growth, development, sexual activities, and health of the entire body.

endocrine system: the bodily system of specialized glands that affect the growth, development, sexual activities, and health of the entire body.

endoderm: (Gr., "inner") deep primary germ layer of the embryo; gives rise to the linings of the pharynx, respiratory tree, digestive tract, urinary bladder, and urethra.

endometrium: the inner membrane of the uterus.

endomysium: individual muscle fibers protected by connective tissue.

endonasal: of, or pertaining to, inside the nose.

endoplasmic reticulum (ER): cytoplasmic organelle composed of a system of interconnected membranous tubules and vesicles; rough ER has ribosomes attached to the side of the membrane facing the cytoplasm and smooth ER does not. Rough ER functions in protein synthesis while smooth ER functions in lipid synthesis.

endoscopic: surgical technique in which an endoscope viewing instrument is employed to allow the procedure to be done via numerous small incisions.

energy fluence: the energy level of a laser, measured in joules.

energy management: a methodology to balance all aspects of body, mind and spirit that includes the practice of assessing one's energy and providing ways to renew and restore balance.

energy nutrients: components of food: carbohydrates, fats, and proteins.

engineering controls: controls that isolate or remove bloodborne pathogens from the workplace; examples include sharps containers, handwashing facilities, eyewash stations, and labels.

enzymes: proteins that regulate and catalyze biological reactions in living organisms; they break down complex food molecules to utilize extracted energy.

eosinophil: white blood cells characterized by the presence of cytoplasmic granules that become stained by an acid (eosin) dye.

epicardium: inner layer of the pericardium, which has direct contact with the heart.

epidermal growth factor (EGF): a hormone involved in the skin repair process.

epidermis: 1. the outermost layer of the skin; a thin, protective layer with many nerve endings. 2. consists of four layers: the basal layer, the spiny layer, the granular layer and the stratum corneum.

epidermolysis bullosa: a blistering congenital disease caused by defects in the keratins 5 and 14 in the basal layer.

epilepsy: neurologic condition characterized by sudden seizures.

epimysium: the connective tissue sheath that surrounds skeletal muscle.

epithelial tissue: 1.) protective covering on body surfaces, such as the skin, mucous membranes, and lining of the heart; digestive and respiratory organs; and glands 2.) capable of constant reproduction which lines other tissue.

epithelium: (Gr., epi, "on, upon" + thele, "nipple") a cellular tissue covering a free surface (internal and external) or lining a tube or cavity; consists of cells joined by small amounts of cementing substances. Epithelial tissue is classified into types based on how many layers deep it is and the shape of the superficial cells.

equation: a chemical reaction such that equal numbers of the same atom are on either side of the reaction.

erector spinae: set of three muscles that run along either side of the spinal column.

erosive esophagitis: erosion of the esophogus; most commonly caused by chronic acid reflux disease.

erythema multiforme: macular eruptions in a patchy formation on the extremities.

erythematotelangiectatic rosacea: a subtype of rosacea that is characterized by diffuse, patchy redness, and a grainy texture.

erythrocyte: (Gr., erythros, "red" + kytos, "hollow vessel") red blood cell that has hemoglobin to carry oxygen from lungs (or gills) to tissues; during their formation in mammals, erythrocytes lose their nuclei, but erythrocytes of other vertebrates retain their nuclei.

ester: a compound structure that is formed through the reaction of an acid with an alcohol.

Estradiol: a steroid made from the hormone estrogen that gives women female characteristics.

estriol: the third estrogen produced by the human body. It is only present in significant amounts during pregnancy. Other than at this time, levels of estriol do not change considerably during a person's life.

estrogen: the hormone that gives women female characteristics.

estrone: an estrogentic hormone secreted by the ovary and the least prevalent of the estrogen hormones. It can be converted by the body to estradiol.

exocrine duct glands: duct glands that produce a substance that travels through small tubelike ducts, such as the sudoriferous (sweat) glands and the sebaceous (oil) glands.

expeller pressed: a mechanical process used to "press" the oil from seeds, nuts, or plant material.

extensor digitorum longus: thin long muscle that runs the length of the side of the tibialis anterior muscle.

external ectoderm: a layer of the ectoderm germ layer that supplies the skin.

external obliques: muscles responsible for the movement of the vertebrae and rotation of the trunk.

external phase: the component of an emulsion that is of the largest concentration.

exudates: fluid oozing from a healing wound.

F

facial bra: protective bandage worn around one's chin and neck after face lifts and liposuction procedures.

Famvir® (famciclovir): antiviral medication that can stop or shorten a recurrent herpes simplex outbreak.

fascia: a thin sheet of fibrous tissue that envelops muscles or groups of muscles.

fatlah: Egyptian word for threading.

fatty acids: lubricant ingredients derived from plant oils or animal fats. Fatty acids are defined by a carboxylic acid group attached to a hydrocarbon chain (an organic aliphatic compound). They are vital factors in the function of the nervous, cardiovascular, immune, and other body systems and hold important roles in the health and protection of the skin. Fatty acids are used as emollients, both as functional spreading agents and texture softeners for creams.

fatty waxes: a fatty acid chain and an alcohol chain with an ester between them.

federal unemployment tax: a joint program between state and federal government that is used to cover employees who lose their jobs and file for unemployment assistance.

fibril: (L. fibra, "thread") a strand of protoplasm produced by a cell and lying within the cell.

fibroblast: a cell that produces protein in the body, such as amino acids and collagen, and originates from the mesechymal tissue. Also known as fibrocyte.

fibroblast growth factor (FGF): a peptide that stimulates fibroblasts to grow.

fibrocyte: a cell that is not fully differentiated for it can go forward or backward in life, makes the most abundant protein in the body called collagen, and originates from the mesechymal tissue, also known as fibroblast.

fibularis muscle group: muscle group consisting of three muscles—the tertius peronaeus, peronaeus longus, and the peronaeus brevis; also called the peronaeus muscle group.

fight or flight response: a brain-stimulated response to stress that prepares the body for trauma.

Fitzpatrick scale: a scale used to measure the skin type's ability to tolerate sun exposure.

5-HT3 antagonists: antienemic which is a selective serotonin inhibitors, which inhibit the binding of serotonin to 5-HT3 receptors.

fixed oil: a nonvolatile fatty oil derived from vegetables and fruits.

flare: an episode in which pimples and redness occur in a person who has rosacea.

flavonoids: active phenylpropanoid compounds with extremely beneficial properties for maintaining health and reversing disease. Foods rich in flavonoids are citrus fruits, grape skins, and tea.

flexation: upward movement.

fluence: irradiance multiplied by the exposure time, measured in Joules/square centimeter.

flushing: sudden facial redness caused by blood rushing to the skin.

follicle-stimulating hormone (FSH): hormone secreted by the pituitary gland that causes the development of the egg, or ovum.

follicular exfoliants: chemical agents that slough the inside of the follicle, shedding debris and dead cells, and preventing cell buildup that can cause comedones and acne lesions.

food sensitivities: a non-allergic, yet negative response to food. Food sensitivities occur when the body cannot properly digest particular foods, but they differ from allergies as the immune system is not involved.

formed elements: red or white blood cells or platelets separated from the fluid part of the blood.

formication: itching and tingling feeling of the skin experienced by some women during menopause.

fourth germ layer: component of the ectoderm known as the *neural crest*.

free fatty acid: a lipid component of the stratum corneum.

free nerve terminals: nerve endings in the skin without myelin sheaths.

free radicals (reactive oxygen species): a major contributor to aging, free radicals are unstable molecules that have broken away from weak molecules. In an attempt to stabilize themselves, they steal electrons from stable molecules, creating more and more unstable molecules. The result is tissue damage, accelerated aging, and vulnerability to disease.

frenulum: tissue that connects one thing to another.

functional group: an atom or group of atoms that bond to a reactive area of an organic compound, giving the compound its overall characteristics.

G

G_0: a stage of DNA synthesis, the resting cell.

G_1: part of interphase that is the time of active metabolism in the cell cycle; also known as Gap 1.

G_2: part of interphase after the synthesis of DNA and before the start of nuclear division; also known as Gap 2.

gap junctions: intercellular channels that allow free passage between the cells of ions and small molecules to pass between cells.

gastrocnemius: the "calf muscle."

gastrula: the name for an embryo during the gastrulation process.

gastrulation: a process during which the cells migrate to the interior of the blastula and form three germ layers.

gellant: an agent that is added to a product to give it a gel-like consistency.

gemstones: gemstones are considered to be any rock, crystal or stone used for jewelry and adornment.

generalized anxiety disorder (GAD): condition characterized by unspecific or unwarranted anxiety.

generally accepted accounting principles (GAAP): the standard procedures established by the accounting profession.

genitourinary: pertaining to the urinary tract.

genuine and authentic: a definition and standard developed several years ago by French insurance companies to label the essential oils suitable for patient reimbursement.

germ layer: in the animal embryo, one of three basic layers (ectoderm, endoderm, mesoderm) from which the various organs and tissues arise in the multicellular animal.

ghee: clarified butter used for massage or for cooking.

glabella: the point above the nose and between the eyes, often subject to dynamic movement.

glial cells: supportive cells closely associated with neurons.

globules: oil droplets in an oil-in-water emulsion.

Glogau scale: a scale used to evaluate the level of sun damage based on wrinkling.

glucans: a saccharide compound found in the cell wall of yeast but can also be found in oats, barley, and other sources. Beta glucans stimulate the immune system, signal tissue repair, and are thought to also stimulate collagen synthesis. They also have antioxidant properties. Also known as beta glucans.

glucose: simple blood sugar which is an important source of energy.

gluteus group of muscles: form the exterior contours of the buttocks.

glycation: a destructive biological process that is the number one cause of premature aging. Under high temperatures, the carbohydrates sugar and starch react to proteins and alter how the body handles food, resulting in the formation of AGE products.

glycolic acid: an alpha hydroxy acid used in skin treatments.

glycosaminoglycans: a water-binding substance such as a polysaccharide (protein and complex sugar) found between the fibers of the dermis with water-binding properties.

Golgi apparatus: organelle of membranous, hollow sacs arranged in a stack; functions in modification, storage, and packaging of secretion materials; may be called *dictyosome* in plants. Also known as the *Golgi apparatus* or *Golgi complex*.

granulocytes: (L. *granulus*, "small grain" + Gr., *kytos*, "hollow vessel") White blood cells (neutrophils, eosinophils, and basophils) bearing granules (vacuoles) in their cytoplasm that stain deeply.

granulomatous rosacea: any form of rosacea that includes hard, nodular papules.

Grave's disease: a form of hyperthyroidism.

gross profit: the total amount of money a business takes in from the sale of products and/or services.

gunas: qualities or attributes given to substances or people such as light, dry or cold. There are 20 fundamental gunas in Ayurveda.

guru: spiritual teacher. Literally guru means one that removes the darkness of ignorance.

H

hair: follicle endings

hallucinations: abnormal visions associated with certain psychoses.

hamstrings: muscle group on the top or posterior side of the thigh.

hantavirus: virus transmitted to humans through mice feces with potentially fatal consequences.

Health Insurance Portability and Accountability Act (HIPAA): a federal act passed in 1996 outlining federal privacy standards for patients. The act covers access to medical records, notice of privacy practices, limitations of use regarding personal medical information, prohibitions on using patient information for marketing, stronger state laws, confidential communication and complaint procedures.

heart disease: any condition that affects the performance of the heart or the cardiovascular system.

hederidform endings: a nerve that occurs in glabrous, or hairless, skin; also called Merkel's discs.

helicobacter pylori: a type of intestinal bacterium that has been associated with rosacea.

helper T cells: cells that serve as managers and direct the immune response; they also secrete lymphokines.

hemidesmosomes: binds the basal layer to the basement membrane through different types of proteins.

hemocytoblast: part of the blood cell line, this multipotential cell can form the white cell series and the red cells and any other cells in the blood.

hemophilia: 1.) disorder characterized by deficiencies of clotting factors reducing the bloods ability to clot. 2.) A recessive genetic disorder occurring almost exclusively in men and boys in which the blood clots much more slowly than normal, resulting in extensive bleeding from even minor injuries.

hemostasis: refers to balance or wellness within the body.

heparin sulfate: a proteoglycan found in the dermis.

heparin: a proteoglycan found in the dermis.

herb wraps: body wrap treatment that includes the soaking of the wrap in an herbal tea blend prior to application.

herbal infusion: the result of using hot water, and sometimes cold, to release the compounds from plant material. For example, tea is an herbal infusion.

hi definition makeup: makeup that is designed to appear like skin when recorded and viewed with HD cameras and TV sets.

hirsutism: excessive growth of an unusual amount of hair on parts of the body normally bearing only downy hair, such as the face, arms, and legs of women or the backs of men.

histamine: amino acid vital to human immunologic response.

holistic: the practice and/or philosophy of treating the person as a whole and remaining alert to all of a client's needs rather than focusing solely on a disease or disorder.

holistic health: the philosophy or practice that sees the body as a whole. The practice takes into consideration the effects of the emotions, lifestyle and the environment on health.

homeostasis: the process of feedback and regulation that keeps the body in a state of equilibrium within its environment.

homogenizers: high-speed mixers used to emulsify products.

hordeolums: infected tear ducts; also called *styes*.

hormone replacement therapy (HRT): oral, topical, implanted or injection methods used to administer female hormones to control or prevent symptoms of menopause. HRT may also help prevent skin changes or osteoporosis in women.

hormones: secretions produced by one of the endocrine glands and carried by the bloodstream or body fluid to another part of the body, or a body organ, to stimulate functional activity or secretion; the internal messengers for most of the body's systems.

human papillomavirus (HPV): a cutaneous viral infection commonly caused by sexual transmission and exhibited by genital warts.

humoral: (L., *humor*, "a fluid") pertaining to an endocrine secretion.

Human Immunodeficiency Virus (HIV): virus that causes AIDS.

hyaluronic acid: a glycosaminoglycan that has no protein component that can hold up to 400 times its own weight in water. A hydrating fluid found in the skin; hydrophilic agent with water-binding properties. Also known as sodium hyalurnate.

hyaluronidase: a self-destruct skin enzyme that destroys hyaluronic acid.

hydrocollators: dry heat units that heat thermal packs to an optimal temperature. Commonly used in massage therapy, chiropractic or physical therapy practices.

hydroquinone: a topical medication that is used for bleaching or reducing excessive melanin lesions in the epidermis.

hydrosol: the water portion, or by-product, of essential oil distillation; used for aromatherapy purposes.

hydrostatic pressure: means of devising fluid pressure by measuring the pressure imposed by an external force.

hydrotherapy: spa treatments that use water.

hydroxy radical: the most dangerous free radicals, which can react with many DNA in the cell nucleus, causing permanent damage to the cell and to the DNA in future cells produced from cell division.

hyperchloremic acidosis: increased chlorine levels resulting in higher acidity levels overall.

hypercholesterolemia: abnormally high levels of cholesterol in the body.

hyperextension: extension of a muscle beyond normal limits.

hyperpigmentation: skin condition characterized by overproduction of melanin resulting in patches of colored skin.

hypertension: high blood pressure.

hyperthyroidism: a condition in which the thyroid gland secretes too much thyroid hormone.

hypertrichosis: excessive hair growth where hair does not normally grow.

hypochlorous acid: chlorine bleach, HOCl

hypopigmentation: skin condition characterized by under production of melanin resulting in patches of non-colored skin.

hypotension: low blood pressure.

hypothalamus: 1.) manufactures hormones that stimulate the pituitary gland to make other hormones. It is also able to detect needs of various parts of the body by chemically monitoring the blood. 2.) regulator of important metabolic functions, hormone release and autonomic function.

hypothalamus gland: controls movement of some involuntary muscles, such as the muscles of the intestines that help move food through the gastrointestinal system.

hypothesis: an educated guess that is based on an observation or study of an issue in question.

hypothyroidism: a condition in which the thyroid glands secretes too little thyroid hormone.

hypoxia: deficiency in the blood's ability to transport oxygen.

I

igneous: rock that forms when magma (liquid rock) cools and solidifies.

immune system: a bodily system made up of lymph, lymph nodes, the thymus gland, the spleen, and lymph vessels; protects the body from the disease by developing immunities and destroying disease-causing microorganisms as well as draining the tissues of excess interstitial fluids to the blood. This system carries waste and impurities away from the cells.

immunization: becoming immune or the process of rendering a person immune.

immunocompromised: refers to limited or reduced functioning of the immune system.

immunologic response: a bodily defense reaction that recognizes an invading substance and produces antibodies specific against that antigen.

impedance: resistance or obstruction of electrical flow; commonly occurs when radiofrequency energy come in contact with tissue.

impetigo: a contagious skin infection caused by staphylococcal or streptococcal bacteria, characterized by clusters of small blisters and often occurring in children.

inactive ingredients: ingredients within a drug that do not specifically cause a physiological change but are necessary for the drug to work.

income statement: a profit and loss statement.

independent contractor: a non-employee service provider in accordance with IRS guidelines who is able to control the means and methods by which they accomplish their work (and is responsible for adhering to all laws set forth by their licensing board and any, local, state, and federal rules and regulations that apply to small business owners in their trade).

individual tax identification number: the number issued by the IRS to a non-resident or resident alien working in the United States to process their tax obligation to the United States government.

inflammatory mediators: chemicals released by inflamed cells that alert the immune system to the irritation.

inframammary crease: place on the female body where the breast meets the chest wall.

infrared: electromagnetic radiation found in the invisible spectrum of light.

ischemia: temporary restriction in normal blood flow.

insertion: the point where the skeletal muscle is attached to a bone or other more movable body parts.

insulin: essential hormone needed for the normal metabolic breakdown of glucose in the body.

insulin-like growth factor (IGF-I): growth regulatory cytokines thought to be responsible for initiating proliferation of fibroblasts and other connective tissue cells.

insurance: provides protection against business casualties; or the transfer of risk to a third party, as in the form of an insurance policy.

integrin: proteins that hold the plaque to the basal lamina.

intense pulsed light (IPL): a polychromatic, noncoherent, dispersive band of light commonly utilizing wavelengths from 500 to 1200 nm; a common photoepilation hair-reduction method.

intercostal muscles: muscles situated between the ribs.

interleukin: cytokines produced by white blood cells and mediating their own activities or those of other white blood cells.

interleukin–1: a cytokine produced by macrophages that stimulates T helper lymphocytes.

interleukin–2: a lymphokine produced by T helper lymphocytes that leads to proliferation of T helper cells and other T lymphocytes.

intermediate filaments: complex fibers that help to maintain cell shape, but also add strength to cells and holds them together.

internal obliques: middle layer of abdominal muscles.

internal phase: component of an emulsion that is of the least concentration.

Internet: a complex communications system that is capable of linking multiple computers worldwide.

irradiance: referred to as power density or wtts/cm^2.

ischemia: temporary restriction in normal blood flow.

islet of Langerhans cells in the pancreas: cell that makes insulin and is responsible for diabetes when it fails to function.

isolates: compounds that are isolated from a plant extract and have an active therapeutic property.

isoprene units: hydrocarbon chains with 5 carbon atoms.

isopropyl alcohol: a fairly strong drying alcohol used as a cleansing and drying agent to remove excess oil.

isotype: in biology, one of several biological types. A physical example or representation of that type.

J

JNK: a pathway used as an intermediate signal as part of the DNA signaling cascade.

joules: units of energy or work. In thermodynamics, joules are defined as a unit of heat energy used to measure the energy change in an object as it warms or cools from temperature T1 to temperature T2. 1 joule = 1 watt per second.

K

kansa vataki: foot massage using a small bowl made from three metals.

kapha dosha: the dosha that gives structure to the body, lubricates tissues, provides strength and supports immune function. This dosha has qualities that are like earth and water.

karma: one's future being determined by present or past actions. Literally karma means "action."

keratin: the major protein made in the epidermis.

keratin proteins: proteins that are made in the skin and hair that resist water and frictions.

keratin sulfate: a proteoglycan found in the dermis.

Keratinocyte: cells composed of keratain; the dominate cell in the epidermis. It is multifunctional but makes proteins and lipids.

keratinocytoblasts: stem cells that do not have a high rate of mitosis but do produce a transient amplifying cell.

keratinohyaline granules: both horny and hyaline, a distinguishing feature of the cells in the granular layer.

keratolytics: also called proteolytic, means "protein dissolving." These agents work by dissolving keratin protein within dead surface cells, helping to remove these cells and making the skin look clearer and smoother.

keratosis pilaris: redness and bumpiness common on the cheeks or upper arms caused by blocked hair follicles. The patches of irritation are accompanied by a rough texture and small pinpoint white papules that look like very small milia.

khite: Arabic word for threading.

Kneipp body wraps: wraps that envelop a body part with wet and dry cloths that are either hot or cold. Effects are achieved through temperature, length of application, and additives.

kundalini: primal energy that is awakened by spiritual practices.

L

lactic acid: an AHA occuring naturally in milk. It is both an exfoliant and a hydrophilic.

Langerhans cell: cell that fixes and processes cutaneous antigens; contains large granules named Birbeck granules. Also known as *dendritic cells*.

laser-generated air contaminates (LGAC): plume or smoke that is generated from an ablative laser device.

laser resurfacing: a laser procedure utilizing the CO_2 or Erbium laser that involves vaporization of the epidermis and/or dermis for facial rejuvenation; used to smooth wrinkles or lighten acne scars and stimulate growth of new collagen.

laser safety officer (LSO): the person responsible for the laser safety program at the facility. The LSO is authorized to monitor, enforce controls, and oversee hazards associated with laser usage.

lateral: to the side.

latissimus dorsal: broad, flat muscle covering the back of the neck and upper and middle region of the back; controls the shoulder blade and the swinging movements of the arm.

Leaky Aura Syndrome: a condition where the aura has developed "energy gaps" from years of leaving bits and pieces of energy behind. This leaves one open to absorbing other energies indiscriminately, resulting in feeling exhausted.

lepas: cleansing pastes or poultices for the skin.

leukemia: disease of the bone marrow characterized by excessive and unwanted white blood cell proliferation.

leukocyte: (Gr., *leukos*, "white" + *kytos*, "hollow vessel") 1. any of several kinds of white blood cells (for example, granulocytes, lymphocytes, and monocytes), so-called because they bear no hemoglobin, unlike red blood cells. 2. specialized cells that work with the immune system to combat disease and infection.

liabilities: the amount of debt or money your business owes to creditors.

ligature: a tying or other binding mechanism.

Light Amplification of the Stimulated Emission of Radiation (LASER): medical device that emits a collimated, coherent, monochromatic radiant energy for therapeutic purposes.

light emitting diode (LED): a device that is made up of panels of tiny diodes that are pulsed at an exclusive array sequence to trigger a photobiochemical response.

limbic system: an important series of brain structures activated by odor, behavior and arousal.

lipase: (Gr., *lipos*, "fat") an enzyme that accelerates the hydrolysis, or synthesis of fats.

lipid bilayer: a molecular structure composed of hydrophilic and hydrophobic components.

lipid peroxide: free radicals formed when the cell membrane is damaged by other free radicals.

lipolysis: the splitting up or destruction of fat cells.

lipophilic: having an affinity or attraction to fats and oils.

liposuction: a surgical procedure used for the removal of stubborn areas of fat.

luteinizing hormone (LH): hormone that causes the actual process of ovulation or the release of the egg from the ovary. It also causes the testes to manufacture testosterone.

lymph: clear, yellowish fluid that circulates in the lymph spaces (lymphatic) of the body; carries waste and impurities from the cells.

lymph nodes: glandlike bodies in the lymphatic vessels that filter lymph products.

lymphatic vessels: reabsorb the lymph, store it in the lymphatic collecting vessels and lymph nodes, and return it to the heart.

lymphocytes: (L., *lympha*, "water, goddess of water" + Gr., *kytos*, "hollow vessel") 1. a type of white blood cell; a component of the immune system produced by stem cells in the bone marrow. 2.) type of white blood cell which is important to the immune system for its ability to digest foreign invaders.

lymphokine: (L., *lympha* + Gr., *kinein*, "to move") a molecule secreted by an activated or stimulated lymphocyte that causes physiological changes in certain other cells.

lymphotoxins: substances that, when released by cytotoxic or killer T cells, causes cell lysis.

lysosome: 1.) cytoplasmic, membrane-bounded organelle that contains digestive and hydrolytic enzymes, which are typically most active at the acid pH found in the lumen of lysosomes. 2.) cell organelle that digests foreign matter considered potentially threatening to the body.

lysozyme: an enzyme capable of dissolving and digesting many types of biochemicals.

M

macrophage: (Gr., *makros*, "long, large" + *phago*, "to eat") a phagocytic cell type in vertebrates that performs crucial functions in the immune response and inflammation, such as presenting antigenic epitopes to T cells and producing several cytokines.

maillard reaction: a term used to describe the chemical reaction produced by browning foods or cooking them at high temperatures, thereby creating AGE products.

malic acid: an AHA derived from apples.

major depression: most severe type of depression characterized by severe and frequent instances of low mood, loss of interest, loss of energy, weight changes, changes in appetite, changes in sleep patterns, fatigue, inability to concentrate, feelings of low self-worth, and possible thoughts of suicide.

malas: body wastes.

mammaplasty: surgery to alter the shape or contours of the breast.

mandala: geometric shaped images used for meditation.

mandibular nerve: a branch of the trigeminal nerve (fifth cranial nerve) that supplies the muscles and skin of the lower part of the face; also, nerve that affects the muscles of the chin and lower lip; carries sensory data from the mandible.

mantra: one or more syllables sung or chanted to help bring balance to the mind body system. The most commonly known and used mantra is OM pronounced AUM.

MAPK: a pathway used as an intermediate signal as part of the DNA signaling cascade.

marketing: a business strategy for how ideas, goods and services are bought, sold or exchanged.

marketing plan: states your marketing goals and objectives and the strategies that you will use to achieve those goals.

marma: sensitive points on the body where there are greater concentrations of the body's life force. There are 108 marma points used therapeutically but thousands of minor marmas. Literary means vital, hidden or secret energy points.

MASER: Microwave Amplification by the Stimulated Emission of Radiation.

mast cell: type of cell in various tissues that releases pharmacologically active substances with a role in inflammation.

mastectomy: a surgical procedure to remove the breast.

mastopexy: breast lift procedures.

maturation promoting factor (MPF): a protein that initiates part of the cellular division known as mitosis. Specifically, it initiates the prophase of mitosis and also functions in the process of mitosis by activating other proteins through the mechanism of phosphorylation, that is, it adds phosphorus to the protein thereby making it an active protein.

maxillary nerve: a branch of the trigeminal nerve (fifth cranial nerve) that carries sensory data from the maxilla; supplies the upper part of the face.

Maximum Permissible Exposure (MPE): the level of laser radiation to which a person may be exposed without hazardous ocular or tissue effects.

medical spa: a medical facility that offers medical aesthetic procedures and traditional spa or esthetic services in a spa-like setting.

medi-spa: a term used interchangeably with medical spa.

Meissner's corpuscles: circular or ovoid structures with a distinct connective tissue capsule that transmit touch, pressure, and cold.

melanocyte: cells that produce pigment granules/melanin in the basal layer of the epidermis.

melanocyte-stimulating hormone (MSH): a hormone that stimulates melanocytes to make melanin.

melanogenesis: the process of making the pigment melanin inside the melanocyte.

melanosomes: pigment granules of melanocyte cells that produce melanin in the basal layer; provides skin's colors.

membrane: in living organisms, a phospholipid bilayer impregnated with protein and certain other compounds that is differentially permeable.

memory T cells: programmed to recognize and respond to a pathogen once it has been invaded and been repelled.

menarche: the first menstrual period.

menopause: the time in a woman's life when the ovaries stop producing ova.

menstruation: process by which the female body rids itself of an unused ovum and accompanying endometrium.

mental body: cognitive intelligence refers to the rational, concrete, learned knowledge. This information is stored in memory and becomes the programmed belief system and perception on life.

mental chatter: constant self-talk in the mind, especially negative or judgmental thoughts that keep you occupied on trivial issues.

mentoplasty: implant to improve the shape of the chin.

Merkel's discs: *see* heder; form endings.

mesenchymal tissue: embryonic connective tissue

mesoderm: (Gr., mesos, "middle" + derma, "skin") the third germ layer, formed in the gastrula between the ectoderm and endoderm; gives rise to connective tissues, muscle, urogenital and vascular systems, and the peritoneum. This tissue from the mesoderm is called mesochymal tissue.

metabolic alkalosis: increased alkalines in the body resulting from decreased acids.

metabolism: 1.) chemical process taking place in living organisms whereby the cells are nourished and carry out their activities. 2.) the process of changing food into forms the body can use as energy. Metabolism consists of two parts: anabolism and catabolism.

metabolites: the products used by living organisms in the process of metabolism.

metamorphosed: the result of a pre-existing rock form undergoing changes. The rock undergoes heat and extreme pressure, resulting in physical and chemical changes.

metastable: describes an apparent state of equilibrium, but are likely to change to a more truly stable state if conditions change.

micelle: a protective sphere that is created by emulsifiers surrounding an internal phase ingredient.

micellized: refers to ingredients encapsulated in a micelle.

micro–thermal zone (MTZ): a column of tissue that is heated up from a fractional laser device.

microampere: a current of .001 ampere or less. Microcurrent treatments typically use a combination of galvanic and faradic current for cosmetic uses of tightening and toning.

microencapsulation: the process of using barrier and intercellular-compatible materials like lipids to form special micro-shells to protect and better penetrate certain ingredients.

microfilaments: protein strands made of actin; responsible for cell movement and cell shape.

micrometer: a unit of length equal to a millionth of a meter or a micron.

microsponge: a variety of specialized microencapsulation that releases a performance ingredient once inside the skin.

microtubules: tiny, cylindrical-shaped tubes composed of a protein called tubulin; its major function is to separate chromosomes during cellular division.

mitochondria: in eucaryotes, subcellular organelles that conduct cellular respiration and produce most of the ATP in aerobic respiration (oxidative phosphorylation).

mitosis: nuclear cells dividing into two new cells called daughter cells; the usual process of cell production of human tissues.

modifies: to qualify or limit the meaning of a word.

modulate: the ability to stimulate or change the cellular function.

moist heat unit: units designed to hold water and to heat linen wraps to an optimal temperature. Commonly herbal blends are added to the water.

monoamine oxidase inhibitors (MAOIs): class of drugs used to treat depression; however, the exact mode of their action is not quite understood.

monochromatic: light consisting of one wavelength that is typically found emitted from a laser system.

monocytes: large white blood cells or leukocytes, which travel the bloodstream neutralizing pathogens; become phagocytic cells (macrophages) after moving into tissues.

monopolar radio-frequency (RF) energy: radio-frequency electrical current that utilizes a dispersive electrode to return the energy back to the generator device.

monosaccharides: a family of saccharides (carbohydrates) made of a single sugar unit that cannot be converted into smaller saccharide molecules.

monounsaturated fatty acids: unsaturated fatty acids that contain one double bond in the carbon chain.

mother cell: a cell capable of multiple divisions, also known as a *stem cell*.

motor (efferent or effector) neuron or nerve: a neuron or nerve that carries an impulse away from the brain or spinal cord to the muscles and organs.

mucosa: epithelial membranes that line internal orificies that lead to the outside of the body; mucous membranes secrete mucous which provides protection and lubrication for the internal surface. Examples are the inside of the nasal cavity or the inside of the intestine.

mucous membrane: membrane-lining passages and cavities communicating with the air. Consists of a surface layer of epithelium, a basement membrane, and an underlying layer of connective tissue. Mucus-secreting cells or glands usually are present in the epithelium but may be absent.

muscle fibers: describes muscle cells.

muscle tissue: tissue that is able to contract and conduct electrical impulses

myelin: (Gr., *myelos*, "marrow") fatty material forming the medullary sheath of nerve fibers.

myeloperoxidase: enzyme used in the killing action of neutrophiles.

myocardial ischemia: temporary restriction in normal blood flow to the heart and cardiac muscles.

myocardium: muscular tissue around the heart.

myofilaments: cells that help muscles contract and shorten.

myosin: (Gr., mys, "muscle" + in, suffix meaning "belonging to") a large protein of contractile tissue that forms the thick myofilaments of striated muscle. During contraction, it combines with actin to form actomyosin.

N

nabhi: navel.

nadi: subtle energy channel. Ayurvedic name for pulse.

nanometer: metric measurement indicating a billionth of a meter.

nare: nostril.

nasal septum: the bone and cartilage that divides the nose into two nostrils.

nasal turbinates: areas of bone and mucosa projecting from the lateral walls of the nasal cavity that warms and humidifies inhaled air; sometimes can cause nasal airway obstruction.

NASHA: non-Animal stabilized hyaluronic acid.

nasolabial folds: the line extending from the nostrils to the corner of the mouth.

nasolabial lines: dynamic wrinkles that connect the nose to the mouth.

natural moisturizing factors (NMFs): natural humectants, lipids, or hydrating agents found within intercellular cement.

necrosis: cell or tissue death.

nervous tissue: a highly specialized tissue used to transport signals to other organs and coordinate all bodily functions.

net profit: the real income of a business after all of the expenses associated with operation are subtracted.

neural crest: early nerve tissue in the embryo; site of origin for melanocytes; a layer of the ectoderm germ layer.

neural tube: a layer of the ectoderm germ layer; provides most of the central nervous system.

neurofilament: an intermediate filament found in nerve cells.

neuroglia: glial cells provide support and nutrition to the tissues.

neuromuscular junction: point at which nerves and muscles connect.

neuron: a nerve cell; basic unit of the nervous system, consisting of a cell body, nucleus, dendrites and axon.

neurotransmitters: 1.) substances that travel across synapses to act on or inhibit a target cell. 2.) chemical messengers, synthesized from food nutrients, transmit instructions from the brain to the nervous system. The health of neurotransmitters is dependent on the quality of nutrients in food.

neutrophils: 1.) most abundant of polymorphonuclear leukocytes; an important phagocyte; so-called because it stains with both acidic and basic. 2.) phagocytic white blood cells.

Nevus of Ota: a deep dermal pigmented lesion usually found on the face in populations of darker-skinned Asians.

nikoliski sign: an epidermal separation caused by lateral pressure on the skin.

nominal hazard zone (NHZ): the direct, reflected, or scattered radiation, during normal operation, exceeds the MPE levels of exposure.

nonablative: a procedure in which the epidermis remains intact and no resulting skin vaporization or trauma occurs.

non-acnegenic: refers to ingredients or products that will not irritate the inside of follicles and cause flares of acne.

non-comedogenic: describes ingredients or products that do not cause comedones or clogged pores to form.

non-immunogenic: unlikely to cause a hypersensitive or antigenic reaction.

nonvolatile: does not evaporate easily.

norephinephrine: neurotransmitter responsible for heartrate and the fight or flight reaction. Overproduction or underproduction are associated with several psychological conditions including depression.

normoblast: a red blood cell with normal development that retains its nucleus; also known as an *erythroblast*.

noun: part of speech that is used to name a person, place, thing, quality or action. It is usually the subject or object of the action in a sentence.

nuclear membrane: membrane surrounding the nucleus of eucaryotic cells.

nucleolus: (diminutive of L. *nucleus*, "kernel") a deeply staining body within the nucleus of a cell and containing RNA; nucleoli (plural) are specialized portions of certain chromosomes that carry multiple copies of the information to synthesize ribosomal RNA.

nucleus: the dense, active protoplasm found in the center of a eukaryotic cell that acts as the genetic control center; plays an important role in cell reproduction and metabolism.

O

obliquely: slanting or inclined.

obsessive-compulsive disorder (OCD): anxiety disorder characterized by perpetual and excessive thoughts and activities that interfere with the normal functioning of the affected individual.

Occupational Safety and Health Administration (OSHA) an agency responsible for workplace safety and health.

ocular rosacea: a subtype of rosacea that affects the eyes, resulting in eye redness, swollen eyelids, and other eye lesions.

ojas: the pure essence of the body that is the power behind immune function and is what gives the body a healthy glow.

olfaction: the sense of smell.

oligohydrosis: condition characterized by excessively low water levels in the body.

open comedones: non-inflammatory acne lesions appearing as large, clogged follicles filled with solidified sebum and dead cell buildup. Often called blackheads.

open rhinoplasty: surgery of the nose involving an incision across the columella between the nostrils which can leave a faint scar.

ophthalmic nerve: a branch of the trigeminal nerve that carries only sensory fibers; supplies the skin of the forehead, upper eyelids, and interior portion of the scalp, orbit, eyeball, and nasal passage.

opportunistic mycoses: fungi that use breaks in the skin or abnormal immunity to infect the body.

Optical Density (OD): the amount of attenuation or a reduction of radiant laser energy as it passes through the filter material in the laser eyewear.

optical resonator cavity: a cavity containing a laser rod or tube made up of 2 reflective mirrors at each end. The mirrors reflect light back and forth to build up amplification of the laser light under external stimulus.

organelle: a body within the cytoplasm of eukaryotic cells. There are several different types of organelles, each with a specialized function, such as the chloroplast, which functions in photosynthesis.

organic compound: compounds that contain the element carbon.

organisms: any living thing, plant, or animal. May be unicellular (bacteria, yeasts, protozoa) or multicellular (all complex organisms including man).

orifice: opening or aperture, such as the mouth or entry to a tube.

oropharynx: pertaining to the throat.

osteoarthritis: joint condition characterized by inflammation of weight-bearing joints.

osteoporosis: a thinning of the bones, leaving them fragile and prone to fractures; caused by the reabsorption of calcium into the blood.

ostium: the opening of a follicle on the skin surface.

other potentially infectious material (OPIM): human body fluids including, but not limited to, semen, vaginal secretions, cerebrospinal fluid, synovial fluid, pleural fluid, pericardial fluid, amniotic fluid, and all body fluids in situations where it is difficult or impossible to differentiate between body fluids.

ovaries: organs in the female reproductive system located just above the uterus and connected to the uterus by two hollow tubes called fallopian tubes.

overactive bladder: condition characterized by abnormally high levels of bladder activity resulting in a frequent need to urinate.

over-the-counter (OTC): any drug that has FDA approval to be sold or consumed without a doctor's order.

owner's equity: the owner's interest in the assets of the company after all of the business' liabilities have been deducted.

oxygenated: rich in oxygen.

oxyhemoglobin: hemoglobin in red blood cells that has been oxygenated; a protein in red blood cells.

oxytalan: elastin-type fiber found in the dermis that contains only microfibrils and is 10-12 nm in diameter.

P

p27 protein: a protein that binds to cyclin and CdK blocking entry into the S phase.

p53 protein: a tumor-suppressor protein with critical functions in normal cells. A mutation in the gene that encodes it, p53, can result in loss of control over cell division and, thus, cancer.

Pacinian corpuscle: a sensory receptor in skin, muscles, body joints, body organs, and tendons that is involved with the vibratory sense and firm pressure on the skin; also called a *lamellated corpuscle*.

Paget's Disease: condition affecting the elderly, characterized by inflammation of the bones.

pain receptor: a modified nerve ending that, when stimulated, gives rise to the sense of pain.

palpebra: the upper or lower eyelid.

panchamahabhutas: the five great elements, space, air, fire, water and earth.

pancreas: organ located in the abdomen; secretes pancreatic enzymes that are delivered into the intestine.

papulopustular rosacea: subtype of rosacea that often resembles acne vulgaris, with large red pustules and papules.

parasympathetic divisions: a major functional division of the autonomic nervous system. It operates under normal nonstressful situations, such as resting, and helps to restore calm and balance to the body after a stressful event.

parathyroid gland: gland responsible for regulating calcium and phosphates in the bloodstream.

parenteral: piercing of mucous membranes or the skin barrier through such events as needlesticks, human bites, and abrasions; any drug delivery route other than through the mouth.

paresthesia: sensation of numbness and prickling; often called "pins and needles."

parfum: scent, fragrance.

Parkinson's disease: nervous system condition characterized by progressive tremors, muscular weakness, and rigidity.

pathogenic fungi: any fungus that results in disease.

pathogens: a microorganism or substance capable of producing disease.

pendulous breasts: large hanging breasts.

peptic ulcer: wearing down of stomach and esphogus tissue resulting in frequent stomach pain, especially after eating.

peptide bond: primary linkage between all proteins. It occurs when the carboxyl molecule of one peptide reacts with the amino group of another peptide.

perifollicular inflammation: inflammation of the follicle walls inside of the follicle.

perimenopause: the time before and around menopause.

perimysium: 1. several muscle fibers are bunched together and wrapped in a fibrous sheathing. 2. thin membrane covering a muscle.

periodic table: chart of all the chemical elements.

perioral dermatitis: an acne-like condition around the mouth. These are mainly small clusters of papules, primarily seen in women of child-bearing age. Must be treated with internal antibiotics.

periorbital fat: the fat supporting the upper and lower eyelids.

peripheral edema: swelling resulting from fluid accumulation in the lower limbs.

personal protective equipment (PPE): specialized clothing or equipment designed for use by an employee in order to minimize, reduce, or eliminate the risk of exposure to bloodborne pathogens and other hazards. Examples include, but are not limited to, disposable latex or nitrile exam gloves, disposable sleeves, disposable aprons, and face and eye protection.

personal selling: a marketing strategy that involves a one to one exchange or dialogue with the consumer.

phagocyte: (G. phagein, to eat + kytos, hollow vessel) any cell that engulfs and devours microorganisms or other particles (process known as phagocytosis).

phenylpropanoid: physiologically active organic compounds containing an aromatic ring and a 3-carbon chain.

phlebitis: inflammation of the wall of a vein.

phobias: anxiety conditions characterized by unwarranted fear such that it interferes with the normal functioning of the affected individual.

phospholipids: compounds that contain fatty acid and phosphoric acid groups.

photodamage: skin damage caused by exposure to the sun's rays; can be as simple as fine lines or as serious as hyperpigmentation, actinic keratosis, deep rhytids, facial laxity and invasive skin cancers.

photodynamic therapy: a beam of light travels along fiberoptics to create light therapy.

photomodulation: LED technology that uses energy-producing packets of light to enhance fibroblast collagen synthesis.

photons: in quantum theory, the element unit of light; a particle of energy that has motion and travels in waves.

photophobia: excessive tearing due to light sensitivity.

photorejuvenation: series of laser or IPL facial treatments conducted to improve vascular and pigmented lesions plus induce collagen stimulation

photosensitivity: responsive to sunlight.

phototoxic: experiencing a toxic effect triggered by exposure of light to the skin; sometimes as a result by topical or oral medications.

phymatous rosacea: a subtype of rosacea in which the nose has a thickened appearance and the individual sometimes has rhinophyma, which is a substantial enlargement of the nose.

physical dependence: chemical dependence in which the body thinks it needs a particular substance to continue to function.

physical emulsions: products emulsified using special blends of emollients and non–surfactant emulsifying agents that are mixed at high speeds.

phytotherapy: the use of plant extracts for therapeutic benefits.

pilosebaceous: the hair follicle.

pineal gland: gland located in the brain. Its function is not well understood, but it is thought to be related to the sex hormones.

pitta dosha: the dosha that is responsible for all metabolic functions and transformations. This dosha has qualities that are like fire and water.

pituitary gland: gland found in the center of the head; serves as the "brain" of the endocrine system.

pityrosporum ovale: a type of yeast sometimes associated with seborrheic dermatitis.

place: refers to the distribution channel or method for delivering your goods and services to clients.

placebo: in research methodology, a substance that appears to be similar but is not the same substance as what is given to the experimental group.

plakoglobin: one of the two proteins that make up the plaques in the cell membrane.

plaques: located in the cell membrane; made up of two proteins: desmoplakin and plakoglobin.

plasma membrane: *see* cellular membrane.

platelet-derived growth factor (PDGF): growth regulatory cytokines thought to be responsible for initiating proliferation of fibroblasts and other connective tissue cells.

platysmal bands: bands around the neck which are a result of dynamic movement of the neck and jaw.

plexuses: network of nerves that branch and rejoin. There are nearly 100 in the body.

plural: form of a word meant to indicate that there is more than one.

pluripotential stem cell: at the start of the blood cell line, this cell is programmed to form all the other cells in the blood stream.

polychromatic: multiple wavelength light, appearing as different colors, as exhibited in Intense Pulsed Light emissions or seen with visible sun light.

polychromatic normoblasts: part of the blood cell line and formed from the basophilic normoblast, this cell (9 to 12 microns diameter) starts to make hemoglobin, but can no longer divide.

polymorphonuclear cells: granulocytes.

polyphenols: antioxidant phytochemicals.

polysaccharides: carbohydrates that contain three or more simple carbohydrate molecules.

polyunsaturated fatty acids: unsaturated fatty acids that contain two or more double bonds.

porphyria: a group of disorders caused by abnormalities in production of heme, a substance important in the creation of blood and bone marrow. Cutaneous porphyrins affect the skin with symptoms of blisters, itching and swelling of the skin when exposed to light.

porphyrins: compound that forms many important substances in the body, including hemoglobin, a part of red blood cells, that carry oxygen in the blood.

positive stool guaiac: test result that indicates the presence of blood in the stool.

post-inflammatory hyperpigmentation: dark melanin splotches caused by trauma to the skin; can result from acne pimples and papules.

post-traumatic stress disorder (PTSD): anxiety condition resulting from stress brought on by a traumatic event.

power density: the rate of energy that is being delivered to tissue by a laser light source.

prakruti: individual or natal constitution. Literary prakruti means ones "nature."

prana: life giving force or vital force.

pranayam: breath control exercises that should be done only with a qualified teacher.

prefixes: parts of Greek or Latin words used at the beginning of a word to alter or modify its meaning.

premenstrual syndrome (PMS): a condition in which some women experience uncomfortable physical changes before menstruation.

pressing agents: ingredients that help powders stay in cake form and also help powder cosmetics adhere or stick to the skin.

preventative maintenance: routine equipment calibration and device checks by qualified, trained biomedical engineers to guarantee that the equipment is in appropriate working order.

price: the monetary value applied to goods and services sold.

primary metabolites: the metabolites required for the growth, structure, and reproduction of a plant.

proanthocyanidins: very strong family of antioxidants found in grapeseed extract and maritme pine extract (pycnogenol).

product: in marketing this term refers to your complete business concept and includes both the tangible and intangible characteristics associated with your marketing strategy.

pro-enzyme: an inactive form of chymotropic enzyme found in the lamellar bodies of the stratum granulosum.

progesterone: hormone that helps prepare the uterus for pregnancy and is an important hormone in the menstrual cycle.

proliferative phase: the phase of wound healing in which there is increased vascularity to supply nutrients and oxygen to the wound.

promissory note: a legal document that defines the terms of a loan agreement between two parties.

promotion: the marketing methods used to persuade others to purchase your products and services.

The Promotion Mix: the communication methods used to promote business in marketing. These include advertising, public relations, publicity, direct marketing, personal selling, and sales promotion.

pronormoblast: part of the blood cell line, formed from the division of the hemocytoblast, this cell (20 microns) continues to divide and forms the basophilic normoblasts.

pronunciation: process of accurately speaking a word as it is meant to be spoken.

Propionibacterium acnes (P. acnes): the scientific name of the bacteria that causes acne vulgaris.

proteases: enzymes that digest proteins; includes proteinases and peptidases.

protectants: ingredients that keep substances from penetrating the skin.

protein: (Gr., from *proteios*, "primary") chains of amino acid molecules used in cell functions and body growth; a macromolecule of carbon, hydrogen, oxygen, and nitrogen, and at times, sulfur and phosphorus.

protein-tyrosine kinase activity: a complex enzyme that catalyze the phosphorylation of tyrosine residues. There are 91 of identified PTK enzymes which are involved in cellular signaling pathways, regulate key cell functions such as proliferation, differentiation, anti-apoptotic signaling and neurite outgrowth. Unregulated activation of these enzymes, through mechanisms such as point mutations or over-expression, can lead to various forms of cancer as well as benign proliferative conditions. The importance of PTKs in health and disease is further underscored by the existence of aberrations in PTK signaling occurring in inflammatory diseases and diabetes. In short, this is a very important enzyme that activates other enzymes.

proteoglycans: a special class of glycoproteins found in the extracellular substance. They vary in size depending on the glycosaminoglycan chains attached to them.

proteolysis: the act of breaking the desmosomal bonds of connecting proteins.

proteolytic enzymes: protein dissolving enzymes.

proton pump inhibitiors (PPIs): type of antacid that works to reduce the production of acid.

psychological dependence: type of chemical dependence characterized by the affected individual thinking he or she needs a substance in order to function.

psychoses: any psychological condition that affects an individuals ability to live their lives in a normal and healthy manner.

ptosis: drooping of the eyelids.

puberty: stage of life when physical changes occur in both sexes and when sexual function of the sex glands begins to take place.

public relations: a marketing strategy that is used to generate positive publicity about your business.

publicity: a marketing strategy used to gain free media attention.

pulmonary circulation: the path deoxygenated blood travels to become oxygenated; through the right ventricle, into the lungs through the pulmonary artery, and into the left atrium via the pulmonary vein.

pulmonary valves: one of the two valves that regulates the flow of blood between the ventricles and the major blood vessel to which it connects.

pulse duration: the duration of an individual pulse of laser light; usually measured in milliseconds. *See* pulse width.

pulse width: the period time in which a pulse of light is emitted. *See* pulse duration.

punctate keratitis: calluses resulting from prolonged and frequent exposure to friction.

Q

quadriceps: muscles located on the anterior, or rear, of the thigh regulate extension.

R

radiant energy (fluence): the energy level of a laser. It is calculated by integrating power with respect to time (joules).

rajasic: energetic, aggressive.

rancid: describes an oxidized cosmetic product that has discoloration and/or odor.

rancidity: condition that is the result of an oxygen reaction at the unsaturated site of a fatty acid, causing a decomposition of the oil and the disagreeable odor associated with it.

receptor: a special protein on a cells surface or within the cell that binds to specific ligands.

receptor sites: a protein on the cell membrane or within the cytoplasm or cell nucleus that binds to a specific molecule (a ligand), such as a neurotransmitter, hormone, or other substance, and initiates the cellular response.

reconstructive rhinoplasty: surgery done to correct or repair abnormal structures.

reconstructive surgeon: a physician who specializes in surgical procedures that are medically necessary and are used to correct abnormalities associated with birth defects, accidents, injuries, and other physical deformities, and the removal of life-threatening diseases such as skin cancer lesions.

rectified: the result of redistilling essential oils to remove color and unwanted compounds from the oil.

rectus abdominis: outermost layer of the abdominal muscle.

reepithelialization: the formation of new epidermis and dermis over an area of injury. The epithelial cells from the wound margin and the philosebaceous units migrate to repair damage.

refined: name given to a plant extract, usually referring to a fixed oil, that has gone through the refinement process of removing colors, odors, or other naturally occurring compounds, such as a refined grapeseed oil.

reflex arc: critical to the autonomic nervous system (ANS), there are two parts of the reflex arc: the sensory (afferent) arm and the motor (efferent or effector) arm.

reflexology: based on the belief that working on areas or reflex points found on the hands, feet, ears and face can reduce tension to the bodies corresponding organs and gland structures. Origin - exact origin is unknown.

Reiki: universal life force energy transmitted through the palms of the hands that helps to lift the spirits and provide balance to the whole self; body, mind and spirit.

Reiki attunement: performed by a Reiki master teacher to open and connect a student to universal healing energy on all levels of the physical, mental, emotional and spirit bodies. The attunement provides a clearing of someone's current energy in order to raise his or her vibration to the next level.

relaxin: hormone manufactured by the ovaries that helps enlarge the pelvic opening during childbirth.

remodeling: the maturation phase of a wound.

resale tax: a tax imposed upon those who sell retail products.

respiratory burst: process that uses oxygen in the killing action of neutrophils.

reticulocyte: part of the blood cell line, formed from the acidophilic normoblast, this cell (8 microns in diameter) contains mitochondria.

rhinophyma: enlarging of the nose, resulting from a severe form of acne rosacea.

rhinoplasty: surgical procedure to correct the shape of the nose or change its appearance.

rhytidectomy: face lift procedure. This procedure removes excess fat at the jawline; tightens loose, atrophic muscles; and removes sagging skin.

ribosomes: small dense organelles that assemble proteins in cells.

risk: the chance of incurring some type of harm, damage or loss.

risk management: the methods used to safeguard your business against loss or damage.

root words: parts of Latin or Greek words that serve as the basis for medical terminology.

rubifacant: an agent that causes the skin to redden.

rubification: inflammation of the skin; chronic congestion primarily on the cheeks and nose, characterized by redness, dilation of blood vessels, and, in severe cases, the formation of papules and pustules.

Rubin scale: evaluates skin based on the depth of the photodamage into the skin.

S

saccharides: any of a various group of organic compounds that contain carbon, hydrogen, and oxygen and includes cellulose, gums, sugars, and starches; also referred to as carbohydrates.

safety plan: a plan for avoiding potential exposure to contaminated fluids and for dealing with it should exposure occur.

sales promotion: a marketing strategy aimed at drawing attention to your products and services with the goal of increasing the volume of business.

samadi: state of pure joy.

Sanskrit: the language in which the root texts of Ayurveda were written. It is sometimes called the language of creation.

sattvic: gentle, calm, nourishing.

saturated fatty acids: fatty acids that contain no double bonds.

scatter: a general physical process involving moving particles that are dispersed through a medium in a non-uniform manner.

scientific method: a philosophy of reasoning that is based on first generating and then testing a hypothesis.

sclerotherapy: injection into a vein of a chemical irritant that causes fibrosis and, later, elimination of the lumen, to treat varicose veins, hemorrhoids, or esophageal varices.

scope of practice: refers to the type of treatments and services one can perform under their license.

scotch hose: hose similar to a fire hose used in water therapy.

SD alcohol: are specially denatured to make them not drinkable. Also known as ethanol.

seaweed wraps: wraps that include application of a seaweed mask followed by a thermal blanket to seal in heat.

seborrheic dermatitis: a skin disorder characterized by flaky, red, patchy skin primarily in the eyebrows, T-zone, and scalp caused by inflammation of the sebaceous gland and resulting in patches of inflamed flakiness in oily areas of the skin; a common form of eczema.

seborrheic keratoses: crusty-looking, slightly raised lesions in mature, sun damaged skin. Often appear in the cheekbone area. They may be black, brown, gray, or sometimes flesh-toned or sallow.

secondary metabolites: metabolites that are not required for the most basic, life sustaining needs. Most secondary metabolites have to do with protection and reproduction.

secreted: synthesized or released by various cells or organs.

sedimentary: a category of rock created by weathering actions of water, ice, wind or other atmospheric actions, or by biological deposits.

select serotonin reuptake inhibitors (SSRIs): type of antidepressant that allows for more productive use of the neurotransmitter serotonin.

selective permeability: the ability of the plasma membrane to let some substances in and keep others out; permeable to small molecules, usually H_2O, O_2, and CO_2, but not permeable to larger molecules or ions.

selective photothermolysis: treatment utilizing an appropriate wavelength, exposure time, and pulse duration with sufficient energy fluence to absorb light into a specific area; allows damage to targeted tissue without involving the surrounding area.

self-employment tax: a tax imposed upon those who are self-employed, which allows them to receive retirement benefits, disability benefits, survivor benefits and hospital insurance or Medicare, in much the same way an employee would.

semilunar valves: valves of the arteries, preventing backflow from arteries into the ventricles.

senescent cell: a cell arrested in G1 that cannot advance or go backward and in some cases is destroyed; a major cause of aging.

sensory (afferent) neuron or nerve: nerve that carries impulses or messages from the sense organs to the brain, where sensations of touch, cold, heat, sight, hearing, taste, smell, pain, and pressure are experienced.

serotonin: neurotransmitter which is associated with many psychoses, especially depression.

sharps: any object that can penetrate the skin, including, but not limited to, needles, razors, scissors, and broken glass.

shiatsu massage: the application of pressure on acupuncture points found throughout the body to balance the body energy flow and to promote health. Origin – a form of physical therapy from Japan.

shirobhyanga: head massage.

shirodhara: a fine warm stream of oil or cool stream of buttermilk is poured over the forehead to deeply calm the nervous system. Shirodhara causes the release of serotonin, which deeply relaxes the body, melting tensions. It alleviates discomfort in the head, neck, and shoulder area, as well as engenders profound feelings of pleasure, inner balance, mental clarity and radiance to the completion.

sidhi: psychic power.

six sense approach: the belief that the health and balance of the body of the body/mind system is influenced by the perceptions of all the senses: sight, smell, taste, touch, hearing and the intuitive sense felt with the heart. Simply put, we are always influenced by the environment in which we find ourselves.

snana: bathing.

snehana: oil massage to lubricate the body.

Social Security number: the number used to identify an individual taxpayer.

sodium PCA: a humectant that helps to bind water in the epidermis

sodium sulfacetamide: topical drug agent sometimes used to treat rosacea or acne.

soleus: located on the back of the leg, this fleshy superficial muscle originates at the fibula, and inserts at the calcaneus tendon at the heel.

soma: nectar.

spa: term originally meaning "health through water." Today it most often refers to day spas or destination spas, where clients can find a wide range of treatments.

spa therapy: a more current term for water treatments provided in a spa.

spasticity: describes spasms or uncontrollable muscle movement.

spirit/energy body: also known as spirit or essence, is the life force energy coming from within and radiating beyond the body. The inner face of the Chakras combined with the outer face of the Aura.

splattering: singed hair

spores: reproductive cells, usually unicellular, produced by plants and some protozoa. Bacterial spores are difficult to destroy because high temperatures are required to destroy them and they are very resistant to heat.

spot sizes: the diameter of the optical or laser light. Beam diameter

srota: channels in the body that carry food, blood, air or energy.

standard precautions: a widely recognized and utilized method of infection control. Under Standard Precautions all blood, other body fluids, secretions, excretions (except sweat), non-intact skin, mucous membranes, dried blood, saliva, and any other body substance are considered contaminated and/or infectious.

stem cell: a cell capable of multiple divisions, also known as the mother cell.

stenciling: use of a template or stencil to prevent color from being applied beyond a certain area.

sterilize: the act of using a physical or chemical procedure to destroy all forms of microbial life, including highly resistant bacterial spores.

stethoscope: device used to magnify the sound of a beating heart.

strabismus: eye disorder in which the optic axes in either eye can not focus on the same object.

stress triggers: situations that bring on a stress response.

striae distensae: stretch marks commonly occurring during pregnancy

subclinical: describes a situation in which normal clinical symptoms are not visible.

subclinical inflammation: biochemical inflammation cannot be seen with the naked eye or a magnifying loop.

subcutaneous mycoses: fungal infections occurring below the skin.

sublingual: below the tongue.

submental: below the mentalis, the area within the anatomic triangular margins of the mandible where the double chin resides.

substantives: ingredients that attach themselves to the surface of the skin to protect and hydrate the surface.

suffixes: parts of Greek or Latin words used at the end of a word to alter or modify its meaning.

sundar: beauty.

supercritical carbon dioxide (CO_2): a modern method of extraction in which the plant material is placed in a high pressure container with CO_2 that is in a state midway between being a liquid and a gas.

superfatted: describes soaps or cleaners that have fat added to buffer their contact with the skin.

superficial: dealing with the outermost parts of the skin.

superficial musculoaponeurotic system: a layer of tissue that covers the deeper structures in the cheek area and is in continuity with the superficial muscle covering the lower face and neck, called the platysma. Some face-lift techniques lift and reposition the SMAS as well as the skin.

superficial mycoses: skin condition that results from the introduction of vegetative matter to an open wound; infection is limited to the dermis.

superoxide: an unstable, reactive single oxygen atom.

superoxide dismutase: an enzyme that helps squelch reactions early in the cascade of reactions.

supination: rotation of the arm.

suppressor T cells: inhibits the production of cytotoxic cells once they are no longer needed so they do not cause more damage than necessary.

supraspinatus: rotator cuff muscle syncope.

sympathetic divisions: the part of the autonomic nervous system which is stimulated by activity and prepares the body for stressful situations, such as running from a dangerous situation or competing in a sports event.

synapse: junction by which a nerve impulse travels.

synergy: two or more agents working as a cooperative whole, producing a result that is greater than the total effect of the individual parts.

synthetic: of, or relating to, being produced by chemical synthesis.

systemic circulation: blood and lymph circulation from the heart, through the arteries, to tissue and cells, and back to the heart by way of the veins; also called general circulation.

systemic mycoses: fungi that affect the internal organs.

systole: blood and lymph circulation from the heart, through the arteries, to tissue and cells, and back to the heart by way of the veins.

T

T cell: type of lymphocyte with a vital regulatory role in immune response; so called because they are processed through the thymus. Subsets of T cells may be stimulatory or inhibitory. They communicate with other cells by protein hormones called cytokines.

tamasic: heavy, dull and destructive.

tartaric acid: an AHA occurring naturally in grapes and passion fruit.

tej: healthy glow or radiant beauty.

telangiectasia: a dilated or distended red capillary

tendons: strong connective tissue which attaches muscle to bone.

terpenoid compounds: lipids made up of multiples of isoprene units.

testes: organs of the male reproductive system; reside in the scrotum and produce sperm.

testosterone: male hormone responsible for development of typical male characteristics.

thalassemia: condition characterized by defective hemoglobin cells, resulting in oxygen deficiency.

thalassotherapy: therapeutic use of sea water.

thermal storage: measure of heat stored in a chromophore.

thermal relaxation time (TRT): the time it takes for the target tissue to dissipate one-half of the heat attained by a laser pulse.

thread lift: a minimally invasive face-lift using special subcutaneous suspension sutures for subtle changes.

threading: hair removal using strands of thread.

thrombocytopenia: abnormal decrease in blood platelet levels.

thrombosis: one or more blood clots that may partially or completely block an artery.

thymidine dinucleotide fragments: fragments produced by damaged DNA, triggering release of MSH, which can then bind to melanocytes to produce melanin.

thymus gland: gland located under the breastbone in the chest; secretes hormones and helps to trigger synthesis of more lymph tissue.

thyroid gland: gland located in the neck; regulates both cellular and body metabolism and produces hormones that stimulate growth.

thyroxine: one of the hormones secreted by the thyroid gland.

tibialis anterior: muscle vital to the control of dorsiflexion of the foot.

tight junction: region of actual fusion of cell membranes between two adjacent cells.

tincture: herbal extract using alcohol or glycerin to extract the compounds from the plant material.

tinnitus: ringing in the ears.

tortuous: taking a twisting, nonlinear path.

Toxic Epidermal Necrolysis (TEN): tissue death on the epidermis.

transient erythema: redness that comes and goes.

transit time: the time it takes for cells to move through the epidermal stages of growth.

trapezius: 1.) diamond shaped coupling of superficial muscles that make up the majority of our upper backs. 2.) muscle that covers the back of the neck and upper and middle region of the back; stabilizes the scapula and shrugs the shoulders.

traverse abdominals: deepest of the abdominal muscles.

tricep brachii: muscles causing extension of the arm and elbow.

tricuspid valve: heart valve which prevents backflow between the right atrium and right ventricle.

tricyclics (TCAs): a strong peel used to diminish sun damage and wrinkles; the most commonly prescribed type of antidepressant used to treat milder cases of depression or anxiety.

trigeminal nerve: the main sensory nerve of the face having three major branches.

triphala: commonly used herb for cleansing and toning the digestive tract.

trophic hormones: chemicals that cause glands to make hormones.

tuberculosis (TB): an infectious disease, most often seen in the lungs, chronic in nature and capable of affecting the lungs, although it may occur in almost any part of the body. The causative agent is mycobacterium tuberculosis (the tubercle bacillus). The most common mode of transmission is the inhalation of infected droplet nuclei.

tubulin: a protein that forms part of the microtubules.

U

ubtan: a blend of flour and powdered herbs used dry or in a paste to remove oil after massage.

ultraviolet: invisible rays that have short wavelengths, are the least penetrating rays, produce chemical effects, and kill germs; also called cold rays or actinic rays.

unicellular: single-celled organism.

unsaturated fatty acids: fatty acids that contain at least one double bond.

U.S. Environmental Protection Agency (EPA): an agency charged with protecting human health as well as air, water and land.

U.S. Food and Drug Administration (FDA): an agency responsible for safety regulation of foods, dietary supplements, medical related items, veterinary items and cosmetics.

V

vacuoles: membrane-bound compartments within some eukaryotic cells that can serve a variety of secretory, excretory, and storage functions.

vaidya: ayurvedic physician.

Valtrex® (Valacyclovir hydrochloride): antiviral medication that can stop or shorten a recurrent outbreak of herpes simplex.

varicose veins: condition characterized by incompetent valves in the veins, most commonly in the legs.

vascular: related to blood vessels.

vascular growth factor (VGF): biochemical within the skin that triggers the growth of capillaries.

vasodilation: vascular dilation of blood vessels; resulting in flushing.

vata dosha: the dosha that is responsible for all movement in the body voluntary and involuntary. This dosha has qualities that are like air and space.

vedas: a collection of root texts of ayurvedic knowledge. Literally means "pure knowledge" or "the principles of creation."

ventricles: the lower, thick-walled chambers of the heart, which force blood to the lungs for oxygenation or throughout to the body.

ventricular arrhythmias: irregular heartbeat originating in the ventricular chambers of the heart.

venture capitalist(s): a private individual (or group of individuals) who invest in businesses with the goal of gaining a return on their investment or profit.

versican sulfate: a proteoglycan found in the dermis, provides the turgor and tautness to the skin by interacting with the elastin and the hyaluronic acid.

vertigo: sensation of moving through space or of having objects float independently around; often synonymous with dizziness.

Vichy shower: overhead shower with adjustable water pressure used in body treatments.

vikruti: imbalance of doshas.

vimentin: an intermediate filament found in fibroblasts.

viscosity: the thickness and liquidity of a solution.

W

watts: measurement of how much electrical energy is being used per second. A unit of power.

wet room: a room lined with tile or other water impervious material and drains to service water treatments such as a Vichy shower.

white blood cell: blood cells responsible for the body's defense mechanisms. They act by destroying disease-causing germs. Also called *white corpuscles* or *leukocytes*.

whole extract: extracts from plant material that have not been changed or altered from their extracted form.

word analysis: process by which the different parts of the words are dissected and interpreted to determine the meaning of the original word.

Y

yantra: geometric symbol that represents a primal sound or syllable.

yoga: exercise that involves postures and breathing techniques. Literally yoga means "union with the divine."

Z

Zithromax Z Pak® (Azithromycin): wide-spectrum antibiotic that is derived from erythromycin. It is highly effective against Staphylococcus aureus, bacteria frequently living on the skin or in the nose of a healthy person, which can cause a wide range of skin infections.

zygote: diploid cell produced by the fusion of an egg and sperm; fertilized egg cell.

Index

Page number references preceeded by an "F" refer to *Milady's Standard Esthetics: Fundamentals*; all other page number references are to *Milady's Standard Esthetics: Advanced*. Page numbers referencing figures are italicized and followed by an "*f*". Page numbers referencing tables are italicized and followed by a "*t*". Page numbers in bold refer to key terms.

A

A (amps), **F148**, *F149f*, **F160**
ABCDE Cancer Checklist, F224
abdominoplasty, **F463**, **F465**, **727**–28, *728f*, **730**
abducent nerve, *F111f*
ablation, **158**, **182**
ablative, **172**, **182**, **736**, **744**
absolutes, **290**, **303**
absorption, **F119**, **F121**, F194–95, **161**, *161f*, **182**
AC. *See* alternating current
access to medical records, 13, 669
accessibility, *F575f*
accessory nerve, *F111f*, **F112**–13, **F122**
accidents, and infection control, 48
Accutane, *F229t*, *F245t*, 11, 231, 273, 373, 377
ACD. *See* allergic contact dermatitis
acetone, 76
acetylcholine, **106**, **119**
acetylsalicylic acid, **443**, **474**
acid mantle, **F135**, **F141**, **F192**, **F208**
acid-alkali neutralization reactions, **F135**, **F141**
acidophilic normoblasts, **71**, **80**
acids, **F134**, **F141**, F447–48, 144, 367–74
acne
  adult, *F242t*, **222**, **227**, **233**, 320
  AHAs and, F352, F354, 373–74
  bacteria and, F216, F226–27, **219**, **234**
  birth control pills and, 223
  causes of, F226–27
  on chin, 97, *97f*, 222, *222f*
  chocolate and, F182
  cosmetics and, F228, 226
  cystic, F227
  defined, **F216**, **F230**
  environmental factors and, 224–25
  excoriée, **F216**, **F230**, 225, *225f*
  exfoliation for, F352
  extractions and, F351
  facials, F351–54
  glycolic acid and, *374f*
  grades of, F228, *F229f*, *F229t*, 220–21, *221f*
  hereditary factors in, 218
  hormones and, F227–28, 221–23
  infection control and, 28
  medicated cleansers for, *F229t*, 309
  nutrition and, 225–26
  oily skin and, 218, 226
  overview of, F225–26
  perimenopausal, 99, 223
  pregnancy and, 223
  progression of, *218f*
  propionibacterium acnes bacteria and, F216, **219**, **234**
  scarring from, 221, *222f*
  skin care and, 320
  stress and, 223
  tanning and, 224
  teenage, 223–24, 320
  treating, F229, F353
  triggers, F227–28
acnegenic products, F228
acquired immune deficiency syndrome (AIDS), **F67**, **F88**, 28, **50**
acquired immunity, **F70**, **F88**
ACS. *See* acute coronary syndrome
actin, **60**, 62, **80**
actin filaments, **73**, **80**
actinic, **F241**, **F251**
actinic keratosis, **F222**, **F230**, *F242t*, **217**, *217f*, **233**, **452**
action plans, F574–76
active electrodes, **F151**, **F160**
active ingredients, **253**, **279**, **280**
active transport, **73**, **80**
acupressure, F366
acupuncture, 242, **402**, **434**
acute, **24**, **50**
acute coronary syndrome (ACS), **331**, **343**
acute hepatitis, 24, **50**
adapalene, *F229t*, *F245t*
Addison's disease, 100
adduction, **111**, **112**, **119**
adductor group of muscles, **115**–16, **119**
adenosine triphosphate (ATP), **F168**, **F184**, **58**–59, **80**
adherens junctions, **73**, **80**
adipose tissue, **F198**, **F208**
adjective, **683**, *683t*, **687**
administrative duties, F558–59
adrenal glands, F118, **91**, 100, **101**
adrenaline, **91**, **101**, **197**, **199**
adult acne, *F242t*, **222**, **227**, **233**, 320
adulteration, **294**, **303**
Advanced Glycation Endproducts (AGE products), **193**, *194f*, **199**
advertising, **F609**, **F616**, **771**–72, 774, **779**
aerosolized, **453**, **474**
aestheticians. *See* estheticians
aesthetics. *See* esthetics
Aesthetics International Association, 14
afferent nerves, F110, F125, F193–94, *F195f*, F200
afferent neurons, **77**, **80**
afferent peripheral system, F108
affirmations, 13, 608
African esthetics, F6, *F7f*
African Karite Butter, 289, *289f*
agate, 619, *619f*
Age of Extravagance esthetics, F7
AGE products. *See* Advanced Glycation Endproducts
age spots, F241
age-management techniques, 9
aging, *F242t*, F406. *See also* mature skin
  AHAs and, *374f*
  cells and, 69
  cosmetic ingredients for, 273–77
  nutrition and, 193–95
  photoaging, *F243f*, 212–13, 367–68, *368f*
agni, **657**
agranulocytes, **125**, **135**
AHAs. *See* alpha hydroxy acids
AIDS. *See* acquired immune deficiency syndrome
air, **F134**, **F141**
air systems, F71
airborne infections, and infection control, 28, 48
airbrush makeup, F522, **546**–51, *547f*, *550f–553f*, **560**
airbrushes, **548**, *548f*, **560**
airlines, F13
Akt, **70**, **80**
ALA. *See* aminolevulinic acid
ala, **111**, **119**

albinism, **F221**, **F230**
albumin, **124**, **135**
alcohol, F204, **F268**, *F268t*, **F290**
alcohol-based antiseptic solutions, 31–32
algae, **F270**, *F270t*, **F290**, 383, 387, 579
algae masks, F282
alipidic skin, **F237**–38, **F251**, 269–70
alkalies, **F134**, **F141**, F447–48
alkaloids, **148**, **153**
allantoin, *F270t*, **F290**, **284**, **303**, 387
allergic contact dermatitis (ACD), F218–20, **31**, 34, **50**
allergic reaction, **743**, **744**
allergies, *F64t*, F172, *F245t*, F267, F272, F282, 697
almond meal, *F270t*
aloe vera, *F270t*, **F290**, *272f*, 273, 286, *286f*, 387
alpha d-tocopherol, **284**, **303**
alpha hydroxy acids (AHAs)
  acne and, F352, F354, 373–74
  aging and, *374f*
  chemical action of, 316–17
  as cosmetic ingredients, 268, 271–73, 277, 576
  defined, **F245**, **F251**, **F263**, **F290**
  exfoliation and, 367–74, *368f*, *370f–372f*
  hyperpigmentation and, 369, 374, *375f*, *376f*
  peels, F447, F449
  safety and, F447
  sunscreen and, 271
  toners and, 272
alpha-linolenic fatty acids, **F170**–71, **F185**
alpha-lipoic acid, F275, *149f*
alternating current (AC), **F148**, **F160**, F390
alternative medicine, 603–4
alum, **F268**, *F268t*, **F290**
aluminum oxide, 270, 453
ama, **657**
amber light, F452
American Cancer Society, F224
American National Standard Institute (ANSI), 164–66, *165f*, 168–71, 440, 505
American Society of Aesthetic Plastic Surgeons, 715
American Society of Plastic Surgeons, 694
American Spa Magazine, 14
American waxing, 493–94
amethyst, 619, *620f*
amino acids, **F167**–68, **F184**, **58**, **80**, 142–**43**, **147**, **153**
aminolevulinic acid (ALA), 452, *452f*
ampoules, **F283**, **F290**, **316**, 352
amps (A), **F148**, *F149f*, **F160**
anabolism, **F97**, **F121**, **189**
anaerobic bacteria, F226
anagen stage, **F403**–4, **F441**
analgesic, **148**
anaphoresis, **F152**, **F160**, **F386**, **F388**, *F389t*, **F396**
anaphylaxis, **333**, **343**
anastomosis, **128**, **135**
anatomy. *See also* muscles
  body systems, F97, *F98t*
  cells, F95–97
  circulatory system, F113–16
  defined, **F95**, **F121**
  digestive system, **F118**–19, **F122**, *F165f*
  endocrine system, **F117**–18, **F122**, *90f*, **291**, **303**
  excretory system, F119, F123
  hair, F199
  heart, **F113**–14, **F123**, 127–28, *127f*
  immune system, F117
  integumentary system, **F120**, **F123**, F191–92, **F208**
  nervous system, F107–13
  organs, **F97**, *F98t*, **F124**
  reasons for studying, F95
  reproductive system, **F120**, **F125**, *91f*
  respiratory system, **F119**–20, **F125**
  skeletal system, F99–102
  tissues, **F97**, **F126**
anchoring system, **74**, **80**
Anderson, Rox, 162
androgen isotypes, 246–47, *246f*
androgens, F227–28, **92**, **101**, *246f*
anecdotal, **272**, **279**
anecdotal evidence, **669**, **671**
anemia, **125**–26, *126t*, **135**
anesthesia
  overview of, 712
  topical, 509, *509f*
anger control, 198
angina, **332**, **343**
angle brushes, F479
angular artery, *F115f*, **F116**, **F121**
anhidrosis, **F217**, **F230**
anhydrous products, **F257**, **F290**
anodes, **F151**, **F160**
anorexia, 100
ANS. *See* autonomic nervous system
ANSI. *See* American National Standard Institute
antacid, **335**, **343**
antagonist, **110**, **119**
anterior auricular artery, *F115f*, **F116**, **F121**
antianginals, **332**, **343**
antianxiety drugs, **328**, **343**
antiasthmatics, **333**, **343**
antibacterial, **30**, **50**
antibiotics, **27**, **50**, 337–38, *338t*, 443
antibodies, **72**, **80**, **124**, 125, **135**
anticholinergics, **334**, **343**
anticonvulsants, **336**, **343**
antidepressants, **328**, **343**
antiemetics, **334**, **343**
antigens, **72**, **80**, **333**, **343**
antihistamines, **333**, **343**
anti-inflammatory properties, 284, 289, 291
antimicrobial properties, 284, 291
antimicrobials, **30**, **51**, 261–62
antioxidants
  broad-spectrum, 275
  defined, **F136**, **F141**, **F245**, **F251**, **F262**, **F264**, **F290**, **190**, *190f*
  as ingredients, 262, 275–76, 284
  mature skin and, F275–76
  skin care products, F265, F275
antipsychotic, **337**, **344**
antiretrovirals, **339**, **344**
antiseptic properties, 291
antiseptics, **F71**, **F88**, F273
antispasmodics, 292, **334**, **344**
antithrombotics, **331**, **344**
antiulcer drugs, **334**, **344**
Antoinette, Marie, F7
aorta, **128**
aortic semilunar valve, **128**, **135**
apatite, 618, *618f*
aperipheral edema, **131**–32
apocrine glands, **F202**, **F208**, **89**, **101**
aponeurosis, **F103**, *F104f*, **F121**, **108**, **119**
apoptosis, **69**, **80**
appearance, personal, F21–23, *F547f*, F553
application forms, for job searches, F549–52, *F550f–552f*
applicators, F79, F413, F498
appointments, scheduling, F46–47, F593–94
apprenticeship, F581
Aquaphor®, **739**, **744**
aqueous calcium, F462
aqueous extract, **285**, **303**
areola repigmentation, 557, *558f*
areolas, **723**, **730**
arms
  circulatory system and, F116
  muscles of, F106–7, 112–14, *113f*, *114f*, *114t*
  nerves of, F113
  skeletal system and, F102
  waxing, 492
arnica montana, *F270t*, 286, *286f*, **741**, **744**
aromatherapy, **F261**, F273–74, **F290**, F366
  Ayurveda and, 630, 649
  botanical practice and, 301–2, *302f*
  essential oils and, 289–91, *299t–300t*
  skin care products and, F273–74
  spas and, *597f*
aromatic properties, F273
aromatic ring, 152, **153**
arrector pili muscles, **F194**, *F195f*, F200, **F208**, **F402**, *F403f*, **F441**
arrhythmia, **332**, **344**
arterial system, 128–30, *129f*
arteries, **F114**, **F121**
arterioles, **124**, 129, **135**
arteriosclerosis, **F171**, **F184**
arthropods, 27
artificial eyelashes, F513–16
ascorbic acid, *F174t*, **F180**, **F185**, **F275**, **F293**, F352, 62, 276–78
asepsis, **29**–30, **51**
aseptic procedures, **F80**–81, **F88**, **29**–30, **51**
ashram, **657**
Asian esthetics, F6
Asian skin, F241
aspartate, **80**
asphyxiated skin, *F242t*
assessment forms, for clients, *F416f*
assets, **752**–54, **762**
asteatosis, **F216**, **F230**
astringents, F273, **F278**, **F290**, 93, 266, 284
asymptomatic, **F84**, **F88**, **25**, **51**
atomic weight, 140
atoms, **F131**, **F141**
atopic dermatitis, **F218**, **F230**
ATP. *See* adenosine triphosphate
atria, *F113f*, **F114**, **F121**, **127**, **135**
atrioventricular valves, **128**, **135**
atrophy, F221
attenuation, **167**, **182**
attitude, F23–24, F553, 36–37
augmentation mammaplasty, 720–21, *720f*, *721f*
augmentation, of lips, *698f*, *699f*, 701
auras, 604, *605f*, **657**
auricularis anterior muscles, **F103**, *F104f*, **F121**
auricularis posterior muscles, **F103**, *F104f*, **F121**
auricularis superior muscles, **F103**, *F104f*, **F121**
auriculotemporal nerve, **F110**, *F112f*, **F121**
Australian sandalwood, 298
autoclaves, **F73**–74, **F88**, *F301f*
  disinfection and, 47
  infection control and, 39–41, 43–49, *45f–47f*, **51**
  manuals for, 46

overview of, *39f–40f*, **41**, 43–49, *45f–47f*, **51**
safety and, 44
autoimmune disorders, *F245t*
defined, **21**, **51**
infection control and, 21, **28**
IPL treatments and, 441
women and, 25
autologous, **698**, **708**
autologous collagen, **698**, **708**
autonomic motor systems, **291**, **303**
autonomic nervous system (ANS), **F108**, **F121**, **77**, **80**
aventurine, 618, *618f*
avian, **697**, **708**
avocado, *F270t*, *F273t*
axons, **F110**, **F121**
Ayurveda
aromatherapy and, 630, 649
defined, **629**, **656**
doshas, **631**–37, *632f*, *634t*, **656**
energy flow and, 242, 630–31
five elements and, 632
herbs of, 637–38, *638t*
marmas and, **639**–40, *640f*, *640t–641t*, *643f–648f*, 655–**56**
shirodhara and, *649f–654f*, 649–50, **657**
treatments, *629f*, 637–55, *641f–643f*
ayurvedic, **F456**, **F465**
azelaic acid, *F229t*
Azelex, *F229t*
azithromycin, **744**
azulene, **F270**, *F270t*, **F290**

B

B cells, 65, **72**–73, **80**
B lymphocyte, **72**, **80**
B vitamins, *F173–74t*, **F178**–79, **F184**
Baby Boomers, F16, 5, 231, 663, 691, 711
baby oil, 254
Bach, Edward, 613
Bach Flower Remedies, 613
bacilli, **F63**, *F64f*, **F88**
back
massage, 400–401, *400f*, *401f*
waxing, F439–40, 501–3, *502f*
back bubble, **550**, **560**
bacteria
acne and, F216, F226–27, **219**, **234**
anaerobic, F226
classifications of pathogenic, F63–65
defined, **F61**, **F88**, **51**
growth and reproduction of, F65
infection control and, F62–67, 27
infections from, F65–67, 337–38
microbiology of, 26
movement of, F65
nonpathogenic, **F63**, **F89**
tuberculosis and, 25
types of, F62–63
bacterial conjunctivitis, **F225**, **F230**
bactericidal disinfectants, **F62**, F74, **F88**
Baker's peel, F447
balance, F21–22, F38, **603**, **625**
balance sheet, **752**, *753f*, **762**
balneology, 7
balneotherapy, **F456**, **F465**, **6**, **15**
bamboo, 286, *287f*
band lashes, **F513**, **F524**
barbae folliculitis, **F356–57**, **F409**, **F441**
barbiturates, **336**, **344**
bariatric surgery, **727**, **730**
barrier function, **F192**, *F193f*, **F208**
basal cell carcinomas, **F223**, **F230–31**, **214**, *214f*, 217
basal lamina, *62f*, *65f*, *67t*, *74f*, 75
basalt, **402**, *410f*, **434**
base colors, F476
bases, **F134**, **F141**, F447–48, **144**–45
basophilic normoblasts, **71**, **80**
basophils, **64**, **80**
bayberry, *F270t*
BDD. *See* body dysmorphic disorder
beauty editors, 10
beds, treatment, F300, F304, *570f*
before and after photos, F42
belly, muscle, **F103**, **F121**
benign, F222
benzene ring structure, **152**, *152f*, **153**
benzodiazepines, **336**, **344**
benzoin, *F272t*
benzoyl peroxide (BP), **F268**, *F268t*, **F290**, F352, F354
benzoyl peroxide gel, 317
bergamot, *F272t*
beriberi, F178–79
beta carotene, 275
beta hydroxy acids (BHAs), **F263**, **F291**, F351–52, F447
chemical action of, 316–17
as cosmetic ingredients, 270, **271**, 576
exfoliation and, 367, *378f–380f*
peels and, F447
beta-carotene, F176–77
beta-glucans, **F264**, **F290–91**
BHAs. *See* beta hydroxy acids
bicep brachii, **112**, **119**
biceps, **F106**, *F107f*, **F121**
bicuspid valve, **127**, **135**
bikini waxing, F435–37, 493–501
binders, **F268**, **F291**
bioavailable, **275**, **279**
biochemistry, **143**, **153**
bioflavonoids, *F174t*, **F180**, **F184**
biohazardous materials, 22
biologically inert, **254**, 270, **279**
biotin, *F173t*, F179
bipolar radio-frequency (RF) energy, **178**, **182**
Birbeck granules, 63
birch leaf, *F270t*, *F272t*
birth control pills
acne and, 223
hormones and, 328–30
hyperpigmentation and, 97–98
melasma and, 97–98
birthmarks, F221, **F221**, **F232**
bismuth oxychloride, 536
Bitters, Patrick, 440
black makeup, F482
black skin, F241
black tourmaline, 617, *617f*
blackheads, F217, *F227f*, *F242t*, F322–23, 217–19, 487, *488f*
blanket wraps, **590**–91, **599**
blastocoel, **70**, **80**
blastoderm, **70**, **80**
blastula, **70**, **80**
bleach, F75
blemishes, *F214f*, F215, *F227f*, F232, *F242t*
blend electrolysis, F407
blending eye makeup, F475
blepharoplasty, **F463**, **F465**, 543, **713**, 715–17, *717f*, **730**
blepharospasm, **693**
blistering, *515f*
blood. *See also* circulatory system
bloodletting, 7
circulatory system and, **F114**–15, **F121**, F202
composition of, F115, 124–25, *124t*
contact with, F84
defined, **F114**, **F121**
disorders of, 125–26, 330–31, *331t*
face and, F115–16
formed elements of, **125**, *125t*, **136**
hands and, F116
head and, F115–16
neck and, F115–16
pressure, **127**, **135**
red cells, **F115**, **F125**
skin nourishment, F202
thinners, *F245t*
vessels, F114
white cells, **F115**, **F126**, **61**, **64**, **86**
bloodborne diseases, 48, 704
bloodborne pathogens, F68–**69**, **F88**, **33**, 37, **48**, **51**
Bloodborne Pathogens Standard, F68, F74, 21–23, 168
blood-brain barrier, **695**, **708**
bloodletting, 7
blue eyes, F484
blue lace agate, 619, *619f*
blue light, **F157**, F159, **F160**, F452
blue makeup, F482
blush, F474–75, F500
blush brushes, F479
BMI. *See* body mass index
board certified, **665**, **671**
bodies
emotional body, **606**–8, **626**
four types of, 605, *606t*
mental body, **605**–7, **626**
physical body, 605–8
spirit/energy body, 606–7, **626**
body contouring, 729
body dysmorphic disorder (BDD), **443**, **474**
body, facials for, 573, *573f–576f*
body fluid, contact with, F84
body hygiene, **F21**, **F32**, F337, 36–38
body masks, **F455**, F458, **F465**, **576**–77, **599**
body mass index (BMI), F171
body movement, types of, *107t*
body scrubs, **F455**, F458, **F465**, *573f–576f*
body systems, F97, *F98t*. *See also* anatomy
body wraps, **F455**, F458, **F465**
blanket wraps, **590**–91, **599**
cellophane, **590**, **599**
elastic, **578**, *579f*, **599**
essential oils and, 589–90, *589t*
herbal, **584**, *585f–588f*, *589f*, *589t*, **599**
Kneipp, **591**, **599**
materials for, 590, *590f*, *590t*
overview of, 566–67, *572f*, 576–78, *578f*
seaweed, **579**, *579f*, *580f–583f*, **599**
boils, **F217**, **F231**
bolsters, F304
bones. *See* skeletal system
bookkeepers, F584
booth rentals, F535, **F573–74**, **F598**
boron nitride, 536
Borrelia burgdorferi, F65
botanicals, **F262**, **F291**
aromatherapy and, 301–2, *302f*
chemistry of, 146–49
methods of extraction of, 284–86
as plant compounds, 283–84
for skin care, 146–49, 272–73, 286–89
Botox. *See* botulinum toxin

botulinum toxin
  defined, **F461**, **F465**
  dermal fillers and, 702, *702f*
  medical interventions and, **693**–96, *694f*, *695f*, *696f*, **708**
boundaries, with clients, F24, F27, F48, 13, 635, 665, 669
bovine collagen, **697**, *697f*, **708**
BP. *See* benzoyl peroxide
brachialis, **113**, **119**
brachii, **113**
brain, **F109**–10, **F121**
brain stem, **F109**, **F121**
branding, private, F10
Brazilian waxing, F437
  for men, 503
  for women, *494f*, 495, *495f*, *496f–500f*
break-even analysis, **752–53**, **762**
breast implants, **720**–21, *720f*, *721f*, 725, **730**
breast reconstruction, 724–27, *725f*, *726f*
breast reduction, 723–24, *724f*
breastbone, *F101f*, **F102**, **F125**
breast-lift, 721–23, *722f*, *723f*
breathing exercises, 13
bridal makeup, F510, *9f*
brighteners, F201, F263–64, F351
broad-spectrum antioxidants, 275
brochure, **774**–75, *775f*, **779**
bromhidrosis, **F217**, **F231**
bronchodilators, **333**, **344**
brow lift, F462, 713, 715–16
brown eyes, F484
brown makeup, F482
brows. *See* eyebrows
brush machines, F301
brushes, F310, F479–80
buccal nerve, **F112**, **F121**
buccinator muscles, **F105**, **F121**, *F367f*
buffering, **262**, 265, **279**
buffering agents, F447
building blocks of treatment, 351–52, *351f*
building clientele, F609–10
bullae, *F214f*, **F215**, **F231**
burns, F85–86, *F86f*
business plans, **F576**–77, **F598**, **749**–51, *750f*, **762**
businesses, skin care. *See also* selling
  action plans, F574–76
  booth rentals, F535, **F573–74**, **F598**
  business plans, **F576**–77, **F598**, **749**–51, *750f*, **762**
  front desks, F591–93
  government regulation of, F578
  leases, F581
  ownership options, F579–80
  personnel, **F588**–91, **F598**
  physical layout of, F586–88
  protecting against mishaps, F581–82
  public relations, F596, **F596**, **F598**, **772**, **779**
  purchasing established salons, F580–81
  record keeping, F584–86
  scheduling appointments, F46–47, F593–94
  strategies, F582–84
  telephone skills, F594–96
butterfly eye pads, F307

C

cacao seed, *287f*
cadherins, **73**, *74f*, **80**
caffeine, 193, 576
cake makeup, **F472**, **F524**
calcium, *F174t*, F180
calendula, **F270**, *F270t*, **F291**, 288
calming ingredients, F273, F350
calories, **F171**–72, **F184**
camouflage makeup, F12, F511, 542–46
camouflage therapy, F12, F511, 542–46
camphor, 576
cancers, skin, F156, F223–24, 213–16, *215f*
Candida albicans, F70
caninus muscles, **F105**, **F123**, *F367f*
cape chamomile, 295, *295f*, 302
capes, F499
capillaries, **F114**, **F122**, F338, 130
capillary bed, *130f*
capital, **F579**, **F598**, **751**, **762**
carbohydrates, **F168**–70, **F184**, 143–44
carbolic acid, F447
carbomers, **F260**, **F291**, 260, 263, 277–78
carbon, chemistry of, 142
carboxylic acid, **149**, **153**
carbuncles, **F217**, **F231**
cardiac fibers, **105**, **119**
cardiac muscles, **F103**, **F122**, **105**, *106f*
cardiovascular system. *See also* circulatory system
  arterial system, 128–30, *129f*
  defined, **124**, **135**
  heart anatomy, **F113**–14, **F123**, 127–28, *127f*
  heart disease, 41, **128**, *128t*, 331–33, *332t*
  heart irregularities, *F245t*
  jugular veins, F116
  varicose veins, 131–**32**, *134f*, **136**
  veins, **F114**, **F126**
  venous system, 130–31, *131f*
careers
  columnist, 10
  compensation, F561–64
  continuing education, F316, F566–67
  cosmetics buyers, F13, 10
  cruise ship estheticians, 9
  employment applications, F549–52, *F550f–552f*
  instructors, of esthetics, 9
  interviews, F542–49, *F545f–547f*
  on the job, F553–57
  job descriptions, **F557**–60, *F559f–560f*, **F569**, **F588**, **F598**
  licensure tests, F529–33
  money management, F564–65, F582
  networking, **F544**, **F569**
  permanent makeup artists, **9**
  planning success, F567–68
  preparing for, F533–35
  resumes, **F535**–39, *F537f*, **F569**
  role models, F21, F566, **F566**, **F569**
  searching for, F540–42
  types of, F10–16
caring attitude, 36–37
carnelian, 617, *617f*
carotenoids, **148**, *148t*, **153**
carpus, **F102**, **F122**
carrier oils, 299–301
carrot, **F270**, *F270t*, **F291**
carts, F301, F305, F412–13
cascade of inflammation, F281, 203–4, *203f*, 274
cash flow statement, **752**, **762**
catabolism, **F97**, **F122**, **189**
catagen stage, **F403**, **F441**
catalyst, **143**, **153**
cataphoresis, **F152**, **F160**, **F388**, *F389t*, **F396**
catechins, **275**, **279**
catenins, **73**, **80**
cathodes, **F151**, **F160**
cautery, **705**, **708**
Cayce, Edgar, 613
CD. *See* cluster of differentiation
CDC. *See* Centers for Disease Control and Prevention
CdK. *See* cyclin-dependent kinase
cedarwood, 295, *295f*
cell cycle, *61f*, **69**–70, **80**
cell mitosis, **F197**, **F208**
cell renewal factor (CRF), F196, **F446**–47, **F465**
cell wall, **73**, **80**
cell-mediated immune system, **72**–73, **80**
cellophane body wrap, **590**, **599**
cells
  aging and, 69
  anatomy of, F95–97
  B cells, 65, **72**–73, **80**
  bonds, 73
  collagen and, 63, **66**–69, *67t*, *68f*
  construction of, F95–96
  cosmetic ingredients for cell metabolism, F264–65
  cycle, *61f*, **69**–70, **80**
  cytotoxic T cells, **73**, **81**
  daughter cells, **60**, **81**
  defined, **F95**, **F122**
  in dermis, 63–65
  DNA and, **69**
  function and histology of, 57–59
  health of, F202–3
  histology, of cell cyle, **69**–70, **81**
  hyaluronic acid and, **67**, *69f*, **83**
  hydroquinone and, 62
  intercellular space and, *68f*
  lysosomes in, **59**
  membrane of, **F96**, **F122**, **57**–58, **80**, 85–86
  metabolism of, **F97**, **F124**, F264–65, **146**, **154**, **189**–90, **329**, 410
  mitochondria of, **58**, 59, **84**
  nerve, F110
  nuclear membrane of, **59**, **85**
  nucleolus of, **59**, **85**
  nucleus of, **59**, *59f*, **85**
  organelles, 58–59, **85**
  plasma and, **72**
  receptor site of, **58**, *58f*, **86**, 89
  red blood cells, **F115**, **F125**
  regenerative properties of, 292
  repair cycle of, *61f*
  replacement of, F203
  reproduction and division of, F96–97
  ribosomes in, **58**, **86**
  structure of, *57f*
  vacuoles in, **59**, **86**
  walls, **73**
  white blood cells, **F115**, **F126**, **61**, **64**, **86**
cellular differentiation, **57**, 60, *65f*, 66
cellular membrane, **F96**, **F122**, **57**–58, **80**, 85–86
cellulite, F455, **F458**, **F465**, 175, 566, 728–29
cellulitis, **454**, **474**
Centers for Disease Control and Prevention (CDC), 21, 26, 30, 41, 559
central nervous system (CNS), **F107**, *F108f*, **F122**
central serous retinopathy, **341**, **344**
ceramides, **F203**, **F208**, **F268**, *F268t*, **F291**, **75**, **80**, 261
cerebellum, **F109**, **F122**
cerebral cortex, F109
cerebrospinal system, **F107**, *F108f*, **F122**
cerebrum, **F109**, **F122**

certificates, F25
certified colors, **F262**, **F291**, 263
cervical cutaneous nerve, **F112**, **F122**
cervical dystonia, **693**, **708**
cervical nerves, **F112**, **F122**
cervical vertebrae, **F101**, **F122**
chain of infection, 28–29
Chakras, **657**
  defined, **625**
  energy management and, 604, **608**, *609f*, *610t–611t*
  healing stones and, 613–20, *614t*, *616t*
chalazia, **230**, **233**
chamomile, **F270**, *F270t*, **F291**, 285, 291, 295, *295t*, 302
charts, for clients, F246–47, *F247f*
checklists
  ABCDE Cancer Checklist, F224
  for facials, F318, *F319f*
  for interviews, *F545f–546f*
  for resumes, F536–38
  for room-cleaning, 49
  for sanitation after facials, F337–39
  for skin analysis, *F248t*, *F319f*
cheek makeup, F484
chelating agents, F261–**62**, **F291**, 262
chemical action, of AHAs, 316–17
chemical changes, **F133**, **F141**
chemical compounds, **F133**, **F141**
chemical exfoliation, **F279**–80, **F291**, 270
chemical peels. *See* peels
chemical properties, **F133**, **F141**
chemical reactions, F135–36, **142**, **153**
chemical sunscreens, F266
chemical terms, for estheticians, 145–46
chemicals, in skin and body
  carbohydrates, **F168**–70, **F184**, 143–44
  lipids, **F170**–72, **F185**, **F192**–93, **F195**, F203, **F208**, **F263**, **F292**, 144
  pH values and, 144–45, *145f*, 272
  polymers and, **F264**, **F292**, **143**, 254
  proteins, **F167**–68, **F185**, **57**–59, **61**, **85**, **143**–45
chemistry
  biochemistry, **143**, **153**
  botanical, 146–49
  of carbon, 142
  of chlorine, 142
  of cosmetics, F136–40, *252f*, 264
  defined, **F130**, **F141**
  equations, **143**, **153**
  of essential oils, 150–52, *150t–151t*, 292, *292t–293t*
  estheticians and, 139
  of galvanic current, 139, 145
  of hydrogen, 140
  matter and, F130–34
  overview of, F130
  of oxygen, 140
  of potential hydrogen, F134–35
  principles of, 139–42
  reactions, F135–36, **142**, **153**
  of sodium, *F175t*, F181, 142
chest
  skeletal system and, F102
  waxing of, 503
chewing, F104
chi, F366, 242–43
chin
  acne on, 97, *97f*, 222, *222f*
  double, F488
  implants, 718–19, *719f*
  long heavy, F488
  receding, F488
  waxing, F430
Chinese esthetics, F6
Chinese medicine, 242–44, 402
Chinese skin analysis method, F248
chin/neck bra, **743**, **744**
chloasma, **F221**, **F231**, 211, *211f*
chlorine, chemistry of, 142
chloroprene, 34
chocolate, and acne, F182
cholesterol, F171, **75**, **81**
choline, *F173t*
chondroitin sulfate, **67**, **81**
chromium, *F174t*, F181
chromophore, **161**, **182**, **503**–4, **517**
chronic, **24**, **51**
chronic hepatitis, 24–25, **51**
chronic stress, *192f*, **197**, **199**
chucking, F363, *F364f*
chymotryptic enzyme (SCCE), 75
CIDESCO International, 14
cilia, **F65**, **F88**
circles under eyes, 317, 542–45, 550, *717f*
circuit breakers, **F149**, **F160**
circuits, complete, **F146**, *F147f*, **F160**
circulatory system
  anatomy of, F113–16
  arms, F116
  blood, **F114**–15, **F121**, F202
  defined, **F113**, **F122**, 130–34, *133f*
  heart, **F113**–14, **F123**, 127–28, *127f*
circumareolar, **722**, **730**
citric acid cycle, 59, 271
citrine, 618, *618f*
classic forehead-lift, **714**, **730**
clavicle, *F101f*, **F102**, **F122**
clay masks, **F281**–82, **F291**, F354
clays, *577t*, 578
cleanliness, F21, F32, F86–87, F337, 22. *See also* sanitation
cleansers, **F260**, F276–77, **F291**
  for combination skin, 93, *93f*, 308–10
  for dry skin, 308–11
  emulsion, 264–66
  foaming, F277, F354, 265, 308-9, 319–20
  lotion, *265f*, 268, *308f*
  medicated, for acne, *F229t*, 309
  milk, 308–10
  for oily skin, 308–10
  rinsable, 308–11, 320
  skin care products and, F276–77
cleansing, F320–21
  deep pore cleansing, F322–23
  facials, F320–21, F328–29
  massage, F366
  products for, F273, F277, F306–7, F328–29
clean-up. *See also* sanitation
  agents for, 38–39, 264–66
  detergents for, 37–38
  end-of-day treatment room, F310
  equipment, 37–38
  after facials, F344
  post facial, F344
  systematically, 48
  ultrasonic technology for, 38, 42
  verifying the process, 39
  water for, 38
  waxing, F419
cleavage, **70**, **81**
cleaving, **697**, **708**
client consultations
  concluding service, F45
  consultation area, F42–43
  defined, **F39**, **F53**
  before exfoliation, 377
  for eyelash extensions, 521
  for facials, F318–20, F338
  forms for, *F247f*, *F416f*
  hair removal, F416–17
  intake forms, F39–40, **F577**, F606, **F606**, **F616**
  before LASER treatment, 507–8, *508f*
  makeup, F494–98
  male issues in, F354
  overview of, F41–42
  preparing for, F42
  skin analysis, F246–47, *F247f*, F248–50, *F248t*, *F319f*, 440
  10-step method, F43–45
  for waxing, F418
clients
  assessment forms for, *F416f*
  boundaries with, F24, F27, F48, 13, 635, 665, 669
  building clientele, F609–10
  charts for, F246–47, *F247f*
  communication with, F41–45, F607
  confidentiality of, F24, F42, F248, 566–67, *566f*
  difficult, F48
  educating, F607–8
  greeting, F39, F317, 12
  health screening of, F182, F246–47, 567, *568f–569f*
  home-care by, *F287t*, 307, *307f*, 514
  information interviews with, **F542**–43, **F569**, F606–7
  makeup charts for, *F497t*
  medications of, 326, 443
  meeting, F39, F317
  new, F39
  preparation procedures, 570–71, *571f*
  questionnaires on makeup for, **F496**, *F496t*, **F577**, **F606**, **F616**
  reactions of, to treatments, 361
  record keeping for, F586, **F606**–7, **F616**
  referrals, F611–12
  release forms for, F246, *F417f*
  retaining, F610–12
  safety of, *F557f*
  self-image of, 10
  service records for, F586, **F606**–7, **F616**
  tardy, F45–46
  unhappy, F47–48
clindamycin, *F229t*
clinic exfoliation treatments, 362–81
clinical estheticians, F464
clinical inflammation, **203**, **233**
clips, for hair, F499
clogged resistive skin treatments, 352
closed comedones, F217, *F227f*, *F242t*, F323, **219**, *219f*, 225, **233**
closed rhinoplasty, **718**, **730**
close-set eyes, F490, F492
closing consultations, **F612**, **F616**
closing sales, F612–15
clotting factors, **124**, **135**
cluster of differentiation (CD), **73**, **81**
CNS. *See* central nervous system
CNs. *See* cranial nerves
cobalamine, *F173t*, F179
cocci, **F63**, **F89**
cocoa, 287, *578f*
cocoa butter, *F270t*
coconut, *F270t*
codes of ethics, **F25**–28, **F32**, 10, 667, 773
coenzyme Q10, **F265**, **F291**
co-enzymes, 146–**47**, **153**

coherent light, **160**, *160f*, **182**
cold sores, **F225**, **F231**
collagen, **F197**–98, **F208**, **F265**, *F268t*, **F291**, F462
  autologous, **698**, **708**
  bovine, **697**, *697f*, **708**
  cells and, 63, **66**–**69**, *67t*, *68f*
  as cosmetic ingredient, 268, 271, 276, 578
  dry collagen sheets, 358, 383, *384f*
  remodeling, **206**, *206f*, **234**, **735**, **744**
  sheet masks, F281, 383, *383f*, *384f*
  shrinkage of, **735**, **744**
  stimulants, F265
  wet collagen eye pads, *383f*
  wet collagen sheets, 358, 383, *383f*
collagenase, **274**, **279**
collarbone, *F101f*, **F102**, **F122**
collateral circulation, **129**, **135**
collimated light, **160**, *160f*, 162
colon, *F165f*
color. *See also* makeup
  agents, F262, 263–64, *263f*
  base colors, F476
  certified colors, **F262**, **F291**, 263
  colorants, F262, **F265**, **F291**
  complementary colors, **F481**, **F524**
  contour colors, F476, F500
  cool colors, *F481f*, **F482**, **F524**
  cosmetics, 251, 535
  exempt colors, F262
  eyebrows, F477
  FDA and, F262, **F262**, **F291**, 263
  hair, F485
  highlights, F476
  lips, F478
  non-certified, **F262**, **F292**
  permanent, for lips, 557, *558f*
  primary colors, **F480**, **F524**
  skin, F200–201, F483–84
  temperatures, F482
  tertiary colors, **F480**, *F481f*, **F524**
  theory of, F480–82
  warm colors, **F481**, **F524**
  wheel, *F480f*, 615, *615f*
colorants, F262, **F265**, **F291**
columnist, 10
comb electrodes, *F392t*
combination skin, F238
  cleansers for, 93, *93f*, 308–10
  toners for, 311, 313
combining form, **676**, **687**
combining vowel, **676**, *677t*, **687**
combustion, **F136**, **F142**
comedogenic products, **F228**, **F231**, F352
comedogenicity, **F259**, **F291**, 255
comedone extractors, F322
comedones, **F217**, F226, *F227f*, **F231**, *F242t*, F322–23, 93, 217, **219**–21, *219f*, 225, **233**
comfrey, *F270t*, 284, 285, 287, *287f*
commission, **F561**, F562, **F569**
common carotid arteries, **F115**, **F122**
communicable diseases, *F64t*, **F66**–67, **F89**, F225
communication
  basics of, F38–41
  with clients, F41–45, F607
  with coworkers, F49–50
  defined, **F38**, **F53**
  during employee evaluation, F52–53, F560–61
  with employees, *F589f*
  human relations, F36–38
  with managers, F50–52
  in salons, F49–53, F560–61
  skills, F24
  special issues in, F45–49
compensation, F561–64
  for employees, 754–55
competency, F553
competition, F575–76
complaints, 13
complement system, in immune system, **73**, **81**
complementary, **615**, **625**
complementary colors, **F481**, **F524**
complementary foods, **F168**, **F184**
complete circuits, **F146**, *F147f*, **F160**
complications
  defined, **701**, **708**
  dermal fillers and, 701–2
  LASER treatments and, 515–16, *516t*
  management of, 472–73, *473t*
compound molecules, **F132**, **F142**
compounding pharmacies, F10
compresses, F306–7
concealer brushes, F479
concealers, **F473**, F500, **F524**, 542–46, *542f*, *544f*, *545f*, 550
conduct, professional, F23–25
conduction, **410**, **434**
conductors, **F146**, **F160**
coneflower, *F270t*, F291
confidence, building, F27
confidentiality, of clients, F24, F42, F248, 566–67, *566f*
congenital leukoderma, **F221**, **F230**
conjunctiva, **716**, **730**
connective tissue, **F97**, **F122**, **72**, **81**
connexins, **74**, **81**
consent forms, F40–41
constructive criticism, F51
consultations. *See* client consultations
consultative selling, **F602**–3, **F616**
Consumer Product Safety Commission (CPSC), 778
consumption supplies, **F585**, **F598**
contact dermatitis, F218, **F218**, **F231**
contagious, 25, **51**
contagious diseases, *F64t*, F66–67, **F89**, F225
contaminants, *F64t*, **F73**, **F89**
contaminate, **51**
contaminated, **F73**, **F89**, 23–24, 28, **29**–**30**, **51**
contamination, versus infection, 26
continuing education, F316, F566–67
contour colors, F476, F500
contract workers, 21
contraindications
  defined, **F237**, **F251**
  for electrodessication, 466
  for electrotherapy, F378
  for essential oils, 150–52, 294–95
  for facial massage, F362
  for facials, *F319f*
  for hair removal, F415–16, *479f*
  IPL treatments and, 443–48
  for LASER treatments, *506t*
  for LED treatments, 449
  for lymphatic massage, 417–18
  for massage, F362, 393
  for medical peels, 707
  for microcurrent facial toning, 469–70
  for microdermabrasion, 454
  overview of, F154, F246
  for peels, F448
  for sensitive skin or redness, F350, 357–58
  for shirodhara, 649
  for skin treatments, F245–46
  for spa therapy, 567
  for stone treatments, 411
  for threading, *481f*
  for waxing, *479f*
control group, **668**, **671**
converters, **F148**, **F160**
cool colors, *F481f*, **F482**, **F524**
cooling device, on LASER, *164f*
cooperation, F555, F583
coping mechanisms, F25
copper, *F174t*, F181, 275
copywriters, F13
corium, **78**, **81**
corneocytes, F196, **60**, 75–76, *76f*, **81**
corneo-desmosomes, 75
cornified, **75**, **81**
cornified envelope, **75**, **81**
corporations, **F579**–80, **F598**
corpus luteum, **94**, **101**
corpuscles of Ruffini, **78**, **81**
corrective makeup
  eyebrows, F491
  for eyes, F489–91
  jawline and neck, F487–89
  lips, F491–94
  overview of, F487
  skin tones, *F483t*, F494
corrugator muscles, **F104**, *F105f*, **F122**, *F367f*
corticosteroids, 341, *342t*
cortisol, **197**, **199**
cosmeceuticals, **F256**, **F291**, 253, 278
cosmetic claim, 253
cosmetic dermatology, **665**, **671**
cosmetic plastic surgeon, **665**, **671**
cosmetic surgery, **F462**–63, **F465**. *See also* plastic surgery
cosmetic tattooing. *See* tattooing
cosmetics. *See also* ingredients, of cosmetics; makeup
  acne and, F228, 226
  buyers of, F13, 10
  chemistry as applied to, F136–40, *252f*, 264
  color cosmetics, 251, 535
  defined, **F255**, **F291**
  detergents for, 76, 257–59, 264
  FDA and, 668
  hormones, F10
  lightening treatment gels, 317
  origin of word, F5
  pH values and, 144–45, *145f*, 272
  representatives, in department stores, 9
cosmetology, F5, 5, 252, 277
Cosmoderm, 698–700
Cosmoplast, 698–700
costs of goods sold, **752**, **762**
cotton compresses, for facials, F340–41
cotton swabs, F322, F499
couperose skin, F206, F219, F242, F251, 212–13, **227**, **233**
cover letters, F539
coverage, by insurance, F578, F581, **754**, **762**
coworkers, communication with, F48–50
CPSC. *See* Consumer Product Safety Commission
cranberries, 287–88, *287f*
cranial nerve V, *118f*
cranial nerve VII, *118f*
cranial nerves (CNs), F110–13, F122–23, F125, 117–18, *117f*
cranium, **F100**–101, **F122**
creams
  day, 312–14
  exfoliants, 380–81
  for eyes, F283–84, 317

foundations, F472
for healing, F352
for masks, F281
for massage, F285, F367
for neck, 318
night, 314–15
nourishing, F284–85
for skin, *312f*
specialty, 316–18
for treatments, F284–85
cream-to-powder foundations, F472
credentials, of estheticians, 663–64
credibility, F27
CRF. *See* cell renewal factor
critical-thinking skills, 10–11, *11f*
cross-contamination, **F78**–79, **F89**, 30, 36, 49, 261, 477
cross-linking, 206, **213**, **233**, **275**, **279**
crow's feet, *698f*, *699f*
cruise ships
companies for, F13, *9f*
estheticians for, 9
crusts, **F215**, *F216f*, **F231**
cryogen, **163**, **182**
cryosurgery, 216
cryotherapy, **214**, 217, **233**
crystals, **614**, **626**
cucumber, *F270t*, *F273t*
Cushing's syndrome, 100, **341**, **344**
custom-designed masks, F283
customer relations, F583–84
customer relationship management, **770**, *770f*, **779**
customer value, 768–69, *770f*
customization, F9
cutaneous, **63**, **81**
cycle, **59**, **81**
cyclin-dependent kinase (CdK), **69**, **81**
cyclins, **69**, **81**
cylindrical, **130**
cystic acne, F227
cysts, **F215**, F227, **F231**, *F242t*, 220, 221
cytochromes, **180**, **182**
cytokines, **61**, 64, 70, **81**, **203**, **233**
cytokinin, **81**
cytophylactic properties, 292
cytoplasm, **F96**, **F122**, **57**, *68f*, **81**
cytoskeleton, **60**, *61f*, **81**
cytotoxic T cells, **73**, **81**

D

daily records, F584–85
damage, from sun, F204–5, 209, 211–12, **440**, **474**
dash method, 549–50, 554
daughter cells, **60**, **81**
day creams and treatments, 312–14
Day Spa Association, 14
day spa estheticians, F10–11
Day Spa Magazine, 14
day spas, F533, F542, 565
DC. *See* direct current
decontaminating equipment, 37
decontamination, **F70**–72, **F89**, **22**, **29**–30, **51**
dedifferentiation, 66
deductive reasoning, **F530**, **F569**
deep breathing, F25
deep exfoliation. *See* superficial peels
deep peels, F446–47
deep pore cleansing, F322–23
deep-set eyes, F490
defatting agents, **264**, **279**
defecation, **F119**, **F122**
dehydrated skin, treatment of, 352
dehydration, F183, **F238**, *F242t*, **F251**. *See also* water
deionization, **253**, **279**
delivery systems, for cosmetic ingredients, **F264**, **F291**
deltoid muscle, **F106**, *F107f*, **F122**, **112**
demodex folliculorum, **228**, **233**
demographics, **F575**, **F598**
dendrites, **F110**, **F122**, **62**, 72, **81**
dendritic cell, **62**–63, **81**
deoxygenated, **124**, **135**
deoxyribonucleic acid (DNA), **F96**–97, **F122**, **F167**, **F185**, 59, **69**, **81**, 142
department store, cosmetics representatives in, 9
dependability, F555
depilation, F408, **F409**, **F441**
depilatories, **F409**, **F441**
depression, **119**, **335**, **344**
depression, scapular, **112**
depressor labii inferioris muscles, **F105**, **F122**, *F367f*
dermabrasion, **F463**, **F465**
dermal fillers, **F461**–62, **F465**
botulinum toxin and, 702, *702f*
complications and, 701–2
hyaluronic acid and, 692, 697, **700**–701, *700t*, *703f*, **708**
medical interventions and, 696–702, *696f*, *698f*, *700f*, *702f*
dermal papillae, **F197**, **F208**
dermal scattering, **512**, **517**
Dermascope Magazine, 14
dermatan sulfate, **67**, **81**
dermatitis, **F218**, **F231**
dermatitis venenata, **F218**, **F231**
dermatoheliosis, **212**, **233**
dermatological surgeon, **665**, **671**
dermatologists, *F11f*, **F213**, **F231**, 9, **665**, **671**
dermatology, **F213**, **F231**
dermatophytes, **F70**, **F89**
dermis
cells in, 63–65
defined, **F208**, **60**, **81**
papillary layer of, **F197**, **F208**
reticular layer of, **F197**–98
subcutaneous layer of, **F198**–99, **F209**
DermLite®, 241, *241f*
desincrustation
defined, **F152**, **F160**, **F351**, **F357**, **F385**, **F396**
electrodes for, F386
galvanic current and, F385–86
overview of, F386–88
procedure for, F322
desmocollins, **74**, *74f*, **81**
desmogleins, **74**, **81**
desmoplakin, **74**, **81**
desmosomes, F196–**97**, **F208**, *65f*, **66**, 73–74, *74f*, **81**
desquamation, F196, F446, 75
destination spas, F535, F542, 565
detergents, **F259**–60, **F291**
for clean-up, 37–38
for cosmetic use, 76, 257–59, 264
enzymatic, 38
detoxifying treatments, F457
development, of products, 318–20
deviated nasal septum, **717**, **730**
device classification, FDA and, 440
DHA (dihydroxyacetone), F285
dhatus, **657**
DHT. *See* dihydrotestosterone
diabetes, *F245t*, **91**, **101**, 337, 442, 704
diagnosing medical conditions, F213
diagnosis, *F64t*
diamond face shape, F486
diamond microdermabrasion, 453–54, *454f*
diaphoretic, **584**, **599**
diaphragm, **F119**, **F122**
diastole, **127**, **135**
diatomic molecule, 140
dictionaries, of cosmetic ingredients, F273
diencephalon, **F109**, **F122**
diet. *See* nutrition
dietitians, F165
differentiation
cellular, **57**, 60, *65f*, 66
cluster of, **73**, **81**
Differin, *F229t*, *F245t*
difficult clients, F36, F48
digestion, **F119**, **F122**
digestive enzymes, **F118**, **F122**
digestive system
defined, **F118**–19, **F122**
and food consumption, *F165f*
overview of, F118–19
digital nerve, *F112f*, **F113**, **F122**
dihydrotestosterone (DHT), **222**, **233**
dihydroxyacetone (DHA), F285
dilution amount, **300**, **303**
dimethylaminoethanol (DMAE), **F275**, **F291**
diminutive, **683**, *683t*, **687**
diopters, F378
diplococci, **F63**, *F64f*, **F89**
diplomacy, F23
direct contact, 28, 40
direct current (DC), **F148**, **F160**
direct high-frequency application, F154
direct mail, *F609f*, 771, *772f*
direct marketing, **772**, 774, **779**
disaccharides, **F169**, **F185**, **144**
discretion, F24
diseases, *F64t*
disinfectants
bactericidal, **F62**, F74, **F88**
choosing, F74
defined, **F61**, **F73**, **F89**
FDA and, **41**, 50
fungicidal, **F62**, F74, **F89**
government regulation of, F61
hospital grade, F61
log, F308
overview of, **40**–42, **51**
prevention of infection and, F74–77
pseudomonacidal, **F74**, **F89**
safety guidelines for, F75–77
sanitation and, F415
toxicity in, 41
tuberculocidal, **F61**, F74, **F90**
types of, F74–75
virucidal, **F62**, F74, **F90**
disinfection, F71, **F72**–73, **F89**
autoclaves and, 47
defined, **28**, **51**
hair removal and, 477–78
infection control and, 28–32, 37–41, 47–49
disorders and diseases. *See also* acne; autoimmune disorders; rosacea; *other specific conditions*
of blood, 125–26, 330–31, *331t*
bloodborne diseases, 48, 704
body dysmorphic disorder (BDD), **443**, **474**
cancers, skin, F156, F223–24, 213–16, *215f*
contagious diseases, *F64t*, F66–67, **F89**, F225
dermatitis, **F218**, **F231**

disorders and diseases *(continued)*
gastrointestinal disorders, 333–35, *334t*
generalized anxiety disorder (GAD), **336**, **344**
of heart, 41, **128**, *128t*, 331–33, *332t*
hypertrophies, **F221**–22, **F231**
inflammations of skin, F218–20
from LASER treatments, 210
lesions, **F214**–16, **F231**, **F232**
lung disorders, 333, *333t*
medical referrals for, 204, 210, 212, 216, 232
mental disorders, 335–37, *335t*
non-cancerous growths, 216–18
obsessive-compulsive disorder (OCD), **336**, **344**
photoaging, *F243f*, 212–13, 367–68, *368f*
pigmentation, F221, F378–80
post-traumatic stress disorder (PTSD), **336**, **345**
psoriasis, **F219**, **F232**
sebaceous hyperplasias, **F217**, **F232**, *F242t*
of skeletal system, 340–41, *341t*
sudoriferous glands, **F194**, *F195f*, *F201f*, **F202**, **F209**, F217–18
sun damage, F204–5, 209, 211–12, **440**, **474**
wound healing, 204–10, *205f*, *206f*, *208f*, *209f*
dispensaries, **F302**, **F311**
dispersing electrode, **178**, **182**
disposables, F79, F310
applicators, *F498f*
asepsis and, 29
extractions and, F310
eye shields, *168f*
disposal, of infected material, 48
distillation, **254**, **279**, **290**, *290f*, **303**
di-tocopherol, **290**, **303**
division, cellular, **F197**, **F208**
DMAE. *See* dimethylaminoethanol
DNA. *See* deoxyribonucleic acid
documentation, F461
dorsum, **719**, **730**
doshas, of Ayurveda
Kapha, **632**, 636–37, **656**
overview of, **631**–33, *632f*, *634t*, **656**
Pitta, **632**, 635–36, **656**
Vata, **631**, 633–35, **656**
dot method, 549, *549f*
double chin, F488
dowager hump, **340**, **344**
Dr. Jacquet movement, **F365**, **F374**
drainage, of lymphatic system, **133**, *134t*, **136**, 420, *420f*, *431f–433f*
draping hair, F320
dressing for success, F22
drinking cures, of water, 7
drooping eyes, F491
drooping lip corners, F493
drugs
antianxiety, **328**, **343**
antiulcer, **334**, **344**
categories of, 328–42, *329t*
claims about, **253**, **279**
defined, **252**, **279**
FDA approval of, 326–27, 693–94
FDA definition of, F256
hormones and, 329–30, *330t*
illegal, F204
oral prescription, *327f*
pain and, 341–42, *342t*
prescription, 327–28, *327f*, *328f*
scope of practice, for estheticians, and, 331, 342
topical prescription, *328f*, 444
viruses and, 338–40, *339t*
dry brushing, *579f*
dry collagen sheets, 358, 383, *384f*
dry skin, F237–38, F345–46
cleansers for, 308–11
facials for, F345–46
masks for, 318
moisturizing products for, F263, **F284**–85, **F292**, F324, 270
toners for, 267–68, 312
duct glands, **F117**, **F123**
ductless glands, **F117**, **F122**
dynamic movement, **693**, **708**
dyschromias, F220, **441**, **474**, **704**–5, **708**
dysmorphic, **344**
dysphagia, **696**, **708**
dysplastic, **216**, **233**
dystonia, **693**, **708**

E

E. coli, 26
ears
muscles of, F103–4
reflexology of, 408–9, *408f–409f*
waxing of, 503
eccrine glands, **F202**, **F208**
echinacea, **F270**, *F270t*, **F291**
ECM. *See* extracellular matrix
ectoderm, **70**–72, **81**
ectoparasites, F69
eczema, **F218**, **F231**
edema, **F218**, **F231**
aperipheral, **131**–32
peripheral, **136**
editors, esthetics, F13
educating clients, F607–8
education opportunities, 8–10, *8f*
educators, F13–14
efferent nerves, **F110**, **F124**, F200
efferent neuron, **77**, **81**
efferent peripheral system, F108
efficacy, **F74**, **F89**
effleurage, **F363**, **F374**
EGF. *See* epidermal growth factor
eggs, *F273t*
Egypt, ancient, 675
Egyptian esthetics, F5
eighth cranial nerve (CN VIII), *F111f*
EIN. *See* Employer Identification Number
Einstein, Albert, 604
elastase, **274**, **279**
elastic body wraps, **578**, *579f*, **599**
elasticity, *369f*
elastin, **F197**, **F208**, 67, 268, 578
elaunin, **67**, **82**
electric blankets, F302
electric current, **F146**, F148, **F160**
electric heat masks, F395
electric mitts and boots, F394
electricity
defined, **F146**, **F160**
electrical equipment safety and, F78, F149–51
electrotherapy, F151–54
light, F154–59
measurements, F148–49
types of electric current, **F146**, F148, **F160**
electrocautery, **716**, **730**
electrodes
active, **F151**, **F160**
comb, *F392t*
defined, **F151**, **F160**
for desincrustation, F386
glass tip, *F392t*
high-frequency machine, F391, *F392t*
inactive, **F151**, **F160**
indirect, *F392t*
large mushroom, *F392t*
rake, *F392t*
small mushroom, *F392t*
sparking, *F392t*
spiral, *F392t*
electrodessication
benefits of, 466
contraindications for, 466
defined, **465**, **474**
devices for, *465f*
treatments using, *466f–468f*
electrolysis
blend, F407
defined, **F406**, **F441**
galvanic, F407
government regulation of, F407
hair removal and, F406–7
high-frequency machine, F390
hirsutism and, 100
thermolysis, F407
electrolytes, **124**, **135**
electromagnetic radiation, **F155**, **F160**
electromagnetic spectrum (EM), physics of, 158–60, **159**, *159f*, **182**
electronic tweezers, F410
electrosurgery, 216
electrotherapy, **F151**–54, **F160**, **F378**, **F396**
elemental molecules, **F131**–32, **F142**
elements, **F131**, *F131f*, **F142**, **140**, *141f*, **154**
elements, five traditional
Ayurveda and, 632
traditional Chinese medicine and, 243–44
eleventh cranial nerve (CN XI), *F111f*, **F112**–13, **F122**
EM. *See* electromagnetic spectrum
embryo, **70**, **82**
embryology, **70**–71, **82**
emergencies, 48
emollients
and comedogenicity, F259, 255
defined, **F257**, **F291**
emulsions and, 260, 266
as functional ingredients, F257–59, 254–57
oils, F258–59
as performance ingredients, 264, 269–70, *269f*, 272
sunscreen and, 254
emotional body, **606**–8, **626**
emotional stability, F23
emotions, negative, 13
employees
communication with, *F589f*
compensation for, 754–55
evaluations of, F52–53, F560–61
manual for, **F588**, **F598**
Employer Identification Number (EIN), **756**, **762**
employment. *See* careers
employment applications, F549–52, *F550f–552f*
emulsifiers, **F260**, *F261f*, **F291**, **301**, **303**, *315f*
emulsions
cleansers, 264–66
defined, **F138**, **F142**
emollients and, 260, 266
gellants and, 263
oil-in-water, *F137f*, **F138**–39, **F142**, F228, 259–60, 266, 270
overview of, F136, F138
physical, **259**, **280**
water-based, 315, *315f*

water-in-oil, *F137f*, F138–40, **F139**, **F142**, F228, 259–60, 270
end-bulbs of Krause, **78**, **82**
endermology, **F457**, **F465**
endocrine glands, **F117**, **F122**, **89**, **101**
endocrine system, **F117**–18, **F122**, *90f*, **291**, **303**
endoderm, **70**–72, **82**
end-of-day treatment room clean-up, F310
endometrium, **94**, *94f*, **101**
endomysium, **106**, **119**
endonasal, **718**, **730**
endoparasites, F69
endoplasmic reticulum (ER), **58**, **82**
endoscopic, **714**, **730**
endospores, 49
energy. *See also* radio-frequency energy
 Ayurveda and, 242, 630–31
 basics of, 604–5
 Chakras and, 604, **608**, *609f*, *610t–611t*
 devices, 158
 fluence, **162**–63, **182**, **512**–13, **517**
 management of, **605**, *606f*, **626**
 medicines for, 612
 nutrients for, **189**, *190f*, **199**
 radiant, **163**, **183**
 rejuvenation procedures for energy balancing, 620, *621f–625f*
 spirit/energy body, 606–**7**, **626**
 treatments, 620, *621f–625f*
engineering controls, 22, **51**
enlarged pores, *F242t*
entertainment industry, F12
entrepreneurship. *See* businesses, skin care
environment, F203–4
environmental factors, acne and, 224–25
Environmental Protection Agency (EPA), F61, 34, 39, **41**, 48, **51**
enzymatic detergents, 38
enzymes
 chymotryptic, 75
 as cosmetic ingredients, 271
 defined, **F172**, **F185**, **147**, **153**
 digestive, **F118**, **F122**
 exfoliation, F263
 as macronutrients, F172
 for peels, **F280**, **F291**, 367
 proteolytic, **271**, **280**
eosinophils, **64**, **82**, 125, **135**
EPA. *See* Environmental Protection Agency
epicardium, **126**, **136**
epicranius, **F103**, *F104f*, **F122**
epidermal growth factor (EGF), **61**, **82**
epidermal separation, *210f*
epidermis
 brick-and-mortar concept, F193
 defined, **F195**, **F208**, **60**, *60f*, **82**
 overview of, **F195**–96
 stratum corneum, **F196**, **F208**, *61f*, **65**–66, 75–76, *76f*, 352
 stratum germinativum, F197, **F208**
 stratum granulosum, F196, **F208**
 stratum lucidum, F196, **F209**
 stratum spinosum, F196–97, **F209**
epidermolysis bullosa, **66**, **82**
epilation, **F408**–10, F414, **F441**
epilepsy, *F245t*, **336**, **344**, 441
epimysium, **119**
epithelial tissue, **F97**, **F122**, **72**, **82**
epithelium, **72**, **82**
Equal Employment Opportunity Commission, F549
equations, chemical, **143**, **153**
equipment
 for clean-up, 37–38
 for decontamination, 37
 estheticians and, 437–40, *438f*
 financing of, 439
 insurability of, 439
 options for, 438–39
 personal protective equipment, 22, 28–29, 37, **51**
 purchasing, F395
 safety and, F78, F149–51
 sanitation, F309
 sterilization of, 39
 for tattooing, *556f*
 treatment room, F300-301, F303–4
ER. *See* endoplasmic reticulum
Erbium device, 739, 744
erector spinae, **112**, **119**
ergonomically correct, **F300**, **F311**
ergonomics, F300, **F305**, **F311**, F412
Er:YAG lasers, 172–73, *175t*
erythema, **F219**, **F231**, *F242t*
 multiforme, **332**, **344**, 701
 transient, **229**, **234**
erythematotelangiectatic rosacea, **229**, **233**
erythrocytes, F115, F125, **71**, **82**, **125**, *125t*, **136**
esophagus, *F165f*
essay questions, F532
essential minerals, F180–81
essential oils, **F261**, *F268t*, *F272t*, F274, **F291**, F384
 application of, 298–99, *298f*, *299t*, *300t*, *301t*
 aromatherapy and, 289–91, *299t–300t*
 body wraps and, 589–90, *589t*
 chemistry of, 150–52, *150t–151t*, 292, *292t–293t*
 contraindications for, 150–52, 294–95
 fragrance and, 264
 massage and, 298–300
 properties of, 291–92
 recipes using, 301
 for skin care, 295–98
ester, **149**, **153**, **257**, **279**
ester C, F275
esthetic surgery, **F462**–63, **F465**. *See also* plastic surgery
estheticians. *See also* careers
 chemical terms for, 145–46
 chemistry and, 139
 credentials of, 663–64
 on cruise ships, 9
 at day spas, F10–11
 defined, **F10**, **F17**, 5, **8**
 equipment for, 437–40, *438f*
 government regulation of, 13–14
 legal considerations for, 21, 302, 439, 516
 medical, F11, **9**, 663–64, 691–92
 for salons, F10–11
 scope of practice of, 189, 193, 214, 232, 331, 342, **664**–65, **671**
 spelling of word, 8
 training of, *440f*, 666–67
esthetician's chair, F300, F305
esthetics
 African, F6, *F7f*
 Age of Extravagance, F7
 Asian, F6
 changes in, 3–16
 Chinese, F6
 defined, **F10**, **F17**
 dermatology and, F213
 editors for, F13
 Egyptian, F5
 Greek, F5, *F6f*
 Hebrew, F5
 instructors of, 9
 Japanese, F6
 medical, **F11**, **F17**, F460–64, 663–70
 of Middle Ages, F6–7
 nutrition and, F182–83
 twentieth century, F8–9
 twenty-first century, F9–10
 Victorian Age, F7–8
 writers on, F13
estradiol, **92**, **101**
estriol, **92**, **131**
estrogen, F206–7, **92**, **101**, *245f*, *246f*
estrogen isotypes, 245–46, *245f*, *246f*
estrone, **92**, **101**
ethanol, 267
ethics, **F25**–28, **F32**, 10, 667, 773
ethmoid bone, *F100f*, **F101**, **F123**
ethnic hair, F405–6
ethnic skin, F240–41
ethyl alcohol, F75
eucalyptus, *F270t*, *F272t*, 295, *295f*
eumelanin, F201
evaluations, employee, F52–53, F560–61
evening makeup, F509
evening primrose, *F270t*, *F272t*
evidence, 11
excoriations, **F215**–16, **F231**
excretion, F194
excretory system, **F119**, **F123**
exempt colors, F262
exercises, for hands and wrists, F305, F362
exfoliants
 creams, 380–81
 follicular, **233**
 as performance ingredients, F263, *270f*, 271–72
 scrubs, 318, *318f*
 skin care products and, F278–80
 toners and, 318
exfoliation
 for acne, F352
 AHAs and, 367–74, *368f*, *370f–372f*
 benefits of, F278–79
 BHAs and, 367, *378f–380f*
 chemical, **F279**–80, **F291**, 270
 client consultations before, 377
 defined, **F263**, **F291**
 enzymes for, F263
 facials, F321
 glycolic acid and, 367–69
 histology of, 73–75
 mechanical, **F279**, **F292**, 270
 microdermabrasion, machine, and, 362, 439, *439f*, 452–60, *453f*, *454f*, *455f–459f*
 microdermabrasion, manual, and, 362, *362f*, *363f–366f*
 peels, F446
 safety and, F449
 superficial peels and, F446, 374–81, *375f*
 treatments, 351, 362–81
exhalation, F120
exocrine glands, **F117**, **F123**, **101**
expectorant properties, 292
expeller pressed, **285**, *285f*, **304**
exposure, to communicable diseases, *F64t*, **F84**, **F89**, 22
extensor digitorium longus, **117**, **119**
extensors, **F106**, *F107f*, **F123**
external carotid artery, **F115**, **F123**
external ectoderm, **70**, **82**

external jugular vein, **F116**, **F123**
external maxillary artery, *F115f*, **F116**, **F123**
external obliques, **112**, **119**
external phase, **259**, **279**
extracellular matrix (ECM), **66**–70, 86
extract, whole, **284**
extractions
  acne facials, F351
  botanical, 284–86
  defined, **F322**, **F357**
  disposables and, F310
  facials and, F322–23, F342–43, 351–52
  government regulation of, F310
  hair removal and, *488f*
  procedure, F342–44
  solvent, 286–87
exudates, **207**, **233**
eye(s)
  blue, F484
  brown, F484
  butterfly pads for, F307
  circles under, 317, 542–46, 550, *717f*
  close-set, F490, F492
  corrective makeup for, F489–91
  creams for, F283–84, 317
  deep-set, F490
  drooping, F491
  eye lifts, 715–17, *716f*, *717f*
  flushes, F86
  glamour, *F509f*
  green, F484
  LASER contact with, 167, *167f*
  makeup colors for, F484
  makeup removal, before facials, F326–27, F476
  muscles of, 108–9, *109f*
  occular protection, 167–68
  pads for, F307
  products in, F320
  protruding, F490
  round, F490
  shadow, F475–76, *F475f*, F500
  shadow brushes, F479
  shapes of, *F490t–491t*
  shields, disposable, *168f*
  small, F490
  smoky eyes makeup, F509
  tabbing of, **F513**, **F524**
  treatments for, F324
  wet collagen pads for, *383f*
  wide-set, F490, F492
eyebrows
  brow lift, F462, 713, 715–16
  color application, F477
  corrective makeup for, F491
  eyebrow design and, 488–91, *490f*, *491f*
  hair removal and, F421–23
  high arch, F492
  ideal, *F491f*
  male, F420, 501, *501f*, *502f*
  muscles of, F104
  pencils for, F500
  shapes of, *F492t*
  tattooing, *555f*, 557, *557f*
  threading of, 478, 481
  tinting, F517–20
  tweezing, F421–23
  waxing, F419–20, F424–27, 486, 488–91, 501
eyelashes
  artificial, F513–16
  client consultations for extensions to, 521
  extension removal, 529–31, *530f–531f*
  extensions, F521
  extensions, semi-permanent, 521–25, *521f*, *523f*, *524f*, *525f–529f*
  life cycle of, 522, *523f*
  perming of, F521, 531–32, *532f–535f*
  safety and, 521–22
  sanitation, of artificial, F516
eyelid excision, *716f*
eyeliner brushes, F479
eyeliners, F476–77, F500, 557
eyewash, 49

F

face. *See also* facial machines; facial massage; facials
  advanced massage movements on, 393–96, *394f*, *395f*, *396f*
  blood supply of, F115–16
  diamond shape, F486
  heart shape, F486
  inverted triangle shape, F486
  long, F492
  muscles of, *F367f*, 108–11, *109f*, *110f*, *470f*
  narrow, F488
  nerves of, F110–13, 117–18
  oblong shape, F486
  oval-shaped, F486–87
  pear-shaped, F486
  powder makeup for, F473–74
  rectangle shape, F486
  reflexology of, 242–45, **407**, *407f*, **434**
  round shape, F486, F488, F492
  shapes and proportions of, F485–87
  skeletal system and, F101
  square shape, F486, F488, F492
  triangular shape, F486, F488
  waxing of, 488–91
  youthful, *691f*
face-lift, 712–13, *713f*, *714f*
facial artery, *F115f*, **F116**, **F123**
facial beds, F300, F304, *570f*
facial bra, **741**, *741f*, 743, **744**
facial implants, 718–19
facial machines
  electric heat mask, F395
  electric mitts and boots, F394
  electrodessication devices, **465**–66, *465f*, *466f–468f*, **474**
  electrotherapy, **F151**–54, **F160**, **F378**, **F396**
  galvanic current, **F151**, *F152t*, **F160**, F385–90, 139, 145
  GentleWaves device, *180f*
  high-frequency machines, F301, **F390**–93, *F392t*, **F396**
  hot towel cabinet, F380
  hyperpigmentation and, *473t*
  IPL treatments and, F159, F407–**8**, **F442**, F452, 440–48, *444f–448f*
  Lucas sprayer, F393–94, F397
  magnifying lamps/lights, *F237f*, F248, F300, F378–79, 237
  microdermabrasion, 362, 439, *439f*, 452–60, *453f*, *454f*, *455f–459f*
  paraffin wax heater, F394
  purchasing equipment, F395
  rotary brush, F380–81, F397
  side effects and, 473, *473t*
  spray machines, F301, **F393**, **F397**
  steamers, F300, F303–4, F381–84
  ultrasonic, F454–55, 460, *460f*
  vacuum machines, F301, **F384**–85, **F397**
  Wood's lamps, **F379**–80, **F397**, 212, 237, 240–41
facial massage
  benefits of, F361
  contraindications for, F362
  Dr. Jacquet movement, **F365**, **F374**
  ear reflexology and, 408
  Shiatsu and, **402**–7, *403f–406f*, **434**
  technical skills, F361–62
  techniques, F365–66, F368–73
  types of movements, F363–65, 393–96, *394f*, *395f*, *396f*
facial nerve, *F111f*, **F112**, **F125**
facials
  acne and, F351–54
  benefits of, F315
  for body, 573, *573f–576f*
  checklist, F318, *F319f*
  cleansing, F320–21, F328–29
  clean-up, F344
  client consultation for, F318–20, F338
  completing service, F324–25
  contraindications for, *F319f*
  cotton compresses, F340–41
  defined, **F315**, **F357**
  draping hair, F320
  for dry skin, F345–46
  exfoliation, F321
  extractions and, F322–23, F342–43, 351–52
  eye makeup removal and, F326–27, F476
  hyperpigmentation, F351
  IPL treatments and, 440–48, *444f–448f*
  lancets, F323, F344
  masks, F324
  for men, F354–56
  mini-facials, F345
  moisturizers, F324
  oily skin, F351
  paraffin wax masks for, **F282**–83, **F292**, F348–49
  philosophies and methods, F325
  procedure for, F332–37
  removing product, F330–31
  rosacea, F350
  salons for, *F587f*
  sanitation after, F337–39
  sensitive skin, F350
  serums, eye and lip treatments, F324
  sunscreen and, F324, 444, 447, 451, 461, 468, 471
  supplies for, *F317t*
  timing of, F30
  toners, F324
  treatment protocol, F316–17
  ultrasonic, F454–55, 460, *461f–465f*
  variations of basic, F325
  warm towels, F321
fact-gathering, 10
fallopian tubes, 91
Famvir® (famciclovir), **739**, **744**
fantasy makeup, 554, *554f*, *555f*
faradic current, **F152**, **F160**
fascia, **727**, **730**
fashion shows, F12
fat tissue, **F198**, **F208**
fatlah, **478**, **517**
fats, **F170**–72, **F185**, 193
fat-soluble vitamins, *F173t–174t*, F175–78
  vitamin A, *F173t*, **F175**–77, **F185**, **F265**, **F293**, F352, 191, 275, 578
  vitamin D, *F173–74t*, **F177**, **F185**, 191, 578
  vitamin E, *F174t*, **F177**–78, **F185**, 191, 260, 262, 275–76, 578
  vitamin K, *F174t*, F178, **F178**, **F185**, **F265**, **F293**

fatty acids, F170–71, **F258**–59, **F291**, **148**, **153**, 255–56, 268
fatty alcohols, **F259**, **F291**, 256
fatty esters, **F259**, **F291**, 257
fatty waxes, **149**, **154**
FDA. *See* Food and Drug Administration
feathering, F366
Federal Packaging and Labeling Act (1977), 668
federal regulation. *See* government regulation
Federal Trade Commission (FTC), 778
Federal Unemployment Tax, **758**, **762**
feedback, F590
feet, muscles of, 116–17, *116f*, *116t*
female reproductive organs, *91f*
ferrule, F480
fever blisters, **F225**, **F231**
FGF. *See* fibroblast growth factor
fiber, F169
fibril, **66**, **82**
fibroblast growth factor (FGF), **70**, **82**
fibroblasts, **F197**, **F208**, **63**, **82**, 276
fibrocytes, **63**, **82**
fibularis muscles, **117**, **119**
fifth cranial nerve (CN V), **F110**–12, **F123**
fight or flight response, **192**, *192f*, 197, **199**
filaments, **61**
filtration masks, and LASER treatments, *169f*
financial planning, 751–53
financing options, for equipment, 439
finger cots, F322
fingernails, F21, F199
fire, F581–82
fire drills, 48
fire extinguishers, *169f*
firming products, 315–16
first aid, F84–86, 48
first cranial nerve (CN I), *F111f*
fissures, **F216**, **F231**
fitness clubs, 566
Fitzpatrick skin typing scale, **F239**–40, **F251**
  IPL treatments and, 442, *442f*
  LASER treatment and, 491, *506t*, 507
  sensitive skin and, **238**–40, *238f*, *238t*, *239t*, **248**
  sun damage and, 211–12
five elements
  Ayurveda and, 632
  traditional Chinese medicine and, 243–44
5-HT3 antagonists, **334**, **343**
fixed costs, **F576**, **F598**
fixed oils, **285**, **304**
flagella, **F65**, **F89**
flare, **228**, *228f*, **233**
flavonoids, **148**, *148t*, **154**
flexation, **113**, **119**
flexors, **F106**, *F107f*, **F123**
fluence, **162**–63, **182**, **512**–13, **517**
fluoride, *F175t*, F181
fluorite, 619, *619f*
fluorouracil, 215
flushing (redness), 99, **227**, **233**, 542
foaming cleansers, F277, F354, 265, 308–9, 319–20
folic acid, *F173t*, F179
follicle endings, **78**, **83**
follicles, **F194**, *F195f*, F199, **F208**, F226, *F227f*, **F401**–2, **F441**
follicle-stimulating hormone (FSH), **92**, **101**
follicular exfoliants, **233**
folliculitis, **F219**, **F231**, **F356–57**
folliculitis barbae, **F356–57**, **F409**, **F441**
follow-up, F614–15, 22
Food and Drug Administration (FDA)
  certified colors and, **F262**, **F291**, 263
  color agent ingredients, F262, 263–64, *263f*,
  cosmetics and, 668
  definition of drugs by, F256
  device classification and, 440
  disinfectants and, **41**, 50
  drug approval and, 326–27, 693–94
  Food, Drug and Cosmetic Act (1938), F255–56, 253, 668
  information on, 14, **51**, 778
  National Organic Program of, 286
  permanent hair removal, F407–8
  product safety, F266–67
  safety and, 164–65
  sunscreen ingredients, F266
food choices, F182–83, F228
food consumption, *F165f*
Food, Drug and Cosmetic Act (1938), F255–56, 253, 668
food pyramids, F165, *F166f*, F167
food sensitivities, **192**, **199**
foot reflexology, **F456**, **F465**, 630
forehead
  low, F492
  narrow, F488
  protruding, F488
forehead-lift, F462
  classic, **714**, **730**
  overview of, 713–15, *715f*
formaldehyde, F74
formalin, F74
formed elements, of blood, **125**, *125t*, **136**
formication, **99**, **101**
forming positive doctor relationships, *6f*
forms
  client assessment, *F416f*
  for client consultations, *F247f*, *F416f*
  client release, F246, *F417f*
  consent, F40–41
  intake, F39–40, **F577**, F606, **F606**, **F616**
  inventory of personal characteristics and technical skills, *F534f*
  job application, F549–52, *F550f–552f*
fortified foods, F177
foundations, F471–73, F500
fourth cranial nerve (CN IV), *F111f*
fourth germ layer, **70**, **82**
fragrance-free products, 264
fragrances, F6, **F261**, F267, F274, **F291**, 264
franchises, F11, **F541**, **F569**
frankincense, *F272t*, 150, 292, 638–39
freckles, 217–18
free fatty acids, **75**, **82**
free nerve terminals, **77**, **82**
free radicals, **F136**, **F142**, **F203**, **F208**, **F274**–75, **F291**
  defined, **279**
  inflammation and, 274
  nutrition and, **190**
  oxidation and, 262
  skin and, **274**–76
  skin care and, F274–75
freelance marketing consultants, *F608f*
French culture, 7
French waxing, 494–95, *494f*, *495f*
frenulum, **110**, **120**
fresheners, **F278**, **F291**
friction, F363–64, **F374**
frisket, 552–54
front desks, F591–93
frontal artery, *F115f*, **F116**, **F123**
frontal bone, *F100f*, **F101**, **F123**
frontalis, **F103**, *F104f–105f*, **F123**, **108**
frontalis muscles, *F367f*
FSH. *See* follicle-stimulating hormone
FTC. *See* Federal Trade Commission
fulling, F363, **F374**
full-service salon, F533, F542, *F587f*
functional groups, **150**, *150f*, *150t*, **154**
functional ingredients, **F256**, **F291**, 252–64
fungal infections, 339–40, *340t*
fungi, **F70**, **F89**, 26–28, 41–42
fungicidal disinfectants, **F62**, F74, **F89**
furniture, treatment room, F300–301, F412
furuncles, **F217**, **F231**
fuses, **F149**, **F160**

G

G_0 (stage of cell cycle), **69**, **82**
G_1 (stage of cell cycle), **69**, **82**
G_2 (stage of cell cycle), **69**, **82**
GAAP. *See* generally accepted accounting principles
GAD. *See* generalized anxiety disorder
Gadberry, Rebecca James, 231
GAGs. *See* glycosaminoglycans
galvanic current
  chemistry of, 139, 145
  defined, **F151**, **F160**, **F385**, **F396**
  desincrustation and, F386–88
  effects of, *F152t*
  galvanic maintenance, F390
  ionto mask, F390
  iontophoresis, F388
  microcurrent technology and, 469, *469f*
  overview of, F385–86
  polarity of solutions, F388–89
galvanic electrolysis, F407
galvanic machines, F301, F386–87, F390
gamma globulin, 23
gap junctions, **74**, **82**
gases, *F132f*, F133
gastrocnemius, **117**, **120**
gastrointestinal disorders, 333–35, *334t*
gastrointestinal system. *See* digestive system
gastrula, **70**, **82**
gastrulation, **70**, **82**
geishas, F6
gel masks, F281
gellants, F260–61, **263**, **279**
gem elixirs, 613
gemstones, **613**, **626**
general circulation, **F114**, **F126**
general infections, **F66**, **F89**
generalized anxiety disorder (GAD), **336**, **344**
generally accepted accounting principles (GAAP), **752**, **762**
genital warts, 478
GentleWaves device, *180f*
genuine and authentic, **294**, *295t*, **304**
geranium, *F270t*, *F272t*, 295–96, *296f*
germ layers, **70**, **82**
germs, *F63t*. *See also* bacteria
ghee, **637**, **657**
glabella, *F461f*, **692**, *698f*, 701
glamour eyes, *F509f*
glamour look, *529f*
glands, **F117**, **F123**, F201–2, F216–18
glass tip electrodes, *F392t*
glial cells, **72**, **82**
globalization, 26
globules, **259**, **280**
Glogau, Richard, 240
Glogau skin typing scale, **240**, *240t*, **248**, 442

glossopharyngeal nerve, *F111f*
gloves, F83, F89, F303, F310, F322, F414
  breakdown characteristics of, 36, *36t*
  infection control and, 22, 33–36, *34t*, 48–49
  latex sensitivity and, 33–34
  safety and, 48
  testing methods for, 35
glucans, **277**, **280**
glucose, F169–70, **337**, **344**
gluteus group of muscles, **115**, **120**
glycation, **193**, **199**
glycerin, **F268**, *F268t*, **F291**, 268
glycolic acid
  acne and, *374f*
  as cosmetic ingredient, 266–68, **270–71**, **280**
  exfoliation and, 367–69
  medical peels and, *F447f*, F461, 705
  wrinkles and, *373f*
glycolic hydrator, *224f*
glycolic peels, *F447f*, F461, 705
glycolipids, F203
glycoproteins, **F265**, **F291**, 277
glycosaminoglycans (GAGs), **F168**, **F185**, F198, 63, **66**–67, **82**
goals, F23, F29, *F30f*, F41
goggles, for LASER treatments, *168f*
Golgi apparatus, *57f*, **59**, *62f*, *65f*, **82**
gommages, **F280**, **F291**, 271
gossip, F51
government regulation, F578. *See also* Occupational Safety and Health Administration
  apprenticeship, F581
  booth rentals, F535, **F573**–74, **F598**
  business operation, F578
  of disinfectants, F61
  electrolysis, F407
  EPA and, F61, 34, 39, **41**, 48, **51**
  of estheticians, 13–14
  ethics, F25, 10
  of extractions, F310
  Federal Packaging and Labeling Act (1977), 668
  Federal Trade Commission (FTC), 778
  HHS and HIPAA, F27, **13**, **15**, 566
  of infection control, F59–62
  lancets, F323, F344
  laws *versus* rules, F62
  of massage, F362
  MSDS, **F59**–61, **F89**, 49
  photoepilation, F408
  regulatory agencies, 21, 438, 516
  sanitation, F310
  state regulation, F61
  tweezing, F430
  waxing, F430
granular scrubs, F279
granulocytes, **64**, **83**, **125**, **136**
granulomatous rosacea, **231**, **233**
grapefruit, 296, *296f*
grapeseed extract, **F270**, *F270t*, **F291**, 275, 578
gratuities, F563–64
Graves' disease, **716**, **730**
greasepaint, **F472**, **F524**
greater auricular nerve, **F112**, **F123**
greater occipital nerve, **F112**, **F123**
Greece, ancient, 6, 676
Greek esthetics, F5, *F6f*
green eyes, F484
green light, F159
green makeup, F482
green tea, **F270**, *F270t*, F276, **F292**, 275–76, *275f*, 288, *288f*, 578
greeting clients, F39, F317, 12
grey makeup, F482
gross profit, **752**, **762**
ground substance, F198
grounding, F149–50
growth, of hair, F403–6
growths, non-cancerous, 216–18
guidelines for success, F28–29
gunas, **657**
guru, **657**

H

H. *See* hydrogen
H_2O. *See* water
H_2O_2. *See* hydrogen peroxide
hacking, F364
hair
  anatomy of, F199
  bulbs, **F402**, *F403f*, **F441**
  clips for, F499
  color, F485
  draping of, F320
  follicle endings, **78**, **83**
  follicles, **F194**, *F195f*, F199, **F208**, F226, *F227f*, **F401**–2, **F441**
  growth of, F403–6
  morphology of, F401–3
  papillae of, **F197**, **F208**, **F402**, *F403f*, **F441**
  roots of, **F402**, *F403f*, **F442**
  shafts of, **F401**, **F442**
  skin and, F199
hair removal. *See also* waxing
  client consultations, F416–17
  contraindications for, F415–16, *479f*
  disinfection and, 477–78
  electrolysis, F406–7
  extractions and, *488f*
  eyebrow tweezing, F421–23
  hair growth and, F403–6
  hydroquinone and, **515**, **517**
  insurance and, 516
  IPL treatments and, 503–16, *504t*, *510f–512f*
  LASER and, F158, F407–**8**, **F442**, 503–16, *504t*, *510f–512f*
  lupus and, 479
  overview of, F401
  permanent and semipermanent, F407–8
  pregnancy and, 478–79
  room preparation, F412–15
  safety and, 477–78
  by sugaring, **F410**, **F442**, 480–86, *482f*, *486f*
  temporary methods, F408–10
  threading, F6, F410, **478**–81, *480f*, *481f*, **517**
hairstyles
  Age of Extravagance, F7
  Middle Ages, F6–7
  Victorian Age, F8
hallucinations, **337**, **344**
hamstring muscles, **116**, **120**
hand washing
  infection control and, F82–83, 22, 28, 30–34, 48
  key points of, 33
  overview of, **30–31**
  solutions for, 31, *36t*
  technique for, *31f–32f*
hands
  blood supply of, F116
  exercises for, F305, F362
  muscles of, F107
  nerves of, F113
  skeletal system and, F102
  waxing of, 493
hantavirus, **339**, **344**
hard sell, F602
hard waxes, F411, F418–19, 486–87, *486f*, *489t*
Hazard Communication Act, F59
hazards
  nominal hazard zone (NHZ), **166**, **182**
  potential, 47–48
HBV (hepatitis B), **22**–24, *23t*, **51**
HCV (hepatitis C), **22**, *23t*, 24, **51**
HDLs (high-density lipoproteins), F171
HDV (hepatitis D), *23t*, **24**–25, **51**
head
  blood supply of, F115–16
  muscles of, *F367f*, 108–11, *109f*, *110f*
  nerves of, F110–13
head lice, *F69f*
healing
  agents, **F262**, **F292**
  creams for, F352
  holistic, **12**–13, **15**
  nutrition and, 209–10
  with stones, 613–20, *614t*, *616t*
  sunscreen and, 209
  of wounds, 204–10, *205f*, *206f*, *208f*, *209f*
health. *See also* Occupational Safety and Health Administration
  of cells, F202–3
  holistic approaches to, **302**, **304**
  screening of clients, F182, F246–47, 567, *568f–569f*
  of skin, F202–4
Health and Human Services (HHS), F27, 13
Health Insurance Portability and Accountability Act (HIPAA), F27, **13**, **15**, 566
heart
  anatomy of, **F113**–14, **F123**, 127–28, *127f*
  cardiovascular system and, **F113**–14, **F123**, *F245t*, 41, 127–28, *127f*, **128**, *128t*, 331–33, *332t*
  circulatory system and, **F113**–14, **F123**, 127–28, *127f*
  disorders and diseases of, 41, **128**, *128t*, 331–33, *332t*
  irregularities, *F245t*
heart face shape, F486
heat regulation, F194
Hebrew esthetics, F5
hederiform endings, **78**, **83**
helichrysum, 291, 296, *296f*, 302
heliobacter pylori, **228**, **233**
helminths, 27
helper T cells, **73**, **83**
hemidesmosomes, **74**, *74f*, **83**
hemocytoblast, **71**, **83**
hemoglobin, **F115**, **F123**
hemophilia, **126**, **136**, *479f*
hemostasis, **204**, **233**
henna, **F5**, **F17**
heparan sulfate, **67**, **83**
heparin, 63, **67**, **83**
hepatitis, **F67**–69, **F89**
  A, *23t*, 24–25
  acute, 24, **50**
  B, **22**–24, *23t*, **51**
  C, **22**, *23t*, 24, **51**
  chronic, 24–25, **51**
  common varieties of, *23t*

D, *23t*, **24**–25, **51**
E, **25**, **51**
G, 25
HIV and, 22–24, 27
infection control and, 21–27
overview of, 23–27
herbal body wraps
ingredients for, *589f*, *589t*
overview of, **584**, *585f–588f*, **599**
herbal bouquet, *283f*
herbal infusion, **285**, **304**
herbs
Ayurvedic, 637–38, *638t*
as ingredients, of skin care products, F272–73
overview of, **F268**, *F268t*, *F272t*, *F273t*, **F292**
herpes simplex
overview of, 212, 477–78, *479f*
virus 1, **F225**, **F231**
virus 2, **F225**, **F231**
herpes zoster, **F225**, **F231**
HEV (hepatitis E), **25**, **51**
HHS. *See* Health and Human Services
hidden lids, F490
high arch eyebrow, F492
high-density lipoproteins (HDLs), F171
high-frequency machines, F301, **F390**–93, *F392t*, **F396**
highlight colors, F476
highlighters, F500
high-tech cosmetic vehicles, 260–61
HIPAA. *See* Health Insurance Portability and Accountability Act
hirsutism, **F405**, **F442**, **100**, **101**, *505f*
histamines, F220, **333**, **344**
histology, **F95**, **F123**, **F191**, **F208**. *See also* skin
of cell cycle, **69**–70, **81**
of cellular functions, 57–59
of embryology, **70**–71, **82**
of exfoliation, 73–75
of immune system, **72**–73
of sensory nerves, 77–78
of skin penetration and permeation, 75–76
of skin structure and function, 60–65
of tissue types, 71–72
history
Africans, F6
Age of Extravagance, F7
Asians, F6
Egypt, ancient, F5, 675
French culture, 7
Greece, ancient, F5, 6, 675
Hebrews, F5
of medical terminology, 675–77
Middle Ages, F6–7
Moors, 7
of peels, F446
Renaissance, F7, 7
Roman Empire, F6, 6, 675
twentieth century, F8–9
twenty-first century, F9–10
Victorian Age, F7–8
World War II, 7–8
HIV. *See* Human Immunodeficiency Virus
hives, F215, F219, F233
holistic approaches. *See also* Ayurveda; traditional Chinese medicine
to healing, **12**–13, **15**
to health, **302**, **304**
Holmes-Rahe Life Stress Inventory, *196f*
home-care
by clients, *F287t*, 307, *307f*, 514
guide, *F614f*
instruction sheet, *F287t*
post-peel, F449–50
skin care products, F286–87
homemade masks, F283
homeostasis, **76**, **83**, **290**, **304**
homogenizers, **260**, **280**
honesty, F553
honey, *F273t*
hordeolums, **233**
hormone replacement therapy (HRT), F206–7, **98**–99, **101**
hormones
acne and, F227–28, 221–23
anorexia and, 100
birth control pills and, 328–30
defined, **F117**, **F123**, **F208**, **89**, **101**
drugs and, 329–30, *330t*
follicle-stimulating, **92**, **101**
hirsutism and, **100**
hyperpigmentation and, 330
of hyperthyroidism, **100**, **101**
of hypothyroidism, **100**, **102**
luteinizing, **92**, **102**
male, F227–28
mature skin and, F206–7
melanocyte-stimulating, **62**, **84**
melasma and, F120
of menstrual cycle, 94–95, *94f*, *95f*
microcirculation, **F206**–7
obesity and, 100
pancreas and, **91**, **102**
phases of life and, 92–99
of pregnancy, 95–96
premenstrual syndrome and, **97**, **102**
skin and, F206–7, 245–47
thyroid gland and, F118, **90**, **102**
trophic, **90**, **102**
use in cosmetics, F10
horsechestnut, **F270**, *F270t*, **F292**
hospital grade disinfectants, F61
'hot cabbies,' F300, F303
hot flashes, 99
hot towel cabinet, F380
hot towels, *354f*
hotel spas, F535, F542
HPV. *See* human papillomavirus
HRT. *See* hormone replacement therapy
Human Immunodeficiency Virus (HIV), **F67**, **F89**
defined, 21–**25**, 27, **51**
hepatitis and, 22–24, 27
OSHA and, **21**–23
human papillomavirus (HPV), **478**, **517**
human relations, F36–38
human resource management, 669
humectants, **F263**, **F292**, 267–68. *See also* moisturizing products, for dry skin
humerus, **F102**, **F123**
humoral immune system, **72**, **83**
hyaluronic acid, **F198**, **F208**, **F268**, *F268t*, **F292**, F462
cells and, **67**, *69f*, **83**
as cosmetic ingredient, 268, 578
as dermal fillers, 692, 697, **700–**701, *700t*, *703f*, **708**
Non-animal Stabilized Hyaluronic Acid, 697, **701**, **708**
sodium hyaluronate, 268
hyaluronidase, **274**, **280**
hybrid pay structures, F562–63
hydration, F183. *See also* water
hydrators, **F263**, **F292**. *See also* moisturizing products, for dry skin
hydrocollators, **584**, *584f*, **599**
hydrogen (H)
chemistry of, 140
defined, **F133**, **F142**
potential, F134–35
hydrogen peroxide (H_2O_2), **F134**, **F142**
hydrolipidic, F193
hydrophilic, **F138**–39, **F142**
hydrophilic ingredients, **F263**, **F292**, **258**, **268**. *See also* moisturizing products, for dry skin
hydropower plants, F147
hydroquinone, F351
cells and, 62
defined, **474**, **738**, **744**
hair removal and, **515**, **517**
hyperpigmentation and, 210, 374
IPL treatments and, **442**, **474**
LASER treatments and, **738**, **744**
hydrosol, **290**, **304**
hydrostatic pressure, **131**, **136**
hydrotherapy, **F456**, **F465**, **6**, **15**, **589**, **599**, 630
hydroxy radicals, **274**, **280**
hyfrecator, 96
hygiene, **F21**, **F32**, F337, 36–38
hyoid bone, **F101**, **F123**
hyperextension, **112**, **120**
hyperhidrosis, **F218**, **F231**
hyperkeratinization, *F242t*
hyperkeratosis, **F222**, **F231**
hyperpigmentation, **F220**, F221, **F231**, F241, *F242t*, F351
AHAs and, 369, 374, *375f*, *376f*
birth control pills and, 97–98
defined, **326**, **344**
facial machines and, *473t*
facials and, F351
hormones and, 330
hydroquinone and, 210, 374
LASER treatments and, 210–14, *210f*, *515f*
photoaging and, 213
pregnancy and, 95, *95f*
self-trauma excoriations and, 225
solar freckles and, 217
sun damage and, 209, 211–12
vitiligo and, 545
hyperproliferation, **61**, **83**
hypersensitivity, 33–34
hypertension, **331**, **344**
hyperthyroidism, **100**, **101**
hypertrichosis, **F405**, **F442**, **335**, **344**
hypertrophies, **F221**–22, **F231**
hypoallergenic, F256
hypochlorous acid, **64**, **83**
hypoglossal nerve, *F111f*
hypoglycemia, **F169**, **F185**
hypopigmentation, **F220**, F221, **F231**, *F242t*, *210f*, **326**, **344**, *473t*
hypothalamus gland, F109, **90**, **101**, **102**, **291**, **304**
hypothesis, **668**, **671**
hypothyroidism, **100**, **102**
hypoxia, **125**, **136**
hyssop, F5

I

ideal eyebrow, *F491f*
IGF-I. *See* insulin-like growth factor
igneous, **410**, **434**
IL-1. *See* interleukin-1
IL-2. *See* interleukin-2
illegal drugs, F204

image, professional. *See* professional image
immiscible liquids, **F137**, **F142**
immune globulin, 23
immune system, **F70**, **F89**, **F117**, **F123**
anatomy of, F117
cell-mediated, **72**–73, **80**
complement system and, **73**, **81**
histology of, **72**–73
humoral, **72**, **83**
infection control and, F70, **26**, 29
lupus and, 72
lysozymes and, **73**, **84**
overview of, **72**–73, **83**
immunization
defined, **24**, **51**
for hepatitis B, 24
immunocompromised, **340**, **344**
immunologic response, **333**, **344**
impedance, **178**, **182**
impetigo, **F225**, **F231**, **454**, **474**
implants
breast, **720**–21, *720f*, *721f*, 725, **730**
chin, 718–19, *719f*
facial, 718–19
implements, **F308**, **F311**
inactive electrodes, **F151**, **F160**
inactive ingredients, **253**, **280**
income statement, *F577t*, **752**, **762**
incoming calls, F595–96
independent contractors, 21, **755**, **762**
independent skin care clinic, F533, F542
indicators, 44
indirect contact, 28
indirect electrodes, *F392t*
indirect high-frequency application, F154
individual lashes, **F513**, **F524**
Individual Tax Identification Number (ITIN), **756**, **762**
inert, biologically, **254**, 270, **279**
infection control
accidents and, 48
acne and, 28
airborne infections and, 28, 48
autoclaves and, 39–41, 43–49, *45f–47f*, **51**
autoimmune disorders and, 21, **28**
bacteria and, F62–67, 27
bloodborne diseases and, 48, 704
bloodborne pathogens and, F68–**69**, **F88**, **33**, 37, **48**, **51**
chain of infection and, 28–29
contamination and, 26
defined, **F65**, **F89**
disinfection and, 28–32, 37–41, 47–49
disposal, of infected material and, 48
first aid, F84–87, 48
fungi and, **F70**, **F89**, 26–28, 41–42
globalization and, 26
gloves and, 22, 33–36, *34t*, 48–49
government regulation, F59–62
hand washing and, F82–83, 22, 28, 30–34, 48
hepatitis and, 21–27
immune system and, F70, **26**, 29
labeling for, 43
nosocomial infections and, 27
OSHA and, 21–22
packaging and, 42–43
parasites and, *F63t*, **F69**, **F89**, 27
pH values and, 40
prevention, F70–79
sterilization and, 29, 37–47, *46f–47f*
storage, of instruments, and, 28–29, 47
transmission of infections and, 28, 32–33
tuberculosis and, **F61**, **F90**, **25**–26, 28–29, 48, **52**
ultrasonic cleaning and, 38, 42
Universal Precautions and, **F84**, **F90**, 22
viruses and, F67–69, 27
infectious agents, *F63t*, F65
infectious diseases, *F64t*, F66–67, F89, F225
inferior labial artery, *F115f*, **F116**, **F123**
inflammation
cascade of, F281, 203–4, *203f*, 274
clinical, **203**, **233**
defined, *F64t*
free radicals and, 274
perifollicular, **222**, **233**
of skin, F218–20
subclinical, **203**, **234**, 274
inflammatory mediators, **203**, **233**
information interviews, with clients, **F542**–43, **F569**, F606–7
information sharing, 13
inframammary crease, **722**, **730**
infraorbital artery, *F115f*, **F116**, **F123**
infraorbital nerve, **F110**, *F112f*, **F123**
infrared rays, F155–57, **F156**, **F160**, F452, 158
infratrochlear nerve, **F111**, *F112f*, **F123**
ingestion, **F119**, **F123**
ingredients, of cosmetics. *See also specific ingredients*
active, **253**, **279**, **280**
for aging skin, 273–77
AHAs, 268, 271–73, 277, 576
antioxidants, 262, 275–76, 284
BHAs, 270, **271**, 576
for cell metabolism, F264–65
chart, F267–72
collagen, 268, 271, 276, 578
color agents, F262, 263–64, *263f*
common components, *F268t–271t*
delivery systems, F264, F291
dictionaries of, F273
emollients, F257–59, 254–57, 264, 269–70, *269f*, 272
enzymes, 271
exfoliants, F263, *270f*, 271–72
fragrances, F6, **F261**, F267, F274, **F291**, 264
functional, **F256**, **F291**, 252–64
gellants and thickeners, F260–61, **263**, **279**
glycolic acid, 266–68, **270–71**, **280**
herbs and plant properties, F272–73
hyaluronic acid, 268, 578
hydrators and moisturizers, F263
hydrophilic, **F263**, **F292**, **258**, **268**
inactive, **253**, **280**
labeling of, 277–78, *308f*
lighteners and brighteners, F241, F263–64
in mineral makeup, F472, 535–39, *538f*, *539f–541f*, 541
natural, *F270–71t*, *F273t*
natural *versus* synthetic, F266
in peels, F449
peptides and collagen stimulants, F265
performance, **F256**, **F292**, 252–53, 264–72, 277
preservatives, **F261**–62, **F293**, 261–62
of sunscreen, F266, 276–77, 312–14, 321
surfactants, F259–60
water, F256–57, 253
waxes, 255
inhalation, F120
injectables, **F461**, F461–62, **F465**
inner beauty, F471, 603, 637
inorganic chemistry, **F130**, **F142**
inositol, *F173t*
in-salon communication
with coworkers, F49–50
during employee evaluation, F52–53, F560–61
with managers, F50–52
insertion, muscular, **F103**, **F123**
insertion, of muscle, **107**, **120**
inspections, by OSHA, 49, 167
instruction manuals, for autoclaves, 46
instructors, of esthetics, 9
instrument lubrication, 38
instruments
lubrication of, 38
positioning of, 41
storage of, 28–29, 47
insulators, **F146**, **F160**
insulin, F169–70, **337**, **344**
insulin-like growth factor (IGF-I), **70**, **83**
insurance issues
coverage, F578, F581, **754**, **762**
equipment insurability, 439
hair removal and, 516
Health Insurance Portability and Accountability Act (HIPAA), F27, **13**, **15**, 566
IPL treatments and, 177
LASER treatments and, 158, 165, 505, 507
liabilities, F266, F557, 516, **752**, **762**
malpractice, F266
intake forms, F39–40, **F577**, F606, **F606**, **F616**
integrators, 44
integrins, **75**, **83**
integumentary system, **F120**, **F123**, F191–92, **F208**. *See also* skin
Intense Pulsed Light (IPL treatments), F159, F407–**8**, **F442**, F452
before and after, *173f*, *178f*, *448f*
autoimmune disorders and, 441
contraindications for, 443–48
cut-off filter for, *176f*
facials with, 440–48, *444f–448f*
Fitzpatrick skin typing scale and, 442, *442f*
hair removal and, 503–16, *504t*, *510f–512f*
hirsutism and, 100
hydroquinone and, **442**, **474**
insurance issues and, 177
Lume 1 device for, *176f*, *441f*
lupus and, 443
overview of, **176**–77, *177f*
physics of, *441f*
pregnancy and, 443
rejuvenation procedures using, 440–48, *444f–448f*
safety and, *171t–172t*
telangiectasias and, **96**
intercellular cement, F192–**93**, **F208**
intercellular space, *68f*
intercostal muscles, **111**, **120**
interferon, *23t*
interleukin-1 (IL-1), **61**, **83**
interleukin-2 (IL-2), **83**
intermediate filaments, **61**, **83**
internal carotid artery, **F115**, **F123**
internal effects on skin, F243
internal jugular vein, **F116**, **F123**
internal obliques, **112**, **120**
internal phase, **259**, **280**
Internal Revenue Service (IRS), F564, 13, 22, 755–57, 759, 762
International Spa Association (ISPA), 8, 565
International Therapy Examination Council, 14
Internet, 774–76, **775**, **779**
interstitial fluids, **F117**, **F123**
interventions. *See* medical interventions

interviews
arranging, F544–45
checklists for, *F545f–546f*
information, **F542**–43, **F569**, F606–7
job searches and, F542–49
legal aspects of, F549
preparing for, F545–47
professional appearance, F21–23, *F547f*, F553
survival tips, F547–49
intestinal epithelial cells, *61f*
intestines, *F165f*
intuitive awareness, 12
inventory, *F585f*
inventory control, F585
inventory of personal characteristics and technical skills, forms for, *F534f*
inverted triangle face shape, F486
involuntary muscles, F103, F124
iodides, F228
iodine, *F174t*, F181–82
ionization, *F152t*, **F160**, **F388**, **F396**
ions, **F388**, **F396**
ionto mask, F390
iontophoresis, **F152**, *F152t*, **F160**, **F385**, **F388**, F389, **F396**, F455
IPL treatments. *See* Intense Pulsed Light
iron, *F174t*, F181
iron oxides, 536
irradiance, **163**, **182**
irritant contact dermatitis, F218, F220, 33
irritation, *F242t*
IRS. *See* Internal Revenue Service
ischemia, **332**, **344**
islet of Langerhans, in the pancreas, **63**, **83**
isolates, **284**, **304**
isoprene units, **150**, **154**
isopropyl alcohol, F75, **256**, 267, **280**
isotypes, **245**, *245f*, *246f*, **248**
isovolemic, 701
ISPA. *See* International Spa Association
ITIN. *See* Individual Tax Identification Number

J

Japanese esthetics, F6
Japanese green tea extract, 275, *275f*
jasmine, *F272t*
jasper, 617, *617f*
jawline, F487–89
Jessner's solution, **F447**, **F465**, 375–80, *378f–380f*, 705
JNK, **70**, **83**
job descriptions, **F557**–60, *F559f–560f*, **F569**, **F588**, **F598**
job searches
application forms, F549–52, *F550f–552f*
employment applications, F549–52, *F550f–552f*
interviews, F542–49
job descriptions, **F557**–60, *F559f–560f*, **F569**, **F588**, **F598**
networking, **F544**, **F569**
options, F541–42
questions to ask, F540–41
jobs. *See* careers
joints, F99–**100**, **F123**
jojoba, **F271**, *F271t*, **F292**, 255, 270, 578, 638
joules, **163**, **182**, **513**, **517**
journalists, F13
journals, F14
jugular veins, F116
junctions (cellular bonds), 73

K

K (kilowatts), **F149**, **F160**
kansa vataki, **655**, **656**
kaolin, 578
Kapha dosha, **632**, 636–37, **656**
karma, **657**
keloids, **F216**, **F231**
kelp, 288, *288f*
Kerastick, *452f*
keratin proteins, **60**, **83**
keratin sulfate, **67**, **83**
keratinocytes, **F195–96**, **F208**, **F222**, **F231**, **60**–62, *62t*, 65–66, **83**
keratinocytoblasts, **66**, **83**
keratins, F70, **F196**, F199, **F208**, **61**, 66, **83**
keratohyaline granules, **66**, **83**
keratolysis, F446
keratolytics, F265, **271**, **280**
keratoma, **F221**–22, **F231**
keratosis, **F222**, **F231**, **F242**, *F242t*, **F251**
actinic, **217**, *217f*, **233**
hyperkeratosis, **F222**, **F231**
keratosis pilaris, **F222**, **F231**, 93, **102**, **224**, *224f*, **233**
retention hyperkeratosis, **F226**, **F232**, **218**, 255
seborrheic, **217**, **234**
Kett Jett, *549f*
khite, **517**
ki, 242
killer T cells, **73**
kilowatts (K), **F149**, **F160**
Kirlian photography, *605f*
Kirlian, Semyon, 605
Kirlian, Valentina, 605
Kligman, Albert M., 242
Kligman rosacea classification, 242, *242t*
Kneipp body wraps, **591**, **599**
Kneipp, Sebastian, 7
kojic acid, **F271**, *F271t*, **F292**
Krebs cycle, 59
kundalini, **657**

L

La Gasse, Antoinette, F446
labeling
of cosmetic ingredients, 277–78, *308f*
of devices, 440
Federal Packaging and Labeling Act (1977), 668
for infection control, 43
private, F10
lacrimal bones, *F100f*, **F101**, **F123**
lactic acid, **271**, **280**, 705
lakes, **F262**, **F292**
lamellar bilayer, 75
lamellar bodies, 75
lancets, F323, F344
Langerhans cells, **60**, 63, **83**
lanolin, **F268**, *F268t*, **F292**
lanugo, **F403**, **F442**
large full lips, F493
large intestine, *F165f*
large macules, F221
large mushroom electrodes, *F392t*
LASER. *See* Light Amplification by Stimulation Emission of Radiation
Laser Safety Officer (LSO), **165**, **182**
laser-generated air contaminates (LGAC), **169**, **182**
lash and brow brushes, F479
lash combs, F498
lash curlers, F498
lash tinting, F517–20
lashes. *See* eyelashes
lateral, **109**, **120**
latex sensitivity, 33–34
latissimus dorsi muscles, **F106**, **F123**, **112**, **120**
laughter, F26
laundry, F309
laundry hampers, F301
lauric acid, *148f*
lavender, *F271t–272t*, **F292**, 296, *296f*, 706
laws. *See* government regulation; legal considerations
layered masks, 388
LDLs (low-density lipoproteins), F171
leadership, F590
Leaky Aura Syndrome, **604**, **626**
leases, F581
LED. *See* Light-Emitting Diode
legal considerations. *See also* government regulation
estheticians and, 21, 302, 439, 516
illegal drugs, F204
of interviews, F549
laws, F62
lawsuits, F581–82
legal counsel and, *F580f*
privacy, F27, 13, 566–67, 572
legs
muscles of, 114–16, *115f*, *116t*
soothing treatment for, 591, *592f–595f*
waxing of, F431–32
lemon, *F272t*
lemon balm, *F272t*
lemongrass, *F272t*
lentigenes, **F221**, **F231**
lentigo, **F221**, **F231**
lepas, **657**
leprosy, 7
lesions
defined, **F214**, **F231**
primary, **F214**–15, **F232**
secondary, **F214**–16, **F232**
vascular, F214
lesser occipital nerve, *F112f*, **F113**, **F125**
leukemia, **126**, **136**
leukocytes, F115, F126, **64**, **83**, **125**, **136**
leukoderma, **F221**, **F231–32**
levator anguli oris muscles, **F105**, **F123**, *F367f*
levator labii superioris muscles, **F105**, **F123**, *F367f*
LGAC. *See* laser-generated air contaminates
LGFB (Look Good . . . Feel Better) public service program, F15, F470
LH. *See* luteinizing hormone
liabilities, F266, F557, 516, **752**, **762**
Licensed Practical Nurse (LPN), 667
licensing, F25, 10, 165, 663–67
licensure tests, F529–33
licorice, **F271**, *F271t*, F276, **F292**
life skills
guidelines for success, F28–29
professional image and, F28–31
setting goals, F23, F29, *F30f*, F41
time management, F30–31
lifestyle
client, F43–44
effect on skin, F204
ligaments, F99
ligature, **129**, **136**
light. *See also* Light Amplification by Stimulation Emission of Radiation
amber, F452
blue, **F157**, F159, **F160**, F452

light *(continued)*
coherent, **160**, *160f*, **182**
collimated, **160**, *160f*, 162
electricity and, F154–59
green, F159
infrared rays, F155–57, **F156**, **F160**, F452, 158
monochromatic, **160**, **182**, **503**, **517**
overview of, F154–55
red, **F157**, F159, **F160**, F452
therapy, **F156**, F159, **F160**, **F452**–53, **F465**
ultraviolet rays, F155–57, **F156**, *F157t*, **F161**, F203–5, 158–59, 312–13
vascular light treatment, *172f*
visible light rays, **F155**, F157, **F161**
visible spectrum of, *159f*
white, **F157**, **F161**
yellow, F159
Light Amplification by Stimulation Emission of Radiation (LASER), **F158**, **F160**, **F451**–52, **F465**
client consultations before, 507–8, *508f*
complications of, 515–16, *516t*
in contact with eye, 167, *167f*
contraindications for, *506t*
with cooling device, *164f*
defined, **158**–59, *158f*
devices, types of, *175t*, *513f*
disorders of skin from, 210
Er:YAG laser devices and, 172–73, *175t*
filtration masks and, *169f*
Fitzpatrick skin typing scale and, 491, *506t*, 507
goggles for, *168f*
hair removal and, F158, F407–**8**, **F442**, 503–16, *504t*, *510f–512f*
hirsutism and, 100
hydroquinone and, **738**, **744**
hyperpigmentation and, 210–14, *210f*, *515f*
insurance issues and, 158, 165, 505, 507
Laser Safety Officer, **165**, **182**
laser technicians, *F11f*
laser-generated air contaminates (LGAC), **169**, **182**
Nd:YAG laser devices and, F452, 160–63, *175t*, 504, 513–14, 739
OSHA and, 164–65, 167, 169–71
physics of, 158–63, *161f*
Q-switched devices, 173–75, *174t*, *175f*, *175t*
resurfacing, **F463**, **F465**, **744**
safety and, 165–72, *167f*, *171t–172t*, 504–5, *505f*
side effects of, 515–16, *515t*
tattoo removal and, *174f*, *174t*
telangiectasias and, 96
therapy and, 172–75, *509t*
treatment consequences, 514, *514t*
window coverings near, *167f*
light and energy devices, 158
light peels, F446–47
Light-Emitting Diode (LED), F159, F452, *F453f*
contraindications for, 449
defined, **448**, **474**
devices for, **180**–81, **182**
treatments using, 449, *449f–451f*
lightening treatment gels, 317
lightening treatments, F241, F263–64
limbic system, **291**, **304**
linens, F78, F414
linoleic acid, **F170**, **F185**
lip brushes, F479
lip gloss, F500
lip liner, F479, F501
lipases, **64**, **83**
lipid bilayer, **57**, **83**
lipid compounds, 76
lipid peroxides, **274**, **280**
lipid replacement, 267
lipid serum, 316
lipids, **F170**–72, **F185**, **F192**–93, **F195**, F203, **F208**, **F263**, **F292**, 144
lipolysis, **175**, **182**
lipophilic, **F138**–39, **F142**, **258**, **280**
lipoplasty, suction-assisted, 728–29, *728f*, *729f*
liposomes, **F264**, *F268t*, **F292**, 261
liposuction, **F463**, **F465**, **728**–29, *729f*, **730**, **744**
lips
augmentation of, *698f*, *699f*, 701
color, F478
color, permanent, 557, *558f*
corrective makeup for, F491–94
fixing fine lines around, F494
shapes of, *F493t–494t*
small, F493
special-occasion makeup, F510
thin, F493
treatments, F284, F324
uneven, F494
waxing, F428–29
lipstick, F327, *F478f*, F501
liquid foundations, F472
liquids, *F132f*, F133
listening skills, F37, F610
liver, *F165f*
local infections, **F66**, **F89**
location, of salon/spa, F574–75
logarithmic scale, **F135**, **F142**
logs
for disinfectants, F308
for treatments, F41
long face, F492
long heavy chin, F488
long-term goals, F29
Look Good . . . Feel Better (LGFB) public service program, F15, F470
lotion cleansers, *265f*, 268, *308f*
loupes, *F237f*, F248, F300, F378–79
low forehead, F492
low-density lipoproteins (LDLs), F171
Lozanov, Georgi, 598
LPN. *See* Licensed Practical Nurse
LSO. *See* Laser Safety Officer
lubricants, **F258**, **F292**
lubrication, of instruments, 38
Lucas sprayers, **F393**–94, **F397**
Lume 1 device, for IPL treatments, *176f*
lung disorders, 333, *333t*
lungs, **F119**, **F124**
lupus
corticosteroids and, 341, *342t*
hair removal and, 479
immune system and, 72
IPL treatments and, 443
sun exposure and, 212
luteinizing hormone (LH), **92**, **102**
lymph, **F117**, **F124**, F202, **132**, **136**
lymphatic system, **F117**, **F123**
capillaries of, **F117**, **F124**
contraindications for massage of, 417–18
drainage, **133**, *134t*, **136**, 420, *420f*, *431f–433f*
lymph nodes and, F117, **F124**, **132**, **136**, *418f*, *419f*
lymph vessels and, **F197**, **F208**, **132**, *134f*, **136**
manual lymph drainage and, **F362**, F366, **F374**, F457–**58**, **F465**
massage for, 417–29, *421f–429f*
massage for, machine-aided, 430–33
overview of, 132–34, *134f*
lymphocytes, **61**, **83**, **337**, **344**
lymphocytic cells, **64**–65
lymphokines, **73**, **83**
lymphotoxins, **73**, **83**
lysis, 162
lysosomes, *57f*, **59**, 63, **83**, **337**, **344**
lysozymes, **73**, **84**

M

M (mitosis), 66, **69**, **84**
machine microdermabrasion, 362, 439, *439f*, 452–60, *453f*, *454f*, *455f–459f*
machine-aided lymphatic massage treatments, 430–33
macronutrients
carbohydrates, **F168**–70, **F184**, 143–44
defined, **F167**, **F185**
enzymes, F172
fats, F170–72, F185, 193
proteins, F167–68, **F185**
macrophage, **73**, **84**
macules, *F214f*, **F215**, F221, **F232**
magnesium, *F174t*, F181
magnifying lamps/lights, *F237f*, F248, F300, F378–79, 237
Maillard Reaction, **193**–94, **199**
maintenance
brushes, F479–80
galvanic machine, F390
high-frequency machine, F391, F393
hot towel cabinet, F380
microdermabrasion equipment, F451
rotary brush, F381
spray machine, F393
steamer, F382–84
vacuum machine, F385
major histocompatibility complex (MHC), 72
makeup. *See also* cosmetics
airbrush, F522
application tips and guidelines, F501
artificial eyelashes, F513–16
artists, F11–12, F522–23, **8**
black, F482
blending, for eyes, F475
blue, F482
blush, F474–75
bridal, F510, *9f*
brown, F482
brushes, F479–80
cake, **F472**, **F524**
as camouflage, F12, F511, 542–46
charts for clients, *F497t*
cheek and lip color, F484
client consultations, F494–98
color theory, F480–82
colors for eyes, F484
concealers, F473
corrective, *F483t*, F487–94
eye shadow, F475–76, *F475f*, F500
eyebrow color, F477
eyelash extensions, F521, 521–25, *521f*, *523f*, *524f*, *525f–529f*
eyelash perming, F521, 531–32, *532f–535f*
eyeliners, F476–77, F500, 557
face powders, F473–74, *F473f*, F500
face shapes and proportions, F485–87
foundation, F471–73, F500

hair color, F485
lash and brow tinting, F517–20
lip color, F478
lip liner, F479, 501
mascara, F477–78, 500
mineral, F472, 535–39, *538f*, *539f–541f*, 541
overview of, F467–70
permanent, F521–22, 9, 554–59, *555f*, *557f*, *558f*
products, F500–501
professional application of, F502–8
psychological aspects of, F470–71
questionnaires on, for clients, **F496**, *F496t*, **F577**, **F606**, **F616**
removers, F277
retailing, F512
reviewing color selections, F485
sanitation, and application of, F498, F508
self-esteem and, F28–29, F470
services, F471
special-occasions, F509–11
stations, *F471f*
supplies and accessories, F498–99
undereye, 317, 542–45, 550
malar bones, *F100f*, F101, F126
malas, **657**
male issues
Brazilian waxing for men, 503
client consultations and, F354
eyebrows, F420, 501, *501f*, *502f*
facials for men, F354–56
hormones, F227–28
melasma in male patient, *96f*
professional treatments, F355–56
reproductive organs, *91f*
skin care for men, F354–55
waxing, F438–40
malic acid, **271**, **280**
malignant, F222
malignant melanoma, **F224**, **F232**
malpractice insurance, F266
mammaplasty, **F463**, **F465**, **730**
management skills, F583
managers, F12–13, F50–52, 10
mandala, **657**
mandible, *F100f*, **F101**, **F124**, **110**
mandibular nerve, **F110**, F112, **F124**, **77**, **84**
manganese, *F175t*, F181
manners, F553, F596
Mantaux (skin test), 25
mantra, **657**
manual lymph drainage (MLD), **F362**, F366, **F374**, F457–**58**, **F465**
manual microdermabrasion, 362, *362f*, *363f–366f*
manuals
for employees, **F588**, **F598**
for use of autoclaves, 46
manufacturers, 9
manufacturer's representatives, F12
MAOIs. *See* monoamine oxidase inhibitors
MAPK. *See* mitosis activating protein
marigold, 288, *288f*
marionette lines, 695
maritime pine extract, 275
marketing, **F608**–9, **F616**
business plans and, 750–51
defined, **767**, **779**
direct, **772**, **779**
freelance consultants, *F608f*
plan, *768f*, **774**, **779**
marmas, of Ayurveda
benefits of, *640t–641t*, *643f–648f*
facial massage and, **639**–40, *640f*, 655–**56**
mascara, F477–78, F500
MASER. *See* Microwave Amplification by Stimulation Emission of Radiation
mask of pregnancy, F221, *95f*
masking fragrances, 264
masks
algae, F282
benefits of, F280
body masks, **F455**, F458, **F465**, **576**–77, **599**
changes due to, *382f*
clay, **F281**–82, **F291**, F354
creams for, F281
custom-designed, F283
defined, **F280**, **F292**
dry collagen sheets, 358, 383, *384f*
for dry skin, 318
electric heat, F395
for facials, F324
filtration masks, for LASER treatment, *169f*
functions of, *382t*
gel, F281
homemade, F283
layered, 388
modelage masks, **F282**–83, **F292**
non-setting, F281
paraffin wax masks, **F282**–83, **F292**, F348–49
powder, 384, *384f–386f*
rubber-type, 387–88, *387f*
seaweed, F282
setting, F281
sheet masks, collagen, F281, 383, *383f*, *384f*
sulfur, F352, F354
therapies using, 352, 381–88
thermal, **F282**–83, **F292**
for treatments, F324
wet collagen sheets, 358, 383, *383f*
massage, F323, F355, **F360**, F365, **F374**. *See also* facial massage; Shiatsu massage
for back, 400–401, *400f*, *401f*
chi and, 243
contraindications for, F362, 393
creams for, F285, F367
essential oils and, 298–300
government regulation of, F362
for lymphatic system, 417–29, *421f–429f*
for lymphatic system, machine-aided, 430–33
for neck, 396–400, *397f*, *398f*, *399f*, *400f*
for pressure points, F366
skin penetration and, F194, 75–76
stones and, **F456**, **F466**, 410–17, *410f*, *412f–417f*
stress and, 393
tables for, 567
treatment variations and, 351
masseter, **F104**, **F124**
mast cells, **63**–64, **84**
mastectomy, **724**, **730**
mastication, muscles for, F104
mastopexy
defined, **722**, **730**
overview of, 721–23, *722f*, *723f*
matching questions, F532
material compatibility, 40
Material Safety Data Sheets (MSDS), **F59**–61, **F89**, 49
matte, **F473**, **F524**
matter, **F130**–34, **F142**
and chemistry, F130–34
maturation phase, 206, *206f*
maturation promoting factor (MPF), **69**, **84**
mature skin
antioxidants and, F275–76
hormones and, F206–7
treatments for, F346–47
maxilla, **110**
maxillary bones, *F100f*, **F101**, **F124**
maxillary nerve, **F110**, *F112f*, **F124**, **77**, **84**
Maximum Permissible Exposure (MPE), **165**–66, **182**
mechanical exfoliation, **F279**, **F292**, 270
MED. *See* minimal erythemal dose
median nerve, *F112f*, **F113**, **F124**
medical asepsis, 29
medical estheticians, F11, **9**, 663–64, 691–92
medical esthetics, **F11**, **F17**, F460–64, 663–70
medical interventions
botulinum toxin, **693**–96, *694f*, *695f*, *696f*, **708**
defined, 691–93
dermal fillers, 696–702, *696f*, *698f*, *700f*, *702f*
medical peels, *F447f*, F461, 704–7, *705f*, *706f*, *706t*
medical micropigmentation, 555
medical peels, *F447f*, F461, 704–7, *705f*, *706f*, *706t*
medical records, 13, 669
medical referrals
for injuries, 210
for skin disorders, 204, 212, 216, 232
Medical Spa Association, 14
Medical Spa Report, 14
medical spas, F10, *F535f*, F542, 565–66, **665**, **671**
medical terminology
basics of, 677–78
history of, 675–77
plurals, 677–78, *677t*, **683**, **687**
prefixes, **675**, 683–84, **687**
pronunciation, **685**–86, *686t*, **687**
root words, **675**, *675f*, *677t*, *678t*, **687**
suffixes, **675**, *675f*, *677t*, 683–85, **687**
word analysis in, **676**, *678t*, *679f–682f*, **687**
medicated cleansers, for acne, *F229t*, 309
medications, of clients, 326, 443. *See also* drugs
medi-spas. *See* medical spas
meditation, 13, 608
medium peels, F446
meeting clients, F39, F317
Meissner's corpuscle, **78**, **84**
melanin, **F193**, **F200**–201, F203, **F208**, 62, 95, 271, 505
melanocytes, **F197**, **F200**, **F208**, 60, **62**, *62f*, **84**
melanocyte-stimulating hormone (MSH), **62**, **84**
melanogenesis, **62**, **84**
melanomas, *F223t*, *F224f*, 214–15, 443
melanosomes, F200, **F240**, **F251**, **62**, *62f*, **84**
melasma, **F120**, **F124**, **F221**, **F232**
birth control pills and, 97–98
hormones and, F120
in male patient, *96f*
as mask of pregnancy, F221, *95f*
melissa, *F272t*
membrane, cell, **F96**, **F122**, 57–58, **80**, 85–86
memory, and scent, 291
memory T cells, **73**, **84**
men. *See* male issues
menarche, **94**, **102**

menopause, F405, **98**–99, **102**, 223
menstrual cycle, 94–95, *94f*, *95f*
menstruation, **94**, **102**
mental body, **605**–7, **626**
mental chatter, **606**, **626**
mental disorders, 335–37, *335t*
mental focus, F361
mental nerve, **F111**, *F112f*, **F124**
mentalis muscles, **F105**, **F124**, *F367f*
mentoplasty, **718**, **730**
menu of services, **774**–75, *775f*, **779**
Merkel cells, F197
Merkel, Friedrich Sigmund, 78
Merkel's discs, **78**, **84**
mesenchymal tissue, **63**, **84**
mesoderm, **70**–72, **84**
mesotherapy, F459
metabolic akalosis, **341**, **344**
metabolism
  of cells, **F97**, **F124**, F264–65, **146**, **154**, **329**, 410
  nutrition and, **189**–90
metabolites, **146**, *147t*, **154**
metacarpus, **F102**, **F124**
metal bone pins/plates, *F245t*
metal salts, **F262**, **F291**
metamorphosed, **410**, **434**
methicillin-resistant *staphylococcus aureus* (MRSA), **F66**, **F89**, 31–32
methyl cellulose, 263
methylparaben, **F268**, *F268t*, **F292**
MHC. *See* major histocompatibility complex
mica, 536
micelle, **260**, **280**
micellized, **260**, **280**
micro thermal zones (MTZ), **173**, *173f*, **182**
microampere, **469**, **474**
microbes, *F63t*. *See also* bacteria
microbiology, 26
microcirculation, F206
microcomedones, *F227f*, 218
microcrystals, F450–51
microcurrent facial toning, **F153**, **F160**, **F454**, **F466**
  contraindications for, 469–70
  devices for, *469f*
  overview of, 469
  treatments using, *470t*, *471f–472f*
microdermabrasion, *F11f*, F446, **F450**–51, F461, **F466**
  contraindications for, 454
  diamond, 453–54, *454f*
  machine, 362, 439, *439f*, 452–60, *453f*, *454f*, *455f–459f*
  manual, 362, *362f*, *363f–366f*
microencapsulation, **260**, 275, **280**
microfilaments, **60**, **84**
micrometer, **159**, **182**
micronutrients
  defined, **F172**, **F185**
  fat-soluble, *F173t–174t*, F175–78
  overview of, F172–75
  water-soluble, *F173–74t*, F178–80
microorganisms, **F62**–63, **F89**, 26–27, 40
micropigmentation, F460, 555
microsponge, **261**, **280**
microtubules, **60**, **84**
Microwave Amplification by Stimulation Emission of Radiation (MASER), **158**, **182**
Middle Ages esthetics, F6–7
middle temporal artery, *F115f*, **F116**, **F124**
mignonette tree, F6
Milady/Cengage Learning, 14
Milady's Skin Care and Cosmetic Ingredients Dictionary, F273
milia, **F217**, **F232**, *F242t*
miliaria rubra, **F218**, **F232**
milk cleansers, 308–10
milliamperes, **F149**, **F160**
mineral makeup, F472, 535–39, *538f*, *539f–541f*, 541
mineral oil, F258, **F268**, *F268t*, **F292**, 254
mineral waters, 7
minerals, *F173–75t*, **F180**–81, **F185**
mini-facials, F345
minimal erythemal dose (MED), F244
mini-meditation, 608
mint, *F271t*
miscible liquids, **F137**, **F142**
mission statement, 14
mitochondria, **58**, 59, **84**
mitosis, F65, **F96**–**97**, **F124**, 66, **69**, *69f*, **84**
mitosis activating protein (MAPK), **70**, **84**
mixed nerves, F110
MLD. *See* manual lymph drainage
modalities, **F151**–54, **F160**
modelage masks, **F282**–83, **F292**
moderately active, F181
modesty towels, *572f*
modifies, **676**, **687**
modulate, **180**, **182**
Mohs, Frederic, 214
Mohs' surgery, 214
moist heat unit, **584**, *584f*, **599**
moisturizing products, for dry skin, F263, **F284**–85, **F292**, F324, 270
moisturizing properties, F273
molecular structure, of water, *142f*
molecular weight, **140**
molecules, **F131**–32, **F142**
moles, F221, **F221**, **F222**, *F224f*, **F232**, 214–17
money management, F564–65, F582
monoamine oxidase inhibitors (MAOIs), **336**, **344**
monochromatic light, **160**, **182**, **503**, **517**
monocytes, 64–**65**, **84**, **136**
monopolar radio-frequency (RF) energy, **178**, *179f*, **182**
monosaccharides, **F168**, **F185**, **144**, **154**
monounsaturated fats, F170
monounsaturated fatty acids, **148**, **154**
monthly records, F585
mood, 12
moodiness, 99
Moors, 7
morphology, of hair, F401–3
mortuary science, F12
mother cells, **60**, **84**
motility, **F65**, **F89**
motor nerves, **F110**, **F124**, F200, **77**, **84**
motor neuron, **70**, **77**, **84**
motor points, *F366f*
mouth, muscles of, F105–6, 109–10, *109t*, *110f*
MPE. *See* Maximum Permissible Exposure
MPF. *See* maturation promoting factor
MSDS. *See* Material Safety Data Sheets
MSH. *See* melanocyte-stimulating hormone
MSRA. *See* methicillin-resistant staphylococcus aureus
MTZ. *See* micro thermal zones
mucolytic properties, 292
mucopolysaccharides, F168, **F185**, **F268**, *F268t*, **F292**, 268
mucosa, **206**, **233**
mucous membrane, **27**–28, **51**
mud therapy, 6, *7f*, *577t*, *591f*
multifunctional machines, F301, F378, F395
multiple choice questions, F531–32
muscles
  adductors, **115**–16, **119**
  of arms, F106–7, 112–14, *113f*, *114f*, *114t*
  arrector pili, **F194**, *F195f*, F200, **F208**, **F402**, *F403f*, **F441**
  auricularis anterior, **F103**, *F104f*, **F121**
  auricularis posterior, **F103**, *F104f*, **F121**
  auricularis superior, **F103**, *F104f*, **F121**
  buccinator, **F105**, **F121**, *F367f*
  caninus, **F105**, **F123**, *F367f*
  cardiac, **F103**, **F122**, **105**, *106f*
  corrugator, **F104**, *F105f*, **F122**, *F367f*
  defined, **F102**, **F124**
  depressor labii inferioris, **F105**, **F122**, *F367f*
  of ears, F103–4
  of eyebrows, F104
  of eyes, 108–9, *109f*
  of face and head, *F367f*, 108–11, *109f*, *110f*, *470f*
  of feet, 116–17, *116f*, *116t*
  fibers of, **105**, **120**
  fibularis, **117**, **119**
  frontalis, *F367f*
  gluteus, **115**, **120**
  hamstrings, **116**, **120**
  of hands, F107
  of head and face, *F367f*, 108–11, *109f*, *110f*
  intercostal, **111**, **120**
  involuntary, F103, F124
  latissimus dorsi, **F106**, **F123**, **112**, **120**
  of legs, 114–16, *115f*, *116t*
  levator anguli oris, **F105**, **F123**, *F367f*
  levator labii superioris, **F105**, **F123**, *F367f*
  for mastication, F104
  mentalis, **F105**, **F124**, *F367f*
  of mouth, F105–6, 109–10, *109t*, *110f*
  of neck, F104, 111, *112f*
  nonstriated, **F103**, **F124**
  of nose, F104–5, 108–9, *110f*, 111
  obicularis oculi, **F104**, *F105f*, **F124**, *F367f*, 470, *470t*, *471f–472f*, **716**
  obicularis oris, **F105**, **F124**, *F367f*
  origins of, F103, **F124**, **107**
  overview of, F102–3
  pectoralis major, **F106**, **F125**, **111**
  pectoralis minor, **F106**, **F125**
  procerus, **F104**, *F105f*, **F125**, *F367f*
  quadratus, **F105**, **F123**, *F367f*
  quadratus labii inferioris, **F105**, **F122**, *F367f*
  quadriceps, **116**, **120**
  risorius, **F105**, **F125**, *F367f*
  of scalp, F103
  serratus anterior, **F106**, **F125**
  of shoulders, F106–7
  skeletal, F103, F125, **106**, *106f*, 106–7
  smooth, F103, F124, **106**, *106f*
  sternocleidomastoids, **F104**, **F125**, *F367f*, **111**, **120**
  striated, **F103**, **F125**
  temporalis, **F104**, **F126**
  tissue of, **F97**, **F124**, **72**, **84**
  triangularis, **F105**, **F126**, *F367f*
  of trunk, 111–12
  types of, *106f*
  visceral, F103, F124
  voluntary, F103, F125
  zygomaticus major and minor, **F105**, **F126**, *F367f*, *470t*
music therapy, 597–98
music volume, 12
Mycobacterium fortuitum furunculosis, F66

mycobacterium tuberculosis, 41, 52
myelin, **72**, **84**
myeloperoxidase, **64**, **84**
myocardial ischemia, **331**, **344**
myocardium, **126**, **136**
myofilaments, **105**, **120**
myosin, **60**, **84**
myrrh, F5, *F272t*

N

N (nitrogen), **F134**, **F142**
nabhi, **657**
nadi, **657**
nail brushes, F304
nails, F21, F199
nanometer, **159**, **182**
nanoparticle technology, 261
nanotechnology, **F9**, **F17**
nare, **111**, **120**
narrow face, F488
narrow forehead, F488
nasal bones, *F100f*, **F101**, **F124**
nasal nerve, **F111**, *F112f*, **F124**
nasal turbinates, **717**, **731**
NASHA. *See* Non-animal Stabilized Hyaluronic Acid
nasolabial folds, *699f*, 701, **712**, **731**
nasolabial lines, **692**, *692f*, **708**
National Accrediting Commission of Cosmetology Arts and Sciences, 14
National Coalition of Estheticians, Manufacturers/Distributors & Associations (NCEA), F26, 14, 158
National Cosmetology Association, 14
National Organic Program, of FDA, 286
National Rosacea Society, 229, 231
National-Interstate Council of State Boards of Cosmetology, 14
natural immunity, **F70**, **F89**
natural ingredients, *F270–71t*, *F273t*
natural moisturizing factors (NMFs), **267**, **280**
natural oils, *255f*, 270
natural rubber latex (NRL), 34
NCEA. *See* National Coalition of Estheticians, Manufacturers/Distributors & Associations
NCEA (National Coalition of Estheticians, Manufacturers/Distributors & Associations), F26
Nd:YAG lasers, F452, 160–63, *175t*, 504, 513–14, 739
neck
- blood supply of, F115–16
- chin/neck bra, **743**
- corrective makeup for, F487–89
- creams for, 318
- massage for, 396–400, *397f*, *398f*, *399f*, *400f*
- muscles of, F104, 111, *112f*
- nerves of, F110–13
- skeletal system and, F101–2
- strips for, F499

necrosis, **700**, **708**, 712
negative emotions, 13
negative nonverbal cues, F38
neoprene, 34
nepotism, 669–70
neroli, *F272t*, 296, *297f*
nerve impulse, *107f*
nerve tissue, **F97**, **F124**
nerves, **F110**, **F124**, F200
- afferent, F110, F125, F193–94, *F195f*, F200
- of arms, F113
- cervical, **F112**, **F122**
- cranial, F110–13, F122–23, F125, 117–18, *117f*
- efferent, **F110**, **F124**, F200
- of face, F110–13, 117–18
- of hands, F113
- of head, F110–13
- mixed, F110
- motor, **F110**, **F124**, F200, **77**, **84**
- sensory, **F110**, **F125**, F193–94, *F195f*, F200, 77–78, **86**
- of skin, F200
- types of, F110

nervous system
- anatomy of, F107–13
- arms, F113
- autonomic, **F108**, **F121**, **77**, **80**
- brain, **F109**–10, F121
- brain stem, **F109**, **F121**
- central, **F107**, *F108f*, **F122**
- defined, **F107**, **F124**
- hands, F113
- head and neck, F110–13
- nerve cells, F110
- parasympathetic divisions of, **F108**, **F125**, **77**, **85**
- peripheral, **F108**, **F125**
- somatic, F108
- spinal cord, F109–**10**, **F125**
- sympathetic, **77**, **86**
- sympathetic divisions of, **F108**, **F126**, **77**, **86**
- tissue of, **F97**, **F124**, **72**, **84**
- types of nerves, F110

net profit, **752**, **762**
networking, **F544**, **F569**
neural crest, **62**, **70**, **84**
neural tube, **70**, **84**
neurofilaments, **61**, **84**
neuroglia, **72**, **85**
neuromuscular junction, **106**, **120**
neurons, **F110**, **F124**, **85**, **106**
neurotransmitters, **106**, **120**, **192**, **199**
neutrophils, **64**, *64f*, **85**, **136**
nevus, F221, **F221**, **F232**
Nevus of Ota, **175**, **182**
new clients, F39
NHZ. *See* nominal hazard zone
niacin, *F173t*, F178
niaouli, 297, *297f*
nicotine, F204
night creams and treatments, 314–15
Nikolski sign, **508**, **517**
ninth cranial nerve (CN IX), *F111f*
nitrile, 34
nitrile gloves, **F83**, **F89**
nitrogen (N), **F134**, **F142**
nmfs. *See* natural moisturizing factors
nodules, *F214f*, **F215**, **F232**
nominal hazard zone (NHZ), **166**, **182**
nonablative, **F461**, **F466**, **440**, **474**
non-acnegenic, **255**, **280**
Non-animal Stabilized Hyaluronic Acid (NASHA), 697, **701**, **708**
non-cancerous growths, 216–18
non-certified colors, **F262**, **F292**, 263
non-comedogenic, F256, **255**, **280**
nonconductors, **F146**, **F160**
nonessential amino acids, **F167**, **F185**
nonimmunogenic, **697**, **708**
nonpathogenic bacteria, **F63**, **F89**
non-setting masks, F281
nonstriated muscles, **F103**, **F124**
nonverbal cues, F38
nonvolatile, **285**, **304**
norepinephrine, **336**, **344**
normal flora, 26
normal skin, F238
normoblast, **71**, **85**
nose
- deviated nasal septum, **717**, **730**
- muscles of, F104–5, 108–9, *110f*, 111
- nasal bones, *F100f*, **F101**, **F124**
- nasal nerve, **F111**, *F112f*, **F124**
- nasal turbinates, **717**, **731**
- rhinoplasty and, **F463**, **F466**, **717**–18, *718f*, **731**
- short, F488
- wide, F488

nosocomial infections, 27
notice of privacy practices, 13
noun, **683**, *683t*, **687**
nourishing creams, F284–85
nourishment, skin, F202
Les Nouvelles Esthetique Magazine, 14
NRL. *See* natural rubber latex
nuclear membrane, of cells, **59**, **85**
nuclei, **F96**, **F124**
nucleolus, of cells, **59**, **85**
nucleoplasm, **F96**, **F124**
nucleus, of cells, **59**, *59f*, **85**
nurse training, 667
nutrition
- acne and, 225–26
- aging and, 193–95
- energy nutrients, **189**, *190f*, **199**
- esthetics and, F182–83
- free radicals and, **190**
- macronutrients and, **F167**–72, **F184**, **F185**, 143–44, 193
- metabolism and, **189**–90
- micronutrients, **F172**–80, *F173t–174t*, **F185**
- minerals, *F173–75t*, F180–81, F185
- recommendations for proper, F165–67
- scope of practice, for estheticians, and, 193
- skin and, F167
- stress and, 190–93
- water, F183
- wound healing and, 209–10

O

O (ohms), **F149**, **F160**
O (oxygen), **F134**, **F142**
O_3 (ozone), F381, F384
oatmeal, *F271t*, *F273t*
obesity, F182, 100
obicularis oculi muscles, **F104**, *F105f*, **F124**, *F367f*, 470, *470t*, *471f–472f*, **716**
obicularis oris muscles, **F105**, **F124**, *F367f*
obliquely, **109**, **120**
oblong face shape, F486
obsessive-compulsive disorder (OCD), **336**, **344**
occipital artery, *F115f*, **F116**, **F124**
occipital bone, **F100**, **F124**
occipitalis, F103, *F104f*, **F124**
occlusion, F257
occlusives, **F238**, **F251**, F346, 269
occupational diseases, *F64t*
Occupational Safety and Health Act of 1970, 21
Occupational Safety and Health Administration (OSHA), F59, F61, F68, F74, F84, F578
- current information on, 14
- guidelines of, **21**–22, **51**, 559
- HIV and, 21–23
- infection control and, 21–22
- inspections by, 49, 167
- LASER regulation by, 164–65, 167, 169–71

OCD. *See* obsessive-compulsive disorder
ocular protection, 167–68
ocular rosacea, **230**, *231f*, **233**
oculomotor nerve, *F111f*
OD. *See* optical density
office culture, 669
ohms (O), **F149**, **F160**
oil glands, **F194**, *F195f*, **F201**–2, **F208**, F216–17
oil soluble substances, **F260**, **F292**
oil-based blush, F475
oil-based foundations, F471
oil-based moisturizers, F284
oil-in-water emulsions, *F137f*, **F138**–39, **F142**, F228, 259–60, 266, 270
oils, F258
oily skin, F238–39, F351
  acne and, 218, 226
  cleansers for, 308–10
  facials for, F351
  sebaceous hyperplasias and, 217
  toners for, 266–67, 311–12
ojas, **657**
oleic acid, *148f*
olfaction, **290**, **304**
olfactory nerve, *F111f*, *290f*
olfactory system, **F274**, **F292**
olive, *F271t*
olive oil, F5
omega-3 fatty acid, **F170**–71, **F185**
omega-6 fatty acid, **F170**, **F185**
Omnilux device, *180f*
onyx, F199
open comedones, F217, *F227f*, *F242t*, F322–23, **219**, *219f*, **233**
open rhinoplasty, **718**, **731**
operator's stools, F300, F305
ophthalmic nerve, **F110**, *F112f*, **F124**, **77**, **85**
OPIM. *See* other potentially infectious materials
opportunistic mycoses, **336**, **344**
optic nerve, *F111f*
optical density (OD), **167**, **182**
optical resonator cavity, **162**, *163f*, **182**
oral prescription drugs, *327f*
orange, *F271t*, *F272t*
organelles, **58**–59, **85**
organic chemistry, **F130**, **F142**
organic compound, **140**, **154**
organisms, **26**–27, **51**
organs, **F97**, *F98t*, **F124**
Oriental reflex zones, of face, 242–45, **407**, *407f*, **434**
orifice, **109**, **120**
origins, of muscles, F103, **F124**, **107**
OSHA. *See* Occupational Safety and Health Administration
osteoarthritis, **340**, **344**
osteoporosis, **F177**, **F185**, **98**, **102**, 340, *341t*
ostium, F226, **219**, **233**
OTC. *See* over-the-counter
other potentially infectious materials (OPIM), 22, 33, 41–42, **51**
outlets, F150
oval-shaped face, F486–87
ovaries, F118, **91**, **102**
overcleaning, 225
over-the-counter (OTC), 264, 311–12, 316–17, **327**–28, *328t*, **344**
owner's equity, **752**, **762**
ownership, salon/spa, F11, F579–80, 9
oxidation, **F135**, **F142**, 262, 276
oxidation-reduction reactions, **F135**–36, **F142**
oxidize, **F136**, **F142**
oxygen (O), **F134**, **F142**, 140
oxygen, chemistry of, 140
oxygen therapy treatments, F352
oxygenated, **127**, **136**
oxygenation, F264–65
oxyhemoglobin, **161**, **182**, **511**, **517**
oxytalan, **67**, **85**
ozone (O_3), F381, F384

P

p27 protein, **69**, **85**
p53 protein, **69**, **85**
PABA, *F173t*
pacemakers, *F245t*
Pacinian corpuscles, **78**, **85**
packaging, and infection control, 42–43
packs, **F280**, **F292**
pain, drugs for, 341–42, *342t*
pain receptor, **85**
palatine bones, *F100f*, **F101**, **F124**
palettes, F499
palmarosa, 297, *297f*
palmitoyl pentapeptide-3, 276
palpebra, **109**, **120**
pancake makeup, **F472**, **F524**
panchamahabhutas, **631**, **656**
pancreas, F118, *F165f*
  hormones and, **91**, **102**
  Langerhans cells and, **63**, **83**
pantothenic acid, *F174t*, F179
papaya, **F271**, *F271t*, *F273t*, **F292**
paper-plastic combinations, 51
papillae, of hair, **F197**, **F208**, **F402**, *F403f*, **F441**
papillary layer, of dermis, **F197**, **F208**
papules, *F214f*, **F215**, *F227f*, **F232**, *F242t*, 220–23, *220f*, 225, 227, 229
papulopustular rosacea, **229**, **233**
parabens, **F268**, *F268t*, **F292**
paraffin wax heaters, F394
paraffin wax masks, **F282**–83, **F292**, F348–49
parasites, *F63t*, **F69**, **F89**, 27
parasitic diseases, *F64t*
parasympathetic divisions, **F108**, **F125**, **77**, **85**
parathyroid glands, F118, **90**, **102**
parenteral, **332**, **344**
parfum, **264**, **280**
parietal artery, *F115f*, **F116**, **F125**
parietal bones, **F100**, **F125**
parking facilities, F575
Parrish, J. A., 162
partnerships, **F579**, **F598**
patch tests, F267, 508, *508f*
patchouli, *F272t*
pathogenic, **F63**, *F64t*, **F89**
pathogenic fungi, **340**, **345**
pathogens, **26**–28, 37, 47, **52**, **337**, **345**
PCV/vinyl. *See* polyvinyl chloride
PDGF. *See* platelet-derived growth factor
PDT. *See* photodynamic therapy
pear-shaped face, F486
pectoralis major muscles, **F106**, **F125**, **111**
pectoralis minor muscles, **F106**, **F125**
pediculosis, **F69**, **F89**
peels
  AHAs, F447, F449
  Baker's, F447
  benefits of, F448
  BHAs, F447
  candidates for, F448–49
  cell renewal factor, F446–47
  contraindications for, F448
  deep *versus* light, F447
  enzyme, **F280**, **F291**, 367
  exfoliation and, F446
  glycolic, *F447f*, F461, 705
  history of, F446
  ingredients to combine with, F449
  Jessner's, **F447**, **F465**
  light, F446–47
  medical, *F447f*, F461, 704–7, *705f*, *706f*, *706t*
  medium, F446
  pH relationships, F447–48
  post-peel home care, F449–50
  safety and, F446, F448
  superficial, F446, 374–81, *375f*
  TCA, **F463**, **F466**, 705, *705f*, *706f*
Pellon, F413
pencils, eyebrow, F500
pencils, makeup, *F477f*, F498
pendulous breasts, **723**, **731**
penetration, of skin, F194, 75–76
peppermint, *F271t*, *F272t*
peptic ulcer, **333**, **345**
peptide bonds, **143**
peptides, **F245**, **F251**, **F265**, **F292**, **61**, 276
percussion, **F364**, **F374**
performance ingredients, **F256**, **F292**, 252–53, 264–72, 277
pericardium, **F113**–14, **F125**
perifollicular inflammation, **222**, **233**
perimenopause, **98**–99, **102**, 223
perimysium, **106**, **120**
periodic table of elements, *F131f*, **140**, *141f*, **154**
perioral dermatitis, **F219**, **F232**, **227**, *227f*, **233**
periorbital fat, **716**, **731**
peripheral edema, **131**, **136**
peripheral nervous system (PNS), **F108**, **F125**
peristalsis, **F119**, **F125**
permanent hair removal, and FDA, F407–8
permanent makeup, F521–22, 9, 554–59, *555f*, *557f*, *558f*
permanent makeup artists, **9**
permeation, of skin, 75–76
perming, of eyelashes, F521, 531–32, *532f–535f*
personal appearance, F21–23, *F547f*, F553
personal budget worksheet, *F565f*
personal consideration, F553
personal hygiene, **F21**, **F32**, F337, 36–38
personal protective equipment (PPE), 22, 28–29, 37, **51**
personal selling, 768–69, 771, **773**–74, **779**
personnel, **F588**–91, **F598**
petrissage, **F363**, **F374**
petrolatum, F258, 254, 269
petroleum jelly, **F268**, *F268t*, **F292**, 254
pH values, **F134**, **F142**, F258, F447–48
  adjusters, **F262**, **F292**
  chemicals, in skin and body, and, 144–45, *145f*, 272
  cosmetics and, 144–45, *145f*, 272
  infection control and, 40
  low pH toner, 93, 266–67, *266f*
  of peels, F447–48
  of water, 38
phagocytes, **64**, **85**, **125**, **136**
phalanges, **F102**, **F125**
phases of life, and hormones, 92–99
phenol, **F75**, **F89**, F447, **F463**, **F466**
phenylpropanoids, *151t*, **152**, **154**, *293t*

pheomelanin, F201
pheromones, F202
phlebitis, **331**, **345**
phlebotomy, 7
phobias, **336**, **345**
phospholipids, **57**, *58f*, **85**, 261
phosphorus, *F175t*, F181
photoaging, *F243f*, 212–13, 367–68, *368f*. *See also* sun
photodamage, F204–5, 211–12, **440**, **474**
photodynamic therapy (PDT), 452
photoepilation, **F407**–8, **F442**
photographers, F12, F510–11
photomodulation, **180**, **183**, **448**, **474**
photons, **159**, **183**
photophobia, **717**, **731**
photorejuvenation, **440**, *444f–448f*, **474**
photosensitivity, **332**, **345**
photosensitizers, F205
phototherapy, **F156**, F159, **F160**, **F452**–53, **F465**
photothermal tissue reactions, 172–73, *172f*
photothermolysis, **F158**, **F160**
phototoxic, **452**, **474**
phymatous rosacea, **229**, **233**
physical body, 605–8
physical changes, **F132**–33, **F142**
physical dependence, **336**, **345**
physical emulsions, **259**, **280**
physical exercise, F22
physical mixtures, **F133**, **F142**
physical presentation, **F22**–23, **F32**
physical properties, **F133**, **F142**
physical salon/spa layout, F586–88
physical sunscreens, F266
physics
  of electromagnetic spectrum, 158–60, **159**, *159f*, **182**
  of IPL treatments, *441f*
  of LASER light, 158–63, *161f*
physiology, **F95**, **F125**, **F191**, **F208**. *See also* anatomy; skin
phytoestrogens, F206
phytotherapy, **F255**, **F274**, **F292**, **283**, **304**
pigmentation, F221, F379–80
pilosebaceous, **204**, **234**
pilosebaceous ducts, F226
pilosebaceous follicles, F401–2
pineal gland, F117, *F118f*, **91**, **102**
pineapple, *F271t*
pink makeup, *F482t*
pinkeye, **F225**, **F230**
Pitta dosha, **632**, 635–36, **656**
pituitary gland, F117, *F118f*, **90**, **102**
pityriasis versicolor, F70, F225, F233
pityrosporum ovale, **226**, **234**
place, **768**, **779**
placebo, **668**, **671**
plakoglobin, **74**, **85**
plant compounds
  in botanicals, 283–84
  in skin care, 147–49, 272–73, 284
plant oils, F258
plaques, **74**, **85**
plasma, **F115**, **F125**
  cells, **72**
  contents of, *125t*
  membrane, **74**, **85**
plastic surgeons, 9, 665
plastic surgery
  abdominoplasty, **F463**, **F465**, **727**–28, *728f*, **730**
  augmentation mammaplasty, 720–21, *720f*, *721f*
  blepharoplasty, **F463**, **F465**, 543, **713**, 715–17, *717f*, **730**
  brow lift, F462, 713, 715–16
  facial implants, 718–19
  forehead-lift, 713–15, **714**, *715f*, **730**
  mammaplasty, **F463**, **F465**, **730**
  mastopexy, 721–23, **722**, *722f*, *723f*, **730**
  reduction mammaplasty, 723–24, *724f*
  rhinoplasty, **F463**, **F466**, **717**–18, *718f*, **731**
  rhytidectomy, **F462**, **F466**, **712**–13, *713f*, *714f*, **731**
  suction-assisted lipoplasty, 728–29, *728f*, *729f*
  transconjunctival blepharoplasty, **F463**, **F466**, 716–17
  for undereye circles, *717f*
platelet-derived growth factor (PDGF), **70**, **85**
platelets, **F115**, **F125**
platysma, **F104**, **F125**, **111**, *111f*, **120**
platysmal bands, **694**, **708**
Plewig, Gerd, 242
plexuses, **130**, **136**
plugs, electrical, **F149**–51, **F160**
plurals, 677–78, *677t*, **683**, **687**
pluripotential stem cells, **71**, **85**
PM. *See* preventative maintenance
PMNs. *See* polymorphonuclear cells
PMS. *See* premenstrual syndrome
pneumonoultramicroscopicsilicovolcanokonio-sis, 683
PNS. *See* peripheral nervous system
pointed upper lip, F493
poison ivy, F220
polarity, **F151**, **F160**, F388–89
policies, F556
policies statements, for salons, *F584f*
pollutants, F203–4
polychromatic, **440**, **474**, **504**, **517**
polychromatic normoblasts, **71**, **85**
polyglucans, **F264**, **F292**
polymers, **F264**, **F292**, **143**, 254
polymorphonuclear cells (PMNs), **64**, **85**
polypeptides, **143**
polyphenols, **275**, **280**
polysaccharides, **F169**, **F185**, **144**, 146, **154**
polyunsaturated fats, F170
polyunsaturated fatty acids, **148**, **154**
polyvinyl chloride (PVC/vinyl), 34
pomegranate, F5, *F271t*
poor elasticity, *F242t*
pores, **F194**, *F195f*, **F208**
port wine stain, F221
positive nonverbal cues, F38
post facial clean-up, F344
posterior auricular artery, *F115f*, **F116**, **F125**
posterior auricular nerve, **F112**, **F125**
post-inflammatory hyperpigmentation, **225**, **234**
postoperative care, F460
post-peel home-care, F449–50
post-traumatic stress disorder (PTSD), **336**, **345**
posture, F22–23
potassium, *F175t*, F181
potassium hydroxide, **F268**, *F268t*, **F293**
potatoes, *F273t*
potential hazards, 47–48
potential hydrogen, chemistry of, F134–35
powder blush, F474
powder brushes, F479
powder foundations, F472
powder masks, 384, *384f–386f*
powders, F473–74, *F473f*, F500
power density, **163**, **183**
PPE. *See* personal protective equipment
PPIs. *See* proton pump inhibitors
PR. *See* public relations
practical examinations, F533
prakruti, **632**, **656**
prana, 242, **657**
pranayam, **657**
pre-exfoliation consultation, 377
prefixes, **675**, 683–84, **687**
pregnancy, *F245t*
  acne and, 223
  hair removal and, 478–79
  hormones of, 95–96
  hyperpigmentation and, 95, *95f*
  IPL treatments and, 443
  mask of, F221, *95f*
  precautions during, 96–97
  skin appearance during, 95–96
  tanning and, 95
premenstrual syndrome (PMS), **97**, **102**
preoperative care, F460
preparation procedures, for clients, 570–71, *571f*
preparing, for interviews, F545–47
preparing treatment rooms, F299
prescription drugs, 327–28, *327f*, *328f*
preservatives, as cosmetic ingredients, **F261**–62, **F293**, 261–62
pressing agents, **254**, **280**
pressotherapy, 430, *430f*
pressure point massage, F366
pressure therapy, 354–57
preventative maintenance (PM), **440**, **474**
prevention, of infection
  cross-contamination, **F78**–79, **F89**, 30, 36, 49, 261, 477
  disinfectants, F74–77
  disinfection, F72–73
  infection control and, F70–79
  linens, F78
  overview of, F70–71
  sanitation, F71–72
  sterilization, F73–74
  workstations, F78
price, F583, **768**, **779**
prickly heat, F218, **F218**, **F232**
primary colors, **F480**, **F524**
primary lesions, **F214**–15, **F232**
primary metabolites, **146**, *147t*, **154**
privacy, F27
  laws on, 13
  notice of, 13
  practices, 566–67, 572
private labeling and branding, F10
private salon owners, F11
proanthocyanidins, **275**, **280**
problem solving, 11–13, 308
procedural guides, **F589**, **F598**
procerus muscles, **F104**, *F105f*, **F125**, *F367f*
product, **767**, **779**
product development, 318–20
product evaluation, 488
product knowledge, *F604f*
product lines, comparing and rating, F288
product recommendations, *F602f*
pro-enzymes, **75**, **85**
professional appearance, F21–23, *F547f*, F553
professional conduct, F23–25
professional image
  balance, creating, F21–22, **603**, **625**
  beauty and wellness, F21
  conduct, F23–25
  defined, **F21**, **F32**

professional image *(continued)*
  dressing for success, F22
  ethics, **F25**–28, **F32**, 10, 667, 773
  life skills, F28–31
  overview of, F299
  personal hygiene and, **F21**, **F32**, F337, 36–38
  physical presentation, F22–23, F32
professional organizations, 13–14
professional products, F286–87
professionalism, F49, F603
profit, **F576**, **F598**
progesterone, **92**, **102**
proliferative phase, **204**–6, *206f*, **234**
promissory note, **763**
promotion mix, **771**–74, **779**
promotions, F604, **F609**, **F616**, **768**, **773**–74, *774f*, 776, **779**
pronators, **F107**, **F125**
pronormoblast, **71**, **85**
pronunciation, **685**–86, *686t*, **687**
propionibacterium acnes bacteria, F216, **219**, **234**
propylene glycol, **F268**, *F268t*, **F293**, 268
proteases, **274**, **280**
protectants, **254**, **280**, 352
protection, skin function, F192–93
protective eyewear, F322
proteins
  chemicals and, **F167**–68, **F185**, **57**–59, **61**, **85**, **143**
  glycoproteins, **F265**, **F291**, 277
  high-density lipoproteins, F171
  keratin proteins, **60**, **83**
  low-density lipoproteins, F171
  as macronutrients, **F167**–68, **F185**
  p27 protein, **69**, **85**
  p53 protein, **69**, **85**
protein-tyrosine kinase activity, **70**, **85**
proteoglycans, **67**–68, **86**
proteolysis, **75**, **86**
proteolytic enzymes, **271**, **280**
proton pump inhibitors (PPIs), **334**, **345**
protoplasm, F65, **F95**, **F125**
protozoa, **F69**, **F89**, 27
protruding eyes, F490
protruding forehead, F488
provitamins, F176
pruitis, **F219**, **F232**
pseudofolliculitis, **F219**, **F232**, **F356–57**, F409
pseudomonacidal disinfectants, **F74**, **F89**
pseudomonas, 26
psoriasis, **F219**, **F232**
psychological aspects, of makeup, F470–71
psychological dependence, **336**, **345**
psychology, of selling, F603–4
psychoses, **345**
ptosis, **693**–96, **708**
PTSD. *See* post-traumatic stress disorder
puberty, **92**, **102**
public relations (PR), **F596**, **F598**, **772**, **779**
publications, professional, 14
publicity, **772**, 774, **779**
pulmonary circulation, **F114**, **F125**, **127**, **136**
pulmonary valves, **128**, **136**
pulse duration, **163**, **183**, **512**–13, **517**
pulse width, **163**, **183**, **513**, **517**
pulsed light. *See* Intense Pulsed Light
punctate keratitis, **696**, **708**
punctuality, F30, F45–46, F553
purchasing
  equipment, F395
  established salons, F580–81
  facial machines, F395
  process of, 437–40
  supplies, F585
purple coneflower, **F270**, *F270t*, **F291**
purple makeup, F482
pus, **F65**, **F89**
pustules, *F214f*, **F215**, *F227f*, **F232**, *F242t*, *218f*, 220, *220f*, 227, 229
pyridoxine, *F173t*, F179

Q

Q-switched LASERS, 173–75, *174t*, *175f*, *175t*
quadratus labii inferioris muscles, **F105**, **F122**, *F367f*
quadratus muscles, **F105**, **F123**, *F367f*
quadriceps, **116**, **120**
quality assurance, 170
quality service, F610
quaternary ammonium compounds, **F74**–75, **F89**
quaternium 15, **F269**, *F269t*, **F293**
quats, **F74**–75, **F89**
questionnaires on makeup, for clients, **F496**, *F496t*, **F577**, **F606**, **F616**
quotas, **F563**, **F569**, **F615–16**

R

radial artery, **F116**, **F125**
radial nerve, *F112f*, **F113**, **F125**
radiant energy, **163**, **183**
radio-frequency (RF) energy. *See also* electrodessication
  bipolar, **178**, **182**
  devices, 465
  monopolar, **178**, *179f*, **182**
  safety and, *171f–172t*
radius, **F102**, **F125**
raindrop therapy, 597
rajasic, **657**
rake electrodes, *F392t*
rancidity, **149**, **154**, **262**, **280**
razor bumps, F219, F232, F356–57, F409
RDAs (recommended daily allowances), F171, *F173t–175t*
reactions, chemical, F135–36
reactions of clients, to treatments, 361
reactive oxygen species, **274**–76, **279**
receding chin, F488
reception area, *F591f–592f*
receptionists, F592–93
receptivity, F23
receptor site, of cells, **58**, *58f*, **86**, 89
recommended daily allowances (RDAs), F171, *F173t–175t*
recommending products, F604–5
reconstructive rhinoplasty, **F463**, **F466**, **717**–18, *718f*, **731**
reconstructive surgeon, **665**, **671**
reconstructive surgery, **F462**–63, **F466**
record keeping
  business, F584–86
  for clients, F586, **F606**–7, **F616**
  medical, 13, 669
rectangle face shape, F486
rectified, **295**, **304**
rectifiers, **F148**, **F160**
rectus abdominis, **112**, **120**
red blood cells, **F115**, **F125**
red jasper, 617, *617f*
red light, **F157**, F159, **F160**, F452
redox reactions, **F135**–36, **F142**
reduction, **F135**, **F142**
reduction mammaplasty, 723–24, *724f*
reduction-oxidation reactions, **F135**–36, **F142**
reepithelialization, **205**, **234**, **739**, **744**
referrals
  of clients, F611–12
  medical, 204, 210, 212, 216, 232
refined, **284**, **304**
reflection, 162
reflective listening, **F44**, **F53**
reflex arc, **77**, *77f*, **86**
reflexes, **F110**, **F125**
reflexology, **F366**, **F374**
  of ears, 408–9, *408f–409f*
  of face, 242–45, **407**, *407f*, **434**
  of foot, 630
regenerative properties, of cells, 292
Registered Nurse (RN), 667
regulation. *See* government regulation
Reiki, **608**–9, 611–12, **626**
Reiki attunement, **612**, **626**
rejuvenation procedures
  energy balancing, 620, *621f–625f*
  IPL treatments for, 440–48, *444f–448f*
  photorejuvenation, **440**, *444f–448f*, **474**
relaxin, **92**, **102**
release forms, for clients, F246, *F417f*
reliability, F590
remodeling, of collagen, **206**, *206f*, **234**, **735**, **744**
removing eye and lip color, F320
Renaissance, F7, 7
Renova, F175–76, F185, *F229t*, *F245t*, F265, *F269t*, F293
repair cycle, of a cell, *61f*
reproduction and division, of cells, F96–97
reproductive system, **F120**, **F125**
  female, *91f*
  male, *91f*
resale tax, **761**, **763**
research, conducting, F28
researchers, F15
resident microorganisms, 26
resolving conflict, F24–25
resort spas, F535, F542, 9, 565
respect, F555
respiratory burst, **64**, **86**
respiratory system, **F119**–20, **F125**
responsibility, F555
restrictions, 8
Restylane, 701
resumes
  checklist for, F536–38
  cover letters, F539
  defined, **F535**, **F569**
  formatting, F535–36
  sample, *F537f*
  writing, F538–39
resurfacing, with LASER device, **F463**, **F465**, **744**
retail areas, *307f*
retail goals, 8
retail supplies, **F585**, **F598**
retailing, F512, **F604**, F605, **F616**. *See also* selling
retaining clients, F610–12
retention hyperkeratosis, **F226**, **F232**, **218**, 255
retention, of sales, F610–12
reticular layer, of dermis, **F197**–98, **F208**
reticulocyte, **71**, **86**

Retin-A, F175–76, F185, *F229t*, *F245t*, F265, *F269t*, F293
retinoic acid, **F175**–76, **F185**, *F229t*, *F245t*, F265, *F269t*, **F293**
retinoids, users of, 361–62
retinol, *F173t*, **F175**–77, **F185**, **F265**, **F293**, F352
revenue, **F576**, **F598**
RF energy. *See* radio-frequency energy
rhinophyma, **229**, *230f*, *231f*, **234**
rhinoplasty, **F463**, **F466**, **717**–18, *718f*, **731**
rhytidectomy, **F462**, **F466**, **712**–13, *713f*, *714f*, **731**
riboflavin, *F173t*, F178
ribosomes, **58**, **86**
ringworm, F225, F233
rinsable cleansers, 308–11, 320
risk
  defined, **749**, **763**
  management of, **753**, **763**
risorius muscles, **F105**, **F125**, *F367f*
RN. *See* Registered Nurse
role models, F21, F566, **F566**, **F569**
roll paper, F414
rolling, F364
roll-on wax, F412
Roman Empire, F6, 6, 675
room temperature, 12
room-cleaning checklist, 49
root words, **675**, *675f*, *677t*, *678t*, **687**
roots, of hair, **F402**, *F403f*, **F442**
rosacea, F206, **F219**, **F232**, *F242t*, F350
  erythematotelangiectatic, **229**, **233**
  facials and, F350
  granulomatous, **231**, **233**
  Kligman classification for, 242, *242t*
  National Rosacea Society, 229, 231
  ocular, **230**, *231f*, **233**
  overview of, 10, **227**–32, *228f*, *229f*, *230f*
  papulopustular, **229**, **233**
  phymatous, **229**, **233**
  skin care products for, 320–22
  treatments for, 357–62
rose, *F271t–272t*, **F293**
rose quartz, 618, *618f*
rosemary, *F272t*, 297, *297f*, 608
rosewood, *F272t*
rotary brushes, **F380**–81, **F397**
round eyes, F490
round face shape, F486, F488, F492
rubber-type masks, 387–88, *387f*
rubifactants, **382**, **389**
Rubin, Mark G., 240
Rubin skin typing scale, **240**–41, *241t*, **248**, 442
ruddy skin, F494
rules and regulations, F62, 21–23. *See also* government regulation

S

S (synthesis), **69**, **86**
saccharides, **144**, *144f*, **154**
safety. *See also* Occupational Safety and Health Administration
  AHAs and, F447
  autoclaves and, 44
  of clients, *F557f*
  Consumer Product Safety Commission, 778
  detoxifying treatments, F457
  disinfectants and, F75–77
  electrical equipment and, F78, F149–51
  exfoliation, F449
  eyelash extensions and, 521–22
  FDA and, F266–67, 164–65
  gloves and, 48
  guidelines for, F75–77, 48–49
  hair removal and, 477–78
  IPL treatments and, *171t–172t*
  Laser Safety Officer (LSO), **165**, **182**
  LASER use and, 165–72, *167f*, *171t–172t*, 504–5, *505f*
  Material Safety Data Sheets, **F59**–61, **F89**, 49
  microcrystals, F451
  peels and, F446, F448
  plans for, **48**, **52**
  radio-frequency energy and, *171f–172t*
  skin care and, F266–67
  waxing and, F417, F419–20, F427, F434, F437
salary, **F561**–62, **F569**
salary-plus-commission model, F562
sales
  closing, F612–15
  management of, 10
  managers, F12–13
  promotions, F604, **F609**, **F616**, **768**, **773**–74, *774f*, 776, **779**
  representatives, 9
  retention, F610–12
  tracking success of, F615, 776–77, *777f*
  training, 773
salespersons, F12–13
salicylic acid, **F269**, *F269t*, **F293**, 270–72, 495, 705
salivary glands, *F165f*
sallow skin, F494
salons
  communication in, F49–53, F560–61
  estheticians for, F10–11
  for facials, *F587f*
  full-service, F533, F542, *F587f*
  location of, F574–75
  ownership, F11, F579–80, 9
  physical layout of, F586–88
  policies statements for, *F584f*
  purchasing, F580–81
salt, F181, 193
salt glow, *F455f*
samadi, **657**
sandalwood, *F271t*, *F272t*, 298, *298f*
sanitary maintenance areas (SMAs), **F304**, **F311**
sanitation
  allergies, F267
  checklist, F337–39
  cleanliness, F21, F32, F86–87, F337, 22
  defined, **F71**, **F89**
  disinfectants and, F415
  disposables, F310
  end-of-day clean-up, F310
  of equipment, F309
  eyelashes, artificial, and, F516
  facials, F337–39
  laundry, F309
  makeup application, F498, F508
  overview of, F70, F71–72, *F72t*
  personal hygiene and, **F21**, **F32**, F337, 36–38
  prevention of infection and, F71–72
  sanitizers and disinfectants, F415
  of treatment rooms, F71, F308–10
sanitizers, **F301**, **F311**
Sanskrit, **657**
saponification, **F386**, **F397**
sattvic, **657**
saturated fats, F170
saturated fatty acids, **148**, *149t*, **154**
SBA. *See* Small Business Administration
SBDC. *See* Small Business Development Centers
SBTN. *See* Small Business Training Network
SC. *See* stratum corneum
scabies, **F69**, **F89**
scales, **F216**, **F232**
scalp, muscles of, F103
scapulae, *F101f*, **F102**, **F125**
scarring, from acne, 221, *222f*
scars, **F216**, **F232**
scatter, **162**, **183**
SCCE. *See* chymotryptic enzyme
scent, and memory, 291
scheduling appointments, F46–47, F593–94
scientific method, **668**, *668t*, **671**
"scissor" movement, F371
sclerotherapy, **F463**, **F466**, **691**–92, 702–4, **708**, *793f*
scope of practice, for estheticians
  drugs and, 331, 342
  limitations on, 189, 214, 232, **664**–65, **671**
  nutrition and, 193
SCORE. *See* Service Core of Retired Executives
Scotch hose, **596**, **599**
scrubs, F446
  body, **F455**, F458, **F465**, *573f–576f*
  exfoliant, 318, *318f*
  granular, F279
scrying, 613
SD alcohols. *See* specially denatured alcohols
sea buckthorn, 288–89, *289f*
seaweeds, **F271**, *F271t*, **F293**
  body wraps, **579**, *579f*, *580f–583f*, **599**
  masks, F282
  uses of, *577t*
sebaceous filaments, **F226**, **F232**
sebaceous follicles, F226, *F227f*
sebaceous glands, **F194**, *F195f*, **F201**–2, **F208**, F216–17
sebaceous hyperplasias, **F217**, **F232**, *F242t*, **217**, 466
seborrhea, **F217**, **F232**, *F242t*
seborrheic dermatitis, F217, **F218**, **F232**, **226**, *226f*, **234**
seborrheic keratosis, **217**, **234**
sebum, **F192**, **F208**, 92
second cranial nerve (CN II), *F111f*
secondary colors, **F480**, **F524**
secondary lesions, **F214**–16, **F232**
secondary metabolites, **146**, *147t*, **154**
secreted, **89**, **102**
secretion, F194
secretory nerve fibers, F200
security, F36
sedative properties, 291
sedimentary, **410**, **434**
seizures, *F245t*
select serotonin reuptake inhibitors (SSRIs), **336**, **345**
selective permeability, **57**, **86**
selective photothermolysis, **162**–63, **183**, **504**, **517**
selenium, *F175t*, F181
self-employment tax, **759**, **763**
self-esteem, F28–29, F470
self-image, of clients, 10
self-tanners, F285–86
self-trauma excoriations, 225
selling. *See also* marketing
  building clientele, F609–10
  client education, F607–8

selling *(continued)*
  closing sales, F612–15
  collecting client information, F606–7
  consultative, **F602**–3, **F616**
  principles of, F602–3
  promotions, F604, **F609**, **F616**, **768**, **773**–74, *774f*, 776, **779**
  psychology of, F603–4
  recommending products, F604–5
  retailing, F512, **F604**, F605, **F616**
  tracking success of, F615, 776–77, *777f*
  upselling, F605–6
  vendor education, F605
semilunar valves, **128**, **136**
seminal vesicle, 91
senescent cell, **69**, **86**
sensation, F192–94
sensitive skin, F239
  contraindications for, F350, 357–58
  facials for, F350
  Fitzpatrick skin typing scale and, **238**–40, *238f*, *238t*, *239t*, **248**
  treatments for, 353, 357–62, *358f–361f*
sensitivity, F23, *F242t*
sensitization, F219
sensory nerves, **F110**, **F125**, F193–94, *F195f*, F200, 77–78, **86**
sensory neurons, **77**, **86**
sensory receptors, 77–78, *78f*
serotonin, **336**, **345**
serratus anterior muscles, **F106**, **F125**
serums, **F283**, **F293**, F324, 316, 352
Service Core of Retired Executives (SCORE), 752
service records, of clients, F586
sesame, *F271t*
setting goals, F23, F29, *F30f*, F41
setting masks, F281
seventh cranial nerve (CN VII), *F111f*, **F112**, **F125**
shafts, of hair, **F401**, **F442**
sharps
  containers for, F84, **F301**, **F311**
  contaminated, **51**
  defined, **52**
  disposal of, **22**, 29, 49
shaving, F355, F409
Shea butter, *F271t*, 289, 578
Shea nut, *289f*
sheet masks, collagen, F281, 383, *383f*, *384f*
Shiatsu massage
  facial massage and, **402**–7, *403f–406f*, **434**
  overview of, **F363**, F366, **F374**
shingles, **F225**, **F231**
shirobhyanga, **657**
shirodhara, *F457f*
  Ayurveda and, 649–50, *649f–654f*, **657**
  contraindications for, 649
short nose, F488
short term goals, F29
shoulders
  muscles of, F106–7
  shoulder blades, *F101f*, **F102**, **F125**
  skeletal system and, F102
shrinkage of collagen, **735**, **744**
side effects
  facial machines and, 473, *473t*
  LASER treatments and, 515–16, *515t*,
sidhi, **657**
silent letters, 685, *685t*
silicones, **F259**, *F269t*, **F293**, 254–55, 259–60
simple sugars, F169
sinus relief, 395
sinusoidal current, **F152**–53, **F160–61**, **F390**, **F397**
sitting posture, F23
six sense approach, 630, *630f*, **657**
sixth cranial nerve (CN VI), *F111f*
skeletal muscles, F103, F125, **106**, *106f*, 106–7
skeletal system
  anatomy and, F99–102
  arms, F102
  chest, F102
  defined, **F99**, **F125**
  disorders of, 340–41, *341t*
  face and, F101
  hands, F102
  neck, F101–2
  overview of, F99–100
  shoulders, F102
  skull, F100–101
Skille, Olave, 598
skin. *See also* disorders and diseases; Fitzpatrick skin typing scale; sensitive skin; skin care
  alipidic, **F237**–38, **F251**, 269–70
  analysis, F246–47, F248–50, 440
  analysis chart, *F247f*
  analysis checklist, *F248t*, *F319f*
  color of, F200–201, F483–84
  conditions and descriptions of, *F242t*
  contraindications for treatments, F245–46
  corneocytes in, F196, **60**, 75–76, *76f*, **81**
  dermis, **F197**–99, **F208**, **60**, 63–65, **81**
  epidermis, F193, **F195**–97, **F208**, **F209**, **60**, *60f*, *61f*, **65**–66, 75–76, *76f*, **82**, 352
  ethnic, F240–41
  free radicals and, **274**–76
  functions of, F192–95
  glands, F201–2
  Glogau typing scale for, **240**, *240t*, **248**, 442
  hair and, F199
  health of, F202–4
  histology of skin penetration and permeation, 75–76
  histology of skin structure and function, 60–65
  hormones and, F206–7, 245–47
  keratinocytes in, **F195–96**, **F208**, **F222**, **F231**, **60**–62, *62t*, 65–66, **83**
  layers of, *F192f*, F195–99
  lifestyle and, F204
  mature, F206–7, F275–76, F346–47
  nails and, F199
  nerves of, F200
  nutrition and, F167
  Oriental perspective on, 243
  overview of, F191–92
  penetration of, F194, 75–76
  Rubin typing scale for, **240**–41, *241t*, **248**, 442
  structure and function of, *F195f*, 60–65
  tags on, **F222**, **F232**
  therapists for, F191
  tones of, *F483t*, F494
  transit time, of cells in, **61**, **86**
  types *versus* conditions, F241–42
  water and, F183
Skin Cancer Foundation, 214–15
skin care. *See also* cleansers; masks; scrubs; sunscreen; toners
  acne and, 320
  ampoules and, **F283**, **F290**, **316**, 352
  antioxidants and, F265, F275
  aromatherapy, F273–74
  botanicals and, 146–49, 272–73, 286–89
  cost, F288
  day creams and treatments, 312–14
  essential oils and, 295–98
  exfoliants, F278–80
  eye creams, F283–84, 317
  free radicals, F274–75
  home-care products, F286–87
  lip treatments, F284, F384
  management program for, *F613f*
  for men, F354–55
  moisturizers for, F263, **F284**–85, **F292**, F324, 270
  night creams and treatments, 314–15
  plant compounds in, 147–49, 272–73, 284
  rosacea and, 320–22
  safety, F266–67
  self-tanners, F285–86
  serums and, **F283**, **F293**, F324, 316, 352
  for young teenagers, 93
Skin Inc. Magazine, 14
skull, bones of, F100–101
slapping, F364
Small Business Administration (SBA), 752
Small Business Development Centers (SBDC), 752
Small Business Training Network (SBTN), 752
small eyes, F490
small lips, F493
small mushroom electrodes, *F392t*
smaller occipital nerve, *F112f*, **F113**, **F125**
SMAS. *See* superficial musculoaponeurotic system
SMAs (sanitary maintenance areas), **F304**, **F311**
smiling, F26, F39, F317
smoke evacuators, *168f*
smoking, F204, 193–95, *195f*, 208–9, 712
smoky eyes makeup, F509
smooth muscles, F103, F124, **106**, *106f*
snana, **657**
snehana, **657**
SOAP notes. *See* Subjective Objective Assessment Procedure notes
soaps, F138, 76, 256–57, *258f*, 265
Social Security Number, **756**, **763**
Society of Permanent Cosmetic Professionals, 14, 555–56
sodalite, 619, *619f*
sodium bicarbonate, **F269**, *F269t*, **F293**
sodium, chemistry of, *F175t*, F181, 142
sodium hyaluronate, 268
sodium hypochlorite, F75
sodium lauryl sulfate, 308–9, 315
sodium PCA, **268**, **280**, 313–14
soft sell, F602
soft skills, 11–13, *12f*
soft waxes, F411, F418–19, 487–88, *487f*, *489t*
solar comedones, *F242t*
solar freckles, 217–18
sole proprietorships, **F579**, **F598**, 49
soleus, **117**, **120**
solids, F132
solutes, **F137**, **F142**
solutions, **F136**–37, **F142**
solvent extraction, 286–87
solvents, **F137**, **F142**, **F262**, **F293**
soma, **657**
somatic nervous system, F108
sonophoresis, F455, 360
sorbitol, **F269**, *F269t*, **F293**, 268
soy, *F271t*
Spa Industry Associations, 14

Spa Magazine, 14
Spa of Bath, England, 6
sparking electrodes, *F392t*
spas
  aromatherapy and, *597f*
  contraindications for therapy at, 567
  defined, **15**
  global evolution of, 6–8
  medical, F10, *F535f*, F542, 565–66, **665**, **671**
  resort style, F535, F542, 9, 565
  services at, *6f*, *565f*
  therapy at, **6**, **15**, 567
  treatments at, F455–57
  types of, 565–66
spatulas, F78, F499
Spaulding Classification System, 41
specialists, F191
specially denatured alcohols (SD alcohols), **267**, **280**
special-occasion makeup, F509–11
specialty creams and treatments, 316–18
speed waxing, 491–501, *492f*
SPF. *See* sun protection factor
sphenoid bone, *F100f*, **F101**, **F125**
sphingolipids, **F269**, *F269t*, **F293**
spider veins, F206, F219, F242, F251
spinal cord, F109–**10**, **F125**
spiral electrodes, *F392t*
spirilla, **F65**, **F89**
spirit/energy body, 606–**7**, **626**
splattering, **514**, **517**
sponges, F498
spores, **27**, **52**
spot blemish treatments, F352
spot sizes, **160**, 163, **183**, 512
spray machines, F301, **F393**, **F397**
squalane, **F269**, *F269t*, **F293**
squalene, **F269**, *F269t*, **F293**
squamous cell carcinomas, **F223**, **F232**, 214, *214f*
square face shape, F486, F488, F492
srota, **657**
SSRIs. *See* select serotonin reuptake inhibitors
staff meetings, *F555f*
stains, **F221**, **F232**
standard precautions, 21, 22, **22**, **52**
standing posture, F22–23
staphylococci, **F63**, F65, **F90**, 26, 76
starches, F169
state board members, F14–15
State Cosmetology Regulatory Agencies, 14
state regulation, F61. *See also* government regulation
  examiners, 10
  licensing examiners/inspectors, F14
  National-Interstate Council of State Boards of Cosmetology, 14
stationary circle technique, 420–26, *421f*
statutes, F62. *See also* government regulation
steam, F321, *7f*, 43–47
steamers, F300, F303–4, F381–84
steatomas, **F217**, **F232**
stem cells, **60**, 63, 70–71, *71f*, **86**
stencils, **554**, **560**
step stools, F301
sterile technique, 29
sterilization, F71–74, **F73**, **F90**
  of equipment, 39
  infection control and, 29, 37–47, *46f–47f*
  prevention of infection and, F73–74
  procedure for, *39f–40f*, 43
  with steam, 43–47
  of water, 254
sterilize, **52**
sternocleidomastoids, **F104**, **F125**, *F367f*, **111**, **120**
sternum, *F101f*, **F102**, **F125**
stethoscope, **127**, **136**
stimulants, collagen, F265
stimulating properties, F273
stockholder, F579
stomach, *F165f*
stones
  Chakras and, 613–20, *614t*, *616t*
  contraindications for treatments with, 411
  gemstones, **613**, **626**
  for healing, 613–20, *614t*, *616t*
  massage and, **F456**, **F466**, 410–17, *410f*, *412f–417f*
stools, F300–301, F305
storage, of instruments, 28–29, 47
strabismus, **693**, **708**
straight upper lip, F494
strategic value, 769
stratum corneum (SC), **F196**, **F208**, *61f*, **65**–66, 75–76, *76f*, 352
stratum germinativum, F197, **F208**
stratum granulosum, F196, **F208**
stratum lucidum, F196, **F209**
stratum spinosum, **F196**–97, **F209**
streptococci, **F63**, *F64f*, **F90**, 26
stress, F228
  acne and, 223
  chronic, *192f*, **197**, **199**
  effects of, on body, 195–97, *196f*
  management of, 197–98, *198f*, *596f*
  massage and, 393
  nutrition and, 190–93
  post-traumatic stress disorder (PTSD), **336**, **345**
  relief properties, 291
  triggers for, **197**, **199**
striae, **96**, **102**
striae distensae, **727**, **731**
striated muscles, **F103**, **F125**
striations, 106
strip lashes, **F513**, **F524**
strip waxes, F411, F418–19
stripless waxes, F411, F418–19
subclinical, **274**, **280**
subclinical inflammation, **203**, **234**, 274
subcutaneous layer, of dermis, **F198**–99, **F209**
subcutaneous mycoses, **340**, **345**
subcuticular (sub-Q), **207**, **234**
subcutis tissue, **F198**, **F208**, **F209**
Subjective Objective Assessment Procedure (SOAP) notes, 11
sublingual, **332**, **345**
submental, **712**, **731**
submental artery, *F115f*, **F116**, **F125**
sub-Q. *See* subcuticular
substantives, **268**, **280**
success
  defining, F25
  dressing for, F22
  guidelines for, F28–29
  planning for, F567–68
  tracking sales for, F615, 776–77, *777f*
suction machines, F301, F384–85, F397
suction-assisted lipoplasty, 728–29, *728f*, *729f*
sudoriferous glands, **F194**, *F195f*, *F201f*, **F202**, **F209**, F217–18
sudoriferous pores, F226
suffixes, **675**, *675f*, *677t*, 683–85, **687**
sugar, 193
sugaring, **F410**, **F442**, 480–86, *482f*, *486f*
sugaring paste, *481f*, 483, *484f*, *484t*, *485f*
sulfur, *F175t*, **F269**, *F269t*, **F293**, 578
sulfur masks, F352, F354
sun
  damage from, F204–5, 209, 211–12, **440**, **474**
  exposure to, F44, F204–5, *F223t*, *F242t*, F243, *239t*
  Fitzpatrick skin typing scale and, 211–12
  hyperpigmentation and, 209, 211–12
  lupus and, 212
sun protection factor (SPF), F285, 538
sun spots, F70, F225, F233
sunblock, F266
sundar, **657**
sunless spray tanning, *F457f*
sunscreen, F266, F284, F285, F324
  AHAs and, 271
  daily use of, 93, 212, 317, 448, 459
  emollients and, 254
  facials and, F324, 444, 447, 451, 461, 468, 471
  FDA and, F266
  healing and, 209
  ingredients of, F266, 276–77, 312–14, 321
  SPF and, F285, 538
supercritical carbon dioxide, **285**, **304**
superfatted, **265**, **280**
superficial, **204**, **234**
superficial musculoaponeurotic system (SMAS), **713**, **731**
superficial mycoses, **340**, **345**
superficial peels, F446, 374–81, *375f*
superficial temporal artery, *F115f*, **F116**, **F126**
superior labial artery, *F115f*, **F116**, **F126**
superoxide, **64**, **86**, **275**
superoxide dismutase, **275**, **280**
supination, **113**, **120**
supinators, **F107**, **F126**
supplies
  consumption, **F585**, **F598**
  facials, *F317t*
  for makeup, F498–99
  purchasing, F585
  retail, **F585**, **F598**
  treatment room, F302–3
  waxing room, F413–14
suppressor T cells, **73**, **86**
supraorbital artery, *F115f*, **F116**, **F126**
supraorbital nerve, **F111**, *F112f*, **F126**
supratrochlear nerve, F111, *F112f*, **F126**
surfactants, **F138**, **F142**, **F259**–60, **F293**, 257–58
surgical asepsis, 29
survival tips, for interviews, F547–49
suspensions, F136–38, **F137**, **F142**
sutures, 207, *207f*, *208t*
sweat glands, F194, *F195f*, *F201f*, F202, F209, F217–18
Swedish massage movements, F363–64
sympathetic divisions, **F108**, **F126**, **77**, **86**
sympathetic nervous system, **77**, **86**
synapse, **106**, *107f*, **120**
synergy, **292**, **304**
synthesis (S), **69**, **86**
synthetic, **718**, **731**
syphilis, 7
systemic circulation, **F114**, **F126**, **127**, **136**
systemic diseases, *F64t*
systemic mycoses, **340**, **345**
systole, **127**, **136**

T

T cells, **72**–73, **86**
tables
massage, 567
for treatments, 567
for waxing, F412
tags, on skin, **F222**, **F232**
tamasic, **657**
tanning, **F221**, *F223t*, **F233**
acne and, 224
habits, *239t*, 443
pregnancy and, 95
self-tanners, F285–86
tapotement, **F364**, **F374**
tardy clients, F45–46
tartaric acid, **271**, **280**
tattooing
equipment for, *556f*
eyebrows and, *555f*, 557, *557f*
LASER removal of, *174f*, *174t*
microorganisms and, 26
as permanent makeup, F521–22, 9, 554–59, *555f*, *557f*, *558f*
tax identification numbers, 756
tax returns, 756–57
taxes, 757–61, *757f*, *758f*, *759f*, *760f*
tazarotene, F175–76, F185, *F229t*, *F245t*, F265, *F269t*, F293, 273
Tazorac, F175–76, F185, *F229t*, *F245t*, F265, *F269t*, F293
TB. *See* tuberculosis
TCA. *See* trichloroacetic acid
TCAs. *See* tricyclics
TCM. *See* traditional Chinese medicine
tea tree, *F271t–272t*, **F293**
teacher training programs, F14
teamwork, F24, *F25f*, F554
technicians, F191
teenage acne, 223–24, 320
teenagers, skin care for, 93
tej, **657**
telangiectases, **227**, **234**
telangiectasias, **F206**, **F209**, **F219**, **F233**, F242, F251, **96**, 212–13, **227**, *227f*, **234**
telephone skills, F594–96
telogen stage, **F403**–4, **F442**
temperatures, of color, F482
temporal bones, *F100f*, **F101**, **F126**
temporal nerve, **F112**, **F126**
temporalis muscles, **F104**, **F126**
TEN. *See* toxic epidermal necrolysis
10-step method, for client consultations, F43–45
tendons, **106**, **120**
tenth cranial nerve (CN X), *F111f*
terpenoid compounds, **150**, *150t*, **154**
tertiary colors, **F480**, *F481f*, **F524**
Tesla high-frequency current (violet ray), **F153**–54, **F161**, F390, F396
testers, F498
testes, F118, **91**, **102**
testosterone, F227, **91**, **102**
test-wise, **F529**, **F569**
TEWL. *See* transepidermal water loss
thalamus, F109
thalassemia, **126**, **136**
thalassotherapy, F459, **589**, **599**
thank-you notes, *F543f*
theatrical makeup, F510
theft, F581–82
theophylline, 578
therapy. *See* treatments; *specific therapies*
thermage unit, *179f*
thermal masks, **F282**–83, **F292**
thermal relaxation time (TRT), **162**, **183**, 513
thermal storage, **512**–13, **517**
thermolysis, **F390**, **F397**, **F407**, **F442**
electrolysis and, F407
photothermolysis, **F158**, **F160**
selective photothermolysis, **162**–63, **183**, **504**, **517**
thermoplastic elastomers, 34
thermoreceptors, **78**
thermotherapy, 352–57, *352f–357f*, 410
thiamine, *F173t*, F178–79
thickeners, F260–61
thin lips, F493
third cranial nerve (CN III), *F111f*
thorax, **F102**, **F126**, 111
thread lift, **713**, **731**
threading, F6, F410
contraindications for, *481f*
defined, **517**
of eyebrows, 478, 481
treatments using, **478**–80, *480f*
thrombocytes, **F115**, **F125**
thymidine dinucleotide fragments, **62**, **86**
thymus gland, **91**, **102**
thyroid gland, F118, **90**, **102**
thyroxine, **89**, **102**
tibialis anterior, **117**, **120**
tight junctions, **73**, **86**
time management, F30–31
tincture, **284**, **304**
tinea, **F225**, **F233**
tinea corporis, **F225**, **F233**
tinea pedis, **F225**
tinea versicolor, F70, F225, **F233**, 212, *212f*
tinnitus, **705**, **708**
tinting, of eyebrows, F517–20
tissue respiratory factor (TRF), F265, **F293**, 277
tissue types, histology of, 71–72
tissues, **F97**, **F126**
titanium dioxide, **F269**, *F269t*, **F293**, F472, 536
tobacco, F204
tocopherol, *F174t*, **F177**–78, **F185**
toners, **F278**, **F293**, F324, F354
AHAs and, 272
for combination skin, 311, 313
for dry skin, 267–68, 312
exfoliants and, 318
for facials, F324
low pH, 93, 266–67, *266f*
for oily skin, 266–67, 311–12
topical anesthesia, 509, *509f*
topical prescription drugs, *328f*, 444
tortuous, **129**, **136**
touch, sense of, F192–94
tourmaline, 617, *617f*
towel techniques, 572–73
towel warmers, F300, F303
toxic epidermal necrolysis (TEN), **340**, **345**
toxicity, in disinfectants, 41
toxins, *F63t*
trace minerals, F181
tracking, of sales, F615, 776–77, *777f*
traditional Chinese medicine (TCM), F248, 242–44, 402
training
of estheticians, *440f*, 666–67
of nurses, 667
of sales staff, 773
Small Business Training Network, 752
trans fatty acids, F171
transconjunctival blepharoplasty, **F463**, **F466**, 716–17
transepidermal water loss (TEWL), **F192**, F194, **F209**, 268
transferable skills, **F538**, **F569**
transgender surgery, 501
transient erythema, **229**, **234**
transient microorganisms, 26
transit time, of skin cells, **61**, **86**
transmission, of infection, 28, 32–33
transverse facial artery, *F115f*, **F116**, **F126**
trapezius, **F106**, **F126**, 111, **112**, **120**
trash cans, F71
travel industry, F13
traverse abdominals, **112**, **120**
treatment rooms
beds, F300, F304, *570f*
equipment, F300–301, F303–4
ergonomics, F300, **F305**, **F311**, F412
furniture and equipment, F300–301, F412
presentation of, F299
professional atmosphere, F299
sanitation, F71, F308–10
setting up, F304–5
supplies, F302–3
treatments
arc and theory of, 353, *353f*
of Ayurveda, *629f*, 637–55, *641f–643f*
beds for, F300, F304, *570f*
building blocks of, 351–52, *351f*
for clogged resistive skin, 352
creams for, F284–85
day creams and, 312–14
for dehydrated skin, 352
electrodessication, *466f–468f*
for energy balancing, 620, *621f–625f*
exfoliation, 351, 362–81
for lips, F284, F324
logs for, F41
masks for, F324
for mature skin, F346–47
microcurrent facial toning, *470t*, *471f–472f*
night creams and, 314–15
pressure therapy, 354–57
reactions to, 361
for rosacea, 357–62
for sensitive skin, 353, 357–62, *358f–361f*
at spas, F455–57
specialty creams and, 316–18
tables for, 567
thermotherapy, 354–57, *354f–357f*, 410
threading, **478**–80, *480f*
variations on, 351
Treponema pallida, F65
Tretinoin, F175–76, F185, *F229t*, *F245t*, F265, *F269t*, F293
TRF. *See* tissue respiratory factor
triangular face shape, F486, F488
triangularis muscles, **F105**, **F126**, *F367f*
tricep brachii, 112, **114**, **120**
triceps, **F106**, *F107f*, **F126**
trichloroacetic acid (TCA) peels, **F463**, **F466**, 705, *705f*, *706f*
trichology, **F401**, **F442**
tricuspid valve, **127**, **136**
tricyclics (TCAs), **336**, **345**
trifacial nerve, **F110**–12, **F123**
trigeminal nerve, **77**, **86**
triphala, **657**
triplet oxygen molecule, 140
tripwires, 320–22
trochlear nerve, *F111f*
trophic hormones, **90**, **102**
trophoblasts, 95

TRT. *See* thermal relaxation time
true or false questions, F530–31
trunk, muscles of, 111–12
tubercles, *F214f*, **F215**, **F233**
tuberculocidal disinfectants, **F61**, F74, **F90**
tuberculosis (TB), **F61**, **F90**, **25**–26, 28–29, 48, **52**
tubulin, **60**, **86**
tummy tuck, 727–28, *728f*
tumors, *F214f*, **F215**, **F233**
turbinal bones, *F100f*, **F101**, **F126**
turnover rate, cellular, F196, **F446**–47, **F465**, 65, 195, 218, 328
tweezers, electronic, F410
tweezing, F7, F409, F413, F420–23, F430
twelfth cranial nerve (CN XII), *F111f*
twentieth century esthetics, F8–9
twenty-first century esthetics, F9–10
tyrosinase, F201, F264
tyrosinase inhibitors, F201
T-zone, **F237**, **F251**, 92, *93f*

U

ubtan, **657**
UL (Underwriter's Laboratory), F149, *F150f*
ulcers, **F216**, **F233**
ulna, **F102**, **F126**
ulnar artery, **F116**, **F126**
ulnar nerve, *F112f*, **F113**, **F126**
ultrasonic technology
  for clean-up, 38, 42
  facial machines using, F454–55, 460, *460f*
  facials using, F454–55, 460, *461f–465f*
  infection control and, 38, 42
  vibrating ultrasonic paddles, 454
ultraviolet (UV) rays, F155–57, **F156**, *F157t*, **F161**, F203–5, 158–59, 312–13
ultraviolet sanitizers, F71, *F301f*
underarm waxing, F433–34
undereye circles
  makeup for, 317, 542–45, 550
  surgery for, *717f*
Underwriter's Laboratory (UL), F149, *F150f*
uneven lips, F494
unhappy clients, F47–48
unicellular, **338**, **345**
uniforms, F22
United States Department of Agriculture (USDA), F165
Universal Precautions, **F84**, **F90**, 22
unsaturated fatty acid, **148**, *149t*, **154**
upselling, **F605**–6, **F616**
urea, **F269**, *F269t*, **F293**
urethra, 91
urticaria, **F215**, **F219**, **F233**
USDA. *See* United States Department of Agriculture
Usui, Mikao, 611–12
utility carts, F301, F305, F412–13
UV. *See* ultraviolet rays
UVA rays, F156, **F205**, **F209**, *F244t*, F285
UVB rays, F156, **F205**, **F209**, *F244t*, F285
UVC rays, F244

V

V (volts), **F148**, **F161**
vacuoles, **59**, **86**
vacuum machines, F301, **F384**–85, **F397**
vaginal opening, *495f*
vagus nerve, *F111f*
vaidya, **657**
Valtrex®, **739**, **744**
values, F23
valves, *F113f*, **F114**, **F126**, *132f*
variable costs, **F576**, **F598**
varicose veins
  cardiovascular system and, 131–**32**, *134f*, **136**
  sclerotherapy and, **F463**, **F466**, **691**–92, 702–4, *703f*, **708**
vas deferens, 91
vascular, **227**, **234**
vascular growth factor (VGF), **228**, **234**
vascular lesions, F214, 172
vascular light treatment, *172f*
vascular system, **F113**, **F126**. *See also* circulatory system
vasoconstricting, **F350**, **F357**
vasodilation, **F219**, **F233**, **228**, **234**
vasospasm, 465
Vata dosha, **631**, 633–35, **656**
vectorborne infection, 28
Vedas, **630**–31, **656**
vegans, F168
vegetarians, F168, F181
vehicles, **F264**, **F293**
vehicles, cosmetic, 253–57, 260–61, 264, 269–70, 272
veins
  jugular, F116
  overview of, **F114**, **F126**
  spider veins, F206, F219, F242, F251
  varicose, 131–**32**, *134f*, **136**, **691**–92, 702–4, *703f*, **708**
Velcro, F309
vellus hair, **F403**, **F442**
vendor education, F605
venous system, 130–31, *131f*
ventricles, *F113f*, **F114**, **F126**, **127**, **136**
venture capitalists, **751**, **763**
verruca, **F222**, **F225**, **F233**
versican, **67**, *69f*, **86**
vesicles, *F214f*, **F215**, **F233**
vestibulocochlear nerve, *F111f*
VGF. *See* vascular growth factor
vibrating ultrasonic paddles, 454
vibration, **F364**–65, **F374**
Vichy shower, *F456f*, **567**, *596f*, **599**
Victorian Age esthetics, F7–8
vikruti, **632**, **656**
vimentin, **61**, **86**
violet ray, F153–54, F161, F390, F396
virucidal disinfectants, **F62**, F74, **F90**
viruses, *F63t*, **F67**–69, **F90**. *See also* hepatitis
  drugs and, 338–40, *339t*
  hantavirus, **339**, **344**
  herpes simplex, **F225**, **F231**, 212, 477–78, *479f*
  herpes zoster, **F225**, **F231**
  HIV, **F67**, **F89**, 21–**25**, 27, **51**
  human papillomavirus (HPV), **478**, **517**
  infection control and, F67–69, 27
visceral muscles, F103, F124
viscosity, **256**, **280**
visibility, *F575f*
visible light rays, **F155**, F157, **F161**
visible light spectrum, *159f*
vitamins
  defined, **F172**
  fat-soluble, *F173t–174t*, F175–78
  overview of, F172–75, 190–91, *190f*
  skin care and, F265
  vitamin A, *F173t*, **F175**–77, **F185**, **F265**, **F293**, F352, 191, 275, 578
  vitamin B_1, *F173t*, F178–79, 191
  vitamin B_2, *F173t*, F178, 191
  vitamin B_3, 191
  vitamin B_5, 191
  vitamin B_6, *F173t*, F179, 191
  vitamin B_7, *F173t*, F179, 191
  vitamin B_9, 191
  vitamin B_{12}, *F173t*, F179, 191
  vitamin B_{15}, *F174t*, F179
  vitamin C, *F174t*, **F180**, **F185**, **F275**, **F293**, F352, 191, 275–76, 578
  vitamin D, *F173–74t*, **F177**, **F185**, 191, 578
  vitamin E, *F174t*, **F177**–78, **F185**, 191, 260, 262, 275–76, 578
  vitamin K, *F174t*, **F178**, **F185**, **F265**, **F293**
  vitamin P, *F174t*, **F180**, **F184**
  water-soluble, *F173–74t*, F178–80
vitiligo, **F221**, **F233**, 545
Vodder, Emil, F458
Vodder, Estrid, F458
voice-mail, F595
volts (V), **F148**, **F161**
voluntary muscles, F103, F125
vomer, *F100f*, **F101**, **F126**

W

W (watts), **F149**, **F161**
warm colors, **F481**, **F524**
warm towels, F321
warts, F222, F225, F233
waste containers, F301
water, F97, **F134**, **F142**, F183, F256–57
  for clean-up, 38
  as cosmetic ingredient, F256–57, 253
  for drinking, 7
  emulsions and, *F137f*, **F138**–40, **F142**, F228, 259–60, 266, 270, 315, *315f*
  hardness of, 40
  molecular structure of, *142f*
  nutrition and, F183
  pH value of, 38
  sterilization of, 254
water-based emulsions, 315, *315f*
water-based foundations, F472
water-based moisturizers, F284
water-in-oil emulsions, *F137f*, F138–40, **F139**, **F142**, F228, 259–60, 266, 270
water-soluble substances, **F260**, **F293**
water-soluble vitamins, *F173–74t*, F178–80
  vitamin B, *F173–74t*, **F178**–79, **F184**, 191
  vitamin C, *F174t*, **F180**, **F185**, **F275**, **F293**, F352, 191, 275–76, 578
watt, **163**
watts (W), **F149**, **F161**
wave therapy, F153, F160, F454, F466
waveforms, *159f*
wavelengths, F154–**55**, **F161**, 513
wax carts, F412–13
wax heaters, F301, *487f*, 496
wax strips, F413–14, 487, 489, 494
waxes
  as cosmetic ingredients, 255
  fatty, **149**, **154**
  hard, F411, F418–19, *486f*, 486–87, *489t*
  roll-on, F412
  soft, F411, F418–19, 487–88, *487f*, *489t*
  strip, F411, F418–19
  stripless, F411, F418–19
waxing
  American, 493–94
  application, F418
  arms, 492
  back, F439–40, 501–3, *502f*
  bikini area, F435–37, 493–501

waxing *(continued)*
Brazilian, F437, *494f*, 495, *495f*, *496f–500f*
chests, 503
chin, F430
clean-up, F419
client consultation for, F418
contraindications for, *479f*
ears, 503
eyebrows, F419–20, F424–27, 486, 488–91, 501
face, 488–91
French, 494–95, *494f*, *495f*
government regulation of, F430
hands, 493
hard wax, F411, F418–19, 486–87, *486f*, *489t*
legs, F431–32
lip, F428–29
lips, F428–29
male Brazilian, 503
males, F438–40
overview of, F410–11
post-wax product application, F419
procedures, F420
product evaluation for, 488
removal, F418–19
roll-on wax, F412
safety precautions, F417, F419–20, F427, F434, F437
soft wax, F411, F418–19, 487–88, *487f*, *489t*
speed waxing, 491–501, *492f*
supplies for, F413–14
tables, F412
underarm, F433–34
weekly records, F585
weight loss, F182
Weiss, Robert, 441
wellness centers, F533, F542, 566
wens, F217, F232
wet collagen eye pads, *383f*
wet collagen sheets, 358, 383, *383f*
wet room, **567**, **599**
wet sanitizers, F75, *F301f*
wheals, *F214f*, **F215**, **F233**
white blood cells, **F115**, **F126**, **61**, **64**, **86**
white light, **F157**, **F161**
white makeup, F482
whiteheads, F217, *F227f*, F232, *F242t*, F323
whole extract, **284**, **304**
wide jaw, F488
wide nose, F488
wide-set eyes, F490, F492
window coverings, near LASER devices, *167f*
witch hazel, **F271**, *F271t*, **F293**
women, and autoimmune disorders, 25
Wood's lamps, **F379**–80, **F397**, 212, 237, 240–41
word analysis, **676**, *678t*, *679f–682f*, **687**
work ethic, F24
work practice controls, 22
workstations, F78, F299, *F318f*
World War II, 7–8
wound healing, 204–10, *205f*, *206f*, *208f*, *209f*
wraps. *See* body wraps
wringing, F364
wrinkles, *F242t*, *373f*
wrists, exercises for, F305, F362
writers, esthetics, F13

X

xanthan gum, 263
xanthophylls, 148, 153
x-rays, 159

Y

yantra, **657**
yeast, 24
yellow light, F159
ylang ylang, *F272t*, 298, *298f*
yoga, **657**
yogurt, *F273t*
Young, D. Gary, 597
youthful face, *691f*

Z

Zelickson, Brian, 441
zinc, *F175t*, F181, 275
zinc oxide, **F269**, *F269t*, **F293**, 536
Zithromax Z Pak® (azithromycin), **739**, **744**
zone therapy, 242–45, 383, *383f*
Zyderm, 693, 697, 699
zygomatic bones, *F100f*, **F101**, **F126**, 109, 405
zygomatic nerve, **F111**, F112, *F112f*, **F126**
zygomaticus major and minor muscles, **F105**, **F126**, *F367f*, *470t*
zygote, **70**, **86**